Lippincott Williams & Wilkins now offers online teaching advice and student tutoring with this textbook!

Instructors – have you ever wanted to:

…get help generating classroom activities or discussion ideas from an expert in your discipline?

…ask questions about the content of your adopted textbook or ancillary package, and have someone get back to you right away?

…have your lesson plans evaluated?

Students – have you ever needed:

…help studying for a test at a time your instructor was not available?

…questions answered outside of class?

…feedback on assignments before turning them in?

If so, Smarthinking™ is the service you need!

Our tutors are handpicked educators that we train to help you. They are very familiar with the textbook you are using in class and the text's ancillary package. You can connect live to a tutor during certain hours of the week, or send e-mail style messages to which the tutor will respond quickly – often within 24 hours.

And the best part - the service is free with the purchase of your textbook!

Instructors – to use this service, please visit http://connection.LWW.com/go/smarthinking

Students – see the codebook in the back of this book for more details. In it you'll find instructions for using this great service, along with your own personal code to log on and get started.

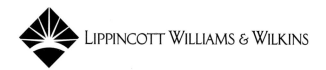

LIPPINCOTT WILLIAMS & WILKINS

Lippincott Williams and Wilkins'

COMPREHENSIVE
Medical Assisting
Second Edition

Lippincott Williams and Wilkins'

COMPREHENSIVE
Medical Assisting
Second Edition

Elizabeth A. Molle, MS, RN
Nurse Educator
Middlesex Hospital
Middletown, Connecticut

Judy Kronenberger, RN, CMA, M.Ed.
Assistant Professor, Medical Assistant Technology
Sinclair Community College
Dayton, Ohio

Laura Southard Durham, BS, CMA
Medical Assisting Program Coordinator
Forsyth Technical Community College
Winston-Salem, North Carolina

Connie West-Stack, M.Ed., MLT, CMA
Medical Assisting Program Director
South Piedmont Community College
Polkton, North Carolina

LIPPINCOTT WILLIAMS & WILKINS
A **Wolters Kluwer** Company
Philadelphia · Baltimore · New York · London
Buenos Aires · Hong Kong · Sydney · Tokyo

Editor: John Goucher
Managing Editor: Rebecca Keifer
Marketing Manager: Hilary Henderson
Production Editor: Christina Remsberg
Compositor: Maryland Composition
Printer: RR Donnelley-Willard

351 West Camden Street
Baltimore, Maryland 21201-2436 USA

530 Walnut Street
Philadelphia, PA 19106

Printed in the United States of America

Library of Congress Cataloging-in-Publication Data

CIP data has been ordered from the Library of Congress and is available upon request.

The publishers have made every effort to trace the copyright holders for borrowed material. If they have inadvertently overlooked any, they will be pleased to make the necessary arrangements at the first opportunity.

To purchase additional copies of this book, call our customer service department at **(800) 638-3030** or fax orders to **(301) 824-7390.** International customers should call **(301) 714-2324.**

Visit Lippincott Williams & Wilkins on the Internet: http://www.LWW.com. Lippincott Williams & Wilkins customer service representatives are available from 8:30 am to 6:00 pm, EST.

04 05 06 07 08
1 2 3 4 5 6 7 8 9 10

This book is dedicated to Ken: Thank you for your love, support, and understanding.
To my friends and colleagues in the Department of Education at Middlesex Hospital,
thank you for your support and encouragement.

ELIZABETH A. MOLLE

I would like to dedicate this book to my children, including Brian, the "first,"
who teaches me how to stay calm no matter how crazy life gets;
Jennifer, my right-brained daughter who teaches me how to be creative;
Brittany, who inspires me to have faith and hope in all people;
and Eric, my youngest, who keeps me focused and laughing.
Most of all, I would like this book to be dedicated to my husband, Joe,
who never gives up on me and will always be the "wind beneath my wings."

JUDY KRONENBERGER

This book is dedicated to all the people who made it possible. To my daughter, Amanda,
who makes me whole. To the rest of my family members who have sacrificed a great deal:
Brad, Susan, Jihad, Dana, Laila, Ramsey, and Ellen. To my parents, Mamie and Joe,
who taught me to work hard. They are proud of me, even from heaven. To Jenifer and
Rhea for getting me through all the ups and downs of the past year. To LeRoy who loves
and encourages me in everything I do. To my students who keep me centered. And espe-
cially to Gracie Ruth Melton, my granddaughter, who gives me wings.

LAURA SOUTHARD DURHAM

I would like to dedicate this text to all of the hard working medical assisting instructors.
Your long hours at work, time missed with family and friends, and your tireless
dedication to your students are truly appreciated. Keep up the good work!

CONNIE WEST-STACK

PREFACE

This is an exciting and challenging time to enter the field of medical assisting. You are uniquely poised to function as the most versatile professional in the medical office. As a medical assistant, you will have the opportunity to perform a variety of clinical and administrative skills. The skills you will perform and your job title will vary among offices. This book was written to help you succeed in performing a variety of administrative medical assisting procedures.

Lippincott Williams & Wilkins' Comprehensive Medical Assisting 2e will define your roles and responsibilities as a professional medical assistant. The book is based on the American Association of Medical Assisting (AAMA) role delineation components for certified medical assistants and the competencies described by the American Medical Technologists (AMT) Registered Medical Assistant Competency Inventory. These roles have evolved and grown over the past decade and will continue to expand to meet the needs of the medical profession.

ORGANIZATION OF THE TEXT

As experienced medical assisting instructors, we understand the complexity of this subject matter can be overwhelming to a new student. Great care and concern were taken to organize this book into a logical and reader friendly presentation. The book is divided into sections:

- Section I, Introduction to Medical Assisting, consists of two units. Unit 1 provides you with a brief history of the medical profession and the practice of medical assisting. Legal and ethical issues governing the medical community and your practice are also discussed. Unit 2 helps you sharpen your communication skills, and its final chapter gives you the tools to deliver effective patient education.
- Section II, The Administrative Medical Assistant, consists of two units. Unit 3 helps you master basic administrative skills. Unit 4 explores financial management of the medical office.
- Section III, The Clinical Medical Assistant, consists of two units. Unit 5 provides you with critical information regarding aseptic technique and infection control. The basic components of patient assessment, which include conducting the patient interview, obtaining vital signs, and assisting with the physical examination are discussed in detail. You will also find an overview of pharmacology as well as information to help you properly prepare and administer medications. The final chapter in this unit will give you the tools to recognize and respond to emergencies in the medical office. Unit 6 focuses on specialty examinations, diagnostic tests, and therapeutic procedures for specific areas of

medicine. Each chapter provides you with a brief overview of the system and common disorders associated with it. Then, the common diagnostic and therapeutic procedures are discussed to help you deliver the proper treatment. The last two chapters in this unit focus on duties relating to special populations.

- Section IV, The Clinical Laboratory, introduces you to the clinical lab, one of medicine's most powerful diagnostic tools. This section provides you with detailed information on collecting and processing specimens. It also explains the process for analyzing blood, urine, and other body samples to facilitate identification of diseases and disorders. In addition, you will learn how to document and maintain a quality assurance program to ensure thorough patient care. Finally, the section will cover a quality control protocol for monitoring and evaluating testing procedures, supplies, and equipment that will ensure accuracy in laboratory performance.
- Section V, Career Strategies, helps you make a smooth transition from the classroom environment to the workforce.

Lippincott Williams & Wilkins' Comprehensive Medical Assisting, 2e is packaged with a complimentary CD-ROM to help you prepare for examinations. The CD-ROM contains questions to help you prepare for CMA and RMA certification and four interactive case studies that place you inside actual situations you will encounter in practice.

FEATURES

Our goal is to make this textbook the most student friendly resource available in the medical assisting field. For students who use English as a second language (ESL), an ESL learning expert reviewed the entire text to ensure the language is appropriate and understandable to non-native English students. To aid these students, an ESL Glossary is provided.

A variety of key features are included to spark interest and promote comprehension. Most chapters include the following:

- A chapter outline
- Learning objectives and performance objectives
- Role delineation components as set forth by AAMA and AMT
- Key terms and key points
- Step-by-step procedure boxes
- Spanish terms and phrases
- Relevant Web addresses
- Critical thinking challenges
- Checkpoint questions
- Unique information boxes, tables, and displays
- Full color illustrations

TEACHING AND LEARNING PACKAGE

This textbook is fully supported with a robust teaching and learning package, each element of which is designed to help you and your instructor get the most out of the textbook. The resource package includes the following:

- A student study guide to enhance learning and comprehension includes competency evaluation forms for each procedure in the textbook, lecture notes, and self-assessment exercises, such as matching, multiple choice, skill drills, critical thinking, and patient teaching.
- A complete instructor's resource kit accompanying the textbook includes suggested classroom activities; chapter quizzes and answer keys; answers to workbook questions; and frequently asked questions about teaching the course, preparing instructional material, and gaining and maintaining accreditation. A CD-ROM with a test generator, image bank, and PowerPoint slides is packaged with the instructor's manual.

As medical assisting instructors, we hope this books exceeds your expectations. May your career in medical assisting be challenging and fulfilling!

Elizabeth A. Molle, MS, RN
Judy Kronenberger, RN, CMA, M.Ed.
Laura Southard Durham, BS, CMA
Connie West-Stack, M.Ed., MLT, CMA

REVIEWERS

We are grateful to the reviewers who read the proposal and drafts of all the chapters. They provided helpful feedback that has resulted in a stronger book. We thank them all. Some of the reviewers wish to remain anonymous. We acknowledge:

Connie Allen
Wallace State Community College
Hanceville, AL

Nancy Akery
North Harris College
Houston, TX

Nina Beaman
Bryant & Stratton College
Richmond, VA

Deborah Bedford
North Seattle Community College,
Seattle, WA

Cindi Brassington
Quinebaug Valley Community College
Danielson, CT

Beth Buchholz
Wichita Area Technical College
Wichita, KS

Michelle Buchman
Springfield College
Springfield, MO

Shirley Buzbee
Modesto Junior College
Modesto, CA

Patricia Davis Christian
Business Office Technology
Southwest Georgia Technical College
Thomasville, GA

Theresa Cyr
Heald College
Honolulu, HI

Pat Csengody
Missouri College
St. Louis, MO

Rose Dovenbarger
Westwood College
Denver, CO

Kent Earley
Dalton State College
Dalton, GA

George Fakhoury
Silicon Valley College
Walnut Creek, CA

Pamela Fleming
Quinsigamond Community College
Worcester, MA

Dr. Eugenia Fulcher
Former Program Director, Swainsboro
   Technical College
Swainsboro, GA

Robyn Gohsman
Medical Careers Institute
Newport News, VA

Glenn Grady
Miller-Motte Technical College
Wilmington, NC

Rene Griffee
Blair College
Colorado Springs, CO

Kris Hardy
Brevard Community College
Titusville, FL

Carol Higuera
East San Gabriel ROP
West Covina, CA

Alicia Hill
Anthis Career Center
Ft. Wayne, IN

Elizabeth Hoffman
Baker College of Clinton Township
Clinton Township, MI

Chris Hollander
Westwood College of Technology
Denver, CO

Michaelea Holten
Concorde Career Institute
Portland, OR

Alexis Jenkins
Chattanooga State Technical Community
   College
Chattanooga, TN

Ray Johns
Medical Careers Institute
Chesapeake, VA

Linda Johnson
Lenoir Community College
Kinston, NC

Marcie Jones
Gwinnett Technical College
Lawrenceville, GA

Kathryn Kalanick
Career Academy
Anchorage, AK

Geri Kale-Smith
William Rainey Harper College
Palatine, IL

Diana Kendrick
Griffin Technical College
Griffin, GA

Sharon Anne Kerber
Instructor
St. Louis, MO

Dorothy Kiel
Rhodes State College
Lima, Ohio

Diane Klieger
Pinellas Area Technical College
St. Petersburg, FL

Wendy Leer
Central Oregon Community College
Bend, OR

Connie Lieseke
Olympic College
Bremerton, WA

Cynthia Lundgren
Houston Community College
Houston, TX

Tanya Mercer
Kaplan Higher Education
Roswell, GA

Pat Moeck
El Centro College
Dallas, TX

Jahangir Moini, MD
Florida Metropolitan University
Melbourne, FL

Ethel Morikis
Ivy Tech State College
Michigan City, MI

Donna Otis
Metro Business College
Rolla, MO

Debra J. Paul
Michiana College,
South Bend, Indiana

Lori Rager
Eagle Gate College
Murray, UT

Deanna Rieke
Montana State University
Billings, MT

Deborah Rojas
College America
St. Petersburg, FL

Suzette Simonson
High-Tech Institute
Las Vegas, NV

Susan Sniffin
Indian River Community College
Fort Pierce, Florida

Cathy Soto
El Paso Community College
El Paso, TX

Nina Thierer
Ivy Tech State College
Fort Wayne, IN

Valeria Truitt
Craven Community College
New Bern, NC

Debra Tymico
Southern Ohio College
Akron, OH

Jane Vallely
Chabot College
Hayward, CA

Deborah Westervelt
Arnold, MO

ACKNOWLEDGMENTS

This book would never have been successfully completed without the assistance, persistence, and hard work of many people. First, we would like to thank John Goucher, the Acquisitions Editor who was there from the beginning to offer support and insight whenever needed. In addition, a special thank-you should go to all of the staff of Lippincott Williams & Wilkins for making this book a reality and supporting the education of medical assistants. In particular, we would like to thank Rebecca Keifer and Nancy Peterson at LWW for their guidance in making this text a reality. We would also like to thank the many reviewers for their hard work and dedication to medical assisting education. Your suggestions and recommendations were invaluable to the accuracy, clarity, and overall quality of this book.

We would like to thank the following people for implementing the reviews and the development editor's comments into selected chapters: Carol Turiello, RN, RDMS, CPC from SUNY Upstate Medical University, Syracuse, NY; Denise Woodson from Bryant and Stratton College, Richmond, VA, Carol Turiello, RN, RDMS, CPC; and Susan Graham, M.S., MT(ASCP)SH, from SUNY Upstate Medical University, Syracuse, NY. Thanks also to Karen Santiago from Nueva Esperanza, Inc., Philadelphia, PA, for developing the ESL Glossary and to Leo Hurst for helping with the Spanish translations. We would also like to thank Melissa Hurley for helping us edit numerous chapters. A special thanks goes to Dr. Rosen and the staff of Ardmore Family Practice for their assistance on various content issues. This book would not have been possible without your contributions.

We would like to express our gratitude to the following: Risa Clow for coordinating the photo shoot; Mark Lozier, Ted Clow, and John Briggs for lending your expertise in photography; Deborah Becker for providing technical guidance and medical expertise; Angela Iorianni-Cimbak from the Mathias J. Brunner Laboratory of the University of Pennsylvania School of Nursing and the staff at Gloucester County Pediatrics in Deptford, New Jersey for allowing us to use their facility and equipment for the photo shoot. We would also like to thank for following people who served as models for the photos: Deborah Becker, Britt Butterfield, Kelli Cambell, Maya Clark, Risa Clow, Ted Clow, Robert Homan, Ramona Hunter, Rebecca Keifer, Mark Lozier, Emily McGee, Jacqui Merrell, Phillip Olive, Rob Randall, Patrick Sheridan, and Shelley Welch. We would thank our colleagues at MICA Information Systems for supplying illustrations. A special thanks goes to Rob Duckwall from Dragonfly Media Group for creating beautiful art to enhance our new edition. Your illustrations convey the concepts beautifully and accurately. This has been an exemplary team effort that is truly commendable.

Finally, we thank all of our medical assisting friends and colleagues at the American Association of Medical Assistants, the Ohio State Society of Medical Assistants, and the Montgomery County Chapter of Medical Assistants for supporting the profession of medical assisting and the education of medical assistants in our states and around the country. We also thank our colleagues and friends with the North Carolina Society of Medical Assistants and Forsyth-Stokes-Davie chapter of Medical Assistants for being an invaluable resource to this book.

The following photos are courtesy of the Mathias J. Brunner Laboratory of the University of Pennsylvania School of Nursing: 19-2, 19-3, 20-2, 21-1, 21-2, 21-6, 21-10, 21-14, 22-1, 22-2, 22-3, 22-7, 22-9, 22-12, 22-13, 24-1, 24-7, 24-8, 24-14, 26-5 (B,C), 26-18 (A), 26-19 (A), 26-20, 27-12, 27-13, 28-6, 29-7, 30-4, 31-4, 32-2, 32-5, 35-4, 36-2, step 3 from Procedure 21-2, step 8 from Procedure 21-5, steps 4, 5, 6 from Procedure 24-1, steps 5, 6 from Procedure 24-6, steps 4, 5, 9, 12, 15, 18 from Procedure 26-8, step 4 from Procedure 32-1, step 2, 8, 9 from Procedure 33-1.

USER'S GUIDE

Lippincott Williams & Wilkins' Comprehensive Medical Assisting **(2nd ed.)** is not just a textbook, it is a complete learning resource that will help you to understand important information, master skills, and become a success in your chosen field of Medical Assisting. To achieve all of this, the authors and publisher have included features and tools throughout the text to help you work through the material presented. Please take a few moments to look through this User's Guide, which will introduce you to the features that will enhance your learning experience.

Chapter Competencies
Learning objectives at the beginning of each chapter tell you the skills you must know by the end of the chapter.

Role Delineation Components
The components from the AAMA's Role Delineation Study that are covered within a chapter are listed at the beginning of each chapter. This list helps you focus on the essential information & skills covered on your certification exam.

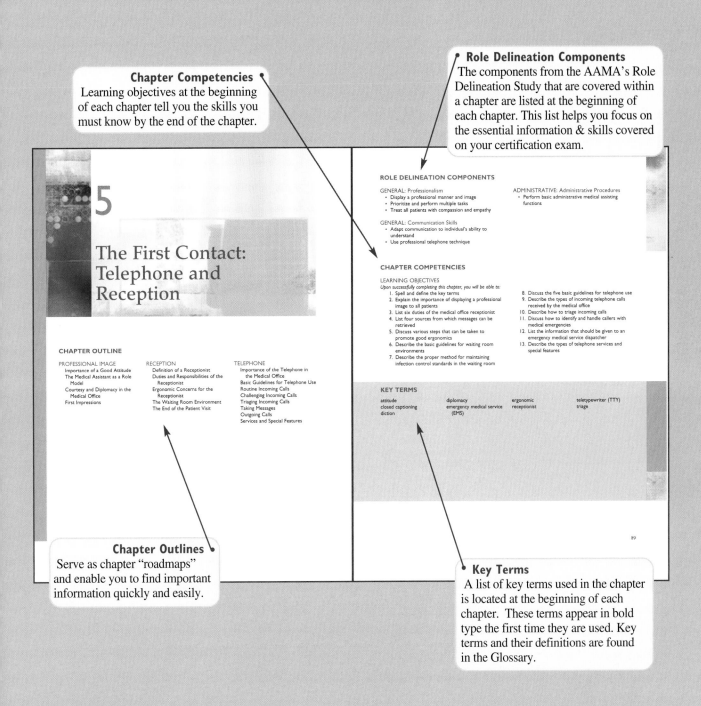

5

The First Contact: Telephone and Reception

CHAPTER OUTLINE

PROFESSIONAL IMAGE
Importance of a Good Attitude
The Medical Assistant as a Role Model
Courtesy and Diplomacy in the Medical Office
First Impressions

RECEPTION
Definition of a Receptionist
Duties and Responsibilities of the Receptionist
Ergonomic Concerns for the Receptionist
The Waiting Room Environment
The End of the Patient Visit

TELEPHONE
Importance of the Telephone in the Medical Office
Basic Guidelines for Telephone Use
Routine Incoming Calls
Challenging Incoming Calls
Triaging Incoming Calls
Taking Messages
Outgoing Calls
Services and Special Features

ROLE DELINEATION COMPONENTS

GENERAL: Professionalism
· Display a professional manner and image
· Prioritize and perform multiple tasks
· Treat all patients with compassion and empathy

GENERAL: Communication Skills
· Adapt communication to individual's ability to understand
· Use professional telephone technique

ADMINISTRATIVE: Administrative Procedures
· Perform basic administrative medical assisting functions

CHAPTER COMPETENCIES

LEARNING OBJECTIVES
Upon successfully completing this chapter, you will be able to:
1. Spell and define the key terms
2. Explain the importance of displaying a professional image to all patients
3. List six duties of the medical office receptionist
4. List four sources from which messages can be retrieved
5. Discuss various steps that can be taken to promote good ergonomics
6. Describe the basic guidelines for waiting room environments
7. Describe the proper method for maintaining infection control standards in the waiting room
8. Discuss the five basic guidelines for telephone use
9. Describe the types of incoming telephone calls received by the medical office
10. Describe how to triage incoming calls
11. Discuss how to identify and handle callers with medical emergencies
12. List the information that should be given to an emergency medical service dispatcher
13. Describe the types of telephone services and special features

KEY TERMS

attitude	diplomacy	ergonomic	teletypewriter (TTY)
closed captioning	emergency medical service (EMS)	receptionist	triage
diction			

89

Chapter Outlines
Serve as chapter "roadmaps" and enable you to find important information quickly and easily.

Key Terms
A list of key terms used in the chapter is located at the beginning of each chapter. These terms appear in bold type the first time they are used. Key terms and their definitions are found in the Glossary.

CALL OUT BOXES

The most important information is emphasized throughout the text in call-out boxes. The following boxes are included:

Patient Education Boxes

One of the most difficult tasks you will face as a Medical Assistant is teaching patients about their health and the health care system. The advice in these boxes will help you to give important information to your patients without confusing or overwhelming them.

What If? Boxes

When a tricky situation comes up in medical practice, the Medical Assistant must be able to think critically. To prepare you to handle any scenario, a variety of situations are defined and explained in these boxes.

Triage Boxes

These boxes contain information and scenarios that will help the Medical Assistant assess and prioritize patient issues that are likely to present themselves in the medical office.

Spanish Terminology

Commonly used Spanish terms & phrases are located in tables throughout the chapter. This will help you communicate effectively with Spanish-speaking patients.

Ethical Tip Boxes

Above all else, a Medical Assistant must adhere to a strict code of ethics. Guidelines in these boxes help you learn and abide by the ethical standards set forth by the AAMA.

Legal Tip Boxes

These boxes contain legal information to help you perform your job duties within the laws governing medical practice.

PATIENT EDUCATION

Television as a Teaching Tool

A television in the reception area can entertain patients while they wait for an appointment, but it can also be a patient education tool. By using a television in conjunction with a VCR, you can play a variety of educational videos. Here are some points to keep in mind:

- Be sure all videos have been previewed by the physician.
- Select videos that are geared toward the specialty of the practice (e.g., a video about heart attacks is appropriate for a cardiologist's office but not for a dermatologist's office).
- Carefully assess the graphic nature of certain videos. (A picture of the birth of a child may interest you but be too much for certain patients.)
- Keep in mind the age of the patients and family members who will be in the waiting room. Caution must be used if small children are often in the area. For example, a video about preventing sexually transmitted diseases may provide information appropriate for a family practice office, but it would not be appropriate to show the video in the reception area.

TRIAGE

While working in a medical office setting, the physician has asked you to call the hospital and schedule Mrs. Roberts for these three tests. What is the correct order for scheduling these tests to be performed?

A. Fiberoptic endoscopic procedure
B. Barium enema
C. Upper GI series

The correct order is fiberoptic endoscopy, upper GI, and finally the barium enema. It is important that procedures be scheduled correctly to ensure optimal results.

WHAT IF

A patient brings in his seeing eye dog and asks, "Can I keep the dog with me in the office?" What would you say?

The Americans with Disabilities Act (ADA) prohibits businesses from banning service animals. A service animal is defined as any guide dog or other animal that is trained to provide assistance to a person with a disability. The animal does not have to be licensed or certified by the state as a service animal. Examples of duties that service animals perform include alerting to sounds patients with hearing impairments, pulling wheelchairs for spinal cord injury patients, picking up items for patients with mobility impairments, sensing smells or auras for seizure patients, and assisting patients with visual impairments. The service animal should not be separated from its owner and must be allowed to enter the examination room with the patient. The ADA law supersedes local health department regulations that ban animals in health care centers. The care of the service animal is the sole responsibility of its owner.

ETHICAL TIPS

All patient communication is confidential. Patient information is sometimes discussed unintentionally, however. To avoid breaching confidentiality, follow these guidelines:

- Do not discuss patients' problems in public places, such as elevators or parking lots. A patient's friends or family members might overhear your conversation and misinterpret what is said.
- The glass window between the waiting room and the reception desk should be kept closed.
- Watch the volume of your voice.
- When calling coworkers over the office intercom, do not use a patient's name or reveal other information. Avoid saying something like, "Bob Smith is on the phone and wants to know if his strep throat culture came back." Instead, say "There's a patient on line 1."
- Before going home, destroy any slips of paper in your uniform pockets that contain patient information (e.g., reminder notes from verbal reports).

LEGAL TIP

The only time an original record should be released is when it is subpoenaed by a court of law. In such situations, the physician may wish to have the judge sign a document stating that he or she will temporarily take charge of the medical record. This signed document should be filed in the medical office until the record is returned. To further ensure the record's safety, a staff member can transport the original record to court on the day it is requested, then return the record at the end of the court session that day. As soon as it is known that a record will be part of a court case, the record should be kept in a locked cabinet. When the court orders that a record be submitted to the court at a given date and time, the legal order is termed *subpoena duces tecum*.

Ñ Spanish Terminology

¡Hola!	Hello!
¿Cómo se llama usted?	What is your name?
¿En qué puedo servirle?	May I help you?
¿Cuál es su dirección?	What is your address?
¿Cuál es el código postal?	What is the zip code?
¿Cuál es su número de teléfono?	What is your phone number?
¿Fecha de nacimiento?	What is your birth date?
¿Cuántos años tiene?	How old are you?
Por favor, siéntese en la sala de espera.	Please have a seat in the waiting roo
Necesito hacerle unas preguntas.	I need to ask you some questions.
Por favor, llene estos papeles.	Please fill out these papers.

Procedure Boxes

Detailed procedures are broken down step-by-step, showing you how to properly perform essential skills. The needed equipment & supplies are listed. Purposes are given for each step to ensure greater understanding.

Handling Incoming Calls

Equipment/Supplies

- Telephone
- Telephone message pad
- Writing utensil (pen or pencil)
- Headset (if applicable)

Steps	Purpose
1. Gather the needed equipment.	Ensures that all materials are available and ready for use.
2. Answer the phone within two rings.	Demonstrates professionalism and courtesy to the caller.
3. Greet caller with proper identification (your name and the name of the office).	Demonstrates professionalism and courtesy to the caller.
4. Identify the nature or reason for the call in a timely manner.	Allows the call to be appropriately managed.
5. Triage the call appropriately.	Prompt identification of emergency calls is important for good patient care.
6. Communicate in a professional manner and with unhurried speech.	Demonstrates compassion and caring for the patient. An unhurried speech pattern is reassuring to the patient.
7. Clarify information as needed.	Prevents errors in communication.
8. Record the message on a message pad. Include name of caller, date, time, telephone number where the caller can be reached, description of the caller's concerns, and person to whom the message is routed.	Promotes good communication between you and the recipient of the message.
9. Give the caller an approximate time for a return call.	Provides reassurance to the patient that the call will be handled promptly and timely.
10. Ask the caller whether he or she has any additional questions or needs any other help.	Confirms that the patient's needs have been met.
11. Allow the caller to disconnect first.	Ensures that the caller has completed the communication.
12. Put the message in an appropriate place.	Ensures that the call will be handled correctly and the intended recipient gets the information.
	nsures that the call is handled promptly and efficiently.

- Insurance representatives regarding billing issues

Facsimile Machines. All physician offices have a fax machine. The most common messages left here are

- Patient referrals
- Consultation reports
- Laboratory and radiology reports

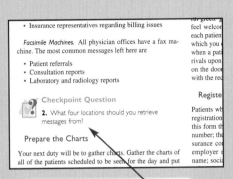

Checkpoint Question

2. What four locations should you retrieve messages from?

Prepare the Charts

Your next duty will be to gather charts. Gather the charts of all of the patients scheduled to be seen for the day and put

Checkpoint Questions

Located throughout the chapter, these questions quiz you on the material covered and reinforce key points in the reading. Answers to these questions are located at the end of each chapter.

Critical Thinking Challenges

Located at the end of each chapter, these challenges encourage you to apply the knowledge gained throughout the chapter in a real-life scenario.

systems for public buildings. These standards can be found on their website.

CHAPTER SUMMARY

As the receptionist, you are the most visible and accessible representative of the medical practice. Duties and responsibilities of a receptionist vary among office settings. The key to being a good receptionist is to demonstrate tact and diplomacy in all interactions with patients. Providing a positive attitude will ease the patient's anxiety and ensure the best and most confident image of the practice is projected. Proper telephone etiquette and manners are essential for good patient care and to achieve effective communication among various health care providers. Triaging incoming calls is a skill that you must master if you are to be an effective receptionist.

Chapter Summary

Each chapter is summarized in a few paragraphs at the end of the chapter. This helps you review important topics covered in the chapter.

Critical Thinking Challenges

1. How would you calm an irate patient on the telephone? Identify some phrases that you might use to calm the caller. What phrases may make the situation worse?
2. Assume you are working in an obstetrician's office. What kinds of educational videos might be appropriate for the waiting room? What if you were working in an orthopedic office or for a surgeon?
3. Here is a triage scenario. Line 1 is a home calling the office with a patient status upd... is a pharmacist questioning a prescription

CD-ROM for
Lippincott Williams & Wilkins'
COMPREHENSIVE
Medical Assisting, 2e

Including
• Certification Exam Preparation
• Interactive Case Studies

Version 1.0

Elizabeth A. Molle, Laura Southard Durham,
Judy L. Kronenberger, and Connie West-Stack

Technical Support: 1-800-638-3030
or at techsupp@lww.com

Copyright 2005   Lippincott Williams & Wilkins
A Wolters Kluwer Company
0-7817-3771-0
All rights reserved.

Back-of-Book CD-ROM

Interactive Case Studies

These computer based, interactive case studies present you with different scenarios that you will face in the medical office. The timely scenarios will encourage you to think critically and apply multiple skills that are taught in the text.

Case study topics include:

- Triage in an emergency situation, communication and documentation
- Patient interviewing, education and confidentiality and specimen handling
- Vital signs, patient education and right of refusal of treatment
- Dealing with a sick patient, infection control, and medication administration

Certification Exam Review Questions

These questions help you prepare for the National Certification exams. A practice exam is included, with questions that closely resemble those that are on the tests.

WWW.GO Websites

These websites can provide you with some additional information:

American Academy of Pediatrics
www.aap.org
American Heart Association
www.americanheart.org
CDC
www.cdc.gov
Federal Communications Commission
www.fcc.gov/cib/dro
Institute for Disabilities Research and Training
www.idrt.com
Online Yellow Pages
www.smartpages.com
OSHA
www.osha.gov
Telecommunications for the Deaf
www.amrad.org
U. S. Department of Justice/Americans with Disabilities Act
www.usdoj.gov/crt/ada

Websites

Listed at the end of each chapter, these online resources will help you to stay up to date in the medical field. Both medical professional sites and patient resources are given.

CONTENTS

SECTION I

INTRODUCTION TO MEDICAL ASSISTING 1

SECTION II

THE ADMINISTRATIVE ASSISTANT 85

SECTION III

THE CLINICAL MEDICAL ASSISTANT 307

EXPANDED CONTENTS

SECTION II

THE ADMINISTRATIVE ASSISTANT, 85

Unit Three
Performing Administrative Duties, 87

SECTION III

THE CLINICAL MEDICAL ASSISTANT 307

Unit Five

Performing Clinical Duties 309

CHAPTER 19: **Medical Asepsis and Infection Control,** 310

SECTION IV

THE CLINICAL LABORATORY 807

Unit Seven

Performing Laboratory Procedures 809

CHAPTER 41: Introduction to the Clinical Laboratory, 810

SECTION V

CAREER STRATEGIES, 977

Unit Eight

Competing in the Job Market, 979

LIST OF PROCEDURES

Introduction to Medical Assisting

Understanding the Profession

Welcome! The world of medicine is an exciting and challenging frontier. This unit consists of two chapters that will introduce you to the field of medicine and medical assisting. In the first chapter, you will learn how medicine has evolved through the years from an era of superstition and magical cures to an age of modern technology. The second chapter introduces you to legal and ethical roles that affect medical professionals. Sometimes, the advances in medicine challenge our laws and ethics. This unit will help you to understand the bond between medicine, law, and ethics. Let the exploration begin!

Medicine and Medical Assisting

CHAPTER OUTLINE

HISTORY OF MEDICINE
  Ancient Medical History
  Modern Medical History
  Recent Medical History

THE AMERICAN HEALTH CARE
SYSTEM

THE MEDICAL OFFICE

MEDICAL SPECIALTIES

THE MEDICAL ASSISTING
PROFESSION
  What Is a Medical Assistant?
  Duties of a Medical Assistant

CHARACTERISTICS OF A
PROFESSIONAL MEDICAL
ASSISTANT

MEMBERS OF THE HEALTH
CARE TEAM
  Physicians
  Physician Assistants
  Nurses
  Nurse Practitioners
  Allied Health Professionals

THE HISTORY OF MEDICAL
ASSISTING

MEDICAL ASSISTING
EDUCATION
  Medical Assisting Program
    Accreditation

MEDICAL ASSISTING
CERTIFICATION
  Certified Medical Assistant
  Registered Medical Assistant

MEDICAL ASSISTING AND
RELATED ALLIED HEALTH
ASSOCIATIONS
  Association Membership

EMPLOYMENT OPPORTUNITIES

ROLE DELINEATION COMPONENTS

GENERAL: Professionalism
- Display a professional manner and image
- Demonstrate initiative and responsibility
- Work as a member of the health care team
- Promote the CMA credential
- Enhance skills through continuing education

GENERAL: Legal Concepts
- Perform within legal and ethical boundaries

CHAPTER COMPETENCIES

LEARNING OBJECTIVES

Upon successfully completing this chapter, you will be able to:

1. Spell and define the key terms
2. Outline a brief history of medicine
3. Identify the key founders of medical science
4. Explain the system of health care in the United States
5. Discuss the typical medical office
6. List medical specialties a medical assistant may encounter
7. List the duties of a medical assistant
8. Describe the desired characteristics of a medical assistant
9. Explain the pathways of education for medical assistants
10. Discuss the importance of program accreditation
11. Name and describe the two nationally recognized accrediting agencies for medical assisting education programs
12. Explain the benefits and avenues of certification for the medical assistant
13. List the benefits of membership in a professional organization
14. Identify members of the health care team
15. List settings in which medical assistants may be employed

KEY TERMS

accreditation	cloning	medical assistant	outpatient
administrative	continuing education units	multidisciplinary	recertification
caduceus	externship	multiskilled health	role delineation chart
certification	inpatient	professional	specialty
clinical	laboratory		

WELCOME TO THE FIELD of medicine and to the medical assisting profession! You have selected a fascinating and challenging career, one of the fastest growing specialties in the medical field. The need for the **multiskilled health professional**—an individual with versatile training in the health care field—will continue to grow within the foreseeable future, and you are now a part of this exciting career direction.

To help you understand the significance of the medical knowledge and skills you will receive during your course of study, we begin by taking a chronological look at the history of medicine and then explore the profession of medical assisting.

HISTORY OF MEDICINE

Tremendous achievements in the general health, comfort, and well-being of patients have been made just within the past 100 to 150 years, with the greatest advances occurring in the 20th century. It is difficult to imagine health care without antibiotics, x-ray machines, or anesthesia, but these developments are fairly new to medicine. For example, penicillin was not produced in large quantities until World War II, and surgery was performed without anesthesia until the mid 1800s.

Ancient Medical History

The earliest recorded evidence of medical history dates to the early Egyptians. Papyrus records of tuberculosis, pneumonia, and arteriosclerosis are still in existence from 4000 B.C. It is evident that during this time the Egyptians performed surgeries, including brain surgery. Fossil remains have shown patients with fractures (broken bones) that were splinted and subsequently healed. Although many cultures practiced primitive forms of surgery, most early practitioners used a combination of religion and superstition to heal ailments. Herbs, roots, and plants were used as medications.

Some of these early medications played a key role in the development of our modern pharmacology. Digitalis, from the common garden plant foxglove, is still in use today for its original purpose of strengthening the heart's action. Opium, from the pods of the poppy plant, is still used to induce stupor and a level of painlessness. Supplemental iron as a method of treating anemia was recognized by the Chinese as early as 2500 B.C. Medical research is constantly uncovering evidence that previously used treatment methods were based on sound theory and are being incorporated into our modern arsenal against illness.

More than 1000 years before Christ, Moses was appointed the first public health officer. He wrote rules for sanitation. He stated that all people preparing and serving public food must be neat and clean. In the days long before refrigeration, it became a religious law that only freshly slaughtered animals could be eaten. Moses also required that serving dishes and cooking utensils be washed between customers at public restaurants.

Aesculapius, Greek god of healing and the son of Apollo, had many followers who used massage and exercise to treat patients. This god is also believed to have used the magical powers of a yellow, nonpoisonous serpent to lick the wounds of surgical patients. Aesculapius was often pictured holding the serpent wrapped around his staff or wand; this staff is a symbol of medicine. Another medical symbol is the **caduceus**, the staff of the Roman god Mercury, shown as a winged staff with two serpents wrapped around it (Fig. 1-1).

Around 400 B.C., Hippocrates practiced medicine and set high behavioral standards for practicing physicians. Hippocrates, called the "Father of Medicine," turned medicine into a science and erased the element of mysticism that it once held. He wrote the Hippocratic Oath, which is still part of medical school graduation ceremonies.

The Greek physician Galen (131–201 A.D.), became known as the "Father of Experimental Physiology." He was the first physician to document a patient's pulse, although he did not know that the pulse was related to the heart. Galen identified many parts of the body. His anatomic findings were mostly incorrect, however, because they were based on the dissection of apes and swine. Postmortem human dissections were illegal and were considered sacrilegious until the Renaissance (1350–1650).

The rule of the Roman Empire, from about 200 B.C. until its dissolution several centuries later, brought great strides in public health. Water was brought from clean mountain streams by way of raised aqueducts that were regularly cleaned and maintained; sewers carried wastes away from the cities; and personal cleanliness was encouraged. One Roman physician Mar-

FIGURE 1-1. (**A**) Staff of Aesculapius. (**B**) Caduceus.

cus Varro (116–21 B.C.) even suggested that there might be creatures too small to be seen that caused illness. This was 1800 years before the invention of the microscope.

During the Dark Ages (400–800 A.D.) and through the Middle Ages (800–1400 A.D.), few advances were made in the medical field. Medicine was practiced primarily in convents and monasteries and consisted of simply comforting patients rather than trying to find a cure for the illness. The population became more mobile, ranging away from traditional homelands for war, crusades, and exploration. Each venture exposed whole cultures to diseases against which they had no immunity. Cities grew larger but without the Roman technology for maintaining sanitation. Ignorance, crowding, and poor health practices led to the eruption of the bubonic plague, which twice swept through Europe and Asia, killing approximately 20 million people. This deadly disease, the greatest killer in our history, spread from rat fleas to humans, killing approximately half of the known population within a few years.

Checkpoint Question

1. Why were Galen's anatomic findings considered incorrect?

Modern Medical History

The Renaissance was a period of enlightenment in all areas of art, science, and education, and it fostered great strides in medicine. The advent of the printing press and the establishment of great universities made the practice of medicine more accessible to larger numbers of practitioners. Great minds collaborated to advance medical and scientific theories and perform experiments that led to discoveries of enormous benefit in the fight against disease.

During this period, Andreas Vesalius (1514–1564) became known as the "Father of Modern Anatomy." He corrected many of Galen's errors and wrote the first relatively correct anatomy textbook. Soon afterward, William Harvey identified the pumping action of the heart. He described circulation as a continuous circuit pumped by the heart to carry blood through the body. Harvey studied the action of the heart using dogs, not humans.

The microscope was invented in the mid 1660s by a Dutch lens maker, Anton von Leeuwenhoek. He was the first person to observe bacteria under a lens, although he had no idea of the significance of the microorganisms to human health. His instrument also allowed him to accurately describe a red blood cell.

John Hunter (1728–1793) became known as the "Father of Scientific Surgery." He developed many surgical techniques that are still used today. Hunter also developed and inserted the first artificial feeding tube into a patient in 1778 and was the first to classify teeth in a scientific manner.

In 1796, Edward Jenner, a physician in England, overheard a young milkmaid explain that she could not catch smallpox because she had already had the very mild cowpox caught while milking her cows. Several weeks later, Jenner inoculated

a small boy with smallpox crusts. The boy did not contract the disease, and the prevention for smallpox was discovered. Jenner's discovery of the smallpox vaccine led to more emphasis on prevention of disease rather than on cures.

The 1800s brought the first notable records of the contributions of women to the medical field. Florence Nightingale (1820–1910) was the founder of modern nursing. She set standards for nurses and developed educational requirements for nurses (Fig. 1-2).

Also during the early 1800s, the importance of the mind as a part of the health care process was becoming a recognized field of medicine. The first extensive work and writing on mental health was published in 1812 by Benjamin Rush, entitled *Medical Inquiries and Observations upon Diseases of the Mind*. He advocated humane treatment of the mentally ill at a time when most were imprisoned, chained, starved, exhibited like animals, or simply killed. Rush's influence began the separate field of study into the working of the mind that became modern psychiatry. The mid 1880s saw a surge in the study of disease transmission. Louis Pasteur (1822–1895) became famous for his work with bacteria. Pasteur discovered that wine turned sour because of the presence of bacteria. He found that when the bacteria were eliminated, the wine lasted longer. Pasteur's discovery that bacteria in liquids could be eliminated by heat led to the process known as pasteurization. This finding led to using heat to sterilize surgical instruments. Pasteur has been called the "Father of Bacteriology" for this accomplishment. Pasteur also focused on preventing the transmission of anthrax and discovered the rabies vaccine and was honored with the title "Father of Preventive Medicine" for this work.

In the mid 1880s, Ignaz Semmelweiss, a Hungarian physician, noticed that women whose babies were born at home with a midwife in attendance had childbed fever less

F I G U R E   1 – 2.   Florence Nightingale.

often than those who delivered in well-respected hospitals with prestigious physicians at the bedside. He was ridiculed by the medical establishment and was fired from his position when he required medical personnel to wash their hands in a solution of chlorinated lime before performing obstetric examinations. He was right, of course, and handwashing is still the most important factor in the fight against disease transmission.

At about the same time, Joseph Lister began to apply antiseptics to wounds to prevent infection. The concept was not clearly understood, but before Lister's practices, as many patients died of infection as died of the primitive surgical techniques of the early part of the century.

Modern anesthesia was discovered in 1842 by Crawford Williamson Long. The effects of nitrous oxide were known by the mid 1700s, but Long discovered its therapeutic use by accident when he observed a group of chemistry students inhaling it for amusement. Before this time, anesthesia consisted of large doses of alcohol or opium, leather straps for patient restraint, or the unconsciousness resulting from pain. Ether and chloroform came into use at about this time.

Elizabeth Blackwell (1821–1910) became the first woman to complete medical school in the United States when she graduated from Geneva Medical College in New York. In 1869, Blackwell established her own medical school in Europe for women only, opening the door for a rapidly expanding role for women in the medical field.

Clara Barton (1821–1912) founded the American Red Cross in 1881 and was its first president. She identified the need for psychological as well as physical support for wounded soldiers in the Civil War.

X-rays were discovered in 1895 by Wilhelm Konrad Roentgen when he observed that a previously unknown ray generated by a cathode tube could pass through soft tissue and outline underlying structures. Medical diagnosis was revolutionized, earning Roentgen a Nobel Prize in 1901 for his discovery. The therapeutic uses of x-rays were recognized much later.

Marie Curie (1867–1934), a brilliant science student, married Pierre Curie, and together they discovered polonium and radium. Their discovery revolutionized the principles of energy and radioactivity. Marie and Pierre Curie shared the Nobel Prize for chemistry in 1903. Marie continued the research after his death and again won the Nobel Prize for physics in 1911.

In 1928, Sir Alexander Fleming, a bacteriologist, accidentally discovered penicillin when his assistant forgot to wash the Petri dishes Fleming had used for experiments. When he noticed the circles of nongrowth around areas of a certain mold, he was able to extract the prototype for one of our most potent weapons against disease. He won the Nobel Prize in 1945 for this accomplishment.

Jonas Edward Salk and Albert Sabin discovered the vaccines for polio in the 1950s, which led to near eradication of one of the 20th century's greatest killers.

Checkpoint Question

2. What did Louis Pasteur discover about bacteria found in liquids?

Recent Medical History

Throughout the next three decades, public health protection improved and advancements continued. Government legislation mandated clean water, and citizens reaped the benefits of preventive medicine and education about health issues.

In the 1980s, advancements in radiology gave doctors ways to see inside a patient with such accuracy that patients no longer had to have exploratory surgery. With computed tomography (CT scan) radiologists can see tumors, cysts, inflammation, and so on, with cross-sectional slices of the patient's body. Magnetic resonance imaging (MRI) uses a strong magnetic field to realign ions to form an image on a screen. MRI is used to detect internal bleeding, tumors, cysts, and so on. Positron emission tomography has further revolutionized radiology.

In July 1998, Ryuzo Yanagimachi of the University of Hawaii announced the **cloning** of mice when 7 of 22 mice were cloned from the cell of a single mouse. In December 1998, researchers from Kinki University in Nara, Japan, cloned 8 calves from a single cell.

On June 26, 2000, after 10 years of work, a team of scientists from both the public and private sectors announced the completion and availability of a rough draft of the identification and mapping of human genes. Mapping the sequence of the letters of the human genome that represent the handbook of a human being is a breakthrough that will revolutionize the practice of medicine by paving the way for new drugs and therapies. The achievement is being hailed as one of the most significant scientific landmarks of all time, comparable to the landing on the moon or splitting the atom. Already many medicines that can be tailored to an individual's genetic makeup are on the market or in development.

New discoveries will continue to expand the parameters of medicine as further research in recombinant DNA, transplantation, immunizations, diagnostic procedures, and so forth push back the boundaries of health care and make today's therapies seem as primitive as those we have just covered. You will be a part of this fascinating evolution of health care. Within the next decade expect to see immunization against or cures for many of the illnesses that continue to plague us.

Your role as a **medical assistant**, the ultimate multiskilled health care professional, will expand as the need for highly trained, versatile medical personnel keeps pace with the ever-changing practice of medicine. Today, heart bypass surgeries and organ transplants are performed routinely. Research continues to search for the cures for cancer, acquired immunodeficiency syndrome, and many other ailments. As a medical assistant, you play a key role in advancing the medical profession in the 21st century.

THE AMERICAN HEALTH CARE SYSTEM

The American health care system is complex and has seen many changes in the past few decades. Twenty years ago, a patient had medical insurance that paid a percentage of his or her medical bills. In today's world of managed care, which is discussed in the chapter on health insurance, patients are a part of a group of covered members of a HMO (health management organization). With this change came new ways of treating patients. The doctor–patient relationship was one of trust and privacy. In today's health care system, patients are treated as outlined by the insurance companies. The purpose of this change was to control health care costs. The government monitors medical finances and controls the Medicare and Medicaid systems through the Centers for Medicare & Medicaid Services (CMS). This government agency was formerly called Health Care Financing Administration (HFCA). It has been estimated that by 2013, 60% of patients being seen in the medical office will be over 65 years of age and will be covered under the Medicare system of insurance for the elderly. The need to adhere to the rules and regulations of the government drives the management practices of the **outpatient** medical facility. The allied health care arena has grown quickly. New professions have been added to the health care team, and each one is an important part of a patient's total care. As an allied health student, you have an exciting course of study ahead of you. Soon you will find yourself among a caring and conscientious group of health care professionals.

THE MEDICAL OFFICE

Today's medical office is quite different from the office of the past, where patients were treated by their family physician, insurance was filed, and reimbursement was based on a percentage of the cost. Large corporations and hospitals now own many medical clinics, and physicians are their employees. Medical practices now have the capability to maintain a patient's record without a single piece of paper. Office employees need a general understanding of the many regulations of insurance carriers. Every employee must be computer literate and should understand the legal aspects of the medical office. Although there are many medical specialties, the skills and basic functions of any medical office will be similar. Many years ago, a physician might teach a neighbor the skills needed to work with him. Those days are over. With the new technology and the need for constant monitoring of regulations and changes, the medical office employee is now expected to acquire a formal education and certification.

The typical medical office employs one or more physicians. To assist with examining and treating patients, the physician may employ physician assistants and/or nurse practitioners. These are the providers, and they need support staff. The goal of any medical practice is to provide quality care while maintaining sound financial practices within the laws and ethics of the medical profession. To achieve this goal, the physician needs a solid team. The administrative staff handles the financial aspects of the practice, and the clinical staff assists the providers with patient care. Both aspects of the office must run smoothly to reach the ultimate goal of the practice. The makeup of the team may differ among specialties. For example, a doctor who treats broken bones may have an x-ray technologist on staff, or an obstetrician may have an on-site sonographer to perform ultrasounds on mothers-to-be. Regardless of the mix of the team, the certified medical assistant is an integral part.

The day-to-day operation of a medical office requires all the skills you learn in your curriculum. The patient's health care encounter can be pleasant or unpleasant, depending on the skills and the attitude of the team.

Checkpoint Question

3. Which members of the health care team are considered providers?

MEDICAL SPECIALTIES

After completion of medical school, physicians choose a **specialty**. Some prefer treating patients of all ages and will choose family medicine or internal medicine. Others choose surgery and further specialize in fields like cosmetic surgery or vascular surgery. Table 1-1 lists the most common surgi-

Table I–I	SURGICAL SPECIALTIES
Surgical Specialty	**Description**
Cardiovascular	Repairs physical dysfunctions of the cardiovascular system
Cosmetic, reconstructive	Restores, repairs, or reconstructs body parts
General	Performs repairs on a variety of body parts
Maxillofacial	Repairs disorders of the face and mouth (a branch of dentistry)
Neurological	Repairs disorders of the nervous system
Orthopedic	Corrects deformities and treats disorders of the musculoskeletal system
Thoracic	Repairs organs within the rib cage
Trauma	Limited to correcting traumatic wounds
Vascular	Repairs disorders of blood vessels, usually excluding the heart

Table 1-2   SPECIALISTS WHO EMPLOY MEDICAL ASSISTANTS

Specialist	Description
Allergist	Performs tests to determine the basis of allergic reactions to eliminate or counteract the offending allergen
Anesthesiologist	Determines the most appropriate anesthesia during surgery for the patient's situation
Cardiologist	Diagnoses and treats disorders of the cardiovascular system, including the heart, arteries, and veins
Dermatologist	Diagnoses and treats skin disorders, including cosmetic treatments for the reversal of aging
Emergency care physician	Usually works in emergency or trauma centers
Endocrinologist	Diagnoses and treats disorders of the endocrine system and its hormone-secreting glands, e.g., diabetes and dwarfism
Epidemiologist	Specializes in epidemics caused by infectious agents, studies toxic agents, air pollution, and other health-related phenomena, and works with sexually transmitted disease control
Family practitioner	Serves a variety of patient age levels, seeing patients for everything from ear infections to school physicals
Gastroenterologist	Diagnoses and treats disorders of the stomach and intestine
Gerontologist	Limits practice to disorders of the aging population and its unique challenges
Gynecologist	Diagnoses and treats disorders of the female reproductive system and may also be an obstetrician or limit the practice to gynecology, including surgery
Hematologist	Diagnoses and treats disorders of the blood and blood-forming organs
Immunologist	Concentrates on the body's immune system and disease incidence, transmission, and prevention
Internist	Limits practice to diagnosis and treatment of disorders of internal organs with medical (drug therapy and lifestyle changes) rather than surgical means
Neonatologist	Limits practice to the care and treatment of infants to about 6 weeks of age
Nephrologist	Diagnoses and treats disorders of the kidneys
Obstetrician	Limits practice to care and treatment for pregnancy, the postpartum period, and fertility issues
Oncologist	Diagnoses and treats tumors, both benign (noncancerous) and malignant (cancerous)
Ophthalmologist	Diagnoses and treats disorders of the eyes, including surgery (an optometrist monitors and measures patients for corrective lenses, and an optician makes the lenses or dispenses contact lenses)
Orthopedist	Diagnoses and treats disorders of the musculoskeletal system, including surgery and care for fractures
Otorhinolaryngologist	Diagnoses and treats disorders of the ear, nose, and throat
Pathologist	Analyzes tissue samples or specimens from surgery, diagnoses abnormalities, and performs autopsies
Pediatrician	Limits practice to childhood disorders or may be further specialized to early childhood or adolescent period
Podiatrist	Diagnoses and treats disorders of the feet and provides routine care for diabetic patients, who may have poor circulation and require extra care
Proctologist	Limits practice to disorders of the colon, rectum, and anus
Psychiatrist	Diagnoses and treats mental disorders
Pulmonologist	Diagnoses and treats disorders of the respiratory system
Radiologist	Interprets x-rays and imaging studies and performs radiation therapy
Rheumatologist	Diagnoses and treats arthritis, gout, and other joint disorders
Urologist	Diagnoses and treats disorders of the urinary system, including the kidneys and bladder, and disorders of the male reproductive system

cal specialties. Table 1-2 lists specialists who may employ medical assistants.

Checkpoint Question

4. What is the specialty that treats newborn babies?

THE MEDICAL ASSISTING PROFESSION

What Is a Medical Assistant?

A medical assistant is a multiskilled allied health professional, a member of the health care delivery team who performs administrative and clinical procedures. **Clinical** tasks generally involve direct patient care; **administrative** tasks usually focus on office procedures. Medical assistants are employed in physicians' offices and ambulatory care settings. Salaries, hours, and benefits depend on experience, size of practice or corporation, and geographic salary ranges. Working conditions for medical assistants vary greatly according to state laws regarding the medical assisting profession and the scope of the certified medical assistant (CMA), specialty of employer, and job responsibilities.

Duties of a Medical Assistant

The duties of a medical assistant are divided into two categories: administrative and clinical, which includes **laboratory** duties. The ratio of administrative to clinical duties varies with your job description. For example, if you work in a family practice office, you may do mostly clinical work; a psychiatric practice will probably require primarily administrative duties.

Administrative Duties

Performing administrative tasks correctly and in a timely manner will make the office more efficient and productive. Conversely, an office that is not managed correctly can result in loss of business, poor patient service, and loss of revenue. Following is a partial list of standard administrative duties:

- Managing and maintaining the waiting room, office, and examining rooms
- Handling telephone calls
- Using written and oral communication
- Maintaining medical records
- Bookkeeping
- Scheduling appointments
- Ensuring good public relations
- Maintaining office supplies
- Screening sales representatives
- Filing insurance forms
- Processing the payroll
- Arranging patient hospitalizations
- Sorting and filing mail
- Instructing new patients regarding office hours and procedures
- Applying computer concepts to office practices
- Implementing ICD-9 and CPT coding for insurance claims
- Completing medical transcriptions

Clinical Duties

Clinical responsibilities vary among employers. State laws regarding the scope of practice for medical assistants also differ. In some states, CMAs are not allowed to perform invasive procedures, such as injections or laboratory testing.

Most states, however, leave the responsibility for the medical assistant's actions with the physician-employer. AAMA has outlined the scope of practice for the medical assistant. Following is a partial list of clinical duties:

- Preparing patients for examinations and treatments
- Assisting other health care providers with procedures
- Preparing and sterilizing instruments
- Completing electrocardiograms
- Applying Holter monitors
- Obtaining medical histories
- Administering medications and immunizations
- Obtaining vital signs (blood pressure, pulse, temperature, respirations)
- Obtaining height and weight measurements
- Documenting in the medical record
- Performing eye and ear irrigations
- Recognizing and treating medical emergencies
- Initiating and implementing patient education

Laboratory Duties

- Low- and moderate-complexity laboratory tests as determined by the Clinical Laboratory Improvement Amendments (CLIA) of 1988
- Collecting and processing laboratory specimens

 Checkpoint Question

5. What are five administrative duties and five clinical or laboratory duties performed by a medical assistant?

CHARACTERISTICS OF A PROFESSIONAL MEDICAL ASSISTANT

Medical assistants play a key role in creating and maintaining a professional image for their employers. Medical assistants must always appear neat and well groomed. Clothing should be clean, pressed, and in good condition. Footwear should be neat, comfortable, and professional. If sneakers are approved by your supervisor, they should be all white. Only minimal makeup and jewelry should be worn. You should wear a watch with a second hand. Fingernails should be clean and at a functional length. If polish is worn, it should be pale or clear.

Medical assistants must be dependable and punctual (Fig. 1-3). Tardiness and frequent absences are not acceptable. If you are not at work, someone must fill in for you. Medical assistants must be flexible and adaptable to meet the constantly changing needs of the office. Weekend and holiday hours may be required in some specialties.

Additional characteristics vital to the profession include the following:

- Excellent written and oral communications skills. You will be required to interact with patients and other health

FIGURE 1-3. Medical assistants play a key role in creating and maintaining a professional image for their employers.

care workers on a professional basis. Only the best spelling and grammar skills are acceptable. (Communication skills are covered in appropriate sections of this text.)

- Maturity. Remaining calm in an emergency or during stressful situations and being able to calm others is a key skill. You must also be able to accept criticism without resentment.
- Accuracy. The physician must be able to trust you to pay close attention to detail because the health and well-being of the patients are at stake. Careless errors could cause harm to the patient and result in legal action against the physician.
- Honesty. If errors are made, they must be admitted, and corrective procedures must be initiated immediately. Covering up errors or blaming others is dishonest. So are using office property for personal business, making telephone calls during work time, and falsifying time records. Such practices can ruin your career and are to be strictly avoided.
- Ability to respect patient confidentiality. Few issues in health care can damage your career as profoundly as divulging confidential patient information.

- Empathy. The ability to care deeply for the health and welfare of your patients is the heart of medical assisting.
- Courtesy. Every patient who enters the office must be treated with respect and gracious manners.
- Good interpersonal skills. Tempers may flare in stressful situations; learn to keep yours in check and work well with all levels of interaction.
- Ability to project a positive self-image. If you are confident in your abilities as a professional, this attitude will reflect in all of your relationships.
- Ability to work as a team player. The patient's return to health is the most important objective of the office. Each staff member must work toward this goal.
- Initiative and responsibility. The entire team expects each of its members to perform assigned responsibilities.
- Tact and diplomacy. The right word at the right moment can calm and soothe anger, depression, and fear and relieve a potentially unsettling situation.
- High moral and ethical standards. Project for your profession the highest level of professionalism.

 Checkpoint Question

6. What are eight characteristics that a professional medical assistant should have?

MEMBERS OF THE HEALTH CARE TEAM

As a medical assistant, you will work with a variety of health care workers. Today's health care team must be **multidisciplinary**. A multidisciplinary team is a group of specialized professionals who are brought together to meet the needs of the patient. Some patients will need the assistance of many individuals, whereas other patients may only need one or two members of the team. The team may be broken into three groups: physicians, nurses, and allied health care providers.

Physicians

Physicians generally are the team leaders. They are responsible for diagnosing and treating the patient. Minimum education for a physician consists of a 4-year undergraduate degree, often consisting of premedical studies, 4 years of medical school, followed by a residency program usually concentrating on a certain specialty. The residency program can vary from 2 to 6 years based on the field of study. Physicians must pass a licensure examination for the state in which they wish to practice.

Physician Assistants

Physician assistants (PAs) are specially trained and usually licensed. They work closely with a physician and may perform many of the tasks traditionally done by physicians. Preliminary physical examinations and basic diagnostic and treatment procedures that do not require an intense medical background may be assigned to a physician's assistant. Their educational levels vary from several months to 2 years, depending on the program and the individual's background in medicine. National certification is available through the American Association of Physician Assistants.

Nurses

Nurses work with physicians and implement various patient care needs in the **inpatient** or hospital setting. Their job descriptions vary according to their experiences, specialties, and certifications. There are several levels of nursing education.

- Bachelor of science in nursing (BSN) — 4 years of education
- Associate degree in nursing (ADN) — 2 years
- Registered nurse (RN) — 2 to 3 years
- Licensed practical nurse (LPN) — 1 year
- Licensed vocational nurse (LVN) — 1 year
- Certified nursing assistant (CNN I and II) — 4- to 6-week certificate

Nurse Practitioners

Nurse practitioners (NPs) may practice medicine independently. In some states, NPs can write prescriptions, operate their own offices, and admit patients to hospitals. In other states, NPs work more closely with a physician. All NPs are experienced RNs and in most cases have a master's degree in nursing with the addition of specialized training as an NP.

Allied Health Professionals

Allied health care professionals make up a large section of the health care team. Box 1-1 lists and describes some of these

---

Box 1-1

ALLIED HEALTH CARE PROFESSIONALS

Chiropractor—Manipulates the musculoskeletal system and spine to relieve symptoms

Dental hygienist—Trained and licensed to work with a dentist by providing preventive care

Dietitian—Trained nutritionist who addresses dietary needs associated with illness

Electrocardiograph technician—Assists with the performance of diagnostic procedures for cardiac electrical activity

Electroencephalograph technician—Assists with the diagnostic procedures for brain wave activity

Emergency medical technician—Trained in techniques of administering emergency care en route to trauma centers

Histologist—Studies cells and tissues for diagnosis

Infection control officer—Identifies risks of transmission of infection and implements preventive measures

Laboratory technician—Trained in performance of laboratory diagnostic procedures

Medical assistant—Trained in administrative, clinical, and laboratory skills for the medical facility

Medical coder—Assigns appropriate codes to report medical services to third party payers for reimbursement

Medical office assistant—Trained in the administrative area of the outpatient medical facility

Medical transcriptionist—Trained in administrative skills; produces printed records of dictated medical information

Nuclear medical technician—Specializes in diagnostic procedures using radionuclides (electromagnetic radiation); works in a radiology department

Occupational therapist—Evaluates and plans programs to relieve physical and mental barriers that interfere with activities

Paramedic—Trained in advanced rescue and emergency procedures

Pharmacist—Prepares and dispenses medications by the physician's order

Phlebotomist—Collects blood specimens for laboratory procedures by performing venipuncture

Physical therapist—Plans and conducts rehabilitation to improve strength and mobility

Psychologist—Trained in methods of psychological assessment and treatment

Radiographer—Works with a radiologist or physician to operate x-ray equipment for diagnosis and treatment

Respiratory therapist—Trained to preserve or improve respiratory function

Risk manager—Identifies and corrects high-risk situations within the health care field

Social worker—Trained to evaluate and correct social, emotional, and environmental problems associated with the medical profession

Speech therapist—Treats and prevents speech and language disorders

Unit clerk—Performs the administrative duties in a hospital patient care unit team members. The educational requirements and responsibilities vary greatly among these professionals. One thing they all have in common is the support of a professional organization. Medical assistants fall into this category.

THE HISTORY OF MEDICAL ASSISTING

Medical assisting as a separate profession dates from the 1930s. In 1934, Dr. M. Mandl recognized the need for a medical professional possessing skills required in an office environment and opened the first school for medical assistants in New York City. Although medical assistants were employed before 1934, no formal schooling was available. Office assistants were trained on the job to perform medical procedures or nurses were trained to perform administrative procedures. The need for a highly trained professional with a background in administrative and clinical skills led to the formation of an alternative field of allied health care. In 1955, the American Association of Medical Assistants (AAMA), a professional organization for medical assistants, was founded during a meeting of medical assistants in Kansas City, Kansas. The resolutions adopted by the group were accepted and commended by the American Medical Association (AMA), the professional association of licensed physicians. In 1959, Illinois recognized the AAMA as a not-for-profit educational organization. The national office was established in Chicago with state and local chapters throughout the United States. The AAMA has guided the practice of medical assisting with strong leadership and vision. With its help, the medical assistant has grown into a highly respected and versatile member of the health care team. In 1963, a certification examination for CMA was developed that would set the standards required for medical assistant education. The first AAMA examinations were given in Kansas, California, and Florida. In the next two decades, the profession grew rapidly. The AMA collaborated in the development of the curriculum and accreditation of educational programs. In 1978, the U. S. Department of Education recognized the AAMA as an official accrediting agency for medical assisting programs in public and private schools.

In 1991, the Board of Trustees of the AAMA approved the current definition of medical assisting: Medical assisting is an allied health profession whose practitioners function as members of the health care delivery team and perform administrative and clinical procedures. Medical assistants continue to be vigilant of threats to their right to practice their profession. Each state mandates the actions of allied health professionals. It is the responsibility of the medical assistant to be familiar with the laws of the state in which he or she is working. The profession has been listed as one of the fastest growing careers of the 1990s, with 74% growth predicted by the U. S. Department of Labor in its 2002 Employment Outlook. Membership in the AAMA reached 18,500, with 525 local chapters in 47 states and the District of Columbia. Today, the organization's membership exceeds 30,000 medical assistants.

Checkpoint Question

7. What prompted the establishment of a school for medical assistants?

MEDICAL ASSISTING EDUCATION

A medical assisting curriculum prepares individuals for entry into the medical assisting profession. Medical assisting programs are found in postsecondary schools, such as private business schools and technical colleges, 2-year colleges, and community colleges. Programs vary in length. Programs of 6 months to a year offer a certificate of graduation or a diploma, and 2-year programs award the graduate an associate degree. The 2-year curriculum usually includes general studies, such as English, mathematics, and computer skills, in addition to the core courses, such as medical terminology and insurance coding. The curriculum in every accredited program must include the skills determined by the accrediting agency. Specific requirements for an accredited program are discussed later.

Accredited programs must include an **externship**. An externship is an educational course offered in the last module or semester during which the student works in the field gaining hands-on experience. It varies in length from 60 to 240 hours. Students are not paid but are awarded credit toward the degree. (See Chapter 19 for more detailed information.) Some schools offer job placement services.

After you finish school, your education should not stop. You should continue to take courses on various related topics. These may include new computer programs, new clinical procedures, new laws and regulations, or pharmaceutical updates. Some employers pay for conferences. In some situations, conference costs may be listed for tax credit when filing your income tax.

Box 1-2 outlines important changes made by the House of Delegates of the AAMA.

Checkpoint Question

8. What is an externship?

Medical Assisting Program Accreditation

In 1995, the AMA House of Delegates voted to require graduation from an accredited medical assisting program for admission to the CMA examination. This change went into effect in January 1998. **Accreditation** is a nongovernmental professional peer review process that provides technical assistance and evaluates educational programs for quality based on preestablished academic and administrative standards. Medical assisting program accreditation is based on a school's adherence to the scientifically grounded occupational analysis known as the AAMA Role Delineation Chart: Occupational Analysis of the Medical Assisting Profession. The **role delineation chart** is a list of the areas of competence expected of the graduate (see Appendix I). Role delineation components covered are listed at the beginning of each chapter of this textbook.

The Commission of Accreditation of Allied Health Education Programs

The Commission on Accreditation of Allied Health Education Programs (CAAHEP) in collaboration with the curriculum review board of the American Association of Medical Assistants' Endowment accredits medical assisting programs in both public and private postsecondary institutions throughout the United States. CAAHEP accredits many allied health education programs included in Box 1-1.

The Accrediting Bureau of Health Education Schools

The Accrediting Bureau of Health Education Schools (ABHES) accredits private postsecondary registered medical assistant (RMA) **certification** through a program review process conducted by the American Medical Technologists (AMT). This body has accredited medical technicians,

medical laboratory technicians, and dental technicians since the late 1930s but offered its first medical assisting examination in 1972.

MEDICAL ASSISTING CERTIFICATION

The AAMA and the AMT have developed certification examinations that test the knowledge of a graduate and indicate entry level competency. After passing the examination, the person can use the initials CMA (certified medical assistant) or RMA (registered medical assistant) after his or her name (Box 1-3).

Certified Medical Assistant

Graduates of medical assisting programs accredited by CAAHEP or ABHES are immediately eligible to take the CMA certification examination of the AAMA. Examinees who pass this test are designated as CMAs. The National Board of Medical Examiners, which administers several medical specialty examinations, serves as test consultant for the CMA certification examination of the AAMA.

Once you pass the examination and become a CMA, you are required to recertify every 5 years. **Recertification** may be obtained either by taking the examination again or by completing 60 **continuing education units** (CEUs) in a 5-year period. CEUs are awarded for attendance at approved local and state AAMA meetings and seminars, completion of guided study courses, and journal articles designed to submit a posttest for CEU credit.

Registered Medical Assistant

In 1972, the AMT offered the first RMA examination. Graduates from ABHES-accredited medical assisting programs are immediately eligible to take the RMA examination. Medical assistants who have been employed in the profession for a minimum of 5 years, no more than 2 of which may have been as an instructor, are also eligible. Those who pass this examination are designated as RMAs.

Although formal recertification is not required by AMT, members and nonmembers are invited to participate in the STEP program, a continuing education home study program for health care practitioners. AMT keeps a record of earned credit and issues annual reports of STEP activities to program participants.

Checkpoint Question

9. What is required to maintain current status as a CMA?

MEDICAL ASSISTING AND RELATED ALLIED HEALTH ASSOCIATIONS

Association Membership

You are not required to join a national organization to work as a medical assistant or to be eligible to take the certification examination. The associations have many benefits, however, for members. These benefits include the following:

- Access to educational seminars
- Access to continuing education units
- Subscription to the professional journals that alert you to new procedures and trends in medicine
- Access to the annual conventions
- Group insurance plans
- Networking opportunities

For further information on these organizations, visit the websites listed at the end of the chapter. Contact your local chapter or speak with your instructor for the procedure for applying for membership. You can download applications and requirements from the AAMA website (http://www.aama-ntl.org) and the AMT website (http://www.amt1.com).

American Association of Medical Assistants

The purpose of the AAMA is to promote the professional identity and stature of its members and the medical assisting profession through education and credentialing. *CMA Today*, which is published and distributed to members of the organization, includes articles of interest to the medical assistant to keep knowledge and skills current. Readers may take a posttest at the end of the article and receive CEU. Accredited continuing education opportunities are available through the national organization, and free transcripts of acquired AAMA-approved CEUs are available online with a member number. Professional benefits, such as insurance, are also made available to AAMA members. Active members are CMAs; non-CMAs, such as some medical assisting educators and those interested in medical assisting, are associate members. Students are encouraged to join and stay active in AAMA. Student members receive a reduced dues rate while in school and for a year following graduation. Figure 1-4 displays the insignia of the AAMA.

American Medical Technologists

The AMT and its governing body are set up similarly to the AAMA, with local, state, and national affiliations, opportunities for continuing education, professional benefits, and a professional journal. Members include medical technologists, medical laboratory technicians, medical assistants, dental assistants, office laboratory technicians, phlebotomy technicians, laboratory consultants, and allied health instructors. To join AMT, you need to be certified by meeting edu-

FIGURE 1–4. Insignia of affiliates of the AAMA.

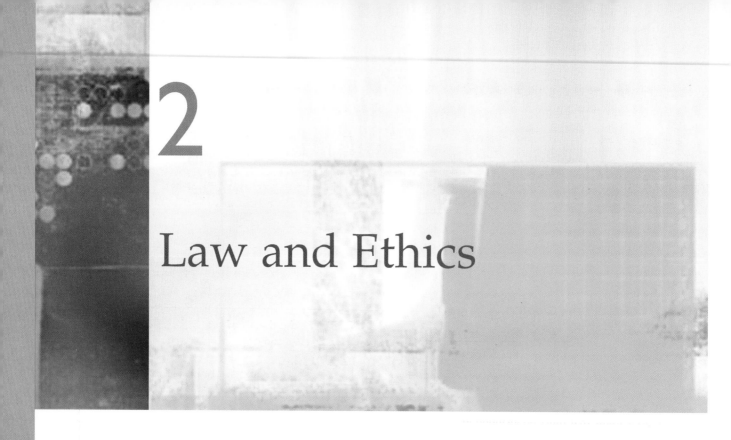

2

Law and Ethics

CHAPTER OUTLINE

ROLE DELINEATION COMPONENTS

GENERAL: Professionalism
- Demonstrate initiative and responsibility
- Treat all patients with compassion and empathy

GENERAL: Legal Concepts
- Perform within legal and ethical boundaries
- Prepare and maintain medical records

- Document accurately
- Follow employer's established policies dealing with the health care contract
- Implement and maintain federal and state health care legislation and regulations

CHAPTER COMPETENCIES

LEARNING OBJECTIVES
Upon successfully completing this chapter, you will be able to:

1. Spell and define the key terms
2. Identify the two branches of the American legal system
3. List the elements and types of contractual agreements and describe the difference in implied and express contracts
4. List four items that must be included in a contract termination or withdrawal letter
5. List six items that must be included in an informed consent form and explain who may sign consent forms
6. List five legally required disclosures that must be reported to specified authorities
7. Describe the purpose of the Self-Determination Act
8. Describe the four elements that must be proven in a medical legal suit
9. Describe four possible defenses against litigation for the medical professional
10. Explain the theory of respondeat superior, or law of agency, and how it applies to the medical assistant
11. List ways that a medical assistant can assist in the prevention of a medical malpractice suit
12. Outline the laws regarding employment and safety issues in the medical office
13. List the requirements of the Americans with Disabilities Act relating to the medical office
14. Differentiate between legal issues and ethical issues
15. List the seven American Medical Association principles of ethics
16. List the five ethical principles of ethical and moral conduct outlined by the American Association of Medical Assistants
17. List 10 opinions of the American Medical Association's Council pertaining to administrative office procedures

KEY TERMS

abandonment	comparative negligence	expert witness	noncompliant
advance directive	confidentiality	expressed consent	plaintiff
age of majority	consent	expressed contracts	precedents
appeal	consideration	fee splitting	protocol
artificial insemination	contract	fraud	registered
assault	contributory negligence	implied consent	res ipsa loquitur
battery	cross-examination	implied contracts	res judicata
bench trial	damages	informed consent	respondeat superior
bioethics	defamation of character	intentional tort	slander
blood-borne pathogens	defendant	legally required disclosure	stare decisis
breach	depositions	libel	statutes
censure	direct examination	licensure	statute of limitations
certification	durable power of attorney	litigation	tort
civil law	duress	locum tenens	unintentional tort
coerce	emancipated minor	malpractice	verdict
common law	ethics	negligence	

DURING YOUR CAREER AS A medical assistant, you will be involved in many medical situations with potential legal implications. You must uphold ethical standards to ensure the patient's well-being. Ethics deals with the concept of right and wrong. Laws are written to carry out these concepts. Physicians may be sued for a variety of reasons, including significant clinical errors (e.g., removing the wrong limb, ordering a toxic dose of medication), claims of improperly touching a patient without consent, or failure to properly diagnose or treat a disease. Medicare **fraud** (concealing the truth) and falsifying medical records can also result in a lawsuit. Medical assistants and other health care workers are included in many of the suits brought to court. You may help to prevent many of these claims against your physician, and to protect yourself, by complying with medical laws, keeping abreast of medical trends, and acting in an ethical manner by maintaining a high level of professionalism at all times.

THE AMERICAN LEGAL SYSTEM

Our legal system is in place to ensure the rights of all citizens. We depend on the legal system to protect us from the wrongdoings of others. Many potential medical suits prove to be unwarranted and never make it into the court system, but even in the best physician–patient relationships, **litigation** (lawsuits) between patients and physicians may occur. Litigation may result from a single medication error or a mistake that costs a person's life. It is essential that you have a basic understanding of the American legal system to protect yourself, your patients, and your physician-employer by following the legal guidelines. You must know your legal duties and understand the legal nature of the physician–patient relationship and your role and responsibilities as the physician's agent.

Sources of Law

Laws are rules of conduct that are enforced by appointed authorities. The foundation of our legal system is our rights outlined in the Constitution and the laws established by our Founding Fathers. These traditional laws are known as **common law**.

Common law is based on the theory of **stare decisis**. This term means "the previous decision stands." Judges usually follow these **precedents** (previous court decisions) but sometimes overrule a previous decision, establishing new precedent. **Statutes** are another source of law. Federal, state, or local legislators make laws or statutes, the police enforce them, and the court system ensures justice. Statutes pertaining to Medicare, Medicaid, and the Food and Drug Administration are common examples in the medical profession.

The third type of law is administrative. These laws are passed by governmental agencies, such as the Internal Revenue Service.

Branches of the Law

The two main branches of the legal system are public law and private or **civil law**.

Public Law

Public law is the branch of law that focuses on issues between the government and its citizens. It can be divided into four subgroups:

1. Criminal law is concerned with issues of citizen welfare and safety. Examples include arson, burglary, murder, and rape. A medical assistant must stay within the boundaries of the profession. Treating patients without the physician's orders could result in a charge of practicing medicine without a license—an act covered under criminal law.
2. Constitutional law is commonly called the law of the land. The United States government has a constitution, and each state has a constitution of its own, laws, and regulations. State laws may be more restrictive than federal laws but may not be more lenient. Two examples of constitutional law are laws on abortion and civil rights.
3. Administrative law is the regulations set forth by governmental agencies. This category includes laws pertaining to the Food and Drug Administration, the Internal Revenue Service, and the Board of Medical Examiners.
4. International law pertains to treaties between countries. Related issues include trade agreements, extradition, boundaries, and international waters.

Private or Civil Law

Private or civil law is the branch of the law that focuses on issues between private citizens. The medical profession is primarily concerned with private law. The subcategories that pertain to the medical profession are contract, commercial, and tort law. Contract and commercial laws concern the rights and obligations of those who enter into contracts, as in a physician–patient relationship. **Tort** law governs the righting of wrongs or injuries suffered by someone because of another person's wrongdoing or misdeeds resulting from a **breach** of legal duty. Tort law is the basis of most lawsuits against physicians and health care workers. Other civil law branches include property, inheritance, and corporation law.

 Checkpoint Question

1. Which branch of law covers a medical assistant charged with practicing medicine without a license?

The Rise in Medical Legal Cases

Since World War II, the number of medical malpractice cases brought to court has increased significantly. **Malpractice** refers to an action by a professional health care worker that harms a patient. A rise in the amounts of settlement awards has had a negative impact on the cost and coverage of malpractice insurance. With this rise, some physicians have actually changed the scope of their practice to reduce their costs. For example, an obstetrician may choose to limit practice to the care of nonpregnant women to avoid the high cost of malpractice insurance for physicians who deliver babies. In an attempt to protect professionals, legislation designed to limit the amount a jury can award has been introduced in Congress. Legal issues involving the medical field are referred to as medicolegal, which combines the words medical and legal.

A government task force found four primary reasons for the rise in malpractice claims:

1. *Scientific advances.* As new and improved medical technology becomes available, the risks and potential for complications of these procedures escalate, making physicians more vulnerable to litigation.
2. *Unrealistic expectations.* Some patients expect miracle cures and file lawsuits because recovery was not as they hoped or expected, even if the physician is not at fault.
3. *Economic factors.* Some patients view lawsuits as a means to obtain quick cash. (In fact, the number of lawsuits filed has increased during economic recessions.)
4. *Poor communication.* Studies show that when patients do not feel a bond with their physician, they are more likely to sue. Attention to customer service helps develop a good rapport between patients, the provider, and the staff.

PHYSICIAN–PATIENT RELATIONSHIP

Rights and Responsibilities of the Patient and Physician

In any contractual relationship, both parties have certain rights and responsibilities. The rights of the patient include the ability to choose a physician. This right may be limited to a list of participating providers under a patient's insurance plan. Patients have the right to determine whether to begin medical treatment and to set limits on that treatment. The patient also has the right to know in advance what the treatment will consist of, what effect it may have, and what dangers are to be expected. The concept of informed consent is discussed later in the chapter.

Physicians have the right to limit their practice to a certain specialty or a certain location. For example, patients may not expect a physician to treat them at home. Physicians also have the right to refuse service to new patients or existing patients with new problems unless they are on emergency room call, in which case they must continue to treat patients seen during this time. The subject of abandonment is discussed later. Doctors have the right to change their policies or availability as long as they give patients reasonable notice of the change. This can be done through a local newspaper advertisement and/or a letter to each patient. Box 2-1 lists the patient's and physician's responsibilities.

Contracts

A **contract** is an agreement between two or more parties with certain factors agreed on among all parties. The physician–patient relationship is reinforced by the formation of a contract. All contractual agreements have three components:

1. Offer (contract initiation)
2. Acceptance (both parties agree to the terms)
3. **Consideration** (the exchange of fees for service)

A contract is not valid unless all three elements are present. A contract offer is made when a patient calls the office to request an appointment. The offer is accepted when you make an appointment for the patient. You have formed a contract that implies that for a fee, the physician will do all in his or her power to address the health concerns of the patient.

Certain individuals, such as children and those who are mentally incompetent or temporarily incapacitated, are not legally able to enter contracts. Patients in this category do not have the capacity to enter into a contract, and therefore decisions about health care should be made by a competent party acting as a health care decision maker for the minor or incompetent person.

The two types of contracts between physicians and patients are implied and expressed.

Implied Contracts

Implied contracts, the most common kind of contract between physicians and patients, are not written but are assumed by the actions of the parties. For example, a patient calls the office and requests to see Dr. Smith for an earache. The patient arrives for the appointment, is seen by the physician, and receives a prescription. It is *implied* that because the patient came on his own and requested care that he wants this physician to care for him. The physician's action of accepting the patient for care *implies* that he acknowledges responsibility for his part of the contract. The patient *implies* by accepting the services that he will render payment even if the price was not discussed.

Expressed Contracts

Expressed contracts, either written or oral, consist of specified details. A mutual sharing of responsibilities is always stated in an expressed contract. The agreement you have

---

Box 2-1

RESPONSIBILITIES OF THE PATIENT AND THE PHYSICIAN

Responsibilities of the Patient	Responsibilities of the Physician
Provide the physician with accurate data about the duration and nature of symptoms	Respect the patient's confidential information
Provide a complete and accurate medical history to the physician	Provide reasonable skill, experience, and knowledge in treating the patient
Follow the physician's instructions for diet, exercise, medications, and appointments	Continue treating the patient until the contract has been withdrawn or as long as the condition requires treatment
Compensate the physician for services rendered	Inform patients of their condition, treatments, and prognosis
	Give complete and accurate information
	Provide competent coverage during time away from practice
	Obtain informed consent before performing procedures (informed consent is a statement of approval from the patient for the physician to perform a given procedure after the patient has been educated about the risks and benefits of the procedure)
	Caution against unneeded or undesirable treatment or surgery

---

with your creditors is an expressed contract. These kinds of contracts are not used as often in the medical setting as implied contracts.

Checkpoint Question

2. An orthopedic surgeon decides to make a change in his services. He wants to limit his practice to nonsurgical patients. What action should the physician take?

Termination or Withdrawal of the Contract

A contract is ideally resolved when the patient is satisfactorily cured of the illness and the physician has been paid for the services. The patient may end the contract at any time, but the physician must follow legal **protocol** to dissolve the contract if the patient still seeks treatment and the physician wishes to end the relationship.

Patient-Initiated Termination. A patient who chooses to terminate the relationship should notify the physician and give the reasons. You must keep this letter in the medical record. After the receipt of this letter, the physician should then send a letter to the patient stating the following:

- The physician accepts the termination.
- Medical records are available on written request.
- Medical referrals are available if needed.

If the patient verbally asks to end this relationship, the physician should send a letter to the patient documenting the conversation and again offering referrals and access to the medical records. Clear documentation is essential.

Physician-Initiated Termination. The physician may find it necessary to end the relationship. A physician may terminate the contract if the patient is **noncompliant** or does not keep appointments or for personal reasons. The physician must send a letter of withdrawal that includes:

- A statement of intent to terminate the relationship
- The reasons for this action
- The termination date at least 30 days from the date of receipt of the letter
- A statement that the medical records will be transferred to another physician at the patient's request
- A strong recommendation that the patient seek additional medical care as warranted

The letter must be sent by certified mail with a return receipt requested. A copy of the termination letter and the return receipt are placed in the patient's record. Figure 2-1

Amy Fine, MD
Charlotte Family Practice
220 NW 3rd Avenue
Charlotte, NC 25673

August 22, 2003

Regina Dodson
Jones Hill Road
Charlotte, NC 25673

Dear Ms. Dodson:

Due to the fact that you have persistently refused to follow my medical advice and treatment of your diabetes, I will no longer be able to provide medical care to you. Since your condition requires ongoing medical care, you must find another physician as soon as possible. I will be available to you until that time, but no longer than 30 days.

To assist you in continuing to receive care, we will make records available to your new physician as soon as you authorize us to send them.

Sincerely,

Amy Fine, MD

FIGURE 2–1. Letter of intent to terminate physician–patient relationship.

shows a sample letter of intent to terminate a physician–patient relationship.

Abandonment. If a contract is not properly terminated, the physician can be sued for abandonment. **Abandonment** may be charged if the physician withdraws from the contractual relationship without proper notification while the patient still needs treatment. Physicians must always arrange coverage when absent from the office for vacations, conferences, and so on. Patients may sue for abandonment in any instance that a suitable substitute is not available for care. Coverage may be provided by a **locum tenens**, a substitute physician.

Other examples of abandonment:

• The physician abruptly and without reasonable notice stops treating a patient whose condition requires additional or continued care.
• The physician fails to see a patient as often as the condition requires or incorrectly advises the patient that further treatment is not needed.

Checkpoint Question

3. What five elements must be in a physician's termination intent letter?

Consent

The law requires that patients must **consent** or agree to being touched, examined, or treated by the physician or agents of the physician involved in the contractual agreement. No treatment may be made without a consent given orally, nonverbally by behavior, or clearly in writing. Patients have the right to appoint a health care surrogate or health care power of attorney who may make health care decisions when the patient is unable to make them. A health care surrogate may be a spouse, a friend, a pastor, or an attorney. A **durable power of attorney** for health care gives the patient's representative the ability to make health care decisions as the health care surrogate. A patient's physician should be aware of the power of attorney agreement, and a copy of the legal documentation should be kept in the office medical record.

Implied Consent

In the typical visit to the physician's office, the patient's actions represent an informal agreement for care to be given. A patient who raises a sleeve to receive an injection implies agreement to the treatment. **Implied consent** also occurs in an emergency. If a patient is in a life-threatening situation and is unable to give verbal permission for treatment, it is implied that the patient would consent to treatment if possible. As soon as possible, informed consent should be signed by either the patient or a family member in this type of situation. When there is no emergency, implied consent should be used only if the procedure poses no significant risk to the patient.

Informed or Expressed Consent

The physician is responsible for obtaining the patient's **informed consent** whenever the treatment involves an invasive procedure such as surgery, use of experimental drugs, potentially dangerous procedures such as stress tests, or any treatment that poses a significant risk to the patient. A federal law discussed later requires that health care providers who administer certain vaccines give the patient a current vaccine information statement (VIS). A VIS provides a standardized way to give objective information about vaccine benefits and adverse events (side effects) to patients. The VIS is available online through the Centers for Disease Control and Prevention (CDC) in 26 languages. Informed consent is also referred to as **expressed consent**.

Informed consent is based on the patient's right to know every possible benefit, risk, or alternative to the suggested treatment and the possible outcome if no treatment is initiated. The patient must voluntarily give permission and must understand the implications of consenting to the treatment. This requires that the physician and patient communicate in a manner understandable to the patient. Patients can be more active in personal health care decisions when they are educated about and understand their treatment and care.

A consent form must include the following information:

1. Name of the procedure to be performed
2. Name of the physician who will perform the procedure
3. Name of the person administering the anesthesia (if applicable)
4. Any potential risks from the procedure
5. Anticipated result or benefit from the procedure
6. Alternatives to the procedure and their risks
7. Probable effect on the patient's condition if the procedure is not performed
8. Any exclusions that the patient requests
9. Statement indicating that all of the patient's questions or concerns regarding the procedure have been answered
10. Patient's and witnesses' signatures and the date

As the medical assistant, you will frequently be required to witness consent signatures. A sample consent form is seen in Figure 2-2.

The informed consent form supplied for the patient's signature must be in the language that the patient speaks. Most physicians who treat multicultural patients have consent

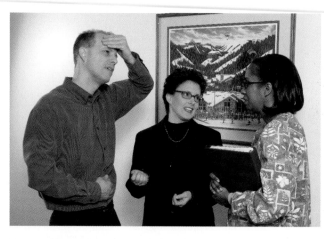

FIGURE 2-3. Using an interpreter, the CMA helps this patient understand the procedure.

forms available in a variety of languages. Never ask a patient to sign a consent form if he or she:

• Does not understand the procedure
• Has unanswered questions regarding the procedure
• Is unable to read the consent form

Never **coerce** (force or compel against his or her wishes) a patient into signing a consent form. Figure 2-3 shows a deaf patient, a signing interpreter, and a certified medical assistant (CMA) with a consent form.

WHAT IF

A well-meaning family member asks for information about her mother's condition. What should you say?

Tell the family member that you are not allowed to discuss the patient without his or her permission. No information should be released to anyone—friends, family, media, or insurance companies—without prior written approval from the patient.

At the first visit, you should establish the patient's wishes about giving information to family members and friends. If there is a particular family member who brings the patient to the office, the patient may sign a release form giving that person the right to receive information. Many physicians provide the patient with a short progress report including the patient's test results, diagnosis, treatment, and next appointment. A form could be designed for this purpose. This gives the patient the opportunity to share complete and accurate information if they choose.

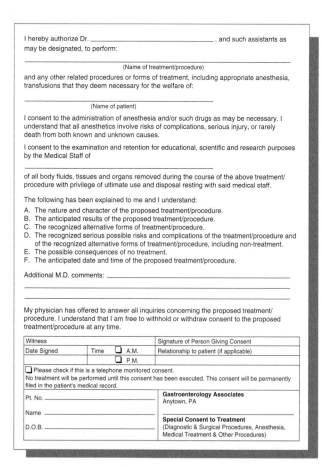

I hereby authorize Dr. _____ , and such assistants as may be designated, to perform:

_____
(Name of treatment/procedure)

and any other related procedures or forms of treatment, including appropriate anesthesia, transfusions that they deem necessary for the welfare of:

_____
(Name of patient)

I consent to the administration of anesthesia and/or such drugs as may be necessary. I understand that all anesthetics involve risks of complications, serious injury, or rarely death from both known and unknown causes.

I consent to the examination and retention for educational, scientific and research purposes by the Medical Staff of

_____

of all body fluids, tissues and organs removed during the course of the above treatment/procedure with privilege of ultimate use and disposal resting with said medical staff.

The following has been explained to me and I understand:

A. The nature and character of the proposed treatment/procedure.
B. The anticipated results of the proposed treatment/procedure.
C. The recognized alternative forms of treatment/procedure.
D. The recognized serious possible risks and complications of the treatment/procedure and of the recognized alternative forms of treatment/procedure, including non-treatment.
E. The possible consequences of no treatment.
F. The anticipated date and time of the proposed treatment/procedure.

Additional M.D. comments: _____
_____
_____

My physician has offered to answer all inquiries concerning the proposed treatment/procedure. I understand that I am free to withhold or withdraw consent to the proposed treatment/procedure at any time.

Witness			Signature of Person Giving Consent
Date Signed	Time	☐ A.M.	Relationship to patient (if applicable)
		☐ P.M.	

☐ Please check if this is a telephone monitored consent.
No treatment will be performed until this consent has been executed. This consent will be permanently filed in the patient's medical record.

Pt. No. _____	**Gastroenterology Associates** Anytown, PA
Name _____	
D.O.B. _____	**Special Consent to Treatment** (Diagnostic & Surgical Procedures, Anesthesia, Medical Treatment & Other Procedures)

FIGURE 2-2. Sample consent form.

Who May Sign a Consent Form?. An adult (usually someone over age 18) who is mentally competent and not under the influence of medication or other substances may sign a consent form. A minor may sign a consent form if he or she is:

- In the armed services
- Requesting treatment for communicable diseases (including sexually transmitted diseases)
- Pregnant
- Requesting information regarding birth control, abortion, or drug or alcohol abuse counseling
- Emancipated

An **emancipated minor** is under the **age of majority** but is either married or self-supporting and is responsible for his or her debts. The age of majority varies from state to state and ranges from 18 to 21. Minors may give consent if any one of the above-listed criteria is present.

Legal guardians may also sign consent forms. A legal guardian is appointed by a judge when the court has ruled an individual to be mentally incompetent. Health care surrogates may also sign consent forms. Health care surrogates are discussed later in the chapter.

Checkpoint Question

4. Under what circumstances should a patient never be asked to sign a consent form?

Refusal of Consent

Patients may refuse treatment for any reason. Sometimes, patients make treatment choices based on religious or personal beliefs and preferences. For instance, a Jehovah's Witness may refuse a blood transfusion on religious grounds, or an elderly person may not want to undergo serious surgery because the potential complications may limit future lifestyle options. In this situation, the patient must sign a refusal of consent form indicating that the patient was instructed regarding the potential risks and benefits of the procedure as well as the risks if the procedure is not allowed. If the patient is a minor, the courts may become involved at the request of the physician or hospital and may award consent for the child. In this situation, the physician should follow legal counsel and document the incident carefully. In any instance that the patient refuses treatment, documentation must be made to protect the physician. The physician has a legal right to refuse to perform elective surgery on a patient who refuses to receive blood if needed.

Releasing Medical Information

The medical record is a legal document. Although the medical record itself belongs to the physician, the information belongs to the patient. Patients have the right to their medical information, and they have the right to deny the sharing of this information.

Requests for medical records are common. Other health care facilities, insurance companies, and patients themselves may need information from the medical chart. Staying within the law when releasing medical information is covered in Chapter 8.

Legally Required Disclosures

Even though patients have the right to limit access to their medical records, health care facilities have a responsibility to report certain events to governmental agencies without the patient's consent, which are referred to as **legally required disclosures**. You and other health care providers must report to the department of public health the situations described in the following sections.

Vital Statistics

All states maintain records of births, deaths, marriages, and divorces. These records include the following:

- Birth certificates.
- Stillbirth reports. Some states have separate stillbirth forms; other states use a regular death certificate.
- Death certificates. These must be signed by a physician. The cause and time of death must be included.

You may assist the physician in completing a death certificate and filing the finished report in the patient's chart.

Medical Examiner's Reports

Each state has laws pertaining to which deaths must be reported to the medical examiner's office. Generally, these include the following:

- Death from an unknown cause
- Death from a suspected criminal or violent act
- Death of a person not attended by a physician at the time of death or for a reasonable period preceding the death
- Death within 24 hours of hospital admission

Infectious or Communicable Diseases

These reports are made to the local health department. The information is used for statistical purposes and for preventing or tracking the spread of these diseases. Although state guidelines vary, there are usually three categories of reports:

- Telephone reports are required for diphtheria, cholera, meningococcal meningitis, and plague, usually within 24 hours of the diagnosis. Telephone reports must always be followed by written reports.
- Written reports are required for hepatitis, leprosy, malaria, rubeola, polio, rheumatic fever, tetanus, and tuberculosis. Sexually transmitted diseases must also

PATIENT EDUCATION

Legally Required Disclosures

Patient's who have conditions that require legal disclosure should be informed about the applicable law. Patients should be assured that all steps to ensure their confidentiality will be followed. Patients should be educated about why the disclosure is necessary, who receives the information, what particular forms will be completed, and any anticipated follow-up from the organization. For example, you are required to report to the local health department the name, address, and condition of a patient with sexually transmitted disease. It is the responsibility of the health department to contact the patient to acquire the names of the patient's sexual contacts. These contacts are notified and counseled by the health department official. Patients who are educated about these legally required disclosures will be more understanding and accepting of the need to file official reports.

be reported. Notification is usually required within 3 days of the date of discovery.

- Trend reports are made when your office notes an unusually high occurrence of influenza, streptococcal infections, or any other infectious diseases. Box 2-2 is a sample of reportable diseases and their time frames.

The CDC keeps a watchful eye on the public health. When necessary, the CDC establishes directives for the protection of the public. For example, when the public appeared to be at risk for contracting anthrax in 2001, the CDC mandated that documented anthrax cases be reported immediately. Fax machines and e-mail help facilitate such urgent public health communication.

National Childhood Vaccine Injury Act of 1986

Health care providers who administer certain vaccines and toxoids must report to the U. S. Department of Health & Human Services (DHHS) the occurrence of any side effects listed in the manufacturer's package insert. In addition, health care providers must record in the patient's record the following information:

1. Date the vaccine was administered
2. Lot number and manufacturer of vaccine
3. Any adverse reactions to the vaccine
4. Name, title, and address of the person who administered the vaccine

Box 2-2

REPORTABLE CONDITIONS

Chapter 19—Health: Epidemiology
Subchapter 19a—Communicable Disease Control
Section .0100—Reporting of Communicable Diseases
.0101 Reportable Diseases and Conditions
(a) The following named diseases and conditions are declared to be dangerous to the public health and are hereby made reportable within the time period specified after the disease or condition is reasonably suspected to exist:

acquired immune deficiency syndrome (AIDS)—
    7 days
amebiasis—7 days
anthrax—24 hours
blastomycosis—7 days
botulism—24 hours
brucellosis—7 days
Campylobacter infection—24 hours
chancroid—24 hours
chlamydial infection (laboratory confirmed)—7 days
cholera—24 hours
dengue—7 days
diphtheria—24 hours
E. coli infection—24 hours
encephalitis—7 days
food-borne disease, including but not limited to
    Clostridium perfringens, staphylococcal, and *Bacillus cereus*—24 hours
gonorrhea—24 hours
granuloma inguinale—24 hours
Haemophilus influenzae, invasive disease—24 hours
hepatitis A—24 hours
hepatitis B—24 hours
hepatitis B carriage—7 days
hepatitis non-A, non-B—7 days
human immunodeficiency virus infection (HIV) confirmed—7 days
legionellosis—7 days
leprosy—7 days
leptospirosis—7 days
Lyme disease—7 days
lymphogranuloma venereum—7 days
malaria—7 days
measles (rubeola)—24 hours
meningitis, pneumococcal—7 days
meningitis, viral (aseptic)—7 days
meningococcal disease—24 hours
mucocutaneous lymph node syndrome (Kawasaki
    syndrome)—7 days
mumps—7 days

Excerpt from the North Carolina Administrative Code Regarding Reporting of Communicable Diseases

Box 2-3

VACCINATIONS REQUIRING VACCINE INFORMATION STATEMENTS

Anthrax
Chickenpox
Diphtheria, tetanus, and pertussis
Hib
Hepatitis A
Hepatitis B
Influenza
Lyme disease
Measles, mumps, and rubella
Meningococcal
Pneumococcal polysaccharide
Pneumococcal conjugate
Polio

Box 2-3 lists the vaccines and toxoids covered by the National Childhood Vaccine Injury Act.

Abuse, Neglect, or Maltreatment

Abuse, neglect, or maltreatment of any person who is incapable of self-protection usually falls under this category and may include the elderly or the mentally incompetent. Each state has its own regulations regarding what must be reported. Patient confidentiality rights are waived when the law requires you to report certain conditions.

Abuse is thought to be the second most common cause of death in children under age 5. The Federal Child Abuse Prevention and Treatment Act mandates that threats to a child's physical and mental welfare be reported. Health care workers, teachers, and social workers who report suspected abuse are not identified to the parents and are protected against liability. State laws vary regarding the procedure for reporting abuse. Local regulations should be outlined in the policies and procedures manuals at any outpatient facility. If you suspect a child is being abused, relay your suspicions to the physician. The physician will make the formal report. When authorities receive a report from a health care provider, they follow up by investigating the situation. For assistance in reporting suspected child abuse, you may call the national 24-hour hotline at 800-4 A CHILD (800-422-4453).

Spousal abuse is on the rise in this country. Many women and children are trapped in a cycle of abuse. Mothers who are financially dependent on their abusers may see no way out. You should record any information gathered in the patient interview or anything observed in the course of dealing with the patient that may indicate abuse. Report these observations to the physician. Most communities have anonymous safe places for victims of domestic abuse, and you should be familiar with these services. With proper referrals, you may be able to help break the cycle of domestic abuse.

This country is also undergoing a rise in elderly parents being cared for by their adult children who also have the responsibility of raising young children. This phenomenon can cause great stress among caregivers. Abuse of the elderly can be in the form of mistreatment or neglect (not providing appropriate care). You should pay attention to observations and information provided by your elderly patients. If mistreatment is suspected, alert the physician. Support groups for those caring for the elderly are useful in dealing with the challenges of caring for others.

Violent Injuries

Health care providers have the legal duty to report suspected criminal acts. Injuries resulting from weapons, assault, attempted suicide, and rape must be reported to local authorities.

Other Reports

A diagnosis of cancer must be reported to assist in tracking malignancies and identifying environmental carcinogens. Just as the CDC keeps track of all communicable diseases reported, a database of treated tumors is kept in hospitals through a tumor registry. Some states also require that epilepsy (a seizure condition) be reported to local motor vehicle departments. The testing of newborns for phenylketonuria (PKU), which can cause mental retardation, is required in all states. Some states require positive PKU results to be reported to the health department so that close observation and follow-up care are ensured to prevent serious complications for the infant. Infantile hypothyroidism is also a reportable condition in some states.

Checkpoint Question

5. What are six situations and conditions you are legally required to report?

SPECIFIC LAWS AND STATUTES THAT APPLY TO HEALTH PROFESSIONALS

Medical Practice Acts

Although each state has its own medical practice act, the following elements are usually included:

- Definition of the practice of medicine.
- Requirements that the physician must have graduated from an accredited medical school and residency program and have passed the state medical examination.
- Description of the procedure for **licensure**.

- Description of the conditions for which a license can be suspended or revoked.
- Description of the renewal process for licensure. Most states require the physician to have attended a certain number of continuing education hours.
- Personal requirements necessary to become a licensed physician. Generally, a licensed physician must be a state resident, of good moral character, a U. S. citizen, and 21 years of age or older.

A physician may have his or her license revoked or suspended by the board of medical examiners in most states for a variety of reasons, including certain criminal offenses, unprofessional conduct, fraud, or professional or personal incompetence. Criminal offenses include but are not limited to murder, manslaughter, robbery, and rape. Examples of unprofessional conduct may include invasion of a patient's privacy, excessive use of alcohol or use of illegal drugs, and **fee splitting** (sharing fees for the referral of patients to certain colleagues). Fraud is a common reason for revoking a license. Fraud may include filing false Medicare or Medicaid claims, falsifying medical records, or professional misrepresentation. Examples of misrepresentation or fraud include advertising a medical cure that does not exist, guaranteeing 100% success of a treatment, or falsifying medical credentials. Incompetence is often a hard charge to prove. The three most common examples are insanity, senility, and other documented mental incompetence.

As a medical assistant, it is your responsibility to report illegal or unethical behavior or signs of incompetence in the medical office. See Box 2-11 and think about how would you handle this difficult situation. (We will discuss ethics later in this chapter.)

Licensure, Certification, and Registration

Medical professionals can be licensed, certified, or **registered**. Licensure is regulated by laws, such as medical practice acts and nursing practice acts. If a particular profession is a licensed one, it is mandatory that one maintain a license in each state where he or she works. Each state determines the qualifications and requirements for licensure of a particular profession. A state agency will be responsible for issuing and renewing licenses. Most professionals are licensed to practice their profession according to certain guidelines and are limited to specific duties. For example, nurses are licensed. In North Carolina, the nursing practice act specifically prohibits a nurse from delegating professional authority to unlicensed personnel.

The term *registered* indicates that a professional has met basic requirements, usually for education, has passed standard testing, and has been approved by a governing body to perform given tasks within a state. X-ray technologists are registered as registered radiologic technologists. A national registry is available to verify a potential employee's status.

Certification is a voluntary process regulated through a professional organization. Standards for certification are set by the organization issuing the certificate. The CMA and registered medical assistant (RMA) credentials are nationally recognized and do not require any action when moving from one state to another. Remember, you must adhere to the laws regarding the CMA or RMA in the state where you work.

As a medical assistant, you are not licensed and therefore not limited to certain duties. The physician-employer has the sole responsibility of setting any limits on the duties of a medical assistant. Although most states do not require certification for employment, employers seek the CMA or RMA because certification indicates the achievement of certain standards of competence. A few states require that you take a test or short course before performing certain clinical duties.

Controlled Substances Act

The Controlled Substances Act of 1970 is a federal law enforced by the Drug Enforcement Agency (DEA). The act regulates the manufacture, distribution, and dispensing of narcotics and nonnarcotic drugs considered to have a high potential for abuse. This act was designed to decrease the illegal use of controlled substances and to prevent substance abuse by medical professionals. The law requires that any physician who dispenses, administers, or prescribes narcotics or other controlled substances be registered with the DEA.

Physicians who maintain a stock of controlled substances in the office for dispensing or administration must use a special triplicate order form available through the DEA. A record of each transaction must be kept and retained for 2 to 3 years. The record must be available for inspection by the DEA at any time. The act requires that all controlled substances be kept in a locked cabinet out of the patients' view and that the keys be kept secure. Theft should be reported immediately to the local police and the nearest DEA office. Prescription pads used for prescribing controlled substances must remain in a safe place at all times. Box 2-4 lists steps you can take to keep these prescription pads safe.

This act also requires a physician to return all registration certificates and any unused order forms to the DEA if the practice is closed or sold. Violation of this act is a criminal offense. Penalties range from fines to imprisonment. Table 2-1 outlines the classification of controlled substances.

Good Samaritan Act

As the number of lawsuits against physicians began to rise, physicians feared that giving emergency care to strangers outside the office could lead to malpractice suits. To combat that fear, all states now have Good Samaritan acts. Good Samaritan acts ensure that caregivers are immune from liability suits as long as they give care in good faith and in a manner that a reasonable and prudent person would in a

PRESCRIPTION PAD SAFETY TIPS

- Keep only one prescription pad in a locked cabinet in the examining room. All other pads should be locked away elsewhere. Do not leave prescription pads unattended.
- Keep a limited supply of pads. It is better to reorder on a regular basis than to overstock.
- Keep track of the number of pads in the office. If a burglary occurs, you will be able to advise the police regarding the number of missing pads.
- Report any prescription pad theft to the police and alert local pharmacies of the theft. If the theft involves the loss of narcotic pads, the Drug Enforcement Agency must be notified.

similar situation. Each state has specific guidelines. Some even set standards for various professional levels, such as one set of standards for a physician and another set of standards for emergency medical technicians. Your state's Good Samaritan Act will not protect you if you are grossly negligent or willfully perform negligent acts.

You are not covered by the Good Samaritan Act while you are working as a medical assistant, nor does it cover physicians in the performance of their duties. Liability and malpractice insurance policies are available to protect you in those situations. If you render emergency care and accept compensation for that care, the act does not apply.

The provisions only cover acts outside of the formal practice of the profession.

BASIS OF MEDICAL LAW

Tort Law

A tort is a wrongful act that results in harm for which restitution must be made. The two forms of torts are intentional and unintentional. An allegation of an **unintentional tort** means that the accuser (the **plaintiff**) believes a mistake has been made; however, the plaintiff believes the caregiver or accused party (the **defendant**) was operating in good faith and did not intend the mistake to occur. Consider this scenario as an example of an unintentional tort: A medical assistant giving a patient a heat treatment for muscle aches inadvertently burns the arm of a patient because the equipment is faulty. This act was not intentional or malicious, but it caused damage to the patient. About 90% of suits against physicians fall into this category.

Table 2-1	**CONTROLLED SUBSTANCES**	
Schedule	**Description**	**Examples**
I	These drugs have the highest potential for abuse and have no currently accepted medical use in the United States. There are no accepted safety standards for use of these drugs or substances even under medical supervision, although some are used experimentally in carefully controlled research projects.	Opium Marijuana Lysergic acid diethylamide (LSD) Peyote Mescaline
II	These drugs have a high potential for abuse. They have accepted medicinal use in the United States but with severe restrictions. Abuse of these drugs can lead to dependence, either psychological or physiological. Schedule II drugs require a written prescription and cannot be refilled or called in to the pharmacy by the medical office. Only in extreme emergencies may the physician call in the prescription. A handwritten prescription must be presented to the pharmacist within 72 hours.	Morphine Codeine Seconal Cocaine Amphetamine Dilaudid Ritalin
III	These drugs have a limited potential for psychological or physiological dependence. The prescription may be called in to the pharmacist by the physician and refilled up to 5 times in a 6-month period.	Paregoric Tylenol with codeine Fiorinal
IV	These drugs have a lower potential for abuse than those in Schedules II and III. They can be called in to the pharmacist by a medical office employee and may be refilled up to 5 times in a 6-month period.	Librium Valium Darvon Phenobarbital
V	These drugs have a lower potential for abuse than those in Schedules I, II, III, and IV.	Lomotil Dimetane expectorant DC Robitussin-DAC

Negligence and Malpractice (Unintentional Torts)

Most unintentional torts involve negligence. These are the most common forms of medical malpractice suits.

Negligence is performing an act that a reasonable health care worker or provider would not have done or the omission of an act that a reasonable professional or provider would have done. Failure to take reasonable precautions to prevent harm to a patient is termed **negligence**. If a physician is involved, the term usually used is malpractice. Malpractice is said to have occurred when the patient is harmed by the professional's actions. There are three types of malpractice:

- Malfeasance—incorrect treatment
- Misfeasance—treatment performed incorrectly
- Nonfeasance—treatment delayed or not attempted

In a legal situation, the standard of care determines what a reasonable professional would have done. Standards of care are written by various professional agencies to clarify what the reasonable and prudent physician or health care worker would do in a given situation. For example, a patient comes to an orthopedist's office after falling from a horse and complains of arm pain. The standard of care for orthopedists would require an x-ray of the injured extremity after trauma. Standards of care vary with the level of the professional. A registered nurse is not held to the same standards of care as a physician, nor is the medical assistant expected to perform by the same standards as the registered nurse. Each must practice within the scope of their training. The representing attorney may seek an **expert witness** to state under oath the standards of care for a specific situation. Expert witnesses may be physicians, nurses, physical therapists, or other specialized practitioners who have excellent reputations in their field.

Expert witnesses are always used in malpractice cases, except when the doctrine of **res ipsa loquitur** is tried. This doctrine means "the thing speaks for itself." In other words, it is obvious that the physician's actions or negligence caused the injury. A judge must preapprove the use of this theory in pretrial hearings. An example of a case tried under this doctrine might be a fracture that occurred when the patient fell from an examining table.

For negligence to be proved, the plaintiff's attorney must prove four elements were present: duty, dereliction of duty, direct cause, and damage. The courts place the burden of proof on the plaintiff; the physician is assumed to have given proper care until proven otherwise.

Duty

Duty is present when the patient and the physician have formed a contract. This is usually straightforward and the easiest of the elements to prove.

Dereliction of Duty

The patient must prove that the physician did not meet the standard of care guidelines, either by performing an act inappropriately or by omitting an act.

Direct Cause

The plaintiff must prove that the derelict act directly caused the patient's injury. This can be difficult to prove if the patient has an extensive medical history that may have contributed to the injury.

Damage

The plaintiff must prove that an injury or **damages** occurred. Documentation must be available to prove a diagnosis of an injury or illness.

Jury Awards

There are three types of awards for damages:

1. *Nominal.* Minimal injuries or damages occurred and compensation is small.
2. *Actual (compensatory).* Money is awarded for the injury, disability, mental suffering, loss of income, or the anticipated future earning loss. This payment is moderate to significant.
3. *Punitive.* Money is awarded to punish the practitioner for reckless or malicious wrongdoing. Punitive damages are the most costly. (Note: A physician may have committed a medical error, but if the patient suffered no injuries or damages, he or she cannot win the suit. Also, if the outcome was not as expected but the physician cannot be shown to be at fault, the patient will not be compensated.)

Checkpoint Question

6. What four elements must be proved in a negligence suit?

Intentional Torts

An **intentional tort** is an act that takes place with malice and with the intent of causing harm. Intentional torts are the deliberate violation of another person's legal rights. Examples of intentional torts are assault and battery, use of duress, invasion of privacy, defamation of character, fraud, tort of outrage, and undue influence. These are described next.

Assault and Battery

Assault is the unauthorized attempt or threat to touch another person without consent. **Battery** is the actual physical touching of a patient without consent; this includes beating and physical abuse. By law, a conscious adult has the right to refuse medical care. An example of battery might be suturing a laceration against the patient's expressed wish.

Duress

If a patient is coerced into an act, the patient can possibly sue for the tort of **duress**. Following is an example in which a patient may be able to sue successfully for assault, battery, and duress: A 22-year-old woman arrives at a pregnancy center. She is receiving public assistance and has five children. Her pregnancy test is positive. The staff persuades her to have an abortion. She signs the consent form, and the abortion is performed. Later she sues, stating that she was verbally coerced into signing the consent form (duress) and that the abortion was performed against her wishes (assault and battery).

Invasion of Privacy

Patients have the right to privacy. Most offices have patients sign an authorization to release information to their insurance company on their first visit. This covers each return visit unless the insurance carrier changes. Written permission must be obtained from the patient to:

- Release medical records or personal data
- Publish case histories in medical journals
- Make photographs of the patient (exception: suspected cases of abuse or maltreatment)
- Allow observers in examination rooms

For example, a 57-year-old woman is seen in your office for a skin biopsy. Her insurance company calls asking for information regarding the bill and asks for the biopsy report. You give the requested information and then find that the patient never signed a release form. She has a valid case for invasion of privacy.

Defamation of Character

Making malicious or false statements about a person's character or reputation is **defamation of character**. **Libel** refers to written statements and **slander** refers to oral statements. For example, a patient asks for a referral to another physician. She states that she has heard "Dr. Rogers is a good surgeon." You have heard that he has a history of alcoholism. You tell the patient that he is probably not a good choice because of his drinking. That is defamation of his character, and you could be sued for saying it.

Fraud

Fraud is any deceitful act with the intention to conceal the truth, such as:

- Intentionally raising false expectations regarding recovery

- Not properly instructing the patient regarding possible side effects of a procedure
- Filing false insurance claims

Tort of Outrage

Tort of outrage is the intentional infliction of emotional distress. For this tort to be proved, the plaintiff's attorney must show that the physician:

- Intended to inflict emotional distress
- Acted in a manner that is not morally or ethically acceptable
- Caused severe emotional distress

Undue Influence

Improperly persuading another to act in a way contrary to that person's free will is termed undue influence. For instance, preying on the elderly or the mentally incompetent is a common type of undue influence. Unethical practitioners who gain the trust of these persons and persuade them to submit to expensive and unnecessary medical procedures are practicing undue influence.

Checkpoint Question

7. What is the difference between assault and battery?

THE LITIGATION PROCESS

The litigation process begins when a patient consults an attorney because he or she believes a health care provider has done wrong or becomes aware of a possible prior injury. The patient's attorney obtains the medical records, which are reviewed by medicolegal consultants. (Such consultants may be nurses or physicians who are considered experts in their field.) Then the plaintiff's attorney files a complaint, a written statement that lists the claim against the physician and the remedy desired, usually monetary compensation.

The defendant and his or her attorney answer the complaint. The discovery phase begins with interrogatories and **depositions**. During this phase, attorneys for both parties gather relevant information.

Next, the trial phase begins. A jury is selected unless the parties agree to a **bench trial**. In a bench trial, the judge hears the case without a jury and renders a **verdict** (decision or judgment). Opening statements are given, first by the plaintiff's attorney, then by the defendant's attorney. The plaintiff's attorney presents the case. Expert witnesses are called, and the evidence is shown. Examination of the witnesses begins. **Direct examination** involves questioning by one's own attorney; **cross-examination** is questioning by the opposing attorney. When the plaintiff's attorney is finished, the defense presents the opposing arguments and evidence. The plaintiff's attorney may cross-examine the defendant's witnesses. Closing arguments are heard. Finally, a verdict is made.

If the defendant is found guilty, damages are awarded. If the defendant is found not guilty, the charges are dismissed. The decision may be appealed to a higher court. An **appeal** is a process by which the higher court reviews the decision of the lower court.

DEFENSES TO PROFESSIONAL LIABILITY SUITS

The objective of all court proceedings is to uncover the truth. Many defenses are available to a health care worker who is being sued. These include the medical record, statute of limitations, assumption of risk, res judicata, contributory negligence, and comparative negligence, discussed next.

Medical Records

The best and most solid defense the caregiver has is the medical record. Every item in the record is considered to be a part of a legal document. Juries may believe a medical record regardless of testimony. Juries tend to believe these records because they are tangible items from the actual time the injury occurred. There is a common saying in the medicolegal world: "If it's not in the chart, it did not happen." This means that even negative findings should be listed. For example, instead of saying that the patient's neurological history is negative, the documentation might say the patient reports no headaches, seizures, one-sided weakness, and so on. Entries in the medical record refresh the memory of the defendant and provide documentation of care. As a medical assistant, you must make sure that all of your documentation is timely, accurate, and legible. (See Chapter 8 for specific information regarding charting practices.)

Statute of Limitations

Each state has a statute that defines the length of time during which a patient may file a suit against a caregiver. When the **statute of limitations** expires, the patient loses the right to file a claim. Generally, the limits vary from 1 to 3 years following the alleged occurrence. Other states use a combination rule. Some states allow 1 to 3 years following the patient's discovery of the occurrence. States vary greatly when an alleged injury involves a minor. The statute may not take effect until the minor reaches the age of majority and then may extend 2 to 3 years past this time. Some states have longer claim periods in wrongful death suits.

Assumption of Risk

In the assumption of risk defense, the physician will claim that the patient was aware of the risks involved before the procedure and fully accepted the potential for damages. For example, a patient is instructed regarding the adverse effects of chemotherapy. The patient fully understands these risks, receives the chemotherapy, and wants to sue for alopecia (hair loss). Alopecia is a given risk with certain forms of chemotherapy. A signed consent form indicating that the patient was informed of all of the risks of a procedure proves this point.

Res Judicata

The doctrine of **res judicata** means "the thing has been decided." Once the suit has been brought against the physician or patient and a settlement has been reached, the losing party may not countersue. If, for instance, the physician sues a patient for not paying bills and the court orders the patient to pay, the patient cannot sue the physician for malpractice. The opposite may occur as well. If the physician is sued for malpractice and loses, he cannot countersue for defamation of character.

Contributory Negligence

With the **contributory negligence** defense, the physician usually admits that negligence has occurred; he or she will claim, however, that the patient aggravated the injury or assisted in making the injury worse. For example, the patient's laceration is stitched with only 3 sutures when 10 were needed. The physician instructs the patient to limit movement of the arm. The patient plays baseball; the laceration reopens, causing infection; and subsequently, extensive scar tissue forms. Both the patient and the physician contributed to the postoperative damages. Most states do not grant damage awards for contributory negligence. If an award is granted, the courts assess **comparative negligence**.

Comparative Negligence

In comparative negligence, the award of damages is based on a percentage of the contribution to the negligence. If the patient contributed 30% to the damage, the damage award is 30% less than what was granted. In the example in the previous paragraph, the courts may decide that the negligence is shared at 50%. Therefore, if the court assessed damages of $20,000, the physician would be responsible for $10,000.

In the past, contributory negligence, such as a patient not returning for appointments, was seen as absolute defense for the physician. Since the 1970s, however, the trend has been toward using the defense of comparative negligence, with the responsibility shared between the physician and the patient.

Immunity

The Federal Tort Claim Act of 1946 prohibits suits against any U. S. governmental facility, such as veterans hospitals or military bases. This provides immunity to all of their employees for ordinary negligence but not for intentional torts.

DEFENSE FOR THE MEDICAL ASSISTANT

Respondeat Superior or Law of Agency

The doctrine of **respondeat superior** literally means "let the master answer." This may also be called law of agency. This doctrine implies that physicians are liable for the actions of their employees. The physician is responsible for your actions as a medical assistant as long as your actions are within your scope of practice. Figure 2-4 features a scope-of-practice decision tree designed to help you make such decisions.

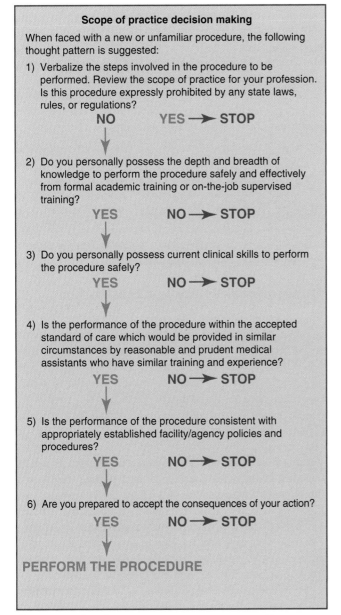

Scope of practice decision making

When faced with a new or unfamiliar procedure, the following thought pattern is suggested:

1) Verbalize the steps involved in the procedure to be performed. Review the scope of practice for your profession. Is this procedure expressly prohibited by any state laws, rules, or regulations?

   NO   **YES ➤ STOP**

2) Do you personally possess the depth and breadth of knowledge to perform the procedure safely and effectively from formal academic training or on-the-job supervised training?

   YES   **NO ➤ STOP**

3) Do you personally possess current clinical skills to perform the procedure safely?

   YES   **NO ➤ STOP**

4) Is the performance of the procedure within the accepted standard of care which would be provided in similar circumstances by reasonable and prudent medical assistants who have similar training and experience?

   YES   **NO ➤ STOP**

5) Is the performance of the procedure consistent with appropriately established facility/agency policies and procedures?

   YES   **NO ➤ STOP**

6) Are you prepared to accept the consequences of your action?

   YES   **NO ➤ STOP**

PERFORM THE PROCEDURE

FIGURE 2–4. Scope of practice decision-making tree. (Adapted from the Washington State Department of Health, Nursing Care Quality Assurance Commission, "Scope of Practice Decision Tree.")

As a new medical assistant, you can use this tool to guard against overconfidence. If your actions exceed your abilities or training, the physician is not generally responsible for any error that you make. You must understand that you can be sued in this instance and that respondeat superior does not guarantee immunity for your actions.

For example, Mrs. Smith is a chronic complainer, calling your office frequently with minor concerns. Today, she calls complaining of tingling in her arms. The physician has left for the day, so you tell Mrs. Smith, "Don't worry about this; take your medication and call us tomorrow." During the night a blood vessel in Mrs. Smith's brain bursts. She has a cerebral hemorrhage (bleeding inside the brain) and dies. The family sues. The physician claims that you were instructed not to give advice over the telephone. You are not covered by respondeat superior because you acted outside of your scope of practice.

To protect yourself from situations such as this, have your job description in written form and always practice within its guidelines. Do not perform tasks that you have not been trained to do. Never hesitate to seek clarification from a physician. If you are not sure about something, such as a medication order, ask!

Malpractice insurance is available to allied health care professionals for further protection. Malpractice premiums are inexpensive and afford protection against losing any personal assets if sued. The insurance company would pay damages as assessed by a jury. Of course, as with any insurance policy, there will be conditions of coverage and maximum amounts the company will pay. Box 2-5 provides some additional tips for preventing lawsuits.

Checkpoint Question

8. What is the law of agency, and how does it apply to the medical assistant?

EMPLOYMENT AND SAFETY LAWS

Civil Rights Act of 1964, Title VII

Title VII of the Civil Rights Act of 1964 protects employees from discrimination in the workplace. The Equal Employment Opportunity Commission (EEOC) enforces the provisions of the act and investigates any possible infractions. Employers may not refuse to hire, limit, segregate or classify, fire, compensate, or provide working conditions and privileges on the basis of race, color, sex, religion, or national origin. This act determines the questions that may be asked in a job interview. For example, a potential employee cannot be asked questions that would reveal age, marital status, religious affiliation, height, weight, or arrest record. It is acceptable, however, to ask if an applicant has ever been convicted of a crime. In the health care setting, employers can require a criminal records check and even drug screening to ensure the safety of the patients. The American Association of Medical Assistants (AAMA) has made recent changes to prohibit convicted felons from taking the CMA examination.

Sexual Harassment

In recent years, Title VII has been expanded to include sexual harassment. Sexual harassment is defined by the EEOC as unwelcome sexual advances or requests for sexual favors in the workplace. The definition includes other verbal or physical conduct of a sexual nature when such conduct is made a condition of an individual's employment, is used as a basis for hiring or promotion, or has the purpose or effect of unreasonably interfering with an individual's work performance. If such behavior creates an intimidating, hostile, or offensive working environment, it is considered sexual harassment. In the past two decades court decisions have confirmed that this form of harassment is a cause for both criminal prosecution and civil litigation.

In the medical office setting, the office manager must be alert for signs of harassment and should have in place a policy for handling complaints.

Americans with Disabilities Act

Title VII also includes the Americans with Disabilities Act (ADA), which prohibits discrimination against people with substantial disabilities in all employment practices, including job application procedures, hiring, firing, advancement, compensation, training, benefits, and all other privileges of employment. The ADA applies to all employers with 15 or more employees. The law covers those with impairments that limit their major life activities. The statute also protects those with AIDS or HIV-positive status and individuals with a history of mental illness or cancer. ADA also requires that employers provide basic accommodations for disabled employees. Those basic accommodations include extra-wide parking spaces close to the door, ramps or elevators, electric or easily opened doors, bathroom facilities designed for the disabled, an accessible break room, and a work area with counters low enough for a person in a wheelchair.

The ADA also takes safety into consideration. Employers are permitted to establish qualification standards that will exclude individuals who pose a direct threat to others if that risk cannot be lowered to an acceptable level by reasonable accommodations. In the medical field, technical standards are established that outline physical requirements of a certain job. For example, a medical assistant needs adequate vision to see the dials on laboratory equipment. If a particular job requires reaching a certain height, it is unreasonable to expect an employer to hire a person who is too short. The law is designed to protect employees, not to require unreasonable accommodations.

The ADA also requires that all public buildings be accessible to physically challenged people. Following is a partial list of ways the medical office can comply with this act:

- Entrance ramps
- Widened rest rooms to be wheelchair accessible
- Elevated toilet bowls for easier transferring from wheelchairs
- Easy-to-reach elevator buttons
- Braille signs
- Access to special telephone services to communicate with hearing-impaired patients

Occupational Safety and Health Act

Employers must provide safe environments for their employees. In accordance with the Occupational Safety and Health Act of 1970, the Occupational Safety and Health Administration (OSHA) controls and monitors safety for workers. Specific OSHA rules and regulations protect the clinical worker from exposure to **blood-borne pathogens**. Blood-borne pathogens are organisms that can be spread through direct contact with blood or body fluids from an infected person. Universal precautions are designed to protect health care workers from blood and body fluids contaminated with HIV, hepatitis, or any contagious "bugs" by requiring that those in direct contact with patients use protective equipment (e.g., gloves, gowns, face mask). In days past, health care workers felt that they needed protection only from patients with known risk factors (sharing needles, having unprotected sexual intercourse). OSHA's regulations ensure protection from contracting a contagious disease from *any* body fluids handled.

Your medical assisting training will include an extensive study of safety issues and protection against accidental exposure to blood-borne pathogens. Box 2-6 outlines OSHA rules governing all free-standing health care providers. Box 2-7 outlines the laws governing employer and employee rights and responsibilities.

Box 2-6

OCCUPATIONAL SAFETY AND HEALTH ACT OF 1970 RULES GOVERNING HEALTH CARE PROVIDERS

OSHA defines body fluids as semen, blood, amniotic fluids, vaginal secretions, synovial fluid (from joint spaces), pleural fluid (from the lungs), pericardial fluid (from the heart), cerebrospinal fluid (from the spinal cord), and saliva. OSHA employs inspectors who may conduct inspections and issue citations for violations and recommend penalties. Under specific rules, OSHA requires that health care facilities provide:

- A list of all employees who might be exposed to blood-borne diseases on either a regular or an occasional basis.
- A written exposure control plan that outlines steps to be taken in the event of an employee's accidental exposure to blood-borne pathogens.
- One employee who is responsible for OSHA compliance.
- Availability of protective clothing that fits properly.
- An employee training program in writing and records of sessions and participants.
- Warning labels and signs denoting biohazards (potentially dangerous materials).
- Written guidelines for identifying, containing, and disposing of medical waste, including housecleaning and laundry decontamination.
- Written guidelines and procedures to follow if any employee is exposed to blood or other potentially infectious materials, as well as a policy for reporting incidents of exposure and maintaining records.
- Postexposure evaluation procedures, including follow-up testing of the exposed employee.
- Material safety data sheets (MSDS) listing each ingredient in a product used in the office Manufacturers provide an MSDS for every product they sell Information included in the sheets includes any hazards involved or necessary precautions that must be taken when handling materials.
- Hepatitis B vaccine free of charge to employees working with body fluids.

Other Legal Considerations

The Clinical Laboratory Improvement Amendments (CLIA) of 1988 contain specific rules and regulations regarding laboratory safety.

The Joint Commission on Accreditation of Healthcare Organizations (JCAHO) is a private organization that sets stan-

dards for health care administration. Each state also has specific laws regarding patient care, insurance billing, collections, and such matters.

Checkpoint Question

9. What are blood-borne pathogens? Which government agency governs their control in the medical office?

Box 2-7

LAWS GOVERNING EMPLOYER AND EMPLOYMENT RIGHTS AND RESPONSIBILITIES

Fair Labor Standards Act of 1939
- Regulates wages and working conditions including
- Federal minimum wage, overtime compensation, equal pay requirements, child labor, hours, requirements for record keeping.

Civil Rights Act of 1964, Title VII
- Applies to employers with 15 or more employees for at least 20 weeks of the year.
- Federal regulation forbids discrimination on the basis of race, color, sex, religion, or national origin. Some state laws also prohibit discrimination for sexual orientation, personal appearance, mental health, mental retardation, marital status, parenthood, and political affiliation.

Americans with Disabilities Act of 1990
- Applies to employers with 15 or more employees.
- Prohibits discrimination against individuals with substantial impairments in all employment practices.

Age Discrimination in Employment Act of 1967
- Applies to employers with 15 or more employees.
- Regulates discrimination against workers on the basis of age. Protects those 40–65.

Family and Medical Leave Act of 1993
- Employees are covered after 1 year or 1,250 hours of employment over the past 12 months.
- Provides up to 12 weeks per year of unpaid, job-protected leave to eligible employees for certain family and medical reasons.

Immigration Reform and Control Act of 1986
- Applies to employers with four or more employees.
- Prohibits employment of illegal aliens and protects legal aliens from discrimination based on national origin or citizenship.

MEDICAL ETHICS

Medical **ethics** are principles of ethical and moral conduct that govern the behavior and conduct of health professionals. These principles define proper medical etiquette, customs, and professional courtesy. Ethics are guidelines specifying right or wrong and are enforced by peer review and professional organizations. Laws are regulations and rules that are enforced by the government. **Bioethics** are issues and problems that affect a patient's life; many bioethical issues have arisen from the advances of modern medicine.

American Medical Association (AMA) Code of Ethics

A code of ethics is a "collective statement from a professional organization that depicts the behavioral expectations for its members. Additionally, a code of ethics allows the organization to set standards by which it may discipline its members." The AMA Code of Ethics states that physicians must recognize and accept their responsibilities for both patients and society. It also states that these are "not laws but standards of conduct by which a physician's professional behavior will be assessed." Box 2-8 outlines the AMA Code of Ethics.

Box 2-8

AMA CODE OF ETHICS

Seven principles in the AMA Code of Ethics state that the physician shall:
1. Practice competent medical care with compassion while respecting human dignity.
2. Remain honest in dealings with patients and colleagues; expose colleagues with character deficiencies or who are incompetent or who engage in fraud or deception.
3. Adhere to all laws, and when needed, be a voice to lawmakers in the best interest of patient care.
4. Respect the rights of patients and other health care professionals; safeguard patient confidentiality (privacy) except within the provisions of the law.
5. Continue appropriate education to remain current; request consultation and obtain the knowledge and skills of other health professionals when needed.
6. Be free to select whom to treat, where to establish a practice, and whom to associate with except in emergency situations.
7. Participate in activities to enhance the community.

Violations of these AMA principles may result in censure, suspension, or expulsion by the state medical board. **Censure**, the least punitive action, is a verbal or written reprimand from the association indicating negative findings regarding a specific incident. Suspension is the temporary removal of privileges and association with the organization. Expulsion is a formal discharge from the professional organization and is the maximum punishment. Many of these issues, however, deal with laws and the patient's rights as established by law. When violations of laws are involved, physicians may lose their license to practice, may be fined, or may be imprisoned. Serious consequences can arise from a breach of this code of ethics.

Medical Assistant's Role in Ethics

As an agent of the physician in the medical office, you are also governed by ethical standards and are responsible for:

- Protecting patient confidentiality
- Following all state and federal laws
- Being honest in all your actions

As a medical assistant, you must apply ethical standards as you perform your duties. You must realize that your personal feelings of right and wrong should be kept separate if they differ from the ethics of your profession. For example, a medical assistant who has a strong opinion against abortion would not be happy working in a medical facility that performs abortions. The care you give patients must be objective, and personal opinions about options must not be shared.

Patient Advocacy

Your primary responsibility as a medical assistant is to be a patient advocate at all times. Advocacy requires that you consider the best interests of the patient above all other concerns. This often means setting aside your own personal beliefs, values, and biases and looking at a given situation in an objective manner. You should never, however, be asked or forced to compromise your own value system.

Patient Confidentiality

Confidentiality of patient information is one of the most important ethical principles to be observed by the medical assistant. As discussed earlier, information obtained in the care of the patient may not be revealed without the permission of the patient unless required by law. Whatever you say to, hear from, or do to a patient is confidential. Patients will reveal some of their innermost thoughts, feelings, and fears. This information is not for public knowledge. Family members, friends, pastors, or others may call the physician's office to inquire about a patient's condition. Many of these calls are made with good intentions; NO INFORMATION, however, should be released to anyone—friends, family, media, or insurance companies—without prior written approval from the patient (see Chapter 8).

Honesty

One of the most important character traits for medical assistants is honesty. We all make mistakes at times; how we handle our mistakes is the indication of our ethical standards. If you make a mistake (e.g., giving the wrong medication) you must immediately report the error to your supervisor and the attending physician. The mark of a true professional is the ability to admit mistakes and take full responsibility for all actions. When speaking to patients concerning medical issues, be honest; give the facts in a straightforward manner. Never offer false expectations or hope. Never minimize or exaggerate the risks or benefits of a procedure. If you do not know the answer to a question, say, "I don't know, but I will find out for you," or refer the question to the physician. Treating the patient with dignity, respect, and honesty in all interactions will build trust in you and your professional abilities.

Checkpoint Question

10. What are the three ethical standards a CMA, as an agent of the physician, should follow?

American Association of Medical Assistants (AAMA) Code of Ethics

Principles

The AAMA has published a set of five principles of ethical and moral conduct that all medical assistants must follow in the practice of the profession. They state that the medical assistant must always strive to:

1. Render services with respect for human dignity
2. Respect patient confidentiality, except when information is required by the law
3. Uphold the honor and high principles set forth by the AAMA
4. Continually improve knowledge and skills for the benefit of patients and the health care team
5. Participate in community services that promote good health and welfare to the general public

These principles are outlined in the AAMA creed seen in the Medical Assistants' Creed.

In 1999, the AAMA adopted *AAMA's Disciplinary Standards & Procedures for CMAs*. For the first time, a policy was established for sanctions against CMAs who violate the disciplinary standards. Possible sanctions include denial of eligibility for the certification examination, probation, reprimand, temporary revocation of the CMA credential, and permanent revocation of the CMA credential. For more information, see the AAMA website.

BIOETHICS

Bioethics deals specifically with the moral issues and problems that affect human life. As a result of advances in medicine and research, many situations require moral decisions for which there are no clear answers. Abortion and genetic engineering are examples. The goal is to make the right decision in each specific instance as it applies to an individual's specific circumstances. What may be right for one patient may be wrong for another; that is the foundation of bioethics.

American Medical Association (AMA) Council on Ethical and Judicial Affairs

Because of the broad scope of medical ethics and bioethical issues, the AMA formed a subcommittee to review AMA principles and to interpret them as they apply to everyday clinical situations. This subcommittee is called the Council on Ethical and Judicial Affairs. The council has formulated a series of opinions on various medical and bioethical issues that are intended to provide the physician with guidelines for professional conduct and responsibilities. These opinions, most recently revised in 1992, are divided into four general categories:

- Social policy issues
- Relations with colleagues and hospitals
- Administrative office procedures
- Professional rights and responsibilities

The following discussion provides a summary of these opinions along with questions designed to promote your ability to use reasoning to examine difficult ethical issues. Your workbook provides some situations for you to consider. These issues are not within the scope of decisions for medical assistants, but you will be faced with their consequences at some time in your career.

Social Policy Issues

The social policy section deals with various issues of societal importance and provides guidelines to aid the physician in making ethical choices. Five common societal topics and the opinion statements from the AMA Council on Ethical and Judicial Affairs follow.

Allocation of Resources

The term *allocate* means set aside or designate for a purpose. Allocation of resources in the medical profession may refer to many health needs:

- *Organs for transplantation.* Who gets this heart, the college professor or the young recovering addict whose heart was damaged by his lifestyle? Should lifestyle or perceived worth be considered in the decision?
- *Funds for research.* Which disease should receive more funding for research, cancer or AIDS?
- *Funds for health care.* Where should the money be spent, for keeping alive extremely premature infants or making preventive health care available for a greater number of poor children?
- *Hospital beds and professional care.* With hospital care at a premium, who will pay for the indigent? How is it decided which patient is entitled to the last bed in the intensive care unit?

Box 2-9 outlines the judicial council's viewpoints on allocation of limited resources.

BOX 2-9

AMA COUNCIL ON ETHICAL AND JUDICIAL AFFAIRS VIEWPOINT STATES:

- When resources are limited, decisions for allocating health care materials should be based on fair and socially acceptable criteria. Economic or social position should not be a factor in the decision.
- Priority care is given to the person or persons who are more likely to receive the greatest long-term benefit from the treatment. Patients with other disease processes or who are not good candidates for treatment for whatever reason will be less likely to receive treatment than otherwise healthy patients. For instance, a patient with cancer in other sites would not be considered for a liver transplant, whereas a patient whose liver was damaged by trauma but who has no other involvement would probably be a good candidate.
- An individual's societal worth must not be a deciding factor during the decision process. A socially or politically prominent patient should not be considered a better recipient of treatment options than a young mother on welfare.
- Age must not be considered in the decision process. If the age of the patient is not a contraindication for the treatment, all ages should be considered on an even basis for most medical resources.

Clinical Investigations and Research

Physicians are frequently involved in studying the effectiveness of new procedures and medications, often called clinical investigations or research. New drugs and treatments are tested on animals first and then considered safe for human testing. The council's viewpoint on research investigation of new drugs and procedures states:

- *A physician may participate in clinical research as long as the project is part of a systematic program with controls for patient evaluation during all phases of the research. At all stages of the testing and at the completion of the study, a protocol must be in place to evaluate the immediate and the long-term effects of the study.*
- *The goal of the research must be to obtain scientifically valid data. The objectives of the study must be available to the physician and the patient, results must be provided to all participants on request, and the testing must serve a medically sound purpose to provide better patient care.*
- *Utmost care and respect must be given to patients involved in clinical research. They are entitled to be treated just as any other patient receiving health care.*

- *Physicians must obtain the patient's permission or consent before enrolling the patient in a research project.*
- *The patient's decision to participate in the program must be completely voluntary.*
- *The patient must be advised of any potential risks, side effects, and benefits of participating in the project.*
- *The patient must be advised that this procedure or drug is experimental. Patients must be made aware that research is not complete, that this is the purpose of the trials, and that risks and benefits are not fully known at this time.*
- *The physician and the institution must have a check and balance system in place to ensure that quality care is always given and ethical standards are followed. Documentation of patient education and instruction for following testing guidelines and patient response to the treatment must be ongoing and thorough.*

Obstetric Dilemmas

Advances in technology have created legal and ethical situations that have polarized opinions and are difficult to bring to consensus. Issues such as the beginning of life, genetic testing and engineering, sex determination, the rights of the fetus, ownership of the fertilized egg, and so forth will not be easily answered. The council formulated an opinion regarding obstetric issues as fairly as possible that states the following:

> ABORTION. *As the law now stands, a physician may perform an abortion as long as state and federal laws are followed regarding the trimester in which an abortion may be performed. A physician who does not want to perform abortions cannot be forced to perform the procedure; that physician, however, should refer the patient to other health care professionals who can assist the patient.*
>
> GENETIC TESTING. *If amniocentesis is performed on a mother and a genetic defect is found, both parents must be told. The parents may request or refuse to have the pregnancy terminated. (Amniocentesis is a procedure in which a needle is inserted in a pregnant woman's abdomen to remove and test amniotic fluid. Many abnormalities and disorders can be diagnosed early in pregnancy by this procedure.)*
>
> ARTIFICIAL INSEMINATION. **Artificial insemination** *involves the insertion of sperm into a woman's vagina for the purpose of conception. The donor may be the husband (artificial insemination by husband [AIH]) or an anonymous donor (artificial insemination by donor [AID]). The council states that both the husband and wife must consent to this procedure. If a donor is used, the sperm must be tested for infectious and genetic disorders. Complete confidentiality for the donor and recipient must be maintained.*

Organ Transplantation

Organ transplantation became a medical option in the mid 1950s, although at that time there were many problems with rejection of the organs by the recipient's immune system. When this postoperative complication was corrected by antirejection drugs, the practice became more common. Organs are viable (able to support life) for varying lengths of time, but most can be used successfully if transplanted within 24 to 48 hours. An organization in Richmond, Virginia, the United Network of Organ Sharing, coordinates local organ procurement teams that will fly to areas where organs are to be harvested to assist with the surgery if needed and to ensure the integrity of the organ. There are far fewer organs available than are needed, and every year thousands of patients die who could have lived if an organ had been available. The scarcity of organs has caused many Third World countries to become sources of organs as poor people sell parts of their bodies to meet their basic needs.

The use of organs from a baby born without a brain (anencephaly) raises serious ethical issues. The council states that everything must be done for the infant until the determination of death can be made. For infant organs to be transplanted, both parents must consent.

The council's views on transplantation state:

- *The rights of the donor and organ recipient must be treated equally. The imminent death of the donor does not release the medical personnel from observing all rights that every patient is due.*
- *Organ donors must be given every medical opportunity for life. Life support is not removed until the patient is determined to have no brain activity and could not live without artificial support.*
- *Death of the donor must be determined by a physician who is not on the transplant team to avoid a charge of conflict of interest.*
- *Consent (permission) must be received from both the donor, if possible, and recipient before the transplant. Family members may give consent if the donor is unable to do so.*
- *Transplants can be performed only by surgeons who are qualified to perform this complex surgery and who are affiliated with institutions that have adequate facilities for the surgery and postoperative care. Box 2-10 highlights the Uniform Anatomical Gift Act.*

Withholding or Withdrawing Treatment

Physicians have a professional and ethical obligation to promote quality of life, which means sustaining life and relieving suffering. Sometimes, these obligations conflict with a patient's wishes. Patients have the right to refuse medical treatment and to request that life support or life-sustaining treatments be withheld or withdrawn. Withholding treatment means that certain medical treatments may not be initiated.

Box 2-10

UNIFORM ANATOMICAL GIFT ACT

Approximately 60 American citizens die each day waiting for an organ transplant. Many organs can be transplanted, including the liver, kidney, cornea, heart, lung, and skin. To meet the growing need for organs and to allay the concern over donor standards, the National Conference of Commissioners for Uniform State Laws passed legislation known as the Uniform Anatomical Gift Act.

All acts include the following clauses:

- Any mentally competent person over age 18 may donate all or part of his or her body for transplantation or research.
- The donor's wishes supersede any other wishes except when state laws require an autopsy.
- Physicians accepting donor organs in good faith are immune from lawsuits against harvesting organs.
- Death of the donor must be determined by a physician not involved with the transplant team.
- Financial compensation may not be given to the donor or survivors.
- Persons wishing to donate organs can revoke permission or change their minds at any time.

In most states the Department of Motor Vehicles asks applicants for a driver's license about organ donation and indicates their wishes on their license. In addition, an individual may declare the wish to donate all or parts of the body in a will or any legal document, including a Uniform Donor Card. Organ donors should make their families aware of their wishes to ensure they will be carried out.

Withdrawing treatment is terminating a treatment that has already begun. In 1991, congress passed the Self-Determination Act, which gave all hospitalized patients the right to make health care decisions on admission to the hospital. These decisions may be referred to as advance directives. Today, everyone is encouraged to participate in his or her own end-of-life decisions. We can go online and complete an advance directive. An **advance directive** is a statement of a person's wishes for medical decisions prior to a critical event. Advance directives may include specific wishes, such as whether a ventilator can be used, whether cardiopulmonary resuscitation (CPR) should be initiated, and whether a feeding tube should be inserted. Just completing an advance directive does not ensure that the patient's wishes will be carried out. It is important to make family members aware of these wishes. The patient's next of kin should keep a copy of the advance directive, and one should be placed in the medical office chart with special notation. Figure 2-5 is a sample of an advance directive.

Checkpoint Question

11. What is an advance directive? How can a patient be sure his or her wishes will be followed?

PROFESSIONAL AND ETHICAL CONDUCT AND BEHAVIOR

The council states that all health care professionals are responsible for reporting unethical practices to the appropriate agencies. No health care professional should engage in any act that he or she feels is ethically or morally wrong. Additionally, the council states:

- *A physician must never assist or allow an unlicensed person to practice medicine.*
- *Hospitals and physicians must work together for the best care for patients. Hospitals should allow physicians staff privileges based on the ability of the physician, educational background, and the needs of the community. (Staff privileges allow physicians to admit their patients to a given hospital.) Issues of a personal nature must never be considered when accepting or declining a physician's application for privileges.*
- *It is unethical for physicians to admit patients to the hospital or to order excessive treatments for the sole purpose of financial rewards.*

ETHICAL ISSUES IN OFFICE MANAGEMENT

As a medical assistant, you are directly involved in some of the council's guidelines regarding administrative issues. In relation to fees, the council states:

- *Financial interests must never come above patient care. Ordering the most expensive tests or not ordering needed tests based on the patient's ability to pay is not acceptable.*
- *If a physician's office routinely charges patients for canceling appointments within 24 hours of the actual scheduled appointment, a warning must be posted to advise patients of this charge.*
- *The medical record must never be held against nonpayment of a bill.*
- *Fees cannot be excessive. They must be based on fair and standard charges for all patients. Guidelines for charges should consider the difficulty and unique nature of the services involved and the use of medical equipment.*
- *Interest on past due accounts can be charged in accordance with state laws and with prior notification to the patient.*

FIGURE 2–5. Sample advance directive.

ADVANCE DIRECTIVE

UNIFORM ADVANCE DIRECTIVE OF [list name of declarant]

To my family, physician, attorney, and anyone else who may become responsible for my health, welfare, or affairs, I make this declaration while I am of sound mind.

If I should ever become in a terminal state and there is no reasonable expectation of my recovery, I direct that I be allowed to die a natural death and that my life not be prolonged by extraordinary measures. I do, however, ask that medication be mercifully administered to me to alleviate suffering, even though this may shorten my remaining life.

This statement is made after full reflection and is in accordance with my full desires. I want the above provisions carried out to the extent permitted by law. Insofar as they are not legally enforceable, I wish that those to whom this will is addressed will regard themselves as morally bound by this instrument.

If permissible in the jurisdiction in which I may be hospitalized I direct that in the event of a terminal diagnosis, the physicians supervising my care discontinue feeding should the continuation of feeding be judged to result in unduly prolonging a natural death.

If permissible in the jurisdiction in which I may be hospitalized I direct that in the event of a terminal diagnosis, the physicians supervising my care discontinue hydration (water) should the continuation of hydration be judged to result in unduly prolonging a natural death.

I herewith authorize my spouse, if any, or any relative who is related to me within the third degree to effectuate my transfer from any hospital or other health care facility in which I may be receiving care should that facility decline or refuse to effectuate the instructions given herein.

I herewith release any and all hospitals, physicians, and others for myself and for my estate from any liability for complying with this instrument.

Signed:

_____
[list name of declarant]

City of residence: _____
[city of residence]

County of residence: _____
[county of residence]

State of residence: _____
[state of residence]

Social Security Number: _____
[social security number]

Date: _____

_____
Witness

_____
Witness

STATE OF _____

COUNTY OF _____

This day personally appeared before me, the undersigned authority, a Notary Public in and for _____County, _____ State,

_____   _____ (Witnesses)

who, being first duly sworn, say that they are the subscribing witnesses to the declaration of [list name of declarant], the declarant, signed, sealed, and published and declared the same as and for his declaration, in the presence of both these affiants; and that these affiants, at the request of said declarant, in the presence of each other, and in the presence of said declarant, all present at the same time, signed their names as attesting witnesses to said declaration.

Affiants further say that this affidavit is made at the request of [list name of declarant], declarant, and in his presence, and that [list name of declarant] at the time the declaration was executed, in the opinion of the affiants, of sound mind and memory, and over the age of eighteen years.

Taken, subscribed and sworn to before me by _____(witness) and

_____ (witness) this _____ day of_____, 20_____.

My commission expires: _____

_____ Notary Public

Box 2-11

ETHICAL DILEMMA

Here is a hypothetical situation that could occur in a medical office. How would you handle it?

You are the office manager for a well-respected family physician in a small town. He is 70 years old and is starting to show signs of senility. He is forgetful and has even been disoriented and confused a few times. No one else seems to have noticed. Should you report your concerns? If so, to whom?

The AMA Principles of Medical Ethics require that physicians, and medical assistants through the law of agency, report unethical behavior among colleagues. The medical profession is also governed by the patient's right to safety and quality care. It is your ethical responsibility to report the doctor's condition to the administration of the hospital where the physician has privileges or to the state board of medicine. The physician's family should be involved in the situation.

- No fees can be charged for physician referrals or for admitting a patient to the hospital.
- A fee should not be charged to the patient for completing or filing a simple insurance form. If the form is extensive, a minimal fee may be charged.
- Caution must be used with computers to maintain patient confidentiality. If patient data are sent via fax machine, utmost care must be used to ensure that the material is received by only the correct recipient.
- If the physician advertises his or her practice, it must be done with the utmost honesty. Misrepresentation of information is never appropriate.
- If a physician closes the practice or dies, all patients must be notified that the office is closing and must be given instructions for retrieving their medical records. Generally, copies of medical records are transferred to another local physician. The originals are stored as directed by state law. Box 2-11 describes an ethical issue that might occur in a medical office. Read it carefully. If you were the physician, how would you handle the problem?

Checkpoint Question

12. What steps should be taken when a physician closes his or her practice?

CHAPTER SUMMARY

The fields of medicine and law are linked in common concern for the patient's health and rights. Increasingly, health care professionals are the object of malpractice lawsuits. You must keep abreast of medicolegal issues to protect yourself and other health care professionals from legal action. You can help prevent medical malpractice by acting professionally, maintaining clinical competency, and properly documenting in the medical record. Promoting good public relations between the patient and the health care team can avoid frivolous or unfounded suits and direct attention and energy toward optimum health care.

Medical ethics and bioethics involve complex issues and controversial topics. There will be no easy or clearcut answers to questions raised by these issues. As a medical assistant, your first priority must be to act as your patients' advocate with their best interests and concerns foremost in your actions and interactions. You must always maintain ethical standards and report the unethical behaviors of others.

Many acts and regulations affect health care organizations and their operations. A medical office must keep current on all legal updates. Most states publish a monthly bulletin that reports on new legislation. Every state has a website that will link you to legislative action. Read these on a regular basis. Each office should have legal counsel who can assist in interpreting legal issues.

Critical Thinking Challenges

1. An acquaintance who knows you work in the medical field asks you to diagnose her rash. What do you say?
2. A patient owes a big bill at your office. She requests copies of her records. What do you do?
3. You suspect that a new employee in the office is misusing narcotics. What do you do?

Spanish Terminology

¿Usted entiende la información que acaba de recibir?	Do you understand the information I have given?
¿Usted nos autoriza a llevar a cabo este procedimiento médico?	Do you give us permission to perform this procedure?
Firme aquí, por favor.	Please sign here.

4. Mrs. Rodriguez has bone cancer. Her doctor has estimated she has 6 months to live. Mrs. Rodriguez wants the physician to withhold all medical treatments. She does not want chemotherapy or any life-sustaining measures. Her family disagrees. Should her family have any input into her health care decisions?

Answers to Checkpoint Questions

1. Criminal law deals with the act of practicing medicine without a license.
2. When a physician changes the scope of his practice, patients should be given advance notice. A letter should be sent to each active patient or an ad may be placed in a local newspaper.
3. The following elements must be in a physician's termination intent letter: statement of intent, explanation of reasons, termination date, availability of medical records, and a recommendation that the patient seek medical help as needed.
4. Never ask a patient to sign a consent form if the patient does not understand the procedure, has questions about the procedure, or is unable to read the consent form.
5. The six situations or conditions legally requiring disclosure are vital statistics, medical examiner reports, infectious diseases, abuse or maltreatment, violent injuries, and others according to state laws.
6. The four elements that must be proved in a negligence suit are duty, dereliction of duty, direct cause, and damages.
7. Assault is the attempt or threat to touch another person without permission; battery is the actual touching.
8. The law of agency implies that physicians are liable for the actions of their employees. The physician is responsible for your actions as a medical assistant, as long as your actions are within your scope of practice and you practice the standard of care required for your assigned duties and responsibilities

9. Blood-borne pathogens are organisms that can be spread through direct contact with blood or body fluids from an infected person. OSHA governs their control in the medical office.
10. The three ethical standards the CMA must follow are protecting patient confidentiality, following laws, and being honest.
11. An advance directive is a statement of a person's wishes for medical decisions prior to a critical event. Letting family know of these wishes and keeping a copy in the medical office chart will help ensure that these wishes are carried out.
12. If a physician closes the practice (or dies), all patients must be notified that the office is closing and must be given instructions for retrieving their medical records. Generally, copies of medical records are transferred to another local physician. The originals are stored as directed by state law.

 ## Websites

To keep abreast of changes in the medical field:

- Go to your state's home page and click on the link to the state legislature to view pending state legislation
- Go to The Library of Congress to view federal legislation to be considered in the coming week via the website http://Thomas.loc.gov

Equal Employment Opportunity Commission
    www.eeoc.gov

For a complete text of Title VII of the Civil Rights Act
    www.eeoc.gov/laws/vii.html

U. S. Department of Labor, Bureau of Labor Statistics
    http://stats.bls.gov

To complete an advance directive
    www.LegalZoom.com

Communicating With Patients

There are two fundamental tasks that you will perform every day when working as a medical assistant. These two tasks are communication and teaching. This unit will introduce you to the skills needed to perform these tasks. Communication is the sharing of ideas between two people. Successful communication ensures that the medical office will run effectively and smoothly. Teaching occurs in all areas of the medical office and is a responsibility shared among all medical professionals. Teaching patients various skills or information helps to ensure that they have received the most comprehensive medical care possible. You will be able to master these skills after completing the next two chapters.

3

Fundamental Communication Skills

CHAPTER OUTLINE

ROLE DELINEATION COMPONENTS

GENERAL: Professionalism
- Display a professional manner and image
- Treat all patients with compassion and empathy

GENERAL: Communication Skills
- Recognize and respect cultural diversity
- Adapt communications to individual's ability to understand

- Use professional telephone technique
- Recognize and respond effectively to verbal, nonverbal, and written communications

ADMINISTRATIVE: Administrative Procedures
- Perform basic administrative medical assisting functions

CHAPTER COMPETENCIES

LEARNING OBJECTIVES

Upon successfully completing this chapter, you will be able to:

1. Spell and define the key terms
2. List two major forms of communication
3. Explain how various components of communication can affect the meaning of verbal messages
4. Define active listening
5. List and describe the six interviewing techniques
6. Give an example of how cultural differences may affect communication
7. Discuss how to handle communication problems caused by language barriers
8. List two methods that you can use to promote communication among hearing-, sight-, and speech-impaired patients
9. List five actions that you can take to improve communication with a child
10. Discuss how to handle an angry or distressed patient
11. Discuss your role in communicating with a grieving patient or family member
12. Discuss the key elements of interdisciplinary communication

KEY TERMS

anacusis	discrimination	messages	presbyacusis
bias	dysphasia	mourning	reflecting
clarification	dysphonia	nonlanguage	stereotyping
cultures	feedback	paralanguage	summarizing
demeanor	grief	paraphrasing	therapeutic

COMMUNICATION IS SENDING and receiving **messages** (information), verbally or otherwise. The ability to communicate effectively is a crucial skill for medical assistants. In your role, you must accurately and appropriately share information with physicians, other professional staff members, and patients. When communicating with patients you must be able to receive messages correctly, interpret them, and respond to the sender appropriately. The medical assistant is usually the first person the patient meets in the medical office. Thus, your positive attitude, pleasant presentation, and use of good communication skills will set the tone for future interactions.

BASIC COMMUNICATION FLOW

Communication requires the following elements:

- A message to be sent
- A person to send the message
- A person to receive the message

During the act of communicating, two or more people will alternate roles as sender and receiver as they seek **feedback** (responses) and **clarification** (understanding) regarding the message. The process of message exchange is a swing moving back and forth between two people. Figure 3-1 illustrates the flow of communication and its common components.

As a medical assistant, you will primarily be communicating in a therapeutic manner. This means that your communication will focus on conversations regarding pertinent topics relating to office procedures, policies, and patient care. Your other responsibilities for ensuring good communication include the following:

- Clarifying confusing messages
- Validating (confirming) the patient's perceptions
- Adapting messages to the patient's level of understanding
- Asking for feedback to ensure that the messages you sent were received by the patient or other persons as intended

Checkpoint Question

1. What three elements must be present for communication to occur?

FORMS OF COMMUNICATION

Verbal Communication

Verbal communication involves an exchange of messages using words or language; it is the most commonly used form and is usually the initial form of communication. You need good verbal communication skills when performing such tasks as making appointments, providing patient education, making referrals, and sharing information with the physician.

Oral communication is sending or receiving messages using spoken language. As a professional, you should use a pleasant and polite manner of speaking. Use proper English and grammar at all times; lapsing into slang and colloquialisms projects an unprofessional image.

Gear your conversation to the patient's educational level. A well-educated patient may resent your using other than the correct terms, yet a less educated patient may be confused and intimidated by the same phrases. Avoid using elaborate medical terminology if you think it might confuse or frighten a patient. Will this patient understand "myocardial infarction," or should you say heart attack? Do not talk down to the patient, but do phrase your communication appropriately.

Be aware, too, that the meaning of spoken messages may be affected by other components of oral communication, including paralanguage and nonlanguage sounds. The cliché that it's not what you say but how you say it is true. Research shows that the primary message is transmitted more by the way it is said than by the words that are used. This refers to paralanguage. **Paralanguage** includes voice tone, quality, volume, pitch, and range. Nonlanguage sounds include laughing, sobbing, sighing, grunting, and so on. Other **nonlanguage** clues to understanding can be found in a speaker's grammatical structure, pronunciation, and general articulation, which can indicate regional or cultural background and level of education. Knowing this information can help you adapt responses and explanations to the patient's level of understanding.

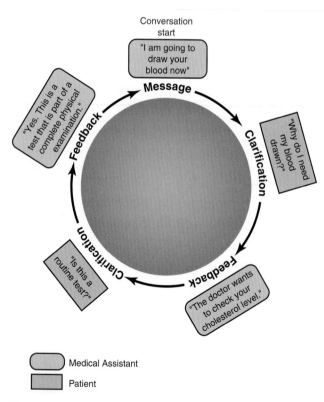

Medical Assistant
Patient

FIGURE 3-1.   Flow of communication.

Box 3-1

EXAMPLE OF WRITTEN DISCHARGE INSTRUCTIONS

Main Street Pediatric Group
343 Main Street, Suite 609
Philadelphia, PA 19106

Discharge Instructions for Otitis Media

Your child has an ear infection. It is easily treated with antibiotics. Get the prescription filled immediately. The first dose should be given as soon as you arrive home. Read the attached information on the antibiotic.

Here are some other important things to remember:
• Ear infections are not contagious.
• Symptoms usually resolve within 24 hours of beginning antibiotics. It is very important to make sure your child takes all of the prescription.
• If the pain persists for more than 48 hours, call the office.
• If you see any blood in the ear canal, call the office.

Make an appointment for a follow-up visit in 2 weeks.

_____   _____
Patient's signature   Physician's signature

Written communication uses written language to exchange messages. The ability to write clearly, concisely, and accurately is important in the health care profession (see Chapter 7). Typically, patients receive oral instructions first, as you or the physician explain key points of concern. These verbal instructions are then reinforced with written instructions (Box 3-1).

If the instructions, oral or written, are not clear, the patient may misinterpret them. This misunderstanding can hinder treatment and recovery and possibly even require the patient to be admitted to the hospital. Here is an example of unclear instruction: "Return to the office if you don't feel better." This provides the patient with no details. Clearer instructions would state, "If your fever and sore throat are not better in 24 hours, call the office to schedule a revisit." Even the most clearly outlined instructions can be misunderstood, particularly by those with deficient hearing or reading abilities. As a medical assistant, you are responsible for asking questions to verify that the patient has correctly understood the information. To verify that the patient understood these instructions, a good question to ask would be, "When should you call the office if you don't feel better?"

Checkpoint Question

2. List five examples of paralanguage.

Nonverbal Communication

Nonverbal communication—exchanging messages without using words—is sometimes called body language. Body language includes several types of behaviors, such as kinesics, proxemics, and the use of touch. Kinesics refers to body movements, including facial expressions, gestures, and eye movements. A patient's face can sometimes reveal inner feelings, such as sadness, happiness, fear, or anger, that may not be mentioned explicitly during a conversation (Fig. 3-2). Gestures also carry various meanings. For instance, shrug-

FIGURE 3-2. Different facial expressions convey different messages.

ging the shoulders can mean simple lack of interest or hopeless resignation. Eyes can often hint at what a person may be thinking or feeling. For example, a patient whose eyes wander away from you while you are talking may be impatient, lack interest, or not understand what you are saying.

Nonverbal communication may more accurately reflect a person's true feelings and attitude than verbal communication. In other words, people may say one thing but show a completely different response with their body language. For example, if the patient says, "The pain in my foot is not too bad," but the patient's face shows pain with each step, the nonverbal clues demonstrate an inconsistent message. Many patients mask their feelings, so you must learn to read their actions and nonverbal clues in addition to what they tell you. Be aware that patients are also acutely attuned to your facial and nonverbal reactions. Responding with an expression of disgust or shaking your head in a negative way can jeopardize communication and rapport between you and the patient.

How and where individuals physically place themselves in relation to others can affect communication as well. Proxemics refers to spatial relationships or physical proximity tolerated by humans. Generally, the area within a 3-foot radius around a person is considered personal space and is not to be invaded by strangers, although this area varies among individuals and people of various **cultures** (societies). To deliver care to a patient, physicians and medical assistants must enter a patient's personal space. After a patient task is completed, it is appropriate to take a few steps back and allow for more space between you and the patient. Because some individuals become uncomfortable when their space is invaded, it is essential to approach the patient in a professional manner and explain what you plan to do. Explanations help ease patient anxiety about what will happen.

Related to proxemics is the use of touch, which can be **therapeutic** (beneficial) for some patients. It can indicate emotional support and convey concern and feeling. For some patients, however, being touched by a stranger is an uncomfortable or even a negative experience. Many patients perceive touch in a medical setting as a prelude to something unpleasant, such as an injection. To change this negative perception, try offering a comforting touch when nothing invasive or painful is imminent (Fig. 3-3). Before comforting a patient by touching, assess the patient's **demeanor** (expressions and behavior) for clues indicating that touch would be acceptable.

ACTIVE LISTENING

Active listening is important to ensure that messages are correctly received and interpreted. Failure to do so can result in poor patient care. To listen actively, you must give your full attention to the patient with whom you are speaking. Interruptions should be kept to a minimum. You need to focus not only on what is being said but also on what is being conveyed through paralanguage, body language, and other aspects of communication. Occasionally, a patient's verbal messages may seem to conflict with the nonverbal messages. For example, a patient who is wringing his hands while telling you that everything is fine is sending conflicting signals that require further exploration. If a patient's verbal response does not correspond to your observations, convey your concern to the physician.

Active listening is a skill that develops with practice. To test your listening ability, try this exercise: Ask another student to speak continuously for 1 to 2 minutes while you listen. (The student should discuss a topic with which you are unfamiliar.) When he or she finishes, wait silently for the same amount of time. Then try to repeat the message. If you have trouble doing this exercise, you need to practice listening.

INTERVIEW TECHNIQUES

As a medical assistant, you are typically responsible for gathering initial information and updating existing information about the patients. This task is accomplished by interviewing the patient. The interview will consist of you asking certain questions and then interpreting the patient's responses. The initial interview includes many areas. The key areas are the patient's medical and family history, a brief review of the body systems, and a social history. Table 3-1 has sample questions that you may ask in each of these areas. The main goal is to obtain accurate and pertinent information. The interview for an established patient, however, is much different. First, you should review the chart to look at the patient's health problems. Make a list of questions regarding the pertinent medical problems. Reconfirm medication usage and any specific treatments the patient is supposed to be doing.

To conduct either type of interview, you must use effective techniques: listen actively, ask the appropriate questions, and record the answers. During the interview, you must demonstrate professionalism. Begin by introducing yourself. Always conduct the interview in a private area.

FIGURE 3-3. Therapeutic touch conveys caring and concern.

Table 3-1   INITIAL PATIENT INTERVIEW COMPONENTS

Area	Sample Questions
Past medical history	Any previous hospitalizations? If so, when? Any previous surgeries? If so, when? Any chronic problems (e.g., asthma, diabetes, heart condition)? Any past pregnancies? Any complications? Any miscarriages, stillbirths, or abortions?
Family history	Age and health of parents? If deceased, what was the cause and at what age did they die? Age and health of siblings? Are there any genetic disorders?
Body system review	General questions regarding all body systems: cardiovascular, pulmonary, integumentary, musculoskeletal, neurological, sensory, gastrointestinal, endocrine, immune, urological, and reproductive
Social history	Alcohol use? Smoking? Drug use? Hobbies? Education? Employment?
Medications	What do you take? When? How much? Any vitamins or herbal supplements?

Know what questions you need to ask and in what order to ask them before you begin the interview. Be organized. It is also helpful to have an extra pen. And most important, do not answer phone calls or attend to other distractions until you have finished the interview. Last, when you leave the room, let patients know who will be in to see them and the approximate time, for example, "Dr. Sanchez will be in to see you in about 10 minutes."

The six interviewing techniques are reflecting, paraphrasing, clarification, asking open-ended questions, summarizing, and allowing silences.

Reflecting

Reflecting is repeating what you have heard the patient say, using open-ended statements. With this technique, you do not complete a sentence, but leave it up to the patient to do so. For example, you might say, "Mrs. Rivera, you were saying that when your back hurts you. . . ." Reflection encourages the patient to make further comments. It also can help bring the patient back to the subject if the conversation begins to drift. (Reflecting is a useful tool, but be careful not to overuse it, because some patients find it annoying to have their words constantly parroted back.)

Paraphrasing or Restatement

Paraphrasing or restatement means repeating what you have heard, using your own words or phrases. Paraphrasing can help verify that you have accurately understood what was said. It also allows patients the opportunity to clarify their thoughts or statements. Typically, a paraphrased statement begins with "You are saying that . . . ," or "It sounds as if . . . ," followed by the rephrased content.

Asking for Examples or Clarification

If you are confused about some of the information you have received, ask the patient to give an example of the situation being described. For instance, "Can you describe one of these dizzy spells?" The patient's example should help you better understand what the patient is saying. It also may give you an insight into how the patient perceives the situation.

Asking Open-Ended Questions

The best way to obtain specific information is to ask open-ended questions that require the patient to formulate an answer and elaborate on the response. Open-ended questions usually begin with what, when, or how. For example, "What medications did you take this morning?" "When did you stop taking your medication?" "How did you get that large bruise on your arm?" Be careful about asking "why" questions, because they can often sound judgmental or accusing. For example, asking "Why did you do that?" or "Why didn't you follow directions?" may imply to patients that you have already made a negative value judgment about their behavior, and they could become defensive and uncooperative. Instead you might ask, "What part of the instructions did you not understand?" or "How can we help you follow these instructions?"

Avoid closed-ended questions that allow the patient to answer with one word, such as yes or no. For example, suppose you ask the patient, "Are you taking your medications?" The patient can easily say yes but may not be taking all of them. However, suppose you ask, "What medications do you take every day?" The patient's answer will give you a clearer understanding of whether the patient is taking the correct medications.

Summarizing

Briefly reviewing the information you have obtained, or **summarizing**, gives the patient another chance to clarify statements or correct misinformation. This technique can also help you organize complex information or events in sequential order. For example, if the patient has been feeling dizzy and stumbling a lot, you might summarize by saying, "You told me that you have been feeling dizzy for the past 3 days and that you frequently stumble as you are walking."

Allowing Silences

Periods of silence sometimes occur during the interview. These can be beneficial. Some people are uncomfortable with prolonged silences and feel a need to break the silence with words in an effort to jump-start a stalled conversation. Silences are natural parts of conversations and can give patients time to formulate their thoughts, reconstruct events, evaluate their feelings, or assess what has already been said. During moments of silence, gather your thoughts and formulate any additional questions that you may have.

Checkpoint Question

3. What are the six interviewing techniques?

FACTORS AFFECTING COMMUNICATION

Sometimes, despite your best efforts, others may not receive your message accurately. A common occurrence that causes messages to be misinterpreted is the use of a cliché. For example, suppose you are teaching a patient to use crutches and she is having difficulty managing them. A cliché comment may be, "Don't worry. Rome wasn't built in a day. This takes time." The cliché is innocent and not meant to be demeaning, but the patient may misinterpret it to mean that she is slow, ancient. A more positive message would be, "I can see that you are making progress. Let's try walking down the hallway."

Here are some reasons for miscommunication:

1. The message may have been unclear or inappropriate to the situation. For example, "I have scheduled you for a PET scan in radiology tomorrow at 8 A.M." Keep in mind that most of your patients do not understand medical abbreviations and terms. Since positron emission tomography (PET) is newer technology, they may confuse it with computed tomography (CT). Also, where is radiology? A better message would be, "The doctor wants you to have a test done tomorrow. It is called a PET scan; here is a brochure that explains it. Go to the second floor of the outpatient center on Main Street. Do you know how to get there?"
2. The person receiving the message may have been distracted, anxious, or confused. A common cause of distraction is pain. For example, teaching a patient how to use crutches cannot be done if the patient's ankle or knee still hurts. The concentration will be on the pain, not on what you are saying. Patients who have just received positive news can also be anxious to contact loved ones. This is commonly seen with patients who have just been told that they are pregnant. The patient's focus is on calling family members and not on your conversation.
3. Environmental elements, such as noise or interruptions, may also distort messages. Environmental noises from staff lounges or break rooms can easily be overheard. Keep the doors to these areas closed. Cleaning staff should not be vacuuming or emptying trash while patients are present.

In addition to these three items, other factors may affect communication. They are discussed next.

Cultural Differences

The way a person perceives situations and other people is greatly influenced by cultural, social, and religious beliefs or firmly held convictions. Personal values (principles or ideals) are commonly developed from these same beliefs. As a medical assistant, you will interact with people from varied ethnic backgrounds and cultural origins who bring with them beliefs and values that may differ from your own. Understanding those differences can aid communication and thereby improve patient care (Table 3-2). It is very important that you not form preconceived ideas about a given culture. Remember that each patient is unique and that their health care needs differ.

Some cultures may be offended by the types of intensely personal questions necessary for a medical history and may

Table 3-2	**CULTURAL FACTORS THAT AFFECT PATIENT CARE**[a]		
Cultural Group	**Family**	**Folk and Traditional Health Care**	**Common Health Problems**
White	Nuclear family is highly valued Elderly family members may live in a nursing home when they can no longer care for themselves	Self-diagnosis of illnesses Use of over-the-counter drugs, especially vitamins and analgesics Dieting, especially fad diets Extensive use of exercise and exercise facilities	Cardiovascular disease Gastrointestinal disease Some forms of cancer Motor vehicle accidents Suicide Mental illness Substance abuse
African American	Close and supportive extended-family relationships Strong kinship ties with nonblood relatives from church or organizational and social groups Family unity, loyalty, and cooperation are important. Frequently matriarchal	Varies extensively and may include spiritualists, herb doctors, root doctors, conjurers, skilled elder family members, voodoo, faith healing	Hypertension Sickle cell anemia Skin disorders; inflammation of hair follicles, various types of dermatitis and excessive growth of scar tissue (keloids) Lactose enzyme deficiency resulting in poor toleration of milk products High rate of tuberculosis Diabetes mellitus Higher infant mortality rate than in the white population
Asian	Welfare of the family is valued above the individual person Extended families are common A person's lineage (ancestors) is respected Sharing among family members is expected	Theoretical basis in Taoism, which seeks balance in all things Good health is achieved through proper balance between yin (feminine, negative, dark, cold) and yang (masculine, positive, light, warm) An imbalance in energy is caused by an improper diet or strong emotions Diseases and food are classified as hot or cold, and a proper balance between them will promote wellness (e.g., treat a cold disease with hot foods) Many Asian health care systems use herbs, diet, and application of hot or cold therapy Many Asians believe some points on the body are on the meridians, or energy pathways; if the energy flow is out of balance, treatment of the pathways may be necessary to restore the energy equilibrium *Acumassage*: Manipulation of points along the energy pathways *Acupressure*: Technique for compressing the energy pathway points *Acupuncture*: Insertion of fine needles into the body at energy pathway points	Tuberculosis Communicable diseases Malnutrition Suicide Various forms of mental illness Lactose enzyme deficiency

(continued)

Table 3–2 CULTURAL FACTORS THAT AFFECT PATIENT CARE[a] *(Continued)*

Cultural Group	Family	Folk and Traditional Health Care	Common Health Problems
Hispanic, Mexican American	Familial role is important *Compadrazgo*: special bond between a child's parents and grandparents Family is the primary unit of society	*Curanderas(os)*: Folk healers who base treatments on humoral pathology: basic functions of the body are controlled by four body fluids, or humors—blood, hot and wet; yellow bile, hot and dry; black bile, cold and dry; and phlegm, cold and wet The secret of good health is to balance hot and cold within the body; therefore, most foods, beverages, herbs, and medications are classified as hot (*caliente*) or cold (*fresco, frio*); a cold disease will be cured with a hot treatment	Diabetes mellitus and its complications Problems of poverty, such as poor nutrition, inadequate medical care, and poor prenatal care Lactose enzyme deficiency
Hispanic, Puerto Rican	*Compadrazgo*: similar to Mexican American culture	Similar to that of other Spanish-speaking cultures	Parasitic diseases, such as dysentery, malaria, filariasis, hookworms Lactose enzyme deficiency
Native American	Families large and extended Grandparents are official and symbolic leaders and decision makers A child's namesake may assume equal parenting authority with biological parents	Medicine men (shamans) are frequently consulted Heavy use of herbs and psychological treatments, ceremonies, fasting, meditation, heat, and massage	Alcoholism Suicide Tuberculosis Malnutrition Communicable diseases Higher maternal and infant mortality rates than in most of the population Diabetes mellitus Hypertension Gallbladder disease

Reprinted with permission from Taylor C, Lillis C, LeMone P. Fundamentals of Nursing, 2nd ed. Philadelphia: Lippincott-Raven, 1996:122–125.

[a] The beliefs and practices vary within each group, and no assumptions should be based on a patient's cultural background alone. The factors in this table are merely a guide to some commonly observed and documented cultural factors.

perceive them as an inexcusable invasion of privacy. If this occurs, your physician may be required to intervene to allay the patient's concerns.

Looking someone else directly in the eyes, or eye contact, is also perceived differently by people of various backgrounds. Eye contact occurs more often among friends and family members than among acquaintances or strangers. In the United States, someone who maintains good eye contact is usually perceived as being honest, believable, and concerned. In contrast, in some Asian and Mideastern cultures, direct eye contact is perceived as sexually suggestive or disrespectful. In other cultures, lack of eye contact or casting the eyes downward is a sign of respect.

In addition to cultural differences in values, many differences occur among individuals. Some people are just more reserved or shy than others and may feel less comfortable in medical settings. To help avoid miscommunication and of-

fending patients, you must be sensitive to these differences in all of your patient interactions.

Stereotyping and Biased Opinions

Medical assisting deals with people of differing ages, races, and sexual orientation. Sometimes, your values may be in stark contrast to those held by a patient, but you should not let your personal values or **bias** (opinions) affect your communication or treatment of a patient. All patients must be treated fairly, respectfully, and with dignity, regardless of their cultural, social, or personal values. To treat them in any other fashion is **discrimination**.

Stereotyping is holding an opinion of all members of a particular culture, race, religion, age group, or other group based on oversimplified or negative characterizations. It is a form of prejudice. Examples of negative stereotypes include

"All old people are frail and senile" and "Those people are always dirty and never bathe." Stereotyping and prejudice are deterrents to establishing therapeutic relationships because they do not allow for patients' individuality and can prevent quality care from being given to everyone on an equal basis.

As a health care professional, you are expected to treat all patients impartially, to guard against discriminatory practices, remain nonjudgmental, avoid stereotypes, and have a professional demeanor. By doing so, you communicate to patients that you accept human differences and that quality health care will be provided to all those who seek it.

Let's suppose Ms. Henry arrives with her 3-year-old daughter for a checkup. The mother says, "I think she has gotten head lice from someone at the shelter." Which response would be most appropriate? "Don't worry about it. The shelter is full of people with lice. Do you know anyone with lice?" or "I will mention to the doctor that you are concerned that she may have lice. Is anyone else in your family being treated for lice?" The latter response demonstrates appropriate caring and concern. It also begins the dialogue for determining additional people who may need to be checked, which is key to preventing community outbreaks. The first response communicates stereotyping of a particular lifestyle and prevents collection of additional data.

Language Barriers

Effective communication depends on the use of language, but some patients cannot speak or understand English well enough for good communication. Because it is crucial for you to give and receive accurate information, you will need to use an interpreter to help bridge any language barriers. A staff person might serve as the interpreter, or an English-speaking member of the patient's family may be able to help. In either case, be sure the interpreter fully understands what you are saying. In the absence of a reliable interpreter, a phrase book of common medical questions with lists of possible answers may be of help. If your area has a large population of non–English-speaking patients, your office should be equipped with an appropriate phrase book (See Appendix II for a list of key health care phrases in English and Spanish).

When choosing an interpreter, try to find someone of the same sex as the patient, because certain cultures prohibit members of the opposite sex (even family members) from discussing personal issues about the body. Some cultures follow religious guidelines dictating how members of the opposite sex should interact with each other.

Use the following suggestions for communicating with non–English-speaking patients:

1. Do not shout. Raising your voice will not increase their understanding.
2. Demonstrate or pantomime as needed. Gestures are usually relatively universal.
3. If you are using an interpreter, speak directly to the patient, with the interpreter in your line of vision, so that the patient can read your facial expressions.
4. Speak slowly with simple sentences and phrases that require simple answers. The patient may comprehend some simple English.
5. Avoid slang; it may not translate well.
6. Avoid distractions and provide a relaxed, quiet interview space.
7. Learn some basic phrases of the most common language used in your area. Patients appreciate your effort.

Spanish Terminology

Hable despacio, por favor.	Please speak slowly.
Sí, hablo español un poco.	Yes, I speak Spanish a little.
No, no comprendo.	No, I don't understand.
¿Comprende?	Do you understand?
¿Cuándo?	When?
¿Qué clase?	What kind?
¿Porqué?	Why?
¿Cuántos?	How many?
¿Qué, Qué tal?	What?
¿En qué puedo ayudarlo?	What can I help you with?
¿Dígame porque esta aquí?	Tell me why you are here?
¿Cómo?	How?

SPECIAL COMMUNICATION CHALLENGES

Many situations present special communication challenges. For instance, hearing- or sight-impaired patients, young children, patients with limited understanding, those who are too ill or sedated to comprehend, and those who are frightened or anxious require particular attention. In each instance, you will need to assess the situation and the patient's ability to comprehend. In some cases, a responsible family member will be with the patient and can be included in the communication process. Never exclude the patient from the exchange, but do ensure that all needed information is communicated, whether you obtain the information through questions about the patient's condition or you give instructions for further care. Patients must feel that they are part of the process even if their condition requires involvement by family members or other caregivers.

Hearing-Impaired Patients

There are many forms of hearing impairments. Impairments can vary from a partial loss to **anacusis**, complete hearing loss. The two types of impairments are conductive and sensorineural. Conductive hearing loss is caused by interference with sound in the external canal or the middle or inner ear. Sensorineural hearing loss is caused by lesions or problems with either nerves or the cochlea. The cochlea is a coiled tubular structure that turns vibrations into sounds. Most patients with anacusis are adept with communicating through sign language, interpreters, or other tools. However, patients with **presbyacusis**, a common hearing impairment in older patients, often have a more difficult time communicating and tend to be in denial about their hearing abilities. Patients with

presbyacusis benefit from hearing aids and other amplification devices.

To communicate with patients who cannot hear what you are saying, you need tact, diplomacy, and patience. These suggestions may help.

1. Touch the patient gently to gain his or her attention.
2. Talk directly face-to-face with the patient, not at an angle and certainly not with your back turned.
3. Turn to the most prominent light so that your face is illuminated.
4. Lower the pitch of your voice, since higher pitches are frequently lost with nerve impairment, but speak distinctly and with force. In most instances, shouting does not help and will only distort what might be heard.
5. Use note pads or demonstration as needed.
6. Pictograms are very helpful and should be readily available. A pictogram is a flash card that shows basic medical terms.
7. Use short sentences with short words. Enunciate clearly but do not exaggerate your facial movements.
8. Eliminate all distractions. Extraneous noises may confuse the patient.

Checkpoint Question

4. What is the term for complete hearing loss?

Sight-Impaired Patients

Sight impairments range from complete blindness to blurred vision. The changes in vision tend to be slow and progressive. Box 3-2 has a list of conditions that can cause visual im-

---

Box 3-2

MEDICAL CONDITIONS THAT CAN CAUSE VISUAL IMPAIRMENT

Below are some common medical conditions that can cause visual impairment:

Cataract
Hyperopia (farsightedness)
Glaucoma
Macular degeneration
Myopia (nearsightedness)
Nyctalopia (night blindness)
Presbyopia
Retinal detachment
Retinopathy
Strabismus

pairment. Patients who can't see lose valuable information from nonverbal communication. To improve communication with a sight impaired patient, try these suggestions.

1. Identify yourself by name each time the patient comes into the office.
2. Do not raise your voice; the patient is not hearing impaired.
3. Let the patient know exactly what you will be doing at all times and alert him or her before touching.
4. Orient the patient spatially by having him or her touch the table, the chair, the counter, and so forth.
5. Assist the patient by offering your arm and escorting him or her to the interview room.
6. Tell the patient when you are leaving the room and knock before entering.
7. Explain the sounds of machines to be used in the examination (e.g., buzzing, whirring) and what each machine will do.

Speech Impairments

Speech impairments can come from a variety of medical conditions. The medical term for difficulty with speech is **dysphasia**. Dysphasia is usually the result of a neurological problem. A common neurological condition can result in dysphasia is a stroke. **Dysphonia** is a voice impairment that is caused by a physical condition, such as oral surgery, cancer of the tongue or voice box, or cleft palate. Stuttering is another medical condition that can impair the patient's ability to communicate.

Here are some suggestions to help you communicate with a patient who has a speech impediment:

- Allow such patients time to gather their thoughts.
- Allow plenty of time for them to communicate.
- Do not rush conversations.
- Offer a note pad to write questions.
- Discuss with the physician the potential benefits for getting a speech therapist referral for the patient.

 Checkpoint Question

5. What is the medical term for difficulty with speech? What does dysphonia mean?

Mental Health Illnesses

Many mental illnesses and psychiatric disorders can impair a patient's ability to communicate. These illnesses produce a broad range of communication challenges. Some illnesses can lead the patient to have uncontrollable outbursts, while others can cause a mute condition in which the patient will not communicate at all. Patients may hear voices that direct their communication to a given topic, while others may see objects that do not exist and will want confirmation from you

that you see the objects. Communicating with patients with moderate to severe psychiatric disorders requires in-depth training. It is important to stress that not all patients with mental illnesses will be challenges. Most mental illnesses can be controlled and treated with medications and other therapies. Here are a few suggestions for communicating with patients who have mental illnesses:

- Tell the patient what to expect and when things will happen.
- Keep conversations focused and professional.
- Do not force or demand answers from patients who are withdrawn or mute.
- If you feel unsafe communicating with a given patient, speak to either your supervisor or the physician regarding your concerns.
- Do not confirm hearing voices or seeing nonexistent objects.
- Orient the patient to reality as appropriate.

Patients with a history of substance abuse, alcoholism, and other addictions can also present a communication challenge. Patients may have euphoria and communicate with a flight of ideas. Or they may demonstrate aggression and agitation while they are withdrawing from the addiction. Your responsibility in communicating with patients who have any of these conditions is to identify the reasons for today's visit and follow your regular assessment duties. It is not the role of the medical assistant to recommend treatments or counseling for these patients. Your communication should be professional, nonjudgmental, and encouraging when appropriate.

Angry or Distressed Patients

Patients' emotions can run the spectrum from polite and cordial to angry and upset. There are numerous reasons for the latter. Prolonged waiting times, financial issues, and illness can spark untoward emotions. At some time in our lives we all have had a cold, felt terrible, and have snapped angrily at an innocent bystander. The key to communicating with upset patients is to prevent an escalation of the problem. Keep your patients informed about waiting times, billing and insurance changes, and other office policies that might trigger untoward emotions.

It is understandable that patients will become upset on hearing sad or unfortunate news about their health. Most patients take sad news in a calm manner. It is important to offer assistance as needed. Provide written instructions and information for the patient to read later. This material should consist of information on the diagnosis, causes of the illness, treatment options, and phone numbers that the patient may call for additional information.

Here are some suggestions that will help you communicate with an angry or distressed patient:

- Be supportive.
- Be open and honest in all communication.

- Do not provide false reassurances.
- Do not belittle the problem or concern.
- Ensure your own safety if the angry patient becomes aggressive or threatening.

Children

Levels of comprehension vary greatly during childhood, and therefore communication needs must be tailored to the specific child's needs. The following suggestions will help facilitate communication:

1. Children are responsive to eye-level contact. Either raise them to your height or lower yourself to theirs.
2. Keep your voice low-pitched and gentle.
3. Make your movements slow and keep them visible. Tell children when you need to touch them.
4. Rephrase your questions until you are sure that the child understands.
5. Be prepared for the child to return to a lower developmental level for comfort during an illness. For example, a child may revert to thumb sucking during a stressful event.
6. Use play to phrase your questions and to gain the child's cooperation. (For example, if the child appears shy and does not want to talk, start by asking the child how a stuffed animal feels today. " How does Teddy feel today?" Follow up on the child's answer with "And how do you feel?" Offering to take the teddy's temperature first may lessen any fear of thermometers.
7. Allow the child to express fear, to cry, and so on.
8. Many adolescents resent authority. During the interview, some teenagers may not want a parent in the room. Assess the situation before including the parent.
9. Never show shock or judgment when dealing with adolescents; this will immediately close communication.

Communicating With a Grieving Patient or Family Member

Occasionally, you will need to support patients who are in grief or great sadness caused by a loss. Grieving starts when a person has a significant loss, such as the loss of a loved one through death or the loss of a relationship, a body part, or personal health. Grief includes such emotional responses as anger, sadness, and depression, and each emotion may trigger certain behaviors. For example, anger may result in outbursts, sadness may cause crying, and depression may lead to unusual quietness or isolation.

Grieving occurs in stages: denial, anger, bargaining, depression, and acceptance. Here are some examples of what a patient in denial may say: "The doctor must have read the test wrong." "I don't have cancer; I feel fine." Anger may be voiced by, "I hate the doctor." "This is a terrible place." Bargaining is a stage in which the patient or family member tries to trade off the sad news, for example, "God, I will be the

best person I can be if you take away this disease." Depression is often expressed through quiet, withdrawn behaviors. The patient may state, "I don't care if I live anymore." Acceptance is the last stage. The patient may state, "I understand that I have terminal disease and am going to die." It is very important to stress that each person grieves in his or her own way and at his or her own pace. These stages may spread over months or years. It is possible to go through stages more than once. Sometimes, the collective signs of grief are referred to as **mourning**.

In medical settings, expect to see grief displayed in many ways. Know, too, that several factors can influence how a patient demonstrates grief and that different cultures and individuals demonstrate their grief in a variety of ways ranging from stoic, impassive responses to loud, prolonged wailing and fainting. Other responses may reflect religious beliefs about the meaning of death. Grieving is a unique and personal process. There is no set time period for grieving, and there is no "right" way to grieve.

Grieving patients may want to talk about their feelings and review events. Terminally ill patients may want to discuss their fears of dying and concerns for surviving loved ones. To support grieving patients, allow time for them to express themselves and actively listen to what they say. When appropriate, consider using touch to convey your understanding. If patients' concerns stem from a lack of understanding about their condition, provide pertinent education for them and for their caregivers (if appropriate). You should also become familiar with available community resources, such as grief or other counseling services and hospice care, so you can suggest these services when necessary.

It is normal for you to feel sad when a patient dies. It is important that your communication focus on empathy, not sympathy. Many psychologists describe sympathy as feeling *for* someone and empathy as feeling *with* someone. In the health care setting, empathy means trying to understand what patients are feeling so you can help them. Empathy can help you recognize a patient's fear and discomfort so you can do everything possible to provide support and reassurance. Sympathy, or pitying your patient, may compromise your professional distance and cause you to become personally involved. Box 3-3 offers suggestions for helping grieving patients.

Checkpoint Question

6. What are the five stages of grieving?

ESTABLISHING POSITIVE PATIENT RELATIONSHIPS

Your approach to patients conveys a message about who you are and how you feel about yourself and your profession. Medical assistants can be role models, earning the trust and admiration of patients. To establish and maintain positive relationships with patients, speak respectfully and exhibit an appropriate demeanor during all interactions.

COMMUNICATING WITH A GRIEVING FAMILY MEMBER OR PATIENT

Patients and families faced with great loss can be helped through a variety of community resources. Hospice is national program that offers support to patients and family members dealing with a loss. Hospice deals with all types of medical conditions and with people of all ages. The earlier the patient is introduced to a hospice program, the more beneficial. Hospice does have a palliative component. Hospice staff and volunteer grief counselors are trained to answer the questions, acknowledge the fears and anger, ease the transition, and offer respite for caregivers. A patient must never be forced to join hospice or other community resources. Grieving is an individual experience. Your local hospital may also have grief counselors or social workers who can help your patients. Other community resources may be available. The knowledgeable medical assistant will, with the physician's permission, direct the patient and the family to the proper organization.

Proper Form of Address

The way you address patients provides clues about your attitude and how you will likely provide care. When greeting patients, use a proper form of address, for example, "Good morning, Mr. Jones!" or "How are you feeling, Mrs. Smith?" This type of address shows respect and sets a professional tone. In contrast, calling patients by pet names, such as sweetie, granny, gramps, or honey, can offend the person. These terms denigrate the individual's dignity and put the interaction on a personal, not professional, level.

Other inappropriate forms of address include referring to the patient as a medical condition, such as "the gallbladder in room 2" or "the broken arm in the waiting room." Patients often come to the medical office feeling anxious, so they may be particularly sensitive to everything they see and hear (or overhear). Referring to the patient as a medical condition sends the message that the staff values the patient as nothing more than an illness, which can lead to heightened anxiety.

Professional Distance

How people interact with each other is influenced by the level of emotional involvement between them. For instance, communication between a husband and wife is more intimate than the personal level of communication between friends or the social level of communication between acquaintances. In the health care setting, you must establish an appropriate level of communication to deliver direct patient care, make objective assessments, and provide quality patient teaching. You should not become too personally involved with patients because doing so may jeopardize your ability to make objective assessments. It is easy to become overattached, especially to elderly patients who are lonely. For example, do not offer to drive patients to appointments, pick up prescriptions, or do their grocery shopping. Keeping a professional distance allows you to deal objectively with patients while creating a therapeutic environment. To keep this distance, avoid revealing intimate information about yourself (e.g., marital woes, financial troubles, family conflict) that might shift the dynamics of the relationship to a more personal level. Often, in an attempt to help a patient, we might say, "My grandmother was diagnosed with cancer too, but she is fine; it's not a big deal. You will be okay too." Every situation is different. The patient may misinterpret this to mean that you don't think that his or her diagnosis of cancer is a big deal. But at that moment it is a very big deal to the patient!

TEACHING PATIENTS

One of the fundamental communication skills you will need is the ability to teach patients about their medical conditions. Teaching patients might involve something as relatively simple as explaining how often they should take a medication or instructing a newly diagnosed diabetic patient about self-injection. The guidelines listed below incorporate such key communication skills as interviewing and active listening. Follow these to provide effective patient education. (See Chapter 4.)

1. Be knowledgeable about current medical issues, discoveries, and trends.
2. Be aware of special services available in your area.
3. Have pertinent handouts or information sheets available.
4. Allow enough teaching time so that you are not interrupted or rushed.
5. Find a quiet room away from the main office flow if at all possible.
6. Give information in a clear, concise, sequential manner; provide written instructions as a follow-up.
7. Allow the patient time to assimilate this new information.
8. Encourage the patient to ask questions.
9. Ask questions in a way that will allow you to know whether the patient understands the material.
10. Invite the patient to call the office with additional questions that may arise.

PROFESSIONAL COMMUNICATION

Communicating With Peers

Communication among your peers must remain professional and appropriate throughout the workday. Discussions of non–work-related topics should be kept to a minimum and occur only during designated break times. It is not appropriate to discuss last night's TV shows, arguments with boyfriends, shopping lists, and so on in front of patients. Excessive laughing, high-pitched voice tones, and whispering can produce an unprofessional atmosphere.

During your career, you may come across a situation that requires communication with your supervisor about another peer's actions. Your communication must always be honest and accurate when reporting facts to a supervisor. Embellishing or hiding information can result in termination of your employment.

An excellent way to promote communication among your peers is to become active in your local professional organization. Your involvement at the local level can spread to national exposure. Involvement in local community organizations and support groups is also beneficial to promoting you and your profession.

Communicating With Physicians

Physicians and other health care practitioners will rely on you to communicate pertinent information to patients in a timely manner to provide quality care. Your communication

ETHICAL TIPS

All patient communication is confidential. Patient information is sometimes discussed unintentionally, however. To avoid breaching confidentiality, follow these guidelines:

- Do not discuss patients' problems in public places, such as elevators or parking lots. A patient's friends or family members might overhear your conversation and misinterpret what is said.
- The glass window between the waiting room and the reception desk should be kept closed.
- Watch the volume of your voice.
- When calling coworkers over the office intercom, do not use a patient's name or reveal other information. Avoid saying something like, "Bob Smith is on the phone and wants to know if his strep throat culture came back." Instead, say "There's a patient on line 1."
- Before going home, destroy any slips of paper in your uniform pockets that contain patient information (e.g., reminder notes from verbal reports).

Box 3-4

TYPES OF REFERRALS

Numerous types of referrals can be made. Here are some of the most common examples:

Cardiac rehabilitation
Diabetes education
Dietitian
Home care services
Laboratory studies
Occupational therapy
Physician specialties (cardiologist, pulmonologist, podiatrist)
Physical therapy
Psychotherapy
Radiology
Social worker
Speech therapy

must always be professional. The physician should always be addressed as doctor unless he specifies otherwise. The use of inappropriate terms is never acceptable. When possible, the correct medical terminology should be used. If you are unsure of the correct medical term, however, explain the condition rather than use a term that you do not understand. For example, if a patient comes into the office with a chief complaint of difficulty urinating, simply say, "Mr. Aramark is complaining of trouble urinating." Never use a slang expression, such as "He is having trouble peeing."

Do not feel intimidated when speaking to a physician. Speak slowly and confidently and you will develop a professional rapport. Be honest. It is better to say, "I am not sure what to do with this specimen" then to assume and make a mistake.

Remember, there is a time and place for everything. The physician may be the biggest jokester or sports fan in the office, but it is not appropriate to draw on these topics in front of patients or family members.

Communicating With Other Facilities

The medical administrative staff often makes referrals to other facilities or physicians. Box 3-4 has examples of various referrals you might make. No matter whom you are contacting, follow these key points:

- Patient confidentiality is always foremost. Make sure you have appropriate patient consent.
- Observe all legal requirements for dispensing patient data.
- Use caution with fax machines, E-mail, and other electronic devices. Make sure the intended receiver is the one who gets the communication.

- Provide only the facts. Do not relay suspicions or assumptions.
- Always be nonjudgmental.
- Confirm that the message was received and that the referral will be handled.

CHAPTER SUMMARY

Communication is a complex and dynamic process involving the sending and receiving of messages. It includes verbal and nonverbal forms of expression and is influenced by personal and societal values, individual beliefs, and cultural orientation. In the medical practice, important aspects of patient communication are interviewing and active listening. You will need to overcome many communication challenges to communicate with all patients. These challenges include patients with hearing, sight, and speech impairments. Children, or angry or distressed patients, and patients with mental illnesses can also present a challenge to communication. To communicate effectively, you must understand the various factors that can affect the exchange of messages and use the communication techniques that are most appropriate for each individual situation.

Critical Thinking Challenges

1. Dr. Rogers has just told a patient she has breast cancer. The words breast cancer can spark many emotions and fears. Write three sample questions that you could ask the patient to promote open communication about her feelings. Suppose the diagnosis made was AIDS. What questions would you ask?
2. Dr. Blanda has just discharged a patient with specific instructions for wound care. How would you determine the patient's understanding of these instructions? Can nonverbal clues help you determine whether the patient is confused?
3. A mother brings in her 3-year-old child for a checkup. The child refuses to have her temperature taken. How would you go about communicating the importance of this? What if the child was 6 years old?
4. List five common clichés. Then select one and draw a picture illustrating how it may be misinterpreted.

5. A patient arrives in your office demanding to see the physician immediately. He is yelling and obviously very angry. The doctor is with another patient. Write three statements that you could say that might help the situation. Write three statements that would escalate the situation.
6. List five local resources that can assist a grieving patient or family member. Include the name of the agency, type of help that it offers, any special information, and its phone number.

Answers to Checkpoint Questions

1. For communication to occur, these three elements must be present: a message to be sent, a person to send the message, and a person to receive the message.
2. Voice tone, quality, volume, pitch, and range are five examples of paralanguage.
3. When interviewing patients, you can use six different techniques. These include reflecting, paraphrasing or restatement, asking for examples or clarification, asking open-ended questions, summarizing, and allowing silences.
4. The medical term for complete hearing loss is anacusis.
5. The medical term for difficulty with speech is dysphasia. Dysphonia is a voice impairment.
6. The five stages of grieving are denial, anger, bargaining, depression, and acceptance.

 Websites

Here are some websites that can give you some additional information:

National Institute of Deafness and Other Communication Disorders
    www.nidcd.nih.gov
American Speech-Language-Hearing Association
    www.asha.org
Hearing, Speech and Deafness Center
    www.hsdc.org
National Hospice and Palliative Care Organization
    www.nhpco.org

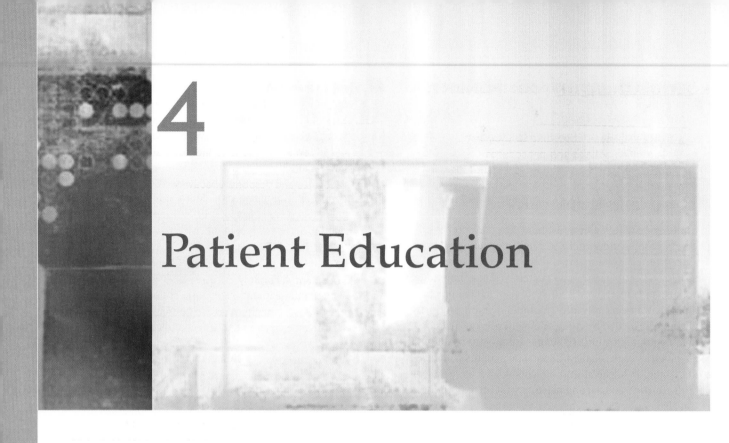

4

Patient Education

CHAPTER OUTLINE

ROLE DELINEATION COMPONENTS

GENERAL: Instruction
- Instruct individuals according to their needs
- Explain office policies and procedures
- Teach methods of health promotion and disease prevention
- Locate community resources and disseminate information
    - Develop educational materials
    - Conduct continuing education activities

GENERAL: Communication Skills
- Recognize and respect cultural diversity
- Adapt communications to individual's ability to understand
- Recognize and respond effectively to verbal, nonverbal, and written communications
- Use medical terminology appropriately

GENERAL: Legal Concepts
- Perform within legal and ethical boundaries
- Document accurately

CHAPTER COMPETENCIES

LEARNING OBJECTIVES

Upon successfully completing this chapter, you will be able to:

1. Spell and define the key terms
2. Explain the medical assistant's role in patient education
3. Define the five steps in the patient education process
4. Identify five conditions that are needed for patient education to occur
5. Explain Maslow's hierarchy of human needs
6. List five factors that may hinder patient education and at least two methods to compensate for each of these factors
7. Discuss five preventive medicine guidelines that you should teach your patients
8. Explain the kinds of information that should be included in patient teaching about medication therapy
9. Identify the components of a healthy diet, and explain how to use a food guide pyramid
10. Explain the importance of teaching range-of-motion exercises to patients
11. Explain your role in teaching patients about alternative medicine therapies
12. List and explain relaxation techniques that you can teach patients to help with stress management
13. List three national organizations that can help patients with smoking cessation
14. Identify a national organization that can assist patients with treating alcoholism
15. Describe how to prepare a teaching plan
16. List potential sources of patient education materials

KEY TERMS

alternative	detoxification	learning objectives	planning
assessment	documentation	noncompliance	psychomotor
carbohydrates	evaluation	nutrition	range-of-motion
coping mechanisms	implementation	placebo	stress

IN THE CURRENT HEALTH care climate of short hospital stays, patients seen in the medical office typically have acute conditions requiring intensive and extensive education from their health care provider. This will be one of your most challenging and rewarding roles as a medical assistant. Of course, you will not be responsible for teaching patients everything they need to know about health care. Patient education is performed under the direction of the physician. The amount and types of education that you will be expected to do will vary greatly from office to office. This chapter will give you the foundation needed for providing patient education.

THE PATIENT EDUCATION PROCESS

Patient education involves more than telling patients which medications they need to take or which lifestyle behaviors they need to change and expecting them to follow these instructions blindly. To educate patients effectively, you need to help them accept their illness, involve them in the process of gaining knowledge, and provide positive reinforcement. Ultimately, that knowledge should lead to a change in behavior or attitudes.

The process of patient education involves five major steps:

- Assessment
- Planning
- Implementation
- Evaluation
- Documentation

These five steps collectively produce the teaching plan. The plan may be formally written as the process is occurring or may be documented after the event. You must follow all these steps to achieve effective patient education.

Assessment

Before you begin to teach, you must assess your feelings and attitudes about the patient and the topic to be taught. Sometime in your career as a medical assistant, you may encounter situations or patients that make you feel uncomfortable. Your role as an educator, however, requires that you set aside your own personal feelings and life experiences to instruct the patient objectively and to the best of your ability. Always consider how your responses and actions will affect the patient and be sure to treat each patient impartially.

Assessment requires gathering information about the patient's present health care needs and abilities. In addition to knowing the present health care needs, you must also look at these other areas:

- Past medical and surgical conditions
- Current understanding and acceptance of health problems
- Needs for additional information

- Feelings about their health care status
- Factors that may hinder learning (covered in detail later in the chapter)

You may obtain this information from a number of sources. The most comprehensive source will be the medical record. The patient's medical record consists of all information regarding current diagnoses, treatments, medications, past medical history, and a variety of other documentation. Most medical records have a problem list on the inside cover. This will provide you with a snapshot of the patient and save you time from reading the entire document. Other sources of information will be the physician, family members, significant others, and other members of the health care team. When you have collected all of the assessment data, you are ready to start the next step of the education process: planning.

 Checkpoint Question

1. What is the purpose of the assessment step during patient education?

Planning

Planning involves using the information you have gathered during the assessment phase to determine how you will approach the patient's learning needs. If possible, involve the patient in this part of the process. Learning goals and objectives that are established with input from the patient are most meaningful. A patient's learning goal is what the patient and educator want to be the outcome of the program. The patient's **learning objectives** include procedures or tasks that will be discussed or performed at various points in the program to help achieve the goal. Make certain the objectives

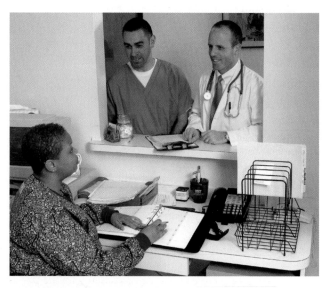

The medical assistant may obtain information regarding the patient's condition from the physician and other members of the health care team.

you establish are specific for each individual patient and are measurable in some manner. If the objectives are measurable, you will be able to evaluate when or whether the patient successfully completed them.

For example, consider a patient who needs to limit his fluid intake. Which of the following objectives is more specific and would allow you to evaluate the patient's progress: (1) the patient understands why he should limit his fluid intake, or (2) the patient is able to prepare a schedule for daily fluid intake and explain why it is important that he limits his fluids? The second objective is more specific and not only evaluates the patient's understanding but also requires the patient to demonstrate understanding. Having patients prepare their own schedule gets them involved in their health care. It allows them to customize the schedule to fit their lifestyle, which is likely to increase compliance.

Implementation

After you establish the need for patient teaching and agree on the goals and objectives, you begin implementation. **Implementation** is the process used to perform the actual teaching. The teaching usually is carried out in several steps. Box 4-1 presents some commonly used teaching strategies.

Box 4-1

IMPLEMENTATION STRATEGIES

Implementing the learning process should be individualized to the patient's best method of comprehension and retention. These may include:

1. *Lecture and demonstration.* This method presents the information in the most basic form but requires no patient participation for reinforcement and retention.
2. *Role playing and demonstration.* The patient watches you perform a medical procedure, then performs it to ensure understanding. Information is more likely to be recalled if the patient actively participates in the process.
3. *Discussion.* This two-way exchange of information and ideas works well for lifestyle changes (e.g., making dietary changes to lower cholesterol) rather than for medical procedures.
4. *Audiovisual material.* Audiocassettes or videos can often be taken home and reviewed by the patient and family members as needed. This allows for reinforcement of teachings and provides both visual and auditory stimulation.
5. *Printed material and programmed instructions.* All information should be discussed with the patient to clarify points and to elicit questions before assuming that the instructions are understood.

For example, you may start by telling the patient how to use crutches, followed by a demonstration, and finally, the patient may do a return demonstration. Patients also benefit from the use of teaching aids (drawings, charts, graphs, pamphlets) that they can take home and use as reference material. You can also use videos and audiocassettes to supplement the implementation process.

Miscommunication or misinterpretation can lead to serious complications or injury. For example, assume you are teaching a patient to use crutches. It is very important that you stress to the patient that the crutch must not press directly into the axilliary area. (There should be a two-finger distance between the crutch and the armpit.) If the patient does not comprehend the dangers of nerve damage to the axillary area from pressing the crutch into the armpit, a serious complication to the patient could occur. Miscommunication about medications can have fatal consequences.

The implementation stage may occur once or over a longer period. The disease process and the patient's ability to comprehend information will dictate the length of teaching. For example, teaching a patient about diabetes takes place over multiple sessions. The first session may focus on what diabetes is, while subsequent teachings may include topics such as diet, foot care, glucose monitoring, and insulin injection.

After implementation of a given skill or knowledge, you must determine whether your teaching was effective. This step is called evaluation.

Evaluation

Is the patient progressing? Did the teaching plan work? Does the plan need any changes? These are a few of the questions you may ask yourself when you begin to evaluate. **Evaluation** is the process that indicates how well patients are adapting or applying new information to their lives.

In the medical setting, where contact with patients is limited, part of the evaluation may have to be done by patients at home. For example, if office visits for direct observation are not scheduled, patients will be responsible for telephoning and reporting their status. In other words, can patients do the task they were taught, or are they having troubles? If they voice concern or appear unclear about their instructions, you should either redirect them on the phone or schedule them for an office appointment.

During the evaluation, you may discover noncompliance. **Noncompliance** is the patient's inability or refusal to follow a prescribed order. After determining that the given order is not being followed, your first step is to determine why the order is not being followed. It may be a misunderstanding. For example, a patient who is to take a certain medication twice a day may be taking it only twice a week because that is what he or she thought you said. If the noncompliance is because the patient refuses to follow these orders, however, you must notify the physician. Remember that the patient has the right to refuse medical treatment unless the patient is determined to be mentally incompetent. The physician will determine the next appropriate action in these cases. Evaluation is an ongoing process, so you should expect to update and modify your plan periodically.

 Checkpoint Question

2. What is the purpose of evaluation during patient education?

Documentation

Documentation includes recording of all teachings that have occurred. It should consist of the following information:

- Date and time of teaching
- What information was taught, e.g., "Diabetes foot care was discussed. It consisted of the proper method for toenail cutting and regular examination by a podiatrist."
- How the information was taught, e.g., "ADA [American Diabetes Association] foot care video shown to the patient."
- Evaluation of teaching. For example, "Patient verbalized the need to make an appointment with a podiatrist."
- Any additional teaching planned, e.g., "Patient will return on Monday to the office with his wife for glucose monitoring instructions."

Box 4-2 has a charting example for patient education. Your signature implies that you performed the teaching. If this is untrue or if another staff member assisted you in teaching, make sure that information is clearly noted. Also include the names of any interpreters who were used.

You must also document all telephone conversations, e.g., "I spoke with this patient via the telephone today and he said he is testing his blood sugar every morning without problem."

Box 4-2

CHARTING EXAMPLE

11/27/04

Patient arrived in the office for teaching on the glucose meter; brought meter from home. Following steps were demonstrated by me: calibration of meter strips, battery change, finger sticks, strip insertion into machine, use of the patient logbook. Normal BGM ranges were reviewed along with the treatment of low blood sugar. Pt returned demonstration without problem. Reviewed glucose meter instructions manual with pt. Pt. instructed to bring logbook to each MD appointment.—Bea Zame, CMA

Documentation is essential because from a legal viewpoint, procedures are only considered to have been done if they are recorded.

CONDITIONS NEEDED FOR PATIENT EDUCATION

Learning is the process of acquiring knowledge, wisdom, or skills through study or instruction. This process does not occur without certain conditions. Learning cannot occur without motivation or a perceived need to learn. For example, suppose you want to teach a patient about the need to adopt a low-sodium diet because of hypertension. Patients who feel that hypertension is not a problem, however, will not be motivated to learn the diet because they have not accepted the need for the teaching. For such patients to be taught, the following steps must occur:

1. The patient must accept that the hypertension has to be managed.
2. The patient must accept that there is a correlation between high sodium intake and hypertension.
3. The patient must accept and be willing to make this dietary change.

Only then can teaching begin.

In addition to patient motivation, basic human needs must be met first.

Maslow's Hierarchy of Needs

Abraham Maslow, an American psychiatrist, recognized that people are motivated by needs and that certain basic needs must be met before people can progress to higher needs, such as taking personal responsibility for their health (self-actualization). Maslow arranged human needs in the form of a pyramid, with basic needs at the bottom and the higher needs at the top. (Fig. 4-1). The patient progresses upward, fulfilling different levels of needs toward the highest level, which results in a state of health and well-being. In your responsibility as an educator, you need to be aware that patients must have the basic needs satisfied before they are willing or able to learn to take care of their own health. Not everyone will start at the bottom of the pyramid. Some patients will never reach the top, while others may be at the top and slide backward as a result of unfortunate circumstances.

Physiologic needs are air, water, food, rest, and comfort. If these basic needs are unmet, the patient cannot begin the process. Everyone has a different tolerance and expectation for these needs. For example, one person may expect that their food is served over three meals with full courses, while another person may accept that they will have one meal a day from a soup kitchen. If the patient perceives that these needs are met, we need to accept that and not judge the situation.

Safety and security needs include a safe environment and

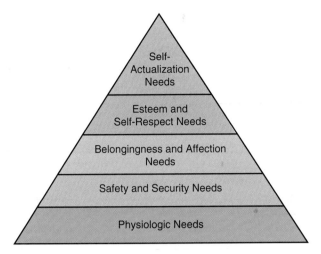

FIGURE 4–1. Maslow's hierarchy pyramid.

freedom from fear and anxiety. Patients are susceptible to fear and anxiety that accompany many medical conditions. For example, patients diagnosed with cancer may be so frightened that they are unable to think of anything but dying. Patients who have undergone some sort of trauma or disaster (hurricane, fire, motor vehicle accident) may place the need to feel safe above all other needs.

Affection needs, or the need for love and belonging, are essential for feeling connected and important to others. A sense of love or belonging can often be a powerful motivation for patients to try to regain good health.

Esteem needs involve our need to feel self-worth. Esteem can be self-generated, or it can come from those who admire us. If others value us or if we value ourselves, we are more likely to strive to maintain good health. Patients who lack self-esteem are less likely to want or accept education that targets improving their health. Thus, they will not see this as important information and will not be motivated to learn.

Self-actualization is the pinnacle of the pyramid, at which a person has satisfied all the other basic needs and feels personal responsibility and control over his or her own life. Self-actualized patients will strive to control their state of wellness by following all health directives and may even help others to achieve wellness. Not all patients will reach this level. Patients who have met this level will be ready to learn a multitude of health care skills and will strive to follow preventive health care maintenance guidelines.

After determining where on the pyramid the patient is, you can determine the appropriateness of education. For example, if the patient has not met the basic physiologic needs, you should help the patient meet these needs before beginning to teach. Patients who are in the middle levels may be able to focus and learn certain skills but may not be ready for complex teachings. If possible, you should involve family members or significant others in the teaching process.

Checkpoint Question

3. What are the basic physiologic needs outlined in Maslow's pyramid?

Environment

The environment where you teach must be conducive to learning. The room should be quiet and well lit and have limited distractions. It is not appropriate to teach patients a skill in a hallway, waiting room, or other high-traffic area. These areas produce distractions and prohibit confidentiality.

For patients to acquire knowledge, they must feel relaxed and comfortable. For example, it would be inappropriate to attempt to teach a patient who is sitting on an examination table with the stirrups in place. She will not feel comfortable. Reset the stirrups and direct the patient to have a seat in a chair. If the patient had a procedure done in the room and bloody dressings or suture equipment is still present, clean the area and then return for teaching.

Equipment

A common type of education is teaching patients to perform a **psychomotor** skill. A psychomotor skill requires the participant to physically perform a task. Some examples include crutch walking, glucose monitoring, eyedrop instillation, and dressing changes. The equipment for the skill must be present and functional. If possible, the equipment should be from the patient's home or be the exact replica of it.

The steps to teach a psychomotor skill are as follows:

1. Demonstrate the entire skill.
2. Demonstrate the skill step by step, explaining each step as you complete it.
3. Have the patient demonstrate the skill with your help.
4. Have the patient demonstrate the skill without your help.

Provide positive reinforcement throughout the steps. Always provide written step-by-step instructions along with the equipment. Always include instructions on maintenance of the equipment.

Knowledge

The person teaching the skill must have a solid knowledge of the material. Imagine how difficult it would be to learn to ski from an instructor who did not know how to put skis on. The same is true in medical assisting. If you are not comfortable or do not feel knowledgeable about the topic, ask for help before starting to teach a patient. Be reassured that you do not have to be an expert on the topic, but you do need to feel comfortable with the information. If you start teaching a given topic and the patient asks you a question that you are not able to answer, state that you are not sure about that specific piece but you will get the answer. Then either research the answer or ask for help from another health care professional. Never guess or imply that you know something that you do not know.

Resources

For patient education to be effective, it must consist of multiple techniques or approaches. The more techniques that are used, the more the patient will learn and retain. The three ways that we can learn are through hearing, seeing, and touch. If you can apply at least two of these senses in your teaching, your patient will be more stimulated to learn and will learn more information. For example, if you were teaching a patient about the dangers of smoking, which of the following would be more effective: (1) giving the patient a pamphlet that explains the dangers of smoking along with statistical data, or (2) showing a patient a diagram of how what a nonsmoker's lung looks like versus a smoker's and providing the patient with pamphlets about local smoking cessation programs? The teaching in the second approach would be more beneficial. The patient sees and hears the dangers of smoking and receives a brochure that contains practical hands-on information. Box 4-3 lists types of resources that you can use to help you teach patients.

In addition to the five conditions already discussed, these factors will be necessary for the patient to learn:

- Family or significant others should be present if the information is complex or if it will require their assistance. Family members are essential if the patient is confused or unreliable.
- Patients should be wearing any sensory devices that they need (glasses, hearing aids).
- Qualified interpreters should be present if needed.

FACTORS THAT CAN HINDER EDUCATION

Many factors or circumstances can hinder learning. It is important to recognize these factors and intervene as appropriate. In certain cases, teaching may have to be delayed, or your teaching plan may have to be revised.

Existing Illnesses

The type of illness that patients have will play a large role in their ability and willingness to learn. Generally, patients with acute short-term illnesses will be motivated to learn a skill that will accelerate healing. Examples of short-term illnesses are orthopedic injuries (uncomplicated fractures, sprains), colds, and viruses.

These are six examples of illnesses or conditions that will affect learning:

- *Any illness in which the patient has moderate to severe pain.* Examples of these illnesses include neuropathies, bone cancer, kidney stones, and recent surgical procedures. The patient's pain level must reach a tolerable stage before teaching can start and the patient can concentrate on learning.
- *Any illness or condition with a poor prognosis or limited rehabilitation potential.* Examples include progressive neurologic disorders, certain cancers, and large traumatic events. It is important that you assess such patients' readiness to learn and their level of acceptance of their illness before you proceed with your teaching.
- *Any illness or condition that results in weakness and general malaise as a primary symptom.* Examples include gastrointestinal disorders that cause vomiting and diarrhea, anemia, Lyme disease, and recent blood transfusion. For these patients, teaching should be limited to the essential information and expanded on as the patient regains strength.
- *Any illness or condition that impairs the patient's mental health or cognitive abilities.* Examples of these conditions include brain tumors, Alzheimer's disease, substance abuse, and psychiatric disorders. In these patients, education should be provided to patients at their ability level. Family members or significant others should be brought in to complement the learning process.
- *Any patient who has more than one chronic illness.* For example, patients with diabetes often have cardiac, renal, and integumentary complications. In patients with multiple system failures, it is important to prioritize the learning needs. Focus your education on the main problem and work from there.
- *Any illness or condition that results in respiratory distress or difficult breathing.* Examples of these conditions include chronic obstructive pulmonary disease, pneumonias, lung cancer, and asthma. The priority goal is first to establish optimal oxygenation for the patient. Once this is met, you can begin teaching. These patients tend to become exhausted easily during acute exacerbations of their illnesses. Keep the teaching time short and to the point and expand teachings as their activity tolerance allows.

Checkpoint Question

4. List six types of conditions or illnesses that may hinder your ability to educate patients effectively.

Communication Barriers

Effective communication skills are essential for patient education. Any barriers to communication must be resolved before you can start teaching the patient. If an interpreter is needed for language translation or for hearing-impaired patients, schedule a time convenient to all parties. (See Chapter 3.)

Age

The age of the patient plays a very important part in the amount and type of education that you can do. Small children need to be educated at an age-appropriate level. For example, it would be inappropriate to teach a 2-year-old child how to assemble an asthma nebulizer. The parent or caregiver must be taught. It would be appropriate, however, to explain to the 2-year-old that the nebulizer is not a toy and that it contains medication. Safety education is a prime teaching focus for small children and their parents. Box 4-4 presents some tips for communicating with and teaching children.

As children mature at different speeds, you should assess what information this child can handle and what information should not be shared with the child. Communication with the parents is essential. They know the child's developmental stage. For example, a 7-year-old child who has just been diagnosed with diabetes needs to know the signs and symptoms of low blood sugar and how to treat it. The child may not be ready, however, to learn about the long-term complications (e.g., blindness, renal failure). It is important to teach the child

---

Box 4-4

TIPS FOR TEACHING CHILDREN

Children require special communication skills and different teaching strategies. Here are a few tips to help you:
- Encourage the child to be part of the teaching process.
- Speak directly to the child.
- Avoid confusing medical terms.
- Avoid using baby language.
- Teach only age-appropriate information.
- Discuss with the parents the child's knowledge base about the illness and any feelings the parent may have regarding what they want the child to know. (This should not be done in front of the child.)
- Demonstrate skills on stuffed animals or dolls.

---

that the disease must be well controlled to prevent future problems, but not to the extent that the child develops fear.

The challenge in teaching adults is that they often have multiple responsibilities to their children, spouses, or aging parents. Obligations at work, school, church, and other activities may also limit their free time. These obligations and responsibilities can interfere with willingness to learn and attentiveness. Your teaching may have to occur in short sessions over long periods. This age group may benefit from electronic resources that they can access on their own time schedule.

Elderly patients can be a challenge to teach for a variety of reasons. These reasons include confusion, lack of interest, and overall poor health. Some older patients, however, can be the most attentive and curious learners. It is fairly common for this age group to address items that they have heard on the news. For example, a patient may hear an advertisement for a new medication for arthritis and request clarification from you regarding its effectiveness.

Checkpoint Question

5. What is the primary teaching focus for small children and their parents?

Educational Background

Most initial health assessment forms ask patients what level of education they have obtained. This information may help you to determine the patient's ability to read. Caution is essential, because graduation alone does not guarantee that the patient can read. You will need to use your tact and diplomacy to evaluate the situation.

Patients who have completed some college courses, however, are likely to be interested in preventive health care. Patients with an educational background in health care will still need the same attention and teaching from you. Do not assume that since the patient is a nurse or a physician, you can skip teaching a skill. Their specialty may be in an unrelated area.

Physical Impairments

Numerous physical impairments may hinder learning. For example, patients with severe arthritis in their hands may have difficulty performing certain psychomotor skills, like giving themselves insulin. An occupational therapist is the best resource to assist you. Speak to the physician to obtain the proper referrals.

Other Factors

Other factors may hinder your ability to teach patients. The patient's culture may affect willingness to learn or the family's involvement in learning. Patients with financial troubles may not be ready to focus on learning new skills or knowledge. It is important that you assess the patient's readiness to learn and remove any obstacles that may be present.

TEACHING SPECIFIC HEALTH CARE TOPICS

Your role in patient education will vary greatly. The topics that you will teach will depend on the patient, type of medical office, and physician's preferences. Next are some topics commonly taught by medical assistants.

Preventive Medicine

Preventing health problems is the key to living a long, healthy life. But the advantages to good preventive medicine extend much further. There are huge economical benefits to preventing illnesses. According to the American Hospital Association, approximately 34 million people are hospitalized each year. Caring for sick patients at home costs Medicare $200 billion annually. These statistics affect everyone. They lead to higher taxes, higher health care insurance premiums, and limited programs for low-income families.

These are some commonly recommended preventive health care tips that you should teach all of your patients:

- Regular physical examinations for all age groups
- Annual flu and regular pneumonia vaccinations
- Adult immunizations for tetanus and hepatitis B
- Childhood immunizations
- Regular dental examinations
- Monthly breast self-examinations for women and regular physician examinations
- Mammograms on a regular basis for certain groups of women
- Annual Papanicolaou tests
- Prostate-specific antigen blood tests for all men, along with need for regular digital rectal examinations

The frequency and age at which these procedures will be recommended to patients vary with the patient's medical history and genetics and the physician's preference. Some insurance will pay for these procedures, while others will not pay unless the procedure is deemed diagnostic. Many hospitals and clinics offer free preventive screenings to patients. Your office should have a list of which free screenings are available. Public health departments may also have this information available for your patients.

Your role as a medical assistant is to promote preventive screenings. The physician you work with will instruct you in his or her recommendations for these tests.

Another large part of preventive medicine is teaching safety tips. Preventable injury is the leading cause of death in persons aged 1 to 21. Approximately 25% of children will require at least one emergency room visit for treatment of a preventable accident during their childhood. Preventable injuries can arise from bicycle and car accidents, poisoning, fires, choking, falls, drownings, firearms, and lawn mowers. Toys can lead to injuries when they are broken or used by a child of an inappropriate age. The American Academy of Pediatrics offers injury prevention tips for parents and health care providers. While working as a medical assistant, you will find valuable teaching tips to give to parents from their website. The AAP also provides numerous educational materials that can be mailed to physician offices and given to your patients.

One in three adults over age 65 will fall. These falls account for most of the 340,000 patients who are admitted to hospitals each year for hip fractures. Hip fractures require long hospitalizations and often rehabilitation in a nursing home. Most falls occur at home and are preventable. Fall prevention tips should be taught to all older patients or any patient who has a problem with maintaining balance or uses an ambulation device (cane, walker). Here are some tips that you can use to teach fall prevention:

- Encourage the patient to remove all scatter rugs in their home. Remind patients to keep hallways clutter free.
- Instruct the patient to ensure adequate lighting in all rooms and hallways.
- Encourage the patient to avoid steps. Encourage one-floor living.
- Ensure that the patient has well-soled shoes or sneakers. Advise the patient to avoid wearing heels.
- Instruct the patient to place nonskid surfaces in bathtubs or purchase a shower chair.
- Instruct the patient to install handrails or grab bars in hallways and stairwells.
- Encourage smoke detector installation and remind the patient to change the batteries twice a year.
- Advise patients taking medications that lower their blood pressure to stand up slowly and get their balance, then begin to walk.
- Advise patients to have regular eye examinations and have their glasses adjusted as needed.
- Encourage patients to have a plan for power outages and severe storms.

 Checkpoint Question

6. Which patients should you teach fall prevention tips?

Medications

With the increasing number of medications available, the possibilities for teaching patients in this area are virtually endless. Pharmaceutical companies offer in-depth medication information for health care providers and patients concerning the chemical makeup of the drug, physiologic reactions in the body, prescribed dosage and route, and possible side effects. This information comes from the pharmaceutical companies either by mail or from the sales support team. In addition, some of this information will come in package inserts. If this information is not available, the patient may not understand the importance of the medication therapy, and this could lead to noncompliance, drug interactions, or other serious side effects. You may be responsible for gathering the information needed and preparing teaching materials for your patients to help prevent such complications.

When preparing a medication therapy teaching tool, you must consider such factors as the patient's financial abilities, social or cultural demands, physical disabilities, and age. Be sure to include the following information in any teaching:

- Medication name (generic or brand)
- Dosage
- Route
- What the medication is for
- Why the medication must be taken as prescribed
- Possible changes in bodily functions (e.g., colored urine)
- Possible side effects
- Other medications (including over-the-counter ones) that might interfere with the action of this medication
- Foods or liquids to be avoided
- Activities to be avoided
- Telephone number to call for any questions or concerns

Figure 4-2 shows a medication therapy teaching tool that incorporates all of these elements.

Medication teaching should also include any over-the-counter medications the patient is taking. This information should consist of the same items listed above. Many patients have the misconception that over-the-counter medications (e.g., aspirin, ibuprofen, cough syrup) are 100% safe and no dangers are associated with them. Some of these medications may interact with their prescribed medications.

After assessing patients' understanding of all of their medications, you may find that scheduling is a prime concern. For example, the patient may be taking several types of medications at different times of the day or week. Before developing a medication schedule, evaluate the patient's daily routine to see how adhering to the schedule may affect the patient's lifestyle. For instance, you might ask the patient:

- How late do you sleep each morning?
- What time do you go to bed?
- When do you usually eat?

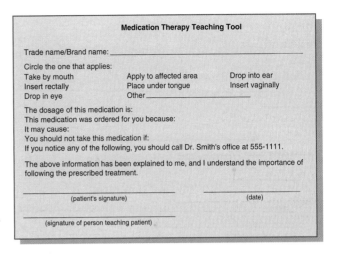

FIGURE 4–2. Medication therapy teaching tool.

Once you have collected this information, you can create a scheduling tool to serve as a reminder to the patient about what medications to take when. Pillboxes can also help to remind patients to take their medication. Pillboxes are plastic containers prelabeled with the days of the week and times. You may instruct the patient in how to fill them. Pillboxes are sold in most pharmacies.

Another patient education area that falls under the category of medication therapy includes how to administer medications—orally, vaginally, rectally, and so on. This information will be taught in the clinical part of your curriculum.

For more patient teaching information regarding safe and effective use of medications, you can contact the National Council on Patient Information and Education (NCPIE), a nonprofit organization, at 666 Eleventh Street, NW, Suite 810, Washington, DC 20001. NCPIE can provide you with literature and referrals to other sources.

Nutrition

Patients seen in the medical office have numerous reasons for being concerned about their **nutrition**. Nutrition is focused not only on what people consume but also on how the body uses the food it ingests to maintain and repair itself. Everyone needs to understand nutrition, not just people

Spanish Terminology

Tres veces al día.	Three times a day.
Antes/después de las comidas.	Before/after meals.
Al acostarse.	At bedtime.
Tómela con la comida.	Take this with food.
Dele la medicina cada cuatro horas.	Give him the medicine every 4 hours.

who are ill. People often turn to the medical profession to sort through the large amount of media hype pertaining to diets that bombards them each day. Whether the information pertains to the values of fast food or fad diets to lose weight, the media should not be the only source of guidelines for your patients. Materials are available to help you instruct patients about healthy eating.

Here are a few basic facts that you can teach all patients:

- There are no quick fixes to weight loss.
- Moderation is key. Total elimination of favorites (chips, ice cream, candy) is not necessary.
- A good dinner or meal will consist of a rainbow of colors.
- Limit salt and sodium intake.
- Eat three balanced meals a day.
- Avoid eating at least 2 hours before going to bed.
- Drink plenty of water. Avoid excessive soda and caffeine ingestion.

The Food Guide Pyramid

The U. S. Department of Agriculture (USDA) has developed a basic food group system and the Food Guide Pyramid (Fig. 4-3). The pyramid consists of five main food group categories and one "other" category:

1. Bread, cereal, grains, and pasta
2. Vegetables
3. Fruits
4. Milk, yogurt, and cheese (dairy)
5. Meat, poultry, fish, dry beans, eggs, and nuts (protein)
6. Fats, oils, sweets (other)

Next are listed some teaching tips for each of these categories.

Bread, Cereal, Grains, and Pasta

- Eat darker breads; avoid white. Avoid croissants, biscuits, sweet rolls, and pastries.
- The best cereals are oat, bran, and whole grain cereal. Avoid frosted or sweet types.
- Graham crackers, melba toast, and saltines are good cracker choices. Avoid cheese and butter crackers.
- Pasta and rice in limited portions are fine, but avoid the sauces.

Vegetables and Fruits

- Fresh or frozen is the best. Avoid dried fruits.
- Eat vegetables without butter or cream sauces.
- Limit boiling time for vegetables to prevent draining out the nutrients.

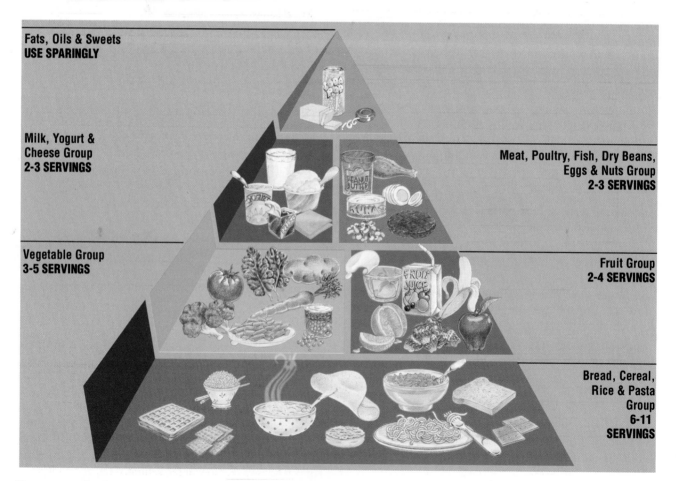

FIGURE 4–3.   General food pyramid.

Milk, Yogurt, and Cheese

- Milk: skim or 1%. Avoid creams and buttermilks.
- Yogurt: low fat or nonfat.
- Eat low-fat cheeses, 1% or 2% cottage cheese.

Meat, Poultry, and Fish

- Use USDA-select grade beef. Avoid beef with large amounts of marbling (indicates fat).
- Limit bacon to small serving sizes and limit its frequency.
- Fish should be fresh. Cook unbreaded and avoid sauces.

Fat, Oil, and Sweets

- Use oil sparingly.
- Avoid mayonnaise and salad dressings (unless low fat).
- Low-fat snacks: air-popped popcorn, pretzels, rice cakes are good choices.

In addition to the traditional food pyramid, the USDA has formed a variety of other pyramids to meet the needs of various groups. There is a special pyramid for children aged 2 to 6 (Fig. 4-4). This pyramid is visually appealing to children and provides parents with realistic serving size portions. The pyramid for people over age 70 focuses on the nutritional

FIGURE 4-5. Food guide pyramid for a Mediterranean diet.

needs of older patients. A variety of ethnic pyramids have also been created to meet the needs of various cultures. For example, the Mediterranean diet pyramid (Fig. 4-5) varies in its recommended daily servings of the basic food groups. When you are teaching nutritional guidelines, provide the patient with a copy of the appropriate pyramid. Copies of pyramids can be obtained from the USDA website.

Checkpoint Question

7. What are the five main food groups listed in the USDA pyramids?

Dietary Guidelines

The USDA and U. S. Department of Health and Human Services also have guidelines to help improve our diets:

1. Eat a variety of foods from each of the five food groups.
2. Maintain a healthy weight by balancing the food you eat with physical activity.
3. Choose a diet low in fat, saturated fat, and cholesterol.

FIGURE 4-4. Food guide pyramid for children.

Spanish Terminology

¿Qué comidas le gustan?	What foods do you like?
De dos a cuatro porciones de leche.	Two to four servings of milk.
De dos a tres porciones de carne, pescado o aves de corral.	Two to three servings of meat, fish, poultry.
De tres a cinco porciones de vegetales.	Three to five servings of vegetables.
Pan de trigo y cereales.	Wheat bread and cereals.

4. Choose a diet with plenty of vegetables, fruits, and grain products.
5. Use sugar and salt (sodium) in moderation.
6. Drink alcoholic beverages in moderation.

Encourage patients to read the labels on food containers; these labels provide important information on the nutritional value of the food, specific ingredients used, or any additives. All information on labels is based on the portion size. If you eat double the portion, you will need to double the nutritional facts. The serving size is at the top of the label. Below the serving size is the number of servings per container.

Total fat will be the first nutritional fact listed. This will give you the total grams of fat in a serving. The average diet consists of 2000 calories per day. On a 2000-calorie diet, the maximum grams of fat per day should be less than 65, with less than 20 g of saturated fat. Teach patients to add their total grams of fat per day. The label will list a percentage number as well. The percentage refers to what percent of the daily allowed fat is contained in one serving. Most patients find it easier to add up their total grams ingested. Explain that an item may be fat free or low fat but not healthy. Food manufacturers often add extra **carbohydrates** to low-fat foods to give them extra flavor and taste.

Total carbohydrates is the next fact listed on labels that patients should understand. This number tells the patient how many carbohydrates are in each serving. Carbohydrates are the prime energy source for our bodies. Carbohydrates are turned into sugar in the body. The unused portion of sugar is stored as fat. Based on a 2,000-calorie diet, the total carbohydrates per day should not exceed 300 g. Again, patients should add their total carbohydrate intake for 24 hours. It is essential that patients with diabetes learn to count carbohydrates.

Sodium, cholesterol, and protein facts are also listed on food labels. Large fast food chains, like McDonald's and Dunkin' Donuts, will have this information available at each of their stores. Patients should be encouraged to read this information.

In certain foods it is easy to determine the serving size. The label may say two cookies or one slice of bread. In other cases, however, it may be more difficult. Generally, serving sizes are listed in ounces. Here is a simple way to teach measuring: A thumb equals 1 ounce, the palm equals 3 ounces, a handful is 2 ounces, and a fist is approximately 1 cup.

After discussing healthy foods, give patients information about healthy food preparation. Here are a few guidelines on how to prepare healthy foods that you can teach your patients:

- Encourage patients to broil, boil, bake, roast, or grill.
- Trim the fat off of beef.
- Use a cooking rack so that fat drips away from the meat.
- Remove the skin from chicken. Use caution with raw chicken. Wash hands and cutting surfaces immediately.
- Homemade soups or gravies should be cooked, then chilled. Skim the fat off and then reheat.
- Use unsaturated oils (canola, corn, safflower). Use nonstick spray when possible. Avoid saturated oils (butter, lard).

Patients may ask you about vegetarian diets. There are three types of vegetarian diets. Lacto-ovovegetarian means that a diet of vegetables is supplemented with milk, eggs, and cheese. Lactovegetarian means the diet is supplemented only with milk and cheese; pure vegetarian is only vegetables and excludes all foods of animal origin. It is possible to eat healthy and obtain necessary nutrients with all three vegetarian diets. The USDA has created a vegetarian pyramid that will provide necessary education to your patients regarding serving sizes and meal planning.

Patients may ask you about vitamin and mineral supplements. If the patient maintains an appropriately balanced diet, adequate vitamins and minerals will be included in the foods consumed. A daily multipurpose vitamin can offer many benefits to patients. A common mineral supplement that patients are urged to take is calcium. Box 4-5 presents some important teaching tips on calcium supplements.

As with any patient teaching, you must consider many factors before sending the patient home with a preprinted diet form. The patient's age, culture, religion, geographic background, and social and financial circumstances may influence how well the patient complies with the diet modification. If necessary, the physician may refer the patient to a registered dietitian for in-depth nutritional education. Patients with diabetes, heart disease, and eating disorders are generally referred to dietitians. Remember to check your patient's progress during each return visit.

Exercise

Exercise is an activity using muscles, voluntary or otherwise, that helps maintain fitness. It is beneficial to the body for several reasons. If done in moderation, exercise can help relieve stress, maintain healthy body weight, and increase circulation and muscle tone. All patients should actively participate in some form of exercise on a regular basis. Box 4-6 discusses some common myths associated with exercising.

Patients who are under age 35 and in good health usually do not need a medical clearance before starting a routine exercise program. A physician consultation is recommended, however, for patients aged 35 or older who have not been active in several years. Patients with known medical disorders (e.g., hypertension, cardiovascular problems, or a family history of strokes) should check with the physician before exercising. Pregnant patients should consult their obstetrician prior to starting an exercise program.

The American Heart Association (AHA) offers information on exercise. The AHA has numerous frequently updated pamphlets available on various exercise activities and programs such as swimming, running, jogging, walking, and biking. Pamphlets cover the following information:

- Benefits of the specific exercise
- How to get started
- How to choose a time to exercise
- How to choose a partner
- What clothing is best suited for the exercise
- How to warm up
- What a target heart rate zone is and how to achieve it
- Training program
- Calories used
- Checklist (a review of highlights from all of the above topics)

After physician clearance (if needed), you should review the information on the pamphlets with the patients. Answer any questions and document the teaching. Patients should be able to take the information in the AHA pamphlets and continue exercising on their own.

If patients are unable to perform exercises without assistance, it may be necessary to instruct them or their family members on **range-of-motion** (ROM) exercises. To perform ROM exercises, the patient moves the affected limb and joint through all of the movements that the joint is capable of making, until resistance is met. In most cases, ROM exercises are ordered by the physician to prevent further loss of motion or disfigurement after a musculoskeletal injury, surgery, or neurological damage.

When a stroke or other type of paralyzing injury is involved, ROM exercises are performed several times a day on each involved joint. If the patient is unable to perform the exercise on the affected area, passive ROM is performed. This requires someone else to perform the exer-

WHAT IF

A patient asks you about "crash" or "fad" diets. What should you say?

Patients often want to try fad diets, but they need to be taught about the potential dangers of these diets. Fad diets are advertised as "quick weight loss" fixes. These diets require precise meal plans and adherence to unhealthy portions and food selections. They are not balanced to meet all food group requirements. Most plans are targeted to a specific food, such as the grapefruit diet. Some of these diet plans can produce cardiac, renal, and digestive complications. Patients who want to lose weight should be instructed about eating regular small, balanced meals, counting calories, monitoring fat intake, and reading food package labels. Patients must also be taught that diet modification alone will not result in a significant long-term weight loss; regular exercise must also be included in any weight reduction plan.

Box 4-6

MYTHS ABOUT EXERCISE

Here are some common myths about exercising that you can correct for your patients:

- "No pain, no gain." Patients should be instructed never to exercise to the point of exhaustion and pain. This can produce serious musculoskeletal injuries and cardiac complications.
- "I'm too old to exercise." Exercising at any age can help improve muscle tone, maintain joint flexibility, and prevent injuries.
- "Weight lifting is a man's sport." Weight lifting has been proved to help with weight reduction and limit the progression of osteoporosis.
- "The only good exercise is aerobic." Although aerobic exercise has many cardiovascular benefits, it can also lead to joint injuries. A combination of weight training, strength and resistance training, and a moderate aerobic workout is often most beneficial.

cises on the patient. Remember, ROM exercises are needed to promote circulation and maintain muscle tone. If they are not performed as ordered, the patient may not be able to regain use of the affected area. Patients with significant loss of motor skills will often be referred to physical therapy or occupational therapy for intense ROM teachings. In these cases, your role as a medical assistant will be to assess their compliance with attendance for physical therapy appointments and to provide positive reinforcement.

Checkpoint Question

8. Why is teaching range-of-motion (ROM) exercises important?

Alternative Medicine

Many ancient remedies that were once considered voodoo and dismissed by Western medicine have proven to be beneficial. Approximately $300 billion a year is spent on **alternative** medicine, and surveys have shown that about 50% of all Americans have used some form of unconventional medicine. In 1998, a federal agency was created to evaluate and monitor alternative medicine therapies. The name of the agency is National Center for Complementary and Alternative Medicine (NCCAM). The NCCAM also conducts clinical trials and training programs for practitioners of alternative medicine.

There are numerous types of alternative medicine therapies. Below is a discussion of four of the most common therapies.

Acupuncture

Acupuncture is one of the oldest forms of Chinese medicine. Acupuncture works on the principle that there are 2,000 acupuncture points in the human body. These 2,000 points are connected throughout the body by 12 pathways called meridians. The meridians conduct energy, or qi, in the body when they are triggered. The trigger comes in the form of a needle. When the meridian is stimulated, it prompts the brain to release certain chemicals and hormones.

Acupuncture is primarily used to treat addictions, fibromyalgia, osteoarthritis, asthma, and chronic back pain. It is sometimes used in treating children with attention-deficit/hyperactivity disorder.

In 1996, the Federal Drug Administration (FDA) required that all acupuncture needles be labeled single use. Only 40 states require that acupuncturists be licensed to practice. Training requirements vary among states.

Acupressure

Acupressure is a similar practice except that it does not use needles. The practitioner applies pressure to the meridians through direct touch. This method has shown great success in treating nausea and vomiting associated with chemotherapy. Some hospitals and clinics offer acupressure on an outpatient basis to cancer patients. Studies have shown that acupressure may help alleviate chronic pains and may even boost the immune system. Requirements for licensure and training vary among states.

Hypnosis

Hypnosis is portrayed on television as a magical method for reaching the inner workings of the brain. There is proof, however, that when conducted properly, it may provide some health care benefits. It is primarily used for weight reduction, for treatment of obsessive-compulsive disorders, and for smoking cessation. The training requirements vary greatly from state to state, and in most areas licensure is not required.

Yoga

Yoga has proved to be very beneficial for relieving stress and improving flexibility. Yoga consists of a comprehensive discipline of physical exercise, posture, breathing exercises, and meditation. There are a variety of types of yoga. Iyengar consists of motionless poses that emphasize posture and form. Once this method is learned, patients are able to practice this at home. This method may help patients who are recovering from injuries. Bikram consists of 26 poses that are conducted at 100°F. This method promotes muscle relaxation and stretching. Perspiration is thought to help cleanse the body of various toxins. Sivananda is a 5-step system that focuses on breathing exercises, relaxation, diet, and meditation.

Herbal Supplements

The use of herbal supplements is a multibillion-dollar business in the United States. The general public views herbal supplements as "natural," hence safe. This is a misconception. Herbal supplements, vitamins, and similar substances are not regulated by the FDA. The patient or consumer must understand that since there has been no formal government testing or approval of these substances, their dosages, side effects, interactions, and possible benefits are unclear. A classic example of an herbal supplement that has been shown to have dangerous side effects is ephedrine. This supplement was once thought to be the weight-loss miracle. It can, however, cause heart attacks and strokes. The FDA has issued many warnings about ephedrine and its dangers.

Furthermore, since these products are not regulated, there is no guarantee that what the label claims is in the bottle is actually there. The quality and the purity of the herbal supplements have shown to vary greatly from manufacturer to manufacturer. Patients should be advised to purchase only supplements that are stamped with a U. S. Pharmacopeia bar code. This bar code means that the manufacture site has met certain standards for distribution but does not mean that the supplement has been tested for health care benefits. Box 4-7 provides some general teaching tips for any patient using an herbal supplement.

Some of these substances have evolved through folklore, various cultures, or clinical research. In some cases, there is an element of **placebo** action involved. Placebo is the power of believing that something will make you better when there is no chemical reaction that warrants such improvement. Other supplements actually have scientific studies to document their effects. Table 4-1 lists some commonly used herbal supplements and their reported benefits.

Your role as a medical assistant is to assess whether patients are using any alternative therapies. Your assessment should include the length of time they have used these treatments and any side effects or benefits that the patient has noted, and you should report such information to the physician. Patients should be advised to verify the training and credentials of the practitioner they are using and to ascertain that the practitioner is appropriately licensed. Patients should be encouraged to look at the NCCAM website for safety updates and for more detailed information about alternative medicine. You should never recommend that a patient start taking herbal supplements or other alterative medicine therapies without a physician's approval.

Box 4-7

GENERAL TEACHING TIPS FOR HERBAL SUPPLEMENTS

Here are a few general teaching points on herbal supplements:

- Explain to patients the importance of always telling the physician or other health care provider about any herbal supplements that they are taking.
- Explain to patients that the fact that a product is "natural" does not mean it is safe. A good example is mushrooms. All mushrooms are natural, but some are very poisonous.
- Teach patients the importance of looking for the USP (United States Pharmacopeia) label. Teach patients to look for expiration dates on all supplements.
- Advise patients not to ask health store clerks for information on supplements but to speak to physicians or pharmacists.
- Advise patients to distrust advertisements that use words like magical or breakthrough or that claim to detoxify the whole body.
- Instruct patients to stop taking all herbal supplements at least 2 weeks prior to surgery and to tell their surgeon what supplement they have been using and how long. (Some supplements can increase bleeding time.)
- Warn diabetic patients that many supplements will interfere with blood sugar levels.
- Advise parents to avoid giving herbal supplements to their children unless approved by a physician.
- Advise pregnant or breast-feeding patients to consult with a pharmacist or physician before taking any supplements.

Checkpoint Question

9. What is a placebo?

Stress Management

Everyone is affected by an illness or injury at some time. Along with this often comes stress. **Stress** can come from forces such as fear, anger, anxiety, crisis, and joy. The stress may produce physiologic changes as well as psychologic effects. When faced with illness or injury, a patient usually must confront:

- Physical pain
- Inability to perform self-care
- Stress of treatments, procedures, and possible hospitalization
- Changes in role identity and self-image
- Loss of control and independence
- Changes in relationships with friends and family

Patients with chronic conditions may need more time to adjust than patients with acute illnesses. If patients are able to deal with stress factors, they are more likely to adapt and adjust to lifestyle changes.

Table 4-1   HERBAL SUPPLEMENTS[a]

Supplement	Reported Benefits
Alfalfa	Relief from arthritis pain; strength
Anise	Relief of dry cough; treatment of flatulence
Black cohosh root	Relief of premenstrual symptoms; rheumatoid arthritis
Camomile	Treatment of migraines, gastric cramps
Cholestin	Lowers cholesterol and triglycerides
Echinacea	Treatment of colds; stimulates immune system; attacks viruses
Garlic	Treatment of colds; diuretic; prevention of cardiac diseases
Ginkgo	Increased blood flow to brain; treatment of Alzheimer's disease
Ginseng	Mood elevator, antihypertensive
Glucosamine	Treats arthritis symptoms; improves joint mobility
Kava	Treatment of anxiety, restlessness; tranquilizer
Licorice	Soothes coughs, treats chronic fatigue syndrome
St. John's wort	Treats depression, premenstrual symptoms; antiviral

[a] This box lists some commonly used herbal supplements and their reported benefits. Research is an ongoing process to document these findings. Some of these herbal supplements may have side effects or may interact with prescribed medications.

Many other causes besides illness or injury can place patients under stress. The best way to cope with stress is by living a healthy lifestyle. When the body is healthy, it can handle stress more easily. Unfortunately, most of the reasons that hinder learning are the same factors that hinder patients' ability to comply with patient education. Patients who are not capable of coping with stress on their own or with the help of instruction provided by the medical office staff may need professional counseling.

Positive and Negative Stress

Two types of stress affect all of us daily: positive stress and negative stress. Positive stress motivates individuals to work efficiently and perform to the best of their abilities. Examples of positive stress include working on a challenging new job or assignment, getting married, and giving a speech or performance. In fact, many people work best under positive stress. Under positive stress the brain releases chemicals that increase the heart rate and breathing capacity. The body also releases stored glucose that gives an energy boost. Once the job (or wedding) is over, though, time must be taken to relax and prepare for the next project. If relaxation techniques are not incorporated into the daily routine, positive stress can become negative stress.

Negative stress is the inability to relax after a stressful encounter. Left unchecked, it can lead to such physiologic responses as

- Headache
- Nausea, diarrhea
- Sweating palms
- Insomnia

- Malaise
- Rapid heart rate

Long-term physical effects of unrelieved stress include increases in blood pressure, glucose levels, metabolism, intraocular pressure, and finally exhaustion. There is also an increased risk of heart attack, stroke, diabetes, certain cancers, and immune system failure. If the stress is not relieved, patients will progress to higher anxiety levels and will require all of their energy and attention to focus solely on the problem at hand. Most mental and physical activity will be directed at relief of the stress to avoid the ultimate anxiety level known as panic—a sudden, overwhelming state of anxiety or terror.

Most people have developed methods of alleviating intense stressors called **coping mechanisms**, which are usually beyond our conscious ability to direct. Coping mechanisms are a psychologic defense against unpleasant situations. Some common coping mechanisms are repression, denial, and rationalization.

It may be difficult to escape completely from stress-causing factors, but management of them is possible. For a patient suffering from the physiologic effects of negative stress, you can offer the following coping strategies:

- Encourage patients to attempt to reduce stressors, but emphasize that it is not possible to remove all stressors. Warn them to avoid attempting to make everything perfect; perfectionism adds its own stress.
- Encourage patients to organize and limit activities as needed.
- Try to lessen patients' fear of failure so they just do the best they can.

- When they are feeling anxious, encourage them to talk to someone about their problems and let off steam.

Any one of these tips may help patients to regain control over stressors. In addition, a number of relaxation techniques described in the following sections may help.

Relaxation Techniques

Patients can use any of several types of relaxation techniques. To determine what works best for them, they must first consider how much time they have and what type of relaxation they need. Next are three examples of relaxation techniques.

Breathing Techniques. Breathing exercises can be done anywhere. Most people are shallow breathers and need to be instructed on deep-breathing techniques. To perform these breathing exercises, the patient should sit up straight with hands placed on the stomach and take a deep breath in through the nose, feeling the hands being pushed away by the stomach. (This may feel awkward because most people do just the opposite.) The patient holds the breath for a few seconds, then exhales through pursed lips as the hands are felt being pulled in. This exercise allows for good control of the rate of exhalation. Sometimes, getting the oxygen flowing through the body at a faster rate is all that is needed to relieve boredom, tension, and stress.

Visualization. Visualization is a relaxation technique that involves allowing the mind to wander and the imagination to run free and focus on positive and relaxing situations. It is similar to daydreaming. It can "remove" the patient from a stressful situation and put him or her in a place where, if nothing else, the mind can relax. Instruct the patient to find a quiet place, close the eyes, and then visualize a soothing scene. Sometimes, background music helps. Remind the patient that it is important to choose appropriate times for this daydreaming technique. For example, it would be dangerous to use this technique when driving a car or operating heavy equipment.

Physical Exercise. There is no better tranquilizer than physical exercise. Most people who exercise regularly say that it helps them reduce tension, relax, and rest better at night.

Smoking Cessation

The health risks associated with smoking have been well documented for many years. Nicotine is highly addictive whether ingested by inhaling or chewing. This drug reaches the brain in 6 seconds, damages the blood vessels, decreases heart strength, and is associated with many cancers. The withdrawal symptoms include anxiety, progressive restlessness, irritability, and sleep disturbances. There are numerous methods to try to stop smoking. The methods vary greatly. Some programs have the patient gradually stop, while other programs seek a total, abrupt stoppage. There is research data to support both methods.

Here are some suggestions to help patients stop smoking:

- Find local smoking cessation support groups. Provide phone numbers and contact names of these groups to your patients.
- If you do not have a local connection, the American Heart Association, American Lung Association, or American Cancer Society may help. Websites are provided at the end of this chapter.
- Discuss with the physician the options of prescribing various patches, gums, or other interventions for the patient. Some products have side effects, and the physician may opt not to order them based on the patient's age or other medical illnesses.

Substance Abuse

Substance abuse is excessive use of and dependency on drugs. Some abused substances are legal (e.g., alcohol, nicotine), whereas others are illegal (e.g., marijuana, cocaine). Patients affected by commonly abused substances usually work with trained specialists or counselors. Substance abuse can be highly detrimental to your patients' health, so it is important that you give them information about substance abuse if they should ask. This information may come from various national organizations. You should have information available for patients on any local chapters or organizations that may help these patients. Following is a brief outline of abused drugs and some of the consequences of using them.

Alcohol is the most commonly abused drug in our society. Alcohol is chemically classified as a mind-altering substance because it contains ethanol, which has the chemical power to depress the action of the central nervous system. This depression affects motor coordination, speech, and vision. In large amounts, alcohol can affect respiration and heart rate. The long-term effects of excessive alcohol use are liver failure, certain cancers, strokes, and nutritional deficiencies.

Alcoholics Anonymous (AA) was founded in 1935 and has approximately 2 million members. It is the leading organization in treating alcoholism. The success of the AA program is based on the patient's completion of a 12-step program. Recovering alcoholics provide many of the support services. The AA has numerous chapters and support services throughout the country for both the patient and the family. There are also special services for teenage alcoholics.

Marijuana and hashish impair short-term memory and comprehension. They alter the user's sense of time and reduce the ability to perform tasks requiring concentration and coordination. They also increase the heart rate and appetite. Long-term users may develop psychologic dependence. Because these drugs are inhaled as unfiltered smoke, users take in more cancer-causing agents and do more damage to the respiratory system than with regular filtered tobacco smoke.

Cocaine and crack cocaine stimulate the central nervous system and are extremely addictive. Crack cocaine is particularly dangerous because this pure form of cocaine is usually smoked and absorbed rapidly in the bloodstream. It can cause sudden death. Use of cocaine can cause psychologic and physical dependency. Side effects include dilated pupils, increased pulse rate, elevated blood pressure, insomnia, loss of appetite, paranoia, and seizures. It can also cause death by disrupting the brain's control of the heart and respiration.

Stimulants and amphetamines can have the same effect as cocaine, causing increased heart rate and blood pressure. Symptoms of stimulant use include dizziness, sleeplessness, and anxiety; these substances can cause psychosis, hallucinations, paranoia, and even physical collapse. The long-term effects of these substances include hypertension, heart disease, stroke, and renal and liver failure.

Depressants and barbiturates can cause physical and psychologic dependence. Abuse of these drugs can lead to respiratory depression, coma, and death, especially when they are taken with alcohol. Withdrawal can lead to restlessness, insomnia, convulsions, and death.

Hallucinogens such as lysergic acid diethylamide (LSD), phencyclidine ("angel dust" or PCP), mescaline, and peyote all interrupt brain messages that control the intellect and keep instincts in check. Large doses can produce seizures, coma, and heart and lung failure. Chronic users complain of persistent memory problems and speech difficulties for up to a year after discontinuing use. Because hallucinogens stop the brain's pain sensors, drug experiences may result in severe self-inflicted injuries.

Narcotics such as heroin, codeine, morphine, and opium are addictive drugs. These drugs can produce euphoria, drowsiness, and blood pressure and pulse fluctuations. An overdose can lead to seizures, coma, cardiac arrest, and death.

Any of these substances can impair a fetus's health. Two such common illnesses are fetal alcohol syndrome and crack baby (cocaine dependency). You will learn more about these conditions in the clinical portion of your program. It is important to teach all pregnant women the damage substance abuse may do to their unborn child and to refer pregnant patients to support services.

Patients with a substance abuse problem may require **detoxification** before counseling. Detoxification is the process of clearing drugs out of the patient's body and treating the withdrawal symptoms. This process varies with the type of substance, length of abusing the substance, and patient's overall health. In certain cases, hospitalization will be needed.

The most important role of the medical assistant in educating patients about any type of substance abuse is to be supportive. Provide positive reinforcements as appropriate. Offer services to patients for cessation programs. Never condemn a patient for not seeking help. Always be nonjudgmental.

Checkpoint Question

10. What is the most commonly abused drug in our society? What does the term detoxification mean?

PATIENT TEACHING PLANS

Developing a Plan

Because medical assistants are usually allotted only minimal time for patient teaching, you may often find yourself teaching without a written plan. To ensure that teaching is done logically, always use the education process to help you formulate a plan in your mind. Also remember to document in the patient's record whatever teaching you perform and the patient's response.

Many facilities use preprinted teaching plans for common problem areas, such as "Controlling Diabetes," "Living With Multiple Sclerosis," and "Coping With Hearing Loss." Although these save time, they are not individualized to the patient. If you use preprinted teaching plans, be sure to adapt them to your particular patient's learning needs and abilities.

If preprinted plans are not an option, consult teaching plan resource books, which contain the necessary information in outline form. You can take the plans from these sources and transfer them as needed to your facility-approved teaching plan format, adding your own comments to fit the patient's needs.

All teaching plans, no matter what the design, should contain the following elements:

- *Learning goal.* A description of what the patient should learn from implementation of the teaching plan.
- *Material to be covered.* All major topics to be discussed.
- *Learning objectives.* Steps or procedures the patient must understand or demonstrate to accomplish the learning goal.
- *Evaluation.* Appraisal of the patient's progress.
- *Comments.* Remarks concerning circumstances that may be preventing successful completion of the objectives.

Teaching plans must also include an area for documenting when the information was presented to the patient and when the patient successfully completed each objective. Figure 4-6 is an example of a teaching plan.

Selecting and Adapting Teaching Material

An enormous amount of teaching material is available. Although the physician or institution may select much of the material you will use, you may be responsible for selecting some teaching aids. Assess your patients' general level of understanding to choose materials appropriately. When using preprinted material, consider the format, headings, illus-

Teaching Plan: 32-year-old female with Iron Deficiency Anemia
Patient Learning Goal: Increase patient's knowledge of Iron Deficiency Anemia, its complications and treatments
Material to be Covered: Description of disorder, complications, diet, medications, procedures

Learning Objectives Comments	Teaching Methods/Tools	Procedure Explained/Demonstrated Date/Initial	PT Demonstrated/ Objectives Met Date/Initial

1. Patient describes what happens when body's demand for oxygen is not met.
  a. oxygen and hgb concentration decrease
  b. signs/symptoms of anemia
  c. anemia occurs only after body stores of iron are depleted
	Instruction		

2. Patient describes complications caused by decrease of oxygen concentration
  a. chronic fatigue
  b. dyspnea
  c. inability to concentrate, think
  d. decrease in tissue repair
  e. increase of infection
  f. increase in heart rate
	Instruction		

3. Patient discusses importance of diet in prevention of iron deficiency anemia
  a. including iron-rich foods in diet (beef, poultry, green vegetables)
  b. including foods that contain ascorbic acid to assist in absorbing iron in body (fruits)
  c. importance of limiting large meals if fatigued; stress importance of several small meals
	Instruction/Video: "Your Diet: Why It Is Important"		

4. Patient describes prescribed medication, its purpose, dosage, route, and side effects	Instruction/Pamphlet: *Taking Your Iron Supplements*		
5. Patient aware of importance of follow-up appointments for evaluation of prescribed plan of treatment	Instruction/Appointment slip with next scheduled appointment		

FIGURE 4-6. Teaching plan.

trations, vocabulary, and writing style for overall clarity and readability. Also, ensure that the information provided on commercial materials is truthful and in agreement with the policies and procedures of your facility. A good rule of thumb is to use commercial material only from nationally recognized organizations or government agencies.

Many patient education textbooks are available from your clinic library. If you do not have access to a library, you can order most texts from local bookstores or through the Internet. Many of these sources list addresses for other patient education materials available from companies or associations. These materials commonly include printed items as well as videos, audiocassettes, and compact discs. Use commercially prepared materials to start a patient teaching library in the physician's office so you will have information at your fingertips when needed.

Developing Your Own Material

Sometimes, you may need to create your own teaching materials. Review available resources and teaching aids and adapt the information to benefit your patients. When developing teaching material, remember to do the following:

- Indicate the objective of the information.
- Personalize the information so the patient wants to learn.
- Make sure information is clear and well organized.
- Use lists and outlines, which are easier to read and remember than paragraphs.
- Avoid medical jargon as much as possible.
- Focus on the key points.
- Select appropriate printing type.
- Use diagrams that are simple, clear, and well labeled.
- Include the names and telephone numbers of people or organizations that patients can call with further questions or concerns.

After patients have been using the material for a while, periodically evaluate its effectiveness and modify your teaching plan as needed.

Not all of the patient teaching materials you create will have to be in print form. Patients must be motivated to read, but many will be more receptive to audiovisual instruction. Take advantage of any opportunity to develop teaching materials in other media.

CHAPTER SUMMARY

Your role in teaching depends on the clinical setting in which you work. Some facilities hire professional staff to teach patients. If that is the case in your facility, your teaching role may be limited. Even so, never pass up an opportunity to teach. Encourage patients to ask questions. Always provide a telephone number that patients can call if they have additional information. Periodically check to ensure that your teaching has been effective.

Remember, do not overstep your role as a medical assistant. The teaching you provide should clarify and complement information provided by the physician. A well-planned patient education program helps ensure that patients receive the high-quality health care they deserve.

Critical Thinking Challenges

1. Look at the Maslow's hierarchy pyramid. What level are you on? What steps can you take to reach the self-actualization level? If you are at that level, what steps can you take to ensure that you remain there?
2. Keep track of all of the food that you consume over a 24-hour period. Calculate your total fat and total carbohydrate intake. Do your meals follow the general food pyramid? If not, what do you need to do to improve your nutritional status? Using pictures from magazines, create well-balanced breakfast, lunch, and dinner plates. Hint: your plate should have many colors in the rainbow.
3. Review the list of information that you should teach patients about their medications. Choose two medications, herbal supplements, or vitamins that you have taken. (The medication can be over-the-counter or prescribed.) Using all available resources, write the information for these two medications or supplements.
4. Review the material on fall prevention and preventing childhood injuries. Make a checklist of at least 10 safety tips for both groups. Take your list and visit your neighbor's home. Review these tips with your neighbor. What safety improvements or recommendations were you able to provide?
5. Make a list of preprinted educational materials that every office should have. What professional organizations (e.g., American Heart Association, American Cancer Society) could help provide these materials?

Answers to Checkpoint Questions

1. The purpose of the assessment step in teaching patients is to allow you to gather information about the patient's health care needs and abilities.
2. The purpose of the evaluation step in teaching patients is to allow you to determine how well patients are adapting or applying the new information to their lives.
3. The basic physiologic needs are for air, food, water, rest, and comfort.
4. Six types of conditions or illnesses that may hinder patients' ability to learn effectively are illnesses with moderate to severe pain; illnesses with a poor prognosis or limited rehabilitation; illnesses resulting in weakness or general malaise as a primary symptom; illnesses that impair the patient's mental health or cognitive ability; more than one chronic illness; illnesses that result in respiratory distress or difficulty in breathing.
5. The primary teaching focus for small children and their parents is safety and injury prevention.
6. Any patient who has trouble maintaining balance or uses an ambulation device should be taught fall prevention tips.
7. The five major food groups are bread, cereals, grains, pasta; vegetables; fruits; meat, poultry, fish; and milk, yogurt, cheese.
8. It is important to teach ROM exercises to patients to prevent further loss of motion or disfigurement to their joints.
9. A placebo is the power in believing that a substance or action will help you when there is no chemical reaction that warrants such improvement.
10. The most commonly abused drug is alcohol. Detoxification is the process of clearing drugs out of the patient's body system and treating the withdrawal symptoms.

 Websites

Here are some websites that you can search for additional information:

Alcoholics Anonymous
  www.alcoholics-anonymous.org
American Academy of Pediatrics
  www.aap.org
American Cancer Society
  www.cancer.org
American Heart Association
  www.americanheart.org
American Lung Association
  www.lungusa.org
Food and Drug Administration
  www.fda.gov
Food and Nutrition Information Center
  www.nal.usda.gov/fnic
National Center for Complementary and Alternative Medicine
  www.nccam.nih.gov
National Institute of Drug Abuse
  www.nida.nih.gov

Section II

The Administrative Assistant

Unit Three

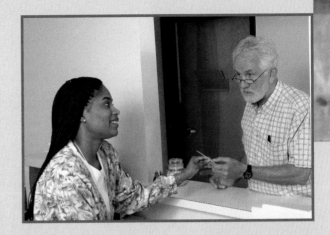

Performing Administrative Duties

A well-run medical office requires that everyone works together as a team. Unit three consists of eight chapters that address administrative duties performed in the medical office. These duties include telephone and reception, appointment management, written communications, medical record management, transcription, computer use, quality improvement, and medical office management. Some of these duties are shared with clinical personnel. This unit will help you to perform these duties whether you work in the front desk area or in the clinical area.

5

The First Contact: Telephone and Reception

CHAPTER OUTLINE

PROFESSIONAL IMAGE
Importance of a Good Attitude
The Medical Assistant as a Role Model
Courtesy and Diplomacy in the Medical Office
First Impressions

RECEPTION
Definition of a Receptionist
Duties and Responsibilities of the Receptionist
Ergonomic Concerns for the Receptionist
The Waiting Room Environment
The End of the Patient Visit

TELEPHONE
Importance of the Telephone in the Medical Office
Basic Guidelines for Telephone Use
Routine Incoming Calls
Challenging Incoming Calls
Triaging Incoming Calls
Taking Messages
Outgoing Calls
Services and Special Features

ROLE DELINEATION COMPONENTS

GENERAL: Professionalism
- Display a professional manner and image
- Prioritize and perform multiple tasks
- Treat all patients with compassion and empathy

GENERAL: Communication Skills
- Adapt communication to individual's ability to understand
- Use professional telephone technique

ADMINISTRATIVE: Administrative Procedures
- Perform basic administrative medical assisting functions

CHAPTER COMPETENCIES

LEARNING OBJECTIVES

Upon successfully completing this chapter, you will be able to:

1. Spell and define the key terms
2. Explain the importance of displaying a professional image to all patients
3. List six duties of the medical office receptionist
4. List four sources from which messages can be retrieved
5. Discuss various steps that can be taken to promote good ergonomics
6. Describe the basic guidelines for waiting room environments
7. Describe the proper method for maintaining infection control standards in the waiting room
8. Discuss the five basic guidelines for telephone use
9. Describe the types of incoming telephone calls received by the medical office
10. Describe how to triage incoming calls
11. Discuss how to identify and handle callers with medical emergencies
12. List the information that should be given to an emergency medical service dispatcher
13. Describe the types of telephone services and special features

KEY TERMS

attitude
closed captioning
diction

diplomacy
emergency medical service (EMS)

ergonomic
receptionist

teletypewriter (TTY)
triage

As a MEDICAL ASSISTANT, YOU are the patient's primary contact with the physician. In certain situations, the patient may spend more time with you than with the physician. Your interaction with the patient sets the tone for the visit and directly influences the patient's perception of the office and the quality of care the patient will receive. Therefore, it is vital that you project a caring and competent professional image at all times. You will have various responsibilities and duties when working as a receptionist. These duties will vary among physician offices. Proper telephone etiquette and use is an essential skill for all medical assistants. You must be able to handle incoming and outgoing calls correctly and efficiently.

PROFESSIONAL IMAGE

Importance of a Good Attitude

An **attitude** is a state of mind or feeling regarding some matter. It can be either positive or negative. Attitudes can be formed by past or present experiences; they can be transmitted from one person to another. How you feel influences how you act; thus, your attitude shapes your behavior. You transmit your attitude to others through your behavior, thereby influencing their attitudes and behaviors.

The medical assistant must be able to transmit a positive attitude to the patient. This requires acceptance of the patient as a unique individual who has the right to be treated with dignity and compassion in a nonjudgmental manner. Ask yourself how you would feel in a similar situation, how you would want to be treated. By demonstrating empathy, interest, and concern, you tell the patient that he or she is important to you and that you care. This exerts a positive influence on the patient's own attitude, behavior, and response.

For example, let's assume that you are working as a receptionist in a busy family practice office. It is the peak of the flu and cold season. Which of the following interactions between the medical assistant and the patient transmits a positive attitude to the patient:

- "I know you feel terrible, Mr. Smith, but so does everyone else in the waiting room. It's the flu season. Just have a seat, and the doctor will see you shortly."
- "I'm sorry you don't feel well. Do you feel well enough to sit in the waiting room for about 10 minutes? The doctor will be ready to see you then."

The second interaction shows the patient that you care about how he feels and reassures him that he will be seen by the physician shortly. In the first interaction, the attitude that was transmitted made Mr. Smith feel like just another sick patient. Your positive attitude will influence the patient's attitude, behavior, and response.

The Medical Assistant as a Role Model

Another way in which you as a medical assistant influence the patient's perception of the medical office is your personal appearance. Good health and good grooming present a positive image to the patient. Taking care of yourself by eating well, exercising regularly, and getting enough rest is important not only for your appearance but also for your job performance. If you are tired or sluggish, you cannot give good patient care.

Pay particular attention to your personal hygiene to avoid offending your patients. A person who is ill is often acutely sensitive to odors, even those normally considered pleasant. A daily bath or shower is essential, followed by an unscented deodorant. Keep your hair clean and styled. Good oral hygiene is important, and during the day you should avoid foods that may give an offensive odor. Keep your fingernails clean and trimmed, with clear or neutral polish. Long nails polished with vivid colors are not appropriate for the medical office. Natural nail tips must be less than a quarter inch long, according to the Centers for Disease Control (CDC). Artificial nails may increase the potential for infection transmission to you and your patients. The CDC recommendation is for health care providers not to wear artificial nails if high-risk patient care is required. If you wear makeup, keep it natural and apply it lightly. Do not wear perfume, cologne, scented lotion, hair spray, or the like.

Most offices have a dress code. Whether you wear a uniform or street clothes, they should be clean, neat, pressed, and in good repair (Fig. 5-1). Wrinkles, missing buttons, split seams, torn hems, and stains project a negative image. Always wear clean, polished shoes. Stockings should be full length, of a neutral shade, and free from runs and holes. Jewelry such as dangling earrings, large rings, long chains, and ornate or multiple bracelets are not appropriate in the health care environment.

FIGURE 5–1.   The properly dressed medical assistant presents a professional and positive image to patients.

Courtesy and Diplomacy in the Medical Office

Being a medical assistant requires excellent human relations skills. In the course of a day you will interact with a variety of personalities in a variety of situations, and you must be able to maintain a positive professional attitude regardless of how difficult the encounter may be. For example, you may have to interact with a person who has done domestic violence to a patient. It is important that you treat him or her with the same courtesy and respect that you offer all patients. Courtesy and diplomacy are fundamental to successful human relations.

Courtesy is based on sensitivity to the needs and feelings of others and demands that everyone be treated with respect and dignity. It is disrespectful to refer to physicians by first name or title only. Always use the title and last name. It is permissible to call a physician by his or her first name outside of clinical areas if the physician so requests. Be courteous to your coworkers as well as your employer and your patients. Do not borrow supplies or use someone else's desk without asking permission. Always knock before entering an office, even if the door is open.

Diplomacy is the art of handling people with tact and genuine concern. Use diplomacy in difficult situations. Patients may be curious about other patients; family members may want to know what the doctor said to the patient—such questions must be met with a polite refusal to disclose confidential information. Pain, worry, and waiting can make a patient unreasonable or irritable. You must exercise self-control and understanding and maintain your professional attitude. Never argue with a patient. Try to calm the patient and communicate your desire to help. Table 5-1 lists three common problems with patients and the diplomatic way to control each situation.

First Impressions

First impressions are lasting. Remember, you have only one chance to make a first impression on patients and other health care professionals. The patient's perception of the medical office is based in part on the impression you make. A negative perception can adversely affect the patient's health. A positive perception contributes to a successful doctor–patient relationship. Patients who feel positive about their relationship with health care providers are likely to follow treatment regimens.

Physician offices must operate as a business to remain financially sound. Patients who are not satisfied with their care may opt to leave the practice. Loss of patients will result in loss of revenue for the practice. As a medical assistant, you play a key role in promoting a positive image for the physician's practice.

Checkpoint Question

1. What are four ways that you can demonstrate a professional image to patients?

RECEPTION

Definition of a Receptionist

The definition of a receptionist will vary greatly among offices. According to the 10th edition of Merriam-Webster's Collegiate Dictionary, a **receptionist** is a person employed to

Table 5-1 DIPLOMACY TABLE		
Common Problem	**Example of What to Say**	**Example of What Not to Say**
Prolonged Waiting Time		
"My appointment was for 9:30, and it is now 10. When am I going to be seen?"	"The doctor will see you in about 30 minutes. Would you like to wait or reschedule your visit?"	"We have had some emergencies." "It's flu season. Everyone is sick. Please sit down."
Patient Confidentiality		
"I am worried about my neighbor. He was seen here yesterday and sent to the hospital by ambulance. What happened?"	"We appreciate your concern, but it is against our office policy to give out patient information."	"He was having some chest pain, but he is fine now." "Yes, we sent him by ambulance because he was very sick."
Patient Discomfort		
"I am in a lot of pain. I want to see the doctor now!" "I have been vomiting all day. I won't sit in the waiting room. I want to be seen now!"	"I can see that you are in pain. Please have a seat for 1 minute. I will find a room for you to lie down."	"You are going to have to wait your turn. There are three patients ahead of you." "If you need to vomit, the rest room is to your left. You will have about a 20-minute wait."

greet telephone callers, visitors, patients, or clients. In certain physician offices the receptionist may be a non–medically trained professional whose primary task is to greet patients, alert staff members when patients are present, and serve as a telephone operator. This situation is generally found in large, multiphysician practices. If you are working in this type of setting, your role as a medical assistant will be to provide coverage while the receptionist is on break or at lunch.

In other office settings, however, you may work as the receptionist. These offices may also have multiple physicians but choose to have a medically trained person as the receptionist. No matter which type of office you work in, you will need to know and be able to assume the duties and responsibilities of a receptionist.

Duties and Responsibilities of the Receptionist

The duties of the receptionist begin long before the first appointment of the day. Most offices have the receptionist arrive at least 30 minutes prior to the first appointment. Your first task will be to prepare the office for patient arrivals.

Prepare the Office

As receptionist, you are responsible for preparing the office for patients and for other employee arrivals. These tasks should be done first:

- Unlock doors as appropriate.
- Disengage the alarm system.
- Turn on appropriate lights.
- Turn on computers, printers, copiers, and other electronic devices.
- If the office uses a drop box to leave specimens for evening pickups, check the box to ensure that the specimens were taken.

After those five tasks are done, do a systematic check of the office. The reception area should be clean and tidy. The reception desk should be free from clutter with confidential material safely out of sight (Fig. 5-2). Restock your desk with necessary forms and office supplies before patients arrive. In smaller offices you may be responsible for checking the examination rooms.

This process should not take long. The office should never be left messy or in disarray at the end of the day. Stocking of supplies and cleaning and disinfecting examination rooms should be done before the staff leaves at night. The office should be left in a professional manner.

Retrieve Messages

Another responsibility you may have as a receptionist is to retrieve messages that were left while the office was closed. All physician offices have a method for communicating with their patients after hours. Most offices leave a voice message

FIGURE 5–2.   The receptionist desk and waiting room area must be easily accessible at all times.

on their main incoming line that directs patients to call a given number (answering service) for acute medical problems. Usually, this message also instructs patients to leave nonemergency messages on the voice mail.

Messages may be obtained from four sources:

- Answering service
- Voice mail system
- Electronic mail
- Facsimile machine

No matter how a message has been sent, however, all information must be treated confidentially.

Messages should be checked as soon as the office opens, at midday, after breaks, and periodically throughout the day. After retrieving the messages, forward them to the appropriate staff for resolution.

Answering Service. Answering services receive calls from patients, hospital staff, and other physicians and communicate the emergency messages to the physician, generally by beeper. Other messages are left for the office staff to obtain the following morning. Examples of messages that could be left here:

- Patients calling the office for a sick appointment (not an emergency) (such as an earache, flulike symptoms)
- Calls from hospitals or skilled nursing facilities about changes in patient status (new wounds or bed sores, patient falls without injury)

Voice Mail Systems. A voice mailbox is a type of answering machine in which the caller can leave a detailed message. You will need to know the security access code to obtain messages. After you obtain the messages, delete them from the recorder unless otherwise directed by office policy. Examples of messages that could be left here are

- Patients wishing to change or cancel their appointment
- Patients requesting prescription refills

- Family members or patients calling to ask for additional information or clarification about their medical care or test results

Electronic Mail. The computer is a vital link for physicians to communicate with all health care professionals. E-mail messages are sent from other physicians, professional organizations, and hospital personnel. Some physician offices provide patients with their E-mail address. Examples of messages left here are

- Memos from professional organizations
- Pharmaceutical representatives' updates or announcements
- Medical staff meeting minutes, announcements from hospital administration
- Upcoming continuing education courses for physicians
- Insurance representatives regarding billing issues

Facsimile Machines. All physician offices have a fax machine. The most common messages left here are

- Patient referrals
- Consultation reports
- Laboratory and radiology reports

Checkpoint Question

2. What four locations should you retrieve messages from?

Prepare the Charts

Your next duty will be to gather charts. Gather the charts of all of the patients scheduled to be seen for the day and put them in order by appointment. Review each chart to ensure

that it is complete and up to date. Check that adequate clinical data sheets are available for the doctor to record any notes. Test results received since the patient's last appointment and any other new information are placed in the front of the chart for the doctor's review. Make up a chart for each new patient and have the appropriate registration forms ready for the patient to complete. Once the charts are prepared, they are usually kept at the reception desk and given to the doctor or clinical assistant as the patient arrives, although some doctors prefer to have all charts on their desk at the start of the day. (See Chapter 8.)

Welcome Patients and Visitors

Make every attempt to greet patients personally and by name, e.g., "Good morning, Ms. Misko." A smile and cheerful greeting promote a positive image and make the patient feel welcome. Try to remember something personal about each patient, such as hobbies, pets, or special interests about which you can ask. Sometimes, you will not be at your desk when a patient arrives. Check the waiting room for new arrivals upon your return. Many offices install a bell or chime on the door and post a sign requesting patients to check in with the receptionist.

Register and Orient Patients

Patients who are new to the office will have to complete a registration form, also called a patient information sheet. On this form the patient provides name, address, and telephone number; the name, address, and telephone number of the insurance company or other party responsible for payment; employer names and addresses; marital status; spouse's name; social security number; and name of the person who referred the patient. Some information sheets include ques-

Spanish Terminology

¡Hola!	Hello!
¿Cómo se llama usted?	What is your name?
¿En qué puedo servirle?	May I help you?
¿Cuál es su dirección?	What is your address?
¿Cuál es el código postal?	What is the zip code?
¿Cuál es su número de teléfono?	What is your phone number?
¿Fecha de nacimiento?	What is your birth date?
¿Cuántos años tiene?	How old are you?
Por favor, sientese en la sala de espera.	Please have a seat in the waiting room.
Necesito hacerle unas preguntas.	I need to ask you some questions.
Por favor, llene estos papeles.	Please fill out these papers.

tions about medical history. In some cases, you may complete the form while interviewing the patient. Most offices have the patients fill in these forms and ask for your help if questions arise.

After registration, orient the patient to the office. Brochures that give the names of the doctor and staff, office hours, and telephone numbers are helpful. Explain any pertinent office policies or procedures, such as billing procedures, how to make or cancel appointments, and parking. Ask if the patient has any questions. Tell the patient where the water fountain and restrooms are, but caution the patient against using the restroom without checking with you to determine whether a urine specimen is needed. Urine specimens are generally needed for pregnant patients, patients with lower back or abdominal pain or back injuries, and patients being seen for drug or preemployment health examinations. At the appropriate time, you may be responsible for taking patients to the examination room unless another health care worker escorts the patients.

Manage Waiting Time

Patients expect to be seen at the appointed time. They have allotted time in their schedule to see the doctor and do not want to be kept waiting. One of the major complaints of patients is the length of time they must wait to see the physician. Be sure to tell the patients if the doctor is behind schedule. If you expect the wait to be 30 minutes or more past the scheduled time, offer waiting patients some choices. Some choose to leave and come back in an hour, and some choose to reschedule the appointment for another time.

Ergonomic Concerns for the Receptionist

For most of the day you will be sitting at your desk performing these tasks. Occasional lifting of delivery boxes, paper supplies, and so on is required. The duties of the receptionist require you to twist from your primary desk to other areas to reach for files or to answer the telephone. These actions can lead to back injuries and other musculoskeletal disorders. Medical professionals are at high risk for such injuries. Having a good **ergonomic** workstation and good body mechanics, however, can prevent most injuries.

An ergonomic workstation is designed specifically to prevent injuries and often results in increased employee satisfaction and work efficiency. The Occupational Safety and Health Administration (OSHA) has many recommendations for preventing such injuries. Box 5-1 offers workstation recommendations. Here are some other suggestions to prevent injuries:

- Keep items that you must lift at waist level when possible. Keep the load close to the body. Bend at your hips.
- Instruct delivery people to place packages in locations that will not require movement.
- Carry only small loads of paper. Make additional trips as needed.

Box 5-1

ERGONOMIC WORKSTATION RECOMMENDATIONS

The following is a list of recommendations to prevent injuries:

- Your head and neck should be upright, not bent down. All desks should lead you to face forward, not twist. Objects should be within reach to allow your arms to stay close to your body, not extended. Forearms, wrists, and hands should be parallel to the ground. Your thighs should be parallel and your legs perpendicular to the floor.
- Chairs should be appropriate size. The backrest should touch the lumbar area and be strong enough to provide lumbar support. Seats should be cushioned and rounded. The seat should press against the back of your legs or knees. Armrests should support both forearms and not interfere with movement. Your feet should rest flat on the floor or on a stable footrest.
- Desks should be large enough to accommodate all needed equipment. There should be clearance between your thighs and the desk. Nothing should be stored under the desk if it limits your mobility.
- Carpets should be flat and not have a thick pile.
- Upper drawers of file cabinets should not be used if they are above your head and require reaching. Lower drawers should not hold files that require constant access, as this causes excessive bending.

- Place items that you frequently use within easy reach. Moves from side to side are safer than twisting to a desk behind you. Avoiding storing charts above chest level to limit reaching over your head. Use a step stool to reach high shelves instead of stretching.
- Telephones with headsets will keep your head upright and allow your shoulders to relax. If you use a stationary phone, a long handset cord can reduce muscle strain. Do not rest the telephone on your shoulder while talking, since this causes neck and back injuries.

 Checkpoint Question

3. What is the purpose of having an ergonomic workstation?

The Waiting Room Environment

General Guidelines for Waiting Rooms

The reception area should be designed for the comfort, safety, and enjoyment of all patients. It should be kept clean and uncluttered, with the furniture arranged to allow ample room for walking. A coat rack and umbrella stand should be present. Restrooms and a water fountain should be easily accessible.

Furniture should be aesthetically pleasing, comfortable, and durable. Chairs are preferable to sofas because most people find sharing a sofa with strangers uncomfortable. Chairs allow patients to maintain a degree of privacy and personal space. There should be a variety of soft chairs and firm chairs and chairs with and without arms. Some patients find it hard to stand up from a soft chair; others prefer the comfort. Some need chair arms to push themselves up, and others are more comfortable without chair arms.

A low-key color scheme is advisable. Muted pastels are preferable to bright primary colors, although the latter work well in pediatric offices. Lighting should be bright but not harsh. The room should be well ventilated and kept at a comfortable temperature. Many offices provide soothing background music.

Landscapes, waterscapes, and floral and animal pictures make better wall décor than abstract art. Lamps and plants can add interest to corners. Keep plants in good condition and remove any dead leaves. An office with dead or dying plants does not project a comforting image.

A good selection of reading material should be available. Have a variety of current magazines that are appropriate for your patients. The doctor's professional journals should not be included. The reception area is a good place to set out patient education materials.

Some offices provide television for patients who prefer not to read. Most patients find television relaxing and entertaining, but other patients find it annoying. Television can serve as an education tool. Here are a few tips that you should follow regarding television:

- The volume should be set to allow a group of people to hear the television but not at a distracting volume for the whole waiting room.
- A simple sign placed on the television, "Please do not touch the controls; see the receptionist for channel changes" will prevent patients from selecting inappropriate programs.
- Only family-oriented programs should be shown. It is acceptable to select a news channel. No shows with violence, strong language, or sexual content should be on. Soap operas are not suitable for medical office waiting rooms.
- Some offices leave the television off unless a patient asks to have it on.
- Patients with hearing impairments must be offered the option of **closed captioning** if they choose to watch television. (Closed captioning is the translation of the spoken word into a written format. Most televisions have this capability under their options menu.)

You should check the waiting room several times during the day to make sure it is clean and tidy. Also check the entrance, hallways, and stairs. These areas too must be well

PATIENT EDUCATION

Television as a Teaching Tool

A television in the reception area can entertain patients while they wait for an appointment, but it can also be a patient education tool. By using a television in conjunction with a VCR, you can play a variety of educational videos. Here are some points to keep in mind:

- Be sure all videos have been previewed by the physician.
- Select videos that are geared toward the specialty of the practice (e.g., a video about heart attacks is appropriate for a cardiologist's office but not for a dermatologist's office).
- Carefully assess the graphic nature of certain videos. (A picture of the birth of a child may interest you but be too much for certain patients.)
- Keep in mind the age of the patients and family members who will be in the waiting room. Caution must be used if small children are often in the area. For example, a video about preventing sexually transmitted diseases may provide information appropriate for a family practice office, but it would not be appropriate to show the video in the reception area.

lighted and maintained. Liability is a concern if patients slip on ice or snow coming into the office.

Checkpoint Question

4. What option should you offer hearing impaired patients if they wish to watch television?

Guidelines for Pediatric Waiting Rooms

Pediatric offices tend to be very busy practices with a multitude of reasons for patient visits. Generally, visits to the pediatrician can be divided into three types: well child checks, sick child visits, and follow-up visits. Because of the large volume of sick child visits, most pediatric waiting room areas are broken into two sections, one for well children and the other for sick children. Parents may have to be instructed by you as to which side of the waiting room they should sit in. According to the American Academy of Pediatrics (AAP), no studies document the effectiveness of segregated waiting room areas. The recommendation of the AAP is to move children with a communicable disease into an examination room as quickly as possible. Your employer will provide you with instructions and guidelines for dealing with sick children.

A children's play area must be closely watched and monitored. Toys should be kept away from the general seating area. Here are some guidelines for toys:

- Toys should be simple and easy to clean, without sharp edges.
- A policy must be in place for routine cleaning of these toys.
- Toys should be checked daily to ensure that they are not broken. Toys that are broken must be thrown away. Toys should never be glued or taped together.
- Battery-powered toys that make loud noises are not permissible.
- Toys can be a choking hazard. According to the American Heart Association, small children should never to be given toys that can fit inside a standard toilet paper roll. Although older children would like to play with toys like Legos, these toys should not be present. Older children should be expected to sit quietly while waiting for their appointment.

A good selection of books should be present for parents to read to their children. Books must be checked periodically to ensure that they are clean and no pages have been torn out. A small table and chairs will give children a place to read or color.

Americans with Disabilities Act Requirements

The U. S. Department of Justice is responsible for ensuring that all people are treated without discrimination of any kind. Under this department is the Americans with Disabilities Act (ADA). This act prohibits discrimination on the basis of a person's disability. The ADA Title III act requires that all public accommodations be accessible to everyone. This includes access into medical facilities. It is important that you be aware of the basic concept of the ADA rules. Table 5-2 lists some of the basic facility requirements. Additional information is available on the ADA website.

The existing structural dimensions are not something that you have control of, but you need to ensure that there is a clear path to the physician's office at all times. Here are some steps that you can take to ensure this:

- Check that deliveries are left in a safe place. They must not be left in the waiting area or block the door.
- Keep toys clear of entrance pathways.
- Check that chairs are not moved, creating obstacles that might limit wheelchair accessibility.
- Ensure that doors are not blocked or propped opened with objects.

Table 5-2   SUMMARY OF ADA REQUIREMENTS FOR PUBLIC BUILDINGS

Area	Specifics
Access	Route must be stable, firm, and slip resistant.
	Route must be 36 inches wide.
Ramps	Ramps longer than 6 feet must have two railings.
	Railings must be 34–38 inches high.
	Ramp must be 36 inches wide.
	Ramps and elevators must be available to all public levels.
Entrance and door	Door must be 32 inches wide.
	Door handle must be no higher than 48 inches and must be operable with a closed fist.
	Interior doors must open without excessive force.
Miscellaneous	Carpeting must be no more than 0.5 inch high.
	Emergency egress system must have flashing lights and audible signals.
	Space for wheelchair seating must be available.
	Tables or counters must be 28–34 inches high.
Restrooms	Tactile signs must identify restrooms.
	Doorway must be at least 32 inches wide.
	All doors (including stall doors), soap dispensers, hand dryers, and faucets must be operable with a closed fist.
	Wheelchair stall is required and must be at least 5 feet by 5 feet.

WHAT IF

A patient brings in his seeing eye dog and asks, "Can I keep the dog with me in the office?" What would you say?

The Americans with Disabilities Act (ADA) prohibits businesses from banning service animals. A service animal is defined as any guide dog or other animal that is trained to provide assistance to a person with a disability. The animal does not have to be licensed or certified by the state as a service animal. Examples of duties that service animals perform include alerting to sounds patients with hearing impairments, pulling wheelchairs for spinal cord injury patients, picking up items for patients with mobility impairments, sensing smells or auras for seizure patients, and assisting patients with visual impairments. The service animal should not be separated from its owner and must be allowed to enter the examination room with the patient. The ADA law supersedes local health department regulations that ban animals in health care centers. The care of the service animal is the sole responsibility of its owner.

- Limit the amount of stacked papers on counters that may limit the patient's access to you.
- Check the restroom regularly to make sure the entrance is open and not obstructed.

 Checkpoint Question

5. What act prohibits discrimination of patients with disabilities?

Infection Control Issues

To prevent the spread of disease, aseptic technique must be used in every aspect of work in the medical office. During the clinical portion of your training, you will learn detailed information about infection control. As a receptionist, however, you need to be aware of a few key points:

- Always follow standard precautions. This means that you must treat all body fluids with precautionary measures.
- Handwashing is the most important practice for preventing the transmission of diseases. You must wash your hands following all direct patient contact (touching the patient) (Fig. 5-3). Since it is not always possible to leave the desk to wash your hands, the CDC has

approved the use of alcohol-based antiseptic handwashing solutions for health care providers.
- Patients are often told to bring specimens to the office. Never touch a specimen container without proper gloves and personal protective equipment.
- Patients who arrive coughing and sneezing should be given tissues and instructed to cover their mouth and nose when coughing. Communicate with the clinical staff to have these patients taken directly into examination rooms. Patients who are vomiting, bleeding, or discharging other body fluids must not be left in the waiting room.

Biohazard Waste. All body fluids must be considered infectious and be managed appropriately. All body fluid spills and blood-stained papers must be disposed of in a biohazard container. The spills must be cleaned with an approved germicidal solution. If you have not been trained in handling such waste, do not touch it. Allow the clinical staff to handle the waste. If possible, contain the spill and prevent other pa-

FIGURE 5–3. Good handwashing skills are essential to prevent disease transmission.

tients from touching the area. Here are some examples of biohazard waste that you may encounter:

- Dressing supplies with bloodstains from cuts or wounds
- Tissues from patients with acute nosebleeds
- Urine-saturated diapers left in the restroom
- Vomit
- Saturated tissues with sputum

Communicable Diseases. Depending on the type of office you work in, the amount of exposure to communicable diseases will vary. Family practice physicians and pediatricians, for example, treat acute communicable diseases regularly. If you work as a receptionist for a pediatrician, you will need to learn how to look at rashes and determine whether they are contagious.

Good communication between you and the clinical staff is essential to manage patients with communicable diseases. The clinical staff is often aware of patients with such diseases and will communicate it to you. Most infectious diseases can't be transmitted with routine physical contact (handshaking, talking, touching, sharing pencils, using the telephone). Examples of infectious diseases that can't be transmitted by routine physical contact include HIV, hepatitis, and the common cold. Some diseases can be easily transmitted, however, and patients with these diseases should not be left in the waiting room. Box 5-2 lists patients who should not be left in the waiting room.

Patients who have an impaired immune system or are taking medications that hinder their immune system (chemotherapy agents) may require immediate placement in an exami-

nation room to prevent exposure to otherwise benign organisms. The clinical staff will alert you to these patients.

Checkpoint Question

6. What is the most antiseptic technique for preventing the transmission of diseases?

The End of the Patient Visit

After physicians have completed the examination or other procedures, they generally direct patients to get dressed and wait for their discharge information. In some offices, physicians provide all discharge instructions, while in other office settings nurses or medical assistants may be assigned to discharge patients. Chapter 4 discusses the information you need to teach your patients. After the medical portion is completed, the patient is escorted to the front desk. It is generally at this time that any fees or copayments are collected by the receptionist. If the doctor has requested a follow-up visit, the appointment should be scheduled. An appointment reminder card is helpful for the patient. You or other administrative personnel may do these tasks. You should bid the patient goodbye in a warm and friendly manner. As patients leave the office, they should feel they have been well cared for by a competent and courteous staff.

TELEPHONE

Importance of the Telephone in the Medical Office

The medical office is filled with expensive scientific equipment used in the diagnosis and treatment of disease, but one of the most important instruments is the telephone. It allows the patient rapid and easy access to medical care. A patient can schedule an appointment, seek medical advice, request prescription refills, obtain test results, question a bill, or report an emergency simply by picking up the telephone. The telephone also links the physician's office to the rest of the medical community, including hospitals, pharmacies, and other doctors.

You must be able to communicate a positive image of the physician and staff over the telephone without the aid of nonverbal cues such as appearance, facial expressions, body language, and gestures. You must be able to use the tone and quality of your voice and speech to project a competent and caring attitude over the telephone.

Basic Guidelines for Telephone Use

Telephone communication is not effective if either party does not fully understand what is being said. Misunderstandings can be embarrassing, frustrating, or even life-threatening. To have effective telephone communication, you must be able to overcome various obstacles, such as a

---

Box 5-2

PATIENTS WHO SHOULD NOT BE LEFT IN THE WAITING ROOM

Patients with any of the following diseases or conditions should not be left in the waiting room. These patients should be taken to an examination room as soon as possible:

- Chickenpox
- Conjunctivitis
- Influenza
- Measles and rubella
- Meningitis (or suspected cases)
- Mumps
- Pertussis
- Pneumonia (if patient is coughing)
- Smallpox
- Tuberculosis
- Wounds (if open and draining)

FIGURE 5−4. While speaking on the telephone, be courteous and professional.

noisy environment, a poor telephone connection, a patient's emotional distress, or a patient's hearing or speech impairments (Fig. 5-4).

Diction

Diction refers to how words are spoken and enunciated. You should speak clearly and distinctly. Talk clearly into the mouthpiece; do not prop the handset between your chin and shoulder. Never chew gum or eat while you speak on the telephone. Speak at a moderate pace to avoid slurring your words.

Pronunciation

Make sure you pronounce words correctly to avoid misunderstandings. Avoid using unfamiliar words, slang, and idiomatic expressions. Most patients do not understand medical terminology, so it is best to use lay terms whenever possible. For example, do not ask the patient, "Are you dyspneic?" Instead ask, "Are you having trouble breathing?"

Expression

Put a smile in your voice by sitting up straight and putting a smile on your lips. Speak with a modulated pitch and volume. Use proper inflection to avoid a droning, monotonous speaking style.

Listening

Be an attentive listener. Focus on the conversation and ignore outside distractions. Do not interrupt the speaker. You may have to ask the caller to repeat what was said. Verify your understanding by repeating the message.

Courtesy

Always speak politely and courteously. Address the caller by title and last name. Although many telephone calls interrupt your work, do not allow your voice to betray impatience or irritation. Remember that you are there to help the patient.

Never answer the telephone and immediately put the caller on hold. If you need to answer another line or finish a task before you can engage in conversation, ask if the caller would mind holding. Courtesy demands that you wait for an answer before you place the call on hold. Also of great importance, you must determine whether the call is an emergency. If you are unable to take the call after 90 seconds, check back with the caller and ask whether he or she would like to continue holding. Again, wait for an answer before you place the call on hold. If the hold exceeds 3 minutes, you should apologize to the caller for the delay and offer to return the call as soon as you are available.

If you are already engaged in a telephone conversation and have to answer another line, ask the party with whom you are speaking if he or she would mind holding. Again, wait for a reply before answering the second call. Explain to the second caller that you are on the other line and need to complete that call. Do not handle the second call while the first party waits unless the second call is an emergency, a long distance call that cannot be referred to another worker, or a physician calling to speak with your physician.

Quite often you will find that you are juggling the telephones and patients who are in the office. Exercise your best judgment in balancing the two tasks. If the call is going to take a long time, ask the caller to wait a moment, address the needs of the patient in the office, and then return to the call. Use caution when talking on the telephone in front of patients. Remember, all information about and conversations with patients are confidential.

Checkpoint Question

7. What are the five basic guidelines for telephone use?

Routine Incoming Calls

An incoming call should be given the same courtesy and attention as an arriving visitor. Just as you would not keep a patient waiting without acknowledging his or her presence, so you must acknowledge an incoming call promptly. Answer the telephone by the second ring if at all possible. Identify both the office and yourself to assure the caller that the correct number has been reached, and offer your assistance. The following are examples of common calls that come into a medical office.

Appointments

New patients call to make appointments and established patients call to schedule return visits. (See Chapter 6.)

Billing Inquiries

In some offices you may be responsible for handling routine inquiries concerning billing, fees, services, and insurance. You may be asked for specific information concerning the cost of services; do not quote exact prices but tell the patient that costs depend on the type of examination and diagnostic tests performed. Sometimes, third-party callers request information about the patient; remember that no patient information can be given to anyone without a specific release from the patient.

Diagnostic Test Results

Many laboratory and radiology reports are called in to the physician's office before the written copy is sent. Record the information and post it on the front of the chart for the physician to review. If the results are needed at once, bring the information to the physician's attention immediately upon receiving the report. Having at hand a blank laboratory slip or specially designed forms listing the most frequently ordered reports for your office will save time and make it easier to accurately record the results as they are relayed from the laboratory or radiology department. Administrative personnel will place a written copy of test results in the patient's chart.

Routine and Satisfactory Progress Reports

At the end of an office visit a patient may be told to call in a progress report within a few days. If the patient says he or she is feeling better or getting stronger or the symptoms have resolved, take down the information, record it in the patient's chart, and place it on the physician's desk for review. You may also handle routine progress reports from hospitals, home health agencies, and other allied health professionals. For example, a home care nurse may call and report that a patient's blood pressure is now within normal limits, or a physical therapist may call the office and to say that a patient's range of motion is improving. Again, record the information and place it on the physician's desk for review.

Test Results

Patients often call for their test results, and many doctors allow the medical assistant to report favorable test results to patients. Your office will have a specific policy for handling these calls. It is illegal to give information to anyone other than the patient without the patient's specific consent.

Unsatisfactory Progress Reports and Test Results

The doctor must speak with patients whose progress or test results are unsatisfactory. The urgency of the patient's condition determines whether the call requires the physician's immediate attention. The physician will discuss serious unsatisfactory test results with the patient. In less serious cases, the physician may ask you to speak with the patient. Never discuss unsatisfactory test results with a patient unless the doctor directs you to do so.

Prescription Refills

As a medical assistant, you can handle requests for prescription refills if they are indicated on the chart. If there is any doubt, tell the pharmacy or the patient that you will check with the doctor and call back.

Other Calls

Other calls you ordinarily handle include requests for referrals to other physicians, clarifying instructions for patients, and calls concerning routine administrative matters.

Ask the physician which calls he or she prefers to have transferred immediately and which calls can be returned later. Calls from other physicians should be directed to the physician immediately or according to office policy. Physicians also receive personal calls. Your employer will tell you which calls should be put through immediately. Otherwise, take a message and tell the caller that the doctor will return the call.

Challenging Incoming Calls

Unidentified Callers

Sometimes, callers who ask to speak with the physician refuse to state their name or the nature of their business. In such instances you should politely but firmly tell the caller that you can't interrupt the physician and politely explain that you would be happy to take a message. If the caller persists, ask the caller to call back at a specific time when the physician will be available. Alert the physician that there will be a call for him or her at the specified time. Unidentified callers may be sales representatives.

Irate Patients

When a caller is angry, you must be careful to keep your own temper in check. Try to calm the patient and offer assurance that you want to help. Listen carefully and take notes. If you cannot resolve the situation, let the patient know you must consult with the physician and offer to call back. The physician will probably want to speak with the patient personally. Always tell the physician about complaints regarding fees or care.

Medical Emergencies

As a medical assistant, you must be able to differentiate between routine calls and emergencies. To do this, first try to calm the caller and ask specific questions concerning the patient's condition. Severe pain, profuse bleeding, respiratory distress, chest pain, loss of consciousness, severe vomiting or diarrhea, and a temperature above 102.0°F are all emergencies, and you should immediately put the call through to the physician or an appropriate health care professional. In some offices, nurses will be assigned to handle these calls.

Determine the patient's name, location, and telephone number as quickly as possible in case you are disconnected or the patient is unable to continue the conversation. This will allow you to direct emergency personnel to the patient's aid. The office should have a policy for handling emergency calls when the doctor is not in the office. Most policies advise you to direct patients to go to the nearest emergency room or walk-in center.

Ask the physician to list instances that might constitute an emergency in his or her specialty and to describe how they should be handled. For example, if you work for a cardiologist, most of your emergency calls will be patients with chest pain and trouble breathing. The cardiologist may instruct you to ask the patient standard questions, have you instruct patients to take certain medications, and then instruct the patient to dial for an ambulance. If you are working for an obstetrician, your emergency calls will be related to patients who have labor concerns or sudden onset of bleeding. Most obstetricians have precise recommendations for when patients in labor should go to the hospital (e.g., contractions lasting more than 1 minute with a frequency of every 5 minutes). Once you have the list of the most common calls and what your response should be, put the list in a prominent place near the telephone.

Triaging Incoming Calls

Usually the office telephone has multiple lines, and frequently several patients call at the same time. You must be able to **triage** (sort) them into a priority order. How would you sort these four calls?

- Line 1: Caller wants to make an appointment for her son, who has a 101.3°F fever.
- Line 2: Caller wants to see the doctor this afternoon because he is having chest pain.
- Line 3: Caller is upset because she has been disconnected 3 times and has a question about her bill.
- Line 4: Caller needs a prescription refill.

Who would you take first? Why? Last? Why?

Any patient with a potentially life-threatening problem needs to be taken first. Therefore, talk first to caller 2. Follow your office policy for emergencies. Sometimes, a nurse will further assess the emergency or the patient may be directed to call 911. The caller on line 3 needs attention next. The longer she waits, the more upset and difficult to please she will be. Explain to the patient that you have to get the bill and chart, and ask for a phone number where you can call her back. Make the appointment for the caller on line 1. Again, follow your office policies regarding patient care issues. Caller 4 is last. Remember, you need to get back to caller 3 promptly. Do not leave messages unresolved.

Taking Messages

Taking messages for the physician or other health care professionals will be a large part of your daily responsibilities. Taking messages is easier using notepads designed for this task. Office supply companies have an assortment of pads, or your physician may choose to design his or her own. Carbonless copies give you a record of the messages taken during the day and the action taken.

The minimum information needed for a telephone message includes the name of the caller, date and time of the call, telephone number where the caller can be reached, a short description of the caller's concern, and the person to whom the message is routed.

Before you end the call, tell the patient when to expect a return call. Callback times vary from office to office. Some physicians return calls only at the end of the day, while others return calls randomly. Learn the policy of the office in which you are working.

The patient's chart must document all calls. If you return the call to the patient, document your conversation in the medical record. Some message pads are designed to be added to the progress note on the patient's chart when the call is complete.

Checkpoint Question

8. What is the minimum information needed for taking messages?

Outgoing Calls

General Guidelines for Outgoing Calls

You will make outgoing calls as well as receive incoming calls. You should prepare for your calls carefully; have all information gathered and know what you want to say before you dial the number. If you are calling a patient to reschedule an appointment, be able to explain why the change is necessary and be prepared to offer a new appointment time.

At times you may have to make long distance calls. Keep in mind the difference in time zones; if you do not know the time zone of the city you are calling, check the front of the telephone directory. Long distance calls should be dialed directly, without operator assistance. If you dial a wrong number or become disconnected during the call, notify the long distance operator immediately to avoid charges.

Your employer may ask you to place a conference call, which connects three or more people. Notify all parties of the date and time the call will be made to ensure that everyone will be available to participate. Participants should be given the access phone number and the access code in advance of the scheduled call.

Calling Emergency Medical Services

Some patients will need immediate transport to a hospital. When emergencies occur in the physician's office, the clinical staff will be busy providing lifesaving procedures to the patient. As a receptionist, you will be directed to call the local **emergency medical service (EMS)** for transport. In most areas of the United States, the emergency number is 911. Prior to placing the call, obtain the following information:

- Patient's name, age, and sex. (Age is important, especially if the patient is a newborn or child. This will allow the dispatcher to send the most appropriate responders.)
- Nature of the medical problem (chest pain, abdominal pain, bleeding).
- Type of service the physician is requesting. Generally, there are two levels of care: basic and advanced life support. Types of services will vary from community to community.
- Any specific instructions or requests the physician may have. Generally, patients are taken to the nearest hospital; the physician may have made arrangements for the patient to be admitted at a specific hospital, however, because of a condition or diagnosis. For example, an patient with a high-risk pregnancy may be sent to a hospital with an appropriate newborn nursery instead of the community hospital. It is important that this information be told to the dispatcher so the appropriate team can be sent.
- The location of the office and any specific instructions for access, e.g., 92 Main Street, Medical Office Group, third floor, last door on the left.

After gathering the information, dial the emergency medical service number. Speak in a slow, calm voice to the dispatcher. Give the information. If the dispatcher has additional questions, answer them. Ask the dispatcher the approximate arrival time for the ambulance. Do not end the call until instructed to do so by the dispatcher.

After placing the call, alert the staff to the approximate arrival time and any other pertinent information. Ensure that the path for the ambulance personnel is unobstructed and accessible. Reassure other patients in the waiting room. If the patient has any family members present, offer them assistance and reassurance.

Checkpoint Question

9. What patient information should you know before calling emergency medical services?

Services and Special Features

The telephone system that is used for physician offices should be large enough to serve the needs of the office. For example, if you are working for a single dermatologist, two incoming phone lines may be enough. If you are a receptionist for a large family practice with multiple physicians and other practitioners, however, the number of incoming lines will be greater. Most offices also have unpublished incoming numbers or lines. Staff members, families, and other physicians primarily use these private lines. In addition, most offices have a direct line to the local hospital. A wide variety of communication equipment is available today, and communications consultants can help determine the appropriate services and equipment for your office. At minimum, the phone system should have recall, volume control, intercom, call forwarding, and caller identification. Cordless headsets prevent neck injuries and allow for mobility.

Most physicians have a cellular telephone. This number should never be given to anyone, although it should be readily accessible for staff members. Physicians and other health care professionals also have pager systems. Most pager systems allow you to send typed messages to the recipient via the computer. These messages are displayed on the pager, e.g., "Kate Larke's blood sugar was 420," or "Please call Dr. Harrison about Patrick Burke." Typing messages directly into a pager system is good time management.

Telecommunication Relay Systems

Patients with hearing or speech impairments often have difficulty communicating with a standard telephone. The ADA requires that telephone companies have telecommunication relay systems (TRS) available 24 hours a day (Fig. 5-5). A relay system allows the caller to type messages into a special telephone that transmits the message across the lines to the other party. The other party reads the message and types a response. The communication continues through written messages. A telephone with an attachment for typing messages is called a **teletypewriter** (TTY). If the other party does not have the capabilities to read the message, an operator can be used to translate the message. Most physician offices have a TTY phone or access to one. The Federal Communication Commission has set minimum standards for TRS and TTY systems for public buildings. These standards can be found on their website.

FIGURE 5–5. Various telephone systems.

Procedure 5-1

Handling Incoming Calls

Equipment/Supplies

- Telephone
- Telephone message pad
- Writing utensil (pen or pencil)
- Headset (if applicable)

Steps	Purpose
1. Gather the needed equipment.	Ensures that all materials are available and ready for use.
2. Answer the phone within two rings.	Demonstrates professionalism and courtesy to the caller.
3. Greet caller with proper identification (your name and the name of the office).	Demonstrates professionalism and courtesy to the caller.
4. Identify the nature or reason for the call in a timely manner.	Allows the call to be appropriately managed.
5. Triage the call appropriately.	Prompt identification of emergency calls is important for good patient care.
6. Communicate in a professional manner and with unhurried speech.	Demonstrates compassion and caring for the patient. An unhurried speech pattern is reassuring to the patient.
7. Clarify information as needed.	Prevents errors in communication.
8. Record the message on a message pad. Include name of caller, date, time, telephone number where the caller can be reached, description of the caller's concerns, and person to whom the message is routed.	Promotes good communication between you and the recipient of the message.
9. Give the caller an approximate time for a return call.	Provides reassurance to the patient that the call will be handled promptly and timely.
10. Ask the caller whether he or she has any additional questions or needs any other help.	Confirms that the patient's needs have been met.
11. Allow the caller to disconnect first.	Ensures that the caller has completed the communication.
12. Put the message in an appropriate place.	Ensures that the call will be handled correctly and the intended recipient gets the information.
13. Complete the task within 10 minutes.	Ensures that the call is handled promptly and efficiently.

Procedure 5-2

Calling Emergency Medical Services

Equipment/Supplies

- Telephone
- Patient information
- Writing utensil (pen, pencil)

Steps	Purpose
1. Obtain the following the information before dialing: patient's name, age, sex, nature of medical condition, type of service the physician is requesting, any special instructions or requests the physician may have, your location and any special information for access.	Information is necessary for quick and correct dispatch of EMS personnel. Certain types of patients require special teams for transport.
2. Dial 911 or other EMS number.	Call can't be placed if number is not dialed correctly.
3. Calmly provide the dispatcher with the above information.	Allows information to be communicated quickly and professionally.
4. Answer the dispatcher's questions calmly and professionally.	Allows dispatcher to obtain any additional information and verify the message.
5. Follow the dispatcher's instructions, if applicable.	Following instructions provides good patient care.
6. End the call as per dispatcher instructions.	Ensures that all communication needs have been met.
7. Complete the task within 10 minutes.	Prompt access to EMS promotes good patient care and is essential for good outcomes.

CHAPTER SUMMARY

As the receptionist, you are the most visible and accessible representative of the medical practice. Duties and responsibilities of a receptionist vary among office settings. The key to being a good receptionist is to demonstrate tact and diplomacy in all interactions with patients. Providing a positive attitude will ease the patient's anxiety and ensure the best and most confident image of the practice is projected. Proper telephone etiquette and manners are essential for good patient care and to achieve effective communication among various health care providers. Triaging incoming calls is a skill that you must master if you are to be an effective receptionist.

Critical Thinking Challenges

1. How would you calm an irate patient on the telephone? Identify some phrases that you might use to calm the caller. What phrases may make the situation worse?

2. Assume you are working in an obstetrician's office. What kinds of educational videos might be appropriate for the waiting room? What if you were working in an orthopedic office or for a surgeon?

3. Here is a triage scenario. Line 1 is a home care nurse calling the office with a patient status update. Line 2 is a pharmacist questioning a prescription. Line 3 is a mother of a 3-year-old child who has been vomiting for 24 hours. Line 4 is a patient who is having trouble breathing. Sort these calls. Who would you take first and last? Why? Explain your choices.

4. Describe how you would handle a patient who is vomiting in the waiting room. What would you do if a patient had a loud, congested cough?

5. Assume you are working for a pediatrician. A mother arrives carrying an 18-month-old child with symptoms of a respiratory illness. As per office policy, you direct her to sit in the sick child area. The mother refuses. What do you do?

Answers to Checkpoint Questions

1. You can demonstrate a professional image by transmitting a positive attitude, acting as a role model, us-

ing courtesy and diplomacy, and making a positive first impression.

2. Messages can be retrieved from answering services, voice mail, electronic mail, and facsimile machines.

3. The purpose of an ergonomic workstation is to prevent injuries to employees and to increase employee satisfaction and work efficiency.

4. Patients who are hearing impaired should be offered closed captioning if they are requesting to watch television.

5. The Americans with Disabilities Act prohibits discrimination against people with disabilities.

6. The most antiseptic technique for preventing the transmission of diseases is handwashing.

7. The five basic guidelines for proper telephone use are good diction, pronunciation, expression, listening, and courtesy.

8. The minimum information needed for a telephone message includes name of the caller, date and time of the call, telephone number where the caller can be reached, a short description of the caller's concern, and the person to whom the message is routed.

9. Before calling emergency medical services, you should know the name, age, and sex of the patient, nature of the medical problem, type of service the physician is requesting, and any special instructions the physician may have.

 ## Websites

These websites can provide you with some additional information:

American Academy of Pediatrics
www.aap.org

American Heart Association
www.americanheart.org

CDC
www.cdc.gov

Federal Communications Commission
www.fcc.gov/cib/dro

Institute for Disabilities Research and Training
www.idrt.com

Online Yellow Pages
www.smartpages.com

OSHA
www.osha.gov

Telecommunications for the Deaf
www.amrad.org

U. S. Department of Justice/Americans with Disabilities Act
www.usdoj.gov/crt/ada

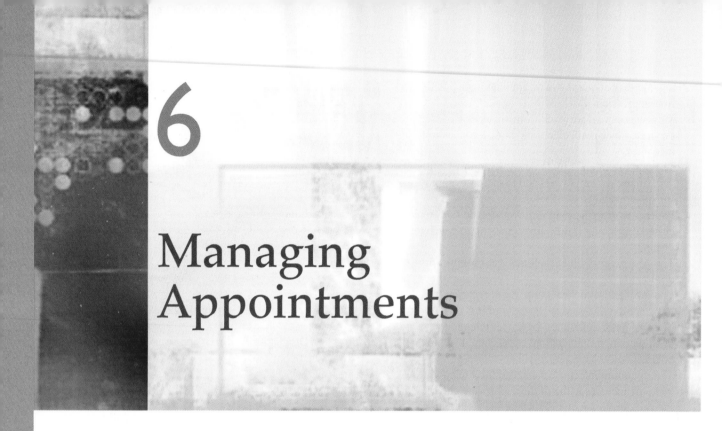

6

Managing Appointments

CHAPTER OUTLINE

ROLE DELINEATION COMPONENTS

GENERAL: Professionalism
- Display a professional manner and image
- Prioritize and perform multiple tasks
- Treat all patients with compassion and empathy

GENERAL: Communication Skills
- Use professional telephone technique
- Utilize electronic technology to receive, organize, prioritize, and transmit information
- Serve as a liaison

GENERAL: Instruction
- Explain office policies and procedures

ADMINISTRATIVE: Administrative Procedures
- Perform basic administrative medical assisting functions
- Schedule, coordinate, and monitor appointments
- Schedule inpatient/outpatient admissions and procedures
- Understand and apply third-party guidance
- Understand and adhere to managed care policies and procedures

CHAPTER COMPETENCIES

LEARNING OBJECTIVES
Upon successfully completing this chapter, you will be able to:

1. Spell and define the key terms
2. Describe the various systems for scheduling patient office visits, including manual and computerized scheduling
3. Identify the factors that affect appointment scheduling
4. Explain guidelines for scheduling appointments for new patients and return visits
5. List three ways to remind patients about appointments
6. Describe how to triage patient emergencies, acutely ill patients, and walk-in patients
7. Describe how to handle late patients and patients who miss their appointments
8. Explain what to do if the physician is delayed
9. Describe how to handle appointment cancellations made by the office or by the patient
10. Schedule an appointment for a new patient
11. Schedule a return appointment
12. Schedule a referral following third-party guidelines

KEY TERMS

acute	constellation of symptoms	precertification	streaming
buffer	consultation	providers	tickler file
chronic	double booking	referral	wave scheduling system
clustering	matrix	STAT	

RESPONSIBILITY FOR SCHEDULING and managing the flow of patient care in a medical office or clinic is one of the most important duties assigned to a medical assistant. As appointment manager, you make the first, last, and most durable impression on the patient and **providers**. Depending on your demeanor and actions, that impression can be favorable or unfavorable. A properly used appointment system helps maintain an efficient office. If improperly used, it can mean confusion and chaos; more important, it can waste precious time for the patient, the provider, and the staff.

To use the office facilities and the physician's availability most efficiently, determine which patients will be seen, when they will be seen, and how much time to allot to each of them, depending on their problems. Of course, every practice will have occasional delays and emergencies. Your responsibility is to manage all of this while maintaining a calm, efficient, and polite attitude.

APPOINTMENT SCHEDULING SYSTEMS

There are two systems of appointment scheduling for outpatient medical facilities: the manual system, which uses an appointment book, and a computerized scheduling system. The choice of systems will depend on the size of the practice, how many providers' schedules must be managed, and the preferences of the staff responsible for the daily schedule. Whether a medical office uses a manual or computerized system, many of the guidelines for effectively scheduling the workday discussed in this chapter are the same.

Manual Appointment Scheduling

Medical offices may choose to use a manual appointment scheduling system even if the other administrative functions in the office are computerized.

The Appointment Book

If your medical office uses a manual system of scheduled appointments for patient office visits, you will need an appointment book. An appointment book provides space for noting appointments for an entire year. It may have a single sheet for each day and a separate page for each provider or show an entire week on two facing pages. Some offices prefer an appointment book with pages showing only one day at a time; others may want to see a whole week at a glance. A different color page for each day may also be desired.

The more information required for scheduling, the larger the pages should be. Make sure the book has enough space for all pertinent information (e.g., patient's name, telephone number, reason for visit), is divided into time units appropriate for your practice (e.g., 10- or 15-minute intervals), can open flat on the desk where it will be used, and fits easily into its storage place when not in use.

Establishing a Matrix

Before you begin using the appointment book, you will have to set up a **matrix**. A matrix is established by crossing out times that providers are unavailable for patient visits (Fig. 6-1). For example, the physician may have a breakfast meeting and not be in the office until 10:00 A.M. This is indicated by crossing out the blocks from 8:00 to 10:00 A.M. Write in the reason for crossing off the space (e.g., vacation, meeting, hospital rounds). Some practices reserve specific times or even days for certain activities, such as physical examinations and surgery. Also, it is advisable to block off 15 to 30 minutes each morning and afternoon to accommodate emergencies, late arrivals, and other delays. Some physicians want their professional or personal obligations noted on the appointment schedule so that patients are not booked immediately before these times.

Once you have acquired and prepared an appointment book, it is not enough to schedule a time and date for a patient visit and hope everything will run smoothly. Before actually making an appointment, you should review the schedule carefully, evaluating the needs of each patient and considering the physician's preferences and availability of the office facilities. At the beginning of each day, copies of the schedule should be distributed to all staff members. Along with the notations in a patient's chart, the pages of

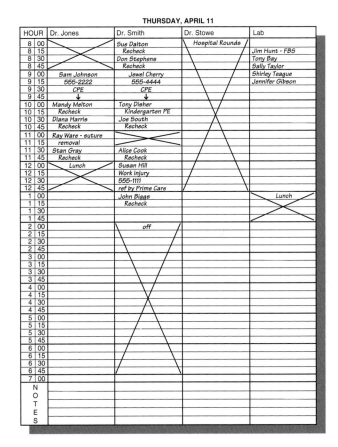

FIGURE 6-1. Sample page from manual appointment book.

```
┌─────────────────────────────────────────────────────┐
│ 5 Visual PRO/5                               _□×     │
│ Settings  Edit  Print  Help                          │
│ PRINT APPOINTMENT SCHEDULES            DATE 06/17/03  │
│ ENTER:  99-CANCEL   CR-MORE                           │
│ ─                                                     │
│           <LEONARD H. MCCOY, MD - 18-Jun-03>          │
│ Time  TOA  Patn# Patient Name       Phone#   Alt.ID#      STS.ID │
│                                                       │
│ 09:00a OV  5020 JOHNSON, CARMEN L.   336/768-5348 []      .SS   │
│ 09:00a                                                │
│ 09:15a OV  5024 JENKINS, RHONDA L.   336/768-5348 []      .SS   │
│ 09:30a OV  2030 MABE, DONNA NELSON   919/765-8912 [ ]     .SS   │
│ 09:45a OV  2056 WRIGHT, HENRY SIMON  919/765-8574 [HMO - B1] .SS │
│ 10:00a WI  2235 SMITH, ASHLEY        003/456-7889 [345]   .SS   │
│ 10:15a OV  5004 SMITH, WILLIAM       336/768-5348 []      .SS   │
│ 10:30a NP  2776 SIMPSON, MARJORIE    336/768-5348 []      .SS   │
│ 10:45a OV  5080 BUNNY, GREY          336/768-5348 []      .SS   │
│ 11:00a                                                │
│ 12:00p                                                │
│ 01:30p NP  2777 COLTRANE, COURTNEY   336/768-5348 []      .SS   │
│ 01:45p OV  2060 THOMAS, JEFFERY LEE  919/768-4110 [2060]  .SS   │
│ 01:45p WI  5024 JENKINS, RHONDA L.   336/768-5348 []      .SS   │
│                                                       │
│ — MORE —                                              │
└─────────────────────────────────────────────────────┘
```

```
┌─────────────────────────────────────────────────────┐
│ 5 Visual PRO/5                               _□×     │
│ Settings  Edit  Print  Help                          │
│ PRINT APPOINTMENT SCHEDULES            DATE 06/17/03  │
│ ENTER:  99-CANCEL   CR-MORE                           │
│ ─                                                     │
│           <LEONARD H. MCCOY, MD - 18-Jun-03>          │
│ Time  TOA  Patn# Patient Name       Phone#   Alt.ID#      STS.ID │
│                                                       │
│ 02:00p CPE  5006 EVANS, RUSSELL      336/768-5348 []      .SS   │
│ 02:15p CPE  5006 EVANS, RUSSELL      336/768-5348 []      .SS   │
│ 02:30p OV   2768 MORRISON, JAMES     336/768-5348 []      .SS   │
│ 02:45p                                                │
│ 03:00p OV   2496 BOWERS, MILLIE E    919/475-2401 [LEXNE] .SS   │
│ 03:15p NP   2778 SAMUEL, MICHAEL     336/768-5348 []      .SS   │
│ 03:45p OV   2015 CARTER, ROY LEE     919/378-2589 [HMO/AMA - B1] .SS │
│ 04:00p RC   2518 CARPENTER, PETER    919/760-0408 []      .SS   │
│ 04:10p RC   2545 ZUCKER, CELIA       910/765-8414 [12487] .SS   │
│ 04:15p                                                │
│ 04:30p OV   2038 RAGEN, ARTHUR CHARLES 919/765-8524 [MCD - B5] .SS │
│                                                       │
│ — END OF DAY —                                        │
└─────────────────────────────────────────────────────┘
```

FIGURE 6–2. A computer-generated appointment schedule with space for all providers of care. (Courtesy of MICA Information Systems, Winston-Salem, North Carolina.)

the appointment book provide documentation of a patient's visits and any changes, such as cancellations and rescheduled appointments. This provides further legal documentation to protect the physician and the patient in case of a dispute, as discussed in Chapter 2.

Computerized Appointment Scheduling

Medical management software designed to assist with administrative functions includes systems for appointment scheduling. Computerized scheduling often saves time. Information used to establish a matrix (e.g., hospital rounds 7:30–8:30, lunch 12:30–1:30) has to be entered only once.

Any medical office software will have an appointment toolbar that requires one click to add a patient, add to the waiting list, see a calendar, or search for available times. Many software packages offer an advanced search that defines the resources required for a certain type of appointment.

This quick method allows you to search for available appointment times. Typically, you enter the desired date, and the computer displays the schedule for that day, showing any available time slots. Another feature allows you to search the

appointment database for the next available time slot. For example, a patient is instructed to return in 3 months and has a preference for the time of day. You can search for the first available afternoon appointment with that particular provider.

Depending on the specific software, you can also print numerous documents, such as the daily or weekly appointment schedule, appointment reminders, or billing slips. Once the daily schedule is printed, this important document is referred to as the daily activity sheet or the day sheet and is the guide for everyone involved in the flow of patient care. Figure 6-2 shows a computer-generated daily activity sheet.

An important advantage to computerized appointment scheduling is the easy access to billing information. For example, a patient may call for an appointment, and the medical assistant can inform the patient that he needs to pay his balance due of $32 when he comes in to be seen. Credit and collections are discussed in Chapter 13.

Checkpoint Question

1. Why is a matrix established?

TYPES OF SCHEDULING

Structured Appointments

Most medical offices use a system of structured or scheduled appointments for office visits. Each patient is assigned a time on the schedule and allotted a specific period for examination and treatment. Box 6-1 shows examples of time allotment. The advantages of this system include good time management and optimum use of the office facility. Additionally, a daily schedule may be developed and charts may be prepared in advance of patient arrival.

Box 6-1

HOW MUCH TIME DO I ALLOT?

Every outpatient medical facility has variables that determine the time allotted for each service. Factors like the number of providers, the number of examination rooms, and the size of the office must be considered when establishing the appointment scheduling guidelines. This partial list of typical outpatient services shows an estimate of the time needed for each.

Service	Time
Complete physical examination	1 hour
School physical	30 minutes
Recheck	15 minutes
Dressing change	10 minutes
Blood pressure check	5 minutes
Patient teaching	30 minutes–1 hour

A disadvantage of this system is that a patient may need more of the physician's time than you have scheduled. Therefore, it is important that you ask the proper questions at the time the appointment is made to anticipate the time needed. Such questions might include "Why do you need to see the doctor?" The patient's reply will tell you how many issues will be addressed. "Do you have a form to be completed for your physical?" The answer to this question will tell you whether this is a school physical or a complete physical.

The practice of adding **buffer** time to the schedule gives extra time to accommodate emergencies, walk-ins, and other demands on the provider's daily time schedule that are not considered direct patient care. Such tasks include returning phone calls, reviewing records, and transcribing reports. For example, you may cross off 30 minutes at the beginning and end of the daily schedule to be used as a buffer.

Methods of scheduling patients include clustering, wave, modified wave, stream, and double booking.

Clustering

Clustering is grouping patients with similar problems or needs. For example, an obstetrics and gynecology practice may see all pregnant patients in the morning and other patients in the afternoon. A pediatrician may schedule vaccinations on certain days of the week. Special tests like sigmoidoscopies may be scheduled one morning a week. Advantages to clustering include maximum use of special equipment, ease in maintaining control of the schedule, the ability to provide many patients with information about their particular situation at the same time, and efficient use of employees' time.

Wave and Modified Wave

Outpatient medical facilities may use the **wave scheduling system** or modify the wave system in ways that work for their particular specialty. With the wave system, several patients are scheduled the first 30 minutes of each hour. They are seen in the order that they arrive at the office. The second half of each hour is left open. This technique works well in large facilities with several departments giving medical care. For example, several patients may arrive for a 9:00 appointment, be seen by the physician, be sent to the laboratory for blood work, and return to the physician 20 minutes later. The physician has the second part of the hour to see these patients after their testing. That second half of each hour is used as a buffer or extra time that can be used for emergencies, walk-ins, returning phone calls, and tasks other than direct patient care. Modifications to this system may include seeing new patients who will have complete physical examinations on the hour with three or four rechecks scheduled on the half hour. For example, a 75-year-old man being seen for a complete physical would be scheduled at 9:00 A.M., with a 22-year-old being seen for a follow-up of strep throat and a 6-year-old being seen for recheck of an ear infection scheduled at 9:30 A.M.

Fixed Scheduling

Fixed scheduling is the most commonly used method. It divides each hour into increments of 15, 30, 45, or 60 minutes. The reason for each patient's visit will determine the length of time assigned. Patients who are late or do not report for their appointment can cause major problems in the flow of the day. It is helpful to schedule chronically late patients at the end of the day. Another tactic is to tell the patient to arrive 30 minutes prior to the time you schedule.

Streaming

Streaming is a method that helps minimize gaps in time and backups. Appointments are given based on the needs of the individual patient. If a patient is being seen for a complete physical, 1 hour may be allotted. The next patient seen may need a blood pressure recheck, which would be allotted a 15-minute slot. Although this method ensures a smooth work flow, the medical assistant scheduling the appointment must understand the procedures and guidelines for deciding the time that should be allotted. Box 6-1 outlines examples of services and their probable time allotments.

Double Booking

With **double booking** two patients are scheduled for the same period with the same physician. This works well when patients are being sent for diagnostic testing because it leaves time to see both patients without keeping either one waiting unnecessarily.

Flexible Hours

Offices that operate with flexible hours are open at different times throughout the week. For example, Monday, Wednesday, and Friday office hours might be from 8 A.M. to 5 P.M., and Tuesday and Thursday office hours might be from 8 A.M. to 8 P.M. Some offices may also be open on Saturdays for all or part of the day. Patients still have scheduled appointments, but this greater range of available appointment times better accommodates work and family schedules. Your main challenge with flexible hours is to determine which patients really need to be scheduled for these special times. For example, Saturday appointments may be reserved only for patients whose work schedules do not permit weekday appointments. Flexible hours are most often used by clinics, group practices, and family physicians.

Open Hours

A medical office that operates with open hours for patient visits is open for specified hours during the day or evening. Patients may arrive at any time during those hours to be seen by the physician in the order of their arrival; there are no scheduled appointments. This system is commonly seen in emergency walk-in clinics and eliminates patient complaints such as "I had an appointment at 2 P.M. but had to wait until 3 P.M. to be seen." Open-hour scheduling, however, has some clear disadvantages:

- Effective time management is almost impossible.
- The facilities may be overloaded at some times and empty at other times.
- Charts must be pulled and prepared as each patient arrives.

So that patients are seen in the order in which they arrive, some offices use sign-in sheets. Some sign-in sheets require that patient's record the reason for their visit. The use of sign-in sheets is prohibited under the Health Insurance Portability and Accountability Act of 1996 regulations, as discussed in Chapter 5. Effective April 2003, sign-in sheets are considered a breach of confidentiality, since patients signing the sheet can see the names and medical conditions of other patients.

Checkpoint Question

2. What are the three systems that can be used for scheduling patient office visits?

FACTORS THAT AFFECT SCHEDULING

Patients' Needs

People express their needs in varied ways. A patient might be feeling uncertainty, embarrassment, shyness, or fear. With a patient in an emotional state, even the slightest real or imagined miscommunication can lead to negative response from the patient. Be courteous and maintain your professionalism.

Before scheduling an appointment, you should determine:

- Why the patient wishes to see the physician
- How long the patient has had the symptoms
- Whether the problem is **acute** (abrupt onset) or **chronic** (longstanding)
- The most convenient time for the patient to come in (e.g., early morning or evenings)
- Any special transportation services the patient requires (community or hospital van services operate only during certain hours)
- Whether the patient needs to see other office staff
- Any third-party payers' constraints
- Receipt of necessary documentation for referrals when the patient is enrolled in a program that requires such documentation (third-party payers are discussed further in Chapter 16)

Control of the appointment schedule is your responsibility. Strive to accommodate a patient's requests whenever possible, but not if it will overload the schedule. For example, if a patient requests a 2 P.M. appointment this Tuesday and you already have patients in that time slot, politely ex-

plain that you cannot schedule the appointment then unless you have a cancellation. You might offer a later time on Tuesday or on another day at 2 P.M.. You can also ask if the patient wishes to be put on a move-up list to be notified if an earlier appointment opens up. In other words, you control the schedule. Do not let it control you.

Providers' Preferences and Needs

The management of the practice depends on the desires and requirements of the providers working in it. Providers in a medical practice may include the physician, nurse practitioner, or physician's assistant. Some providers often run behind schedule; others are extremely punctual. Recognize your providers' habits and communicate any problems to a supervisor. The physician may allow you to adjust the schedule to accommodate his or her habits. If you are employed to assist the physician with clinical duties (e.g., removing sutures, performing electrocardiograms, giving injections), the schedule can be adjusted to accommodate a larger number of patients while still allowing the provider enough time to give each patient personal attention.

As discussed earlier, the physician also needs time to receive and return telephone calls, review laboratory and pathology reports, dictate chart notes or correspondence, and so on. If your physician is on the staff of a teaching hospital, you may also have to block off time for clinic conferences and other teaching duties.

The physician will need time to meet with unscheduled office visitors other than patients. Such visitors might include other physicians and sales representatives from medical supply or pharmaceutical companies. You should determine in advance how the physician wants you to handle these visitors. For example, the physician may want to be notified immediately if another physician comes to the office. With salespersons or pharmaceutical representatives, however, the physician may have another staff member meet with them or may request that an appointment be scheduled for a more convenient time.

Physical Facilities

The physical facilities available in the medical office will affect the management of the appointment schedule. Consider these points: How many providers use the facility? How many examination rooms are there? Is it necessary to resterilize instruments between procedures, or is more than one set of instruments available? You would not want to schedule two sigmoidoscopies at the same time, for example, if the office has only one appropriately equipped examination room. You must thoroughly understand the requirements for procedures to be performed in the office to schedule appointments accurately.

Checkpoint Question

3. What are three factors that can affect appointment scheduling?

SCHEDULING GUIDELINES

Whether the patient is making an appointment by telephone or in person, be pleasant and maintain a helpful attitude. Always write the patient's telephone number on the schedule when making appointments. Emergencies and delays are unavoidable, and schedule corrections can be made quickly if the telephone number is handy. Leave some time slots open during each day, perhaps 15 to 20 minutes in the morning and in the afternoon. Invariably problems will arise (e.g., late patients, emergencies) and disrupt the regular appointment schedule. These open blocks can allow the schedule to catch up. Also, patients calling for appointments will not appreciate being told that no time is available for 2 or 3 weeks. Open slots can be used to schedule brief appointments as needed. Procedure 6-1 describes the steps for scheduling appointments for new patients.

New Patients

Most appointments for new patients are made by telephone. The information you exchange at this encounter is crucial, and entering the patient's data accurately is imperative. The first encounter with a new patient is discussed in Procedure 6-1.

An office brochure can be mailed to the patient in advance of the appointment. Some offices send new-patient forms to be filled out and brought in at the appointment. When scheduling an appointment for a new patient, follow these guidelines:

1. Allow an adequate amount of time for the appointment. To do so, obtain as much information as possible from the patient:
   • Full name and correct spelling
   • Mailing address
   • Day and evening telephone numbers
   • Reason for the visit
   • Name of the referring physician or individual
   • Responsible party and third party payer (insurance plan)
2. Explain the office's payment policy. Most offices require full or partial payment at the time of an initial visit, and patients must understand this policy. Instruct patients to bring all pertinent insurance information.
3. Be sure patients know your office location; if needed, give them concise directions. You may also want to tell patients how long they can expect to be at the office.
4. Some patients are sensitive about messages left on an answering machine or given to a coworker. To avoid violating confidentiality, ask the patient if it is permissible to call at home or at work and include this information in the patient's chart.
5. Before ending the call, confirm the time and date of the appointment. You might say, "Thank you for calling Mr. Brown. We look forward to seeing you on Tuesday, December 10, at 2 P.M."

6. Always check your appointment system or book to be sure that you have placed the appointment on the correct day in the right time slot.
7. If the patient was referred by another physician, you may need to call that physician's office in advance of the appointment for copies of laboratory work, radiology and pathology reports, and so on. Remember, the patient must give authorization to release medical documents (see Chapter 8). Give these reports to the physician prior to the patient's appointment.

Established Patients

Established patients will be given return appointments when necessary. Most return appointments are made before the patient leaves the office. Procedure 6-2 describes the steps for scheduling a return appointment.

When making a return appointment, follow these guidelines:

1. Carefully check your appointment book or screen before offering an appointment time. If a specific examination, test, or x-ray is to be performed on the return visit, avoid scheduling two patients for the same examination at the same time.
2. Offer the patient a specific time and date. For example, you might say, "Mrs. Hernandez, I have next Tuesday, the 15th, available at 3:30 P.M." (Avoid asking the patient when he or she would like to return, as this can elicit indecision.) If the offered appointment is not convenient, offer another specific time and date.
3. Write the patient's name and telephone number in the appointment book or enter in the information on the appointment screen.
4. Transfer the pertinent information to an appointment card and give it to the patient. Computerized systems print an appointment card. Repeat aloud the appointment day, date, and time to the patient as you hand over the card (Fig. 6-3).

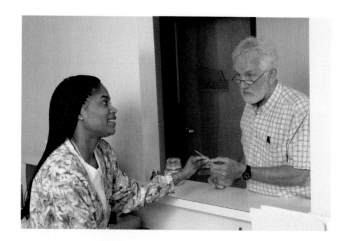

FIGURE 6–3. Photograph of a medical assistant handing a patient an appointment card.

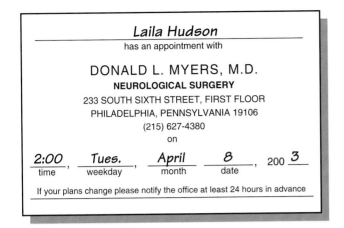

Laila Hudson
has an appointment with

DONALD L. MYERS, M.D.
NEUROLOGICAL SURGERY
233 SOUTH SIXTH STREET, FIRST FLOOR
PHILADELPHIA, PENNSYLVANIA 19106
(215) 627-4380
on

2:00 , Tues. , April 8 , 200 3
time   weekday   month   date

If your plans change please notify the office at least 24 hours in advance

F I G U R E 6 – 4 . Sample reminder postcard.

5. Double-check your book or screen to be sure you have not made an error.
6. End your conversation with a pleasant word and a smile.

PREPARING A DAILY OR WEEKLY SCHEDULE

In most offices, as medical assistant you are responsible for preparing a daily and weekly schedule of appointments. Make a copy for the providers and other office staff members. When there are changes in the schedule, ensure that corrections are made on all copies. Place the next day's schedule on the physician's desk before he or she leaves for the day. Give the next week's schedule to the physician before he or she leaves on Friday. Schedules should include not only patients' appointments but also hospital rounds, surgeries, meetings, and any personal engagements on the schedule. Computer systems print a daily or weekly schedule, but you must remember to make changes manually as the day progresses.

PATIENT REMINDERS

Offices use various kinds of reminders to tell a patient about an appointment that should be made or to remind them that an appointment has been made on a specific date and time. These reminders are the appointment card, the telephone call, and the mailed card.

Appointment Cards

An appointment card is given to the patient when he or she leaves the office. It should have the following information:

- Patient's name
- Day, date, and time of the return visit
- Physician's name and telephone number

If the patient requires a series of appointments, try to make them on the same day of the week and at the same time of day. This will make it easier for the patient to remember the appointments. Unless your appointment card allows you to list the complete series of appointments, however, give the patient a card for the next appointment only and repeat this procedure after each subsequent visit. When the patient has to save several cards, they can easily be lost or cause confusion. If using a manual system, write on the card with ink so that it cannot be altered. Computer appointment scheduling software provides appointment cards that can be printed on special perforated paper.

Telephone Reminders

All new patients and patients with appointments scheduled in advance should receive a telephone reminder the day before their appointment. Computer systems can place the call to the programmed number and remind the patient of the appointment with a prerecorded message. Remember, do not call a patient at work or leave a message unless you have been given permission to do so. Make the telephone reminder simple. Identify your office, yourself, and state the date and time of the appointment. For example, you might say, "This is Ms. Palmer from Dr. Reid's office. I'm calling to confirm your appointment for tomorrow, Thursday, February 10, at 3:30 P.M." Unless the patient has a question, then say, "Thank you and good-bye." This reminder helps jog the patient's memory, and if the patient must cancel or reschedule an appointment, you will have time to fill the slot. Keep a list with the names and phone numbers of patients who have asked to be called or who need to be seen sooner than their next appointment. This list may be called a cancellation list, a waiting list, or a move-up list. Make a notation on the appointment schedule, such as confirmed, left message, or no answer.

Box 6-2

A TICKLER FILE CAN TICKLE YOUR MEMORY

A **tickler file** helps remind you to do something by a certain time in the future. It can be something as simple as a card file box (like a recipe box) or an accordion folder with insert guides in chronological order. The guides may be in weekly or monthly divisions. Put patient appointment reminder cards in the appropriate location in the file. Check the file each week or month, depending on the divisions, then mail the reminders.

Medical office computer software often offers help with patient reminders. With a search of the database, a report of every female patient over age 50, for example, could be generated. Some systems even generate patient reminders based on preprogrammed criteria.

Mailed Reminder Cards

Some offices send reminder cards instead of making phone calls. Reminder cards are also used to remind patients who could not be reached by phone that it is time to keep an upcoming scheduled appointment. These should be mailed at least a week before the date of the appointment. In addition, reminder cards are sent after a set period since a patient's last appointment. Reminder cards are often used to alert patients to the need for annual examinations (e.g., Pap smears, mammograms, prostate examinations).

To handle this kind of reminder, keep a supply of preprinted postcards in the office (Fig. 6-4). The cards should have a simple one- or two-sentence message, such as, "According to our records, you are due for your annual physical. If you would kindly call the office, we will be glad to arrange an appointment for you." The physician's name, address, and telephone number should be printed on the card. Place the card in a tickler file (Box 6-2) and mail it at the appropriate time. Some medical management software packages produce a list that can be used to alert patients of necessary services.

Checkpoint Question

4. What are the three types of patient reminders?

ADAPTING THE SCHEDULE

Emergencies

When a patient calls with an emergency (Fig. 6-5) , your first responsibility is to determine whether the problem can be treated in the office. The office should have a policy for evaluation of the situation. The word **STAT** is used in the medical field to indicate that something should be done immediately (Box 6-3). You also should have a list of appropriate questions to ask the patient, such as "Are you having chest pain? Are you having difficulty breathing? How long

FIGURE 6–5.   Patient at home making an emergency call.

Box 6-3

WHEN DOES THE PATIENT NEED TO BE SEEN NOW?

When the patient calls with any of the following complaints:

- Shortness of breath
- Severe chest pain
- Uncontrollable bleeding
- Large open wounds
- Potential accidental poisoning
- Bleeding in a pregnant patient

- Injury to a pregnant patient
- Shock
- Serious burns
- Severe bleeding
- Any symptoms of internal bleeding (dark, tarry stools; discoloration of the skin)

Note: Remember to check with the physician for proper procedures concerning triage.

---

have you had the symptoms?" (Box 6-4). When several symptoms occur together, they may indicate a particular problem. This group of complaints is referred to as a **constellation of symptoms**. One group of symptoms found to indicate a certain disorder is severe right lower quadrant pain, nausea, and fever. A physician who sees this constellation of symptoms considers appendicitis.

Patients Who Are Acutely Ill

Patients who are acutely ill often have serious though not life-threatening conditions. These patients need to be seen as soon as possible but not necessarily on that same day. Obtain as much information about the patient's medical problem as you can so your message to the physician will allow him or her to decide how soon the patient should be seen. Place the chart with a note in the location selected by the physician, and tell the patient you will call back as soon as the physician makes a decision.

Walk-in Patients

Walk-in patients are those who arrive at the office without a scheduled appointment and expect to see the physician that day. Typically, the physician will have a set protocol, or prescribed list of steps, for handling such situations. In general, you must first determine the reason for the walk-in. Patients with medical emergencies need to be seen immediately. Other patients can be asked to have a seat in the waiting room while you inform the physician of the patient's presence. The physician can then make the decision to see the patient or not.

If the patient is to be seen, explain that you will work him or her into the schedule as soon as possible for a brief examination. When the patient leaves the office, you might apol-

COULD IT BE A HEART ATTACK?

When a patient calls complaining of the following constellation of symptoms, you should assume that this is a potential heart attack:

- Shortness of breath
- Arm or neck pain
- Chest pain
- Nausea and/or vomiting

Studies have shown that in women, early symptoms of a heart attack are different from those in men. These symptoms include jaw, neck, and back pain and severe fatigue. Keep this in mind when questioning the patient.

Call 911 and stay on the line with the patient. Do not advise the patient to drive to the hospital. Follow office policies for such an emergency.

ogize for the delay, then ask the patient to schedule an appointment for the next visit.

If the physician decides not to see a walk-in patient, you will have to ask the patient to schedule an appointment and to return later.

Late Patients

Patients who are late cause problems in the schedule. You should gently but firmly apologize for any delay but tell the patient, "You were late and Dr. Wooten is seeing another patient now. The doctor should be able to see you in about 15 minutes." Patients who are routinely late should be politely advised that "according to our office policy, patients who are more than 15 minutes late will have to be rescheduled." Some offices have found that scheduling the habitually late patient at the end of the day is helpful. In addition, ask patients to call the office if they know ahead of time they are going to be late.

Physician Delays

Of course, sometimes the physician calls in to say he or she has been delayed and will be in the office later. If office hours have not yet begun, call patients with appointments scheduled early, and give them the option of coming in later in the day or rescheduling the appointment for another day. If patients are waiting in the office, inform them immediately if the physician will be delayed. For example, you might say, "Dr. Franklin has been delayed and will probably be 20 to 30 minutes late. Would you like to wait, or would you prefer to reschedule for another time?" Always keep your patients informed; most people will understand if they know you have not ignored or forgotten them. Most patients appreciate the fact that the physician would also be available to them in an emergency. If you reschedule an appointment, note in the patient's chart the reason for the cancellation or rescheduling.

Missed Appointments

A missed appointment, or no-show, occurs when a patient neglects to keep an appointment and does not notify the office. When this happens, call the patient to try to determine why the appointment was missed and to reschedule for another time. If you are unable to reach the patient by telephone, send a card asking the patient to call the office to reschedule. Note in the patient's chart the missed appointment and that you have either rescheduled the appointment or mailed a card to schedule another appointment. Even if the facility does not routinely remind patients of appointments, be sure to call and remind habitually late patients the day before the appointment.

Continued failure to keep appointments should be brought to the attention of the physician, who may want to call the patient personally (particularly if the patient is seriously ill) or send a letter expressing concern for the patient's welfare. In extreme cases, the physician may choose to terminate the physician–patient relationship. See Chapter 2 for the proper procedure for this action. Notations of all actions and copies of any letters sent to the patient should become a permanent part of the individual's medical record. Box 6-5 is a sample of a chart note.

CANCELLATIONS

Cancellations by the Office

You may have to cancel a patient's appointment if the physician is ill, has an emergency, or has personal time off. Patients who must be rescheduled need not be told the specific reason for the physician's absence. These cancellations should be noted in the patient's medical record.

When you have advance notice, write a letter to patients with appointments you must cancel, indicating that the physician will be away from the office but will return by a certain date. Patients should be alerted to cancellations a week before their appointments. Ask the patient to call the office to reschedule. If you have to cancel on the day of the appointment, call the patient and explain. For example, you

CHARTING EXAMPLE

05/12/03–1530

Mrs. Parrish was called regarding missing scheduled appointment for today at 9:30 A.M. Patient said she forgot about the appointment. Appointment was rescheduled for 05/14/03 at 10:00 A.M. Patient was advised of the need to have regular prenatal checkups. Patient verbalized understanding. Dr. Wong was notified that appointment was missed and rescheduled.—Norreen Brooks, CMA might say, "Dr. Flora has been called out of the office unexpectedly. Would it be convenient to reschedule your appointment for sometime next week?" If the patient arrives at the office before you can contact him or her, apologize and politely explain the situation. Most patients will be understanding. When a physician is unavailable for an extended period, another physician must cover the practice or be on call. Everyone in the office should have a list of names and addresses of on-call physicians, and you should give this information to your patients, according to your office policy. When a locum tenens, or substitute physician, is employed, the office appointments will not be interrupted (see Chapter 2).

Cancellations by the Patient

When a patient cancels an appointment, ask the reason for the cancellation and mark it on your appointment schedule and in the patient's chart. Offer to reschedule at another time. If the patient is being seen for a continuing problem, be sure he or she understands the necessity for the follow-up visit. If the patient wants to call back for an appointment, make a note to yourself to check on the call-back in a few days. If a patient cancels appointments frequently, bring this to the physician's attention.

If a patient cancels an appointment and you have a full schedule, no action is needed. If your schedule is light, however, refer to your move-up list to try to fill the vacancy.

MAKING APPOINTMENTS FOR PATIENTS IN OTHER FACILITIES

Referrals and Consultations

When the provider requests assistance from another physician in **consultation** or makes a **referral** to another physician for the patient, make certain that the referral meets the requirements of any third-party payers. Managed care companies like HMOs have strict requirements regarding **precertification** and documentation for referrals to specialists and other facilities. (See Chapter 16.) Be sure the physician you are calling is on the preferred provider list for the patient's insurance company. Patients should be given a choice when being referred to a specialist.

When calling another physician's office for an appointment for your patient (Procedure 6-3), provide the following information:

- Physician's name and telephone number
- Patient's name, address, and telephone number
- Reason for the referral
- Degree of urgency
- Whether the patient is being sent for consultation or referral (see Box 6-6 for an explanation of the terms referral and consultation)

Box 6-6

REFERRAL OR CONSULTATION?

It is important to know the difference between a referral and a consultation. According to the coding guidelines in the *Current Procedural Coding Terminology*, a consultation is a request for the opinion of a colleague. A letter is provided to the referring physician by the consultant and contains the consulting physician's impression and recommendations for the patient, but the patient returns to the referring physician for treatment. For example, an orthopedist may send a patient with rheumatoid arthritis to a rheumatologist for medication management, but the orthopedist will continue the patient's care based on the rheumatologist's recommendations.

A referral usually involves a specialist and requires that the patient's care be transferred to that specialist. For example, a patient may see a physician for an ingrown toenail but be referred to a podiatrist for care.

Record in the patient's chart the time and date of the call and the person who received your call. Tell the person you are calling that you wish to be notified if your patient does not keep the appointment. If this occurs, be sure to tell the physician and enter this information in the patient's record.

Write the name, address, and telephone number of the referral doctor on your office stationery and include the date and time of the appointment. Give or mail this information to your patient. The patient may call the referring physician to make his or her own appointment. If this is the situation, ask the patient to call you with the appointment date and document it in the chart.

Diagnostic Testing

Sometimes, patients are sent for diagnostic testing or treatment at another facility. Such testing includes laboratory tests, radiology, computed tomography, magnetic resonance imaging, and nuclear medicine studies. These appointments are usually made while the patient is still in the office. Before scheduling, determine the exact test or tests the physician requires and how soon the results are needed. (Be sure to indicate to the facility if the results are needed immediately, or STAT.) Also, check with the patient for any time restrictions he or she may have. Give the facility the patient's name, address, telephone number, the exact test or tests required, and any other special instructions from the physician. Give the patient a laboratory or x-ray referral slip with the time and date of the appointment and the name, address, and telephone number of the outside facility.

Some laboratory studies or x-ray tests require advance preparation by the patient. Give your patient a written and verbal explanation of the required preparation, and be sure he or she understands the importance of following the instructions. On the patient's chart, note the name of the outside facility and the date and time of the appointment. Also place a reminder in your tickler file or on your appointment schedule to be sure the test results are received as requested.

Surgery

You also assist with the scheduling of procedures in a hospital operating room or an outpatient surgical facility. Determine the patient's need for precertification with the insurance carrier. You may have to call the number on the back of the patient's insurance card for a precertification number. Call the participating facility chosen by the patient and specify the time and date the physician has requested. The operating facility will need to know the exact procedure, the amount of time needed, the type of anesthesia required, and any other special instructions your physician may have. The facility will also need the patient's name, age, address, telephone number, insurance information, and the precertification number if required.

If the hospital has supplied your office with preadmission forms, give a copy to the patient and make sure he or she understands the need to complete and return the form in a timely manner. Follow the policies of the surgical facility regarding preadmission testing, which may include laboratory studies, x-rays, or autologous blood donation (donation of a person's own blood in advance). Write down all appointment dates, times, and locations for the patient and be certain he or she understands where to go and when.

Finally, note in the patient's record the name of the operating facility and the date and time the surgery is scheduled. You may also need to arrange for hospital admission by providing the same information to the hospital admitting department.

Ñ Spanish Terminology

¿A qué se debe su visita?	Why do you need to see the doctor?
¿Desde cuándo se siente mal?	How long has this being going on?
¿Prefiere la cita en la mañana o en la tarde?	Would you prefer morning or afternoon?
Llamo para recordarle su cita.	I am calling to remind you of your appointment.
Le daré una cita para que vea al Doctor nuevamente.	I will give you an appointment to return to see the doctor.
Para su próxima visita, por favor traiga su tarjeta del seguro y todas las medicinas que esté tomando.	Please bring your insurance card and medicine bottles with you for your appointment.

Días de la semana	Days of the week	Horas del día	Times of the Day
Domingo	Sunday	A la una	One o'clock
Lunes	Monday	El medio pasado uno	1:30
Martes	Tuesday	Dos en punto	2:00
Miércoles	Wednesday	Son las dos y media	2:30
Jueves	Thursday	Tres en punto	3:00
Viernes	Friday	Son las tres y media	3:30
Sábado	Saturday	Siete en punto	7:00
		Son las siete y media	7:30
		Ocho en punto	8:00
		Son las ocho y media	8:30
		Nueve en punto	9:00
		Son las nueve y media	9:30

Checkpoint Question

5. What information should be readily available when calling to schedule a patient for surgery in another facility?

WHEN THE APPOINTMENT SCHEDULE DOES NOT WORK

No appointment schedule runs smoothly all the time, and an occasional glitch is to be expected. If, however, you find that your schedule is chaotic nearly every day, you should determine the cause. Evaluate the schedule over time, generally 2 to 3 months. For example, make a list of all patients seen, their arrival times, the amount of time they spent with the physician, the time they left, and the amount of time needed to perform each examination or treatment. Since the work flow of the office affects every staff member, involve all employees in your study.

Office meetings are an ideal way to identify scheduling problems. Your evaluation may reveal that many of your patients are arriving late or that you have not allotted enough time for certain procedures. Sometimes, a habitually delayed physician is the problem. You may find that too many staff people are making appointments. If this is the case, you can assign only one staff person to handle all scheduling. Some problems may never be completely solved. If they are identified, however, you can often make adjustments to avoid causing frustration for both patients and office personnel.

Procedure 6-1

Making an Appointment for a New Patient

Steps	Reason
1. Obtain as much information as possible from the patient, such as: • Full name and correct spelling • Mailing address (not all offices require this) • Day and evening telephone numbers • Reason for the visit • Name of the referring person	To stay on schedule, you must allow enough time for the appointment. This information will help determine appointment needs and save time at the first visit.
2. Explain the payment policy of the practice. Most offices require payment at the time of an initial visit. Instruct patients to bring all pertinent insurance information.	Patients must understand this policy if they are to follow it
3. Be sure patients know your office location; give concise directions if needed. You may also want to give patients an idea of how long they can expect to be at the office.	Helps patients arrive on time and lets them budget their time.
4. To avoid violating confidentiality, ask the patient if it is permissible to call at home or at work.	Some patients are sensitive about messages left on an answering machine or given to a coworker.
5. Before ending the call, confirm the time and date of the appointment. Say, "Thank you for calling, Mr. Brown. We look forward to seeing you on Tuesday, December 10, at 2 P.M."	Repeating the appointment time will ensure that effective communication has taken place and increase the likelihood that the patient will be there on time.
6. Always check your appointment book to be sure that you have placed the appointment on the correct day in the right time slot.	Failure to record every appointment in the proper location can cause overbooking, frustrated physicians and staff, and irate patients.
7. If the patient was referred by another physician, you may have to call that physician's office before the appointment for copies of laboratory work, radiology and pathology reports, and so on. Remember, the patient must give authorization to release medical documents (see Chapter 8). Give this information to the physician prior to the patient's appointment.	Having the necessary information will eliminate ordering of tests that have already been done and will give the physician the tools to care for the patient.

Procedure 6-2

Making an Appointment for an Established Patient

Steps	Reason
1. Determine what will be done at the return visit. Check your appointment book or computer system before offering an appointment.	If a specific examination, test, or scan is to be performed, you will want to avoid scheduling two patients for the same examination at the same time.
2. Offer the patient a specific time and date. Avoid asking the patient when he or she would like to return, as this can cause indecision.	Give the patient a choice, and if neither time is convenient, offer another specific time and date. Giving a patient a choice is good practice. "Mrs. Chang, we can see you next Tuesday, the 15th, at 3:30 P.M. or Wednesday, the 16th, at 9:00 A.M."
3. Write the patient's name and telephone number in the appointment book or enter it in the computer.	Writing the phone number in the appointment book or making a notation in the computer will give you a quick reference if you need to call the patient to change the appointment.
4. Transfer the pertinent information to an appointment card and give it to the patient. Repeat aloud the appointment day, date, and time to the patient as you hand over the card (Fig. 6-4).	Repeating the information reinforces the patient's memory and helps ensure that the appointment will be kept.
5. Double-check your book or computer to be sure you have not made an error.	Errors in appointments waste the patient's, staff's, and physician's time.
6. Whether in person or on the phone, end your conversation with a pleasant word and a smile.	A smile always feels good to a patient who may be apprehensive about needing to return to the doctor.

Procedure 6-3

Making an Appointment for a Referral to Another Provider

Steps	Reason
1. Make certain that the requirements of any third-party payers are met.	Some third-party payers require that referrals be precertified. Preexisting conditions may not be covered for referral. Most companies require that only the patient's primary care physician (PCP) or gatekeeper make referrals. It is important to research each situation. Telephone numbers for precertification and questions will be printed on the back of the insurance card.
2. Refer to the preferred provider list for the patient's insurance company. Allow the patient to choose a provider from the list.	Managed care companies have strict requirements for precertification and documentation for referrals (see Chapter 16). If there is more than one provider with the same qualifications, the patient should always be given a choice.
3. Have the following information available when you make the call: • Physician's name and telephone number • Patient's name, address, and telephone number • Reason for the call • Degree of urgency • Whether the patient is being sent for consultation or referral	The referred or consulting physician's office needs to know these things to serve the patient well.
4. Record in the patient's chart the time and date of the call and the name of the person who received your call.	This is necessary for proper documentation of the patient's care.
5. Tell the person you are calling that you wish to be notified if your patient does not keep the appointment. If this occurs, be sure to tell your physician and enter this information in the patient's record.	This is necessary for proper documentation of the patient's care.
6. Write down the name, address, and telephone number of the doctor you are referring your patient to and include the date and time of the appointment. Give or mail this information to your patient.	It is important that the patient have a reminder so the appointment will be kept.
7. If the patient is to call the referring physician to make the appointment, ask the patient to call you with the appointment date, then document this in the chart.	Recording the appointment information in the patient's chart completes the transaction and proves that the physician's order was carried out.

CHAPTER SUMMARY

The outpatient medical facility can be chaos without an efficient appointment system. Moving patients through the facility while treating each person equally and thoroughly is one of the biggest challenges in the medical office. It is difficult for a busy practice to run smoothly all of the time. You need structure, but you must be flexible. Available times, equipment and room usage, and personnel coverage must be considered when finding just the right formula for a well-run and efficient office.

The goals of the outpatient medical facility are to provide quality patient care and maintain financial stability. To reach those goals, an office must have a plan for the efficient scheduling and carrying out of the daily activities. Appointment scheduling systems include manual systems using appointment books and computerized systems that render helpful reports and daily activity sheets. The size of a practice, the number of physicians, the types of services, and so on are considered when establishing an appointment scheduling system. Sick patients calling to make appointments should be given priority, and there are established guidelines for determining the urgency of a patient's problem. Other functions, such as phone calls, reviewing records, and lunch breaks, are also scheduled into the daily activities of the office. An established protocol or list of steps should be in place to handle pharmaceutical representatives and other visitors to the office. As the medical assistant at the front desk, you will be one of the most important factors in the daily operation of the outpatient medical facility. As a medical assistant, you will make appointments, document encounters with patients that deal with appointments, and make referrals to other health care facilities. Learning the issues involved in successful appointment scheduling will help you make sure your facility runs smoothly.

Critical Thinking Challenges

1. Assume that you are the office manager in a physician's office. Create a policy and procedure for scheduling patients.
2. Sign-in sheets can cause a breach in patient confidentiality. What other methods could you use that would limit the potential for invasion of patient privacy?
3. You notice that patients typically wait 30 to 45 minutes past their scheduled appointment times because of the physician. How would you approach a physician who chronically runs late?

Answers to Checkpoint Questions

1. A matrix is established to indicate times of each day that are not available for patient appointments.
2. The three systems that can be used for patient office visits include scheduled appointments, flexible hours, and open hours.
3. The three factors that can affect scheduling are patients' needs, physicians' preferences, and the physical facilities.
4. The three types of reminders are appointment cards, telephone reminders, and mailed reminder cards.
5. When scheduling a patient for surgery, the following information is needed: demographic and insurance information, the patient's name, age, address, telephone number, precertification number (if required), diagnosis, surgery planned, and any special instructions.

7

Written Communications

CHAPTER OUTLINE

ROLE DELINEATION COMPONENTS

GENERAL: Communication Skills
- Adapt communications to individual's ability to understand
- Recognize and respond effectively to verbal, nonverbal, and written communications
- Utilize electronic technology to receive, organize, prioritize, and transmit information

GENERAL: Legal Concepts
- Perform within legal and ethical boundaries

ADMINISTRATIVE: Administrative Procedures
- Perform basic administrative medical assisting functions

CHAPTER COMPETENCIES

LEARNING OBJECTIVES

Upon successfully completing this chapter, you will be able to:
1. Spell and define the key terms
2. Discuss the basic guidelines for grammar, punctuation, and spelling
3. Describe six key guidelines for medical writing
4. Discuss the eleven key components of a business letter
5. Describe the three steps to writing a business letter
6. Describe the process of writing a memorandum
7. Discuss the various mailing options
8. Identify the types of incoming written communication seen in a physician's office
9. List the items that must be included in an agenda
10. Identify the items that must be included when typing minutes

PERFORMANCE OBJECTIVES

Upon completing this chapter, you will be able to:
1. Write a business letter
2. Write a memorandum
3. Address and send written communication
4. Open and sort mail

KEY TERMS

agenda	enclosure	margin	salutation
annotation	font	memorandum	semiblock
BiCaps	full block	proofread	template
block	intercaps		

THE ABILITY TO WRITE WELL IS an important skill for medical assistants. Your written communication must be clear, concise, and correct. Poorly written documents reflect negatively both on the physician's practice and on you. You will be responsible for creating and handling many types of written communication. Examples of written communication include letters, consultation reports, agendas, and minutes from meetings. Written communication may be sent or received through the postal service, facsimile machines, or electronic mail. This chapter discusses guidelines for professional writing, letter development, memorandum writing, sending written communication, handling incoming mail, and composing agendas and minutes.

PROFESSIONAL WRITING

Professional writing is different from writing letters to your friends or family members. The goal of professional writing is get information communicated in a concise, accurate, and comprehensible manner. Slang or idiomatic terms that are commonly used in writing letters to friends are not appropriate for business letters. For example, "Drop by and say hi" is not suitable for a professional letter, even if you know the recipient personally.

Basic Grammar and Punctuation Guidelines

Grammatical rules seem to be an endless maze of twists and turns! And each rule comes with numerous exceptions. You must be familiar with these rules and be able to apply them to your writing. Key rules of punctuation and grammar are listed in Box 7-1.

Basic Spelling Guidelines

Good spelling skills take time to acquire. Box 7-2 gives you basic tips for spelling. Many words sound exactly alike but are spelled differently and have different meanings. Be very careful with these words. Which of the following sentences has a spelling error?

- Wound cultures were taken from the left lower leg site.
- Wound cultures were taken from the left lower leg cite.

The first sentence is correct. Site and cite sound alike, and both are spelled correctly, but in the second sentence, the wrong word was used. These types of errors occur as a result of poor word usage and poor spelling. Appendix E lists words that are most likely to be misused or misspelled.

Guidelines for Medical Writing

Writing letters to medical professionals follows many of the standard guidelines. There are, however, some specific guidelines about which you need to be aware. They are discussed next.

Box 7-1

BASIC GRAMMAR AND PUNCTUATION TIPS

Punctuation
- Period (.)—Used at end of sentences and following abbreviations.
- Comma (,)—Used to separate words or phrases that are part of a series of three or more. The final comma before the "and" may be omitted. A comma can also be used after a long introductory clause or to separate independent clauses joined by and, but, yet, or, and nor.
- Semicolon (;)—Used to separate a long list of items in a series and to separate independent clauses not joined by a conjunction (e.g., and, but, or).
- Colon (:)—Used to introduce a series of items, to follow formal salutations, and to separate the hours from minutes indicating time.
- Apostrophe (')—Used to denote omissions of letters and to denote the possessive case of nouns.
- Quotation marks (" ")—Used to set off spoken dialogue, some titles (e.g., journal articles, newspaper articles, television and radio program episodes), and words used in a special way.
- Parentheses [( )]—Used to indicate a part of a sentence that is not part of the main sentence but is essential for the meaning of the sentence. Also used to enclose a number, for confirmation, that is spelled out in a sentence.
- Ellipsis (. . .)—Used in place of a period to indicate a prolonged continuation of a conversation or list. Also used to display individual items or to connect phrases that are loosely connected.
- Diagonal (/)—Used in abbreviations (c/o), dates (2003/2004), fractions (3/4), and to indicate two or more options (AM/FM).

Sentence Structure
- Avoid long, run-on sentences.
- A verb must always agree with its subject in number and person.
- Ensure that the proper pronoun (he or she) is used.
- Adjectives should be used when they add an important message. Don't overuse adjectives or adverbs. Remember, double negatives used in one sentence make the sentence positive.

Capitalization
- Capitalize the first word in a sentence, proper nouns, the pronoun "I," book titles, and known geographical names.
- Names of persons, holidays, and trademark items should be capitalized.
- Expressions of time (a.m. and p.m.) should not be capitalized.

Box 7-2

BASIC SPELLING TIPS

When in doubt about the spelling of a word, always use a dictionary or a spell check. Keep in mind that a computer spell check will check for spelling but will not alert you to inappropriate word usage.

- Remember this rhyme: I comes before e, except after c, or when sounded like a as in neighbor and weigh. Examples: achieve, receive. (The exceptions are either, neither, weird, leisure, and conscience.)
- Words ending in -ie drop the e and change the i to y before adding -ing. Examples: die, dying; lie, lying.
- Words ending in -o that are preceded by a vowel are made plural by adding s. Example: studio, studios; trio, trios. Words ending in o that are preceded by a consonant form the plural by adding es. Examples: potato, potatoes; hero, heroes.
- Words ending in -y preceded by a vowel form the plural by adding s. Examples: attorney, attorneys; day, days. Words ending in -y that are preceded by a consonant change the y to i and add es. Examples: berry, berries; lady, ladies.
- The final consonant of a one-syllable word is doubled before adding a suffix beginning with a vowel. Examples: run, running; pin, pinning. If the final consonant is preceded by another consonant or by two vowels, do not double the consonant. Examples: look, looked; act, acting.
- Words ending in a silent -e generally drop the e before adding a suffix beginning with a vowel. Examples: ice, icing; judge, judging. The exceptions are dye, eye, shoe, and toe. The e is not dropped, however, in suffixes beginning with a consonant unless another vowel precedes the final e. Examples: pale, paleness; argue, argument.
- For all words ending in -c, insert a k before adding a suffix beginning with e, i, or y. Examples: picnic, picnicking; traffic, trafficker.

Accuracy

Many of the medical documents or letters that you will write contain information that requires precision, accuracy, and careful attention to details. Inaccurate information in some letters can lead to injury of a patient and lawsuits and can harm the physician's practice. Some of your letters will be placed in the patient's permanent medical record. Most letters will start with the physician asking you to draft a letter. He may or may not give you some notes to follow. Either way, your responsibility in typing the letter is to be as accurate as possible and to question anything about which you are unsure. Here are some examples of inaccuracy:

- You wrote, "The patient was started on the MVP chemotherapy regimen." The physician, however, had written "MVPP." These are two completely different regimens. MVP is used for treating lung cancer, and MVPP is used for Hodgkin's lymphoma.
- The physician wrote, "Patient was told to take Dristan Cold tablets." You rearranged the sentence, however, and wrote "The patient had a cold and was told to take Dristan tablets." Dristan Cold contains an antihistamine medication that plain Dristan does not. Never edit a physician's sentence unless you are sure that it will not affect the meaning.
- The physician wrote, "There is no reason for him to start radiation therapy at this time." You wrote, however, "There is reason for him to start radiation therapy at this time." The simple elimination of the word "no" completely changes the meaning of the sentence and can lead to errors in patient care.
- The physician wrote, "Hospitalization is needed because the patient continues to be violent." You typed, however, "Hospitalization is needed because the patient continues to be violet." The meaning of the sentence has been changed by the elimination of one "n" in violent.

 Checkpoint Question

1. What are three consequences that could arise from inaccurate information in a business letter?

Spelling

Spell check in word processing programs can be a great asset, but it has limitations. Medical terminology spell check software should be added to your computer and be updated frequently.

You can add medical terms into your computer's spell check dictionary, but make sure that any word you add is spelled correctly! Spell checks can never be 100% stocked with all the needed terms, especially in the medical profession, as new technologies, medications, and treatments arise daily. Remember, spell check will not recognize words that are spelled correctly but misused. Which of the following sentences has a spelling error?

- The patient's mucus was yellow.
- The patient's mucous was yellow.

Mucus (noun) refers to a sticky secretion. Mucous is a type of membrane that secretes mucus. The second sentence is wrong. Here is another example:

- The physician received a plague.
- The physician received a plaque.

There is a big difference between plaque (commemorative item) and plague (bacterial disease)! Box 7-3 lists some commonly used medical words that can easily be misspelled or misused.

Box 7-3

COMMONLY MISUSED OR MISSPELLED MEDICAL TERMS

- anoxia and anorexia
- aphagia and aphasia
- bowl and bowel
- emphysema and empyema
- fundus and fungus
- lactose and lactase
- metatarsals and metacarpals
- mucus and mucous
- parental and parenteral
- postnatal and postnasal
- pubic and pubis
- rubella and rubeola
- serum and sebum
- uvula and vulva

Capitalization

Pay particular attention to how words, names, and abbreviations are capitalized. Words or phrases with unusual capitalization are called **intercaps** or **BiCaps**. Never change how a word is capitalized unless directed to do so. Ask for clarification and mark the proof letter with a question mark for the physician to answer. For example m-BACOD is a very different medication regimen from M-BACOD. Here are some other common medical intercaps: pH, RhoGam, rPA, ReoPro, aVR.

Abbreviations and Symbols

Abbreviations and symbols can save time in long handwriting and with typing. Use abbreviations sparingly. When typing professional letters, you should spell out all abbreviations that are not universally accepted (e.g., P.M.). Become familiar with the abbreviations and symbols that are used where you work. Most offices have a policy listing their approved ones. Appendix D lists the most common abbreviations. Following are some ways abbreviations can be misinterpreted:

- The physician wrote, "The patient had good BS." You assumed that BS meant bowel sounds, so you typed "The patient had good bowel sounds," but the physician meant the abbreviation BS to mean breath sounds.
- Do not change < or > signs to *less than* or *greater than* unless you are sure of what the statement is saying. For example, "The patient will not be admitted to the hospital until her hemoglobin is less than 13." If you made a mistake and typed "greater than 13," confusion could occur.
- The symbols for male (♂) and female (♀) are commonly used in handwritten notes, but you should re-

place these symbols with words when writing a business or professional letter.

Plural and Possessive

Converting words to plural or possessive form can be tricky in English. Refer to your medical terminology book or a dictionary when you are unsure. Which of the following sentences is correct?

- The patient had multiple bullas.
- The patient had multiple bullae.

The second sentence is correct. *Bullae* means multiple blisters; *bulla* is one blister.

Numbers

In general, numbers one to ten should be spelled out, except when used with units of measurement (e.g., 5 mg), and those over 10 may be expressed as a numeral. Here are some important tips you will need to remember about numbers:

- Numbers referring to an obstetrical patient's medical history are not written out: "The patient is a gravida 3, para 2." Do not convert these numbers.
- Watch decimal point placement. There is a huge difference in medication between 12.5 mg and 1.25 mg.
- Double-check that you have not transposed numbers. For example, you typed, "The patient's red blood cell count was 5.1," but it was actually 1.5. A red blood cell count of 1.5 is incompatible with life.

WHAT IF

You are writing a letter and can't find out how to spell a word. What should you do?

Begin with your computer's spell check software. Spell check is generally under the heading Tools at the top of the screen. Most programs offer suggestions for the misspelled word. Be very careful that you do not select the wrong word on the suggestion list. You may also either look up the word in a dictionary or use an online dictionary. Two Web addresses that offer online dictionaries are given in this chapter. You may ask a colleague for spelling assistance. An option is to exchange the word for another word from a thesaurus. Be sure that the meaning of the sentence does not change if you use a different word. If these steps do not work, print the letter, mark the word with a question mark, and leave it for the physician. Never mail a letter with a spelling error.

- Roman numerals should never be changed to words. For example, "lead II of the patient's electrocardiogram" should never be changed to "lead two of the patient's electrocardiogram."
- Many health care professionals use military time. Time that is written in military style does not have to be changed if the recipient of the letter is familiar with it (doctors, nurses). If the letter is going to a patient or other person who may not be able to interpret it, however, either convert the time or express the standard time in parenthesis; for example, "The patient's next appointment is at 1430 hours (2:30 P.M.)." No colons are used in military time.
- Temperatures must always have the correct symbol for Celsius or Fahrenheit included (98.6°F or 37°C).
- Telephone numbers should include the area code in parentheses or followed by a hyphen, then the number with a hyphen. Add extensions to the number by placing a comma after the last digit of the number, then type Ext. and the number: (800) 555-0000, Ext. 6480. Periods may replace hyphens and parentheses: 800.555.0000.

LETTER DEVELOPMENT

Writing effective business letters is a skill that requires practice and careful attention to detail. To write a professional business letter, you must:

- Understand the components of a letter
- Use the correct letter format
- Ensure that the message is clear, concise, and accurate

These skills are described in the following sections.

Components of a Letter

A typical business letter has 11 components. We will explore each one, beginning at the top of the page. For easy reference, Figure 7-1 displays a sample business letter with these components marked.

1. *Letterhead.* The letterhead consists of the name of the practice or physician, address, telephone number, fax number, and sometimes the company logo. The letterhead is often embossed in color and centered on the top of the page. The letterhead may also be preset into a **template**. (Templates are discussed later in the chapter).
2. *Date.* The date includes the month, day, and year. It should be positioned two to four spaces below the letterhead. The date must be typed on only one line and abbreviations should not be used.
3. *Inside address.* The inside address refers to the name and address of the person to whom the letter is being sent. A nine-digit zip code should be used if available. The inside address is placed four spaces down from the date unless the letter is being mailed with a window envelope and it will not be aligned correctly. Never abbreviate city or town names. States can be abbreviated. (See Appendix C for a list of abbreviations approved by the postal service.) Never abbreviate business titles (e.g., President, Chief Executive Officer). Here are some other points to remember:
   - If the letter is going to a business, type the name of the addressee, followed by his or her title, name of the business on the next line, then the address.
   - If the letter is being addressed to two or more people at different addresses, type the individual address block one line space under the other or place the addresses side by side.
   - If the letter is going to two people at the same address but with different last names, type the woman's name on the first line, man's name on the second line, then the address. If the sexes are the same, do them in alphabetical order, followed by the address.
4. *Subject line.* The subject line, an optional component, is used to state the intent of a letter or to indicate what the letter is regarding. It is placed on the third line below the inside address and is written as Re: (an abbreviation for regarding) followed by the subject. For example, Re: Blood tests.
5. *Salutation.* The **salutation** is the greeting of the letter. It is placed two spaces down from the inside address or the subject line. Capitalize the first letter of each word in the phrase and end the phrase with a colon. It is permissible to eliminate the salutation if the letter is informal or if a subject line has been used. When writing to a physician, write out the word doctor. Here are some recommendations when writing salutations:
   - If the letter is going to one person and the gender is known write, Dear Mr. Rogers.
   - If the letter is going to one person and the gender is *not* known, write, Dear Pat Smith (use the person's first name).
   - If the letter is going to a woman and a man with different last names, always address the woman first: Dear Ms. Ray and Mr. Oscar.
   - If the letter is going to several people, place them in alphabetical order: Dear Mr. Andersen, Mr. Cats, Ms. Dart, and Mr. Raymond.
   - To Whom It May Concern, Dear Sir, or Dear Madam should not be used.
6. *Body of the letter.* The body of the letter contains the message. It should be single-spaced with double spacing between the paragraphs. Here are some guidelines for writing the body of the letter:
   - If the letter is more than one page long, try to avoid dividing a paragraph at the end of a page. If you must, leave at least two sentences at the bot-

Benjamin Matthews, M.D.
999 Oak Road, Suite 313
Middletown, Connecticut 06457
860-344-6000
①

February 2, 2003 ②

Dr. Adam Meza
Medical Director   ③
Family Practice Associates
134 N. Tater Drive
West Hartford, Connecticut 06157

Re: Ms. Beatrice Suess ④

Dear Doctor Meza: ⑤

Thank you for asking me to evaluate Ms. Suess. I agree with your diagnosis of rheumatoid arthritis. Her prodromal symptoms include vague articular pain and stiffness, weight loss and general malaise. Ms. Suess states that the joint discomfort is most prominent in the mornings, gradually improving throughout the day.

My physical examination shows a 40-year-old female patient in good health. Heart sounds normal, no murmurs or gallops noted. Lung sounds clear. Enlarged lymph nodes were noted. Abdomen soft, bowel sounds present, and the spleen was not enlarged. Extremities showed subcutaneous nodules and flexion contractures on both hands.

⑥

Laboratory findings were indicative of rheumatoid arthritis. See attached laboratory data. I do not feel x-rays are warranted at this time.

My recommendations are to continue Ms. Suess on salicylate therapy, rest and physical therapy. I suggest that you have Ms. Suess attend physical therapy at the American Rehabilitation Center on Main Street.

Thank you for this interesting consultation.

Yours truly, ⑦

Benjamin Matthews, MD
}⑧
Benjamin Matthews, MD

BM/es ⑨

Enc. (2) ⑩

cc: Dr. Samuel Adams ⑪

F I G U R E   7 – 1 .   Components of a business letter. This letter is done in full block format and contains these elements: (1) letterhead, (2) date, (3) inside address, (4) subject line, (5) salutation, (6) body, (7) closing, (8) signature and typed name, (9) identification line, (10) enclosure, (11) copy.

tom of the first page. Use the widow and orphan control feature of your word processor program to prevent orphan lines from appearing.

- Tables and graphs should not be broken. They should appear on one page only.
- Web addresses and e-mail addresses should fit on one line and never be continued to another page.
- If the letter is more than one page long, page numbers should be used.
- Use a bulleted format to highlight key points for the reader. For example, "The possible side effects of this medication are:" (then list them vertically with a bullet symbol).
- Letterhead is used only on the first page of the letter. The second page should be the same quality paper as the letterhead. Start the second page with a continuation line (name of person the letter is going to and the date of the letter). Continue the letter two lines down from the continuation line. Your margins must be the same as those on page 1. Most templates type the continuation line for you.

7. *Closing.* The closing concludes the letter. Some common closings are: Sincerely, Yours truly, Regards, Respectfully, and Cordially yours. Only the first word is capitalized and a comma follows the phrase. Closings are placed two spaces down from the end of the letter. Never put the closing alone on a page.

8. *Signature and typed name.* The name of the person sending the document is typed four spaces below the closing, with the person's title typed directly below. The physician will read and sign the letter above the typed name. If you are instructed to sign the letter, sign the physician's name followed by a slash mark and your name, e.g., Susan James, MD/Raymond Smith, RMA.

9. *Identification line.* The identification line, an optional component, indicates who dictated the letter and who wrote it. It consists of abbreviations only. The initials of the person who dictated the letter are capitalized (generally the physician); the initials of the writer of the letter are in lower case (generally these will be yours). The identification line can also be called the reference line.

10. *Enclosure.* An **enclosure** is something that is included with a letter. It is abbreviated Enc. and is placed two spaces down from the identification line. The number of documents included is placed in parentheses; if only one document is included, just the abbreviation Enc. is used.

11. *Copy.* The abbreviation c is used to indicate that a duplicate letter has been sent. It is typed two spaces below the enclosure line. Usually, letters are copied to managers, supervisors, or to the physician who requested that the given information be dispersed.

Checkpoint Question

2. Whose address is typed as the inside address? What is the purpose of the salutation? What is the purpose of the identification line?

Letter Formats

There are three basic types of letter formats: *full block*, *semiblock*, and *block*. Office policy or the physician preference's will dictate which format you use.

Full Block

In **full block** format, each line is flush left. Full block is the most formal format and is most commonly used for professional letters. Figure 7-1 shows a letter in full block format.

Block

In **block** format, the date, subject line, closing, and signatures are flush right. All other lines are flush left (Fig. 7-2).

Semiblock

In **semiblock** format, the first sentence of each paragraph is indented five spaces, if done on a typewriter, or is tabbed, if done on a computer (Fig. 7-3). Semiblock is also referred to as modified block.

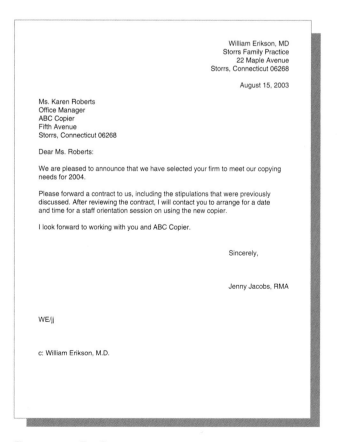

FIGURE 7–2. Sample block letter.

Elizabeth Jones, M.D.
750 East Street, Suite 205
Hialeah, Florida 33013
305-311-2666

June 12, 2003

Margaret Trent
18 Cambridge Street
Hialeah, Florida 33013

Dear Ms. Trent:

As per our phone conversation, your blood glucose level remains elevated. It is essential that we stabilize your blood sugar level.

In order to achieve normal blood sugar levels, you must follow the enclosed diet. A meeting with a Registered Dietitian can be arranged for you to discuss any dietary concerns you may have.

I am also enclosing patient education instructions for the use of a glucometer. You must test your blood sugar every morning and keep a diary of your results. Glucometers can be purchased from any pharmacy. If you need assistance in using the glucometer, please contact Raymond Smith, CMA, at 555-6423.

Presently, I do not wish to prescribe any medications. If we are unable to get your blood sugar under control, I will prescribe an oral diabetic medication.

Please call my office and schedule an appointment for the week of June 20 for a blood draw and a follow-up visit.

Sincerely,

Elizabeth Jones, M.D.

EJ/rs

enc. (2)

FIGURE 7–3. Sample semiblock letter.

Writing a Business Letter

To create a professional business letter, follow these three steps: preparation, composition, and editing. Box 7-4 gives you some guidelines for starting to write a letter.

Preparation

Good preparation is a key element in writing professional business letters. Preparation consists of planning the content and the mechanics of the letter.

Mental Preparation. Before you begin to compose a letter, mentally prepare your message. You might start formulating the message by envisioning yourself talking to the person to whom you are sending the letter. Preparation offers three benefits:

1. It helps eliminate writer's block.
2. It gets you to focus on the message, not the mechanics (e.g., spelling, grammar, punctuation).
3. It enhances your organization.

Using cue cards or note cards will help ensure all the necessary information is covered in the letter.

Mechanics of the Letter. Before you begin to type the letter, select the appropriate *template*, *margin*, and *font*. A template

---

BOX 7-4

HOW TO START WRITING A LETTER

By determining the answers to these four questions, you can better prepare the message of your letter.

1. Who is my reader?
   It is very important that you use proper gender identification. Be especially careful with names that can be used for males or females (eg, Sam, Kelly, Ronnie, Alex, Tracy). Determine the reader's comprehension level. Letters to physicians will be more technical and will use medical terminology. Letters to patients will be less technical and use medical terminology sparingly.

2. What do I want my reader to do?
   This is your call to action; make it clear and specific. For example, you might write, "Please complete the enclosed insurance form (2 pages). Be sure to include all necessary information and sign your name. Place the form in the enclosed envelope and return it to our office by June 15, 2003." Avoid using "at your earliest convenience"; include a date for the required action. If possible, include a response mechanism, such as a self-addressed, stamped envelope.

3. What do I want to say?
   Briefly list the necessary information. To help you remember all of the necessary information, ask yourself who, what, where, when, why, and how.

4. How will I organize my message?
   Here are three basic ways that you can organize your message:
   • *Chronological:* Discuss items in a sequential manner, beginning with the earliest date and proceeding to the most recent date. For example, when discussing the physician's career, list his or her earlier experiences before the most recent career achievements.
   • *Problem oriented:* Let the reader know about a specific problem and provide instructions for correcting the problem. For example, if a patient's blood work came back with abnormal findings, a letter would be sent, identifying the problem (e.g., low hematocrit) and advising the patient on the possible causes, treatments, and follow-up procedures.
   • *Comparison:* Evaluate the effectiveness of two or more items. For example, as an office manager, you may have to write to the physician comparing two service contracts or two sample computer software packages.

Box 7-5

FONTS

Here are fonts that would be suitable for a business letter:

- This is 12-point Times New Roman.
- This is 10-point Times New Roman.
- This is 12-point Garamond.
- **This is 12-point Arial.**

Here are fonts and sizes that would not be appropriate:

- This is 8-point Times New Roman.
- **This is 12-point Colossalis Black.**
- THIS IS 12-POINT COTTONWOOD.
- This is 12-point Tekton.
- **This is 12-point impact.**

provides you with the skeleton of the letter. The key elements are already set and spaced correctly, so you just type in the pertinent information. Most computers have numerous letter templates or a letter wizard. These programs will make the process of letter writing easy, fast, and professional. You may use macros in your template to make repetitive tasks faster.

The **margin** is the blank space around the letter. A 1-inch margin is used for both left and right sides of the letter and the bottom. Margins are used to center the components of the letter in a standarized manner. If you select a template, your margins will be set for you.

Next, select the font. A **font** is the typeface; it affects the way words look and how easy it will be to read the letter. Choose a font that is easy to read and that is appropriate in size. Avoid cute or elegant fonts that can be difficult to read or see. The most common fonts used in business letters are Times New Roman, Garamond, and Arial. Box 7-5 gives you some examples of fonts and their sizes.

Checkpoint Question

3. Before you begin to type a letter, name three mechanics that you need to select.

Composition

The goal of composition is to ensure that your message is transmitted clearly, concisely, and accurately to your reader. As you did during preparation, focus on the message, not on the mechanics.

A clear message ensures that your reader knows precisely what is expected; an unclear message leaves room for doubt.

Unclear: Please contact me.
Clear: Please contact me by Thursday, October 1.
Unclear: You need to make an appointment for blood work.

Clear: Call Temple Hospital laboratories (555-4010) and make an appointment for a blood glucose test on March 13.

A concise message is short and to the point. Wordy phrases with many adjectives should not be used.

Not concise: Please enclose a check in an envelope for exactly $50.
Concise: Please enclose a $50 check.

An accurate message includes the correct date, time, figures, and information. Inaccurate messages cause delays and confusion and can lead to poor public relations.

Editing

After you have composed the letter, edit it for both grammatical errors and factual information. Editing is a key step in making your letter a success. Editing entails two steps: proofreading and corrections.

Proofreading. Whenever possible, have a colleague **proofread** (read text and check for accuracy) your letter and provide constructive criticism. Be sure to maintain confidentiality. If you are using a computer, consider printing out a hard copy of your document for proofreading; some individuals find it difficult to proofread a document on the computer screen. Check for the following items:

- Accuracy of all information
- Clarity and conciseness
- Grammar
- Spelling
- Punctuation
- Paragraphs appropriate in length and limited to one subject
- Capitalization
- Logical organization and flow

Use proofreaders marks (Box 7-6) to speed up the editing process. These are standard marks used to indicate corrections. You should become familiar with the basic marks.

Checkpoint Question

4. What is the purpose of proofreading?

Corrections. After making corrections, print a final copy of the letter. As discussed earlier in the chapter, a computer spell check should be used with caution, as it highlights misspelled words but not incorrectly used words.

Types of Business Letters

You will be asked to create and type various letters. Letters that you write will be sent to patients, insurance companies, other health care providers, pharmaceutical companies, and

Box 7-6

STANDARD PROOFREADER MARKS

$\mathcal{S}$ or $\mathcal{V}$ or $\mathcal{V}$ delete; take it out

⊃ close up; print as o ne word

$\widetilde{\mathcal{S}}$ delete and close up

∧ or > or ⋀ caret; insert here ⌒ (something

insert a space

eq # space evenly where indicated

stet let marked text stand as set

tr transpose; change order the

/ used to separate two or more marks and often as a concluding stroke at the end of an insertion

[set farther to the left

] set farther to the right

⌒ set æ or fl as ligatures æ or fl

═ straighten alignment

|| straighten or align

X imperfect or broken character

□ indent or insert em quad space

¶ begin a new paragraph

sp spell out (set 5 lbs. as five pounds)

cap set in capitals (CAPITALS)

sm cap or s.c. set in small capitals (SMALL CAPITALS)

lc set in lowercase (lowercase)

ital set in italic (*italic*)

rom set in roman (roman)

bf set in boldface (**boldface**)

═ or -/ or ⌒ or ⊔/hyphen

$\frac{1}{N}$ or en or /N/ en dash (1965–72)

$\frac{1}{M}$ or em or /M/ em—or long—dash

∨ superscript or superior ($\overset{2}{\vee}$ as in πr^2)

∧ subscript or inferior ($\overset{}{\wedge}$ as in H_2O)

◇ or X centered (◇ for a centered dot in $p \cdot q$)

⌃ comma

⌄ apostrophe

⊙ period

; or ;/ semicolon

: or ⊙ colon

quotation marks

(/) parentheses

[/] brackets

OK/? query to author: has this been set as intended

↓ or ∧[1] push down a work-up

∅[1] turn over an inverted letter

wf[1] wrong font; a character of the wrong size or esp. style

[1] The last three symbols are unlikely to be needed in making proofs of photocomposed matter.

---

various businesses. Here are some common types of letters that you may write:

- Letters welcoming new patients to the practice
- Letters to patients regarding their test results
- Consultation reports to other health care professionals
- Workers' compensation letters verifying the patient's injury or treatment
- Justification or explanation of treatments to insurance companies
- Cover letters for transferring patients' records to another practice
- Clarification or explanation to patients regarding fees or billing concerns
- Thank you letters to sales representatives
- Physician changes for on-call schedules (generally sent to the hospital and covering physicians)
- Announcements of new services, hours, or office location changes.

MEMORANDUM DEVELOPMENT

A **memorandum** (often called a memo) is for communication within the office or with another department only; it is never sent to patients. It is less formal than a letter and is generally used for brief announcements.

Components of a Memorandum

A memorandum contains the standard elements in the following list. Use these guidelines to complete each element. Figure 7-4 shows a sample memorandum.

1. *Heading.* The word Memorandum is typed across the top of the page.
2. *Date.* Use the same rules for letters when typing the date for memorandums.
3. *To.* List the names of all recipients in either alphabetic or hierarchic order. If the memorandum is going to a particular group (e.g., all department managers, all employees), it can be addressed to the group.
4. *From.* List the name and title of the person sending the memorandum.
5. *Subject.* Insert a brief phrase describing the purpose of the memorandum.
6. *Body.* Write the message of the memorandum here.
7. *Copy (c).* Use the same rules as for letters when sending duplicate copies of memorandums.

Salutations and closings are not used in memorandums. All lines in a memorandum are justified left, and 1-inch margins are used. Writing a memorandum entails the same steps (preparation, composition, editing) as writing a business letter. The memorandum should be read and initialed by the physician before it is distributed. Your computer software will have a memorandum template.

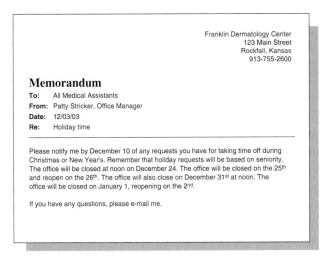

F I G U R E 7 – 4 . Sample memorandum.

 Checkpoint Question

5. What are memorandums used for?

SENDING WRITTEN COMMUNICATION

After the document has been written, proofread, and signed, it is ready for you to send it to its receiver. Fold the letter in thirds and place it in an envelope. Procedure 7-1 explains how to do this. Procedure 7-2 shows you how to fold a letter into a envelope with a window. Most professional letters are sent through the postal service. Other types of written communications are sent through facsimile machines or by electronic mail. Here are two key steps to remember when sending any type of written communication:

- All attempts must be made to ensure patient confidentiality. The outside of envelopes should be marked confidential when the correspondence contains information about a patient. Send letters only to known or confirmed addresses.
- Return addresses must be used so that mail can be returned if the recipient is no longer at the given address.

Facsimile Machines

Facsimile, or fax, machines allow the medical office to send and receive printed material over a phone line. These machines offer a convenient and cost-effective way to transmit records, orders, prescriptions, test results, and other materials that require quick receipt. Always use a cover sheet (Fig. 7-5) when sending papers through a fax machine. At minimum a cover sheet should have the following information:

- Name, address, telephone, and fax number of the physician's practice

- Name of the intended receiver of the fax
- Number of pages being sent, counting the cover sheet
- Telephone number of the fax machine of the intended recipient
- Date and time the fax was sent
- Confidentiality statement (e.g., "The information in the facsimile message and any accompanying documents is confidential. This information is intended only for use by the individual or entity name above. If you are not the intended recipient of this information you are hereby notified that any disclosure, copying or distribution of this information is strictly prohibited. Please notify the sender immediately by telephone").

When you receive a fax, photocopy it if it is printed on thermal paper (text printed on thermal paper fades quickly), then forward it to the appropriate person. The fax machine should be checked regularly throughout the day, and all items should be sorted quickly.

Sometimes when you fax a given letter, the fax machine may be busy or the number dialed may be busy. If the number is busy, it is not acceptable to leave the fax papers in the machine for redial unless you are sure that no one else will have access to that document. Never leave documents unattended.

F I G U R E 7 – 5 . Sample fax cover sheet.

Electronic Mail

Electronic mail, or e-mail, allows computer-to-computer communication, whether within the same facility or anywhere throughout the world. The communication occurs through a modem. Each computer must be linked to an online service provider. Chapter 10 discusses electronic mail in more detail. Here are a few things you should remember about sending letters via electronic mail:

- Confidentiality cannot be guaranteed.
- Follow the usual steps of preparation, composition, and editing.
- You can attach letters to an e-mail by clicking on the file attachment icon, locating the letter, and inserting it. It is always a good idea to open the attachment to make sure that you are attaching the correct letter or version.

United States Postal Service

Written communication is commonly sent via the United States Postal Service (USPS). Envelopes must be correctly prepared so that the optical character readers (OCR) used by the USPS can sort the mail quickly and efficiently. The OCR reads the envelope, scanning for information. The OCR scans all envelopes using these margins: ½ inch on either side and ⅝ inch from the top or bottom of the envelope. Addresses or notations outside of these margins will not be read.

Addressing Envelopes

The standard business envelope is no. 10. USPS regulations state that the minimal size of an envelope is 3½ × 5 inches. It must be rectangular and no less than 0.007 inch thick. The standard no. 10 business envelope is 4⅛ × 9½ inches.

The return address is placed in the upper left hand corner. It should not exceed five lines. The return address is typed with the same guidelines as for letters and is single spaced. Often, medical offices have the return address preprinted on the envelope.

The recipient's address is typed 12 spaces down from the top and centered on the face of the envelope. All words of the address should begin with a capital letter. Only postal abbreviations for states should be used, and no punctuation is used between the postal abbreviation and the zip code. All addresses must include the five-digit zip code; whenever possible, the four-digit expanded zip code should also be used. The expanded zip code allows the USPS to sort and route the mail faster and more accurately. Envelopes should not be handwritten, as this does not portray a professional image. The entire address should not exceed five lines. Your software may allow you to insert a USPS PostNet bar code. This is generally inserted two to three lines below the address. This bar code accelerates USPS sorting. Always check your software to make sure it is certified by the USPS.

Special notations such as "confidential" or "personal" are placed on the left-hand side of the envelope two lines below the return address. Notations for hand canceling and special delivery are made in the upper right-hand corner of the envelope below the postage. Nothing should be printed in the right lower corner of the envelope, because the USPS uses that space for its bar codes. Figure 7-6 displays a properly addressed envelope.

Here are some additional things to remember regarding envelopes:

- Be sure that graphics or logos do not impede the OCR's ability to read the address.
- Do not use fancy fonts that may impede the OCR's ability to read the address.
- A minimum of eight-point type is recommended by the USPS.
- Do not use dark envelopes.
- White or tan envelope with black type is preferred.
- Do not use the # sign; if it cannot be avoided, leave one space between the # sign and the number (this is a USPS recommendation).
- If you are using an envelope with a window frame, there should be an eighth-inch clearance around the address.

Checkpoint Question

6. What does an optical character reader do?

Affixing Postage

Proper postage must be affixed to the envelope by a stamp, permit imprint, or a postage meter machine. Postal meter machines are in-house machines that are regulated by the USPS. They contain a prepaid amount of postage and can imprint the postage stamp either directly on the envelope or onto an adhesive tape that is applied to the envelope. Some machines weigh, stuff, and seal the envelopes. The date on the postal machine must be changed daily, and the ink roller must be kept full.

The physician may opt to use the USPS permit imprint program. In this case, you take the mail, sealed and ready to be sent, to the post office. The postal clerk passes your letters through the USPS machine, and a permit stamp is placed on the envelope. The postal clerk deducts the postage charges from your prepaid account. The advantages to this

The Women's Health Center
24 Crescent Street
Phoenix, Arizona 03210

Robin Harrison
000 Main Street
Anytown, AA 12345

FIGURE 7-6. Properly addressed envelope.

ñ̃Spanish Terminology

¿Donde está la oficina de correos?	Where is the post office?
Tengo que enviar esta carta.	I need to mail this letter.
¿Cuanto cuesta el franqueo?	How much does the postage cost?

system are that is saves time and does not require the office to care for the postal meter machine.

USPS Mailing Options

Mail can be sent in a variety of ways based on its urgency and value. The following is a brief description of the services offered by the USPS:

- Express mail, the fastest service, ensures delivery of your package by the next day (by noon in most areas). Express mail is delivered 7 days a week. The rate starts at $13.65, and fees increase by weight and destination. Express mail is automatically insured for $500. Additional insurance is available.
- Priority mail, the second fastest service, offers 2-day delivery to most destinations. The maximum weight is 70 pounds, and the maximum size is 108 inches combined length and girth. The rate is based on the weight of the package. You can purchase up to $5,000 of insurance for packages.
- First-class mail is the service used for sending standard mail (letters and postcards) weighing up to 13 ounces. Mail weighing more than 13 ounces will be considered priority mail.
- Standard mail (A) is used by companies to mail books and catalogs. Standard mail (B) is used to mail packages weighing more than 1 pound. The maximum weight is 70 pounds, and the maximum measurement is 130 inches combined length and girth.
- Postal rates, fees, and services are subject to change.

You must stay abreast of the latest information. Use the USPS website for additional information and updates.

USPS Special Services

A certificate of mailing is used to prove that a document was mailed. No record is kept at the post office. It does not provide proof that the letter was received by the addressee.

Certified mail provides a mailing receipt and a record of the mailing at the local post office (Fig. 7-7). This service is available only for first-class and priority mail. Return receipts can be purchased in conjunction with this. Return receipts are used to prove that the recipient received the document (Fig. 7-8).

Registered mail provides the most protection for valuables. It is available only for priority and first-class mail. The maximum insurance that can be obtained is $25,000. This service can be combined with return receipts.

International rates are available from your local post office. Type the address as discussed earlier, and type the name of the country on the last line without abbreviations (Japan, Korea), All physician offices should have a supply of express and priority mail envelopes along with a current fee schedule.

Other Delivery Options

Many other companies specialize in document and package delivery, particularly with next-day or second-day delivery services. Examples of these companies include Airborne Ex-

FIGURE 7-7. Certified mail receipt.

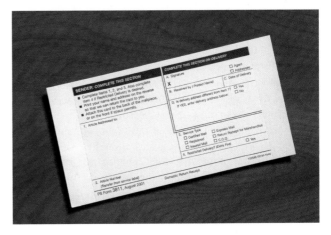

FIGURE 7-8. Return receipt.

press, Federal Express, and United Parcel Service (UPS). Use the company with which the physician has an account. Fees vary, so you may have to contact each company for prices and available services. These companies offer services such as tracking, pick-up services, money back guarantees, and proof of delivery. The tracking service can be done through their websites.

RECEIVING AND HANDLING INCOMING MAIL

Part of the daily routine for a medical assistant is handling the incoming mail. Sort the mail quickly and promptly to ensure efficient functioning of the office.

Types of Incoming Mail

Many types of mail are received daily in a physician's office:

- Advertisements
- Bills for office services
- Consultation letters
- Hospital communications and newsletters
- Laboratory and radiographic reports
- Office supply magazines
- Patient correspondence
- Payments from insurance companies and patients
- Professional journals
- Literature from professional organizations
- Samples (drugs, laboratory test kits)
- Waiting room magazines

Opening and Sorting Mail

Each physician will have an individual policy on which mail you should open and how you should process it. Any mail marked urgent should be handled first, followed by mail about patient-related issues. Promotional materials should be handled last. Some physicians will have you sort, file, and respond to mail without their review. In some practices, however, all mail is placed in a special file folder and handled only by the physician or office manager. Box 7-7 lists general guidelines for opening and sorting the mail. Most physicians will open and handle their own e-mail. If the physician is on vacation, he or she will apply an auto reply response to his or her e-mail address.

When the physician is away, personal mail is placed on his or her desk and left for the physician to handle. Mail that pertains to patient care issues should be opened and handled appropriately. Ask your supervisor if you are unsure which pieces of mail you should open. If the mail requires an urgent response, the covering physician should be contacted unless otherwise directed. Mail should never be allowed to accumulate in outside mailboxes because patient information is confidential.

Box 7-7

OPENING AND SORTING MAIL

1. Gather the necessary equipment: a letter opener, paper clips, and a date stamp.
2. Open all letters and check for enclosures; paper clip these to the letter. If the letter states that enclosures were sent but they are not in the envelope, contact the sender and request them. Indicate on the letter that the enclosures were missing and the name of the person you contacted.
3. Date-stamp each item.
4. Sort the mail into categories and deal with it appropriately. Generally, you should handle the following types of mail as noted:
   - Use a paper clip to attach test results to the patient's chart; place the chart in a pile for the physician to review.
   - Record promptly all insurance payments and checks and deposit them according to office policy.
   - Account for all drug samples and appropriately log them into the sample book.
   - Dispose of miscellaneous advertisements unless otherwise directed.
5. Distribute the mail to the appropriate staff members. For example, mail can be for the physician, nurse manager, office manager, billing clerk, or other personnel.

 Checkpoint Question

7. What mail must be opened first?

Annotation

Some physicians request that letters be annotated. **Annotation** involves reading a document and highlighting the key points. If the letter is very detailed, a summary of the key points should be written in the margins. The summary should be factual and not editorialized.

COMPOSING AGENDAS AND MINUTES

Two other forms of written communication are agendas and minutes. The purpose of an **agenda** (Figure 7-9) is to outline briefly the topics to be discussed at a meeting.

It allows the meeting participants to prepare any necessary reports before the meeting and to anticipate questions. Agendas usually begin with a call to order, followed by a review

```
Quality Improvement Committee
February 15, 2003
Agenda

  I.  Call to order
 II.  Review and acceptance of the minutes from
      January 10, 2003
III.  Old business
      A. Copy machine updates
      B. Insurance updates for overdue accounts
 IV.  New business
      A. New contract for laboratory supplies
      B. Scheduling guidelines for summer vacations
  V.  Adjournment
```

FIGURE 7–9. Agenda.

of previous meeting minutes, old business updates, then new business. Adjournment is the last item on the agenda.

You should type the minutes of a meeting as soon as possible, including the following:

- List of members present
- List of members absent
- Date and time the meeting was called to order
- Statement regarding the acceptance of the previous minutes
- Brief description of discussions
- List of reports that were submitted
- Date and time of the next meeting
- Adjournment time
- Signature of the person who prepared the minutes and the chairperson's signature

Procedure 7-1

How to Fold a Letter for a No. 10 Envelope

Equipment/Supplies

- Letter, 8.5 × 11
- Envelope, no. 10

Steps	Purpose
1. Place the letter right side up and flat on a table.	Ensures that the letter will be folded correctly and neatly.
2. Bring the bottom third of the letter up and make a solid crease line.	Divides the letter into equal thirds. Solid crease displays a professional look.
3. Fold the top third of the letter down to within three eighths of an inch of the first fold. Make a solid crease.	Ensures that the second fold does not interfere with the first fold. A solid crease displays a professional look.
4. Place the letter in the envelope with the last fold at the top of the envelope.	Allows the recipient to open the letter easily. Ensures that the letterhead is seen first.

Procedure 7-2

How to Fold a Letter for an Envelope With a Window

Equipment/Supplies

- Letter, 8.5 × 11
- Envelope, no. 10 with a window

Steps	Purpose
1. Place the letter face down on a flat surface.	Ensures that the letter will be folded correctly and neatly.
2. Bring the bottom third of the letter up. Make a solid crease line.	Divides the letter into equal thirds. Solid crease displays a professional look.
3. Fold the top third of the letter down to within three eighths of an inch of the first fold. Make a solid crease.	Ensures that the second fold does not interfere with the first fold. A solid crease displays a professional look.
4. Place the letter in the envelope. Turn the envelope over and look at the window.	Makes sure the letter is correctly seated in the envelope and the address can be read.

Chapter Summary

As a medical assistant, you need excellent written communication skills. Careful attention to detail is essential. Good grammar, punctuation, and spelling are key skills. Be careful when you use your computer spell check. It will not recognize words that are misused. You will use these skills to write letters, memorandums, and other correspondence. These letters will be sent to patients, physicians, and businesses. After writing these documents, you must be able to select the appropriate service for mailing your letters. Your primary goal with all written communication is to get your message across in a clear, concise, and accurate manner.

Critical Thinking Challenges

1. Create a business letter. Include all the components and use the full block format. Print your unedited copy and, using proofreaders marks, indicate your corrections. Make the corrections and reprint a final copy. Ask your instructor to review both copies.
2. Write 10 sentences using terms from Box 7-3. Use some terms correctly and others incorrectly. Exchange your sentences with another student. Correct your peer's sentences.
3. Collect five pieces of mail that you have received at home. What method of affixing postage did they use?

Go to your local USPS office. Obtain either a priority mail or express mail envelope. Correctly address the envelope.

4. Suppose the physician told you to read his e-mails while he was on vacation. In doing so, you come across a personal piece of information that you know he would not want you to see. How would you handle it? Would you tell anyone that you saw it? Would you question the physician about it?

Answers to Checkpoint Questions

1. Inaccurate information in a business letter can lead to injuries to the patient and lawsuits and can harm the physician's practice.
2. The inside address is the address of the person to whom the letter is going. The salutation is the greeting. The identification line shows the initials of the person who dictated the letters and the initials of the person who typed the letter.
3. Before you begin to type a letter, select the template, font, and margins that you will use.
4. Proofreading allows you to check the accuracy and content of the letter.
5. Memorandums are used for communication within the office and with other departments.
6. The USPS uses optical character readers to quickly and efficiently sort the mail.
7. Any mail marked urgent must be opened first.

Websites

Here are some Web addresses that may help you:

Airborne Express
www.airborne.com

Medical dictionary
www.medical-dictionary.com

Merriam-Webster's Dictionary
www.m-w.com

United Parcel Service
www.ups.com

United States Postal Service
www.usps.com

8

Medical Records and Record Management

CHAPTER OUTLINE

ROLE DELINEATION COMPONENTS

GENERAL: Legal Concepts
- Perform within legal and ethical boundaries
- Prepare and maintain medical records
- Document accurately
- Implement and maintain federal and state health care legislation and regulations

ADMINISTRATIVE: Administrative Procedures
- Perform basic administrative medical assisting functions

CHAPTER COMPETENCIES

LEARNING OBJECTIVES
Upon successfully completing this chapter, you will be able to:

1. Spell and define the key terms
2. Describe standard and electronic medical record systems
3. Explain the process for releasing medical records to third-party payers and individual patients
4. List and explain the EMR guidelines established to protect computerized records
5. List the standard information included in medical records
6. Identify and describe the types of formats used for documenting patient information in outpatient settings
7. Explain how to make an entry in a patient's medical record, using abbreviations when appropriate
8. Explain how to make a correction in a standard and electronic medical record
9. Identify the various ways medical records can be stored
10. Compare and contrast the differences between alphabetic and numeric filing systems and give an example of each
11. Explain the purpose of the Health Insurance Portability and Accountability Act

PERFORMANCE OBJECTIVE
Upon successfully completing this chapter, you will be able to:

1. Prepare and file a medical record file folder

KEY TERMS

alphabetic filing
chief complaint
chronological order
cross-reference
demographic data

electronic medical records (EMR)
flow sheet
medical history forms
microfiche

microfilm
narrative
numeric filing
present illness
problem-oriented medical record (POMR)

reverse chronological order
SOAP
subject filing
workers' compensation

MEDICAL RECORDS HAVE A VITAL role in ensuring quality patient care. Proper medical records management requires adherence to certain legal, moral, and ethical standards. If these standards are disregarded, a breach of contract between patient and physician may occur, exposing the patient to potential embarrassment and making the physician vulnerable to lawsuits. (See Chapter 2.)

Medical records have many uses, including research, quality assurance, and patient education. Information gathered from medical records aids the government in planning for future health care needs and protecting the health of the public.

A thorough and accurate medical record furnishes documented evidence of the patient's evaluation, treatment, change in condition, and communication with the physician and staff.

STANDARD MEDICAL RECORDS

The standard practice of recording and filing patient information in a folder and labeling it with the patient's name or a number is gradually being replaced by the use of **electronic medical records (EMR)**, but in the meantime, a physician accumulates mounds of paper every day. A medical facility has a variety of options for record keeping. The best systems are those that have been tried, revised, and revised again. No matter how the records are stored, make sure that the information is:

- Easily retrievable
- Kept in an orderly manner
- Complete
- Legible
- Accurate
- Brief

Whether a record is on paper or a computer disk, all medical records have the same contents.

Contents of the Record

A medical record in an outpatient facility, often called a chart or a file, contains confidential clinical information about the patient's health and treatment in addition to the billing and insurance information discussed in Chapter 13.

General information such as name, address, telephone number, date of birth, social security number, credit history, and next of kin is vital to a complete chart but should never be intermingled with the clinical information. Metal fasteners can be used to keep certain pages on one side of the chart. For a thorough discussion and samples of typical medical reports found in the medical record, see Chapter 9.

The following information is typically found in the clinical section of the medical chart:

- *Chief complaint*—A description of the symptoms that led the patient to seek the physician's care. This information is supplied by the patient during the interview at the beginning of the visit. It is usually stated in the patient's own words in quotation marks. For example, the patient complains of "something stuck in my throat."
- *Present illness*—A more specific account of the chief complaint, including time frames and characteristics. For example, the patient says it started 2 days ago. She describes the pain as severe and stabbing and reports taking Tylenol with no relief.
- *Family and personal history*—A review of any major illnesses of family members, including grandparents, parents, siblings, aunts, and uncles. Any previous major illnesses and surgeries of the patient are listed under personal history.
- *Review of systems*—A systematic review of the body's ten systems to detect problems not yet identified. For example, problems with the integumentary system (skin) may be identified if the patient reports a rash, areas of discoloration, or change in a mole.
- *Progress notes*—Documentation of each patient encounter, including information obtained in phone calls and refills of prescriptions.
- *Radiographic reports*— Reports of any x-ray studies performed in the office. If patients are sent to other facilities for radiographs, a report of that study is placed in the chart.
- *Laboratory results*—A copy of the results of any laboratory work done in the office or a report from an outside facility.
- *Consultation reports*—Any reports from other physicians regarding consultations with the patient.
- *Medication administration*—Some facilities use a separate sheet to log medications given in the office. If an opioid is given, still another form is completed, as discussed in Chapter 2.
- *Diagnosis or medical impression*—The most recent entry on the progress note will contain the provider's opinion of the patient's problems.
- *Physician's and/or medical assistant's identification and signature*—Experts have suggested that you sign your entire name instead of initials, with your credentials written after the name, e.g., Susan Jones, CMA.
- *Documented advance directives, such as living will and power of attorney for medical care*—A copy of any instructions from the patient regarding end-of-life decisions or the appointment of another person who can give consent for treatment for the patient.
- *All correspondence pertaining to the patient*—Any letters or memos generated in the facility and sent out are copied and placed in the chart. Correspondence from other physicians is also included in the chart.

Checkpoint Question

1. What is the chief complaint?

ELECTRONIC MEDICAL RECORDS

Outpatient medical facilities often use computers for storing patient **demographic data** (e.g., address, phone number), insurance billing, printing statements, managing appointments, and word processing. Data are saved, backed up, and stored electronically. In addition to accounting and tracking, computer charting in the clinical area is becoming more common in physician offices. Such systems often use a touch screen, making it easy to store a patient's history, vital signs, and any other information. Documents such as letters from other providers are scanned and become a part of the permanent electronic record. Computer record keeping has many advantages, including legibility, easy storage and retrieval, and improved documentation. Documentation is improved because the computer will require that specific information be inserted. For example, when completing a patient history form, the computer will ask, "Is this patient male or female?" The question must be answered before you can move to the next screen, which prevents missed documentation. A paperless system eliminates the need for paper and storage space, and the possibility of losing a chart is nonexistent. Computer charting takes less time than handwriting notes. Medical record software will continue to expand and integrate data in ways that will further revolutionize medical documentation.

Computers do have some disadvantages, however, including downtime, cost, security issues, equipment failure, and the need for more in-depth staff training. In the medical office, the setup may consist of a mainframe with various terminals placed throughout the office.

Electronic Medical Record Security

With computer records, confidential health information is at risk for being seen by unauthorized persons. The Health Insurance Portability and Accountability Act of 1996 (HIPAA) was passed to ensure the privacy of patients' records without creating problems transferring information between health professionals, which might harm the quality of care. HIPAA's privacy rule applies to health insurance plans, insurance clearinghouses, and health care providers who perform administrative transactions electronically (e.g., electronic billing, electronic claims submission). After review and some changes, HIPAA's final rule took effect in April 2003.

The American Medical Association (AMA) and many risk management companies have published guidelines for the EMR. Following are suggestions and guidelines based on HIPAA's requirements for practices using computers to transfer or store patient information. Experts advise physicians and office managers considering software programs to look for the following capabilities:

- User friendly commands that allow users to move easily within the system.
- Spell check, free text fields for inserting corrections and late entries. The electronic record is corrected by

using the same rules as in the standard record. Entries are not deleted but corrected, with an explanation to avoid the appearance of hiding information.
- Security levels to limit entry to all functions. For example, a receptionist does not need access to the physician's personal taxes.
- A system to repel hackers. Evidence shows that persons with access to technology can invade patients' records stored on computer databases. This is a gross breach of confidentiality and is illegal.

To maintain security, facilities are urged to do the following:

- Keep all computer backup disks in a safe place away from the practice.
- Store disks in a bank safe-deposit box.
- Use passwords with characters other than letters and encrypt the passwords.
- Change log-in codes and passwords every 30 days.
- Prepare a backup plan for use when the computer system is down.
- Turn terminals away from areas where information may be seen by patients.
- Keep the fax machines and printers that receive personal medical information in a private place.
- Ensure that each user is restricted to the information needed to do his or her job.
- Train employees on confidentiality and each person's responsibility. With HIPAA's final rule, effective April 2003, training is available from vendors of medical software.
- Design a written confidentiality policy that employees sign.
- Conduct routine audits that produce a trail of each employee's movement through the EMR system.
- Include disciplinary measures for breaches of confidentiality.

In this era of paperless medical offices, care must be taken to protect the privacy of the patient as carefully as in the world of paper.

Other Technologies for Medical Record Maintenance

Providers may use a handheld personal data device (PDA), laptop, or personal computer (PC) in central areas or examination rooms. The same security measures apply to these items. Patients should not have access to computer screens in the examination room. The physician should take care in keeping a personal data system, just as he or she protects the prescription pad. The personal data device may contain the entire *Physicians' Desk Record*, giving the provider information needed for prescribing drugs at the fingertips. Other applications of the PDA include downloading patient education materials and documenting and transferring information about patient encounters when the office is closed.

MEDICAL RECORD ORGANIZATION

Information in the paper medical record is usually organized in a standard chart order and placed in a specially designed folder. The order in which documents are placed in the medical record depends on the physician's preference. As mentioned earlier, the demographic information is kept separate from the clinical information. The clinical portion of the medical record is organized in either a source-oriented or a problem-oriented format. In source-oriented medical records, all similar categories or sources of information are grouped together. The typical groupings:

- Billing and insurance information
- Physician orders
- Progress notes
- Laboratory results
- Radiographic results (magnetic resonance imaging, computed tomography, ultrasound)
- Patient education

All documentation in these categories is placed in **reverse chronological order**; that is, the most recent documents are placed on top of previous sheets.

Provider Encounters

Whether the patient is seen by a physician assistant, nurse practitioner, or physician, the visit is documented.

Narrative Format

Some providers document visits in the narrative form. **Narrative** is the oldest documentation form and the least structured. It is simply a paragraph indicating the contact with the patient, what was done for the patient, and the outcome of any action. In the sample page shown in Figure 8-1, the chart entries made by the CMA are in narrative format.

Some offices record new patients' encounters in the history and physical format, which is discussed in Chapter 9. Visits of established patients returning for follow-up are documented in a different format. Although some offices use the same format for new and established patients, the most common formats used to document each established patient encounter are narrative, SOAP, and POMR.

SOAP Format

The **SOAP** (subjective-objective-assessment-plan) format is one of the most common methods for documenting patient visits. The *subjective* component is a statement of what the patient says. Whenever possible, actual quotations by the patient should be used. The *objective* component is what is observed about the patient when the medical assistant begins the assessment and when the provider does the examination. The *assessment* portion is a phrase stating the impression of

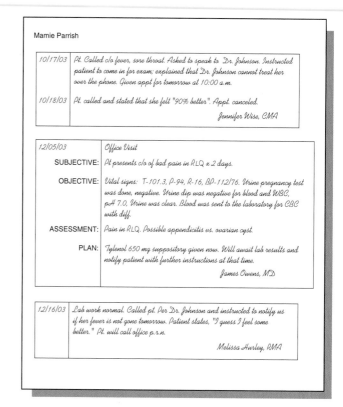

FIGURE 8-1.   Sample page from patient's progress record.

what is wrong or the patient's diagnosis. If a final diagnosis cannot be made yet, the provider lists possible disorders to be ruled out, called the differential diagnosis. The *plan* is a list of interventions that are to be carried out. In Box 8-1, the note is written in the SOAP format.

POMR Format

The **problem-oriented medical record (POMR)** lists each problem of the patient, usually at the beginning of the folder, and references each problem with a number throughout the folder. This method was developed by Dr. Lawrence Week and is a common method of compiling information because of its logical flow and the ease with which information can be reviewed. In group practices where patients may be seen by more than one physician, the POMR format makes it easier to track the patient's treatment and progress. For instance, if Mr. Jones has hypertension and hyperglycemia, each diagnosis will be assigned a problem number as soon as the diagnosis is made:

2/4/9 #1. Hypertension
2/4/9 #2. Hyperglycemia

At each subsequent visit made by Mr. Jones, these problems will be referenced by these numbers. If a problem develops and is resolved, the problem number will be terminated by a single strike-through with a date beside it or by adding an X to a heading that indicates resolution of problems. Chronic problems, such as hypertension and hyperglycemia, will be retained by number for as long as the patient remains with the practice. These may be divided by headings of acute and chronic or short-term and long-term for convenience.

POMR documents are divided into four components:

1. *Database.* This contains the following:
   - Chief complaint (Fig. 8-2 shows charting for a chief complaint and history of present illness)
   - Present illness
   - Patient profile
   - Review of systems
   - Physical examination
   - Laboratory reports
2. *Problem list.* This includes every problem the patient has that requires evaluation, including social, demographic, medical, and surgical problems. (Demographic problems relate to statistical characteristics of certain populations.)

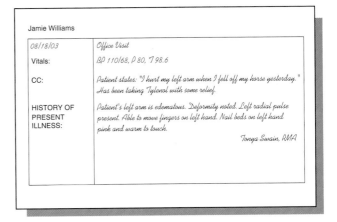

Jamie Williams	
08/18/03	*Office Visit*
Vitals:	*BP 110/68, P 80, T 98.6*
CC:	*Patient states: "I hurt my left arm when I fell off my horse yesterday." Has been taking Tylenol with some relief.*
HISTORY OF PRESENT ILLNESS:	*Patient's left arm is edematous. Deformity noted. Left radial pulse present. Able to move fingers on left hand. Nail beds on left hand pink and warm to touch.*
	Tonya Swain, RMA

FIGURE 8–2. Charting a chief complaint and history of present illness.

3. *Treatment plan.* This includes management, additional workups that may be necessary, and therapy.
4. *Progress notes.* These are structured notes corresponding to each problem.

 Checkpoint Question

2. What are three common formats used to document patient–provider encounters?

DOCUMENTATION FORMS

Using printed forms and flowcharts in the medical record saves space and time and allows for easy retrieval of information. They are usually customized to meet the needs of the individual practice. Some forms, like vaccination records, are required by federal law. In the paperless office, these forms are completed by the patient and transferred to the patient's electronic record by data entry, and then the completed form is shredded.

Medical History Forms

Medical history forms are commonly used to gather information from the patient before the visit with the physician. Many medical offices mail these forms to new patients and have them bring the completed form to their visit. This gives the patient the opportunity to concentrate on the questions, gather information about the family history, and give a more complete history. Whether the patient brings the completed form or fills out the history form in the office, you will review the information with the patient to clarify any questions and add additional information gathered in the interview. Specialty practices use forms designed to gather the type of information they will need to manage the patient's care. For example, an orthopedist's history form might include fields for prior orthopedic injuries, accident information, and flow sheets for physical therapy visits.

Box 8-1

SOAP METHOD TO DOCUMENT PATIENT INFORMATION

Jennifer Mosley states that her daughter Melissa has been vomiting all night. She also states that Melissa had diarrhea for 2 days before her appointment and has only eaten crackers and bananas since 6 P.M. last night. Dr. Gibson's notes indicate that Melissa has lost 3 pounds since her last visit and that she appears pale, weak, and slightly dehydrated. He suspects a viral infection.

Dr. Gibson ordered a stool culture along with a complete blood count (CBC) with differential. He prescribed the BRAT diet and suggested that Mrs. Mosley give Melissa Imodium D for the next 48 hours. He also told Mrs. Mosley to call the office if Melissa's symptoms worsen and to bring her back for a recheck if the symptoms are not cleared up by the end of the week.

S: According to the patient's mother, the patient has been vomiting all night and has had diarrhea for the past 2 days. She has eaten only crackers and bananas since 6 P.M. the night before.

O: Patient appears pale, weak, and slightly dehydrated and has lost 3 pounds since her last visit.

A: Possible viral infection.

P: Stool culture, CBC with diff, BRAT diet, and Imodium for the next 48 hours. Call office if symptoms worsen; return to office if patient not well by the end of the week.

Flow Sheets

The **flow sheet** is designed to limit the need for long, hand-written care notes by allowing information to be recorded in either graphic or table form. Generally, flow sheets are designed for a given task. Color-coded sheets for medication administration, vital signs, pediatric growth charts, and so on eliminate the need to read through the pages of a chart to retrieve information. For example, if the physician asks you what the baby weighed 3 months ago, you find the pink growth chart, which saves time and frustration. An advantage of using electronic medical records is the capability of converting such information to charts, graphs, and flow sheets. In a computer medical record, clicking an icon for a growth chart takes you to a screen that allows you to enter the information. The software transfers the numbers to a graph. Figure 8-3 shows the growth chart that appears on the screen. When you refill a patient's daily blood pressure medication, you enter the information into the computer record, and it is transferred to the medication record. The record of all entries related to the patient's medications can then be easily retrieved by clicking on the medication icon. Figure 8-4 is an example of a medication flow chart from a fictitious patient's electronic chart.

Progress Notes

Progress notes are written statements about various aspects of patient care. Some facilities use a lined piece of paper with two columns. The left column is used to document the date and time, and the right column is used to write the note. Oth-ers use a plain or lined piece of paper without columns. The progress notes will reflect each encounter with the patient chronologically, whether by phone, by e-mail, or in person. No matter what form is used for documenting, you must always include the date, time, your signature, and credential.

Checkpoint Question

3. List three advantages of using flow sheets in a medical chart.

MEDICAL RECORD ENTRIES

Proper medical record entries are necessary for efficient communication and for legal considerations. The medical record allows health care practitioners to communicate among themselves and therefore provide the best care possible for the patient. Good communication fosters continuity of patient care.

The medical record is a legal document that can be subpoenaed in a malpractice suit. If the documentation is accurate, timely, and legible, it can help win a lawsuit or prevent one altogether. If the documentation is messy, inaccurate, or improperly done, however, it can raise questions that might cause the practice to lose a malpractice suit. Figure 8-5 shows the difference between a well-written chart note and one that leaves in question what really happened. The golden rule in documentation is that if it is not documented, it was not done. Therefore, all patient procedures, assessments, interventions, evaluations, teachings, and communications must be documented.

Follow these guidelines for documenting in patients' medical records:

1. Make sure you know the office policy regarding charting. Find out who is allowed to write in the chart and the procedures for doing so.
2. Make sure you have the correct patient chart. If the patient's name is common, ask for a birth date or social security number as a double check.
3. Always document in ink.
4. Always sign your complete name and credential.
5. Always record the date of each entry. Some outpatient facilities record the time as well. Using military time will eliminate the need to use A.M. and P.M. (Fig. 8-6).
6. Write legibly. Printing is more legible than cursive writing.
7. Check spelling, especially medical terms, before entering them into the chart. Chapter 7 offers help with spelling.
8. Use only abbreviations that are accepted by your facility. Abbreviations can cause confusion and errors in patient care if they are overused, used incorrectly, or open to interpretation. For instance, the abbreviation BS might stand for bowel sounds,

FIGURE 8-3. Growth chart from electronic medical record.

Ardmore Family Practice, P.A.
2805 Lyndhurst Avenue
Winston-Salem, NC 27103
PHONE: 336-659-0076
FAX: 336-659-0272

Patient: MICHAEL FIELDS   **Date:** 02-12-2003 9:06 AM

MEDICATIONS

Date	Drug Name	Strength/Form	Dispense	Refill	Sig	Last Dose/ Disc Date	Status
1/28/03	SINGULAIR	10 MG TABS	5	0	1 PO BID		NEW
1/28/03	ZITHROMAX	200 MG/5ML SUSR	5	0	1 P.O Q DAY		NEW
1/22/03	ACCUPRIL	10 MG TABS	34	4	1 PO QD	1/28/03	CONTINUE
1/22/03	ADVIL	200 MG TABS	1	1	1/2 Q A.M.	1/25/03	NEW
1/22/03	ALTACE	5 MG CAPS	60	5	ONE TWICE DAILY	1/28/03	CONTINUE
1/22/03	MACROBID	100 MG CAPS	14	0	1 PO BID	1/28/03	CONTINUE
8/26/02	ALTACE	5 MG CAPS	60	5	ONE TWICE DAILY		CONTINUE
8/7/02	PRECOSE	25 MG CAPS	60	0	1/2 B.I.D.	10/5/02	NEW
5/2/01	ACCUPRIL	10 MG TABS	34	4	1 PO QD		NEW
5/2/01	ACCUPRIL	20 MG TABS	30	0	1 PO QD		NEW
5/2/01	ACCUPRIL	40 MG TABS	30	5	1 PO QD		NEW
4/25/01	ACCUPRIL	20 MG TABS	30	0	1 PO QD	4/25/01	NEW
4/25/01	ACCUPRIL	40 MG TABS	30	5	1 PO QD		NEW
4/25/01	MACROBID	100 MG TABS	14	0	1 PO BID	5/1/01	NEW
3/2/01	ACIPHEX 20 MG	TABS	30	6	1 PO QD		NEW
3/2/01	ACTOS 30 MG	TABS	30	2	1 PO QD		NEW
1/23/01	ENTEX PSE	120-600 MG TB12	45	0	1 PO BID		NEW
1/23/01	NASONEX	50 MCG/ACT SUSP	1	3	2 SPRAYS EACH NOSTRIL QD		NEW
8/24/99	ADALAT CC	60 MG TBCR	34	5	1 PO QD	8/24/99	NEW
7/8/99	NITROGLYCERIN	0.4 MG/DOSE AERS	100	1	1 TAB SL Q 5 MIN X 3, IF CHEST PAIN PERS	7/8/99	NEW
6/26/99	CLARITIN	10 MG TABS	30	5	ONE EVERY MORNING		NEW
6/23/99	CELEBREX 100 MG	CAPS	90	3	1 PO Q AM AND 2 PO Q PM		NEW
6/3/99	GLUCOPHAGE	850 MG TABS	90	6	ONE 3 TIMES DAILY	6/3/99	NEW
6/3/99	HYTRIN	5 MG CAPS	30	6	ONE EVERY DAY	6/3/99	NEW

F I G U R E 8 – 4 . Medication administration flow sheet.

Correct	
9-15-03	*Pt. Called to cancel appt. for recheck of UTI on 9-16-03. States she is feeling better. Advised to keep appointment, since Dr. Smith wants to repeat a urinalysis to see if her bladder infection has cleared up. Pt. states, "I don't see any sense in that; I'm not coming". Advised Dr. Smith.* *Fred Lane, CMA*

Incorrect	
9-15-03	*Pt. Called to cancel appt.* *Fred Lane, CMA*

FIGURE 8–5. Right and wrong chart entries.

breath sounds, or blood sugar. Box 8-2 shows abbreviations used in charting, and Appendix D has a general list of commonly used abbreviations. Chapter 9 fully explains the use of abbreviations in medical documentation.

9. When charting the patient's statements, use quotation marks to signify the patient's own words.
10. Do not attempt to make a diagnosis. For example, if the patient says, "My throat is sore," do not write pharyngitis. It is not within the scope of your training to diagnose.
11. Document as soon as possible after completing a task to promote accuracy.
12. Document missed appointments in the patient's chart. Chart your attempts to reach the patient to remind him or her of the appointment.
13. Document any telephone conversations with the patient in the chart.
14. Be honest. If you have given a wrong medication or performed the wrong procedure, as soon as the appropriate supervisor is notified, document it, then complete an incident report (see Chapter 11). State only the facts; do not draw any conclusions or place blame.
15. Never document for someone else, and never ask someone else to document for you.
16. Never document false information.
17. Never delete, erase, scribble over, or white-out information in the medical record because this can be construed as attempting to cover the truth and tampering with a legal document. If you do make an error, draw a single line through it, initial it, and date it. Then write the word "correction" and document the correct information (Fig. 8-7). You can click on an icon to make a correction in the electronic chart, but the original information is not deleted. For example, if you discover that you have entered the wrong date of birth after the patient's information has been saved, you can correct it, but most systems allow only certain users to make changes in the saved database.

Charting Communications With Patients

In addition to documenting patient visits to the facility, other encounters and communications may occur and should become a part of the permanent record. To ensure continuity of care and patient safety, charts should contain a progress sheet or some sort of tool to record each communication with a patient. Actions taken by the physician or employees as directed by the physician on behalf of the patient should be charted. For example, when a prescription is phoned to a pharmacy, the action is recorded. The physician may give instructions to be carried out regarding a patient, such as calling the patient with normal test results. This should be concisely explained in the chart. These entries should appear in **chronological order**. Dates that are out of order and gaps between entries may confuse the reader and give the appearance of poor service. For this reason, entries should be made immediately after communications with the patient.

Telephone communications with patients are typically recorded in a narrative manner. When a patient calls or e-mails the office, the conversation must be documented in the chart immediately. Phone calls should be documented with the time and date of the call, patient's problem or request, and actions taken by the person making the entry. If special telephone message pads are used, a copy should be placed in the patient's chart. E-mails from patients should be printed and kept in the chart. Replies to a patient's e-mail should be printed out and included with the progress sheet. Remember, care must be taken to protect the patient's privacy when using electronic means to communicate.

FIGURE 8–6. Military time.

Box 8-2

ABBREVIATIONS USED IN CHARTING

In office charting, use these common abbreviations to save time and space.

Abbreviation	Meaning
ā	before
abd	abdomen
ant.	anterior
AP	anteroposterior
Ax	axillary
b.i.d.	twice a day
BP	blood pressure
C	Celsius
c̄	with
CC	chief complaint
C/o	complains of
CPX	complete physical examination
Cx	canceled
D/C	discontinue
F	Fahrenheit
Fx	fracture
h.s.	bedtime, hour of sleep
Hx	history
L	left
LLE	left lower extremity
LLQ	left lower quadrant
LUE	left upper extremity
LUQ	left upper quadrant
NKDA	no known drug allergies
noct.	nocturnal
p̄	after
p.c.	after a meal
PE	physical examination
p.r.n.	as needed
pt.	patient
q.i.d.	4 times a day
R	right
R/O	rule out
RLE	right lower extremity
RUE	right upper extremity
RLQ	right lower quadrant
RUQ	right upper quadrant
R/s	rescheduled
s̄	without
SOB	shortness of breath
spec	specimen
s/p	status post
STAT	immediately
t.i.d.	3 times a day
TPR	temperature, pulse, respiration

When correcting a charting error, draw a single line through the error, initial it, date it, and document the correct information.

left 05/15/03 TW

05/15/03 Patient presents today complaining of pain in ~~right~~ eye. Tracy Wiles, CMA

FIGURE 8–7. Correcting an error.

Additions to Medical Records

Any additions to a medical record, such as laboratory re-sults, that are smaller than the standard 8.5 × 11 inches should be transcribed onto a full sheet of paper or shingled and placed in the appropriate area of the chart. Shingling is taping the paper across the top to a regular-size sheet. Each sheet is then added under the current one with a piece of tape across the top. Each sheet can be lifted to view the entire document. Most laboratory reports are computer generated and will come ready to insert into the chart. All additions to the medical record (e.g., laboratory results, radiographic reports, consultation reports) should be read and initialed by the physician before you put them in the chart.

Checkpoint Question

4. What is the golden rule in documentation?

WORKERS' COMPENSATION RECORDS

From time to time, a patient who is active in your practice may seek treatment for a **workers' compensation** case or an injury or illness related to employment. The government requires em-ployers to provide insurance for care when an injury occurs at work. Workers' compensation is discussed in Chapter 17. When this occurs, do not simply add the information to the pa-tient's medical record. Instead, start a new record. A workers' compensation medical record actually belongs to the employer, so the data in that record can be reviewed by the employer's in-surance carrier. No information about the patient's previous health or family history that is not pertinent to the workplace incident should be made available to the insurance carrier.

Before treating a patient for a possible workers' compen-sation case, you must first obtain verification from the em-ployer unless the situation is life-threatening. Be sure to doc-ument the name of the person who authorizes treatment as well as any other information that becomes available during the verification process.

Workers' compensation cases are kept open for 2 years af-ter the last date of treatment for any follow-up care that may be required. After that time, care may not be covered under the same case. Even after the care is complete, the separate record is kept with the patient's other record, and informa-tion is incorporated into the original record as needed.

MEDICAL RECORD PREPARATION

To start filing, you need folders, labels, and any other appropriate supplies. Keep these supplies on hand and follow the same steps every time you put together and file a medical record. Procedure 8-1 outlines the steps for preparing a medical record file. Over the course of many years, you may have to replace worn-out folders or peeling labels and stickers. Do so before the folder tears or the labels fall off.

After preparing the folders, you may also want to prepare several out guides, that is, plastic sheets with a tab (projection) and a pocket for index cards. Type "Out guide" on the tabbed edge of the sheet. Then, when you remove a chart, write the date, name of the patient, your initials, and where the chart can be found on an index card. Place the card inside the out guide, and put the out guide in the spot in the file cabinet where the chart was. An out guide indicates that the chart has been removed and where it can be found. Hospitals and larger clinics often use a wand to keep track of charts and radiographs. When a chart arrives in a certain location, a wand is passed over a bar code. When the patient's number is entered into the computer, the screen shows the location of the patient's chart at the moment. If it is in the file cabinet, that is also indicated.

FILING PROCEDURES

Every day in the medical office, information is added to a patient's chart. It is best to keep this information filed on a daily basis. Pieces of paper to be added can be kept in a central location until filed so that employees can retrieve it if needed before the patient's next visit. This holding area should be used only until the daily filing can be done. In a paperless office, these additions to the medical record are scanned into the system and the original paper is shredded.

To ensure efficient and speedy filing and document retrieval, follow these four steps:

1. *Condition.* Prepare items by removing loose pieces of tape or paper clips. Make sure each sheet of paper includes the patient's name in case a second page gets separated from the first page.
2. *Index.* Separate business records from patient records.
3. *Sort.* Put each group of records in proper order to be filed on shelves, either alphabetic or numeric. This makes actual filing go much faster because you are not moving up and down and back and forth to find the proper letter area; you will just move down in order.
4. *Store.* Place each record in the proper storage area, as described next.

Checkpoint Question

5. Why is it necessary to make a new chart for an established patient who is being seen for an injury sustained at work?

FILING SYSTEMS

The two main filing systems are alphabetic and numeric. In some practices you may use both systems, each for different types of files.

Alphabetic Filing

As the name implies, **alphabetic filing** is a system using letters. Begin alphabetic filing by distinguishing the first, second, and third unit as described in Box 8-3. (A unit is each part of a name or title that is used in indexing.) Using the first letter of the first unit, place your records in small groups in order from A to Z. After that, take each small group and gradually work through the second and consecutive letters to put the small groups in order. Using this process allows you to work in a progressive order as you add records to existing files.

If the entire first unit is the same, move onto the second unit. If the second unit is still the same, move onto the third unit. Occasionally, you will have records whose units one, two, and three are identical. In such cases, it does not matter which one is filed first; use extreme caution, however, when retrieving records with identical units to prevent errors. Asking the patient to provide his or her birthday will ensure that you have the right patient and avoid confusion.

With alphabetic filing, color coding may also be used. Letters of the alphabet are color-coded and affixed to each folder, or a color-coded bar is placed next to the label with the patient's name. For example, names beginning with A to F may be blue; G to L, green; M to T, yellow; and U to Z, purple. Using this system, Michele Beals would have a blue strip, Laurie Palmer would have a yellow strip, Lauren Kayser's would be green, and Dana Warbeck would have purple. Finding misfiled charts is easier. With one glance at the cabinet, for example, you can spot one purple tab in the middle of the green ones.

Numeric Filing

Numeric filing uses digits, usually six. The digits are typically run together but read as three groups of two digits. For example, the record filed as 324478 is read as 32, 44, 78. Commas are not placed or any separation used when applying the labels to the tabbed edge of the file folder. The records are placed in numeric order without concern for duplication, which may sometimes happen with the alphabetic system. If you use this technique, it is called straight digit filing because you are reading the number straight out from left to right.

Sometimes, the file label will look the same, 324478, but will be read in the reverse order: 78, 44, 32. This technique is called terminal digit filing; that is, the groups of numbers are read in pairs from right to left. Be careful not to mix the two filing systems. If using both techniques within your office, be sure to keep them separate by changing the folder color or some other means to prevent errors. The chart is filed by using the last pairs of digits.

Numeric filing plays an important role in the medical office. With tests for human immunodeficiency virus (HIV) and acquired immunodeficiency syndrome (AIDS) and their results being held in strict confidence, the use of numeric filing is becoming even more popular. When this technique is used, it is important to keep a **cross-reference** in a secure area, away

---

Box 8-3

INDEXING RULES FOR ALPHABETIC FILING

When filing records alphabetically, use these indexing rules to help you decide the placement of each record. Indexing rules apply whether you use the title of the record's contents or a person's name.

File by name according to last name, first name, and middle initial, and treat each letter in the name as a separate unit. For example, Jamey L. Crowell should be filed as Crowell, Jamey L. and should come before Crowell, Jamie L.

- Make sure professional initials are placed after a full name. John P. Bonnet, D.O., should be filed as Bonnet, John P., D.O.
- Treat hyphenated names as one unit. Bernadette M. Ryan-Nardone should be filed as Ryan-Nardone, Bernadette M. not as Nardone, Bernadette M. Ryan.
- File abbreviated names as if they were spelled out. Finnigan, Wm. should be filed as Finnigan, William, and St. James should be filed as Saint James.
- File last names beginning with Mac and Mc in regular order or grouped together, depending on your preference, but be consistent with either approach.
- File a married woman's record by using her own first name. Helen Johnston (Mrs. Kevin Johnston) should be filed as Johnston, Helen, not as Johnston, Kevin Mrs.
- Jr. and Sr. should be used in indexing and labeling the record. Many times a father and son are patients at the same facility.
- When names are identical, use the next unit, such as birth dates or the mother's maiden name. Use Durham, Iran (2-4-94) and Durham, Iran (4-5-45).
- Disregard apostrophes.
- Disregard articles (a, the), conjunctions (and, or), and prepositions (in, of) in filing. File *The Cat in the Hat* under Cat in Hat.
- Treat letters in a company name as separate units. For ASM, Inc., "A" is the first unit, "S" is the second unit, and "M" is the third unit.

Box 8-4

ALPHABETIC FILING EXAMPLES

The following patient records are to be filed alphabetically:

Mary P. Martin
Floyd Pigg, Sr.
Susan Bailey
Ellen Eisel-Parrish
Anita Putrosky
Susan R. Hill
Sister Mary Catherine
Cher
Stephen Dorsky, MD
Mrs. John Moser (Donna)

The proper order is:

Susan Bailey
Cher
Stephen Dorsky
Ellen Eisel-Parrish
Susan R. Hill
Mary P. Martin
Donna Moser
Floyd D. Pigg
Anita Putrosky
Sister Mary Catherine

---

from patient areas, listing the numeric code and the name of the patient. Such a reference is called a master patient index. This way limited numbers of people know who the patient is, which maintains privacy. Boxes 8-4 and 8-5 show how to file patient records alphabetically or numerically.

Other Filing Systems

The medical office keeps files other than patient records. An office manager keeps files on employees, insurance policies, accounts payable, and so on. For this type of filing, systems include **subject filing**, in which documents are arranged alphabetically according to subject (e.g., insurance, medications, referrals); geographic filing, in which documents are grouped alphabetically according to locations, such as state, county, or city; and chronological filing, in which documents are grouped in the order of their date.

Box 8-5

NUMERIC FILING EXAMPLES

The following patient records are to be filed numerically:

LeRoy Flora	213456
Ramsey Curtis	334387
Sharon Moore	979779
Cathy King	321138

In straight digit filing, the proper order is:

213456
321138
334387
979779

In terminal digit filing, the proper order is:

321138
213456
979779
334387

With files in which one or two groups of numbers are the same numbers, you refer to the second or third groups or numbers. For example, in straight digit filing (reading from left to right) the number 003491 comes before 004592. The first group of numbers (00) is the same for both files, so you determine the order of filing by the second group of numbers; in this case, 34 comes before 45.

In terminal digit filing (reading from right to left), 456128 would come before 926128. The first two groups of numbers (28 and 61) are the same for both files, so you go to the third group of numbers; in this case, 45 comes before 92.

Checkpoint Question

6. What are the two main filing systems? Briefly describe each.

CLASSIFYING MEDICAL RECORDS

Records are classified in three categories: active, inactive, or closed. Active records are those of patients who have been seen within the past few years. The exact amount of time is designated within each practice; it usually ranges from 1 to 5 years. Keep these records in the most accessible storage spot available because you will be using them regularly.

Inactive records are those of patients who have not been seen in more than the designated time set aside for active records. You will still keep these records in the office, but

they do not have to be as accessible as the active files. Usually, they are placed on bottom shelves to eliminate constant bending when reaching for active files, or they may be stored in another room within the office. "Inactive" patients have not formally terminated their contact with the physician, but they have either not needed the physician's services or have not informed the office regarding a move, change in physician, or death.

Closed records are those of patients who have terminated their relationship with the physician. Reasons for such termination might include the patient moving, termination of physician–patient relationship by letter, no further treatment necessary, or death of the patient.

INACTIVE RECORD STORAGE

Inactive records can be stored in the office in an out-of-the-way area, such as a basement or attic. They may even be kept in the physician's home. This practice is permitted because the records belong to the physician, but it is not recommended because at any time the office staff may need access to these records. Many practices use **microfilm** or **microfiche** to store closed records. Microfilm and microfiche are ways to photograph documents and store them in a reduced form. Microfilm, a popular method for storing large volumes of records, particularly in hospitals and clinics, uses a photographic process that develops medical records in miniature on film. Information is stored on cards holding single film frames or in reels or strips for projection on compact electric viewers placed at convenient office locations. The cost of the equipment is declining, making this a more practical method for storing and retrieving inactive files.

Microfiche is a miniature photographic system that stores rows of images in reduced size on cards with clear plastic sleeves rather than on film strips. Information can be handled manually, examined on a viewer that enlarges the record, or reproduced as hard copy on a high-speed photocopier. A standard microfiche card holds more than 60 pages of information. The microfiche process allows 3,200 papers to be reduced to fit on a single 4 × 6-inch transparency.

Checkpoint Question

7. What are the three classifications of medical records? Describe each.

STORING ACTIVE MEDICAL RECORDS

Medical offices use a variety of storage methods for active files that are used on a daily basis. Shelf files are stationary shelves. Shelving units are stacked on each other or placed side by side. These shelves may also be custom-ordered to the width you need. Records are stored horizontally, and labels are read from the side. Figure 8-8 shows such shelving units.

Drawer files are a type of filing cabinet. The drawer pulls

F IGURE 8 – 8 .   File cabinets.

out for easy access and visibility of all records. This type of filing system allows you easier access to all sides of files, which can help in searches for missing files that may have been pushed to the back or behind other files. Drawer files also allow easier filing because you can read from above the files, rather than squatting to read the labels from the sides as you work your way down to the lower shelves. A disadvantage is that these files take up a great deal of space.

Rotary circular or lateral files allow records to be stored in units that either spin in a circle or stack one behind the other, enabling you to rotate different units to the front. This system allows for maximum use of office space and is suggested for a medical office with large quantities of records to be stored. With shelf or drawer units, more wall space is needed to spread out each unit, but with rotary files, less wall space is needed.

Even the paperless medical office must consider storage because backup copies of computerized records must be made daily and stored in a safe, fireproof location. Security experts advise storing backup disks off-site.

Record Retention

As discussed in Chapter 2, the statute of limitations is the legal time limit set for filing suit against an alleged wrongdoer. The time limit varies from state to state. You must observe the statute of limitations in your particular state to know how long medical and business records should be kept in storage.

It is recommended that medical records be stored permanently, because in some states malpractice lawsuits can be filed within 2 years of the date of discovery of the alleged malpractice. The statute of limitations for minors is extended until the child reaches legal age in every state; the time given past the legal age varies, however.

Tax records and liability plans, including old and new policies, should be permanently stored in a fireproof cabinet. Older liability plans may provide coverage should a mal-

practice lawsuit be filed later, after that policy expires and a new policy takes effect.

Insurance policies should also be stored in a fireproof cabinet. You can keep the newest policy and discard the older one.

Canceled checks should be kept in fireproof storage for at least 3 years. After that, keep them indefinitely in regular storage.

Receipts for equipment should be kept until each item listed on the receipt is no longer being used.

Checkpoint Question

8. How long should medical records be kept?

RELEASING MEDICAL RECORDS

Although the physical medical record legally belongs to the physician, the information belongs to the patient. Any release of records must first be authorized by the patient or the patient's legal guardian. When releasing a medical record, provide a copy only. *Never* release the original medical record except in limited circumstances (see the Legal Tip nearby).

Insurance companies, lawyers, other health care practitioners, and patients themselves may request copies of medical records. All requests should be made in writing, stating the patient's name, address, and social security number, and must contain the patient's *original* signature authorizing the release of records. Never release information over the telephone. You will have no way of verifying that the person with whom you are speaking is actually the person who has authorization.

Unless the request is made by the patient, state laws allow facilities to charge a fee for copying the medical record. The AMA published guidelines for physicians to ensure ethical

LEGAL TIP

The only time an original record should be released is when it is subpoenaed by a court of law. In such situations, the physician may wish to have the judge sign a document stating that he or she will temporarily take charge of the medical record. This signed document should be filed in the medical office until the record is returned. To further ensure the record's safety, a staff member can transport the original record to court on the day it is requested, then return the record at the end of the court session that day. As soon as it is known that a record will be part of a court case, the record should be kept in a locked cabinet. When the court orders that a record be submitted to the court at a given date and time, the legal order is termed *subpoena duces tecum*.

business practices. They recommend a reasonable fee for re-production of records to be no more than $1 per page or $100 for the entire record, whichever is less. If the record is less than 10 pages, the office may charge up to $10 to cover postage and miscellaneous costs associated with the retrieval process. Laws may vary from state to state.

You must follow certain guidelines even with a signed authorization release form (Fig. 8-9). The authorization form must give the patient the opportunity to limit the information to be released. Patients may release only information relating to a specific disorder, or they may specify a time limit. They may not, however, ask that the physician leave out information pertinent to the situation. References to mental health diagnosis or treatments, drug or alcohol abuse, HIV, AIDS, or any other sexually transmitted disease may not be released without specific mention on the signed authorization form. If it is not specifically requested, when you are copying the record, place a piece of blank white paper over any such areas of information. Never white-out these areas on the original document or mention what these blank areas are.

Releasing Records to Patients

For a thorough discussion of releasing medical records, see Chapter 2. When patients request copies of their own records, the doctor makes the decision about what to copy. Patients aged 17 and under cannot get copies of their own medical records without a signed consent from a parent or legal guardian, except for emancipated minors. They may obtain certain services independently (check your state's law regarding treatment of minors), however; in such cases, under the law, you are not permitted to contact the parent or guardian. Some states allow minors to seek treatment for sexually transmitted diseases and birth control without parental knowledge or consent. Sometimes, the parent or guardian may still be billed for these services without the bill

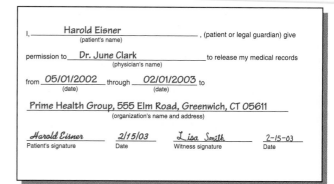

FIGURE 8-9.   Sample authorization to release information.

being itemized. The billing statement should include only the treatment dates and amount due.

Checkpoint Question

9. What is required for a legal disclosure of a patient's HIV status?

Reporting Obligations

Although patients' records are confidential, in certain situations concerning the public's health and safety, the law requires reporting information to particular authorities. Requirements for reporting vary among states. Generally, the following types of items must be reported: vital statistics, communicable diseases, child and elderly abuse or maltreatment, and certain violent injuries (see Chapter 2).

Spanish Terminology

Por firmar aquí, usted nos da permiso de compartir su información medical con su compañía de seguro.	By signing here, you are giving us permission to share your medical information with your insurance company.
Necesitaremos copias de su historia medical de los archivos de su médico anterior.	We will need copies of your medical records from your previous doctor.

Procedure 8-1

Preparing a Medical File

Equipment/Supplies

- File folder
- Title, year, and alphabetic or numeric labels

Step	Reason
1. Decide the name of the file (a patient's name, company name, or name of the type of information to be stored).	Properly naming a file allows for easy retrieval.
2. Type a label with the title *in unit order* (e.g., Lynn, Laila S., *not* Laila S. Lynn).	Typing the label in unit order helps avoid filing errors.
3. Place the label along the tabbed edge of the folder so that the title extends out beyond the folder itself. (Tabs can be either the length of the folder or tabbed in various positions, such as left, center, and right.)	This ensures easy readability.
4. Place a year label along the top edge of the tab before the label with the title. This will be changed each year the patient has been seen. *Note:* Do not automatically replace these labels at the start of a new year; remove the old year and replace with a new one only when the patient comes in for the first visit of the new year.	Doing this makes removing inactive files more time efficient. At the beginning of each new year, you can easily spot the records that are years beyond your storage time limit in the active file area. Doing this also can help you locate inactive files if patients return years later. (By determining the last year the patient was seen, you can narrow your search to files with a matching year label.)
5. Place the appropriate alphabetic or numeric labels below the title.	This aids in accurate filing and retrieval.
6. Apply any additional labels that your office may decide to use.	Labels noting special information (e.g., insurance, drug allergies, advanced directives) act as quick and easy reminders.

CHAPTER SUMMARY

Medical records not only are a means of communication among health care providers but also are legal documents depicting the quality of patient care. Preparing and maintaining medical records is an important responsibility. To ensure efficient recording and retrieval, you must be familiar with the varied documentation forms as well as the different kinds of filing systems. In addition, you must adhere to strict guidelines when releasing any information in patients' medical records. Electronic medical records are giving rise to new issues in protecting medical records. The patient's privacy must be protected at all times. The quality, use, and care of the medical record are reflections of the quality of the outpatient facility itself.

Critical Thinking Challenges

1. Interview a fellow student with a hypothetical injury. Document the incident with the chief complaint and the present illness.
2. Compare and contrast alphabetic filing with numeric filling. Which system do you think works better? Explain your response.
3. Instruct a fellow student in the requirements of your office regarding the release of medical records.
4. Write an office policy for maintaining confidentiality with electronic modalities, such as fax machines, printers, laptops, and computer screens.

Answers to Checkpoint Questions

1. The patient's chief complaint is the reason the patient is seeing the physician.

2. Narrative, SOAP, and POMR are three common formats for recording patient–provider encounters.

3. The advantages of using flow sheets in the medical chart are that they limit the need for long handwritten notes, save time and space, and make it easier to locate information.

4. The golden rule in documenting is that if it is not documented, it was not done.

5. The chart of the patient injured on the job has information that should not be available to the employer, who has access only to the information about the worker's injury.

6. The two main filing systems are alphabetic (using letters to file records) and numeric (using digits to file records).

7. The three classifications of medical records are active (seen within the past few years), inactive (not currently being seen but still patients), and closed (relationship is terminated because of death, patient moved, or change in physician).

8. Medical records should be kept forever.

9. Permission to release information about a patient's HIV status must be specifically given on the release form that is signed by the patient.

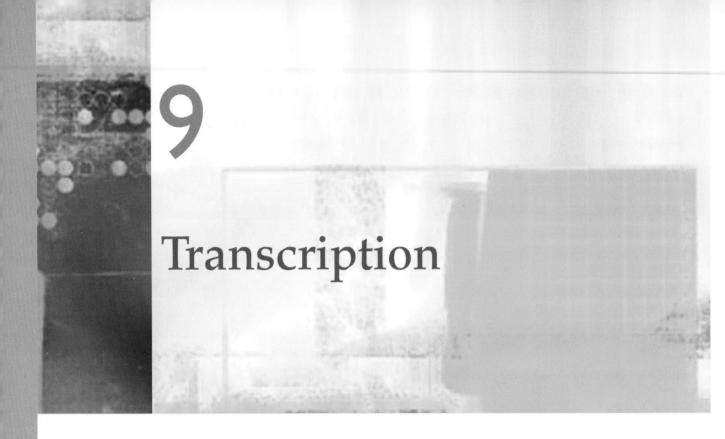

9

Transcription

CHAPTER OUTLINE

ROLE DELINEATION COMPONENTS

GENERAL: Communication Skills
- Recognize and respond effectively to verbal, nonverbal, and written communications
- Use electronic technology to receive, organize, prioritize, and transmit information

GENERAL: Legal Concepts
- Prepare and maintain medical records
- Document accurately

ADMINISTRATIVE: Administrative Procedures
- Perform basic administrative medical assisting functions

CHAPTER COMPETENCIES

LEARNING OBJECTIVES

Upon successfully completing the chapter, you will be able to:
1. Explain the role of the medical assistant in performing medical transcription
2. Explain the roles of the JCAHO and HIPAA on medical transcription
3. List the various reports generated in inpatient and outpatient medical facilities
4. List the rules of medical transcription as outlined by the AAMT
5. Discuss the various medical transcription systems

PERFORMANCE OBJECTIVES

Upon successfully completing the chapter, you will be able to:
1. Transcribe various medical reports from taped dictation
2. Use proper punctuation, grammar, and spelling

KEY TERMS

analogue   digital   transcription

MEDICAL TRANSCRIPTION

Transcription is the process of typing a dictated message. The word *transcript* is from Latin and translates literally to "across writing," meaning to change the spoken word to written word. In the medical office, certified medical assistants (CMAs) often use the skills taught in this chapter. The role delineation chart by the American Association of Medical Assistants (AAMA) discussed in Chapter 1 reveals that medical transcription is a function of the practicing medical assistant (Fig. 9-1). Therefore, as with all topics covered in this text, accrediting agencies require that this skill be taught in accredited medical assisting educational programs.

Those who choose to focus their education on medical transcription are trained to transcribe both inpatient and outpatient reports. The types of reports you will transcribe in a physician's office are different from those seen in the inpatient or hospital facility. The transcription training you receive as a medical assistant focuses on outpatient documents. Most hospitals employ certified medical transcriptionists. Some physicians' offices use outside medical transcription companies, and this is another employment opportunity for the trained medical assistant. In today's computerized world, with a modem and sound privacy protection practices, a transcriptionist could conceivably generate and transmit reports from anywhere in the world.

To transcribe well, you must

- Be a fast and accurate typist
- Have a strong vocabulary in medical terminology
- Have a thorough knowledge of grammar, spelling, and punctuation rules
- Have excellent listening skills
- Have good editing skills

FIGURE 9–1. A transcriptionist must have good communications and computer skills.

The Transcription Process

When a patient visits a physician's office, the provider either writes the findings or dictates a report into a handheld microphone. The provider places the cassette tape and the charts from that day in a designated area. The employee responsible for transcription listens to the tape on a machine called a transcriber. A foot pedal controls play, rewind, and fast forward. The words are typed into a word processor, proofread, and printed. The printed copy is placed on the chart and given to the provider for review. Corrections are made and a final copy is printed and given to the provider for final review and signature. Copies of the report are distributed to anyone the provider names to receive a copy, and a copy is placed in the chart. As tapes are transcribed, they are erased and given back to the provider to use again.

When an office is paperless, the process is the same, but the document is entered into the record instead of being printed. A visual signal can alert the provider as reports become ready for edit. The provider accesses the report and makes edits or marks errors. When the provider is ready to authenticate the report, the stroke of a key "signs" the report. The software allows the provider to check the status of a report at any time.

Off-site Transcription

Many medical offices outsource their transcription through various types of services. Individuals or companies offer services to physicians ranging from picking up tapes and delivering the work on hard copy to transmitting the documents through e-mail.

Several large transcription companies operate solely on the Internet. These websites can be found at the end of the chapter. You can log on, and after passing an online examination, you may begin receiving dictation via modem. The report is transmitted back to the company, which sends it to the provider. Usually, the transcriptionist must buy the necessary equipment. The new regulations of the HIPAA (Health Insurance Portability and Accountability Act) discussed in earlier chapters will require changes in practices for transmission of confidential information via modem.

REPORT FORMATTING

There is no set format for each type of medical document. Every facility has its own format and design, but any professional document should be well balanced and attractive, with single spacing, double spacing between headings, and 1-inch margins. Being familiar with the logical sequence and proper sorting of information for each type of document will help you adapt to any prescribed format. Headings and subheadings are used to report the information gathered in the course of a patient encounter. These general headings are seen in the sample reports in Figures 9-2 to 9-9.

History and Physical Examination Reports

In the inpatient setting, the H&P is a vital part of the quality of patient care. The JCAHO (Joint Commission on Accreditation of Healthcare Organizations) accredits and regulates every aspect of the policies and practices of hospitals and physician offices owned by hospital organizations.

The JCAHO guidelines require hospitals to provide a H&P on a patient's chart within 24 hours of admission in a facility. This report is dictated by the admitting physician and must be signed or authenticated electronically within a specified time. Many times the patient is seen in the office, and the physician makes the decision to admit. The examination takes place in the office, but the report is dictated to the hospital, which is responsible for transcription. Many physicians use the H&P format to record a patient's annual physical examination in the office as well.

The H&P is divided into two sections: the history, which gives an overview of the patient's medical, family, and social history; and the report on the physical examination, which reviews the results of the examination. Figure 9-2 is a sample history and physical examination report.

Checkpoint Question

2. List two requirements of the JCAHO regarding H&Ps.

Consultation Reports

When one provider refers a patient to another, usually a specialist, the consulting physician prepares a consultation report to report the findings of the encounter. A consultation

WHAT IF

You are transcribing notes and hear an unfamiliar word or phrase on the tape. What should you do?

You should have a selection of reference materials available at your workstation. Examples of useful reference books include a standard dictionary, a general medical dictionary, a medical dictionary specific to your specialty, a drug reference such as the *Physicians' Desk Reference* (PDR), and a medical textbook on anatomy, physiology, and disease processes. Remember, software that provides a medical dictionary to interact with your word processing spell check is available. If you cannot find the word, leave a blank large enough for the physician to write in the word. The report can be edited before being signed.

LEGAL TIP

Legal Aspects of Transcription

Health care facilities are expected to adhere to general standards to ensure patient rights and safety. The JCAHO, Joint Commission on Accreditation of Healthcare Organizations, requires that all hospitals and hospital-owned physician practices:
- Use abbreviations from an approved list and provide a key to the reader (if requested.) For a list of accepted abbreviations used in charting, see Chapter 8.
- Adhere to a specific time frame for review and completion (signing) by physicians.

In addition, as discussed in Chapter 8, HIPAA establishes specific regulations to safeguard the privacy of patient information when using electronic means for medical transcription.

Checkpoint Question

1. List four requirements of any professional document.

TYPES OF MEDICAL REPORTS

Hospital (inpatient) documents and medical office (outpatient) documents are different. The most common documents transcribed in a medical office are history and physical examination (H&P) reports, consultation reports, and progress reports. Practices that offer diagnostic tests are required to generate a report of the findings. For example, a neurologist's practice may perform electroencephalography (EEG) to measure the electrical activity in the brain. The medical assistant transcribes a dictated report of the findings. Other types of documents in outpatient facilities are reports of minor surgical procedures, legal abstracts, and general office correspondence.

Documents that are seen in the hospital setting include H&Ps, consultation reports, radiology and pathology reports, transfer summaries, discharge and death summaries, and autopsies. Many radiologists who work in hospitals also have a private practices and will dictate a report for each radiology procedure done in the office. You need to become familiar with the reports generated in a hospital because they become a part of the office chart and are used for insurance. Figures 9-6 to 9-9 are samples of typical reports generated in a hospital or inpatient setting.

CENTRAL MEDICAL GROUP, INC.
Department of Internal Medicine

201 Medical Center Drive • Central City, US 90000-1234 • PHONE: (012) 125-8888 • FAX: (012) 125-3434

PATIENT: COHEN, SARA E.   DATE: April 8, 20xx

HISTORY

CHIEF COMPLAINT: Epigastric distress

HISTORY OF PRESENT ILLNESS: This 33-year-old Caucasian female comes in because of excessive burping, epigastric distress and nausea for several weeks. Coffee makes it worse. She complains that it is worse at night when lying down. She gets an acid-like taste in her mouth. She has tried antacids, to no avail.

PAST MEDICAL HISTORY: The patient states that she had the usual childhood diseases. She has had no serious medical illnesses and has been involved in no accidents. Family History: There is some diabetes on her mother's side. Her mother is 52 and has hypertension. Her father, age 56, is living and well. She has a sister who is anemic and a brother who has ulcers. Social History: The patient discontinued smoking ten years ago. Drinks alcohol socially. Allergies: NKDA. Current Medications: Medications at this time consist of Entex, Guaifed, birth control pills, iron and vitamin supplements.

REVIEW OF SYSTEMS: HEENT: Chronic sinusitis. She sees an ENT specialist and an allergist. Respiratory: Negative. Cardiac: Occasional flutters. Gastrointestinal: As stated above. Genitourinary: Occasional infections. Pap smear is up-to-date and negative. She has had no mammogram at this point. Neuromuscular: Negative.

PHYSICAL EXAMINATION

GENERAL APPEARANCE: Reveals a well-developed, well-nourished female in no acute distress.

VITAL SIGNS: Blood Pressure: 120/80. Pulse: 76 and regular.

HEENT: Head normocephalic. Eyes: Pupils are equal, round, and reactive to light and accommodation. Fundi are benign. Ears, nose and throat are negative. NECK: No thyromegaly. No carotid bruits.

CHEST: Clear to percussion and auscultation. BREASTS: Reveal no masses. HEART: Normal sinus rhythm. No murmurs.

ABDOMEN: Liver, spleen and kidneys could not be felt. Femorals pulsate well, no bruits.

EXTREMITIES: No edema. Pulses are good and equal.

PELVIC & RECTAL EXAMS: Deferred to gynecologist.

NEUROLOGIC EXAM: Physiologic.

IMPRESSION: 1. PROBABLE PEPTIC ULCER DISEASE WITH GASTROESOPHAGEAL REFLUX.
                  2. POSSIBLE GALLBLADDER DISEASE.

PLAN: Patient started on Pepcid 40 mg, 1 at night. She is given Gaviscon tablets so she can carry them with her. Schedule routine lab work and upper GI series. If negative, schedule ultrasound of the gallbladder.

D. Everley, M.D.

DE:mc
D: 4/8/20xx
T: 4/9/20xx

F I G U R E   9 – 2 .   Sample history and physical examination report. (Reprinted with permission from Willis MC. Medical Terminology: The Language of Health Care, 1st ed. Baltimore: Williams & Wilkins, 1996.)

report contains a detailed account of the consulting physician's findings and recommendations regarding the patient. These reports are often written in the format of the H&P but are structured as a letter to the physician who referred the patient. Chapter 6 discusses the use of the terms *referral* and *consultation*. Figure 9-3 is a sample consultation report.

Progress Reports

In the outpatient medical facility, the patient's progress is recorded on an ongoing sheet in the chart (see Chapter 8). When the notes are transcribed, they are printed either directly on this sheet or on special paper with perforations and adhesive backing. The reports are separated and stuck on the progress sheet. Remember, the entries in the medical record must be consecutive. This presents a problem if the transcription is not on the chart when the next entry is made. Entries that are out of order give the appearance of disorganization, improper record keeping, or even an attempt to cover up negligence.

Progress notes are formatted in several ways. These are discussed in Chapter 8. The SOAP (subjective, objective, assessment, plan) method of reporting a patient's visit is the most common format used in medical offices. The report is dictated in narrative form using general headings. In the outpatient medical facility, you will transcribe this information. Refer to Figure 9-4 as we examine each part of the report.

SOAP Notes

Subjective. The subjective portion of the report includes information that cannot be detected or measured. This information can only be provided by the patient. Pain and nausea are examples of subjective information. This heading also includes the *chief complaint* (CC), the reason the patient is at the facility. In the subjective section, the provider explains the chief complaint in detail, including how long the symptoms have been present and what remedies the patient has tried, along with their results. This is sometimes called the *history of present illness* (HPI). A subheading titled *Medication* may be included in this section to report medications that the patient is taking.

Objective. The objective information in this section comes from the physical examination, laboratory data, diagnostic test results, and other data that can be measured or observed. The patient's appearance, vital signs, any rash, and results of laboratory tests are examples of objective information. For example, the narrative report might say, "EEG is normal."

Assessment. As discussed earlier, the assessment portion of the report refers to the established or possible diagnosis based on the subjective and objective information provided and gathered. Other subheading titles include *Diagnosis*, *Evaluation*, *Impression*, and *Differential Diagnoses*.

Plan. The plan is the steps the physician intends to take. They are usually typed in a numbered list. Medications pre-

scribed, diagnostic tests ordered, referrals to other physicians, and return appointments are included in this section.

Checkpoint Question

3. Compare subjective and objective information. Give two examples of each.

Hospital Reports

H&Ps, consultation reports, operative reports, pathology reports, radiology reports, discharge summaries, and death summaries are generated primarily in inpatient facilities. Every document generated by a hospital transcription department is "copied to," that is, copied and sent to the physician who dictated it. These documents are kept in the physician's office chart.

Operative Report

Each surgical procedure performed in a hospital is documented. Physicians dictate an operative note immediately after the procedure. It is typed and put on the chart as soon as possible so that others caring for the patient have access to the information. When physicians perform surgery in their outpatient offices, the operative report is transcribed in the physician's office. The terms used in operative reports are often difficult. Many sutures and instruments are named for the person who developed them. A reference book for surgical terms is essential for transcribing. Information included in the operative reports includes the patient's preoperative and postoperative diagnoses, the type of anesthesia used, step-by-step details of the procedure, estimated blood loss, results of sponge and instrument counts, and the condition of the patient at the end of the procedure. The subheadings usually follow that format. Figure 9-5 is a sample operative report.

Pathology Report

Any organ or tissue removed from a patient in the operating room is examined by a pathologist. A pathology report outlines the findings of gross and microscopic examinations performed on organs, lesions, and tissue samples removed in surgery. Figure 9-6 is an example of a typical pathology report on a specimen.

Autopsy Report

Pathologists also dictate autopsy reports. An autopsy report, also called necropsy report or medical examiner report, is generated as the autopsy is performed. Autopsies are done to find the cause of death of a patient or to find or confirm diseases present. As discussed in Chapter 2, the law requires that autopsies be performed in certain situations. The autopsy report includes a preliminary diagnosis, a brief history of the

(text continues on page 167)

CENTRAL MEDICAL GROUP, INC.
Department of Otorhinolaryngology
201 Medical Center Drive • Central City, US 90000-1234 • PHONE: (012) 125-8888 • FAX: (012) 125-3434

Patient: Perron, Carleen   DATE: February 17, 20xx

Referring Physician: C. Camarillo, M.D.

CONSULTATION

REASON FOR CONSULTATION: This 28-year-old white female presents with a one week history of upper respiratory infection (URI), sinusitis, and some periorbital headaches in recent weeks. She also has expectorated yellow-green mucus occasionally and has had a history of tonsillitis.

MEDICATIONS: None. **ALLERGIES:** No known allergies (NKA). **SURGERIES:** None. **HOSPITALIZATIONS:** None.

PAST MEDICAL HISTORY/REVIEW OF SYSTEMS: Cardiopulmonary: There is no history of angina, dyspnea, hemoptysis, emphysema, asthma, chronic obstructive pulmonary disease (COPD), hypertension, or heart murmurs. Cardiovascular: There is no history of high blood pressure. Renal: There is no history of dysuria, polyuria, nocturia, hematuria, or cystoliths. Gastrointestinal: There is no history of gallbladder disease, hepatitis, pancreatitis, or colitis. Musculoskeletal: There is no history of arthritis. Endocrine: There is no history of diabetes. Hematologic: There is no history of anemia, blood transfusion, or easy bruising. Gynecological: The patient states her menses are regular, and the start of her last menstrual cycle occurred 15 days ago.

FAMILY HISTORY: The patient states her maternal grandmother has diabetes.

SOCIAL HISTORY: The patient is single and has no children. She denies smoking tobacco. She denies drinking alcoholic beverages. She denies taking drugs.

CHILDHOOD DISEASES: The patient has had the usual childhood diseases.

OTOLARYNGOLOGIC EXAMINATION: Otoscopy: Tympanic membranes (TMs) are dull and slightly congested. Sinuses: There is maxillary fullness. Rhinoscopic examination reveals mild nasoseptal deviation (NSD). Pharynx: There is moderate inflammation; no exudates. Oropharynx: No masses. Nasopharynx: No masses. Larynx: Clear. Neck: Supple. Cervical Adenopathy: There is mild adenopathy.

IMPRESSION:
1. MAXILLARY SINUSITIS.
2. PHARYNGITIS.
3. CHRONIC TONSILLITIS.

DISPOSITION:
1. Warm salt water gargle (WSWG).
2. Ery-Tab 333, #24, 1 t.i.d. p.c.
3. Robitussin.
4. Return to office (RTO) in one week.

P. Rodden MD
PATRICK RODDEN, M.D.

JR:ti
D: 2/17/20xx
T: 2/18/20xx

FIGURE 9-3. Sample consultation report. (Reprinted with permission from Willis MC. Medical Terminology: The Language of Health Care, 1st ed. Baltimore: Williams & Wilkins, 1996.)

CENTRAL MEDICAL GROUP, INC.

Department of Otorhinolaryngology

201 Medical Center Drive • Central City, US 90000-1234 • PHONE: (012) 125-8888 • FAX: (012) 125-3434

PROGRESS NOTES

Patient: PERRON, CARLEEN

03/30/20xx

S: The patient presents with a sore throat x 2 weeks.

O: Sinus exam: Maxillary and frontal congestion. Hypopharynx/adenoids: No inflammation.

A: Recurrent pharyngitis/sinusitis x 2 weeks.

P:
1) Ceftin 250 mg, #21, 1 t.i.d. p.o. p.c.

2) Entex LA, #30, 1 b.i.d. p.o.

3) Warm salt water gargle.

P Rodden MD
PATRICK RODDEN, M.D.

05/25/20xx

S: Recurrent sore throat every month.

O: Recurrent tonsillitis, cryptic tonsillitis. Sinus exam: Maxillary and frontal congestion. Neck: Supple; no masses. Hypopharynx/Adenoids: No inflammation. Paranasal Sinus X-ray: Bilateral frontal and maxillary sinusitis.

A: Recurrent tonsillitis, 8-10 times per year. Chronic maxillary and frontal sinusitis.

P:
1) Tonsillectomy discussed with the patient. The risks of general and local anesthesia, as well as the surgical procedure, were discussed with the patient. The consent form was signed.

2) An admitting order was given to the patient for CBC, UA, and BCP-7 to be done one day prior to being admitted.

3) Ceftin 250 mg, #21, 1 t.i.d. p.o. p.c.

4) Entex LA, #30, 1 b.i.d. p.o.

5) Beconase nasal inhaler, 2 sprays each nostril b.i.d.

6) Warm salt water gargle.

P Rodden MD
PATRICK RODDEN, M.D.

F I G U R E 9 – 4 . Sample progress report. (Reprinted with permission from Willis MC. Medical Terminology: The Language of Health Care, 1st ed. Baltimore: Williams & Wilkins, 1996.)

CENTRAL MEDICAL CENTER

211 Medical Center Drive • Central City, US 90000-1234 • PHONE: (012) 125-6784 • FAX: (012) 125-9999

OPERATIVE REPORT

DATE OF OPERATION: June 3, 20xx

PREOPERATIVE DIAGNOSIS: Chronic tonsillitis.

POSTOPERATIVE DIAGNOSIS: Frequent, recurrent tonsillitis.

SURGEON: Patrick Rodden, M.D.

ASSISTANT SURGEON: None

ANESTHESIOLOGIST: Robert Jung, M.D.

ANESTHESIA: General.

SURGERY PERFORMED: Tonsillectomy.

DESCRIPTION OF OPERATION: After general anesthesia induction, with intubation, the McGivor mouth gag and tongue retractor were utilized for exposure of the oropharynx. Local anesthetic consisting of 6 cc of 0.5% Xylocaine with 1:100,000 epinephrine was utilized. Tonsillectomy was carried out using dissection and air technique. The right tonsillectomy electrocoagulation Bovie suction was utilized for hemostasis. Examination of the nasopharynx was normal.

The patient tolerated the procedure well and went to the recovery room in good condition.

P. Rodden MD
PATRICK RODDEN, M.D.

JR:as
D: 6/3/20xx
T: 6/4/20xx

OPERATIVE REPORT	PT. NAME:	PERRON, CARLEEN
	ID NO:	672894017
	ROOM NO:	312
	ATT. PHYS:	PATRICK RODDEN, M.D.

FIGURE 9-5. Sample operative report. (Reprinted with permission from Willis MC. Medical Terminology: A Programmed Learning Approach to the Language of Health Care, 1st ed. Baltimore: Lippincott Williams & Wilkins, 2002.)

CENTRAL MEDICAL CENTER

211 Medical Center Drive • Central City, US 90000-1234 • PHONE: (012) 125-6784 • FAX: (012) 125-9999

PATHOLOGY REPORT

PATIENT: PERRON, CARLEEN
28 Y (FEMALE)

DATE RECEIVED: June 3, 20xx   DATE REPORTED: June 4, 20xx

GROSS:

Received are two tonsils each 2.5 cm in greatest diameter.

MICROSCOPIC:

The sections show deep tonsillar crypts associated with follicular lymphoid hyperplasia. No bacterial granules are seen.

DIAGNOSIS:

CHRONIC LYMPHOID HYPERPLASIA OF RIGHT AND LEFT TONSILS.

MARY NEEDHAM, M.D.

MN:gds

D: 6/4/20xx
T: 6/5/20xx

F I G U R E 9 – 6 . Sample pathology report. (Reprinted with permission from Willis MC. Medical Terminology: A Programmed Learning Approach to the Language of Health Care, 1st ed. Baltimore: Lippincott Williams & Wilkins, 2002.)

patient, findings from the examination of the gross anatomy of the body and its organs, findings of the microscopic examination of the cells, and a determination of cause of death.

Radiology Report

Each radiograph must be interpreted by a radiologist. Even when radiological procedures are performed in an emergency room or walk-in clinic, a radiologist must read the film and dictate a formal report. Radiology reports include the title of the procedure, any contrast medium or nuclear medicine given, and an interpretation of the film (Fig. 9-7).

Discharge Summary

The discharge summary is a chronological account of the patient's hospital stay. If the patient is being transferred to another facility, this report may be titled *Transfer Summary*. It is a concise report of the reason for the patient's admission, tests performed, treatments given, results of those tests and treat-

CENTRAL MEDICAL CENTER

211 Medical Center Drive • Central City, US 90000-1234 • PHONE: (012) 125-6784 • FAX: (012) 125-9999

X-RAY REPORT

LUMBOSACRAL SPINE:
Multiple views reveal no evidence of fracture. There is slight lumbar spondylosis with slight lipping and minimal bridging. The disc spaces appear maintained except for slight narrowing at L4-L5 and L5-S1. There is also a Grade I spondylolisthesis of L5 on S1 and evidence of spondylolysis at L5 on the left. There is also slight dextroscoliosis in the lumbar region and slight increased lordosis in the lumbosacral region. The bony architecture is unremarkable except for eburnation between the articulating facets at L5-S1. The SI joints appear unremarkable. Incidentally noted are slight osteoarthritic changes involving both hips.

CONCLUSION:

1. Slight lumbar spondylosis with hypertrophic lipping and slight narrowing of the L4-L5 and L5-S1 disc spaces, 'rule out discogenic disease. If clinically indicated, CT of the lumbosacral spine may prove helpful in further evaluation.

2. Grade I spondylolisthesis of L5 on S1 with evidence of spondylolysis at L5 on the left.

3. Slight dextroscoliosis in the lumbar region and slight increased lordosis in the lumbosacral region.

M. Volz, MD

M. Volz, M.D.

MV:ti

D: 10/19/20xx
T: 10/20/20xx

X-RAY REPORT	PT. NAME:	DORN, JAY F.
	ID NO:	RL-483091
	ATT. PHYS:	T. LIGHT, M.D.

F I G U R E   9 – 7 .   Sample radiology report. (Reprinted with permission from Willis MC. Medical Terminology: The Language of Health Care, 1st ed. Baltimore: Williams & Wilkins, 1996.)

ments, procedures performed, improvements, setbacks, and, finally, the condition of the patient at the time of discharge.

The discharge summary is an excellent tool for members of the health care team involved in the patient's posthospital care. A patient who is recovering from a stroke may receive services from a home health nurse, a physical therapist, and a speech therapist. The discharge summary provides a snapshot of the patient's situation in one document.

Figure 9-8 is a sample discharge summary. Be sure it is in the office chart for the patient's first visit after hospitalization.

CENTRAL MEDICAL CENTER

211 Medical Center Drive • Central City, US 90000-1234 • PHONE: (012) 125-6784 • FAX: (012) 125-9999

DISCHARGE SUMMARY

DATE OF ADMISSION: 10/25/20xx   DATE OF DISCHARGE: 10/29/20xx

ADMITTING DIAGNOSIS:
Left ureteropelvic junction obstruction.

DISCHARGE DIAGNOSIS:
Left ureteropelvic junction obstruction.

PROCEDURE PERFORMED:
Left dismembered pyeloplasty and placement of stent.

BRIEF SUMMARY:
The patient is a 19-year-old male who was admitted to the hospital a month ago with left pyelonephritis. He was found to have a left ureteropelvic junction obstruction. The patient was brought to the hospital at this time for repair of the moderately to severely obstructed left kidney. A preoperative urine culture was sterile. The patient underwent the procedure without complication. A double-J stent was placed. The Jackson-Pratt drain was removed on the second postoperative day because of minimal drainage. The patient initially had urinary retention, but this resolved by the third postoperative day. He was doing fine at the time of discharge. His condition on discharge is good.

INSTRUCTIONS TO THE PATIENT:
1) Regular diet. 2) No heavy lifting, straining, or driving an automobile for six weeks from the day of surgery. He should also keep the incision relatively dry this week. 3) Follow up in my office in three weeks. 4) It is anticipated the stent will remain indwelling for six weeks and then will be removed cystoscopically at that time. 5) Discharge medication is Tylenol #3, 1-2 q 4 h p.r.n. pain.

L. Zlatkin, M.D.

LZ:mr

D: 10/29/20xx
T: 10/30/20xx

DISCHARGE SUMMARY	PT. NAME: MERCIER, CHARLES F.
	ID NO: IP-392689
	ROOM NO: 444
	ATT. PHYS: L.ZLATKIN, M.D.

FIGURE 9–8. Sample discharge summary. (Reprinted with permission from Willis MC. *Medical Terminology: A Programmed Learning Approach to the Language of Health Care*, 1st ed. Baltimore: Lippincott Williams & Wilkins, 2002.)

Checkpoint Question

4. List the information found in a discharge or transfer summary.

TRANSCRIPTION RULES

The following section is not intended to be a complete list of rules, but it includes most of the general rules necessary in medical transcription. Different texts give different rules for punctuation, so it is recommended that you follow the guidelines of the American Association of Medical Transcription (AAMT), the source of these rules.

Abbreviations

When you use abbreviations in medical documents, your reader must be able to recognize or translate the abbreviation. Every licensed medical facility is required to keep a list of approved abbreviations, and this list should be updated regularly. Some facilities have local abbreviations that are specific to the facility. Like words in English, many abbreviations have two meanings. The use of capital letters can change the meaning entirely. For example, CC means chief complaint, but cc means cubic centimeters. For this reason, be very cautious in using abbreviations. Some abbreviations have become accepted because they are used more than the long form. BP has come to be easily recognized as blood pressure when used in the vital sign section of the report. In a hospital setting, the use of abbreviations in typed reports is forbidden. For example, you are not allowed to abbreviate the diagnosis on an operative report.

Most doctors' offices use standard abbreviations in the patients' charts, but when you are typing a formal report, it is risky to use abbreviations. If it is the policy of your facility to use abbreviations in letters and formal reports, spell out the words the first time the abbreviation is used, with the abbreviation following in parentheses. In general, "when in doubt, spell it out."

Capitalization

Knowing when to capitalize and when to use lowercase letters is a mark of an excellent transcriptionist. The rules about using capital letters you learned in grammar school still apply, but when you are transcribing medical records, capitals are used in additional situations.

Use capital letters:

1. For headings.
   CHIEF COMPLAINT or Chief Complaint
2. For eponyms (terms formed using the name of a person, usually the name of the researcher or physician who identified a disorder or the inventor of equipment, instruments, supplies, and so on), the second word in the phrase is not capitalized. *Note*: Recent revisions in punctuation guidelines eliminate the possessive apostrophe.
   Down syndrome   Foley catheter   Healy clamp
3. For trade or brand names of drugs and products. Do not capitalize generic names of drugs and products.
   diazepam   Valium
   tissue   Kleenex
4. For the genus of an organism. An example of this classification system of living organisms is *Staphylococcus aureus*. *Staphylococcus* is the genus and *aureus* is the species. A singular genus is capitalized and italicized. If the genus is plural or used as an adjective, it is lower case and not italicized. Use lowercase letters and italics for the species.
   as noun: *Staphylococcus aureus*
   as adjective: staphylococcal infection
5. For a department name when the name is the proper title of a place, but not for department names within a facility.
   The patient was taken to the emergency room.
   The patient was taken to the Forsyth Medical Center Emergency Room.
6. For proper names of languages, races, and religions.
   She is a 23-year-old Hispanic woman.
   Do not capitalize informal designations such as white or black.
7. For acronyms (words formed from initials of words in a phrase).
   NKDA (no known drug allergies)
   CABG (coronary artery bypass graft)
8. To draw attention to vital information, such as allergies.
   ALLERGIES: The patient is allergic to PENICILLIN.

Numbers

Traditional office technology courses teach the rules for using numbers, but many of those rules do not apply to medical documents. When those guidelines have the potential to cause confusion or harm a patient, you must be flexible enough to bend them. The safety of the patient is a goal of the transcriptionist.

Follow these guidelines for using numbers in medical reports:

1. Spell out the numbers one through nine in a narrative report (see guidelines 3 and 6 below). Ten and above are keyed as numerals (e.g., 10, 11) unless they begin a sentence, as in this sentence.
2. If you are using two numbers in one sentence, be consistent. It does not matter whether you choose numerals or words, but they should be consistent.
   Dr. Smith saw 14 patients today; one of them was only 2 days old.
   If using more than one number could cause confusion, spell out the one that is easiest and shortest.
   The patient states that she drinks 12 two-liter sodas per week.

3. Always use numerals with symbols. Do not key a space between the number and the symbol.
   100% oxygen
   $14.27 balance due
   #2 specimen
4. For balance and clarity, add a zero before and after a decimal point. The provider will say, "The specimen measures eight by five and a half by point six."
   Clear: The specimen measures $8.0 \times 5.5 \times 0.6$.
   Unclear: The specimen measures $8 \times 5.5 \times .6$.
5. Key a space between numerals and a unit of measurement, abbreviation, or symbol.
   10 mg%   40 mL   20 mm Hg
6. Use numerals for measurements of vital signs, laboratory values, age, height, weight, and so on.
   BP 110/70   Respirations 20
   Temperature 98.7°F   Wt. 140 lb.
   Pulse 80   Ht. 60 inch.
   FBS (fasting blood sugar) 98
7. Spell out ordinal numbers except in dates.
   She began feeling better the third day after surgery.
   The patient was seen on May 3.
8. Roman numerals are used with cranial nerves, obstetric history, electrocardiographic leads, types and factors, and cancer stages.
   Cranial nerves II through XII are intact.
   Limb leads II through V on the electrocardiogram were not making contact.
   The carcinoma is stage II.

Punctuation

One of the most important skills necessary to be an efficient and productive transcriptionist is the ability to punctuate without direction. Some physicians dictate punctuation, but you should not automatically type these directions unless they follow the AAMT's *Guidelines for Transcription.*

Apostrophes

Use an apostrophe:

1. To show possession
   The patient's appointment is Wednesday.
2. To form contractions
   She's having flu symptoms. (The apostrophe contracts *she* and *is.*)
   Note: "It is" can be shortened to "it's," but there is no apostrophe in the possessive:
   Its length is 4 cm.
3. With units of time and money when they are possessive
   We will give him a week's worth of medication.
   Nine months' gestation is standard.
   He bought 10 dollars' worth of gas.

4. For clarity when using one letter as a word
   The I's were not dotted.
   But not to form plurals
   DRGs
   WBCs
   I've had this dress since the 1970s.
   Unless it is possessive
   The CMA's uniform is neat and clean.

Commas

Use a comma:

1. Between items in a series (the last comma is optional).
   The patient is alert, oriented and talkative.
   Or
   The pain is bilateral, severe, and stabbing.
   Note: Do not use commas between items that modify each other. Even though this seems like a series of adjectives, it is really one unit.
   There is severe, stabbing, bilateral pain in the lower abdominal region.
   The first three adjectives modify *pain* and are separated by commas. "Lower" refers to the abdomen, not the region, so no comma is used.
2. To link two complete sentences that are separated by a conjunction.
   She is a very sick patient, and I will admit her immediately.
   But not when both clauses lack a subject and a predicate
   She is a very sick patient and needs to be admitted.
   "Needs to be admitted" does not contain its own subject. Therefore, no comma is needed.
3. After the conjunctive adverb.
   The medical assistant is in great demand; therefore, most schools have a waiting list.
4. After an introductory phrase or clause with a subject and a verb.
   After she has her chest radiograph, she will come back to the office.
   NO comma is needed when the sentence is reversed.
   She will come back to the office after she has her chest x-ray.
   Lightheaded, she sat down on the floor.
5. To set off clauses within a sentence that provide additional information.
   Electroencephalography, a test that assesses the electrical activity in the brain, is a diagnostic tool used by neurologists.
6. To set off parenthetical expressions.
   The pain, according to the patient, measures 10 on the pain scale.

7. With dates when using the year, place names, and long numbers.

> The patient was seen last on May 2, 2003.
> *But*: The patient was seen last on May 2 at 2:00 p.m.
> Duke University Medical Center is in Durham, North Carolina.

Numbers over five figures:

> 4500
> 567,158,230

8. With quotations.

> The patient said, "I will quit smoking tomorrow."

9. To prevent confusion.

> "The physician came in, in order to see the patient."

Semicolons

Use a semicolon:

1. To separate main clauses that do not have a conjunction such as *and* or *but*

> The patient arrived 10 minutes late; she had car trouble.

2. To separate two main clauses if they are long or you need other commas within the sentence

> She had chest pain, nausea, and headache; and her daughter took her to the emergency room.

Colons

Use a colon:

1. After headings

> FAMILY HISTORY: The patient reports no family history of cancer.

2. To introduce a series after a complete clause but not after a verb

> The physician prescribed the following medications: Keflex, Darvocet-N 100, K Tabs and Prinivil.
> The physician prescribed Keflex, Darvocet-N 100, K-Tabs, and Prinivil.

3. To separate hours from minutes

> Your appointment is scheduled for 10:30 a.m.

4. After a salutation in a business letter

> Dear Dr. Johnsen:

Periods

In addition to ending sentences, periods are used:

1. With lowercase abbreviations

> a.m., p.m.   *But:* AM, PM   PhD

Metric measurements do not use periods.

> They had to remove 3 ft. of her colon.
> We removed 15 mL of pleural fluid.

2. After an abbreviation that is a shortened part of a word

> American Association of Medical Assistants, Inc.

3. After a person's initials

> J. T. Weaver, MD

Quotation Marks

Quotation marks enclose:

1. A direct quotation

> The patient stated, "My friend recommended your office to me."

2. Words that are slang or thought to be a quotation.

> The patient stated he was "blown away" by his improved cholesterol reading.
> Jessica thinks her new boyfriend is "Prince Charming."

3. Titles of articles, short stories, subdivisions, and so on

> Please read "Making the Patient Comfortable" in the most recent issue of our professional journal. Table 9-1 presents rules for using other punctuation with quotation marks.

Slash Marks

In medical transcription, the slash mark is used:

1. In place of the word *per*. The provider says, "Give the patient one hundred percent oxygen at two liters per minute." You type:

> Give the patient 100% oxygen at 2 liters/minute.

In some cases, the provider may not say "per," but you insert a slash.

> The student took the class on a pass/fail basis.

2. To separate options and alternatives.

> This is a pass/fail course.

Hyphens

Hyphens are used:

1. In compound words. The general rule is that when two words are used together to form a word, they are joined by a hyphen. Many compound nouns have been used long enough to be consolidated and are now accepted words in their own right. For example, spread-sheet has become spreadsheet.

> mother-in-law   figure-of-eight sutures

2. A hyphen can clear up confusion or ambiguity. For example, re-creation is quite different from recreation. Without the hyphen, the reader would misinterpret the meaning.

> We will *re-treat* with a different antibiotic.

As opposed to

> We went on a weekend *retreat*.

Table 9–1 THE USE OF OTHER PUNCTUATION WITH QUOTATION MARKS

Rule	Example
Place commas and periods inside quotation marks.	"Your bill, explained the patient, "has not come in the mail."
Place colons and semicolons outside quotation marks.	She said, "The doctor told me to come back on Friday"; however, he has no openings.
Place other punctuation inside quotation marks only if they belong in the quotation.	The student asked, "Is that going to be on the test?" *But* Did the patient say, "Yes, I'll come"?
Place commas and periods outside quotation marks when used with single letters or single words.	Even though she made an "A," she felt it was not her best work.

3. When joining the two words would result in two or more identical letters.

   post-traumatic   pre-enteric   pre-existing

   Note: Otherwise, the hyphen is not used with these prefixes.

   postoperative infection   prehistoric

4. When spelling out the compound numbers twenty-one to ninety-nine.

   Fifty-eight percent of our patients are over sixty-five years old.

5. When using compound adjectives before a noun.

   high-frequency hearing loss

   well-developed frame

   22-gauge needle

   6-month-old infant

   Remember, the hyphen is not used when the compound adjective follows the noun it modifies:

   The patient is 6 months old.

6. The hyphen is not used when adverbs modify adjectives.

   very high fever   quickly spreading cancer

7. When a compound adjective contains the suffix -free.

   symptom-free

8. When the compound includes an acronym.

   post-CABG care   pre-ICU lab results

9. When keying suture sizes.

   2-0 Prolene

Grammar

When a physician dictates a report using incorrect grammar, it is your job to correct the mistake. The physician expects you to produce an error-free report, even though he or she may overlook basic parts of speech and rules of sentence grammar. Although a thorough discussion of the grammar rules in the English language is outside the scope of this text, some basic rules should be mentioned. The most common errors made in medical transcription are those dealing with verb tense.

Always be sure that subjects and verbs agree in number.

One patient: The patient *is* alert.

More than one vital sign: His vital signs *are* normal

Always make sentences within a paragraph agree in tense and subject. Suppose the provider dictates, "The patient was seen in clinic today for pain in the left knee. The examination *is* negative." You will key, "The patient was seen in clinic today for pain in the left knee. The examination *was* negative."

Spelling

When in doubt about the spelling of a word or drug, always use a reference book, dictionary, or spell check to confirm the spelling. Keep in mind that computer spell check will check for spelling only, and a misused word will not be caught if it is spelled correctly. For example, "the patient was late four his appointment" will pass the spell check because "four" is spelled correctly, even though the transcriptionist meant to key "for."

Here are some basic spelling tips:

1. I comes before e except after c or when sounded like a as in neighbor and weigh.

   Examples: achieve, receive (the exceptions are either, neither, weird, leisure, and conscience)

2. For words ending in ie, drop the e and change the i to y before adding ing.

   Examples: die, dying; lie, lying

3. Words ending in o that are preceded by a vowel are made plural by adding s.

   Examples: studio, studios; trio, trios

   Words ending in o that are preceded by a consonant form the plural by adding es.

   Examples: hero, heroes; potato, potatoes

4. Words ending in y preceded by a vowel form the plural by adding s.

   Examples: attorney, attorneys; day, days

   Words ending in y that are preceded by a consonant change the y to i and add es.

   Examples: berry, berries; lady, ladies

5. The final consonant of a one-syllable word is doubled before adding a suffix beginning with a vowel.

   Examples: pin, pinning; run, running

   If the final consonant is preceded by another consonant or by two vowels, do not double the consonant.

   Examples: act, acting; look, looked

6. Words ending in a silent e generally drop the e before adding a suffix beginning with a vowel.
> Examples: ice, icing; judge, judging

The exceptions are dye, eye, shoe, and toe. The e is not dropped in suffixes beginning with a consonant, however, unless another vowel precedes the final e.
> Examples: argue, argument; pale, paleness

7. For all words ending in c, insert a k before adding a suffix beginning with e, i, or y.
> Examples: picnic, picnicking; traffic, trafficker

You must pay close attention to spelling when transcribing medical documents. Remember, in the medical world a misspelled drug or word can be dangerous.

TRANSCRIPTION SYSTEMS

Vast improvements have been made in dictating and transcribing capabilities and equipment over the past decade. Traditionally, the physician or health care provider uses a dictation machine with a handheld microphone to tape a report of a patient encounter or other correspondence. With the **analogue** or tape system, after the message is taped, the cassette tape will be removed and marked with some form of identification. Cassette tapes range in size from micro to standard.

Traditional Tape Dictation Systems

Each model of transcription machine is slightly different; however, most have the basic parts described next (Fig. 9-9).

- The foot pedal is used to start, stop, fast-forward, and rewind the tape.
- The speed control regulates the speed at which the tape plays. As a beginner, you want to keep the speed slow. As your listening and typing coordination improve, you will be able to increase the speed of the tape. When you become experienced with a particular

provider's voice speed, you will be able to set the speed control to match his or her voice speed and your typing speed.
- The tone dial can be adjusted to change the bass or treble of a provider's voice.
- The volume control is used to adjust the sound level.
- The headset is used to eliminate distracting external noises. It is not a good habit to share headset earplugs with fellow colleagues because an ear infection may be transmitted. Ear cushions that attach to the headsets should be used and washed or replaced often.
- The speaker allows the sound to be heard from a speaker in the transcriber instead of the headset. This feature is handy when the transcriptionist needs assistance or clarification in interpreting the dictation.
- Counters are available on most machines for ease in locating certain reports and to judge the length of a document.

Because every transcription machine is slightly different, you should read the instruction manual before you begin working on a unfamiliar machine. All instruction manuals should be kept in one central location in the office for easy access.

Tapes are usually transcribed in or near the medical records department. Tapes should be erased after the material has been transcribed, reviewed, and signed by the provider. Before discarding a worn-out tape, erase it completely to maintain confidentiality.

Digital Systems

The industry is moving toward a **digital** system, which converts the voice into digits, decodes it, and sends the voice directly to a transcriber through the telephone lines. The system integrates with a computer at the transcriptionist's desk, where a certain code is entered. This code will automatically produce the information and report format on the screen of the computer. In hospitals, most patient care units have dictation phones or ports for digital systems.

Voice Recognition Systems

Voice recognition software and digital voice recording systems have expanded and improved medical transcription. Some people predicted that the invention of voice recognition software would eliminate the need for medical transcriptionists, but the medical community has been slow to respond to the technology. Some limitations are difficult to overcome. For example, if the provider says "there," how does the computer know whether to type "there," "their," or "they're"? Accents, dialects, proper names, and garbled speech are challenges for transcriptionists no matter which system is being used. These same challenges face the inventors of voice recognition software. Even with sophisticated voice recognition systems, there will always be a need for

FIGURE 9-9. Transcription machines vary. Speed control is an important function of the machine.

WHAT IF

You are having trouble understanding a particular physician's dictation tapes because of a dialect or foreign accent. How should you handle this situation?

First, rewind the tape and listen again to the phrase. You can try to adjust the speed control to slow the pronunciation of the word. Consider what a word would sound like with the accent on a different syllable or using a short sound instead of a long sound of a vowel. Being familiar with the type of report being dictated will help you anticipate what the provider might be saying. If you are still uncertain about the word or phrase, leave a blank space for that word and continue transcribing. Edit the report to fill in the blank. Never guess! If you have difficulty understanding a provider, discuss the problem with him or her. Open communication will help you both make adjustments. Neither of you wants to take the chance of producing an erroneous report.

transcriptionists or medical language specialists to proofread, punctuate, and edit medical documents.

Transcription With Word Processing Software

When using word processing programs, you may use macros, templates, and other functions that record keystrokes or provide a blank format to speed the process of transcribing reports that contain the same text over and over again. For example, the format for a certain type of report or letterhead and normal dictation for ordinary examinations can be recorded for playback with a quick keystroke. Legal experts warn providers not just to report examination results as "normal." Instead, they should describe the negative findings. For example, when a patient's throat appears normal to the examiner, he or she should report, "The throat appears normal, with no redness or exudate" (pus).

Checkpoint Question

5. Describe the main difference between analogue and digital transcription equipment.

ñ Spanish Terminology

Esto es una máquina de transcripción.	This is a transcription machine.
Yo no lo podría oír con los auriculares.	I couldn't hear you with the headphones on.
¿Qué escucha usted?	What are you listening to?
Escucho y escribo a máquina cartas para el doctor.	I am listening and typing letters for the doctor.

Transcribing a Medical Document

Steps	Purpose
1. Prepare the equipment: transcribing machine, headphones, transcription (dictation) tapes, computer or typewriter, paper, letterhead, and envelopes.	Having everything ready will cut down on interruptions and will help you focus. Concentration is key to being productive.
2. Select a transcription tape with the oldest date, unless there are special requests for priority reports.	Most dictation systems have the capability of *marking* a document for priority status. This alerts you to complete marked dictation first.
3. Turn on the transcriber, and insert and rewind the tape.	Always rewind the tape so that the document starts in the beginning.
4. Put on the headset and position the foot pedal in a comfortable location.	The foot pedal is operated by pressing a certain area for a certain function. In some machines, pressing the left side of the pedal rewinds the tape, pressing the right side fast-forwards it, and pressing the center plays the tape.
5. Play a sample of the tape. Adjust the volume, speed, and tone dials to your comfort.	This promotes efficiency and speed.
6. Select the appropriate format and place proper patient identification on the page.	Proper patient identification is essential for legal and ethical reasons.
7. Play a short segment of the tape by pressing the foot pedal, stop the tape, and type the message.	As your speed and skills progress, you will not need to stop the tape as often.
8. If you come across an unfamiliar term, leave enough blank space for the provider to write it in and continue transcribing. When you have finished the document, contact the physician or colleague or use a reference book to fill in the blank.	A thorough knowledge of medical terminology will minimize time spent looking up words.
9. When you are finished, place the initials of the provider, followed by a slash and your initials, on the bottom of the page. The date that each was done should be added.	The reader must know who dictated the report and who transcribed the document and the dates each was carried out.
10. Spell check the document by using medical spell check software.	The spell checker of standard word processing programs does not recognize most medical terms. Medical spell check software is available to ensure accuracy.
11. Print and proofread the document.	Spell checkers mark only misspelled words, not errors. You need to proofread the hard copy for other errors. After typing a lengthy report, it is common to overlook errors. It is helpful to have a coworker also proofread.
12. Leave the document, along with the tape, in a designated area for review.	After reviewing the document, the provider will sign it, indicating that the report is accurate. If corrections are necessary later, a revised copy must be placed with the original report. The final copy should include a notation to identify it as a revised copy.
13. After the provider has reviewed and approved the document, make a copy of the report for the patient's chart.	Reports can be mailed, faxed, or e-mailed. Be careful to follow the guidelines for protecting patients' privacy outlined in Chapter 8.
14. Send the report to the recipient.	This allows the report to be filed.
15. Erase the tape and return it to the dictation area.	Tapes that are not erased cause confusion to the provider when they are recording and may infringe on a patient's right to privacy.

CHAPTER SUMMARY

Medical transcription is a growing industry. The person who possesses the necessary skills transforms vital information about a patient's care and treatment and is an important member of the health care team. Many medical assistants perform this important function in the medical office. The training you receive in your medical assisting education will enable you to perform at entry-level competency, but experience in transcribing will enhance your skills and make you a more desirable employee for medical offices. Medical information is crucial to patient care and must be prepared with proper grammar, punctuation, and spelling. Physicians depend on timely and accurate preparation of their reports to make decisions. This information is confidential and must be handled with great caution and integrity.

Answers to the Checkpoint Questions

1. A professional document should be well balanced and attractive with single spacing, double spacing between headings, and one-inch margins.
2. JCAHO requires that results of the H&P be placed on a patient's chart within 24 hours of admission to a hospital facility. The physician must sign the H&P report within a prescribed amount of time as well.
3. Subjective information is provided by the patient and is information that cannot be seen or measured. Examples are pain and nausea. Objective findings are reported by the examiner and can be observed or detected. Examples are rash and blood pressure.
4. The discharge, transfer, or death summary is a concise report of the reason for the patient's admission, tests performed, treatments given, results of those tests and treatments, procedures performed, improvements, setbacks, and, finally, the condition of the patient at the time of discharge.
5. The analogue system uses cassette tapes to record the voice, and the digital system uses digits that are converted and sent across the telephone lines.

 Websites

American Association of Medical Transcription
www.aamt.org
Medical Transcription Jobs
www.mtjobs.com
Medical Transcription Daily
www.mtdaily.com

10

Computer Applications in the Medical Office

CHAPTER OUTLINE

ROLE DELINEATION COMPONENTS

GENERAL: Communication Skills
- Recognize and respond effectively to verbal, nonverbal, and written communication
- Use electronic technology to receive, organize, prioritize, and transmit information

GENERAL: Operational Functions
- Perform routine maintenance of administrative and clinical equipment
- Apply computer techniques to support office operations

GENERAL: Instruction
- Locate community resources and disseminate information

GENERAL: Legal Concepts
- Perform within legal and ethical boundaries

ADMINISTRATIVE: Administrative Procedures
- Perform basic administrative medical assisting functions

CHAPTER COMPETENCIES

LEARNING OBJECTIVES

Upon successfully completing this chapter, you will be able to:

1. Spell and define the key words
2. Identify the basic computer components
3. Explain the basics of connecting to the Internet
4. Discuss the safety concerns for online searching
5. Describe how to use a search engine
6. List sites that can be used by professionals and sites geared for patients
7. Describe the benefits of an intranet and explain how it differs from the Internet
8. Describe the various types of clinical software that might be used in a physician's office
9. Describe the various types of administrative software that might be used in a physician's office
10. Describe the benefits of a handheld computer
11. Describe the considerations for purchasing a computer
12. Describe various training options
13. Discuss the ethics related to computer access

PERFORMANCE OBJECTIVES

Upon successfully completing this chapter, you will be able to:

1. Search a given topic on the Internet
2. Conduct a basic literary search

KEY TERMS

cookies	Ethernet	literary search	virus
downloading	Internet	search engine	virtual
encryption	intranet	surfing	

COMPUTERS PLAY A MAJOR ROLE in the physician's office. Computers are used for both clinical and administrative applications. A few examples of administrative applications are appointment scheduling, billing, staff scheduling, and insurance fillings. Clinical software programs are used for many areas, such as reading laboratory and radiology reports and helping the physician to prescribe medications. Computers promote communication among health care professionals and provide access to new treatment options. You will need excellent computer skills to work as a medical assistant. This chapter will help you to improve your existing skills. It provides a basic review of computer components. You will learn how the Internet is used in health care settings and some precautions. Various medical software applications will also be discussed. You will learn about training options and how to purchase a computer.

THE COMPUTER

A computer system is roughly divided into two areas, hardware and peripherals.

Hardware

Computer hardware consists of seven key elements (Fig. 10-1). Here is a review of their parts:

FIGURE 10–1. The computer consists of the CPU, keyboard, monitor, hard drive, printer, and secondary storage systems. Additional peripherals include the mouse, battery backup and modems.

- *Central processing unit.* The central processing unit (CPU), or microprocessor, is the circuitry imprinted on a silicon chip that processes information. The CPU consists of a variety of electronic and magnetic cells. These cells read, analyze, and process data and instruct the computer how to operate a given program. All CPUs function basically the same way, but chips differ dramatically in capabilities and speeds. Your CPU has many ports to connect the printer, mouse, and speakers. At minimum, it has two serial ports, one parallel port, and two universal serial bus (USB) ports. Serial ports are used for items like modems; parallel ports are used for connecting printers and backup drives to the CPU; and USB ports allow the computer to connect with various instruments.
- *Keyboard.* The keyboard is the primary means by which information is entered into the computer. Besides the typical letter and number keys, you will find special function keys that provide increased capabilities. Examples of special function keys are Alt, Ctrl, Insert, and Esc. Each of these keys has a specific function that is determined by the software program. These functions may include searching for and replacing words, moving blocks of text, indenting or centering text, and spell checking.
- *Monitor.* Monitors, also called the visual display terminals, come in various sizes and qualities. The quality of the image is based on the DPIs (dots per inch). The more DPIs, the clearer the picture. There are adjustment dials for brightness and contrast.
- *Hard drive.* The hard drive provides storage for programs, data, and files. The capacity of a hard drive (i.e., the quantity of program and data it can hold) is measured in megabytes or gigabytes. Originally, hard drives could hold 5 MB (equivalent to about 2,000 typed pages), but today they have much more capacity.
- *Printer.* The printer transfers information to paper (hard copy). Printers use various technologies, operate at various speeds, and print in either black or color. The printer allows you to generate bills, print letters, and produce a daily schedule. The two types of printers used in physicians' offices are dot matrix and laser. Dot matrix printers are used primarily for printing insurance forms. They should not be used to print patient discharge instructions unless the instructions can be clearly read. You should print all business letters on a laser printer.
- *Scanner.* A scanner allows you to take a picture or report and read it into the computer. You may scan laboratory reports, radiology reports, and discharge summaries into a patient's file. This is very helpful when a new patient arrives with reports from a previous physician. Patient education materials can also be scanned into the computer and then adjusted to meet the needs of your office. Keep in mind that you need to adhere to copyright laws.

- *Secondary storage systems.* All computers have multiple methods for saving data. Examples include floppy diskettes, compact disks, digital video disks, and zip drives. Cartridges are used by hospital for large storage systems. When saving any type of data, remember that good organization skills are essential. Name your files appropriately and place files in properly identified folders. Most computers have preset timing systems that automatically save data. Check your default setting and readjust as needed.

Checkpoint Question

1. What do the CPU cells do?

Peripherals

Computers can have many peripheral connections. Three key computer peripherals that you need to know are:

- *Mouse.* The mouse can be used to control the cursor on the display screen. Although you cannot type in characters using the mouse, you can move or delete individual characters, words, or entire blocks of text with it. The track ball is an alternative to a mouse. Your finger rotates the ball to move the pointer. It takes less space than a mouse and is used based on personal preference.
- *Battery backup.* A battery backup allows the computer system to function in the event of a power failure. Batteries come in various sizes depending on the size of your computer and the amount of work to be done during a power failure.
- *Modem.* A modem is a communication device that connects your computer with other computers, including the Internet, online services such as bulletin boards, and electronic mail systems. The faster the modem, the faster the transmission. Modems may be connected through cable systems or through the telephone. Digital subscriber line (DSL) is the preferred method. To use a cable or DSL connection, your computer must have an **Ethernet** port or an Ethernet interface card.

Checkpoint Question

2. Why should your computer have an Ethernet port or Ethernet interface card?

Care and Maintenance of the System and Equipment

As with any piece of equipment in the medical office, it is necessary to maintain your computer on a regular basis. Some general care guidelines follow:

- Place the monitor, keyboard, and printer in a cool dry area out of direct sunlight.

Box 10-1

BASIC CARE OF DISKS

Whether you are using a floppy diskette, CD or DVD disk, follow these guidelines:
- Always handle the disk by the label or jacket.
- Do not touch the inside of the disk.
- Store in a safe, cool dry place. Avoid high-moisture areas.
- Keep all food and liquids away.
- Never store near a magnetic field, such as a television screen or cellular telephone.
- Store in a vertical container designed for that purpose.
- Always label before storing. Write on the label sticker before sticking the label to the disk.

- Static electricity can cause memory loss, inaccurate data collection, and other adverse reactions. To control this problem, place the computer desk on an antistatic floor mat or carpet, or purchase a specific antistatic device.
- Use available accessories to care for your system. For example, use dust covers for the keyboard and the monitor when they are not in use. Antistatic wipes are available to use on the screen, and they should be used as an alternative to glass cleaners.
- When moving the computer, lock the hard drive to protect the CPU and disk drives.
- Keep keyboards free of debris and liquids, which can be hazardous to the keyboard, as it is directly plugged into the computer. Vacuum the keyboard periodically to eliminate dust particles under the key pads. Do not eat or drink while working on the computer.
- Be aware of any maintenance and warranty contracts for the computer system and do not hesitate to contact the service representative when needed. Some maintenance agreements require that a service representative clean and inspect the system on a regular basis.
- Handle data storage disks with special care. Box 10-1 provides some general guidelines.

INTERNET BASICS

Most physicians' offices can connect to the **Internet**. The Internet is used for both clinical and administrative reasons. The first thing you need to know is how to get your computer connected.

Getting Started and Connected

The Internet is used for access to the World Wide Web (www) and for electronic mail. To get connected, you will need an Internet connection company and appropriate Internet software.

There are three ways that your computer can connect to the Internet. One is an Internet service provider (ISP). The ISP is a company that connects your computer's modem to the Internet through the phone line. It is often called a dial-up service. This method provides the slowest service but is the cheapest. The second option is your cable television company. This system provides a faster connection. The third option is a digital subscriber line (DSL). This is the fastest connection but is not available in all areas. DSL is the most expensive connection system. If you need to download large files through the Internet, you should use either a DSL or cable connection. If you are having trouble accessing the Internet because of either slow service or connection troubles, speak to the physician or office manager to determine whether a different connection or ISP is needed.

Second, your computer will need a Web browser. A Web browser is software that communicates with your computer and the Internet. Two common examples are Internet Explorer and Netscape Navigator. Most computers are pre-loaded with a Web browser.

Clicking on the Web browser icon makes the actual connection to the Internet. Depending on how your system is set up, you may have to use a password. Box 10-2 gives you some guidelines on password use.

Checkpoint Question

3. Which two types of Internet connection are recommended for downloading large files?

Security

If you choose correct sites and follow some general safety tips, the Internet is a safe way to obtain and transfer patient information. Here are a few key points:

Box 10-2

PASSWORD USE

Here are some guidelines for passwords:
- Make unique passwords (combine letters and numbers)
- Do not use your initials, birth date, or phone number.
- Systemwide passwords that allow access to the computer should be changed after an employee has been fired.
- Do not share your password with your colleagues.
- Do not tape your password on the computer monitor or leave it on your desk.
- It is a good idea to have additional password verifications for certain secure sites (laboratory reports).

- Never send **any** patient information over the Internet to a site that does not have a secure sockets layer (SSL). This scrambles your information as it leaves your computer and unscrambles it when it arrives at its designated address.
- Look for a lock icon on the status bar.
- Set limits on your Web browser for **cookies**. A cookie is a tiny file left on your computer's hard drive from a website without your permission. By examining your cookies, a website can learn what sites you have visited, products that you have been searching, and files that you have downloaded. You may control your computer's cookies by setting limits on your Web browser software. Limit setters can generally be found on your toolbar under Internet options, then under either privacy or security.

Viruses

Virus protection is an important security issue. A virus is dangerous invader that enters your computer through some source and can destroy your files, software programs, and possibly even the hard drive. A worm is a specific type of virus that affects e-mail. Most computers come with virus protection software. This software will identify and stop harmful transmission. No virus protection is, however, 100% guaranteed. Some ways that you can protect your computer are:

- Do not open any attachments that are from unknown or suspicious sites.
- Update your virus protection software regularly. Most virus protection programs offer an updating service. Virus protection updates address new worms, as well.
- Remember, new viruses are detected daily.

Downloading Information

The Internet is filled with great patient teaching resources and other information. You may decide to copy some of this material into your computer. This is **downloading**. Downloading transfers information from an outside location to your computer's hard drive. Download only files that pertain to work. Do not download screen savers, news releases, recipes, or other personal information. Do not assume that you can photocopy any material that you have downloaded and distribute it. Always ask for permission from the author. Some government and professional medical websites state that their material can be freely copied and used. A good example of this is the United States Department of Agriculture (USDA) website that allows the food pyramids to be copied and used for teaching.

Working Offline

It is possible to access Web pages without connecting your computer to the Internet. To do this, save your commonly accessed sites on your Web browser. (If you are unsure how to do this, search your help topics for working offline). Then, to view the pages off line, click on the connection icon, select work off line, and locate your file. Remember, Web pages are regularly updated, and a page that you have saved to view off line may not be the latest version. Periodically view the online site and resave the site.

ELECTRONIC MAIL

Electronic mail (e-mail) provides many benefits to the health care system. It is estimated that about 6.6 trillion e-mail messages are sent every year. E-mail promotes good patient care, enhances communication, promotes teamwork, eliminates phone tag, and provides written documentation of messages. E-mail messages can't be guaranteed to provide confidentiality. Some general tips for using e-mail follow:

- Use the office e-mail address only to send work-related messages. Do not send personal messages.
- Do not participate in chain letters.
- Download your e-mail and read it off line unless you are using a DSL or cable connection.
- All e-mail messages should be professional.
- Read your e-mail's **encryption** feature and activate it. Encryption is a process of scrambling messages so that they cannot be read until they reach the recipient.
- Always leave a message on your e-mail system when you will be out of the office for a vacation or other reason. This message is automatically sent to the incoming e-mail senders. This alerts the sender that you will not be reading their message. Include the date when you will be returning to the office and instructions on whom they should contact in case of emergencies. This feature is often called "out-of-office assistant." An example of a good message: "I will be out of the office from 1/20 through 1/28. If this e-mail requires immediate attention, please forward it to Barbara Smith. I will respond to your e-mail when I return."

Checkpoint Question

4. What does the encryption feature do?

Access

Access to your e-mail account is through either Internet or intranet. The intranet is discussed later in the chapter. To access your e-mail, locate the mail icon, double-click it, and enter appropriate information. A password is generally required.

Composing Messages

When composing a message, follow the guidelines in Chapter 7 for writing business letters. Here are a few additional tips:

- Check your spelling, grammar, and punctuation before sending any messages.

- Keep messages short, concise, and to the point.
- Flag messages of high importance. This will alert the recipient that the message is important and should be read first. Do not overuse this feature. Flag only messages that warrant immediate response or attention. Never send an e-mail about a patient who is having an emergency. Always call or page the physician instead. An example of inappropriate e-mail is, "Ms. Smith's water broke. Do you want her to go the hospital or come into the office?"
- Use appropriate fonts and an appropriate font size.
- Generic or plain stationery should be used. Do not use stationery that has cute figures or looks busy.
- Always complete the subject line. Keep the subject line short and use only a few key words, for example, Staff meeting tomorrow.
- It is a good idea to restrict e-mail messages to only one topic.
- Paragraphs are not indented on e-mail messages. Skip a line between paragraphs.
- You can add a permanent signature to all outgoing e-mails. Your signature should include your name and phone number.

Address Books

Your e-mail software will allow you to create address books. An address book is a collection of e-mail addresses. Additional information, such as phone numbers, fax numbers, and street addresses, can be added. A few tips regarding address books are:

- Keep your addresses up to date.
- Organize your addresses in folders or categories. For example, one folder may contain all the cardiologists in the area, and another may contain just insurance-related addresses.

Attachments

An attachment is a file that is sent along with an e-mail. You attach a single file (letter) or several documents at one time. Remember these guidelines:

- When you receive an e-mail with an attachment, open the attached file or letter. File it in an appropriate place on your computer. If appropriate, print the attachment and distribute it as needed.
- If you are sending an e-mail and need to attach a file, compose your message first. Then attach the file by going into the tool bar and locating the menu for file attachments. Find the file on your computer and click to attach it. It is a good idea before sending the attachment to open it to be sure that you have selected the correct file or version of the document.

Opening Electronic Mail

Some general guidelines regarding opening an e-mail message follow:

- Open only your own e-mail messages unless otherwise instructed.
- After reading the e-mail, either delete it or place it in a folder. Do not allow multiple e-mails to clog your inbox.
- Always open flagged messages first and respond to them immediately.
- If you receive a message that you cannot address or resolve, forward the message to your supervisor and alert the sender that the message has been forwarded.
- If you start receiving bulk mail, either block the sender or ask to be deleted from that mailing list. This can be accomplished by clicking on "unsubscribe," usually at the end of the message.

Checkpoint Question

5. Can you be 100% guaranteed that your e-mail transmissions are safe?

MEDICAL APPLICATIONS OF THE INTERNET

Besides e-mail, the Internet offers the World Wide Web, which provides health care professionals with great resources and information. Navigating through the Web quickly and efficiently takes skill and practice. The process of searching the Internet is called **surfing**. Surfing that is unorganized and not focused can be time consuming and unproductive.

Before surfing for information, you need to remember one important rule: Not all of the information on the Web is accurate or truthful. Anyone can post anything or make any claim. Since the information that you obtain from the Web will affect patient care, all steps must be taken to ensure that only accurate information is found and used. First, look for the HON (Health on the Net) seal. The HON seal (*www.hon.ch*) is a voluntary seal that indicates that the site has met certain standards for reliability and credibility. It does not certify that the information is correct or truthful, but it is a good starting point. Keep in mind that many good sites, for example governmental sites, do not have this seal. Box 10-3 provides you with some guidelines for selecting safe sites.

Search Engines

A **search engine** allows you to find sites that have the information that you need. There are numerous search engines (Google, Yahoo, Lycos, Excite, Dogpile). These sites are best used for searching out general information. Once you arrive at the search engine page, you must enter some

---

Box 10-3

SAFE SITE SELECTION GUIDELINES

Remember these key points when reading information on a website:
- Beware of phrases like breakthrough, medical miracle, secret formula.
- Avoid sites that advertise that they have cured a disease.
- Use caution when you see the phrase "ancient remedy."
- Use caution when you find a site that will treat a whole list of diseases with the same treatment.
- Do not believe every testimonial that you read.
- If the sites claims that the government is hiding information to cure a disease, use extreme caution.
- Use caution when the treatment can "only be bought here."
- If the site suggests that you not tell your doctor about it, stay away.
- See *www.quackwatch.com*.
- You can send complaints to the Federal Trade Commission at *www.ftc.gov* about sites that provide information that is misleading and wrong.
- Do not try to learn lifesaving skills, such as cardiopulmonary resuscitation, on the Internet. No matter how good the information or site is, you need to take a professional class.

---

key words. Your key words should be focused to limit the number of responses that you will get. For example, if you type in the key word "heart," you will get thousands of sites that pertain to the heart. Some of these sites will be referring to the heart as an organ and other sites will address how to mend a broken heart. If you had selected your key words to be "heart attack," however, you would narrow your search tremendously. To further narrow your search use the advanced search feature. Click on advance search and use the key words "heart and attack and prevention." By doing this, you will obtain the information you want faster and more efficiently. Unless you are using a medical search engine, avoid using medical terms. For example, use the word lung instead of pulmonary. When you need to find medical information, use a medical search or a megamedical site with links. Procedure 10-1 lists the steps necessary to search the Internet. See the listing of websites at the end of this chapter for some good places to start searching for medical information.

Checkpoint Question

6. What is a search engine?

Professional Medical Sites

At the end of the chapters in this book you see various Web addresses listed that provide you with more information on that chapter's content. These are good starting points for - professional topics. But keep in mind that Web addresses change frequently. If you are unable to access a site, try eliminating the letters and symbols after a slash (/). Use the primary site address. For example, suppose you want to enter this site: *www.fda.gov/cder/drug/consumer/buyonline/guide.htm.* If you cannot access that site, try *www.fda.gov* and advance from there. Most sites will link you automatically to a new home page. Also, depending on your Web browser, you may not have to type in **www**. In this case, you would just type in fda.gov.

The Internet can help you communicate with patients who speak a foreign language. Some websites translate phrases and words. Box 10-4 lists sites that physicians are most likely to use. All medical specialties have their own special site. Hospitals have their own sites also. When you start working as a medical assistant, learn the Web addresses of the specialty of your physician and of local hospitals *(www.hospitalselect.com)*. For example, if you work for a neurologist, you will frequently use *www.aan.com* (American Academy of Neurology).

These sites will help you translate between English and Spanish:

- AltaVista
  www.altavista.com (click on translate)
- Free English to Spanish translations
  www.freetranslation.com

The CDC site is also available in Spanish. You can give this address to patients: *www.cdc.gov/ncidod/EID/spanish.htm.*

Literary Searches

According to the American Medical Association, approximately 80% of practicing physicians regularly surf the Internet for medical research information. Most research information is found through a **literary search**. A literary search involves finding journal articles that present new facts or data about a given topic. Physicians who specialize in a given area and have conducted a controlled research study write these articles. Various databases can be used to do a literary search:

- OVID will search for articles as far back as 1966. It contains access to more than 4,000 professional journals. Its address is *www.gateway.ovid.com.*
- PubMed will search for journal articles back to 1966 from the National Library of Medicine.
- CINAHL contains journal articles published since 1982. It has primarily journals for nurses and other allied health care professionals.

Most literary search databases require an annual subscription fee. Once you arrive at the site, you can start to search for the information. First, enter your key words. To narrow the search, you can request journal articles from all countries or limit it to the United States. You can also limit the search by selecting a time line, such as the past 6 months. Once you have done your search, a list of articles will be displayed, and you can highlight the ones you wish to see. You will be asked whether you want to see the whole article or only the abstract. An abstract is a summary of the article. It is always a good idea to print only the abstracts and allow the physician to decide which full articles he or she will want to see. Fees for downloading the complete journal article vary. Abstracts can generally be downloaded free. Your local hospital librarian is often available to assist you with literary searches and may be able to get the article for free. Some libraries will do searches for physicians on staff at no charge. Use this service if it is available.

Checkpoint Question

7. How is a literary search different from a search on an internet website?

Health-Related Calculators

The Web has numerous calculators that can be used for various health care topics:

- Basal metabolic rate calculator
  www.global-fitness.com/BMR_calc.html
- Due date calculator
  www.babycenter.com/calculators/duedate
- Ovulation calculator
  www.babycenter.com/calculators/ovulation
- Target heart rate
  www.webmd.com/heartrate

Box 10-4

SITES PHYSICIANS USE

Physicians and other health care professionals are likely to use these sites:

Journal of the American Medical Association	*www.jama.com*
New England Journal of Medicine	*www.nejm.org*
Lancet	*www.lancet.org*
Annals of Internal Medicine	*www.annals.org*
AMA	*www.ama-assn.org*
JCAHO	*www.jcaho.org*
CDC	*www.cdc.org*
Clinical trials	*www.clinicaltrials.gov*

Insurance-Related Sites

The insurance world can seem like an endless maze of papers and regulations. The Internet can help you sort through and clarify some information. Your first stop should be the patient's insurance company. Its Web address is usually listed on the back of the patient's insurance card. Bookmark these sites. Chapter 16 will get into more details on this issue. A few sites that can also help you and your patients follow:

- For information on buying health insurance online: *www.ehealthinsurance.com.*
- The Medicare site (*www.medicare.gov*) discusses the basics of Medicare programs, eligibility, enrollment, drug assistance programs, and many frequently asked questions. This site will link you to various other options. You will also find links to report Medicare fraud and abuse.
- Patients who express concern about their health records being red-flagged because of an illness (HIV, cancer) can check a database that alerts insurance companies to "red-flagged" patients. This site is *www.mib.com.* There is a fee for using this site.

Patient Teaching Issues Regarding the Internet

Some of your patients will be very skilled at using the Internet. They can find enormous amounts of information regarding their disease, treatment options, medications. The guidelines discussed in Box 10-3 pertain to patients who surf the Internet. You cannot stop or limit the information that patients will search and find. Keep in mind that patients often turn to the Internet when they feel confused or hopeless about their disease or anger about the medical profession. If a patient communicates any such feelings, alert the physician.

Teach patients to acquire reliable medical information and advise them of the dangers on the Web. Some physician offices print brochures with recommended Web addresses. This is a very good education tool for patients. Box 10-5 gives you some good patient education sites. Some areas you should be aware of are discussed below.

Buying Medications Online

As the cost of prescription medications soar, patients look for options. It is possible to buy prescription medications over the Internet. A good Internet pharmacy will provide information on what the medication is used for, possible side effects, dosage recommendation, and safety concerns. If patients want to purchase prescriptions online, advise them to use only sites that are certified by the Verified Internet Pharmacy Practice Site (VIPPS). This certification comes from the National Association of Boards of Pharmacy and indicates that the site has been checked and is monitored for safety and quality care. Advise patients

to purchase only medications that have been prescribed by the physician. Warn patients never to purchase medications from sites outside of the United States. These sites may not meet safety standards of the Food and Drug Administration (FDA). In addition, the FDA warns patients never to buy certain medications online because of their inherent dangers. Advise patients to use *www.fda.gov/cder/drug/consumer/buyonline/guide.htm* for consumer safety tips. Box 10-6 lists medications that the FDA warns people never to purchase online.

Some sites offer virtual prescribing. This means that the Internet user provides some information and asks for a prescription. For example, the patient may type in, "My cholesterol is too high. What medication will get it down?" The site will then ask the patient a few questions and select a medication. In other cases, the patient may simply request a medication: "I want some amoxicillin." In either case, the prescription is filled and mailed to the patient. Warn patients about the dangers of self-prescribing medications and alert the physician to any communication you have with the patient regarding this practice. Serious health risks can arise.

 Checkpoint Question

8. Name three safety tips to teach patients about buying medications on the Internet.

Box 10-5

GOOD PATIENT EDUCATION SITES

These sites provide good patient information:
American Dental Association
   www.ada.org/public/index.asp
American Sleep Apnea Association
   www.sleepapnea.org
Consumer Health Publications
   www.health.nih.gov
Merck Manual Home Edition
   www.merckhomeedition.com
National Attention Deficit Disorder Association
   www.add.org
Hotlines of National Library of Science
   www.nlm.nih.gov/hotlines
American Association of Poison Control Centers
   www.aapcc.org
Smoking cessation
   www.QuitNet.org
Sources for children with cancer
   www.cancersourcekids.com
Travel health
   www.cdc.gov/travel

Financial Assistance for Medications

Patients who are having trouble paying for their prescription medications can find many financial resources on the Web. First, you should advise patients to search the drug company's home page, for example, *www.Pfizer.com*. Patients on Medicare will find assistance on *www.medicare.gov/prescription/home.asp*. Another good site is *www.needymeds.com/Mainpage.htlm*. Physicians can access *www.Rxhope.com* to find local financial resources for patients.

Medical Records

Patients may choose to create their own "medical records" and store personal health information on sites. Patients who travel frequently may opt for this. Two sites that offer this are *www.personalmd.com* and *www.mywebmd.com*. Patients can store information about their medications, immunizations, laboratory tests, surgeries, and so on. For their own protection, patients should be discouraged from doing this. Instead, advise patients to download medical record forms, complete the printed copy, and store them safely.

Medical Record Forms

The American Health Information and Management Association provides forms online for patients to record their health histories. This is available at *www.ahima.org/consumer/index.html*. The American College of Emergency Physicians has an emergency consent form (*www.acep.org*) that parents can sign giving permission for another person to consent to their child to be treated in case of an emergency. This is valuable for parents who travel on business and have their child stay with a relative or friend.

Advance directives and legal forms for medical power of attorney are also available online. Patients should be advised to seek legal counsel and speak to the physician before completing these forms. The federal government does have cards available online for patients to complete and carry with them regarding their wishes to be an organ and tissue donor at *www.organdonor.gov/signup1.html*.

Injury Prevention

Injuries are a leading cause of death for children. The American Academy of Pediatrics (*www.aap.org*) has reference materials that can help parents with safety tips. The federal government sites (*www.cdc.gov and www.nih.gov*) also have good information that you can direct parents to search. The National Safe Kids foundation is another excellent resource (*www.safekids.org*). Questions regarding product recalls can be found at *www.cpsc.org*.

INTRANET

An **intranet** is a private network of computers that share data. Intranets, sometimes called internal webs, are used in large multiphysician practices. The only people with access to an intranet home page are people with an affiliation to the practice. Access may be limited to those within the offices or may allow for access from home computer systems. The benefits of an intranet are enhanced communication, quick access to needed information, and increased productivity. Common examples of data found on an intranet are:

- Policy and procedure manuals
- Marketing information

WHAT IF

Parents ask you how to keep their child safe on the Internet. What should you say?

First and foremost, explain to the parent that direct parental observation is the best method. Encourage parents to have an open and honest discussion with their child regarding the dangers on the Internet. Computers should be kept in living rooms or family rooms. Advise parents not to let children have a computer with Internet access in their bedroom. Parents can require a password to be entered for Internet access. This prevents access when the parent is not present. Most Web browser programs let the parent allow access only to "safe" sites. A few sites can add filters or safety nets to a child's computer. These sites are *www.netnanny.com*, Internet Guard Dog (*www.mcafee.com*), and CyberPatrol (*www.cyberpatrol.com*)

- Minutes from meetings and upcoming agendas
- Staff schedules
- Local hospital announcements or information
- Commonly used forms
- Internal newsletters
- Internal job postings
- Phone lists
- Video conference support
- Links to specialty sites

Checkpoint Question

9. How does an intranet differ from the Internet?

MEDICAL SOFTWARE APPLICATIONS

The types of medical applications and their possibilities are endless. Every day, thousands of new software packages are released into the market. Upgrades and new versions of existing packages are also released daily. Each type of software program will have good benefits and will lack some features. The type of software that you will use will vary among different physician offices. The selection of software is based on the size of the practice, number of physicians, specialty, and the affiliated hospital's software. If the hospital software is compatible, interchanging information is relatively easy. Physician and office manager preferences play a role in the software selection. Other factors include how many users can use software at one time, can the software be used with multiple windows open, and how often does the company plan to update it.

Never buy or install a new software program or update an existing version without permission from either the office manager or the physician.

Learning to use a particular software program and navigate quickly and efficiently through its features takes time. Most programs come with a tutorial program. On-site training is often included in the purchase price of major software applications. Training options will be discussed later in the chapter.

Medical software applications can be divided into two main groups: clinical and administrative. Clinical software packages help the physician or health care professional provide the best possible medical care to patients. Administrative software packages focus on tasks to keep the office flowing efficiently and financially strong. The next sections introduce you to what types of software capabilities are available and most commonly used. Keep in mind that new technologies are emerging every day. Box 10-7 lists some companies that sell medical software.

Clinical Applications

Clinical software is designed to help the physician, nurse, medical assistant, or other health care professional provide

the most efficient, safest, and most reliable health care available. Here are some examples of the benefits that clinical software programs can bring into the physician's office:

1. Create a **virtual** patient chart. A virtual chart is a paperless chart in which all documentation is stored on computer. Some offices create dual charts (virtual and paper), and other offices will keep one or the other. The advantages to a virtual charting system are that it saves filing space, increases access to patients' charts for all staff members, eliminates hunting for misplaced charts, and keeps the charts better organized and neater. Since the charting is done through keyboarding, the notes are always readable.

2. Clinical software can maintain an up-to-date list of clinical tasks organized by employee's name. For example, suppose you just discharged a patient and made a note on his chart that you need to check his laboratory tests tomorrow. The task manager would automatically assign this task to your list of duties for tomorrow. Or a physician may discharge a patient and want you to call that patient in the morning for a follow-up. The physician could assign this task to your list. This promotes organization and decreases the potential for tasks to get overlooked or forgotten.

3. The software available for prescription management and drug information is tremendous. A good program that focuses on pharmaceutical information will decrease medication errors, increase patient satisfaction, and provide better patient care, and it can be financially beneficial to the patient and to the practice. At minimum, the software should enable the physician to find the patient's name in a database, virtually write the prescription, and download it directly to the patient's pharmacy. This allows the pharmacist to fill the prescription before the patient arrives. Thus the patient gets the medication much faster. More important, since most prescription filling errors are due to physicians' poor handwriting, this potentially lethal error is prevented. Most medication software packages red-flag the physician if the prescription is contraindicated for the patient. Medications can be contraindicated because of a particular disease (e.g., asthma or diabetes), interaction with other medications the patient is taking, or an allergy. For example, assume the physician has written a prescription for Bactrim, which contains a sulfonamide. The software would find in the patient's medical record that the patient is allergic to sulfonamides. The computer would alert the physician, and the physician would select a different medication. Software also allows the physician to save the patient money. Each insurance company and hospital has a formulary of medications that it reimburses. If the physician orders a medication that is on the patient's insurance formulary, the patient saves money. If the physician selects a medication

Box 10-7

MEDICAL SOFTWARE COMPANIES

Numerous companies sell medical office software programs. Here are a few sites that you can visit:

Advanced Medical Management
www.amdsoftware.com

AltaPoint Practice Management
www.altapoint.com

American Medical software
www.americanmedical.com

EZ Claim medical billing
www.ezclaim.org

Find Medical Billing Software
www.findaccountingsoftware.com

Medical Manager
www.medicalmanager.com

Medical Software products
www.medsoftware.com

NextGen
www.nextgen.com

Plexis Health Care
www.plexisweb.com

SoftAid
www.soft-aid.com

Web-based appointment scheduling
www.compassscheduling.com

outside the formulary, the insurance company may refuse to pay some or all of the cost of the medication.

4. Computer programs can insert laboratory reports directly into the patient's records. This is more time efficient than faxing or manually recording the results. It also eliminates transcription errors. Most software will alert the physician when a new laboratory report has been received. Laboratory reports of serious or life-threatening findings will still be telephoned to the office.

5. Perhaps one of the greatest technologies is the importing of the actual imaging study into a patient's chart. Some software allows the physician to see the radiograph or computed tomograph from the office. Without this program, the physician gets a typed written report, such as "chest radiograph shows left lower lobe infiltrate." With this technology the physician can see the radiograph itself and thus make better clinical decisions.

6. Plastic surgeons use a wide variety of image reconstruction programs in their office. This software allows the physician to insert a picture of the patient and contrast it with the expected outcomes of the surgery. This helps patients both to decide whether the

surgery is warranted and to develop realistic expectations of the surgery.

7. Many physicians' offices have a special defibrillator called an automated external defibrillator (AED). Once the AED is used on a patient, the information from the machine must be downloaded to the patient's chart for legal documentation. After use, the AED is attached to a desktop computer, and the AED sends the report into the computer and then into the patient's record. If the patient's chart is not on computer, the data can be printed on paper and placed in a conventional chart.

8. Some programs can help you with telephone triage. Triage is sorting patients. The software allows you to select a caller's topic and displays a list of relevant questions. The software also provides you some instructions for the patient. For example, assume you have a caller with abdominal pain. You type the key words abdominal pain, and a list of questions appears. These programs log the calls with the date, time, and instructions. This provides legal protection for you.

Checkpoint Question

10. What is a virtual chart?

Administrative Applications

There are hundreds of administrative software packages available for physician offices. Most systems have a combination of features. At present, the Medical Manager system is the most commonly used software in physician offices. Some examples of benefits administrative software can bring to the physician's office follow:

1. Appointment making and tracking are more efficient with a computer program than with a book format. Good appointment software will allow you to enter appointments quickly and make changes more easily. It should allow for an unlimited comment area near the patient's name. The comment area allows you to add special notes, such as "patient is requesting a pregnancy test." Appointment software can keep a waiting list of patients who are looking for appointments or wanting to move their appointment date and time to the first available. Appointment software can also automatically print notices to remind patients of the need to make appointments. For example, the program can be set to alert patients who have an annual Pap smear to be sent a letter each year reminding them when it is time for the next one. Appointment software can be integrated with other physicians' offices to allow you to have access to their appointment books. This allows you to see when the next available appointment is. For example, assume your physician makes a referral for

Mr. Mannual to see a dermatologist. You would be able to view the schedule of the dermatologist and see when he could get an appointment and then later see if he went for his appointment. Software programs allow appointments to be made only when certain equipment is available. For example, the patient needs a biopsy that is done with a particular laser machine. The machine is available only on Tuesdays, so the program would automatically set the appointment for the patient on a Tuesday.

2. Software can allow you or the office manager to track patient flows. This can be helpful to adjust staff scheduling needs, with more help at the busiest hours or days and less staff on slower days. It can alert managers to productivity of staff members. For example, one physician may average 45 minutes per patient, while another may average 30 minutes. This allows you to schedule appointments at various intervals and thus promotes patient flow. It can track the time patients wait in the waiting room or examination room. Examining such information allows the staff to change the office flow to decrease waiting times or to indicate the need for additional staff. It can also highlight the days when patients are most likely to cancel their appointments. Patient demographics can be obtained, used for marketing, and allow the office to apply for special funding based on patient demographics.

3. Software programs are needed to send insurance claims electronically. You will be able to send claims and track their progress. This allows for faster reimbursement to the practice and can identify problems of reimbursement earlier. The programs that you will use should have access to numerous plans and can be updated frequently and easily.

4. Software programs can allow integration with insurance companies and other businesses to allow for automatic quick payment and posting. This saves time and is less complicated to use them traditional accounting books.

5. Physicians' offices should have software that allows for credit card authorization. A variety of card types should be available (Visa, MasterCard, American Express).

6. Insurance software can allow you to check for patient eligibility. Most programs have enough room for the addresses and phone numbers of the primary, secondary, and tertiary providers. Case manager names should be added when available. Software can also allow for preadmission certifications to completed and electronically submitted. Preadmission or preauthorization allows you and the patient to verify that the insurance company will cover the procedure or admission. Some software programs come with codes (ICD-9, CPT, HCPCS) and anesthesia codes preinstalled.

7. Some programs aim to comply with the Health Insurance Portability and Accountability Act (HIPAA). HIPAA is a federal act that requires all health care professionals to follow a variety of privacy and confidentiality rules; these programs allow you to document your adherence to these rules and regulations. For more information on HIPAA, visit *www.hipaa.org*.

8. Other programs alert you to send collection letters. These programs have a variety of template collection letters. Always double-check the information before sending a collection letter. More information on how to collect past due accounts is discussed in Chapter 13.

9. A variety of financial software programs track accounts receivable and accounts payable. You may need to adjust the billing cycles to meet the needs of the office in which you are working. Software programs can also automate the tickler system.

10. Automated payroll software can automatically calculate tax deductions and other deductions. You will be able to arrange for direct deposit of employee checks through these software programs.

11. You will find transcription systems in most physicians' offices. These programs help you transcribe various medical reports quickly and effectively. Transcription is covered in Chapter 9.

12. A medical office can't effectively run without a word processing system. These systems help you write letters and other types of documentation.

13. An important part of any administrative software is the section that handles the personnel records. Contracts, disciplinary reports, performance evaluations, and so on can all be stored in a virtual personnel record.

Paging System Software

Most physicians carry a pager. In some offices, other staff members may also be assigned pagers. **Always double-check to make sure that the physician you are paging is the one on call.** Most paging systems allow you to type alphabetic (alpha) messages versus a numerical code. A numerical message is simply a telephone number. An alpha message is a written message that is displayed on the pager; for example, "Call the office regarding Ms. Home's blood gas results." Here are some guidelines regarding paging:

- Always provide a return phone number unless you are asking the physician to call the office.
- Watch your spelling on alpha pages.
- Keep the message short and concise.
- Keep track of what time the message was sent and repage if there is no response.
- If it is an emergency page and there is no response, repage or page another physician as per office policy.
- Never give out pager numbers to patients or sales representatives.
- If you are given a pager, do not give the pager number

to anyone. Insert fresh batteries when the battery icon is first showing; treat the pager with care and respect. Notify the office manager immediately if is lost or stolen.

Checkpoint Question

11. What is an alpha page message?

PowerPoint

Physicians are often asked to do formal presentations. These presentations may be made to other physicians, support group meetings, hospital staff meetings, and professional inservices. The most popular program used to write presentations is PowerPoint. Using this software, the physician will create slides. The slides can then be shown on a projection screen by connecting a computer to a projector. Most often a laptop computer is used. You may be asked to print slides or handouts for the program or to transfer files. Use the tutorial software for tips on making presentations.

Meeting Maker

Meeting Maker is a common package that promotes internal coordination of meetings and calendars. This system is primarily used in large practices with multiple offices and multiple administrative personnel. This is how the system works: Everyone is listed as user. Each user enters his or her schedule into a personal calendar. Calendars can be seen daily, weekly, or monthly. For example, you may type in, "Monday, Middletown office, 8 A.M.–4 P.M.; Tuesday, Southside office, 10A.M.–5 P.M.." The system allows you to view other people's calendars. It is possible to allow other people to enter data to your calendar. You can also maintain a list of tasks and print your schedule. If you are asked to arrange a staff meeting, you enter the names of the people who should come, and the computer will select a date and time that is convenient for everyone.

HANDHELD COMPUTERS

According to the American Medical Association, approximately 23% of physicians use a handheld computer, or personal digital assistant (PDA). A handheld device can do almost anything that your desktop computer can do. Companies that make PDA software can be found at these three Web addresses: *www.pdacortex.com, www.skyscape.com,* and *www.handheldmed.com.* At minimum, handheld computers come with software that can do these functions:

- Address book
- Calendar
- Memo pad
- E-mail
- Word processing

Information can be entered into the handheld device either with a stylus (pen) or on a small keyboard. It is possible to attach a regular-size keyboard to a PDA. Information can be sent back and forth between a PDA and a desktop computer in either of two ways. The PDA can be placed in a cradle that is connected via a cable to the desktop ("hot sync"), or information can be sent via e-mail. PDAs can beam information among themselves (business cards, memos) and can attach their modem through a cellular phone for Internet access.

Physicians often add software that allows them to:

- Access patients' charts
- Set up a virtual office
- View financial data
- Use pharmacy and formulary dosing tools
- Access Micromedx (drug information, toxicology, databases)
- View procedures that they may not routinely do, enhancing lifesaving skills

PURCHASING A COMPUTER

Purchasing a new office computer system or updating an existing one is a very important business decision. All key members of the staff should be consulted prior to such a purchase and should be actively involved in selecting the hardware and software. Here are some general guidelines to follow when shopping for a computer and software:

- Determine your specific needs. For example, do you need both clinical and administrative applications?
- Visit physicians' offices and clinics to see what other medical office staff are using. Ask questions: How user friendly are the programs? How long did it take to educate the staff? What does the staff like and dislike about the programs?
- Try out many software packages. Most have demonstrator disks that can be used to evaluate the system.
- Interview and compare different computer vendors. Find out:
  1. How long they have been in service
  2. How many service representatives they have and whether they are available 24 hours a day
  3. Specifics of the system
  4. Specifics of any service and warranty contracts they provide
  5. What training they provide and at what additional cost
  6. How to transfer data into the new system
  7. How much the system costs
  8. Whether the software can be customized and at what cost
  9. What is their response time for service or technical support calls

Independent computer consultants can be hired to evaluate your particular office and make specific recommendations. This option is often more expensive initially but can save money in the long run.

TRAINING OPTIONS

To achieve the optimal benefit from any computer or software package, you must be trained in its use. There are a number of ways that this can be accomplished:

- The company from which the computer was purchased may provide personnel to train you and other staff members.
- A user manual will come with your system. You can refer to it when you have problems.
- Help screens installed with every software package allow the user to self-teach. The disadvantage of this method is that it is often time consuming.
- Most software packages come with a tutorial. This is an on-screen short course on the use of the software.
- Most computer manufacturers and software programs will have a service called a help desk, which provides technical support. It is usually accessed by calling a toll-free number and is manned by computer professionals who can answer your questions concerning the system.

A combination of these methods is the best approach to learning about your computer and software.

COMPUTER ETHICS

The computer is a must in all physicians' offices. Its capabilities are endless. It can, however, lead to invasion of patients' privacy and unethical behavior. Some key points to keep in mind are:

- Never give out your login password. New employees must be issued their own password.
- Never leave a screen open with patient information and walk away from the computer. Exit the file.

- Only key people need access to sensitive patient information. Some programs, such as those with laboratory results, should have individual passwords.
- Physicians can often access patient data (e.g., radiology and laboratory reports) from the hospital computers. The hospital gives the physician a special code. It is not appropriate for the physician to share this with staff members. If you are using another person's password to get patient information, you should contact the administrator of the program and get your own code.
- Do not use the office Internet access for your own pleasure. It is inappropriate to surf the Internet for personal reasons while at work.
- E-mails should be read only by the person to whom they were sent. To avoid conflicts, the physician should have his or her own e-mail account, and the practice should have a generic e-mail address. It is never appropriate for you to receive personal e-mail messages on the office's e-mail address. It is also inappropriate to access your personal e-mail while at work.
- Sensitive patient data should not be sent via e-mail from one office to the other unless it is clearly known that the recipient of the e-mail is the only one with access to it. It is a common practice to send patient information to the consulting physician. This information may include cancer diagnosis, HIV testing, and drug abuse reports. Extreme caution must be used.
- If you are allowed access to local laboratories to obtain laboratory results, it is to be used only on patients in your practice. It is unethical and illegal to obtain other people's reports. For example, if your son had a throat culture done at the pediatrician's office and sent to the laboratory you have access to, you should not look up his results.
- Do not take advantage of your position in the medical field. Remember, you have a legal and ethical responsibility to protect patient information.

Procedure 10-1

Searching on the Internet

Equipment/Supplies

- Computer with Web browser software
- Modem
- Active Internet connection account

Steps	Purpose
1. Connect your computer to the Internet.	An Internet connection is necessary to search the Internet.
2. Locate a search engine.	A search engine is necessary to find information on the Internet.
3. Select two or three key words and type them at the appropriate place on the Web page.	Key words tell the search engine what to look for.
4. View the number of search results. If no sites were found, check spelling and retype or choose new key words.	The search engine was unable to find sites that can provide the information you requested.
5. If the search produced a long list, do an advanced search and refine your key words.	Reading through numerous sites is not time efficient.
6. Select an appropriate site and open its home page.	This allows you to view the information on the website.
7. If you are satisfied with the site's information, either download the material or bookmark the page. If you are unsatisfied with its information, either visit a site listed on the results page or return to the search engine.	Downloading or bookmarking the information gives you access to it in the future.
8. Complete this task within 10 minutes.	Quickly and effectively searching the Internet is necessary for good time management.

CHAPTER SUMMARY

Computers are an essential piece of technology in the medical office. As a medical assistant, you will use the computer for both clinical and administrative tasks. Computers will help you perform your job more efficiently, timely, and professionally. Computers also promote good patient care. You will be able to communicate with various health care professionals by using electronic mail. The Internet plays a key role in medicine. Patients, physicians, and medical assistants use the Internet to find new medical cures and for seeking current information about various health topics. You will need to be able to navigate the Web quickly and safely. It is essential that you stay abreast of computer technology, as it changes and improves daily.

Critical Thinking Challenges

1. Log on to the Internet and locate a search engine. Search for a medical topic. It can be administrative or clinical. What are your key words? How many sites are listed? Now, using the same key words, use the advanced search engine. How many sites are listed? What are the benefits of using the advanced search method?
2. Select any five Web addresses listed in this chapter. View their home page. What benefits did the sites offer? What information or topics were missing or appeared inaccurate?
3. Review Box 10-3 about how to select a site safely. Find three websites that use these types of phrases or words. Do you think these sites are misleading? Do you think they pose a danger to patients?

4. Formulate a list of questions that you can ask a vendor before buying a computer system. Include questions regarding software applications.

5. Create a patient education pamphlet about the Internet. The pamphlet may focus on a particular disease process or contain broad information. Make sure you provide at least six Web addresses.

Answers to Checkpoint Questions

1. The CPU cells read, analyze, and process data and instruct the computer how to operate a given program.

2. Your computer should have an Ethernet port or Ethernet interface card so that it can be connected to a cable or DSL provider.

3. The two types of Internet connections that are recommended for downloading large files are DSL and cable.

4. The encryption feature scrambles messages as they leave your site and unscrambles them when they arrive at the receiver's site.

5. You cannot be 100% guaranteed that your e-mail messages are secure, but you can take many steps to safeguard them.

6. A search engine allows you to find the sites that will have the information that you need quickly and efficiently.

7. A literary search is different because it is searching for a professional journal article that addresses a topic versus searching for general information.

8. Three safety tips that you need to teach patients about buying medications online are: (1) buy medications only from a site with a VIPPS certification; (2) buy only medications for which they have prescriptions; and (3) buy medications only from sites within the United States.

9. The intranet is a private network of computers; the Internet is a global network of computers.

10. A virtual chart is a paperless chart that holds all necessary documents on the computer.

11. An alpha paging message is a written message that is displayed on the pager.

 Websites

OSHA ergonomics
 www.osha-slc.gov/SLTC/ergonomics/index.html
Websites that offer additional information
 www.tifaq.com
 www.healthfinder.gov
 www.medlineplus.gov
 www.healthcentral.com
 www.mywebmd.com
 www.Mayoclinic.com
 www.familydoctor.org
 www.raredisease.org (this site has a database of over 1,000 rare diseases and over 900 drugs that can be used to treat rare diseases)

11

Quality Improvement and Risk Management

CHAPTER OUTLINE

QUALITY IMPROVEMENT
    PROGRAMS IN THE MEDICAL
    OFFICE SETTING
    Regulatory Agencies

DEVELOPING A QUALITY
    IMPROVEMENT PROGRAM
    Seven Steps for a Successful
        Program

RISK MANAGEMENT
    Incident Reports
    When to Complete an Incident
        Report
    Information Included on an Incident
        Report

Guidelines for Completing an
    Incident Report
Trending Incident Reports

PUTTING IT ALL TOGETHER:
    A CASE REVIEW

ROLE DELINEATION COMPONENTS

GENERAL: Professionalism
- Display a professional manner and image
- Demonstrate initiative and responsibility
- Work as a member of the health care team
- Adapt to change
- Enhance skills through continuing education

GENERAL: Legal Concepts
- Perform within legal and ethical boundaries
- Document accurately
- Implement and maintain federal and state health care legislation and regulations
- Comply with established risk management and safety procedures

CHAPTER COMPETENCIES

LEARNING OBJECTIVES
Upon successfully completing this chapter, you will be able to:
1. Spell and define the key terms
2. List four regulatory agencies that require medical offices to have quality improvement programs
3. Describe the accreditation process of the Joint Commission on Accreditation of Healthcare Organizations
4. Describe the intent of the Clinical Laboratory Improvement Amendments Act
5. Describe the intent of the Health Insurance Portability and Accountability Act
6. Describe the steps to developing a quality improvement program
7. List five guidelines for completing incident reports
8. Explain how quality improvement programs and risk management work together in a medical office to improve overall patient care and employee needs

PERFORMANCE OBJECTIVE
Upon successfully completing this chapter, you will be able to:
1. Complete an incident report

KEY TERMS

Centers for Medicare & Medicaid
Clinical Laboratory Improvement Amendments Act

expected threshold
incident reports
Health Insurance Portability and Accountability Act

Joint Commission on Accreditation of Healthcare Organizations
Occupational Safety and Health Administration

outcomes
quality improvement
sentinel event
task force

QUALITY IMPROVEMENT (QI) is the commitment and plan to improve every part of an organization. Its goal is both to meet and to exceed customers' (patients') expectations and employees' needs. QI plans examine the way care is delivered, analyze problems in the delivery system, and investigate methods to correct the problems. Although quality medical care has been a concern of health care providers for many years, formal QI plans were not always required. In the mid 1980s, health care settings were required to develop quality assurance (QA) plans. The purpose of a QA plan was to "assure" patients that they received good medical care. QA plans often created mounds of statistical data to prove that the physicians and staff were doing a good job. QA plans did not focus on improving care, only on acquiring statistical data. Therefore, physician offices now focus on QI plans. These plans require that you collect the data and then use the information to improve and provide quality health care.

In this chapter, we discuss why health care organizations have QI programs, the process for developing and maintaining QI plans in a medical office setting, and risk management. We also discuss the agencies that mandate physician offices to have QI programs.

QUALITY IMPROVEMENT PROGRAMS IN THE MEDICAL OFFICE SETTING

Quality improvement programs let an organization scientifically measure the quality of its products and services. A health care organization's success depends on patient satisfaction and patient **outcomes**. The patient's outcome is the final result of the care that he or she received. For example, Mrs. Brown arrives in the office with a laceration on her leg. The cut is sutured, and in 6 days she returns for suture removal. The wound healed without complications. The patient's outcome was acceptable. Patient outcomes are reported to various regulatory agencies. At present, only hospitals are required to post report cards about patient outcomes. Legislative bills now in Congress would require all health care settings to report patient outcomes. Patients can review report cards and other regulatory agencies' reports on various websites. Then, patients can select the health care organization that best meets their needs in terms of professional services and personal care.

Quality improvement programs have many other benefits for all health care organizations. These benefits include the following:

- Identifying system failures or delays in patient care
- Improving patient and family customer service
- Improving patient outcomes and satisfaction
- Improving employee efficiency and productivity
- Improving company morale
- Encouraging teamwork within the institution or organization

Regulatory Agencies

Quality improvement programs exist in medical office settings because of these benefits and because regulatory agencies require such programs. The primary regulatory agencies that mandate QI programs are the **Joint Commission on Accreditation of Healthcare Organizations** (JCAHO), **Occupational Safety and Health Administration** (OSHA), **Centers for Medicare & Medicaid** (CMS), and state public health departments. Some other organizations and associations have requirements for QI programs. These associations require QI data along with applications for research or grant money and for specific accreditation of services. For example, the American Diabetes Association may require an endocrinologist to receive a certification in diabetes care to provide QI data on diabetic patient outcomes. The three major agencies are discussed next.

Joint Commission on Accreditation of Healthcare Organizations (JCAHO)

The JCAHO is a private agency that sets health care standards and evaluates an organization's implementation of these standards for health care settings. Prior to the mid 1990s, the primary focus of the JCAHO was on evaluating hospitals and in-patient care institutions such as nursing homes. In 1996, the JCAHO expanded its jurisdiction to outpatient and ambulatory care settings. This change was, in part, due to the shift of patient care from inpatient to outpatient services. The JCAHO sets standards and evaluates the care in the various health care settings. Box 11-1 lists various types of freestanding facilities for which the JCAHO sets standards and provides accreditation.

The JCAHO surveys these centers and then assigns them an accreditation title. A survey is on-site evaluation of the organizations facility and policies. Participation in the JCAHO is voluntary for health care organizations; without accreditation, however, the health care organization may not be eligible to participate in particular federal and state funding programs, such as Medicare and Medicaid. In addition, accreditation indicates to the community that an organization has met basic practice standards, which is important for marketing its services.

 Checkpoint Question

I. What are the benefits to a health care organization that has obtained an accreditation from the JCAHO?

JCAHO Accreditation Process. The process of obtaining and maintaining accreditation by the JCAHO occurs in various stages:

1. The health care organization files a survey application and a business associate agreement with the JCAHO. The business associate agreement is a new require-

Box 11-1

TYPES OF FACILITIES

The Joint Commission on Accreditation of Healthcare Organizations accredits a variety of health care settings. These are some types of centers that can be accredited:

- Ambulatory care centers
- Birthing centers
- Chiropractic clinics
- Community health organizations
- Corporate health services
- County jail infirmaries
- Dental clinics
- Dialysis centers
- Endoscopy centers
- Group practices
- Imaging centers
- Independent practitioner practices
- Lithotripsy centers
- Magnetic resonance imaging centers
- Oncology centers
- Ophthalmology surgery centers
- Pain management centers
- Podiatry centers
- Physician offices
- Rehabilitative centers
- Research centers
- Sleep centers
- Student health centers
- Women's health centers

---

ment that is part of the Health Insurance Portability and Accountability Act regulations. These regulations are discussed later in the chapter. The application, which is sent from the JCAHO headquarters, consists of inquiries regarding the following:

- Ownership of the organization
- Demographics (e.g., address and phone number)
- Types of services provided
- Volume of patients served per year

2. The health care organization prepares for the survey by reviewing each JCAHO standard and assessing its own compliance. JCAHO standards can be found in its publications or on its website. In addition, the organization to be inspected reviews and updates all policy and procedure manuals. Personnel records are checked for accuracy and completion. Staff members are taught about the survey process and provided with sample questions that they may be asked during the survey.

3. The JCAHO informs the health care organization of the date, time, and duration of the survey. The length of the survey depends on the size and complexity of the setting. A first-time survey visit usually lasts 2 to 4 days. The JCAHO surveyors who specialize in health care standards conduct the survey.

4. The JCAHO conducts the survey, which consists of reviewing patient records, interviewing patients and family members, and touring the facility. Employees are interviewed to determine whether they know where the policy and procedure manuals are kept, what is in the manuals, and safety rules. An exit conference in which preliminary findings are discussed is held between the surveyors and the administration (leadership) of the health care organization.

5. The JCAHO mails the accreditation decision to the health care organization within 60 days after the survey. An organization can appeal to the JCAHO for reevaluation of its assigned title. The organization receives a certificate indicating the level of accreditation that it has achieved. The certificate is posted at the facility.

6. If the initial site review identified some unsatisfactory areas, a second survey, called a focus survey, may be required to prove that corrections have been made. This type of survey generally lasts 1 to 2 days.

After 3 years (the period for which accreditation by the JCAHO is valid), the health care organization submits a renewal application, resuming the cycle. Approximately 50% of the JCAHO standards are directly related to patient safety issues. As of January 2003, all site surveys are based on a new set of national goals aimed at improving the overall safety of patient care in hospitals and in other health care settings. All settings must show that they have reached these six goals:

- Improved accuracy of patient identification. (Always use two methods to identify patients.)
- Improved effectiveness of communication among caregivers. (Physician offices and hospitals must standardize abbreviations, acronyms, and symbols used in documentation. All sites must also have a policy stating what abbreviations and symbols cannot be used.)
- Improved safety of using high-alert medications. (These medications are given only in hospitals by registered nurses. Examples of high-alert medications are chemotherapy agents and potassium injections.)
- Eliminate wrong-site, wrong-patient, and wrong-procedure surgeries. (All steps must be taken to prevent procedures on a wrong patient. Wrong procedures can be simple errors, such as drawing blood from a wrong patient, to serious life-changing mistakes.)
- Improved safety of infusion pumps. (Examples of infusion pumps are pain management devices and insulin administration devices.)
- Improved effectiveness of clinical alarm systems. (All alarms must be checked on a regular basis and must be audible to everyone.)

In addition, the JCAHO requires accredited health care organizations to have a **sentinel event** policy and alert forms. **A sentinel event is an unexpected death or serious physical or psychological injury to a patient.** Box 11-2 lists some examples of sentinel events. Anytime a sentinel event occurs, the organization must determine the cause, implement

EXAMPLES OF SENTINEL EVENTS

These are examples of sentinel events that are reportable to the JCAHO:

- Any patient's death, paralysis, coma, or other major loss of function associated with a medication error
- Any suicide of a patient in a setting where the patient is housed around the clock, including suicides following elopement from such a setting
- Any procedure on the wrong patient, wrong side of the body, or wrong organ
- Any intrapartum maternal death and any death of a newborn weighing more than 2500 g that is not due to a congenital condition
- Any fall by a patient that directly results in death or major permanent loss of function
- Hemolytic transfusion reactions involving major blood group incompatibilities

improvements to prevent a repeat occurrence, and monitor the effectiveness of its plan. The JCAHO publishes a newsletter, *The Sentinel Event Alert*, discussing reported events to alert other facilities to potential problems, and copies can be viewed on its website. The sentinel event alert has raised awareness in the health care community and in the federal

government about the occurrences of adverse events and ways these events can be prevented.

Physicians who perform office-based surgery need to follow the standards set forth by the JCAHO in the *Standards Manual for Office-Based Surgery*. The manual addresses certain standards, such as customer service, quality of care, qualified and competent staff levels, patient safety, leadership, and improving care and health. The manual provides the standards, the intent or purpose of the standards, and some tips for compliance. Box 11-3 displays a sample standard. If office-based surgeries are performed where you work, you should be familiar with these standards. Questions on how to implement these standards can be answered via the JCAHO website or through its hotline.

Checkpoint Question

2. What is a sentinel event?

Occupational Safety and Health Administration

OSHA is a federal agency that regulates health and safety concerns in the workplace. OSHA requires that QI programs be in place to protect the health and welfare of patients and employees. OSHA's mission is to save lives, prevent injuries, and protect the health of America's workers. Many rules under OSHA affect your job. Examples are rules for bloodborne pathogen protection, use of personal protective equipment (PPE), tuberculosis prevention, management of bio-

SAMPLE STANDARD

The practice demonstrates respect for the following needs of patients:

Standard	Intent	Tips for Compliance
RI.1.5 Privacy	Confidentiality of information gathered during treatment	Private examination rooms and treatment areas
	Privacy during care	Staff members who demonstrate concern for patients' privacy
	Security of self and property	Gowns provided when clothing must be changed
RI.1.6 Communication	Effective communication that considers hearing, speech, and visual impairments	Interpreters available when needed
		Staff age-specific training
		Patient information packets, educational materials, and consent forms available in the patients' languages
RI 1.7 Resolution of complaints	The right to complain about care and to have complaints reviewed and resolved	Documentation on investigation of patients' complaints or issues regarding care

hazardous waste, ergonomics, and laser protection. Laser protection is needed if you are working with a physician who is operating a laser in the office. These rules and other guidelines can be found on the OSHA website. Unlike the JCAHO, compliance with OSHA regulations is not voluntary. Noncompliance with OSHA regulations can result in fines and closure of the health care organization.

Checkpoint Question

3. What is the mission of OSHA?

Centers for Medicare & Medicaid Services

The Centers for Medicare & Medicaid Services (CMS) [formerly the Health Care Financing Administration (HCFA)], a division of the United States Department of Health and Human Services, regulates and runs various departments and programs, including Medicare and Medicaid. This group is assigned to monitor and follow two key regulations that will affect your job as a medical assistant. These two laws are the **Clinical Laboratory Improvement Amendments Act** (CLIA) and the **Health Insurance Portability and Accountability Act** (HIPAA).

Clinical Laboratory Improvement Amendments Act. CLIA (Public Law 100-578) was originally written in 1988 and was aimed a streamlining the standards and quality of all laboratory settings. There are three levels of testing complexity. Laboratory sites and physician offices may perform tests only to the level of their certification. The three levels are low complexity, moderate complexity, and high complexity. Most physician offices perform only low- to moderate-complexity tests. Examples of low-complexity tests are urine dipsticks, fecal occult blood packets, urine pregnancy tests, ovulation kits, centrifuged microhematocrits, and certain blood glucose determinations. Examples of moderate-complexity tests are white blood cell counts, Gram staining, packaged rapid strep test, and automated cholesterol testing.

As the CMS has expanded, many amendments have occurred, with the latest one (CMS-2226F) occurring on January 24, 2003. The amendments aim at further reducing the potential for errors. Most laboratory errors occur in specimen collection and handling. Laboratory settings must have a complete and comprehensive QI program that studies and corrects problems associated with specimen collection and handling. Box 11-4 lists examples of errors in collecting and handling specimens.

Health Insurance Portability and Accountability Act. The HIPAA has four main objectives. They are to ensure health insurance portability for all people, reduce health care fraud and abuse, enforce standards of health information, and guarantee security and privacy of health information. Health insurance portability ensures that all working Americans

---

Box 11-4

ERRORS IN SPECIMEN COLLECTION

Errors in handling specimens or collecting them can occur in many ways. These errors can lead to errors in patient care. In most of these cases, the laboratory will not do the test and will dispose of the specimen. Another specimen will have to be collected from the patient. Here are some common errors:

- Wrong container used for specimen
- Container's expiration date passed
- Wrong patient's name on the label
- Wrong physician's name on the label
- No date or time on the label
- Patient's identification number not matched to laboratory slip
- Messy or illegible label
- Specimen label not matched to laboratory slip
- Specimen not stored at right temperature
- Laboratory slip not completely filled out

---

have access to health insurance and can take that insurance along if they leave the job. Some key requirements of the HIPAA are:

- Each physician practice must designate a privacy officer. This person is responsible for maintaining the privacy and security of all patients and ensuring compliance with the HIPAA.
- Physician offices must post a note in all waiting room areas that explains the practice's privacy policies.
- Policies and procedures must ensure that patients' safety and confidentiality are protected.

You will need to focus and guarantee security and privacy of all patient health information. There are specific guidelines on how you can transmit electronic transactions. Information must be encrypted before it is sent electronically. Many software programs can help physician offices to comply with these new regulations. The government is planning on implementing new laws that will require digital signatures to be sent with electronic data to decrease the potential for fraudulent Medicare claims. You can stay abreast of these new changes and regulations through the CMS website.

Physician offices must take appropriate steps to ensure that any company they are associated with also follows HIPAA regulations. Physician offices often have a variety of business partnerships that help keep the office flowing professionally and effectively. Some examples of business partnerships are cleaning services, document-shredding companies, laboratory and specimen transport personnel, and temporary staffing agencies. Contracts among physicians and their business partners should reflect that the business adheres to HIPAA regulations. For the JCAHO to meet HIPAA regulations and ensure security and privacy of patient information during the site visit, health care settings being surveyed must sign a business associate agreement prior to inspection.

Checkpoint Question

4. What governmental agency would you look to for additional information on HIPAA and CLIA regulations?

State Health Departments

Each state has a specific agency to license and monitor health care organizations. Each state has specific guidelines for required QI programs. As in participation with OSHA regulations, participation with state regulations is not optional. The rules and regulations vary among states. It is important that you be aware of the regulations in your state. For example, in some states medical assistants cannot administer medications, while in other states they can. Using your Internet search engine, type in key words "public health department" and look for your state's health department website.

DEVELOPING A QUALITY IMPROVEMENT PROGRAM

The size and complexity of an organization's QI program depends on the organization's particular needs. In large hospitals, numerous committees may be assigned to monitor and implement QI plans. Examples of QI plans are fall prevention, needlestick surveillance, and laboratory contamination rates. The committees will consist of staff members, including physicians. Most hospitals have a specific person assigned to oversee all of these committees.

In the medical office and ambulatory care settings, QI programs tend to be more informal. Usually the office manager or senior physician is responsible for monitoring and implementing QI plans. As more outpatient centers become accredited by the JCAHO, however, QI programs have become more structured. A few examples of quality issues that can be monitored in the physician offices are:

- Patient waiting times
- Unplanned returned patient visits for the same ailment or illness
- Misdiagnosed illnesses that are detected by another partner in the practice
- Patient or family complaints
- Timely follow-up telephone calls to patients
- Patient falls in physician's office or office building
- Mislabeled specimens sent to the laboratory
- Blood specimens that are coagulated or contaminated

Seven Steps for a Successful Program

The following seven steps are essential for creating an effective QI program:

1. *Identify the problem or potential problem.* All organizations can improve their delivery of patient care. Suggestions for improving care can come from many resources, including the following:
   - Office managers
   - Physicians (recommendations and complaints)
   - Other employees (e.g., nurses and medical assistants)
   - Patients (interviews)
   - Incident report trending (discussed later)

   The person responsible for QI in the medical office reviews all QI problems or potential problems and selects the one to be addressed first. Problems given top priority are those that are high risk (most likely to occur) and those that are most likely to cause injury to patients, family members, or employees.

2. *Form a task force.* A **task force** is a group of employees with different roles within the organization brought together to solve a given problem. In a medical office, the task force usually consists of a physician, nurse, medical assistant, and office manager. In large hospitals, various department managers are generally involved.

3. *Assign an expected threshold.* The task force establishes an **expected threshold** (numerical goal) for a given problem. Thresholds must be realistic and achievable. For example, if the problem is needlestick injuries, the expected threshold is a realistic number of employee needlestick injuries that the task force considers acceptable in a given period. For instance, the threshold may be one employee stick per month. It is not realistic to set the goal at zero; this may be optimal but is not achievable.

4. *Explore the problem and propose solutions.* The task force investigates the problem thoroughly to determine all potential causes and possible solutions. After various solutions are discussed, the task force decides what solution or solutions are to be implemented.

5. *Implement the solution.* The key to successful implementation of the solution is staff education. All staff members must be taught about the problem and the plan to decrease the problem. The type of implementation will be based on the problem. For example, if the problem is patients falling at the entrance to the building, fixing the problem is likely to be complex and expensive. It may involve reengineering and construction of new walkways. If the problem is mislabeling or misspelling patient's names on laboratory specimens, the implementation will be simpler, possibly printing labels from the computer database.

6. *Establish a QI monitoring plan.* After implementation, the solution must be evaluated to determine

whether it worked and if so, how well. QI monitoring plans have three elements:
- Source of monitoring, that is, where the numerical data will be obtained (e.g., medical record review, incident reports, laboratory reports, office logs)
- Frequency of monitoring, that is, how often the data will be monitored and tallied (e.g., once a week, once a month)
- Person responsible for monitoring, that is, who collects the data and presents the results in graphic form, allowing for easy comparison of data from before and after implementation of the solution

7. *Obtain feedback.* The members of the task force must review the graphs in relation to their expected threshold. Did they meet the threshold? If yes, the problem has been resolved. If the threshold was not met, the task force must determine whether the expected threshold was unrealistic or the solutions were inadequate. In either case, the problem has not been resolved; therefore, the task force must review each of the steps and make appropriate changes.

Checkpoint Question

5. How does an organization select problems for a QI program?

RISK MANAGEMENT

Risk management is an internal process geared to identifying potential problems before they cause injury to patients or employees. Potential problems are related to risk factors. A risk factor is any situation or condition that poses a safety or liability concern for a given practice. Examples of risk factors are poor lighting, unlocked medication cabinets, failure to dispose of needles properly, and faulty patient identification procedures. Such factors may lead to patient falls, medication errors, employee needlesticks, and mistakes in therapeutic intervention. Risk factors for a particular health care organization are identified through the trending of incident reports.

One of the most challenging problems for risk managers is to prevent noncompliance with regulatory agencies. As discussed earlier, numerous agencies regulate health care settings, and these rules and regulations change frequently. You can stay up-to-date with new changes by reading newsletters from these organizations, attending your state and local professional meetings, and frequently visiting various professional websites.

Incident Reports

Incident reports, sometimes referred to as occurrence reports, are written accounts of untoward (negative) patient, visitor, or staff events. Such events may be minor or life or limb threatening. The insurance company that provides the institution's liability insurance often requires incident reports.

An incident report is written or completed by the staff member involved in or at the scene of the incident. The report is reviewed by a supervisor for completion and accuracy and is then sent to a central location. In a hospital, incident reports are sent to the risk manager. In a medical office, incident reports are usually given to the office manager or the physician. Depending on the type of event and organizational policy, a physician may or may not document the event on the incident report. If an unusual event happens to a patient, however, the physician should assess the patient and document the findings on the incident report.

Checkpoint Question

6. What is an incident report?

When to Complete an Incident Report

Even in the safest settings, undesirable things can happen to patients. These events sometimes result from human error (e.g., giving the wrong medication), or they may be idiopathic. Idiopathic means that something occurred for unknown reasons and was unavoidable (e.g., an allergic reaction). Incident reports must be completed even if no injury resulted from an event. A few examples of situations requiring an incident report are:

- All medication errors
- All patient, visitor, and employee falls
- Drawing blood from a wrong patient
- Mislabeling of blood tubes or specimens
- Incorrect surgical instrument counts following surgery
- Employee needlesticks
- Workers' compensation injuries

The rule of thumb is, when in doubt, always complete an incident report. Many health care professionals are reluctant to complete incident reports, owing to various myths, which are discussed in Box 11-5.

Information Included on an Incident Report

Although every agency has its own form, the following data are always included on an incident report (Fig. 11-1):

- Name, address, and phone number of the injured party
- Date of birth and sex of the injured party
- Date, time, and location of the incident
- Brief description of the incident and what was done to correct it
- Any diagnostic procedures or treatments that were needed
- Patient examination findings, if applicable
- Names and addresses of witnesses, if applicable
- Signature and title of person completing form
- Physician's and supervisor's signatures as per policy

Box 11-5

MYTHS ABOUT COMPLETING AN INCIDENT REPORT

Myth	Fact
If I complete an incident report, I will get fired.	Employers want incident reports to be completed for documentation of events. You are more likely to get fired for *not* completing one.
Incident reports go into my personnel file.	They are not placed in your file. They are stored separately. Supervisors may document discussions or education that you were given about the incident.
If I complete the incident report, I am admitting that I am at fault.	Incident reports do not imply fault. They document the evidence.
I need to photocopy the incident report and save it at home for my own legal protection.	You may find yourself in more trouble if you copy the document and store it at home. Most incident reports contain confidential patient information, and it is illegal to copy private patient information and store it at home.

Guidelines for Completing an Incident Report

When completing an incident report, follow these guidelines:

1. State only the facts. Do not draw conclusions or summarize the event. For example, if you walk into the reception room and find a patient on the floor, do not write, "Patient tripped and fell in reception area," because that draws a conclusion. Instead, document the incident as follows: "Patient found on the floor in the reception area. Patient states that he fell" (Fig. 11-2).
2. Write legibly and sign your name legibly. Be sure to include your title.
3. Complete the form in a timely fashion. In general, incident reports should be completed within 24 hours of the event.
4. Do not leave any blank spaces on the form. If a particular section of the report does not apply, write n/a (not applicable).
5. Never photocopy an incident report for your own personal record.
6. Never place the incident report in the patient's chart. Never document in the patient's chart that an incident report was completed. Only document the event in the patient's chart. (By writing in the medical record that an incident report was completed, it opens the potential for lawyers to subpoena the incident report, should there be a lawsuit.)

Trending Incident Reports

After incident reports are completed, they are reviewed and tracked to highlight specific patterns. The resulting statistical data can be used to identify problem areas, which can be corrected through QI programs. Examples of statistical data that can be found in incident reports follow:

- Particular days of the week when most negative events happen (if most events occur on Friday afternoons, perhaps staffing on Friday afternoon should be reevaluated)
- Most common area for patient falls (if most falls happen in the lobby, a QI program may need to be established to assess why falls occur there)
- Medications that are routinely given incorrectly (educating staff and using colored labels to highlight similar drug names may correct this)
- The age group most likely to have problems (if most of your incident reports reflect problems in the geriatric population, a QI program focusing on geriatric care may be needed)
- Incident reports should be kept in a special file in the manager's office (some managers file these reports

WHAT IF

You give the wrong medication, and the patient has a bad reaction to it. Would you be better off not documenting the medication error?

NO! By not documenting the incident, you place yourself at risk. These risks can include allegations of falsifying medical records, tampering with medical records, and failing to follow reporting policies and procedures. On the incident report, do not say, "I gave the wrong medication"; just state the facts: "X medication was ordered. I gave Y medication." Then document whom you told and when, what you were advised to do, and any other pertinent information. Your supervisor or the risk manager may call the medical office's insurance company to alert them to the incident. If the incident results in a malpractice lawsuit, an accurately completed incident report can prove helpful to your organization's attorney.

INCIDENT REPORT FORM
PRIVILEGED & CONFIDENTIAL

Patient Stamp

☐ Inpatient ☐ Outpatient ☐ Visitor ☐ Volunteer ☐ Other   *NOT A PART OF THE MEDICAL RECORD–FORWARD TO RISK MANAGER WITHIN 72 HOURS*

Name	Age	Sex	Admit Date	Location of Incident	Room #

Diagnosis	Date of Incident	Time AM/PM	Date of Report	Person Reporting & Title (print)

CONDITION BEFORE INCIDENT
☐ Alert ☐ Disoriented ☐ Unconscious ☐ Agitated
☐ Confused ☐ Sedated ☐ Uncooperative ☐ Other

Activity Orders
☐ Adib ☐ BRP ☐ BRP c help
☐ With assist ☐ CBR
☐ Up in chair ☐ BSC

Signature

INCIDENT (please check all items that apply)   FALLS

FALLS	PREFALL FACTORS	RESTRAINTS	RISK CONDITIONS	CURRENT MEDICATIONS
☐ Fall from Bed ☐ Fall from Chair ☐ Fall from Bedside Commode ☐ Fall from Stretcher ☐ Fall from Wheelchair ☐ Fall from Toilet ☐ Fall while Ambulatory ☐ Other_____	☐ Bed Up ☐ Bed Down ☐ Brake On ☐Y ☐N ☐ Not working ☐ Siderails Down ___ 2 Up ___ 3 Up ___ 4 Up ___ Climbed Out	Restraints Ordered ☐Y ☐N Restraints in Use ☐Y ☐N Type: ☐ Vest ☐ Wrist ☐ Ankle ☐ Secured Mittens ☐ Tied ☐ Untied by: ___ Staff ___ Patient ___ Family/S.O. Call light in reach ☐Y ☐N Fall follow-up program initiated prior to fall ☐Y ☐N	☐ Weakness ☐ Decreased Mobility ☐ Confusion ☐ Neuro/ortho diagnosis ☐ Cardiovascular diagnosis ☐ Inpaired Vision ☐ History of Syncope ☐ Poor Nutritional Status ☐ Incontinence ☐ History of fall last 6 months Safety Education given prior to fall: ☐ None ☐ Patient ☐ Family/S.O.	☐ None ☐ NTG ☐ Diuretics ☐ Cathartic preps/enemas ☐ Antihypertensives ☐ Antiseizure ☐ Antidepressants ☐ Antiemetics ☐ Antipsychotics ☐ Analgesics/Hypnotics ☐ Narcotics ☐ Cardiovascular

Environment: ☐ Floor wet ☐Y ☐N   ☐ Free from obstacles ☐Y ☐N   Describe: _____
☐ Night light on ☐Y ☐N ☐N/A   ☐ Objects not in reach-searching for _____

MEDICATION VARIANCE, Including IV & Blood Product(s)	PROCEDURE VARIANCE		MISCELLANEOUS

☐ Incorrect Pt. Identification ☐ Incorrect IV Solution
☐ Incorrect Dosage ☐ Incorrect IV Rate
☐ Incorrect Route ☐ Incorrect Count/Missing Med
☐ Incorrect Time ☐ Topical Substance Reaction,
☐ Incorrect Med Given   including Tape
☐ Incorrect Med Dispensed ☐ Allergy Not Documented
☐ Med Omitted ☐ Contrast Reaction/Complication
☐ Med Transcription Error ☐ Medication Past Due 1 hour
☐ Incorrect Blood Given   or more
☐ Pharmacy Notified ☐ Other_____
☐ Infiltration
☐ Blood Reaction
☐ Med Reaction
	☐ Record Error ☐ Transcription
	☐ Incorrect Pt. Identification
	☐ Omitted Treatment
	☐ Delayed Treatment
	☐ Omitted Diagnostic/Lab
	☐ Delayed Diagnostic/Lab
	☐ Traumatic Venipuncture
	☐ Break in Sterile Technique
	☐ Incorrect Surgical Count–Sponge
	☐ Incorrect Surgical Count–Needle
	☐ Incorrect Surgical Count–Instrument
	☐ Retained Foreign Body
	☐ Other:
		☐ Documentation Error
		☐ Consent Variance
		☐ Improper Prep of Pt.
		☐ NPO Violated
		☐ Radiation/Toxic Chemical Exposure
		☐ X-ray Interpretation Discrepancy
		☐ Airway/Intubation Problem
		☐ Incorrect Level of Heat/Cold Applied
		☐ Incorrect Procedure/Treatment
		☐ Unordered Procedure/Treatment
		☐ Equip./Product Malfunction
		☐ User Error
		☐ Equipment Unavailable
			☐ AMA/Elopement
			☐ Admitted c Pressure Sore
			☐ Damaged/Lost Teeth/
			   Denture
			☐ Injury During Transport
			☐ Self Inflicted Injury/Suicide
			☐ Malpositioning/Incorrect
			   Body Alignment
			☐ Pt. Self Extubation
			☐ Tube/IV Catheter Out
			☐ Accidental Strking Against
			   an Object
			☐ Fainted
			☐ Pt. Dissatisfied/Pt.
			   Threatened Law Suit
			☐ Transfer to Critical Care
			   p incident
			☐ Behavior Out of Norm.
			☐ Other: _____

INJURY (please check all items that apply) All serious/significant injuries must be described on reverse side

SERIOUS	SIGNIFICANT	SUPERFICIAL	PROCEDURE/LABOR & DELIVERY/NURSERY
☐ None ☐ Spinal Cord Injury ☐ Injury to Nerves ☐ Brain Injury ☐ Surgery to Wrong Pt. ☐ Incorrect Surgical Procedure ☐ Shock ☐ Trauma Causing Internal Injury ☐ Hemorrhage ☐ Death ☐ Unscheduled Return to OR ☐ Other:	☐ None ☐ Major Infiltration ☐ Hospital Acquired Decubiti ☐ Burn ☐ Fracture ☐ Sprain/Strain Joint/Muscle ☐ Injury to Blood Vessel ☐ Dislocation of Joint ☐ Open Wound Needing Medical Care ☐ Adverse Effect Due to Med/Anesthesia/Transfusion ☐ Adverse Effect Due to Exposure to Toxic Chemical ☐ Complication Due to Mechanical Device ☐ Prolongation of Hospital Stay ☐ Anoxia/Respiratory Distress ☐ Cancellation of or after induction of anesthesia	☐ None ☐ Unknown ☐ Abrasion ☐ Bruising ☐ Blister/Skin Tear ☐ Skin Prick ☐ Laceration ☐ Rash/Hives ☐ Other:	☐ Newborn with apparent Cerebral dysfunction ☐ Newborn with APGAR of four (4) or less at five (5) minutes ☐ Newborn with serious birth trauma ☐ Precipitous Delivery ☐ Unattended Delivery **MEDICAL DEVICE/EQUIPMENT RELATED** Equipment involved: _____ Manufacturer: _____ Serial #: _____ Asset #: _____ Biomedical Dept. Notified: _____ Date Tagged & Removed from Service: _____ Date/Time **Maintain all components of device such as connectors, adaptors, tubings, etc. Document all readings/settings.** **DO NOT ADJUST OR CLEAR ANY READINGS.**

AMA FOLLOW-UP

Reason for leaving: _____
Patient admitted <24 hours ☐ Yes ☐ No
Patient/S.O. Teaching: ☐ Completed ☐ Partial ☐ None ☐ Patient Uncooperative

FIGURE 11–1. Sample incident report.

(continued)

Description of event: _____

_____

_____

_____

_____

_____

_____

_____

_____

_____

_____

_____

_____

_____

_____

_____

Physician notified: ☐ Yes ☐ No   Name of Physician (print): _____

Physician Remarks: _____

_____

_____

_____

_____

_____

_____

_____

_____

| _____ | |
| Physician Signature | Date |

Supervisor/Manager Investigation/Follow-up Action: _____

_____

_____

_____

_____

_____

_____

| _____ | |
| Supervisor/Manager Signature | Date |

Witness: Name (print)	Department/Shift	Address	Phone

| _____ | |
| Risk Manager Signature | Date |

F IGURE 11–1. *(Continued)*

FIGURE 11–2. When writing an incident report, document only the facts. Do not draw conclusions. Always be honest, and never falsify the information.

according to dates, whereas others file them according to the problem)

PUTTING IT ALL TOGETHER: A CASE REVIEW

Following is a case study in which the elements of successful QI and risk management programs are put into action.

You are working in a busy family practice. The average number of patients seen daily is 92. The physicians, nurses, and medical assistants are responsible for labeling specimen containers before they go to the laboratory. On the average, 15 specimens are collected daily. The hospital laboratory that analyzes the specimens reports that an average of seven specimens are mislabeled monthly.

The office manager brings to a staff meeting a graph (Fig. 11-3) depicting the number of mislabeled specimens that occurred over a 4-month period. She notes that most mislabelings occurred on Monday and Friday afternoons. It is decided that this is a significant patient care issue and that a QI program to address and resolve the problem is needed.

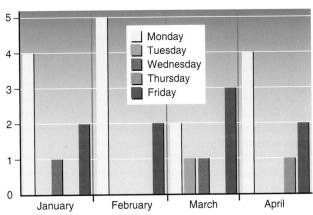

FIGURE 11–3. Frequency of mislabeled specimens by day of the week and by month.

A task force is formed. It includes a physician, a nurse, and a medical assistant. The task force identifies the problem as a high-risk issue and assigns the expected threshold to be fewer than two mislabeled specimens per month. The task force identifies the factors related to the problem, which includes lack of sufficient labels in patient rooms, high patient volumes on Monday and Friday afternoons, and overall need for educating all staff members about the importance of labeling specimens correctly.

Solutions to these three problems are created:

Problem: *insufficient labels in the rooms.*
Solution: *Additional specimen labels are placed in every room. Also, specimen labels will be already printed and waiting for patients who arrive for an anticipated specimen collection (stool, urine, skin biopsy).*
Problem: *large volume on Monday and Friday afternoons.*
Solution: *The medical assistant's hours will change to 10:00 A.M. to 6:30 P.M. on Monday and Fridays instead of 8 A.M. to 4:30 P.M. This creates more staff coverage during peak hours.*
Problem: *lack of knowledge.*
Solution: *A representative for the hospital laboratory will conduct an in-service for all staff members. He or she will explain the implication of mislabeled specimens and how they can impair patient care. Lets say*

Spanish Terminology

¿Vio usted lo que pasó?	Did you see what happened?
¿Cayo usted?	Did you fall?
¿Está lastimado usted?	Are you hurt?
¿Quiere usted ver un doctor?	Do you want to see a doctor?
Usted necesita obtener una radiografía.	You need an x-ray.

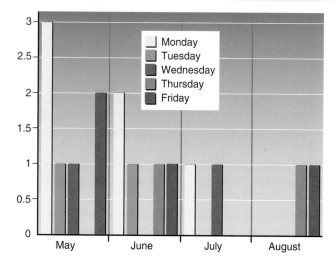

FIGURE 11-4. Frequency of mislabeled specimens by day of the week and by month after a QI plan was carried out. Note the change in the numerical system on the graph.

that both Mrs. Brown and Mrs. Lisien came into the office for skin biopsies. The specimens were taken and placed in bottles. The bottles were put next to each other on the shelf. The name labels were reversed on the specimens. One specimen showed a malignancy. Which patient would get treated? The wrong patient would be treated, causing unnecessary expense and distress, while the patient with the malignancy would not be treated and might get sicker.

After these steps were taken, a new graph was developed showing the improvement (Fig. 11-4). Because the threshold has been met, the task force does not think any more changes are needed, and the QI mislabeling program is ended.

CHAPTER SUMMARY

Quality improvement programs have many benefits to heath care organizations. They can identify potential problems for patients and employees. After identifying the problem, the task force can create solutions to resolve them. QI programs are also required by various agencies. Four important agencies are the JCAHO, OSHA, CMS, and your state health department. You must stay alert to new regulations from these agencies. More information about various health care regulations can be found through their websites, newsletters, and professional organizations. Patients place trust in all health care workers and health care settings. We must all work hard to provide good quality care to all patients every time they are treated.

Critical Thinking Challenges

1. Create a list of potential patient or employee problems that could be solved with a QI program. Be sure to include some administrative, clinical, and laboratory examples. Then select three problems and develop a list of solutions for each problem.
2. List 10 reasons to complete an incident report. Select one of these reasons and complete the incident report. (Photocopy the incident report from the chapter.) Be sure to review the guidelines for completing an incident report. Make sure your description of events on page 2 follows these guidelines.
3. Search the JCAHO website. What information can you find regarding sentinel events? What steps can be taken to prevent them?
4. Privacy of patient information is essential. Write a policy that aims at protecting patients' privacy. What steps can you take to ensure patients' privacy? Would you make a good privacy officer? Why or why not?

Answers to Checkpoint Questions

1. The benefits of being accredited by the JCAHO are that the health care organization is eligible for state and federal funding programs and that accreditation proves to the community that the facility has met basic standards of care.
2. A sentinel event is an unexpected occurrence involving a death or serious physical or physiological injury to a patient.
3. OSHA's mission is to save lives, prevent injuries, and protect the health of America's workers.
4. Centers for Medicare & Medicaid (CMS) are responsible for HIPAA and CLIA regulations.
5. QI programs should be selected to address problems that are high risk and those most likely to cause injury to patients, family members, or employees.
6. An incident report is a written account of untoward or negative events involving patients, visitors, or employees.

 Websites

Centers for Medicare & Medicaid Services
www.cms.gov
Clinical Laboratory Improvement Amendments Act
www.cms.hhs.gov/clia/
Health Care Report Cards
www.healthgrades.com
Health Insurance Portability and Accountability Act
www.cms.hhs.gov/hipaa
Joint Commission on Accreditation of Healthcare Organizations
www.jcaho.org
Occupational Health and Safety Administration
www.osha.gov

12

Management of the Medical Office Team

CHAPTER OUTLINE

OVERVIEW OF MEDICAL
  OFFICE MANAGEMENT
  Organizational Structure
  The Medical Office Manager

RESPONSIBILITIES OF THE
  MEDICAL OFFICE MANAGER
  Communication
  Staffing Issues
  Policy and Procedures Manuals
  Developing Promotional Materials
  Financial Concerns
  Maintenance and Inventory of
    Supplies
  Education

LEGAL ISSUES REGARDING
  OFFICE MANAGEMENT
  Americans with Disabilities Act
  Sexual Harassment
  Family and Medical Leave Act
  Other Legal Considerations

ROLE DELINEATION COMPONENTS

GENERAL: Professionalism
- Demonstrate initiative and responsibility
- Work as a member of the health care team
- Adapt to change
- Enhance skills through continuing education
- Promote the practice through positive public relations

GENERAL: Legal Concepts
- Perform within legal and ethical boundaries
- Follow employer's established policies dealing with the health care contract
- Implement and maintain federal and state health care legislation and regulations
- Comply with established risk management and safety procedures
- Recognize professional credentialing criteria
- Develop and maintain personnel, policy, and procedures manuals

GENERAL: Communication Skills
- Recognize and respond effectively to verbal, nonverbal, and written communications
- Serve as a liaison

GENERAL: Operational Functions
- Perform inventory of supplies and equipment
- Perform routine maintenance of administrative and clinical equipment
- Apply computer techniques to support office operations
- Perform personnel management functions
- Negotiate leases and prices for equipment and supply contracts

ADMINISTRATIVE: Administrative Procedures
- Perform basic administrative medical assisting functions
- Understand and adhere to manage care policies and procedures
- Negotiate managed care contracts

ADMINISTRATIVE: Practice Finances
- Manage accounts receivable
- Develop and maintain fee schedules
- Manage renewals of business and professional insurance policies
- Manage personnel benefits and maintain records
- Perform marketing, financial and strategic planning

CHAPTER COMPETENCIES

LEARNING OBJECTIVES
Upon successfully completing this chapter, you will be able to:

1. Spell and define the key terms
2. Describe what is meant by organizational structure
3. List seven responsibilities of the medical office manager
4. Explain the five staffing issues that a medical office manager will be responsible for handling
5. List the types of policies and procedures that should be included in a medical office's policy and procedures manual
6. List five types of promotional materials that a medical office may distribute
7. Discuss three financial concerns that the medical office manager must be capable of addressing
8. Discuss four legal issues that affect medical office management

PERFORMANCE OBJECTIVES
Upon successfully completing this chapter, you will be able to:

1. Write a job description
2. Create policy and procedures manuals

KEY TERMS

Americans with Disabilities Act	compliance officer	job description	policy
budget	Family and Medical Leave Act	mission statement	procedure
		organizational chart	

A SUCCESSFUL MEDICAL practice needs an effective medical office management process. This process must be a team effort among the physicians, nurse managers, and the office manager. This chapter provides an overview of medical office management as well as a discussion of a medical office manager's specific responsibilities.

OVERVIEW OF MEDICAL OFFICE MANAGEMENT

Each medical office is organized in a slightly different manner, depending on the size and complexity of the setting.

Organizational Structure

The medical office's organizational structure, or chain of command, is depicted in an **organizational chart**, a flow sheet that allows the manager and employees to identify their team members and to see where they fit into the team. Figure 12-1 displays a sample organizational chart for a physician's office in which there is a partnership between two physicians. In this example, it is assumed that the physicians have an equal partnership in the practice.

Checkpoint Question

1. What is the purpose of an organizational chart?

The Medical Office Manager

The medical office manager must be multiskilled, multitalented, and able to prioritize a variety of issues, juggle responsibilities, and communicate effectively with patients, staff, and physicians. In some settings, the medical office manager may be referred to as the business manager. Managers may be nurses, medical assistants, or administrative support personnel. Although the qualifications and educational requirements for the position vary greatly among health care organizations, a successful medical office manager must be:

- Flexible
- A positive role model for employees
- Honest and fair
- A good communicator
- A resource person for employees
- Supportive of all management decisions
- Well organized
- Able to focus on a given task
- Able to resolve conflicts
- Able to see the big picture

A medical office manager's responsibilities include varied tasks:

- Communicating with patients, physicians, and staff
- Handling staffing issues

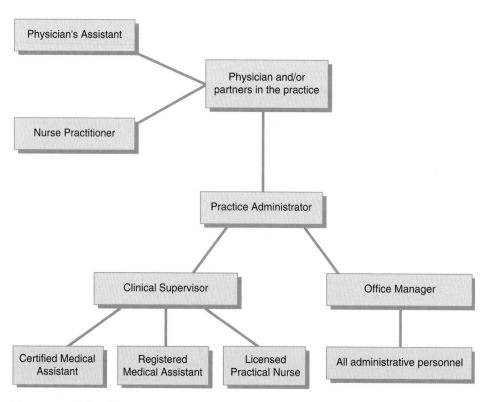

FIGURE 12-1.   Sample organizational chart.

- Writing and revising policy and procedures manuals
- Developing promotional materials
- Handling financial concerns
- Handling maintenance and inventory
- Ensuring that the staff receives appropriate education

RESPONSIBILITIES OF THE MEDICAL OFFICE MANAGER

Communication

Perhaps one of the hardest and yet most important aspects of being an effective manager is being able to communicate with fellow employees, colleagues, physicians, and patients. (The techniques for effective communication are discussed in Chapter 3.) You must be a good listener, have good interpersonal skills, and be aware of your own nonverbal language.

Communicating With Patients

Communication with patients on a management level can often be challenging. Patients come to you with a variety of complaints, such as incorrect billing, poor care, or long waits to see physicians. Of course, you must always be diplomatic. Your goal should be to correct the problem in a timely and professional manner and to alleviate any negative feelings the patient may have.

Communicating With Staff

Communication with staff members can be difficult, depending on the number of employees, number and locations of satellite centers, and the variety of shifts that are in place. There are three ways to promote communication with staff members: staff meetings, bulletin boards, and communication notebooks.

Staff Meetings. Staff meetings should be scheduled at a predictable frequency and time to allow the staff to plan (e.g., they might be held the first Monday of every month at 8 A.M.) Meetings should never be canceled except in a true emergency.

Staff meetings must be well organized and should begin and end on time. Agendas should be created prior to the meeting and posted for staff review. (See Chapter 7 for information on agendas.) The agenda should be followed as closely as possible. Individual staff concerns or complaints should not be handled during a general staff meeting; the meeting should remain focused and constructive and not turn into a battleground for staff disagreements. Minutes should be taken and kept in a notebook for staff to review as needed. (See Chapter 7 for information on minutes.)

Staff meetings should be conducted in a private area out of patients' sight and hearing (Fig. 12-2). All interruptions except for emergencies should be avoided.

Have the telephone covered by an answering service or a prerecorded message informing callers of the time the staff will be unavailable. Lock the door and place a sign with the time the office will reopen. Of course, you will give clear instructions to callers or visitors who have an emergency. The personnel manual should clearly state the attendance policy for staff meetings. In addition, some offices include attendance as a duty in each employee's job description (statement of work-related responsibilities). To improve attendance at staff meetings, consider serving food or including an educational presentation.

Bulletin Boards. Bulletin board postings allow employees to get a quick and easy look at new polices or procedures. To encourage staff members to read the postings, make sure the bulletin boards are attractive, well organized, and updated regularly. It is a good idea to have employees initial all messages on the bulletin board after reading them.

Communication Notebooks. A simple notebook can serve as a two-way communication tool: You can write messages to employees, and they can write back to you. Such a notebook is usually kept in the staff lounge. Again, staff members should initial any important messages after reading them. If the message is directed to you, be sure to respond as soon as possible.

Communicating Electronically

E-mail has become popular and is an easy and time-saving way to communicate with staff. Messages can be printed and kept in a binder for easy reference. E-mail messages eliminate the need for memos that must be posted or circulated. Your e-mail system will provide you with an address book that can be customized to include groups such as all employees, all clinical employees, employees and physicians, and so on.

Sometimes, the stress of daily duties prevents managers from communicating with staff members on a personal level. To be an effective manager, you should communicate not

FIGURE 12-2. Staff meeting being conducted in a private area.

only bad news but also positive messages to your employees. You can communicate positive messages through birthday and holiday cards and employee recognition awards.

Checkpoint Question

2. What are three ways to promote communication with staff members?

Staffing Issues

Staffing issues will occupy most of your time as an office manager. These concerns include writing job descriptions, hiring new employees, evaluating present employees, taking disciplinary actions, handling terminations, and scheduling.

Writing Job Descriptions

Each job must have a description. The purpose of a **job description** is to inform the employee about the duties and expectations for a given position. Job descriptions also help you in interviewing applicants and evaluating existing employees.

Each employee should receive a copy of his or her job description at the time of hiring and after any revisions to the description are made. Some medical offices have a policy requiring the employee to read and sign the job description at the time of hiring.

Formats for writing job descriptions vary among offices. In general, the following elements are included: job title, supervisor, position summary, hours, location, employment requirements, physical requirements, duties, and the evaluation process (Fig. 12-3). The description should also include the date it was written and date of any revisions.

If possible, involve staff members in writing and revising their job descriptions. Employee participation leads to greater cooperation.

Hiring and Interviewing Employees

Only after creating or reviewing an existing job description can you begin the process of interviewing and hiring a new employee. Finding applicants for most medical office positions is usually not a problem. You can seek applicants through advertising in local newspaper classified sections,

placement personnel at local schools that offer medical assisting programs, networking, and employment agencies.

All applicants should complete an application. State laws vary regarding the types of questions that can be asked on applications. In general, you must avoid any questions pertaining to an applicant's age, sex, race, religion, and physical or mental disabilities. If your medical facility requires a criminal background check and drug testing, the form should include this information with a place for the applicant to give necessary permission with a signature. Any employee application form should be reviewed by legal counsel prior to its use. It is always a good idea to request that the applicant bring a résumé to the interview.

Before interviewing an applicant, prepare a list of questions. Again, use caution; under law you are not permitted to ask about some topics. During the interview, assess the applicant's ability to do the following:

- Perform technical skills
- Treat patients in a caring manner
- Fit into your organization
- Communicate in a professional yet friendly manner
- Remain flexible

Evaluating Employees

All employees must be evaluated annually. The evaluation should be a positive experience for the employee. Employee evaluations must be fair, accurate, and objective. Some type

Spanish Terminology

Busco un trabajo.	*I am looking for a job.*
¿Tiene usted cualquier abierto?	*Do you have any openings?*
¿Dónde estan las aplicaciones?	*Where are the applications?*
Soy el director.	*I am the manager.*

Job Description

Title: Medical Assistant

Supervisor(s): Clinical Supervisor

Office Manager for Administrative Duties

Position summary: This is a 40-hour position that will require the employee to perform various duties including administrative, clinical, and laboratory procedures. Scheduling will be variable to meet the needs of the office.

Hours: Hours will vary to meet the needs of the office. Hours will rotate from 8:00 AM–4:30 PM and 10:00 AM–6:30 PM. You will be expected to work one Saturday per month.

Location: Our main office is located at 129 South Main Street. The satellite office is located at 56 West Road, Suite 102. This position will primarily require you to work at our main office. However, occasional days may be assigned at the satellite office.

Employment Requirements: The employee must have graduated from a medical assisting program. CMA or RMA is preferred. The employee must have a current CPR and First Aid card. One year of experience or completion of an externship is preferred.

• *Language skills:* The employee must be able to read and interpret documents and respond appropriately (verbally and/or in writing). Must be able to document in a professional manner.

• *Mathematical skills:* The employee must be able to add, subtract, multiply, and divide whole numbers and fractions.

Physical requirements: The following are physical requirements for this job: Standing: 6–8 hours/day; Sitting: 6–8 hours/day; Lifting: 50 pounds; Twisting and rotating: 45 degrees; Squatting: As needed to assist patients or to perform office tasks.

Duties: You will be expected to perform the following duties after completing the orientation process. This is a partial list; and other duties can be added as necessary.

Administrative:

Scheduling appointments	Processing mail
Transcribing documents	Operating the telephone
Filing	Providing patient education
Completing insurance forms	

Clinical/Laboratory:

Operating centrifuge	Obtaining vital signs
Performing phlebotomy	Administering vaccines and other medications
Performing HCT/HGB/CBC	as ordered
Performing pregnancy and monospot tests	Providing patient education
Obtaining visual acuities	Assisting the physician as directed

Evaluation process: Three evaluations will be conducted in the first year. Thirty days from start date, ninety days from start date, and then at the one-year anniversary date. Following the first year of employment, annual evaluations will be done.

I have read my job description, and I understand what is expected of me. I am able to physically perform all the required duties.

Signature of employee: _____   Date: _____

Signature of supervisor: _____   Date: _____

Signature of supervisor: _____   Date: _____

Dates: original JD - 1977, revised March 1998.

FIGURE 12–3.   Sample job description.

of written evaluation should be given to the employee to read, sign, and comment on. Most forms ask employees to list their objectives and goals for the coming year. Figure12-4 displays a sample evaluation form. Some organizations call evaluations performance appraisals.

New employees should be evaluated 1 month after their start date, again in 90 days, and then at their 1-year anniver-

sary date. This process helps new employees gain confidence and improve weaknesses.

Taking Disciplinary Action

Most offices have policies regarding documentation of disciplinary action. Disciplinary actions can be verbal or

Employee Evaluation Form

Employee: _____

Evaluation Date: _____

Job Title: _____

Ratings:

Traits	Score
Appearance	
Communication Skills	
Attendance	
Quality of work	
Reliability	
Initiative	
Other:	
Total Score:	

Rating scale:

5—excellent

4—above average

3—meets job expectations

2—below job expectations

1—does not meet job expectations

Supervisor comments:

_____

_____

Employee goals for the next year (to be completed by employee):

_____

_____

_____

Employee Comments:

_____

_____

_____

Supervisor signature: _____   Date: _____

Employee signature: _____   Date: _____

FIGURE 12–4.   Sample employee evaluation form.

written. Verbal warnings are generally done for a first-time minor occurrence (e.g., not showing up for work and not calling in). A note should go into the employee's file stating that a verbal warning was given, the date, any actions that were taken, and any comments that the employee made.

Written notices are used for more serious problems (e.g., breaching patient confidentiality, substance abuse) or recurrent minor ones. Employees should sign any written warning notices. These documents can be used as evidence in the event that the person is fired and brings a lawsuit for wrongful discharge. Figure 12-5 shows a sample written disciplinary action form. Determine whether the employee's credentialing agency should be notified of serious infractions.

Terminating Employees

Having to terminate (fire) an employee is never an easy or pleasant task. It is essential that policies regarding termination be followed precisely. All disciplinary actions must be clearly and objectively stated. Terminating employees for unlawful reasons or failing to follow the organization's termination policy can result in lawsuits against you and the office. Some reasons for termination:

- Excessive tardiness or absenteeism
- Inappropriate dress or behavior
- Alcohol or drug use
- Endangering patients

- Lying or stealing
- Falsifying medical records or time sheets
- Breaching patient confidentiality

Scheduling

The primary goal of scheduling is to meet the needs of the office. The secondary goal is to meet the requests of your employees. You must be fair in scheduling and always follow your organization's policies for weekend and holiday or personal day requests. If possible, employees should be given time off with pay when attending seminars and meetings of their professional organization. This practice will keep morale high and encourage employees to stay current with their skills. Depending on the number of employees that you have to schedule and the complexity of the hours or shifts, you can either schedule by hand or use a computer program. If your organization is small and cohesive, you may want to assign a senior staff member to do the scheduling, or you might allow the employees to self-schedule. No matter what scheduling format is used, you are ultimately responsible for ensuring that the appropriate number and type of employees needed are scheduled.

Requests for time off should be put in writing. Depending on the size of the organization, such requests may have to be received by a given date or time. For example, the policy may read, "A request for a day off in May may have to be submitted by April 15. Any requests for time off filed after the cutoff date will be approved whenever possible." This eliminates repeated adjustment of the staffing schedule.

Checkpoint Question

3. What is the medical office manager's primary goal in scheduling?

Policy and Procedures Manuals

Every business needs written rules and regulations to ensure that its practices are within legal and ethical boundaries. Employees need written procedures to ensure consistency in the practices of the business. In the outpatient medical facility, these written policies and procedures are *required* by regulatory and accrediting agencies.

It is the office manager's responsibility to coordinate the orientation and training of any new employee. A personnel manual that includes the organization's policies and out-

---

Discipline Record

Employee Name: _____ #: _____ Date of Warning: _____

Warning

Date of Violation: _____ Time: _____ Place: _____

Description of Violation:

_____

_____

_____

_____

_____

_____

_____ Verbal Warning	Action To Be Taken:
_____ Written Warning	_____
_____ Probation _____ Days	_____
_____ Suspension _____ Days	_____
_____ Termination	_____
Supervisor's Signature	Date

Employee's Remarks

Do you agree with the details above: Yes: _____   No: _____

Comments: _____

_____

_____

Employee's Signature: _____   Date: _____

FIGURE 12-5. Sample disciplinary action form.

WHAT IF

You receive a call requesting a reference for an employee who was fired. What should you say?

Be careful! This situation can turn into a legal nightmare if not handled appropriately. If you give a wonderful report to the potential employer and say, "She was great; never had any problems," you and the office may be sued by the former employee for wrongful discharge. In court, you would be asked: "If she was so wonderful, why did you fire her?" On the other hand, if you say, "She was a terrible employee, and we fired her," you can be sued for defamation of character. Because of the legal concerns in providing employment references, most organizations have a policy stating that the only information to be released is verification of employment dates and job titles. When in doubt, give no information. Ask for the caller's name and phone number; discuss the issue with the physician in charge, and then return the phone call.

North Shore Family Practice is a group practice dedicated to providing quality care through compassion, innovation, performance and education. It is our goal to provide medical care to the community of Rochester, New York. The physicians, nurse practitioners, and all staff members are committed to working together as a team to provide the patient with the best care possible.

FIGURE 12–6. Sample mission statement.

lines step-by-step procedures for each task performed in the facility becomes the new employee's information source. Even veteran employees may have to refer to the proper procedure for a task. As new procedures become available or existing procedures are changed, this is added to the procedures manual.

Most organizations create *a policy and procedures manual* that is written, maintained, and regarded as one document. A **policy** is a statement regarding the organization's rules on a given topic. A **procedure** is a series of steps required to perform a given task. Policies and procedures must be written in a clear, concise, and understandable format. Each policy or procedure is signed by the employees, indicating they have read, understand, and will adhere to the policy or procedure. Policies regarding medical office management are signed by the physician and supervisory staff.

Tips for Writing Personnel Manuals

- Form a personnel committee. If staff members help develop the policies and procedures, they are more likely to follow them.
- Determine the rules and regulations of the office with the physician and managers.
- Contact local organizations, medical offices, or ambulatory care centers and ask for copies of their personnel manuals including policies and procedures.
- Research state and federal laws that regulate the medical office.
- Ensure compliance by appointing a **compliance officer**.
- Personnel manuals must be kept in a central location and be available to each employee for review.
- Review all policies and procedures annually to assess for currentness and accuracy.

Types of Policies and Procedures. There are many types of policies and procedures. In general, the following areas are included in a policy and procedures manual:

1. Mission statement
2. Organizational structure
3. Human resources, or personnel
4. Quality improvement and risk management
5. Clinical procedures
6. Administrative procedures
7. Infection control

Box 12-1

TYPES OF HUMAN RESOURCES POLICIES

Absentee policies	Jury duty
Cafeteria plans	Office hours
Confidentiality policy	Orientation
Continuing education requirements	Overtime reports
Disciplinary action procedures	Parking
	Payroll
Emergency procedures	Personal phone calls
Employee benefits (health and dental insurance)	Resignations
	Sexual harassment
	Sick leave and family leave
Evaluation and performance appraisals	Staff meetings
	Tardiness
Grievance procedures	Termination process
Grooming, uniforms, appearance	Time recording
	Vacation days
Holiday coverage and compensation for holidays	

Section 1: mission statement. A **mission statement** describes the goals of the practice and whom it serves. Often a mission statement provides a philosophical look at an organization. It is generally one to two paragraphs long (Fig. 12-6).

The mission statement should not only be included in the policy and procedures manual; it should also be available to patients. Often it is framed and placed in the waiting room or printed in the practice brochure.

Section 2: organizational structure. The organizational chart is included in this section along with policies regarding the following:

- Chain of command
- How and when to contact various members of the team
- Coverage for managers
- Physician on-call policies

Section 3: human resources, or personnel. This section consists of policies relating to staff responsibilities, benefits, and rules and regulations for employees. Box 12-1 lists the kinds of policies found in this section of the manual. A sample human resources policy is displayed in Figure 12-7.

Section 4: quality improvement and risk management. This section includes policies outlining who is in charge of quality improvement, the steps for developing a quality improvement plan, and explanations of incident reporting. (See Chapter 11.)

Section 5: clinical procedures. Any task that requires intervention with a patient should be listed in this section. (Some offices separate laboratory procedures into a different section for convenience.) In addition, clinical procedures should include specific infection control guidelines for the particular procedure, patient education guidelines, and instructions for documentation. Sample documentation forms should be included in this section. It is a good idea to complete the sample form correctly so that it can serve as a model. In the medical office, these procedures may vary slightly to meet the needs of the office, physicians' requests, or manufacturers' guidelines.

Section 6: administrative procedures. This section includes procedures on all tasks that the administrative office staff must perform. Sample forms should also be included and updated as necessary. Examples of administrative tasks follow:

- Accounting and bookkeeping
- Appointment scheduling
- Collections
- Computer care and operations
- Insurance filings
- Medical records management
- Mail and postal machines operations

Section 7: infection control. Depending on the length of this section, some offices opt for a separate manual dedicated to infection control and prevention. Examples of these policies are:

Benjamin William, MD
2295 Matthews Drive
Boca Raton, Florida 33432
POLICY AND PROCEDURE MANUAL

Policy title: Human Resources, Call offs
Purpose: The purpose of this policy is to advise all employees of the policy for call offs and to prewarn employees regarding the disciplinary steps that will be taken as a result of not complying with this policy.
Equipment/Forms necessary: No equipment or forms are required.
Explanation:

- If you are going to call in sick, you must call in two hours prior to your assigned time. Messages should be left with the answering service if the office is not open.
- If you have personal days accrued, you can use them for compensation.
- If you are going to be out sick for more than three consecutive working days, you will need to obtain a physician's note to document the illness.
- Employees are allowed six (6) call offs per year without disciplinary action. Seven (7) call offs will result in a verbal warning regarding attendance. Eight (8) call offs will result in a written warning. Nine (9) call offs will result in termination. Exceptions to disciplinary action will be reviewed on an individual basis and are at the joint discretion of the office manager and physician.

Susan Rogers, RMA
Office Manager

Benjamin William, MD

date: original policy - 06/96, revised 07/98
HR: 14

FIGURE 12-7. Sample human resources policy.

- Types of personal protection equipment available
- Biohazardous waste disposal
- Handling of various disease identities
- Handling of employee exposures and needlesticks
- Documentation required by the Occupational Safety and Health Administration (OSHA)
- Employee education for infection control

Checkpoint Question

4. Which seven elements must be included when writing a policy or procedure?

Developing Promotional Materials

The medical office manager is often responsible for developing and distributing promotional literature for the practice. Depending on the budget, promotional materials can be created and produced at commercial printing shops or done in the office with desktop publishing programs. Examples of promotional materials follow:

- Education pamphlets and booklets for patients
- Practice brochure
- Newsletters
- Holiday cards
- Birthday cards (usually used by pediatricians)
- Newspaper articles
- Yellow pages
- Direct mail
- Business cards

Follow these guidelines when creating promotional materials:

- Double-check all spelling and grammar.
- Ensure accuracy.
- Use clear and specific language.
- Avoid abbreviations and complex medical terms.
- Use brightly colored materials.

If you are using a commercial printer, be sure to review the proofs carefully before the final printing.

Financial Concerns

Budgets

A **budget** is a financial planning tool that helps an organization estimate its anticipated expenditures and revenues. Budgeting has many purposes for an organization:

- Forcing the manager and physician to plan
- Causing managers and staff to become cost conscious
- Promoting communication among staff and managers
- Helping the organization achieve a financial goal

The medical office generally has both an operating and a capital budget. Operating budgets consist of all costs to run the office. These include but are not limited to payroll, office and medical supplies, education, promotional materials, and electricity and telephone services. Capital budgets consist of large outlays of money. These usually include large purchases (usually over $500), building maintenance, property management, and equipment.

Developing and writing a budget takes practice and instructions from the financial officer or physician. In general, the previous year's expense report is reviewed, revenues are projected for the following year, and figures are assigned to ensure that income balances with the outgoing expenses.

Checkpoint Question

5. What are the two basic types of budgets?

Payroll

Another financial concern for the manager is payroll. All employees expect to receive the correct amount of pay on time, and those expectations must be met. Payroll is a complex task that must satisfy state and federal laws regarding deductions for Social Security and other taxes. Because of this and because payroll is so time-consuming, some offices outsource this service (see Chapter 15).

Petty Cash

Most offices keep a small amount of cash in the office. Petty cash is used to purchase small items (e.g., postage, emergency office supplies) or to reimburse employees for small items. It is essential that the office manager keep close tallies on the petty cash fund. Most offices have some form of a petty cash receipt. Petty cash must be kept in a separate drawer from the change box (see Chapter 14).

Maintenance and Inventory of Supplies

One of the medical office manager's key responsibilities is to keep the office neat, clean, and well organized. Most offices have an outside cleaning agency to maintain the lobby, examination rooms, and offices. Special attention to waiting room toys is necessary because they can pose a safety threat to children (see Chapter 5). Staff should be encouraged to check the lobby periodically for neatness and to assist in routine cleaning and straightening.

Service Contracts

The medical office manager is responsible for keeping track of all service contracts. A service contract is an agreement between the medical organization and a service company in which the company agrees to perform regular inspections of and care for a specific piece of equipment. Service contracts are usually obtained for copiers, computers, fax machines, and other large and expensive pieces of equipment.

Inventory

Extensive amounts of supplies are needed to run a medical office. As a medical office manager, you must develop a logical system to keep track of them. There should be a policy outlining who is responsible for ordering supplies and the procedure for ordering. There also must be some process to check that deliveries of supplies are complete and accurate.

Education

Staff Education

The medical office manager must keep the staff up to date on medical procedures, drugs and vaccines, insurance coding and billing regulations, and any other topics that promote good patient care. In addition to these topics, annual education is usually conducted on cardiopulmonary resuscitation (CPR), infection control, and fire and electrical safety. Most allied health professionals are required to accumulate continuing education units (CEUs). CMAs must receive 60 CEUs every 5 years to retain the CMA credential. The office manager may choose to keep a file for each employee with the necessary documentation. This will assist the staff in the recertification process.

As the medical office manager, you should select an educational topic for each month. In some offices, the educational topic is covered during the monthly staff meetings, whereas other offices have separate educational programs. After choosing the monthly topic, select an appropriate presenter. Suggestions for presenters include colleagues, physicians, sales representatives, local hospital staff development coordinators, and specialists. Presenters for CPR classes must be CPR instructors who are approved by a national organization. To promote attendance, create informative flyers and distribute them to all staff members. Keep attendance records for all classes given.

In addition to formal educational programs, there are other ways to keep your staff up to date. For instance, educational videos can be rented or purchased for staff viewing; consider developing a posttest to assess for comprehension. Also, many professional magazines have continuing education articles on various topics, usually accompanied by a posttest. Finally, staff members should be sent to one or two seminars a year. Outside seminars help increase employee productivity, self-esteem, and retention.

Patient Education

All members of the health care team must constantly contribute to educating patients. As a manager, you may not provide patient education directly, but you are responsible for assisting the staff in performing this task. You can help the staff with patient education by creating booklets, developing posters, and by teaching your staff how, when, and what to teach patients and families.

Patient education brochures should be colorful and easy to read. Close attention to spelling, grammar, punctuation, and accuracy is essential. All brochures should be reviewed by a physician. Depending on your office's clientele, the brochures should be printed in various languages. Refer to Chapter 4 for more details on creating patient education brochures.

Manager Education

Managers should attend workshops and conferences and read appropriate printed materials to enhance their knowledge and skills in managing a medical office. All new managers can benefit from courses on time management, stress management, solving personnel conflicts, and budget preparation. Memberships in professional organizations can also assist the new office manager. Two such organizations are:

Medical Office Management Association
1355 South Colorado Boulevard, Suite 900
Denver, CO 80222-3331

Professional Association of Health Care—Office Managers
Suite 102
2929 Langley Avenue
Pensacola, FL 32504-7355

LEGAL ISSUES REGARDING OFFICE MANAGEMENT

Americans with Disabilities Act

Formerly called the Rehabilitation Act, the **Americans with Disabilities Act** (ADA) was expanded in 1994. All companies with more than 15 employees must comply with regula-

LEGAL TIP

Many acts and regulations affect health care organizations and their operations. As a medical office manager, you must keep current on all legal updates. Most states publish a monthly bulletin that reports new legislation. Every state has a website that will link you to legislative action. Read these regularly. Each office should have legal counsel who can assist in interpreting legal issues. It is important for a new manager to meet with the medical office's attorney to discuss legal concerns for the practice.

tions designed to meet the needs of people with physical and mental disabilities. This act requires that all buildings be accessible to physically challenged people. Following is a partial list of ways the medical office can comply with this act:

- Entrance ramps
- Widened rest rooms and doors to be wheelchair accessible
- Elevated toilet bowls for easier transferring from wheelchairs
- Easy-to-reach elevator buttons
- Braille signs
- Access to special telephone services to communicate with hearing-impaired patients

Sexual Harassment

Sexual harassment of any employee or patient is illegal. Sexual harassment comes in many forms. As a medical office manager, it is your responsibility to be alert for signs of harassment and to have in place a policy for handling complaints regarding this.

Family and Medical Leave Act

The **Family and Medical Leave Act**, approved in 1993, allows an employee to leave his or her job for up to 12 weeks (unpaid) to meet family needs (e.g., the birth or adoption of a child; serious illness of a child, parent, spouse, or self). Employers must hold the employee's job position or offer the employee a position of similar nature on return.

Other Legal Considerations

The Clinical Laboratory Improvement Amendments (CLIA) of 1988 contain specific rules and regulations regarding laboratory safety.

OSHA is a federal agency that sets standards for employee safety. OSHA regulations are also discussed in Chapter 11.

The Joint Commission on Accreditation of Healthcare Organizations (JCAHO) is a private organization that sets standards for health care administration. The JCAHO is discussed in Chapter 11.

Each state also has specific laws regarding patient care, insurance billing, payroll management, and so forth that a medical office manager must understand.

Checkpoint Question

6. What are some legal issues of concern to the medical office manager?

Procedure 12-1

Creating a Procedures Manual

Equipment/Supplies

- Word processor
- 3-ring binder
- Paper

Steps	Reason
1. Gather product information; consult government agencies, as needed. If the procedure is for using new equipment, ask the sales representative for educational pamphlets. Some companies offer printed sample procedures.	This ensures that you are using products and equipment according to the manufacturer's suggestions and that you are practicing within legal and ethical boundaries.
2. Title the procedure, e.g., Infection Control Procedure for Handwashing.	A logical, easily identifiable format will allow easy retrieval.
3. Number the procedure, e.g., "HR 14" means human resource section, policy 14.	All policies and procedures should be numbered to allow for easy access and identification.
4. Define the overall purpose of the policy. This should be a sentence or two at most explaining the intent of the procedure.	Provides the staff with a rationale for the policy.
5. List any necessary equipment or forms. Include everything needed to complete the task. Also indicate so if no special equipment or forms are necessary.	The employee will be prepared before beginning the procedure if he or she has everything needed at hand.
6. List each step with its rationale. The steps must be complete and in order. Never assume the reader knows how or when to perform a given step, such as handwashing. The employee will be able to follow specific steps, ensuring patient safety.	Listing the steps in order promotes compliance and accuracy for policy completion.
7. Provide spaces for signatures. Administrative procedures are signed by the physician and office manager. Clinical procedures usually are signed by the clinical manager and a physician. Employees must have a space to sign.	The employee's signature will verify that he or she has read and understands the policy.
8. Record the date the policy was written. If changes are needed, the procedure is rewritten, signed, and dated again. The previous dates also are generally listed.	By recording the date, you ensure that you are reading the most current revision. It will also help you know when a new revision should be considered.

CHAPTER SUMMARY

Effective management of the medical office is essential for a health care organization to succeed in the competitive marketplace. A good manager must be able to perform a variety of tasks in an organized and efficient manner. These tasks include communicating with patients and staff, handling staffing issues, developing policy and procedures manuals, creating promotional materials, preparing budgets, and overseeing educational programs. In addition, the medical office manager must keep current on legal requirements related to office operations.

Critical Thinking Challenges

1. Review the list of qualities that a manager should have. Which ones do you have? How would you acquire the others? Should any other qualities be listed?
2. Review the types of sections that are often included in policy and procedures manuals. Now assume that you are to help a physician set up a practice. How would you organize your policy and procedures manual? Create one sample sheet for each section of your manual. Be sure to include all necessary elements when you write your policies and procedures.
3. Write a description of your ideal job. How would you go about finding this position?

Answers to Checkpoint Questions

1. An organizational chart is a flow sheet that allows the manager and employees to identify their team members and to see where they fit into the team.
2. Three ways to communicate with staff members are through bulletin boards, staff meetings, and communication notebooks.
3. The primary goal of scheduling is to ensure that the needs of the office are met.
4. The elements that must be in a policy or procedure are document name, purpose, equipment or forms needed, steps or explanations, signatures, numbering system, and dates.
5. The two basic types of budgets are operating and capital.
6. Some of the legal issues are the Americans with Disabilities Act, sexual harassment laws, Family and Medical Leave Act, CLIA, and OSHA.

 Websites

Medical Group Management Association
    www.mgma.org
Physician Practice Group
    www.physicianspractice.com
Family Leave Act/Department of Labor
    www.dol.gov
Americans with Disabilities Act/U. S. Department of Justice
    www.ada.gov
    www.usaoj.gov

Managing the Finances in the Practice

Good management of finances is essential for a medical practice to succeed. This unit introduces you to various aspects of medical office finances, beginning with a chapter on credit and collections, in which you learn the process of collecting fees. Next, you will learn bookkeeping and banking skills to register the fees that you have collected. Medical offices must also pay various people, and this information is covered in the following chapter. Most of the income for the physician's practice is through insurance reimbursements. To be able to collect fees from insurance companies, you must understand coding. This information is covered in the last three chapters. A financially strong practice is good for the patients, the community, and you.

13

Credit and Collections

CHAPTER OUTLINE

ROLE DELINEATION COMPONENTS

GENERAL: Legal Concepts
- Perform within legal and ethical boundaries

ADMINISTRATIVE: Administrative Procedures
- Perform basic administrative medical assisting functions

ADMINISTRATIVE: Practice Finances
- Apply bookkeeping principles
- Manage accounts receivable
- Manage accounts payable
- Document and maintain accounting and banking record

CHAPTER COMPETENCIES

LEARNING OBJECTIVES

Upon successfully completing this chapter, you will be able to:
1. Spell and define the key terms
2. Explain the physician fee schedule
3. Discuss forms of payment
4. Explain the legal considerations in extending credit
5. Discuss the legal implications of credit collection
6. Describe three methods of debt collection

PERFORMANCE OBJECTIVES

Upon successfully completing this chapter, you will be able to:
1. Use an aging schedule
2. Write a collection letter

KEY TERMS

adjustment	credit	participating providers	professional courtesy
aging schedule	installment	patient co-payment	write-off
collections			

THE MEDICAL PRACTICE MUST operate in a financially sound manner to continue to serve the patient's need. The office depends on the fees generated by patient visits, laboratory work, and in-office procedures. Without these fees, the medical office would be unable to pay for staff, office space, and supplies. Therefore, collecting fees, whether paid by the patient, an insurer, or a third party, is essential for the medical practice to succeed. Box 13-1 shows how to determine whether your office is collecting fees satisfactorily.

FEES

Fee Schedules

Generally, the physician sets the fees for office visits, laboratory work, and in-office procedures based on the UCR concept: (1) U (usual) fair value of the service; (2) C (customary) competitive rates charged by other physicians; and (3) R (reasonable), that which meets the other two criteria. Fee setting also considers the resource-based relative value scale (RBRVS), by which fees are based on the relative value of a particular service and adjusted for geographical differences. (See Chapter 16 for more information about UCR fees and Chapter 18 for more information about RBRVS.) A physician's fee schedule also takes into consideration the costs of operating the office, such as rent, utilities, malpractice insurance, salaries, and so on. A list of the services and procedures

Code	Key	Mod	Par Fee	Non Par Fee	Limiting Charge
50010			$690.30	$655.79	$754.16
50010			$690.30	$655.79	$754.16
50020			$1,112.72	$1,057.08	$1,215.64
50021			$522.30	$496.19	$570.62
50040			$1,009.84	$959.35	$1,103.25
50045			$921.52	$875.44	$1,006.76
50060			$1,116.74	$1,060.90	$1,220.04
50065			$1,128.28	$1,071.87	$1,232.65
50070			$1,172.52	$1,113.89	$1,280.97
50075			$1,451.88	$1,379.29	$1,586.18
50080			$976.28	$927.47	$1,066.59
50081			$1,336.92	$1,270.07	$1,460.58
50100			$1,033.66	$981.98	$1,129.28
50120			$945.54	$898.26	$1,033.00
50125			$980.30	$931.29	$1,070.98
50130			$1,010.09	$959.59	$1,103.53
50135			$1,110.42	$1,054.90	$1,213.14
50200			$138.72	$131.78	$151.55
50205			$696.55	$661.72	$760.98
50220			$1,015.02	$964.27	$1,108.91
50225			$1,168.36	$1,109.94	$1,276.43

FIGURE 13–1.   Sample Medicare fee schedule.

offered in an office along with descriptions, procedure codes, and prices must be available to patients. Federal regulations require that a sign to this effect be posted in the office.

There may be several fee schedules based on the reimbursement schedules of different insurance companies. **Participating providers** are those who agree to participate with managed care contracts and other third-party payers in exchange for building a solid patient base. Patients covered under participating plans will have a different fee schedule from patients who are private pay (paying with no money from insurance). Each managed care plan, workers' compensation company, Medicaid carrier, and Medicare has a different fee schedule. See Chapter 16 for further discussion of third-party payers.

A Medicare fee schedule has three columns. A participating fee is the amount paid to physicians who participate or agree to accept a certain fee. A nonparticipating fee is the amount paid to physicians who do not have agreements with Medicare. A limiting charge is the amount a physician can charge a Medicare patient. Figure 13-1 is a sample Medicare fee schedule.

Discussing Fees in Advance

It is always a good policy to discuss fees with patients in advance. This ensures that patients are aware of the charges. Patients will need to know in advance whether the medical office is a participating provider with their insurance carrier. Managed care companies usually require that the patient pay

---

Box 13-1

DETERMINING A PRACTICE'S COLLECTION PERCENTAGE

Medical practices should evaluate their method of collections periodically to determine the effectiveness of their practices. A collection analysis lets you identify the strengths and weaknesses of the system.

To do a collection analysis, determine the monthly production from the first day of each month to the last day. This will be the total charges posted to all patients' accounts. Next determine the revenues the practice received. Computer systems will automatically total payments received during a specified time. Divide revenue by production to determine the collection percentage. Analysis of the collection percentage should reveal the percentage of the collection of all outstanding debts to the practice.

Collection percentage =
monthly production ÷ monthly revenue received

Most medical practices average 8 to 20% loss yearly. Experts consider a collection percentage above 80% to be reasonable. Performing a 2-year collection percentage comparison analysis will help you evaluate past collection effectiveness.

a certain share of the bill, known as the **patient co-payment,** or co-pay. A good and easy way to initiate a discussion of fees is by providing an office brochure that lists not only the office's address, telephone number, and hours but also office policies regarding fees and collections, third-party payments, and how they are handled. Patients should understand that co-pays are to be paid at the time of service. Such information should be included in the office brochure. Many offices post a sign in the waiting area stating this.

Always collect the entire amount due from a new patient on the first visit. Most problems associated with collection (acquiring funds that are due) come from patients who go from one practice to another. Be sure you get a picture identification, such as a driver's license, on a patient's first visit.

Forms of Payment

Depending on the medical office's policies, the patient can usually pay for services in one of two ways: with cash or by personal check. If a new patient is paying by check, get two forms of identification. Many larger practices accept credit and debit cards (Visa, MasterCard, Discover) also. By agreeing to accept a credit card payment, the medical office also agrees to pay the credit card company a percentage (usually 1.8%) of the total charge. Although this may seem costly, it is sometimes more cost effective to receive payment by credit card than to receive it in installments—or not at all—from the patient.

Payment by Insurance Companies

By far the largest proportions of fees are paid by insurance companies. Therefore, it is imperative that patients' insurance information be kept current. Most medical practices require that a patient submit a medical insurance card for each visit; this way, changes in insurance can quickly and easily be noted. Always make a copy of both sides of the patient's insurance card and staple it to the appropriate section of the chart for billing reference.

Adjusting Fees

Sometimes, **adjustments** (changes in a posted account) must be made to a standard fee, as when the medical office accepts a set insurance rate for a service that is lower than the practice's rate. You must charge the patient the normal fee for the service; when the insurance carrier sends payment, however, the explanation of benefits (EOB) will show how much you may collect for the service. The difference between the physician's normal fee and the insurance carrier's allowed fee will be adjusted in the credit adjustment column on the patient's account.

Other fee adjustments include **professional courtesy** fees, in which other health care professionals are charged a reduced rate. The physician may choose not to charge a fee at all; this too is considered a professional courtesy and should not be confused with writing off a fee. (A **write-off** is cancellation of

an unpaid debt; these generally can be claimed on the practice's federal taxes.) Again, you charge the normal fee and then adjust the designated amount in the adjustment column with "professional courtesy" in the description column.

Checkpoint Question

1. To avoid collection problems, what should you get from a new patient on the first visit?

CREDIT

Extending Credit

It is not always possible for patients to pay the entire bill when such costs are incurred. Depending on the medical office's policy, **credit** may be extended to patients on an installment plan. Collection experts have estimated that billing one patient costs the practice about $8 per month. This total includes the time it takes to prepare the statements, the supplies needed, and so on. Extension of credit to a patient is a decision that is often made solely by the physician.

Legal Considerations

When a medical practice extends credit to a patient, it may charge interest on the patient's unpaid balance. If this is the case, the medical office is legally required to disclose this information to the patient, along with any other fees or charges incurred by the patient's acceptance of credit. This legal documentation, called a truth-in-lending statement, must be filed in the patient's medical chart.

Different states have different laws concerning the extension of credit. Generally, credit cannot be denied based on age, gender, race, marital status, religion, national origin, or source of income (e.g., if a patient receives public assistance). If your facility has given credit to one patient, you typically may not refuse the same arrangement to another patient. Some states have laws limiting the amount of interest that can be charged. The practice's accountant should be able to provide the information required by the state and municipality.

Checkpoint Question

2. On what grounds should credit *not* be denied?

COLLECTIONS

When a patient has an unpaid bill or has not paid an installment per a credit agreement, those funds must be collected. Collecting an unpaid debt is costly to any business. Collecting fees can also be time consuming, and collecting practices are regulated by a variety of consumer protection laws. Many medical practices outsource their billing to companies specializing in billing and debt collection.

RULES FOR TELEPHONE DEBT COLLECTION

When attempting to collect a debt by telephone, a debt collector may not:

1. Contact the patient at his or her place of employment if the employer objects
2. Tell anyone other than the patient or responsible party about a debt without court authorization
3. Contact the patient before 8:00 A.M. or after 9:00 P.M.
4. Contact the patient at all if the patient has filed for bankruptcy
5. Harass or intimidate the patient; that is, use abusive language, provide false or misleading information, or pose as someone other than a debt collector

COLLECTING DEBTS FROM A PATIENT'S ESTATE

When a patient dies, the family needs time to grieve and accept the death. Collecting debts from an estate requires professionalism and tact. Never contact the family regarding a debt immediately after a patient's death. Most offices have a policy stating that family members of deceased patients will not be contacted until a week after the funeral. At the appropriate time, call the next of kin listed in the patient's chart. Offer your sympathy and ask for the name of the patient's executor, the individual responsible for handling the patient's affairs after death. The executor may be an attorney, spouse, friend, or other relative. Call the executor and introduce yourself. Obtain the executor's address and send a final bill. It is important that all claims on a patient's estate be made promptly. In case the estate does not have enough funds to meet all of its debts, the probate court will decide the priority list for debt collection.

Legal Considerations

Certain procedures should be followed in attempts to collect a debt. A debt collector—in this case, the administrative medical assistant or billing clerk—must exercise reasonable restraint when contacting a patient about a bill. Box 13-2 displays guidelines for collection attempts by phone.

Attempting to collect a debt from a patient's estate requires particular diplomacy. Box 13-3 offers some guidelines to follow in such a situation.

Collecting a Debt

Monthly Billings

The easiest way to collect a debt or an installment is by monthly billing. Once a month, the medical office sends bills to its patients who have unpaid balances. Larger offices set up a billing cycle and divide the alphabet, sending statements once a week to each selected group. For example, patients with names beginning with the letters A to G might be billed

on the 1st of the month, H to N on the 8th, O to S on the 15th, and T to Z on the 22nd. If your facility changes a billing cycle, you are legally required to notify patients of the change 3 months before the change takes effect.

The uncomputerized office normally just copies the ledger cards of the patients who owe balances. It is important to make each entry on the ledger card with consistency and provide a key for office codes or abbreviations. The patient should be able to understand each entry. When a practice is computerized, the staff can easily send statements. Medical office software usually gives the option of printing a separate message at the bottom. For instance, you may add "Happy Holidays" to every patient's December statement or "Time for your flu shot" in the September statements.

If the account is on an **installment** plan, the patient receives a bill that lists the amount due for that month, any third-party payments or adjustments applied to the account, the total amount due, and the amount the patient owes. This

ñSpanish Terminology

Necesito recoger el total en su cuenta.	I need to collect the balance on your account.
¿Puede pagar usted algunos de su deuda?	Can you pay some of your balance?
Esto es una carta de la colección.	This is a collection letter.
Usted debe este dinero a esta oficina.	You owe this office money.

way, the patient has the option of paying more than is due for that particular month (and thereby reducing the amount of any interest charged) and is aware of the current balance.

Aging Accounts

Unpaid accounts must be monitored to determine how far overdue or in arrears they are. Aging of an account is calculated from the first date of billing, not by the procedure date. For example, a patient has an office visit on January 5 and the first statement is sent on February 1. The account will not be past due until March 1.

For this purpose, the medical office keeps an **aging schedule** that lists the patient's name, balance, any payments, and comments, such as reminders or second notices sent. Such a schedule can be kept on a large sheet of paper or by a comprehensive computer billing program. Figure 13-2 is a sample of a manual report. Figure 13-3 shows a computer screen that automatically places the amounts charged under the proper heading based on the age of the account. This account shows that $132 of the charges are current, or less than 30 days old. The $95 represents charges that were incurred and posted at least 120 days ago.

Aging of accounts is a measure of the practice's ability to collect its fees. Nearly all fees (80%) should be collected within 30 days. If the aging shows a high percentage (50%) of fees being collected 30 days or more after billing, the practice's billing and collection procedures should be reviewed.

Collecting Overdue Accounts

The three most common ways of collecting an overdue account are sending an overdue notice to the patient, telephoning the patient to let him or her know the account is overdue, and informing the patient at the next office visit.

Overdue Notices. With a manual system, overdue notices are fairly simple to prepare. Often, they consist of a copy of the patient's monthly billing with the words "overdue" or "second notice" stamped in red. Alternatively, a form letter with spaces for the patient's particulars may be sent. Figure 13-4 is a sample collection letter. If a computer billing program is used, the computer often can automatically generate overdue notices.

Telephoning the Patient. If written notices bring no response, you may have to telephone the patient to inquire about an overdue account. Always ask when payment may be forthcoming and document the reply on the patient's account. If payment is not received as promised, contact the patient again.

Aging of Accounts Receivable Report: April 30, 2003

Patient Name	Account Number	Due Date	Amount
Accounts 30 Days Past Due:			
Doe, John C.	000-00-0000	3/6/03	625.00
Graham, Paula R.	000-00-0000	3/29/03	450.00
O'Toole, William Q.	000-00-0000	3/13/03	25.00
Parker, Mary W.	000-00-0000	3/25/03	299.00
Reeves, Chris A.	000-00-0000	3/11/03	58.00
South, Cheryl C.	000-00-0000	3/8/03	385.00
Yarkony, Ralph M.	000-00-0000	3/11/03	108.00
Accounts 60 Days Past Due:			
Forest, Patricia L.	000-00-0000	2/19/03	476.00
Heany, Beverly O.	000-00-0000	2/13/03	57.00
Thomas, Walter T.	000-00-0000	2/27/03	185.00
Accounts 90 Days Past Due:			
Glick, Rhonda K	000-00-0000	1/4/03	28.00
Payne, Robert A.	000-00-0000	1/25/03	456.00
Accounts 120 Days or More Past Due:			
Baird, Jane C.	000-00-0000	10/3/02	45.00
Wallace, Michael S.	000-00-0000	12/15/02	349.00
Total Overdue Accounts Receivable			**$3,546.00**

FIGURE 13–2. Sample aging of accounts receivable report.

```
PRO 5 Visual PRO/5                                        _ □ ✕
 Settings   Edit   Print   Help
ACCOUNT LEDGER                                    DATE 03/27/03
                                                  Post Date: 03/28/03

ENTER:  1-HISTORICAL DETAIL   2-VISIT DETAIL   'CR'-END
        3-EDIT COLLECTION NOTES   4-LEDGER NOTE PAD

 Name/#    WALKER, DONNA (#  2070)        Bs. Phone# 919/768-5348
 Addr1     3400 HEALY DRIVE              Alt. Rec#   2000
 Addr2                                   Account Codes -
 Addr3     WINSTON-SALEM, NC 27103-0000   PC  HP  CS  SM  OC
                                          BC  R1  SO  __  __
 P-  2  STATE EMPLOYEES-  S-VAD  MEDICAID OF VIRGI
- - - - - - - - - - - - - - - - - - - - - - - - - - - - - - - - - - -
     Last Statement Date  04/16/02      Last Statement Date  03/28/03
     Last Statement Amt=  95.00         Last Statement Amt=  45.00(per)
- - - - - - - - Current - - 30 Days- - -60 Days- - - 90 Days - - -120 Days - - - -·Total - - - -
 Ins. Bal=    90.00     0.00     0.00     0.00     0.00     90.00
 Per. Bal=    42.00     0.00     0.00     0.00    95.00    137.00
 Pending=      0.00     0.00     0.00     0.00     0.00      0.00
 Act. Bal=   132.00     0.00     0.00     0.00    95.00    227.00
- - - - - - - - - - - - - - - - - - - - - - - - - - - - - - - - - - -
 Notes:   SEE LEDGER NOTE PAD




                   MICA-MED PRACTICE MANAGEMENT SYSTEM
```

FIGURE 13–3.
Sample computer screen.

Family Practice Associates
2345 Oak Street
Forest, OR 77777
(234) 567-8900

June 23, 2003

Mary W. Parker
300 Red Bird Lane
Lake, OR 77771

Dear Ms. Parker:

It has recently come to our attention that your account with our office is slightly overdue. Your balance of $299.00 is over 30 days past due. Please pay this amount as soon as possible. If you are having trouble paying this amount, please call our office and make arrangements to pay your balance.

If you have recently paid this amount and your payment is on the way to us in the mail, please disregard this letter. If you have any questions or concerns, feel free to contact me at the phone number above.

Sincerely,

Kathy Porter
Accounting Manager

FIGURE 13–4.
Sample collection letter.

WHAT IF

A patient who has an overdue account wants to schedule an appointment. What should you do?

As a medical assistant, you are not responsible for deciding whether a patient who has an outstanding balance gets to be seen by the physician. Schedule the appointment, then discuss the issue privately with the physician. Ethically, the physician may opt to care for the patient until the disorder is resolved. Legally, the physician is obligated to care for this patient until the physician–patient relationship is terminated (see Chapter 2).

In-Office Reminders. A patient can be reminded of an overdue balance when he or she comes to the office to see the physician. To handle this situation discreetly, simply give the patient a copy of the most recent overdue notice. Once again, ask when payment may be forthcoming and follow through. Computer systems may offer the option of a flashing computer screen when the patient's overdue account is retrieved. This alerts anyone working with the patient either to discuss payment or to refer the patient to someone in the office who will explain that payment is expected.

Collection Alternatives

Sometimes, it is more cost effective for **collections** to be handled outside the medical office. Three common options include collection agencies, small claims court, and credit bureaus. Collection agencies specialize in collecting debts. For either a fee or a percentage of the debt, the collection agency attempts to collect the monies due by the methods listed earlier. In addition, the collection agency can represent the medical practice in small claims court and can have the bad debt listed with credit-reporting agencies.

LEGAL TIP

The Fair Debt Collection Act
The Fair Debt Collection Act is a federal law that states how and when a collector can attempt to collect a debt. It is a violation of the law to threaten to send a patient to a collection agency if you do not intend to do so. Unlawful threats can result in a lawsuit for harassment against the caller. Box 13-2 shows the guidelines for telephoning patients to attempt to collect a debt.

The medical practice can, of course, sue patients in small claims court or list patients with credit bureaus itself, but it is often more time and cost effective to hire an outside agency.

Checkpoint Question

3. What are three ways of collecting overdue accounts?

CHAPTER SUMMARY

The financial status of a medical office is based on the ability of the staff to collect the physician's fees. This must be done in a professional manner and in accordance with state and federal laws. Technology affords the medical office the ability to streamline procedures, and collection practices are more efficient with computer systems. Aging accounts and communicating with patients in a fair and professional manner ensures a constant cash flow and success in managing the finances of the outpatient medical practice.

Critical Thinking Challenges

1. Under what circumstances might a patient need credit? To what local resources could you refer this patient?
2. A patient has an overdue account balance. What steps would you take to collect the debt?
3. Create a collection letter for a patient account that is 60 days' overdue. Create a collection letter that you would send to a patient's executor or patient's estate.

Answers to Checkpoint Questions

1. On a new patient's first visit, collect the entire amount due and get a picture identification.
2. Credit cannot be denied based on age, gender, race, marital status, religion, national origin, or source of income.
3. Overdue accounts can be collected by sending overdue notices, telephoning patients, and informing patients at the next office visit.

 Websites

Credit and Collections World
www.collectionsworld.com
Fair Debt Collection Practice/Federal Trade Commission Statutes
www.ftc.gov
National Credit Systems
www.nationalcredit.com

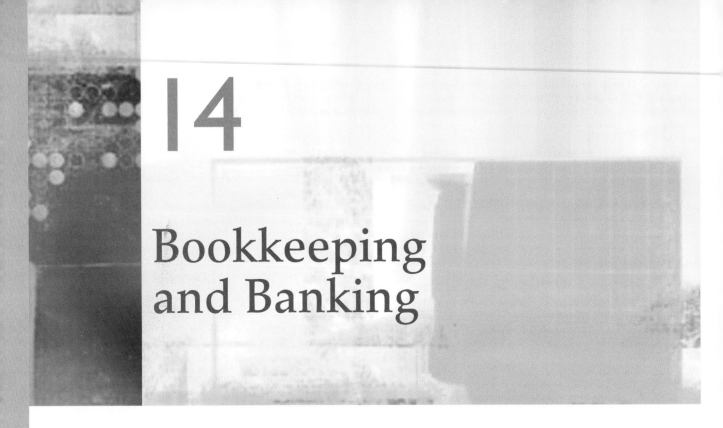

14

Bookkeeping and Banking

CHAPTER OUTLINE

ROLE DELINEATION COMPONENTS

GENERAL: Legal Concepts
- Perform within legal and ethical boundaries

ADMINISTRATIVE: Administrative Procedures
- Perform basic administrative medical assisting functions

ADMINISTRATIVE: Practice Finances
- Apply bookkeeping principles
- Manage accounts receivable
- Manage accounts payable
- Document and maintain accounting and banking records

CHAPTER COMPETENCIES

LEARNING OBJECTIVES

Upon successfully completing this chapter, you will be able to:
1. Spell and define the key terms
2. Explain the concept of the pegboard bookkeeping system
3. Describe the components of the pegboard system
4. Identify and discuss the special features of the pegboard day sheet
5. Describe the functions of a computer accounting system
6. List the uses and components of computer accounting reports
7. Explain the services and procedures of the bank

PERFORMANCE OBJECTIVES

Upon successfully completing this chapter, you will be able to:
1. Record financial transactions, such as charges, payments, credits, and adjustments to patient ledger cards
2. Balance a day sheet
3. Complete a bank deposit slip and make a deposit
4. Reconcile a bank statement
5. Write a check
6. Maintain a petty cash account

KEY TERMS

accounts payable	bookkeeping	debit	posting
accounts receivable	charge slip	encounter form	returned check fee
adjustment	credit	ledger card	service charge
balance	day sheet		

BOOKKEEPING AND BANKING are important facets of medical office management. In most medical practices, bookkeeping and banking involve maintaining both patient and office account records, including petty cash, **accounts receivable** (money owed to the practice), and **accounts payable** (money owed by the practice). Most medical practices use computer accounting systems, although some smaller practices and satellite offices still use manual systems. In large outpatient medical conglomerates with many sites, a central billing office may handle bookkeeping and billing. Some practices outsource their billing and related accounting functions. Although daily bookkeeping practices are handled in the office, the office also employs an accountant who receives reports of the daily financial functions.

FIGURE 14–1.   Sample day sheet with ledger card and charge slip. (Courtesy of Control-o-fax, Waterloo, IA.)

DAILY BOOKKEEPING

Bookkeeping is defined as an organized and accurate record-keeping system of financial transactions for a business. The daily financial transactions of a medical office include patient payments that arrive through the mail, patient payments from patients seen in the office, and patient charges that are added to the accounts receivable. Most medical practices use the single-entry bookkeeping system.

The foundation of accounting is this equation:

$$\text{Assets} = \text{liabilities} + \text{equity}$$

Assets are all things of value owned by or relating to the practice. Liabilities are monies owed. Equity refers to the amount of capital the physician has invested in the practice. Because the two sides of the accounting equation must always **balance** (be equal), each transaction requires a **debit** (charge) on one side of the equation and a **credit** (payment) on the other side of the equation; the amount of the debit and credit must be equal. Double-entry systems are usually used by accounting firms and corporations.

Most medical facilities use the *cash basis* type of accounting, which means that income is considered as income only when money is collected and that payables (money owed) are considered expenses only when money is paid.

The most popular formats for daily bookkeeping are the manual pegboard system and computer systems.

MANUAL ACCOUNTING
Pegboard Bookkeeping System

The pegboard, or write-it-once, bookkeeping system uses a board with pegs running down the left side. The pegs hold a **day sheet**, or daily journal, in place on the board. All transactions for the day are recorded on this day sheet. Each patient has a ledger card (record of the patient's financial activities). When a patient transaction occurs, the bookkeeper places the ledger card over the day sheet and the **charge slip** (preprinted patient bill) over the ledger card on the next available entry line and makes the appropriate entry on the ledger card. Figure 14-1 is a sample day sheet.

Day sheets come with a sheet of carbon paper; thus, the entry recorded on the ledger card, even when a charge slip is not used, is also recorded on the day sheet. When a payment received in the mail is posted, for example, no charge slip is needed. As the day progresses, each patient's ledger card is placed on the next available line on the day sheet, so that the day's entries appear consecutively. At the end of the day, all of the transactions are added.

The various components used in a pegboard system and the specific steps for recording patient transactions are discussed in greater detail next.

Day Sheet

The day sheet keeps track of daily patient transactions, such as charges for services to patients, payments received from pa-

Spanish Terminology

Esto es su total.	This is your balance.
Esto es su crédito.	This is your credit.
No pague esta cuenta.	Do not pay this bill.
Su cheque se volvió para fondos de insuficiente.	Your check was returned for insufficient funds.
Su cuenta ha sido mandada a una agencia de la colección.	Your account has been sent to a collection agency.

tients and insurance carriers, and adjustments to patient accounts. A day sheet should be kept for each day that the physician sees patients; on busy days or for practices with more than one physician, more than one day sheet may be required.

The day sheet has several sections: a deposit slip, distribution columns, a section for payments, a section for adjustments, and a section for **posting** proofs (listing financial transactions in a ledger).

The deposit slip is a detachable portion of the day sheet. All payments received are noted on the deposit slip, and at the end of the day it is separated from the day sheet and deposited with that day's payments.

The distribution columns are used to assign charges for various services. How these columns are used depends on the needs of the individual practice. In a group practice, each practitioner has his or her own column. Some practices may assign columns to the various insurance plans they accept. Finally, these columns can be used to provide information on quality improvement issues. The distribution columns, regardless of how they are assigned, provide the physician with important information about how the practice earns its income.

An **adjustment** is an entry to change an account. The adjustments section allows for reductions in office fees, as with professional courtesy discounts and insurance disallowances. The adjustments section also allows for crediting an account for uncollectible monies without using the payment column. It can also be used to return charges to an account if the patient's payment has been returned by the bank for insufficient funds.

The posting proofs section is where the day's totals are entered and the day sheet is balanced, much as one would balance a checkbook. Once the day sheet is complete, each column or section is totaled individually. It is best to total each column twice to make sure that no errors have been made. After all the columns have been totaled, the posting proofs section is filled out.

If the posting proofs do not balance, an error has been made on the day sheet. To locate the error, go over each transaction one by one. Add the previous balance to the fee or subtract the payment from the previous balance to check whether the new balance listed is correct. If the posted charges are correct, total each column again. Do not erase

---

---

or white-out errors, but draw a line through the erroneous entry and enter the transaction on a new line. When you reenter a transaction on the day sheet, use the ledger card again. Box 14-1 outlines some basic bookkeeping tips.

The day sheet is important because it keeps track of accounts receivable. The accounts receivable total changes every time a charge, payment, or adjustment is made to an account. You should perform a trial balance at the end of each month. Add the totals of each ledger card with an outstanding balance. The total should match the running total kept on the day sheet. This practice ensures the accuracy of your financial records.

Completed day sheets are filed chronologically in a ledger (a book of accounts) with the most recent day sheet on top. Completed day sheets are important legal documents and must be kept for at least 7 years for tax purposes. They should be stored in a safe, dark area to avoid loss or fading.

Checkpoint Question

1. What are five sections of a pegboard day sheet?

Ledger Cards

The **ledger card** is a financial record for each patient. Most ledger cards include areas for the responsible person's name, address, telephone number, and insurance information. Fig. 14-2 is a sample ledger card. Other information, such as employment information and primary and secondary insurance information, may appear on the ledger card. Patient information appears on the top of the ledger card; the bottom portion is used to record the patient's financial activities.

Many practices use photocopies of an individual's ledger card as a bill, mailing the photocopy to the patient each time payment is required. If you use a copy of the ledger card for billing, make sure that no information other than the billing name and address is visible through the window

---

Box 14-1

BASIC BOOKKEEPING TIPS

- Always use black ink; do not use pencil.
- Write legibly.
- *Never* erase or white-out errors. Draw a single line through the incorrect entry, record the correct information, and initial the change.
- Always double-check each entry.

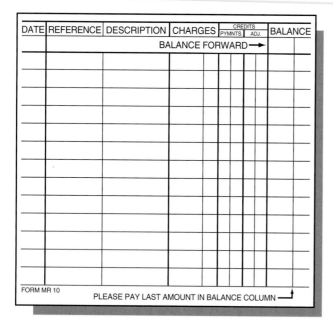

DATE	REFERENCE	DESCRIPTION	CHARGES	CREDITS PYMNTS.	ADJ.	BALANCE
BALANCE FORWARD ➝						

FORM MR 10   PLEASE PAY LAST AMOUNT IN BALANCE COLUMN ➝

FIGURE 14–2. Sample ledger card.

of the envelope. Allowing other information to be visible is a breach of privacy.

The ledger card is a legal document and should be kept for the same length of time as the patient's medical record. Ledger cards are filed alphabetically in a ledger tray. A medical practice may require more than one ledger tray. Ledger cards with outstanding balances are kept separate from paid ledger cards; this makes it easier to photocopy the monthly bills or find a ledger card when a patient calls about an outstanding bill. If the office uses only one ledger tray, the ledger cards with outstanding balances are filed alphabetically in the front of the ledger tray, with the paid ledger cards filed alphabetically in the back.

Encounter Forms and Charge Slips

The **encounter form** and the charge slip are preprinted patient statements that list codes for basic office charges and have sections for the patient's current balance and next appointment. Most encounter forms and charge slips have three-part copies:

1. The first copy is kept by the facility for auditing purposes (all are numbered).
2. The second copy is given to the patient for insurance filing (if the patient files the insurance claims).
3. The third copy, which has a carbon line at the top to match your ledgers and day sheets, is given to the patient as a receipt of services.

Charge slips are smaller versions of an encounter form and are designed to be used in conjunction with ledger cards. They often have different-colored no-carbon-required

(NCR) copies. Figure 14-3 shows a computer-generated encounter form and a charge slip used in a manual system.

> ## Checkpoint Question
>
> **2.** How do ledger cards and encounter forms differ?

Posting a Charge

The charge column of the day sheet is for original charges incurred for services received by the patient from the physician or staff on a specific date. Examples include office visits, electrocardiogram, blood work, hospital visits, consultations, and fees for returned checks. Charges in a medical office are based on a fee schedule or list of charges determined by the usual, customary, and reasonable charges of similar providers in similar localities who practice under similar circumstances. Fee schedules are discussed further in Chapter 16. Procedure 14-2 outlines the steps for posting a charge.

Posting a Payment

Payments received by the practice may include insurance checks received in the mail, money orders, credit card payments, or cash received from patients. Procedure 14-3 outlines the steps for posting payments and adjustments.

Posting a Credit

Sometimes an account is overpaid, either by the patient or the insurance company. Such an overpayment is termed a credit (money owed to the patient or insurance carrier). This will show on the patient's ledger card as the last balance, with brackets (e.g., [25]) indicating a credit. Brackets are used to show the opposite of the column's normal meaning. For example, the balance column normally shows patients' debits, or amounts patients owe to the doctor. Brackets around an amount indicate the opposite, namely, that the doctor owes the patient money.

Credits are handled in one of two ways: (1) the credit stays on the account and is subtracted from the charges on the patient's next visit, or (2) the patient is mailed a refund for the amount of the overpayment. How an overpayment is handled depends on office policy and the amount of the overpayment. Generally, overpayments under $5 are left on account as a credit, whereas overpayments over $5 are refunded.

Posting a Credit Adjustment

The adjustments section is used to indicate nonstandard office fees and to credit an account for uncollectible monies. Below are three specific situations that require a credit adjustment.

Patient Name: _____

Patient ID #: _____ DOB: _____ Sex: _____

PCP: _____

SSN: _____ Financial Class: _____

Phone: _____ (home) _____ (work)

Medical Record #: _____ Date of Service: _____

Benefit Pkg: _____ Copay $ _____

Encounter #: _____

Service Provider: _____

Appt. Status: ☐ Scheduled ☐ Same Day ☐ Walk-in

Check-in Time: _____ Check-out Time: _____
Escorted to Exam Room: _____ Time Patient Seen: _____

Appointment Time: _____

Is Patient Being Seen in Relation to:
☐ Motor Vehicle Accident ☐ Workman's Compensation

Appointment Failure Reason:
☐ Patient Cancel ☐ No Show ☐ Walk Out ☐ PHA Cancel

TYPE OF VISIT

✓	CODE	DESCRIPTION	FEE	✓	CODE	DESCRIPTION	FEE	✓	CODE	DESCRIPTION	FEE	✓	CODE	DESCRIPTION	FE
		OFFICE VISITS-EST.				**OFFICE VISITS-NEW CONT.**				**PREVENTATIVE, NEW**				**COUNSELING**	
	99211	Minimal			99204	Compreh.			99385	E&M 18-39			99401	15 Min.	
	99212	Focused			99205	Comp. & Complex			99386	E&M 40-64			99402	30 Min.	
	99213	Expanded				**NURSE VISIT**			99387	E&M 65 & over			99403	45 Min.	
	99214	Detailed			99211	Minimal				**CONSULTATION**			99404	60 Min.	
	99215	Compreh.				**PREVENTATIVE, EST.**			99241	Focused					
		OFFICE VISITS-NEW			99395	E&M 18-39			99242	Pre-Op Consult					
	99201	Focused			99396	E&M 40-64			99244	2nd Opinion					
	99202	Expanded			99397	E&M 65 & over									
	99203	Detailed													

PROCEDURES

✓	CODE	DESCRIPTION	FEE	✓	CODE	DESCRIPTION	FEE	✓	CODE	DESCRIPTION	FEE	✓	CODE	DESCRIPTION	FE
	88170	Aspiration - Cyst			11200	Skin Tag Removal				**IMMUNIZATIONS/INJECTIONS**				**IMMUNIZATIONS/INJECTIONS CONT**	
	20600	Aspiration - Joint (Small)			20550	Trigger point/Tendon Inj.			G0009	Administration Fee - Pneumovax			J2203	Triamcinolone Inj.	
	20605	Aspiration - Joint (Interm.)							G0010	Administration Fee - Hepatitis B			J3420	Vitamin B₁₂	
	20610	Aspiration - Joint (Large)				**SPECIALTY SERVICES**			95115	Allergy Injection Single				**IN-HOUSE LABORATORY**	
	16020	Burn Dressing			99070	Ace Bandage			95117	Allergy Injection Multiple			89050	Cell Count, except blood	
	69210	Ear Irrigation			E0110	Crutches			90788	Antibiotic IM			89060	Crystalanalysis	
	10120	Foreign Body Removal, Skin			29130	Finger Splint			J2910	Aurothioglucose			82948	Glucose	
	10060	I&D Abscess, simple			29125	Wrist Splint			G0008	Flu Vaccine			85013	HCT	
	90780	IV Infusion Therapy			99080	Form Completion			J1600	Gold Injection			85018	Hemoglobin Screen	
	12001	Laceration Repair, Simple				**TESTING/SCREENING**			90731	Hepatitis B			81025	Pregnancy	
	13160	Laceration Repair, Extens.			95004	Allergy - Skin Test			90741	Immune Globulin			81002	Urinalysis, Dipstick	
	64450	Medial Nerve Infiltration			92557	Audiometry			90724	Influenza			81000	Urinalysis, Full	
	17110	Molluscum/Wart Rmvl			93000	EKG			J9217	Lupron 3.75 mg			G0001	Venipuncture	
	94640	Nebulizer			92506	Hearing Screen			J9217	Lupron 7.5 mg				**OTHER PROCEDURES**	
	82270	Stool for Blood (Hemocult)			86580	PPD			J9250	Methotrexate 2-5 mg					
	12001	Suturing, Superficial			94010	Pulmonary Function			90732	Pneumovax					
	13100	Suturing, Complex			94760	Pulse Oximetry, Single			90718	Td					
	11050	Skin Les./Wart Cautery			45330	Sigmoidoscopy, Flexible			90782	Therapeutic SQ or IM					

P = PRIMARY   S = SECONDARY   S1-S9 = NUMBERED SECONDARY

DIAGNOSIS

✓	CODE	DESCRIPTION	✓	CODE	DESCRIPTION	✓	CODE	DESCRIPTION
	789.0	Abdominal Pain		780.6	Fever		462	Pharyngitis (sore throat)
	879.8	Abrasion/Laceration		704.8	Folliculitis		486	Pneumonia
	995.3	Allergic Reaction		535.5	Gastritis		V70.3	Pre-Marital Testing
	477.9	Allergic Rhinitis		558.9	Gastroenteritis		V72.81	Pre-op Cardiac Exam
	285.9	Anemia		274.9	Gout		V72.83	Pre-op Exam, Other
	413.9	Angina		V72.3	Gyn Exam		601.0	Prostatits
	300.00	Anxiety		784.0	Headache		600	Prostatism
	716.9	Arthritis		389.9	Hearing Loss		782.1	Rash
	427.9	Arrhythmia		536.8	Heartburn/Indigestion		569.3	Rectal Bleeding
	493.90	Asthma		573.3	Hepatitis		530.81	Reflux
	611.72	Breast Lump		455.6	Hemorrhoids		V81.2	Screening for Cardiac Condition
	490	Bronchitis		553.9	Hernia		780.3	Seizure Disorder
	727.3	Bursitis		401.9	Hypertension (NOS)		473.9	Sinusitis
	354.0	Carpal Tunnel Syndrome		272.4	Hyperlipidemia		848.9	Strain/Sprain
	682.9	Cellulitis		242.00	Hyperthyroidism		438	Stroke
	786.50	Chest Pain		251.2	Hypoglycemia		305.90	Substance Abuse
	575.1	Cholecystitis		380.4	Impacted Cerumen		099.9	STD
	372.3	Conjunctivitis		780.52	Insomnia		727.00	Tenosynovitis, Tendonitis
	496	COPD		564.1	Irritable Bowel Syndrome		451.9	Thrombophlebitis
	414.9	Coronary Artery Disease		719.40	Joint Pain		246.9	Thyroid Disease
	290.9	Dementia		592.0	Kidney Stones		435.9	TIA
	311	Depression		464.0	Laryngitis		463	Tonsillitis
	692.9	Dermatitis		724.2	Low Back Pain		011.90	Tuberculosis
	250.01	Diabetes, IDDM		710.0	Lupus		465.9	Upper Respiratory Infection
	250.00	Diabetes, NIDDM		V70.0	Medical Exam/Physical		599.0	Urinary Tract Infection
	558.9	Diarrhea		346.9	Migraine		V04.8	Vaccination, Flu
	562.10	Diverticular Disease		278.0	Obesity		V03.9	Vaccination, Pneumovax
	780.4	Dizziness		382.9	Otitis Media		616.10	Vaginitis
	995.2	Drug Reaction		614.9	Pelvic Inflammatory Disease		424.9	Valvular Heart Disease
	782.3	Edema		533.9	Peptic Ulcer Disease		079.9	Viral Syndrome
	780.7	Fatigue/Tiredness/Malaise		443.9	Peripheral Vascular Disease			

Comments:

PREVIOUS BALANCE	$
TODAY'S CHARGES	$
PAYMENT	$
BALANCE	$

RETURN APPOINTMENT:
_____ Days   _____ Weeks   _____ Months
APPT. LENGTH: _____ PROVIDER: _____

APPT. REASON:

PROVIDER SIGNATURE:

Adult

Philadelphia
Health Associates
Tax ID #23-2350500
PHA Group # PH75923

☐ 3550 Market Street
Philadelphia, PA 1910
(215) 823-8660

☐ The Bourse Building
111 S. Independence
East • 7th Floor
Philadelphia, PA 1910
(215) 625-9100

OTHER DIAGNOSIS

✓	CODE	DESCRIPTION	✓	CODE	DESCRIPTION

FIGURE 14-3. Sample encounter form and charge slip.

Example 1. The physician wishes to give a registered nurse a 25% professional discount on charges incurred for an office visit. You enter the fee from the fee schedule in the charge column, show in the description column an office visit with a professional discount of 25%, and put the 25% in the adjustment column. Assume an office visit is $40. You put $40 in the charge column and $10 (25% of $40) in the adjustment column. The patient owes your facility $30 for this visit.

Example 2. Most medical offices participate with certain insurance groups, which means the physician has signed an agreement with the insurance carrier to accept the fee for services set by that carrier instead of the physician's normal fee. Again, you must charge the same fee for the same procedure. When payment is received, however, the explanation of benefits from that carrier will show the agreed-on amount for that procedure. You will post the payment in the normal way, but you must write off the difference between the physician's standard fee for this procedure and the agreed-on amount. Assume the doctor charged $40 for an office visit and the insurance carrier's agreed-on amount was $35. You would post $40 in the payment column and $5 in the adjustment column to arrive at the agreed-on amount.

Example 3. Most facilities request that you write off the balance of an account when you turn it over to a collection agency to keep better control of the accounts receivable. Therefore, if the patient's balance is $1200, you would show "collection agency" in the description column of the ledger and put the $1200 in the adjustment column, which would bring the balance to 0. Procedure 14-4 lists the steps for posting an adjustment.

Checkpoint Question

3. What do brackets around an amount listed in a column indicate?

Posting a Debit Adjustment

Generally, a credit adjustment reduces the patient's account balance, whereas a debit adjustment adds to the patient's account balance. Below are three specific situations that require a debit adjustment.

Example 1. You receive an insufficient funds (NSF) check from the bank today from a payment made earlier by a patient and posted as such to his account. The previous payment is no longer valid. Therefore, you must eliminate that payment because the patient now owes it again. Because this is not an original charge, you may not use the charge column for this entry. To post this debit adjustment to the patient's account, you will show NSF in the description column and the amount of the NSF check in the adjustment column with brackets.

Example 2. Assume that you have turned over an account to a collection agency and the patient comes in later to pay

the amount owed. You must first put the money back on the account, or you will create a credit balance. Place the ledger card on the day sheet and in the description column write "reverse collection." Again, this is not an original or new charge, so you do not use the charge column. Show the amount in the adjustment column in brackets because you are adding the amount to the patient's balance. You may now show the payment in the payment column.

Example 3. Your office requires that you refund all money over $5 to the patient or insurance carrier. You must also post this to eliminate the credit balance on the account. Place the ledger card on the day sheet and in the description column write "refund to patient" (or insurance carrier). To eliminate a credit balance, you must debit the account. You put the amount of the refund in the adjustment column in brackets, indicating that it is a debit, not a credit adjustment.

Checkpoint Question

4. How does a credit adjustment differ from a debit adjustment?

Posting to Cash-Paid-Out Section of Day Sheet

Sometimes, the physician may take cash from the day's receipts. When this happens, your bank deposit for that day will be short by the amount taken out. The best way to account for this is to have the physician sign in the cash-paid-out section of the day sheet for the amount. This documents the transaction and prevents anybody else from being able to do this.

Some insurance carriers adjust for money overpaid to your facility by holding that amount out of money they are paying your facility for other patients. Although you are posting the correct amounts in the payment column for each patient, the check amount from the insurance carrier is short the refund or kept-out money. You write this in the cash-paid-out section of the day sheet, explaining, "insurance refund on account of [patient's name]." It is also a good idea to make a copy of the explanation of benefits and staple it to the back of your day sheet for future reference.

COMPUTER ACCOUNTING

Most medical office accounting software available today is easy to use and requires a minimum of computer skills. Computer programs fulfill many of the same functions as a pegboard system but do so much faster. Instead of recording entries on a day sheet, you key entries into a computer. You can print out invoices and receipts for patients and insurance companies. Since most practices have computer stations in several locations, the patient's account can be quickly and easily retrieved in all areas of the office, enabling everyone involved in the patient's care to access information about third-party coverage, co-payments required, and so on.

Computer bookkeeping programs have a variety of advantages over pegboard bookkeeping. Computer programs work as expanded calculators and perform the arithmetic functions, such as balancing individual accounts and the day's totals. Many bookkeeping programs also can write checks. Some programs manage electronic banking between the office and bank. The office may have computerized many functions, including bookkeeping, making appointments, and generating other office reports, such as forms for insurance reimbursement. It is essential that data stored on computer be backed up in a reliable way in case the computer crashes.

Posting to Computer Accounts

If you understand the fundamentals of accounting and how to post entries manually, you will be able to use a computer system with ease. To post payments, first retrieve the patient's account. The software will take you through the process. You enter the source and amount of the payment, the allowed amount for the service, and any necessary adjustments. As in a manual system, this information is provided on the insurance carrier's explanation of benefits (EOB). Calculations are automatic and error free.

When you post charges into the computer database, in most systems you use a local code to indicate a certain procedure or service. For example, you may enter 211 to post a level 2 office visit for a new patient. When the information prints on the claim form, the CPT (current procedural terminology) code 99212 will appear (see Chapter 18).

Computer Accounting Reports

Depending on the software package, you can easily generate daily, monthly, and yearly reports or reports on transactions of an individual physician in a group practice. Daily and weekly reports provide the same information found on the bottom of a day sheet in a manual accounting system. At any given time, you can request a report that displays the practice's period-to-date and year-to-date financial status.

Computer systems record the daily activities described earlier for the manual system, and bookkeeping software enables you to create a closing report that prints a list of the day's financial activities. You may run a trial daily report or a final daily report. In a trial report, the information keyed in that day is printed for review. You correct any errors before running a final report. As on the day sheet, you categorize receipts as cash, check, and so on. A check register report can print the amount of the daily deposit and a list of checks for the day.

BANKING

Banks and Their Services

Besides physical location, several factors are important when choosing a bank for the office business account. These factors include the monthly service fees, overdraft protection programs (protection against bouncing checks), interest-bearing accounts, and returned check fees.

Checking Accounts

A checking account allows you to write checks for funds that are deposited in the account. Each day you will deposit to a checking account the money collected in the office. At the time a new checking account is opened, checks are ordered with a check order form. The administrative medical assistant must maintain the checkbook and ensure that checks are reordered as needed.

Banks offer a variety of options for checking accounts. Variables include monthly service charges, maximum amounts of checks written, minimum balance requirements, and so on. Interest-bearing checking accounts pay interest if the balance is kept above a certain amount. Most banks set the minimum checking account balance at $500 to $2500. The bank pays this interest in exchange for the use of your money for loans and other transactions. If you drop below the minimum balance, however, you will not earn interest. Most banks also charge a monthly service fee and a fee for each check written for the period the balance was below the limit. Some banks waive the monthly service fee if the office agrees to maintain a minimum balance in another account, such as a savings account.

Savings Accounts

The medical practice may use a savings account for money that is put aside for long-term plans or money that is not needed for writing checks. A savings account pays interest at a higher percentage rate than a checking account, allowing the money to grow. Funds can be transferred to the checking account as needed.

Money Market Accounts

Money market accounts are a combination of a savings account and an interest-bearing checking account. The minimum balance is usually much higher than that of a checking account (as much as $2500), but the interest rate also is much higher. These accounts offer limited check-writing privileges, including an initial deposit of $2000 and minimum balance of $500 per check.

Bank Fees

Banks charge fees for services. In an effort to get new business, banks offer special services and plans for small business, including the medical office.

Monthly Service Fees

Bank policies concerning monthly fees or service charges vary widely. A **service charge** is a fee charged monthly for using an account. The charge can be a fixed amount or may be an individual charge for each check written on the account. As discussed, some banks do not levy a service charge if a specific minimum balance is maintained for the account.

Overdraft Protection

Overdraft protection guarantees that checks written against the account will be paid even when there is not enough money in the account at the time. Usually, the bank pays the checks and retrieves the money owed to it when the account balance is restored. Many banks offer overdraft protection only up to a certain dollar amount.

Returned Check Fee

Some banks charge a **returned check fee**, which is a fee charged for any check that is deposited into the checking account but that is later returned to the bank because the account it was issued from had insufficient funds with which to pay the check. Such a check is often referred to as a bounced check. Most facilities charge this amount to the patient. Because this is an original charge, the bad check fee is listed in the charge column of the patient ledger and day sheet, with the amount of the check being recorded as a debit adjustment.

Types of Checks

Most medical offices use the standard business check, but when certain circumstances require, there are other types available:

- Certified checks are stamped and signed by the bank to verify that the amount of the check is being held in the account for payment. The check is written from the customer's account.
- Cashier's checks are sold to a customer for cash or a personal check. The check is written by the bank, giving the recipient the added guarantee that the check is good.
- Traveler's checks are a convenient and safe way to carry cash when traveling. They are available in denominations of $10, $20, and $50, and if lost, they can be replaced. Traveler's checks are signed when bought and are countersigned (signed again) in the presence of the payee.
- Money orders, although not checks, can be purchased with cash from a bank or the U. S. Postal Service. Money orders, which guarantee payment to the recipient, are often used for mailing payments, since it is not safe to mail cash.

Box 14-2 highlights other terms used in the language of banking.

Box 14-2

DO YOU SPEAK "BANKING?"

ABA number: A number originated by the American Bankers Association to identify the bank on which the check is written. It is written in the form of a fraction and is usually found above or below the check number. The top number of the fraction indicates the geographic location, and the bottom number identifies the bank.

ATM: Automated teller machines have made 24-hour banking possible. With the use of a card you insert in a slot and a personal identification number (PIN), you can make deposits, withdrawals, and transfers at an ATM. If your bank owns the ATM, this convenience is usually free. If you use any other ATM, a service fee of up to $3.50 is charged. The ATM screen gives you the opportunity to cancel the transaction if you are not willing to pay the service fee.

Debit card: A card with a magnetic strip that is presented for payment directly from your checking account. When a transaction occurs, you record it in your check registry.

Online banking: Electronic or online banking gives you the opportunity to view your account at any time. Withdrawals and deposits are listed and can be printed, and transfers can be made.

Stale check: A check that has not been cashed within a certain time, usually 6 months. Some checks must be cashed within a shorter time, but that requirement must be printed on the check.

Checkpoint Question

5. List three types of checks available through banks.

Writing Checks for Accounts Payable

Another financial duty of the medical assistant may be to handle accounts payable, or pay the bills. The accounts payable in a medical office usually include rent, utilities, taxes, salaries, vendors of supplies and services, patient refunds, and petty cash reimbursement. The accounts are usually paid by check. Banks require signature cards for each person authorized to sign checks. In most cases, this is limited to the physician or physicians. Some medical offices require two signatures, especially if the check is over a certain amount. Computer systems allow you to enter information in the proper field and print checks. Software systems also keep track of every transaction using a check. When using a manual system, type or write legibly. Use the current date and write the amount of the payment in both figures and words and the name of the payee. Complete the memo line for reference. Record the date, check number, amount of the check, and payee on the check registry. Post this transaction to the appropriate account in the general ledger or apply it to the

```
ENDORSE HERE

FOR DEPOSIT ONLY

WILLIAM BROWN, M.D.

#00-00000

DO NOT SIGN / WRITE / STAMP BELOW THIS LINE
   FOR FINANCIAL INSTITUTION USAGE ONLY*
```

F I G U R E 1 4 – 4 . An endorsed check.

proper category in a computer system by entering the type of payment on the proper screen. Recording transactions in the proper account or category is important when preparing the office taxes. Subtract each amount from the check register balance.

Receiving Checks and Making Deposits

When checks are received in the office, they are first endorsed. To endorse a check requires writing (or rubber stamping) on the back of the check the name and number of the account into which it will be deposited (Fig. 14-4). This way, if the payments are lost or stolen, no one else can cash them. It also ensures that the bank deposits the payments to the correct account. An endorsement stamp can be purchased from your bank or a stationery store.

After all payments are posted, total all of the checks and all cash received that day. This total should match the totals of the payments column on your day sheet. Detach the deposit sheet from the day sheet and stamp the back with the endorsement check stamp. If a computer program is used, print out a deposit slip. Wrap the deposit slip around the checks and complete a bank deposit slip for the account to which the deposit is made. The deposit can be hand-delivered or mailed to the bank.

A hand-delivered deposit may be taken to a teller, who will issue a deposit receipt, or dropped in a depository. If the deposit is mailed, make sure sufficient postage has been affixed to the envelope. Never include cash payments in a deposit that is mailed or placed in a depository. Cash deposits should always be hand-delivered, and a teller's receipt should always be obtained.

Reconciling Bank Statements

All banks mail monthly statements to account holders on which are listed all transactions since the last closing date. This bank statement must be reconciled, or compared for accuracy, with your records each month.

The statement consists of a list of all checks written and their amounts, all deposits made and their amounts, any electronic transactions, and any service charges. Verify that all checks and deposits are listed correctly. Make a check mark on the checkbook stub of each check that has been paid by the bank. On the back of the statement is a worksheet that explains how to balance the account (Fig. 14-5). Following the steps listed on the worksheet makes balancing the account fairly easy. The steps for reconciling a bank statement are listed in Procedure 14-5.

Checkpoint Question

6. What information is found on a bank statement?

1. Subtract any fees or charges that appear on this statement from your checkbook balance.
2. Add any interest paid on your checking account to your checkbook balance.
3. List the checks you have written that have not been paid (these checks did not yet appear on your bank statement). You can also include in this list any withdrawals you have made since the ending date of the banking statement that do not appear on the statement.

Check Number	Amount
_____	_____
_____	_____
_____	_____
_____	_____
Total	_____

4. If you have entered deposits or other additions to your checkbook that do not appear on the statement, list them there:

Date	Amount
_____	_____
_____	_____
Total	_____

5. Enter the ending balance from your statement here: _____
   Add the total deposits from Step 4: + _____
   Subtract the total from Step 3: – _____
   Total (this should equal your checkbook balance): _____

If these balances do not equal your checkbook balance:
• Check the addition and subtraction in your checkbook
• Check the amount of each transaction in your checkbook with the amount shown on your statement
• Check to see that all transactions from your previous statement have been accounted for
• Call your bank manager for assistance

FIGURE 14–5. Bank statement reconciling worksheet.

PETTY CASH RECEIPT

_____ 20 ____

To Office Manager:
   Please furnish for_____

Supplies:	
Postage:	
Travel Expenses:	
Other:	
Approved	
TOTAL	

Received Above Amount

_____

FIGURE 14–6. Petty cash voucher.

PETTY CASH

A petty cash account is a cash fund kept in the office specifically for small purchases, such as buying postage stamps or office supplies. The value of the petty cash account should always remain the same. A petty cash fund is always a designated sum of money. When money is taken from the fund, a voucher (Fig. 14-6) or receipt is placed in the fund to verify the purchase. The remaining cash and the sum of the vouchers should always equal the designated sum; for example, a petty cash fund of $40 with $13 in actual cash should have receipts that amount to $27.

Petty cash funds should be kept separate from patient cash payments. All cash should be kept in a securely locked area. One person should be designated to maintain the petty cash fund and issue vouchers. A voucher with an attached receipt should always be placed in the petty cash box, both to provide proof of the purchase and to keep the account balanced. The petty cash fund normally is replenished once a month. To replenish the fund, cash a check in the amount of the total of the vouchers. The money is placed in the fund, and the vouchers are removed and filed.

Some offices keep a petty cash expense record. This record is similar to a checkbook that keeps track of the account balance as checks are written, such as personal checkbook. This expense record also categorizes purchases so that they can be included with the monthly office expenses. Purchases such as stamps and office and medical supplies can be deducted as office expenses and added to the accounts payable expense record.

 Checkpoint Question

7. List six guidelines for managing petty cash.

Procedure 14-1

Balancing the Day Sheet

Equipment/Supplies

- Calculator
- Current day sheet with yesterday's previous balance total
- Carbon
- All ledger cards with transactions on the day sheet
- Pencil
- Pen

Steps	Reason
1. Determine if all entries are complete.	If all charge slips listed on the day sheet are not returned to you, the day sheet will not balance. Make sure you have finished the transaction on each account.
2. Add each column with a calculator and place the total in pencil in the appropriate column.	Day sheets include a portion for performing a daily proof (verifying the accuracy of the entries). Using pencil will enable changes if needed.
3. Add the totals from today to the totals from the previous day sheet.	A running total is kept by placing the ending figure for each day under the column for the beginning figure on the next day's sheet. This gives you a total accounts receivable amount at any time.
4. To verify the accuracy of the entries: • Add the total of the previous balance column to the total of the current balance column • From this total, subtract the totals of the payment and adjustment columns • This amount equals the current balance	This allows for double verification of current totals.
5. When the totals are verified, go back over them in pen.	Day sheets are legal documents that are retained. They must be written in ink.

Posting Charges to the Patient's Account

Equipment/Supplies

- Day sheet
- Carbon paper
- Pegboard
- Ledger card
- Charge slip and/or encounter form
- Calculator
- Form
- Pen

Steps	Purpose
1. Take the charge slip from the patient and check to be sure it is complete, signed by the provider, and belongs to the patient whose ledger card or account is in hand.	It is difficult to undo entries to the wrong account. It's best to be accurate the first time. Just as in the clinical area, identify your patient.
2. If using a ledger card, post the total amount of today's charges in the charge column on the ledger card. Each service can be listed in the description column by using abbreviations such as OV, INJ, LAB for office visit, injection, and laboratory services, respectively.	Since the manual billing system uses a copy of the ledger card for a statement, it is important that patients be able to understand your abbreviations. Provide a key at the bottom of the ledger card.
3. If using a computer, post each charge separately on the charge screen. Most programs require a local code for a particular service. When you enable this code or the CPT code, the computer will automatically post the appropriate charge in the proper field.	Proper computer entry allows for accurate financial records to be maintained.

Posting Payments to a Patient's Account

Equipment/Supplies

- Day sheet
- Carbon paper
- Pegboard
- Ledger card
- Charge slip and/or encounter form
- Calculator
- Form
- Pen

Steps

1. Align the patient's ledger card on the day sheet. If the patient is paying for services received by the physician today, the charge slip that shows today's charges should also be in place on the day sheet.

2. Enter the patient's name and previous balance in the appropriate columns. If using a charge slip, make sure you place the charge slip number in the receipt number column. Enter the posting date in the date column.

3. Enter the type of payment being made in the description column, whether personal check (pers. ck.), money order (m. o.), credit card (MC, VISA), or insurance check (ins. ck.). Enter the amount of payment in the payment column and on the deposit section of the day sheet in the cash or checks column.

4. Subtract the payment amount from the previous balance and record the new balance. If only a payment is being posted, no entry is made in the fee area. If an entry has been made in the fee area, you will start with the previous balance, add the charges, subtract the payment, and record the new balance.

Procedure 14-4

Posting a Credit Adjustment

Equipment/Supplies

- Day sheet
- Carbon
- Pegboard
- Ledger card
- Calculator

Steps	Reason
1. Align the patient's ledger card on the day sheet.	Proper alignment is needed for accurate record keeping.
2. Record the patient's name, previous balance, and the date in the appropriate columns.	Payments and adjustments can be posted at the same time. The payment is recorded in the payment column, and the adjustment is entered in the adjustment column. Both are subtracted from the previous balance, and the new balance is recorded in the new balance column.
3. Record [in brackets][a] the amount of the adjustment in the adjustment column of the ledger card. Enter a description of the adjustment in the professional service column, that is, insurance adjustment or correction adjustment.	A description of the adjustment is needed for proper financial record keeping and quality assurance.
4. Subtract the amount of the adjustment from the previous balance and record the new balance in the balance column.	Knowing the balance of an account is essential for the financial stability and growth of a business.

[a]Brackets indicate that the amount is subtracted.

Procedure 14-5

Reconciling a Bank Statement

Equipment/Supplies

- Monthly bank statement
- Check register
- Calculator
- Pen

Steps	Reason
1. Determine which portion of the checkbook is covered on this bank statement.	You must know where your last bank statement ended and where the current one begins.
2. Find the ending balance and the list of checks and deposits on the bank statement.	
3. Check your checkbook register or record of disbursements against the bank statement and place a check mark against each check and deposit on your record that has been recorded on the bank statement.	To balance the account, you must identify which checks or deposits are recorded by the bank and which ones are outstanding.
4. Total all checks not listed on the bank statement. Place this total in the space provided on the back of the bank statement (outstanding checks).	Since there is no standard form, each bank's worksheet may be different, but there will be a space reserved for the total of all outstanding checks and withdrawals.
5. Total all deposits that do no appear on the bank statement and place this total in the space provided on the worksheet (outstanding deposits).	Outstanding deposits must be accounted for to balance the bank statement.
6. Note any additional charges, such as for services, ATM use, or returned checks.	Miscellaneous charges must be taken into account when balancing the checkbook
7. Calculate the correct balance by starting with the ending balance from the bank. Then, add the outstanding deposits to that balance (from Step # 5). Then, subtract the outstanding withdrawals (from Step # 4).	Outstanding deposits and withdrawals must be accounted for to reconcile the bank statement.
8. Verify that the correct balance (from Step # 7) matches with your checking account amount.	This allows verification that, as of today, your checking account balance agrees with your bank statement.
9. If the figure is not the same, recheck your work. If the two numbers still do not match, contact the bank to check for possible bank errors.	This allows you to verify your records with the bank's record. It is easy to transpose numbers or misread figures when using a calculator. You should add the columns again. It is helpful to have a coworker add the columns also.

CHAPTER SUMMARY

Whether a medical practice uses a manual bookkeeping system, such as the pegboard system, or a computer system, you may be responsible for keeping records of accounts payable, accounts receivable, and petty cash. You may also be responsible for banking functions, such as receiving checks, making deposits, and reconciling monthly bank statements. To carry out these responsibilities effectively, you must record all transactions accurately and promptly. Computers have made the daily bookkeeping practices much easier, but you must understand the principles of accounting applied in the manual system if you are to use the computer system. Using the appropriate banking services will allow the day-to-day financial operations to be efficient, accurate, and secure.

Critical Thinking Challenges

1. Your day sheet deposit slip and your posting proofs do not agree. How do you find the error?
2. An employee is prosecuted for stealing money for more than a year from her physician employer's funds. Investigation reveals that she was stealing any cash payments given to her. How could she do this for so long without being caught? What necessary monthly action would make this crime impossible?
3. Your office is considering going from a pegboard system to a computer bookkeeping system. What features should you look for in the software?

Answers to Checkpoint Questions

1. Five sections of a pegboard day sheet include the distribution columns, adjustment column, deposit slip, payments section, and posting proofs section.
2. Ledger cards provide an overall financial record of a patient; encounter forms provide documentation of today's financial activity.
3. Brackets indicate the opposite of the normal meaning of that column.
4. Generally, a credit adjustment reduces the patient's account balance, whereas a debit adjustment increases the patient's account balance.
5. Three types of checks offered by banks include cashier's checks, certified checks, and traveler's checks.
6. The statement consists of one or more pages that lists all checks written and their amounts, all deposits made and their amounts, any electronic transactions, and any service charges.
7. These are the six guidelines for managing petty cash:
   - Keep petty cash separate from patient cash payments.
   - Keep in a secure, locked area.
   - Designate one person to maintain the petty cash fund and issue vouchers.
   - Place a voucher with an attached receipt in the petty cash fund.
   - Replenish the petty cash fund once a month.
   - Remove and file all vouchers.

 Websites

Superbill Forms and Creations
www.physicianshelp.com
Comptroller of Currency Administrator of National Banks
www.occ.treas.gov
Maximum Returned Check Fees allowed by state
www.checkagain.com/statefees.asp

15

Accounts Payable and Payroll

CHAPTER OUTLINE

ACCOUNTING CYCLE

RECORD-KEEPING
  COMPONENTS

ACCOUNTS PAYABLE
  Ordering Goods and Services
  Receiving Supplies
  Paying Invoices

PAYROLL
  Types of Payroll Systems
  Employee Records
  Tax Withholdings

PREPARATION OF REPORTS

ASSISTING WITH AUDITS

ROLE DELINEATION COMPONENTS

GENERAL: Legal Concepts
- Perform within legal and ethical boundaries

ADMINISTRATIVE: Administrative Procedures
- Perform basic administrative medical assisting functions

ADMINISTRATIVE: Practice Finances
- Apply bookkeeping principles
- Manage accounts receivable
- Manage accounts payable
- Process payroll
- Document and maintain accounting and banking records

CHAPTER COMPETENCIES

LEARNING OBJECTIVES

Upon successfully completing this chapter, you will be able to:
1. Spell and define the key terms
2. Describe the accounting cycle
3. Describe the components of a record-keeping system
4. Explain the process of ordering supplies and paying invoices
5. Discuss the types of payroll records
6. Explain which taxes are withheld from paychecks

PERFORMANCE OBJECTIVES

Upon successfully completing this chapter, you will be able to:
1. Issue a payroll check, using the pegboard system
2. Calculate the amount of an employee's payroll check for a given pay period

KEY TERMS

accounting cycle	federal unemployment tax	liabilities	profit-and-loss statement
audit	gross income	net pay	purchase order
check register	Internal Revenue Service	packing slip	summation report
check stub	(IRS)	payroll	withholding
FICA	invoice	payroll journal	

ACCOUNTING IS THE compilation of a business's financial records. It is necessary for assessment of the practice's financial history and current financial stakes, which serves as the basis for sound financial management. The medical office, like other businesses, requires strict adherence to sound record-keeping practices. Records must be maintained in an orderly fashion so you can retrieve financial information at any time and to present an organized picture of the business's finances. A system of checks and balances is an integral part of record management. Generally, the check-and-balance status of accounts is examined monthly by comparing the total of all accounts with outstanding balances against the running total taken from the daily logs of all financial transactions. The practice's accountant will also closely scrutinize these records at scheduled intervals for tax-reporting purposes.

Although manual accounting systems are still used widely, computer accounting is available as part of most medical software packages, and the many advantages include efficient tracking and analysis of critical information, improved productivity, and smarter business decisions. General ledger, payables, receivables, inventory, purchasing, cash flow, bank reconciliation, collections, fixed assets, and many other applications integrate with each other so you can manage the office's core processes efficiently and effectively.

ACCOUNTING CYCLE

The finances of medical practices operate in one of two 12-month intervals or durations. The office **accounting cycle** follows either a fiscal year (a consecutive 12-month period starting with a specified date) or a calendar year (January through December). The yearly interval used depends on the way the practice's accountant has structured the business. For example, the medical practice can exist as a sole proprietorship or as a professional corporation.

The federal **Internal Revenue Service** (IRS) examines a business's income statements for the amount of profit and owed tax four times a year by quarterly estimated tax returns. The practice's annual tax return is a summary of the quarterly returns and reports the final year-end profit or loss (income minus expenses equals profit or loss) for the fiscal or calendar reporting period. If financial records are scrupulously maintained all year, preparation of the annual income tax return should merely be a summation of existing accounting facts. Well-maintained office records not only facilitate IRS returns but also provide data that define the practice's business picture.

There are many reasons for a physician along with an accountant to review financial data on a regular basis. Financial records reflect growing expenditures and growth in the business. Conclusions drawn from financial data can affect future financial decisions. For example, analysis of the practice's accounts receivable can predict the amount of salary increases. Tax records must be available in case of an IRS inquiry or **audit** (review of accounts). Records such as receipts should be retained for 7 years, but records such as bank statements, canceled checks, and IRS tax returns should be kept for the duration of the business.

RECORD-KEEPING COMPONENTS

The practice's financial records should include a running record of income, accounts receivable, and total expenditures, including **payroll** (employee salaries), cash on hand, and **liabilities** (amounts the practice owes). Expenditures can be broken down into categories (Box 15-1). This is important because it enables the record keeper to track the practice's expenses and provide the physician and accountant with a cohesive picture of the practice's expenses at tax time.

Categories can be accommodated by several types of bookkeeping systems; a simple business checkbook does not allow this. Pegboard systems allow the bookkeeper to write the check once over the **check register** (a place to record checks) or the ledger sheet and then have multiple pages with columns to distribute an expense into categories, including a back sheet for payroll. These columns are totaled and balanced at the completion of each check register sheet and can be subtotaled monthly, quarterly, and annually (discussed later in the chapter). Keeping a monthly accounts payable disbursement sheet lets the administrative medical assistant easily compare past years' expenses for the same part of the year.

Box 15-1

CATEGORIES OF EXPENDITURES

- Office supplies: items used by the facility's employees, such as paper, pencils, day sheets, ledger cards
- Medical supplies: items used for patients, such as examination gowns, electrocardiograph paper, syringes, tongue depressors
- Drugs: drug purchases, such as injectables; some facilities keep a separate column for these purchases and others put this amount in the medical supplies category
- Payroll: gross amount paid to employees
- Taxes: taxes paid, such as FICA, Medicare, federal withholding, state withholding, listed separately
- Rent: amount paid to rent the facility
- Utilities: gas, electric, telephone
- Maintenance: routine care of the facility, such as cleaning personnel
- Travel: physician's car lease payment, gas mileage if paid to employees, and so on
- Personal: any money used personally by the physician

Software packages offer the most sophisticated way to maintain financial records, not just for the categorization of expenses but also for the rapid formation of financial reports. Automating accounts payable does, however, require a personal computer (PC), software, and the training to use it.

There are advantages and disadvantages to both computer systems and paper records. Each practice should make this decision based on its particular volume and needs. Either system (pegboard or computer) can provide the practice and its accountant with the ability to pay and track expenses and to furnish the financial data necessary to create reports.

Multiple **summation reports**, such as the payroll report, itemized category report, account balances, and the **profit-and-loss statement**, must be prepared for the practice's accountant. If financial data are entered diligently into the bookkeeping system, preparing monthly, quarterly, or yearly reports should not be a daunting task. Income tax accounting cycles are divided into quarters: January through March, April through June, July through September, and October through December. Payroll reports show the amount of taxes being withheld and made monthly, quarterly, or annually. Normally, the practice's accountant will send you necessary reports and have you mail the checks.

ACCOUNTS PAYABLE

Ordering Goods and Services

There are many economical ways to purchase office supplies or equipment. For instance, purchasing cooperatives (co-ops) offer bulk rate discounts by allowing physicians to order in a pool with other purchasers. Vendors may offer discounts for buying in volume or for paying promptly. Large warehouse-type merchandisers and companies with discount catalogs also offer competitive prices. Researching and cost-comparing office products and medical supplies can be time consuming, but it is worth the effort, especially for items used frequently. Compare past invoices with prices in new catalogs.

Besides cost, other considerations come to bear when purchasing office supplies. For example, office supply companies often provide free delivery, but office warehouse chains may charge a fee or require a minimum order for free delivery. Quality also plays a role. Supplies should be of standard quality as well as economical. It is common to use several office supply vendors according to quality or pricing of specific goods.

Office supplies or equipment can be ordered in a number of ways. Once an account is set up, offices can place orders by telephone, fax, mail, or e-mail. These orders can be paid monthly by check or by credit card. It is preferable to pay for supplies by check or credit card rather than by cash, but when cash purchases are necessary, retain a detailed receipt for tax purposes. Credit card purchases can be made over the telephone or by mail, but for security reasons, credit card account numbers should not be faxed.

When placing orders for supplies, give the office's account number to the vendor or write it on the order form. It is a good idea to use a **purchase order** that lists the supplies ordered and their order numbers, so that order numbers for frequently ordered items can be pulled from the previous purchase order; this saves time with subsequent orders. Be sure to record the charges for your order and verify them against the bill later. It is also handy to keep a list of all vendors, telephone numbers, and account numbers.

Checkpoint Question

1. When purchasing office supplies, what factors besides price should you consider?

Receiving Supplies

When goods are delivered to the office, a receipt or **packing slip** listing the enclosed items should always accompany the order. The office staff member who receives the supplies must check the packing slip against the actual contents to ensure that all supplies are in the shipment. The person should initial the packing slip, which shows that all goods were received. When it is time to issue checks for payables, the assistant can then pay the **invoice** or bill. These receipts or packing slips should be placed in a bills pending file, so that they may be compared to the bill when it arrives. If the bill has already been paid by check or credit card, the invoice should be placed in the appropriate accounts paid file; there should be such a file for each fiscal or calendar year.

Paying Invoices

Invoices for supplies and other types of bills payable by the practice should be kept together in a bills pending file to avoid loss or misplacement of a bill. Bills can be paid daily, weekly, biweekly, or monthly.

Manual Payment

Manual payment of bills requires a checkbook and checks. The practice's accountant may recommend use of a log or record book into which is entered information about each check, such as payroll taxes or the breakdown of expenses for a monthly credit card bill. The large checks and checkbooks available from banks and business printers offer more space for writing memos or itemizing a check. Each check, once written, is detached from a **check stub**, which remains in the checkbook. If you make a mistake while writing a check, void the check and stub and staple the voided check to the stub. Never make corrections on the facility's checks. Check stubs should be filed with other fiscal or calendar year records and kept for the life of the practice.

The information recorded on the check stub includes the check number, the date the check was issued, the payee (the party to whom the check was written), and the full amount of the check. Notes should be written on both the memo section of the check and on the check stub. For example, when entering the purchase of a new beeper, the note might read, "payee: Office Communications" or "new beeper for Dr. Smith." The check is then attached to the bill or invoice and signed by an authorized individual.

Memos or notations on check stubs can be referenced later if a question arises concerning payment by a particular check. A log or record book enables the bookkeeper to make entries for each expense, categorize expenses, and maintain detailed payroll records. Unlike one-write (pegboard) or computer systems, multiple entries must be made by hand to track office bill paying. This can seem laborious when compared to other bookkeeping systems, but it may be ideal for smaller practices.

Pegboard Payment

The same pegboard system that is used for accounts receivable (see Chapter 14) may be used for bill paying; it has several advantages over the ordinary manual method of paying bills. Instead of using a day sheet, a **check register** page is used to record the checks that have been written. The check is then aligned on the pegboard over the register page and is filled out as with any other check (Fig. 15-1). Pegboard checks have a carbon or transfer strip, and on this strip is written the date, the payee, the check number, and the amount. The information written on the strip is recorded automatically on the check register. These check-writing systems are referred to as one-write systems for this reason. The check can be addressed directly beneath the payee line and mailed in a window envelope, which saves the time it would take to address an envelope.

The pegboard check register has approximately 20 columns that can be used to categorize expenses, such as rent, insurance, office supplies, utilities, service contracts, postage, and any other applicable categories. All entries on the check register are totaled when the register is completed;

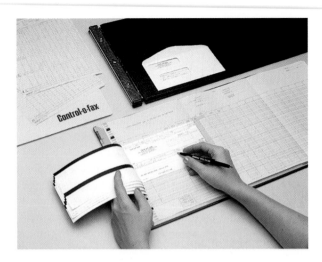

FIGURE 15–1. Sample pegboard check and check register. (Courtesy of Control-o-fax, Waterloo, IA.)

these totals are carried forward to the new register page. Each fiscal or calendar year begins with a new first page (page 1), and the last check register page will have totals for the entire year. The check register provides a system of checks and balances even before the bank statement arrives because the check register must be balanced, as with a bank statement.

The check register also allows entries for bank deposits, and the back page of the register is used for payroll record keeping. As with pegboard accounts receivable, completed pegboard check registers are filed in a separate binder in chronological order, with the most recent register on top.

Computer Payment

A computer accounts payable system has all the advantages that a pegboard system offers: access at a glance to check registers, itemized categories and their totals, payroll records, and entries for bank deposits. To use such a system, you must have a PC, accounts payable program software, printer, and bank checks that are compatible with the software and printer. The initial expense with a computer system is much higher than that of manual or pegboard systems. Office personnel will need computer training to use the program. Also, since it runs on electricity, a computer may not work during power failures. A good computer accounting program will, however, provide functions for both accounts receivable and accounts payable. Financial data should be recorded in three forms: on the computer's hard drive, on a magnetic tape or floppy disk, and in printout form (hard copy).

Although entering data in the computer at first may be time consuming, this becomes less of a concern with practice. Furthermore, financial reports can be compiled and printed in a fraction of the time required with manual or pegboard systems. The computer program can also perform the record-keeping arithmetic; as a result, mathematical errors are practically nonexistent.

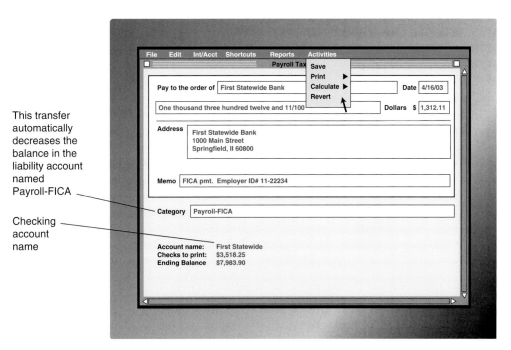

FIGURE 15–2.
Computer screen showing a check for payroll taxes.

This transfer automatically decreases the balance in the liability account named Payroll-FICA

Checking account name

Paying bills by computer requires using the software to open the check-writing file. Checks are presented on the computer screen in the same way that a paper check would normally appear (Fig. 15-2), and the information that is required to appear on the check is entered on the computer keyboard. The information is stored and the check is printed out; the computer program automatically subtracts the amount of the check from the account's balance. The bookkeeper can print one check at a time or a batch of checks together.

The computer can "memorize" checks so that the information on them can be recalled and reprinted without reentering it; this is especially helpful with payroll checks. A good accounting program also allows for bill reminders and disk or magnetic tape backup reminders. Of course, it is essential to back up financial data on magnetic tapes or floppy disks in case of computer problems.

Checkpoint Question

2. Whether using a manual, pegboard, or computer accounts payable system, two steps must always occur when ordering and receiving supplies. What are they?

PAYROLL

Types of Payroll Systems

The medical office will have payroll obligations to its staff, and federal, state, and, possibly, local payroll taxes will be due. The administrative medical assistant may issue payroll checks for the practice's entire staff, including the physician, or just for the office staff. Or an outside payroll service may be retained to issue the checks and keep the records. These payroll services specialize in computing, withholding, and paying taxes and payroll for businesses. Such a firm can provide all of these services for considerably less than it would cost for office time and personnel or for an accountant. The larger the practice's staff, the more economical a payroll service becomes. Firms that provide payroll services are especially cost effective, in that they are highly accurate, aware of changes in tax laws, and legally liable.

Generally, payroll checks for the medical office will be issued at one of the following intervals:

- Weekly (52 pay periods per year)
- Biweekly (26 pay periods per year)
- Monthly (12 pay periods per year)

The pay period is set up by your employer and is the same for all employees.

There are various ways to record payroll expenditures, depending on what type of bookkeeping system is used by the office.

Manual Payroll Systems

When payroll checks are issued manually without a pegboard system, separate payroll records must be kept. The check stub will indicate to whom the check was issued, in what amount, and on what date. A separate record or log book must be maintained to keep track of gross income and tax withholdings for each employee. These withholdings should be totaled monthly, quarterly, and annually; for this reason, it is advisable to maintain payroll records in a timely manner throughout the year.

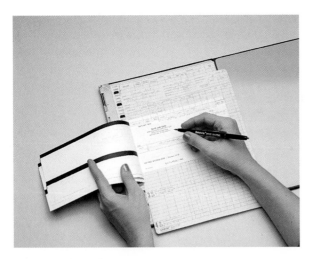

FIGURE 15–3. Sample pegboard payroll journal. (Courtesy of Control-o-fax, Waterloo, IA.)

Pegboard Payroll Systems

The pegboard system allows for payroll entries as well as the accumulation of payroll data by using an employee payroll record form and the correlating back page of each check register, called the **payroll journal** (Fig. 15-3). Procedure 15-1 outlines the steps in issuing a payroll check using the pegboard system.

Computer Payroll Systems

Payroll records can be maintained with various software packages; many such packages integrate payroll with other accounting functions, such as accounts receivable and accounts payable. Computer programs can calculate tax withholdings automatically, record payroll data, and print payroll checks. In most cases, a computer program provides substantial time savings over manual and pegboard payroll systems.

Employee Records

Regardless of the payroll system used, it is necessary to maintain an individual file for each employee that contains pertinent employment information. The personnel file should include the following information:

- Employee's original résumé or completed job application
- Job references
- Hourly rate or salary at the time of hire
- Dates and amounts of pay raises
- Job evaluations
- All employee withholding authorization forms, such as W-4 forms (discussed later)
- Pension plan, health, and life insurance paperwork
- Vital facts about the employee (e.g., date of birth, name of spouse, Social Security number, address and telephone number, name and daytime phone number of emergency contact person)

Tax Withholdings

Federal, state, and, possibly, local taxes must be withheld from employees' paychecks; for this reason, each employee must complete a W-4 form on the first day of hire. This form must be completed by the employee before the first pay period; otherwise, you are required to withhold taxes at the highest rate, which classifies the person as single with no dependents. The W-4 form lists the employee's name, Social Security number, address, marital status, and the number of exemptions to be used in the calculation of tax withholding. If any of the information contained on an employee's W-4 form changes, the employee must fill out a new form, which is placed in the personnel file.

The federally mandated taxes are Social Security (**FICA**), Medicare, and federal income tax. Each of these taxes is based on a percentage of total gross income; the federal income tax also factors in marital status and the number of withholding exemptions claimed on the W-4 form.

Box 15-2 features the information needed to calculate employee withholding manually by using the combination method found on the IRS website. Procedure 15-2 outlines the steps for calculating the amount of an employee's paycheck.

The employer must match the amount withheld from each employee's paycheck for Social Security and Medicare taxes. For example, if $150 is withheld from an employee's paycheck for Medicare and Social Security taxes, the employer must pay $300 to the IRS ($150 withheld from the employee plus $150 matching amount). The employer does not match federal, state, or local taxes. The practice's accountant should inform the office bookkeeper of tax rates and withholdings. Usually, each pay period or at least monthly you will deposit the federal taxes withheld from all employees plus doubled FICA in an account at a federal depository (normally the facility's bank). Your accountant normally will send you the estimated federal depository slips for this purpose.

The employer must also pay a **federal unemployment tax** (FUTA) for each employee based on that employee's gross income. The amount of this tax is calculated by the practice's accountant and paid either quarterly or annually. Individual states may levy their own unemployment tax. The practice's accountant calculates this tax.

Other withholdings from an employee's paycheck might include health, life, or disability premiums; pension plan contributions; or court-ordered garnishment of wages owed to a third party.

Checkpoint Question

3. What taxes must be withheld from an employee's paycheck?

Box 15-2

CALCULATING PAYROLL WITHHOLDING USING THE COMBINATION METHOD

Combined Income Tax, Employee Social Security Tax, and Employee Medicare Tax Withholding Tables

If you want to combine amounts to be withheld as income tax, employee Social Security tax, and employee Medicare tax, you may use the combined tables found in the IRS publications for businesses. Combined withholding tables for single and married taxpayers are provided for weekly, biweekly, semimonthly, monthly, and daily or miscellaneous payroll periods. The payroll period and marital status of the employee determine the table to be used.

If the wages are greater than the highest wage bracket in the applicable table, you must use one of the other methods for figuring income tax withholding described in the publication or in circular E. For wages that do not exceed $84,900, the combined Social Security tax rate and Medicare tax rate is 7.65% each for the employee and the employer for wages paid in 2002. You can figure the employee Social Security tax by multiplying the wages by 6.2%, and you can figure the employee Medicare tax by multiplying the wages by 1.45%.

The combined tables give the correct total withholding only if wages for Social Security and Medicare taxes and income tax withholding are the same. When you have paid more than the maximum amount of wages subject to Social Security tax ($84,900 in 2003) in a calendar year, you may not use the combined tables.

If you use the combined withholding tables, use the following steps to find the amounts to report on your form 941, employer's quarterly federal tax return:

1. Employee Social Security tax withheld: Multiply the wages by 6.2%.
2. Employee Medicare tax withheld: Multiply the wages by 1.45%.
3. Income tax withheld: Subtract the amounts from steps 1 and 2 from the total tax withheld.
4. You can figure the amounts to be shown on form W-2, wage and tax statement, in the same way.

Courtesy of the IRS website.

Payment of Taxes

Payroll taxes are paid according to different schedules as determined by the IRS and the state and local tax authorities. Federal taxes, such as Social Security, Medicare, and federal income tax, must be paid monthly, bimonthly, or more frequently, depending on the size of the gross payroll. Always re-

member to match the Medicare and Social Security payments withheld from the employee's check (the amount withheld × 2). These payments are made on IRS form 941 for deposit requirements; the IRS furnishes these forms free of charge.

If the total federal taxes due are more than $3000, these payroll taxes must be paid within 3 calendar days of the time the payroll check was issued. State taxes that are withheld from the employee's pay check are usually paid by mail and must be paid and mailed before the tax due date to avoid penalties.

The IRS also requires the employer to file quarterly returns for all federal taxes withheld; these returns are due by April 30, July 31, October 31, and January 31 each year. This quarterly return is a summary of the Social Security, Medicare, and federal wage taxes paid. State quarterly returns have the same due dates and are usually paid by mail. Your accountant will keep you informed of taxes due.

W-2 Forms

At the end of the calendar year, all pertinent payroll information should be summarized for each employee and made available to the practice's accountant. The W-2 statement provided to the employee by January 31 of each year should list the following information:

- Total gross income for the previous year
- Total federal, state, and local taxes withheld
- Any taxable fringe benefits
- The employee's total net income

Checkpoint Question

4. What information does the employee list on the W-4 form? What happens if this information changes?

PREPARATION OF REPORTS

The bookkeeper must also prepare reports for the practice's accountant or the IRS, based on financial data stored in the office's bookkeeping system. For this reason, care should always be taken when recording financial data.

WHAT IF

The medical practice where you work did not pay its payroll taxes. What can happen?

The IRS charges penalties and interest on all unpaid taxes. The IRS can attach the business and its assets and close the business.

Ñ Spanish Terminology

Los impuestos deben ser sacados de su cheque.	Taxes must be taken out of your paycheck.
Usted necesita completar estas formas.	You need to complete these forms.
Gracias para su pago.	Thank you for your payment.
Gracias para su cheque.	Thank you for your check.
Esto es su recibo.	This is your receipt.

The manual system, when assisted by the use of a log or record book, should be able to provide monthly, quarterly, and annual summaries for income, expenditures, and payroll. It is advisable to have subtotals and totals for these periods for tax payment purposes.

The pegboard system is also practical for providing summaries of income, expenses, and payroll and can be totaled monthly, quarterly, and yearly. Each day sheet, check register, and payroll journal is individually totaled, with all balances forwarded to the next page. These records are stored in binders and kept for future reference.

A computer system of accounting offers all of the previously mentioned reports along with other more complicated reports that generally require more advanced accounting skills. The great advantage with report generating by computer is that the computer will perform all of the mathematical calculations for the time frame requested.

ASSISTING WITH AUDITS

An **audit** may be informal (in-house) and used to assist the practice's accountant with tax preparation, or it may be formal audits by the IRS. If meticulous attention to record keeping has been paid throughout the year, the preparation time needed for such an audit should be minimal. It is important to save all bank statements, copies of annual and quarterly tax returns, and receipts for expenditures. Canceled checks and payroll records should be readily available.

Manual and pegboard systems can provide spending category and payroll summaries in addition to examination of the actual entries for the period being audited. A computer accounting system can provide all of this plus reports such as profit-and-loss statements, which normally would be compiled by an accountant.

Procedure 15-1

Issuing a Payroll Check Using the Pegboard System

Equipment/Supplies

- Pegboard with checks
- Carbon paper
- Payroll register
- Tax tables
- Calculator
- Time card

Steps	Reason
1. Align the carbon or transfer strip at the top of the check on the employee's payroll record, then align both on the payroll journal.	The write-it-once system will eliminate the need to post information more than one time.
2. Enter the employee's name first, followed by the check number, the payroll period, and the **gross income** (the amount of money an employee earned before taxes are withheld) plus any additional earnings.	The employee's name must be entered to issue a payroll check. The pay period indicates to the employee the time frame of the checks.
3. From the gross income, subtract federal, state, and local taxes and Social Security; this is called tax **withholding**. See Procedure 15-2.	Witholdings must be subtracted from gross income to issue a payroll check.
4. Enter the **net pay** (amount of money an employee is paid after taxes are withheld) on the detachable payroll slip. Fold this slip behind the check.	When the check is placed in the envelope, this information will not be visible, which will protect the employee's privacy.
5. Total the payroll journal as each page is completed.	Total amounts of income and tax withholdings should be accrued for each quarter for tax-reporting purposes.

Procedure 15-2

Calculate the Amount of an Employee's Payroll Check

Equipment/Supplies

- Calculator
- W-4 form

Steps	Reason
1. Calculate the number of hours worked from the employee's time card or record.	The employee's payroll check is based on the number of hours worked.
2. Calculate the employee's annual gross wage using this formula: Hourly wage × number of hours worked per week × 52 (number of weeks in a year) = gross annual wage Assume an employee earns $7 per hour and works 40 hours per week: $7 × 40 × 52 = $14,560 annual gross wage	The annual gross wage must be calculated to determine the employee's payroll check amount.
3. If your pay period is • Biweekly, then ÷ this sum by 26 • Monthly, then ÷ this sum by 12 • Weekly, then ÷ this sum by 52	This converts the gross wage into paycheck amounts.
4. Divide by 52 weeks in a year and then divide by 5 (work days in a week) to get the amount of a day's pay.	Always go to the yearly gross wage when figuring deductions or increases to gross wages; you will get the exact amount.
5. Deduct this amount from the gross wage to get the adjusted gross wage from which you will withhold taxes. Using the example above, the calculation would be as follows: ($14,560 ÷ 52) = $280 = week's pay $280 ÷ 5 = $56 = day's pay $280 − $56 = $224 (adjusted gross wage)	The adjusted gross wage is needed to calculate withholding taxes.
6. Calculate any overtime worked.	Overtime is defined as hours worked over the normal for the pay period. Overtime is calculated by paying 1.5 times the normal hourly wage. If the employee earns $7 per hour, overtime pay would be calculated by dividing $7 in half ($3.50) and adding that amount to the hourly wage: the hourly pay rate for overtime would be $10.50.
7. Refer to the appropriate tax tables (e.g., federal, FICA, Medicare, state taxes) for the deductions for taxes.	The tax tables will specify the amount of withholdings.
8. Subtract the taxes from the gross or adjusted gross wages to obtain net pay.	The net pay amount is the result of the gross wages minus the withholdings
9. Write the payroll check for this amount.	The net pay is the amount of the payroll check.

CHAPTER SUMMARY

Accounting is a complex process involving many legal issues. As a medical assistant, you must keep neat and well-organized accounting records. You also will be expected to understand how to order goods and services efficiently and economically and how to pay invoices. In addition, you must understand the payroll process. With the computer being used for many administrative medical office functions, it is imperative that you keep abreast of changes and new opportunities to make this process more efficient and up-to-date.

Critical Thinking Challenges

1. Explain the advantages of manual, pegboard, and computer accounting systems. In what instances would each be the preferred method?
2. A vendor continually mixes up your orders, and the physician asks you to look for a new vendor. How do you decide which one to recommend? What factors influence your choice of one office supply vendor over another?
3. An employee gets divorced. She is irate when she gets her W-2 form and discovers that her deductions were still being based on her married filing status. What is your response? What should you do now?
4. The physician asks you, the office manager, how much money is owed to him. How do you gather the information needed to answer his question?

Answers to Checkpoint Questions

1. Besides cost, consider delivery charges and product quality when purchasing office supplies.
2. The bookkeeper must write out a purchase order and compare the packing slip and final invoice to the purchase order.
3. Social Security, Medicare, and federal, state, and local wage taxes must be withheld from an employee's paycheck.
4. The employee provides his or her name, Social Security number, marital status, current address, and number of withholding exemptions. If any of this information changes, the employee must complete a new W-4 form.

 ### Websites

The Accounting Library (TAL)
    www.accountinglibrary.com
Quickbooks Online
    www.quickbooks.com
Microsoft Business Solutions
    www.microsoft.com/businesssolutions
Internal Revenue Services
    www.irs.gov
Payroll Taxes
    www.payroll.com

16

Health Insurance

CHAPTER OUTLINE

ROLE DELINEATION COMPONENTS

ADMINISTRATIVE: Administrative Procedures
- Perform basic administrative medical assisting functions
- Understand and apply third-party guidance
- Obtain reimbursement through accurate claims submission
- Monitor third-party reimbursement
- Understand and adhere to managed care policies and procedures

ADMINISTRATIVE: Practice Finances
- Apply bookkeeping principles
- Manage accounts receivable
- Manage accounts payable
- Document and maintain accounting and banking records

CHAPTER COMPETENCIES

LEARNING OBJECTIVES
Upon successfully completing this chapter, you will be able to:
1. Spell and define the key terms
2. Describe group, individual, and government-sponsored (public) health benefits and explain the differences between them
3. Explain the differences between Medicare and Medicaid
4. List the information required on a medical claim form and explain why each piece of information is needed
5. Name two legal issues affecting claims submissions
6. Explain how managed care programs work
7. Explain the differences between health maintenance organizations, preferred provider organizations, and physician hospital organizations

PERFORMANCE OBJECTIVES
Upon successfully completing this chapter, you will be able to:
1. Fill out a CMS-1500 claim form

KEY TERMS

assignment of benefits
balance billing
birthday rule
capitation
carrier
claims
claims administrator
coinsurance
coordination of benefits
co-payments

crossover claim
deductible
dependent
eligibility
employee
explanation of benefits (EOB)
fee-for-service
fee schedule
group member

health maintenance organization (HMO)
independent practice association (IPA)
insurance
insured
managed care
Medicare
peer review organization
physician hospital organization

plan maximum
preexisting condition
preferred provider organization (PPO)
third-party administrator
unbundling
usual, customary, and reasonable (UCR)
utilization review

BEFORE 1930, ACCESS TO medical care in the United States was based on ability to pay. In 1929, Baylor University introduced a plan to provide schoolteachers 21 days of hospital care for $6 per year. The idea quickly spread to other Dallas employers, and the organization known as Blue Cross was born. Health plans were originally designed to protect families from catastrophic financial burdens in the event of a serious illness or accident. By 1939, the Blue Cross symbol was adopted by the American Hospital Association as an endorsement that health plans met guidelines established by its member hospitals.

In the Pacific Northwest, lumber and mining companies wanted to provide outpatient care to their employees as well. They paid monthly fees to groups of physicians to provide care for their employees. This model led to the first Blue Shield plan, founded in California.

Blue Cross and Blue Shield as we know them today are actually a federation of more than 42 independent companies that insure about 30% of the U. S. population.

While the **insurance** industry was developing in the United States, other countries took a different approach to providing health care to their residents. Canada, for example, established publicly funded universal health insurance. This type of coverage provides hospital and physician services with no deductibles, **co-payments**, or dollar limits on coverage for insured services and is funded by tax revenues.

In the United States, health insurance is funded by a combination of employer and employee contributions and tax-funded coverage.

Today, virtually every state has a Blue Cross and a Blue Shield plan. Health benefits also are provided by insurance companies, self-funded group plans, and government plans such as Medicare and Medicaid. The benefits vary with each plan and from state to state. Approximately 80% of Americans are enrolled in health benefits plans of one sort or another. Consequently, most of the patients you will encounter in the physician's office have some type of health insurance. As a medical assistant, you will need to understand the differences in health benefits plans and the requirements of each so that you can complete and file claim forms appropriately. You will also need to learn the special terminology associated with health insurance claims. In addition, you may need to instruct patients about insurance matters.

HEALTH BENEFITS PLANS

Group Health Benefits

Group health benefits are sponsored by an organization, such as an employer, a union, or an association. A person covered by group health benefits is either an **employee** or a **group member**, who by virtue of employment or membership in an organization may participate in and receive benefits from a health plan. Coverage in health plans differs greatly, so you need to know the **eligibility** of the patient for services being provided by your office. For example, birth control is frequently not covered unless there is medical necessity.

Benefits may be either **insured** or self-funded. Commonly, health benefits are referred to as insurance. It is, however, important to distinguish between the actual benefits and the vehicle used to fund and provide them.

With insured benefits, the employer, employee, or both pay a monthly premium to an insurance company. The insurance company, in turn, is obligated to pay for any eligible health benefits. Self-funded benefits on the surface appear the same as insured benefits. They are paid for in the same manner as group health benefits, but instead of the employer paying the insurance company to invest the money to cover payments, they invest it themselves. They pay an insurance company or other agency to process **claims** and make payments on their behalf. Any payment for medical services that are not paid by the patient or physician is said to be paid by a *third-party payer*. In this case, the payer is an agent for the self-funded plan and is, therefore, known as a **third-party administrator** (TPA). Many employers now choose to self-fund their group benefit plans rather than insure them.

You will need to be aware of these funding differences as they relate to state and federal regulations. For instance, insured benefit plans are subject to state regulations. Many states mandate that certain types of benefits be included in any insurance plan. These mandated benefits vary from state to state but often include such medical services as childhood immunizations, routine diagnostic care, and treatment for substance abuse.

Although it would seem that these are routine medical services, many insurance companies consider them outside the scope of treating physical illness. Screening for illness, psychiatric illness, and prevention of illness by immunization are not routinely covered.

For a group benefit plan to cover (pay for) eligible expenses, the patient must meet several criteria, called eligibility requirements. These are defined in the policy or plan document and may include a minimum number of hours worked per week and a waiting period from the date of employment before benefits become effective.

The eligibility of a **dependent** (spouse, children) is based on the employee's eligibility. Certain eligibility limitations apply to dependent children. For example, children are usually eligible until they reach the limiting age defined by the plan. The age limitation is usually extended if the child is a full-time student. Eligibility usually requires that children be the unmarried natural or adopted children of the employee, unmarried stepchildren, or children for whom the employee has legal guardianship.

To confirm a patient's eligibility, call the **claims administrator** for the health benefits plan. A provider inquiry telephone number is commonly included on the patient's identification (ID) card (Fig. 16-1).

Group and individual health benefits describe contractual agreements and how the policies are paid. Both group and in-

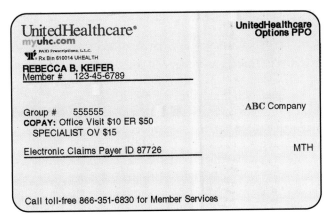

FIGURE 16-1. Sample identification card for a managed care plan.

dividual policies can be many different types of plans, such as traditional, HMO, and PPO. These types are further discussed later in this chapter.

 Checkpoint Question

1. What is the difference between an insured benefits plan and one that is self-funded?

Individual Health Benefits

Individual health benefits policies are purchased by an individual from an insurance company. The individual pays premiums directly to the insurance company, and the insurance company pays either the doctor or the hospital directly if they are a participating provider or reimburses the individual for eligible medical expenses.

For patients with individual health benefits, the criteria for completing and filing claims are the same as for patients with group health benefits. Individual health policies commonly have less generous coverage, however, than group health plans have. An individual policy may also have a rider that limits or eliminates benefits for certain illnesses or injuries, based on the determination of the underwriter at the time the policy was issued. Box 16-1 outlines the requirements of the Health Insurance Portability and Accountability Act of 1996 (HIPAA), which include a provision to protect employees changing jobs from being denied benefits for preexisting conditions.

With the cost of health care skyrocketing and more insurance companies limiting what they will cover, many people have more than one health care insurance policy. It is extremely important that you know which insurance you bill first (primary) and which to bill the remainder of the charges (secondary).

Government-Sponsored (Public) Health Benefits

Government-sponsored benefit programs are funded and regulated by the federal government or individual states. Government programs have been developed over the years to assist persons who do not otherwise have health benefits, such as the elderly, the indigent, and others unable to obtain benefits. Government programs include Medicare, Medicaid, TRICARE/CHAMPVA, and workers' compensation.

Box 16-1

REQUIREMENTS OF HIPAA

As discussed in earlier chapters, the Health Insurance Portability and Accountability Act of 1996 brought about changes in the health care industry that protect patients and health care providers. According to the HIPAA website, **www.cms.gov/hipaa**, the following provisions are now in effect:

- HIPAA contains provisions for insured persons enrolled in employer-sponsored insurance programs without regard to their health status if they change employment.
- HIPAA prohibits the use of genetic testing information to deny health insurance coverage.
- HIPAA provides tax incentives for the purchase of long-term care insurance.
- HIPAA requires the adoption of new standards for financial and administrative electronic transmission of claims, new standards for claims attachments, and standardization of diagnostic and procedure coding.
- HIPAA strengthens existing regulations for fraud and abuse in the system.
- HIPAA Administrative Simplification: These HIPAA requirements, which are separate from the insurance portability requirements, are intended to reduce the costs and administrative burdens of health care by making possible the standardized electronic transmission of many administrative and financial transactions.
- HIPAA adds guidelines for confidentiality issues in electronic medical records, as discussed in Chapter 8.

Medicare

In 1965, the Social Security Act established **Medicare** to provide health insurance for the elderly. Elderly persons were defined as Social Security recipients age 65 or older. In 1972, amendments to the Social Security Act expanded Medicare coverage to two additional high-risk groups: disabled persons who have been receiving Social Security benefits for 24 months and persons suffering from end-stage renal disease.

Medicare Part A covers hospital expenses and is provided at no additional charge to persons eligible for Social Security benefits. Medicare Part B pays for physician fees, both inpatient and outpatient, diagnostic testing, certain immunizations (influenza and pneumonia), and specific screening tests (PSA, mammograms, Pap smears, bone density testing, colorectal screening). Part B Medicare is optional, and the participant is charged a monthly fee. The fee is deducted from the monthly Social Security payment.

Persons signing up for or receiving Social Security benefits are automatically enrolled in both Part A and Part B Medicare when they reach 65. If they do not wish to participate in Part B, they must decline it. Both Part A and Part B of Medicare have deductibles and co-payments, and as with most health insurance policies, these generally increase yearly.

A patient with Medicare coverage who is actively employed and covered by the employer's plan will have secondary Medicare benefits. A retired person age 65 or over who has health insurance in addition to Medicare will have primary Medicare benefits. Physicians are required to submit claims to Medicare on behalf of Medicare patients. These claims must be filed within 1 year of the time the service is incurred. (See section on filing claims for more information.)

After the **deductible** has been met, Medicare Part B reimburses the physician 80% of the Medicare-approved charges. The patient is responsible for the remaining 20% of the Medicare-approved fee. Under certain circumstances, if paying the 20% causes undue financial hardship, the physician may not charge the remaining 20%. The Centers for Medicare & Medicaid Services (CMS) can provide forms with the requirements, and the forms should always be used. In addition to Medicare, the Social Security Act of 1965 established Medicaid, a program of health care coverage for the poor. If patients are financially unable to pay the 20%, they may be eligible for Medicaid. This is referred to as a **crossover claim** because the patient is eligible under both Medicare and Medicaid and the claim crosses over automatically from one coverage to the other. In this situation, Medicare is primary and Medicaid is secondary. Medicare will accept original claims (no copies) filed on CMS-1500 universal claim forms only.

The CMS, which was known as the Health Care Financing Administration (HCFA) prior to July 1, 2001, is a government agency that oversees the financial aspects of health care in the United States (Box 16-2). The CMS has adopted a revised Current Procedural Terminology (CPT) coding

system that must be used for Medicare claims. Medicare B claims use the standard CPT codes. For equipment, supplies, and services not listed in the CPT code, the CMS has established the Healthcare Common Procedure Coding System (HCPCS) codes. (See Chapters 17 and 18.)

It is important to inquire of the patient regarding supplemental or secondary coverage. This policy, which patients may purchase on their own, covers charges not covered by Medicare. In this case, filing a second claim is necessary.

Checkpoint Question

2. What is the difference between parts A and B of Medicare coverage?

Medicaid

Medicaid provides health benefits to low-income or indigent persons of all ages. Often, eligibility for Medicaid is based on a patient's eligibility for other state programs, such as welfare assistance. The federal government provides funds to each state for Medicaid costs; each state is required to provide a Medicaid program. Although the federal government

---

Box 16-2

WHAT IS THE CMS?

In 1977, the administration of the Medicare and Medicaid programs were combined under a single administrative agency. The administrator is appointed by the president of the United States and reports directly to the Secretary of Health and Human Services. Formerly known as HCFA, the CMS has become a big influence in the health care industry.

According to its website, **www.cms.gov**, the CMS is the federal agency that administers Medicare, Medicaid, and the State Children's Health Insurance Program (SCHIP). It provides health insurance for more than 74 million Americans. It also performs quality-focused activities, including regulation of laboratory testing, development of coverage policies, and quality-of-care improvement. The CMS maintains oversight of the survey and certification of nursing homes and continuing care providers, including home health agencies and intermediate-care facilities for the mentally retarded. It makes available to beneficiaries, providers, researchers, and state surveyors information about these activities and nursing home quality.

To ensure public and expert involvement in running their programs, the HCFA maintains a number of chartered advisory committees. These committees, whose meetings are open to the pubic, provide advice or make recommendations on a variety of issues relating to HCFA's responsibilities and activities.

Spanish Terminology

¿Tiene usted seguro médico?	*Do you have medical insurance?*
¿Qué es el nombre del seguro?	*What is the name of the insurance?*
¿Qué es el número de su póliza?	*What is the number of your policy?*
¿Va a pagar el hospital?	*Will it pay for the hospital?*
¿Tiene Medicare?	*Do you have Medicare?*
¿Tiene su tarjeta de Medicare?	*Do you have your Medicare card?*

stipulates the minimum health care coverage, states can provide coverage beyond the minimum. Therefore, Medicaid eligibility and benefits vary from state to state. At a minimum, Medicaid provides 100% coverage for the following:

- Inpatient hospital care
- Outpatient treatment and services
- Diagnostic services
- Family planning
- Skilled nursing facilities
- Diagnostic screenings for children

Many states have gone to a managed care type of Medicaid coverage in which recipients make a co-payment based on their income and are assigned a primary care physician as a gatekeeper.

Since circumstances that make recipients eligible for coverage change from month to month (i.e., employment), Medicaid patients receive a new ID card each month. Make a photocopy of the card for the patient's file on the first visit of each month. Most states require prior authorization by the Medicaid **carrier** before any services are rendered. Because reimbursement is considerably less than other insurances, not all physicians accept Medicaid patients, nor are they required to do so. If Medicaid patients are accepted, you need to be familiar with Medicaid as administered in your state.

Checkpoint Question

3. How often do Medicaid recipients receive a new card?

TRICARE/CHAMPVA

TRICARE, the new name for CHAMPUS, is administered by the U. S. Department of Defense and provides medical coverage for dependents of active service personnel, dependents of service personnel who died during active duty, and retired service personnel. When Congress realized that CHAMPUS costs could be controlled with managed care, they mandated that HMOs and PPOs (discussed later in this chapter) be added to the coverage. This three-part system is now called TRICARE. This system requires that participants

be assigned a primary care manager (PCM). The PCM is named on the beneficiary's card.

If a patient lives within 40 miles of a uniformed services hospital and that facility is unable to handle the needs of patients covered by TRICARE, a statement of unavailability is required for treatment by a physician's office or civilian hospital. Patients who live more than 40 miles from a uniformed services hospital do not need this statement to be treated in a physician's office or civilian hospital and for the physician or hospital to be reimbursed.

The Civilian Health and Medical Program of the Veterans Administration (CHAMPVA) covers dependents of veterans who have total and permanent service-connected disabilities. CHAMPVA is administered by the area Veterans Administration hospital. Once admitted to the CHAMPVA program, patients select their own physician; this allows them the same benefits as private insurance.

MANAGED CARE

Over the past 3 decades, health care costs in the United States have grown at about twice the general rate of inflation. As a result, the United States now spends more for health care services than any other industrialized nation, both as a percentage of gross national product and per person. At the same time, a smaller percentage of our population has health insurance coverage than in other advanced nations.

In the United States, most people obtain health coverage through their employer. The exceptions are Medicare for the

ETHICAL TIP

All patients must be treated equally and fairly. Financial issues regarding the patient's type of insurance or lack of insurance should have no bearing on the care provided. As a medical assistant, you must avoid stereotyping and care for the patient in an objective, professional manner.

elderly, TRICARE for the retired military and their dependents, Medicaid for low-income Americans, and those who do not have access to group coverage and buy coverage directly from insurers. In total, these programs cover fewer people than employment-based health plans.

The rapid rate of health care inflation has encouraged employers to begin offering **managed care** programs, which are typically less costly than traditional insurance coverage systems. Managed care programs vary greatly, but all involve a different relationship between the insurer, health care provider, and covered individual from that of traditional insurance programs. To understand this difference, we first discuss the traditional insurance system.

In traditional insurance systems, the covered patient may seek care from any provider. Normally, the patient and physician decide what care is needed. Then, services are rendered and the insurer pays a portion of the provider's bills (after deductibles and coinsurance). The insurer has no relationship with the provider.

In managed care systems, however, the insurer has a contractual relationship with the provider. The contract usually establishes what prices will be charged for each service and the conditions under which a service would be covered. Most managed care programs contain the following elements:

- *Precertification of hospital admissions* (often also called utilization management [UM] or utilization review [UR]). A patient can be admitted to a hospital for certain conditions only if that admission has been certified (approved) by the insurer. The goal of this requirement is to ensure that a patient's care is provided in the most cost-effective setting. For example, many surgical procedures that used to require an inpatient hospital stay can now be performed in an outpatient setting if proper education and support are available to the patient. Conflict between a UR guideline and the physician's requirements for the patient should be appealed to an impartial **peer review organization** composed of physicians and specialists who will review the case and make the final recommendation.
- *Approved referrals.* In many managed care plans a specialty physician can provide services to a managed care patient only on referral from the patient's primary care physician. The purpose is to ensure that the services provided by the specialist are medically necessary and, again, provided in the most cost-effective setting.
- *Network.* A network consists of providers (physicians, hospitals, pharmacies, and other providers and suppliers) who have signed contracts with the insurer or **health maintenance organization (HMO)** to provide services to covered persons in individual, group, or public health plans. A patient is normally required to use network providers to receive full coverage. The financial penalties (lost coverage) are often very high if a patient does not use these providers.
- *Assignment of benefits.* By contract, the network provider cannot bill the patient for any amounts not paid by the insurer (no **balance billing**) except for copayments, coinsurance, and deductibles. If payment for a service provided by a network physician or hospital is denied by the insurer because it was not properly authorized, the provider cannot bill the patient for these services unless the contract does not contain a hold-harmless clause for the patient. This puts teeth in the control features of the managed care program.

Most physicians have contracts with more than one managed care program, and each of these programs has it own requirements and reimbursement schedules. So that the physician can provide the patient with needed health care services, while ensuring that the physician is paid for his or her services, it is necessary to consider the requirements of each patient's program. UM or precertification requirements are extremely important. Check the patient's ID card for details. UM requirements may apply to inpatient services or to a variety of outpatient and doctor office services.

Until you are very familiar with the requirements of each of your patient's managed care programs, you should call the number on the ID card before a patient is admitted to a hospital (on a nonemergency basis), referred to another physician, or scheduled for specific laboratory, radiological, or other test or evaluation. For inpatient admissions, the UM firm may ask for the diagnosis, the procedure or procedures to be performed, and other related information before approving the admission. Once the procedure is approved, the UM firm may only approve a specified length of stay in the hospital. Failure to comply with the precertification requirements results in a financial penalty for the patient and possibly also for the physician and the hospital.

It is important to be familiar with physicians within the network. The physician, hospital, laboratory, or other provider you normally refer a patient to may not be in the patient's managed care network. By calling the UM number to check, you can avoid penalties and improve the satisfaction of the patient with your services.

 Checkpoint Question

4. What are the four key elements of a managed care program?

Health Maintenance Organizations

It is easiest to understand how a HMO functions if we contrast it with a traditional health insurance program. In the traditional insurance system, the relationship between the covered individual and the insurer or self-insurer is purely financial. In return for receiving a paid monthly premium, the insurer promises to reimburse (indemnify) the individual if he or she incurs certain types of covered medical expense. There are often limits to coverage (exclusions and limitations), and normally the coverage has a **deductible** (amount below which services are not reimbursable) and **coinsur-**

ance (the patient pays a percentage of the medical expense after the deductible is satisfied). For example, the patient pays the first $200 (deductible) in physician charges each year starting January 1; then insurance pays 80% of covered charges, and the patient must pay the other 20%.

The covered individual seeks medical services and thereby incurs an expense. The individual, not the insurer, must pay for this expense. If the medical treatment is covered as defined in the insurance policy, the insurer will reimburse the patient a portion of the amount incurred after deductibles and coinsurance.

In contrast to traditional insurance companies, a HMO promises to provide covered services rather than pay for them. In this respect, the HMO acts as both an insurer and a provider of service. HMO policies are written differently from insurance policies. The HMO policy lists the medical services that the member is entitled to receive and the physicians and hospitals that will provide these services. The HMO has a contract with both the patient and provider. It must provide covered services to the member either directly from its own physician staff and hospitals or indirectly from physicians and hospitals contracted to provide the services promised to the member. The HMO, rather than the patient, is responsible for the costs of medical services, and providers bill the HMO rather than the patient when a reimbursable service is rendered to a HMO member.

This is one reason HMOs do not normally use deductibles and coinsurance, which are standard features of health insurance programs. A patient does not receive a provider's bill, so deductibles and coinsurance cannot apply. Instead, HMOs use predetermined co-payments (e.g., $10 per physician office visit) to reduce premium prices.

Health maintenance organizations come in many forms. Kaiser Permanente Health Plan is generally recognized as the nation's first HMO (there were earlier organizational forms but none that lasted into the modern era). In the early 1930s, Kaiser Industries needed to provide physician services for its employees in remote areas where no physicians were available. Kaiser sought the services of a physician to build a medical group that would provide the necessary services. Rather than paying for these services on a **fee-for-service** basis, the company paid the physicians per employee (as the company did for workers' compensation coverage).

Over time, the physician group grew and became the Permanente Medical Group. Coverage was expanded first to include non–work-related illness and injury for employees and then services for the dependents and spouses of employees. Finally, the program was expanded to allow other employers to purchase care for their employees from the Permanente Medical Group. The organization was restructured into three mutually dependent entities: Kaiser Permanente Health Plan, Permanente Medical Group (a very large multispecialty group practice), and Kaiser Foundation Hospitals. This company, the best example of the group model HMO, serves more than 6 million members. The HMO contracts with employers to cover their employees. The medical group and hospitals contract with the health plan to provide the services required in the health plan's contract with employers.

Consistent with its history, the health plan does not pay the medical group a fee for each service provided. Instead, it pays each party based on the number of members enrolled in the health plan. This is often called **capitation** because there is one payment per capita. Capitation payments are also used by other types of HMOs.

As group model HMOs developed (they were called prepaid group practices until 1973 federal legislation changed their names), nongroup physicians organized into an entity called an **independent practice association (IPA)**. The early IPA HMOs were often sponsored by a local medical society and were developed to allow independent physicians to compete with prepaid group practices.

IPA HMOs contract with employers in the same manner as group model HMOs, and their members receive covered services from IPA physicians. The HMO's contracts with physicians are different, however, because these physicians are not organized into a single multispecialty group practice. IPA physicians are paid in a number of ways. Some are paid on a capitation basis, and some may be paid on a fee-for-service basis using a **fee schedule** established by the HMO. Often, a portion of any reimbursement is withheld by the HMO and paid only if the HMO's total medical expense is within budget; this encourages the physician to be cost conscious in caring for patients.

In some of these HMOs, the IPA is a separate corporation, often owned by physicians. With this structure (still called an IPA HMO), the IPA contracts with physicians, and the HMO contracts with the IPA instead of directly with each physician.

Over the years, HMOs have continued to evolve, and many are now a mixture of these discussed models. As a medical assistant, you must know what type of relationship the practice has with a HMO before you can determine how the practice is reimbursed. Most HMOs require claims to be submitted even if payment is capitation rather than fee-for-service. Many HMOs also require the collection and transmission of other patient information, which is not required in the traditional insurance industry.

Checkpoint Question

5. How does a HMO differ from a traditional health insurance program?

Preferred Provider Organizations

Whereas HMOs promise to provide services and have a financial risk in their relationships with subscribers, a **preferred provider organization (PPO)** is a type of health benefit program whose purpose is simply to contract with providers, then lease this network of contracted providers to health care plans. The PPO network is not risk bearing; it does not have any financial involvement in the health plan.

PPOs are typically developed by hospitals and physicians as a vehicle to attract patients, although some are developed and managed by insurance carriers.

PPOs contract with participating providers, including hospitals and physicians. These contracts allow the PPO to contract with insurers and other purchasers of health care services on behalf of the participating providers, who typically accept less than their normal charges and agree to follow the UM and other administrative protocols as specified by the PPO.

Typically, a health plan with a PPO offers benefits at two levels, commonly referred to as in network and out of network. Unlike in a HMO, patients may visit any provider they wish for services. If the provider is in network (a participating provider), the levels of benefits for the patient are greater than if the patient receives services from an out-of-network (nonparticipating) provider.

A typical health plan with a PPO may look like the breakdown shown in Figure 16-2.

As you can see from the example, each time the patient sees an in-network provider, he or she receives significantly better benefits. A primary difference between a HMO and PPO, therefore, is that patients can see any physician of their choice and receive benefits; they simply have an incentive in the form of higher benefits when they see an in-network provider.

As part of your responsibilities, you should identify the PPOs with which the physician has contracted and determine the administrative requirements set forth by each PPO in the contract. To understand the necessary administrative procedures agreed to by the physician, review all managed care contracts carefully. Also be aware that most PPOs have a provider relations representative who works with the contracted providers (physicians) to answer questions and clarify procedures. The PPO is typically operated by a group of hospitals or physicians or by an insurance company or independent organization. Physicians agree to participate in PPOs to serve their existing patients who now have PPO plans and sometimes to gain additional patients who seek the services of a PPO physician.

Participating physicians have agreed to perform certain administrative services for PPO patients. Commonly, the physician's office must accept assignment of benefits and provide claims filing services for the patient. The physician agrees to accept the reimbursement by the claims administrator as payment in full and agrees not to bill the patient for any difference between the physician's usual charge and the PPO-negotiated charge for the service. The participating physician is responsible for collecting any co-pay amount at the time of service. The physician also agrees to comply with any precertification requirements stipulated by the plan.

Checkpoint Question

6. What is the primary difference between a HMO and a PPO?

Physician Hospital Organizations

Physicians and hospitals have become more active in developing managed care alternatives. A **physician hospital organization (PHO)** is a coalition of physicians and a hospital contracting with large employers, insurance carriers, and other benefits groups to provide discounted health services. There are numerous variations of PHOs. A PHO may look much like a PPO with no risk-bearing elements, in which case the network of providers constituting the PHO are under no financial obligation to subscribers. A PHO may be more like a HMO, wherein the participating providers in the PHO do have a risk-bearing contract and assume responsibility for the overall medical budget of subscribing units. Physician organizations (POs) are such groups consisting of physicians only. As with any managed care program, it is important to know and understand the particulars of each managed care contract and requirements of the provider and obligations to patients and the managed care entity.

Other Managed Care Programs

Although HMOs, PPOs, and increasingly PHOs are the most common managed care programs, many others cover patients today and still more are being developed.

Although requirements vary, a gatekeeper provision is common. A gatekeeper is a primary care physician. Participants are required to see a primary care physician for all nonemergency services. That physician will either treat the patient or, if necessary, refer the patient to a specialist. The physician must complete and submit a referral form or call the claims administrator for approval of the referral.

The gatekeeper provision seeks to reduce the plan cost of specialists. For example, without such a provision, a patient might see a specialist first at a more costly fee, even though the condition may have been adequately treated by a less costly primary care physician. The gatekeeper approach also encourages patients to establish a relationship with a primary care physician, who is then in a position to manage the patient's care.

Example of a Health Plan With a PPO		
Benefit	In-network	Out-of-network
Deductible	$100	$300
Coinsurance	90%	70%
Routine care	$200 per calendar year	-0-
Mental health	80%	50%
Office visit	$10 co-pay; no deductible	70%

FIGURE 16–2. A health plan with a PPO.

The Future of Managed Care

Managed care has changed the organizational structure of medicine. To form risk-bearing organizations, physicians and hospitals are combining into new relationships. Hospitals are buying physician practices, and small-group or solo-practice physicians are combining into larger group practices. Some of these are forming public companies and raising investment capital to foster even more rapid growth in size and geographic scope. The size of medical practices is increasing and is expected to continue to increase in the foreseeable future.

The role of primary care physicians is changing relative to subspecialty physicians. In many managed care programs, primary care physicians act as patient care managers. Services authorized by these gatekeepers are covered, whereas those not authorized by the patient's primary physician may be denied or paid at a lower rate. Patients often join managed care organizations only if their primary care physician is a participant in a particular plan.

As coverage changes from an insured fee-for-service system to a managed care system with incentives to decrease the cost of patient care, employers and other purchasers have become much more interested in measuring the quality of care provided by managed care organizations. The very largest employers worked with leading HMOs to develop a report called HEDIS (Healthplan Employer Data Information Set). This uniform data set (reporting many indicators of health care quality, such as immunization rates and cesarean section rates) is now required of any HMO that wishes to serve the largest employers in the nation. HEDIS is upgraded continually and is being adopted by governmental agencies and many smaller employers as a prerequisite for a HMO to cover employees and governmental populations. This is only a start. Demands for increasingly sophisticated medical information will intensify.

The new demands to reduce the cost of care while measuring quality and improving it over time have led many organizations to develop increasingly sophisticated patient care protocols. These require documentation of efficacy and quality using information contained in patients' medical records. These demands are leading to increased automation of medical records. With automated medical records, a patient's medical history can be immediately available to any provider in virtually any location. Not only will it be easier to document quality and measure improvement over time, but a complete medical record that is available to any provider (with the patient's permission) will improve coordination among physicians and reduce illness. This alone can lead to substantial improvement in the quality of care.

Physicians are no longer isolated practitioners but are continuously involved with and accountable to community standards of practice. Protocols for patient care are becoming common and will change further as knowledge increases. Quality measurement and reporting will become more public, and the best medical care systems may be rewarded with higher patient volume for attaining the highest standards of patient care quality and satisfaction.

How does the progression of managed care affect you as a medical assistant? Managed care will continue to evolve and be refined. These trends in managed care will continue to affect individual physician practices as the face of health care continues to change. There will be increasing cooperative efforts by groups of physicians contracting together, with or without hospitals, carriers, or other parties. Family practice physicians will accept expanded responsibilities in managing the total care of a patient, managing specialist care and hospitalizations. These coalitions of providers will result in more uniform protocols of care and the application of outcome measurements in physician practices. The collection of data will become increasingly important to the practice. That collection and the management of the data will be a vital responsibility for you.

WORKERS' COMPENSATION

Employees in every state are covered by a workers' compensation program administered by the state. Workers' compensation benefits were developed to cover the expenses resulting from a work-related illness or injury.

ETHICAL TIP

The following scenario may occur in a medical office:

While you are filing an insurance claim, the physician tells you to "readjust" the laceration length from 4 cm to 9 cm. (The physician can bill more for a 9-cm laceration.) When you question him about this, he says, "Don't worry. The patient isn't paying the difference, the insurance company is, and they have plenty of money." How should you handle this situation?

Ethically and legally, you cannot change the length of a laceration on the medical record or the bill. This is fraud. You must explain to the physician that you are uncomfortable with this request and that you are ethically and legally bound to truthful billing. Any requests to alter or misrepresent the medical records or claims of a patient must be firmly denied.

A physician who operates in an unethical manner should be reported. If he or she is a partner in a practice, alert the other physicians about the suspect actions. You can also contact your state medical association, the American Medical Association, or the institutional review board at the hospital where your physician is affiliated.

PLEASE
DO NOT
STAPLE
IN THIS
AREA

HEALTH INSURANCE CLAIM FORM

PICA		PICA

1. MEDICARE   MEDICAID   CHAMPUS   CHAMPVA   GROUP HEALTH PLAN   FECA BLK LUNG   OTHER   1a. INSURED'S I.D. NUMBER   (FOR PROGRAM IN ITEM 1)
(Medicare #)   (Medicaid #)   (Sponsor's SSN)   (VA File #)   (SSN or ID)   (SSN)   (ID)

2. PATIENT'S NAME (Last Name, First Name, Middle Initial)

3. PATIENT'S BIRTH DATE MM DD YY   SEX   M   F

4. INSURED'S NAME (Last Name, First Name, Middle Initial)

5. PATIENT'S ADDRESS (No., Street)

6. PATIENT RELATIONSHIP TO INSURED   Self   Spouse   Child   Other

7. INSURED'S ADDRESS (No., Street)

CITY   STATE

8. PATIENT STATUS   Single   Married   Other   Employed   Full-Time Student   Part-Time Student

CITY   STATE

ZIP CODE   TELEPHONE (Include Area Code) (   )

ZIP CODE   TELEPHONE (INCLUDE AREA CODE) (   )

9. OTHER INSURED'S NAME (Last Name, First Name, Middle Initial)

10. IS PATIENT'S CONDITION RELATED TO:

11. INSURED'S POLICY GROUP OR FECA NUMBER

a. OTHER INSURED'S POLICY OR GROUP NUMBER

a. EMPLOYMENT? (CURRENT OR PREVIOUS)   YES   NO

a. INSURED'S DATE OF BIRTH MM DD YY   SEX   M   F

b. OTHER INSURED'S DATE OF BIRTH MM DD YY   SEX   M   F

b. AUTO ACCIDENT?   PLACE (State)   YES   NO

b. EMPLOYER'S NAME OR SCHOOL NAME

c. EMPLOYER'S NAME OR SCHOOL NAME

c. OTHER ACCIDENT?   YES   NO

c. INSURANCE PLAN NAME OR PROGRAM NAME

d. INSURANCE PLAN NAME OR PROGRAM NAME

10d. RESERVED FOR LOCAL USE

d. IS THERE ANOTHER HEALTH BENEFIT PLAN?   YES   NO   If yes, return to and complete item 9 a-d.

READ BACK OF FORM BEFORE COMPLETING & SIGNING THIS FORM.
12. PATIENT'S OR AUTHORIZED PERSON'S SIGNATURE I authorize the release of any medical or other information necessary to process this claim. I also request payment of government benefits either to myself or to the party who accepts assignment below.
SIGNED   DATE

13. INSURED'S OR AUTHORIZED PERSON'S SIGNATURE I authorize payment of medical benefits to the undersigned physician or supplier for services described below.
SIGNED

14. DATE OF CURRENT: ILLNESS (First symptom) OR INJURY (Accident) OR PREGNANCY(LMP) MM DD YY

15. IF PATIENT HAS HAD SAME OR SIMILAR ILLNESS. GIVE FIRST DATE MM DD YY

16. DATES PATIENT UNABLE TO WORK IN CURRENT OCCUPATION FROM MM DD YY   TO MM DD YY

17. NAME OF REFERRING PHYSICIAN OR OTHER SOURCE

17a. I.D. NUMBER OF REFERRING PHYSICIAN

18. HOSPITALIZATION DATES RELATED TO CURRENT SERVICES FROM MM DD YY   TO MM DD YY

19. RESERVED FOR LOCAL USE

20. OUTSIDE LAB?   YES   NO $ CHARGES

21. DIAGNOSIS OR NATURE OF ILLNESS OR INJURY. (RELATE ITEMS 1,2,3 OR 4 TO ITEM 24E BY LINE)
1. ___ . ___   3. ___ . ___
2. ___ . ___   4. ___ . ___

22. MEDICAID RESUBMISSION CODE   ORIGINAL REF. NO.

23. PRIOR AUTHORIZATION NUMBER

24. A DATE(S) OF SERVICE From MM DD YY To MM DD YY	B Place of Service	C Type of Service	D PROCEDURES, SERVICES, OR SUPPLIES (Explain Unusual Circumstances) CPT/HCPCS MODIFIER	E DIAGNOSIS CODE	F $ CHARGES	G DAYS OR UNITS	H EPSDT Family Plan	I EMG	J COB	K RESERVED FOR LOCAL USE
1										
2										
3										
4										
5										
6										

25. FEDERAL TAX I.D. NUMBER   SSN EIN

26. PATIENT'S ACCOUNT NO.

27. ACCEPT ASSIGNMENT? (For govt. claims, see back)   YES   NO

28. TOTAL CHARGE $

29. AMOUNT PAID $

30. BALANCE DUE $

31. SIGNATURE OF PHYSICIAN OR SUPPLIER INCLUDING DEGREES OR CREDENTIALS (I certify that the statements on the reverse apply to this bill and are made a part thereof.)
SIGNED   DATE

32. NAME AND ADDRESS OF FACILITY WHERE SERVICES WERE RENDERED (If other than home or office)

33. PHYSICIAN'S, SUPPLIER'S BILLING NAME, ADDRESS, ZIP CODE & PHONE #
PIN#   GRP#

(APPROVED BY AMA COUNCIL ON MEDICAL SERVICE 8/88)   PLEASE PRINT OR TYPE   APPROVED OMB-0938-0008 FORM CMS-1500 (12-90), FORM RRB-1500, APPROVED OMB-1215-0055 FORM OWCP-1500, APPROVED OMB-0720-0001 (CHAMPUS)

CARRIER   PATIENT AND INSURED INFORMATION   PHYSICIAN OR SUPPLIER INFORMATION

FIGURE 16–3. CMS-1500 claim form. This is the most commonly used insurance claim form. On the facing page you will find a detailed list explaining how to complete each line of the form. The form should be clearly and neatly typed.

Box Number	Information to Be Entered	Comments
1	Where the claim is being submitted	Confirm the patient's coverage and accuracy of your file information. A change in the patient's coverage will change how the claim is filed.
1a	The insured's ID number	Important: Enter the ID number of the insured (or employee), not the patient. This frequent filing error will cause rejection of the claim. The ID number is often the SSN, but check the ID card; the ID number may differ from the SSN.
2	Name of patient	The correct order (last, first, middle initial) is important.
3	Patient's date of birth	
4	Name of insured	Again, be sure to enter the name of the insured (or employee), not the patient.
5	Address of patient	
6	Patient's relationship to the insured	
7	Address of the insured	Check and update regularly.
8	Patient's status	Check and update frequently.
	Name of other insured	If the patient is covered under more than one plan, enter second plan here. For example, if a patient's claim is being submitted for her employer but she is also covered under her husband's plan, list the husband's name here.
9	Other insured's name	
9a	Other insured's policy or group number	Husband's policy number
9b	Other insured's date of birth	Husband's date of birth and sex
9c	Employer's name or school	Husband's employer
9d	Insurance plan name or program name	Husband's insurance company
10	Patient's condition	
10a	Patient's condition related to employment?	If yes, claim should be submitted to the workers' compensation carrier.
10b	Related to an auto accident?	If yes, the claim will not be processed unless a police report is attached.
10c	Other accident?	If yes, details of that accident must be attached.
11	Insured's policy group or FECA number	Very important. Some payers automatically return claim if group number is not indicated here. Group number is on patient's ID card.
11a	Insured's date of birth	Again, this is insured person, not patient.
11b	Employer's name	The insured's employer or school.
11c	Insurance plan name or program name	
11d	Is there another health plan?	If the patient is covered under more than one plan, check yes. If yes, the coverage will be coordinated between the plans covering the patient.
12	Patient's or authorized person's signature	This signature authorizes the release of information necessary to process the claim. If the patient's signature is in his or her file in your office, "signature on file" may be entered here.
13	Insured's signature	
14	Date of current	This is not date of service but the date the illness began or accident occurred.
15	If patient has had same or similar illness	If the patient has had this illness before, enter the date of the first occurrence.
16	Is patient unable to work	This information is required for the patient to receive disability payments.
17	Name of referring physician	If this patient was referred by another physician, enter name here.
17a	ID number of referring physician	EIN of the physician who referred the patient
18	Hospitalization dates	If the patient has been hospitalized for this illness or reason for visit, enter dates here.
20	Outside lab	If charges were incurred by an outside lab, check yes and enter amount. If not, check no.
21–24	Codes	Accuracy of this information determines accuracy of reimbursement. Thorough understanding of coding is essential for completing this section. See Chapters 17 and 18.
25	Tax ID number	Enter the EIN of the physician
26	Patient's account number	If you have assigned an account number to the patient, enter it here.
27	Accept assignment?	If you will accept assignment of the benefits, check yes. If not, check no.
28	Total charge	Enter the total amount of charges for this visit or service
29	Amount paid	Enter here any amount paid by the patient.
30	Balance due	Subtract any amount paid from the total charge and enter that amount here.
31	Signature of physician	
32	Name and address of facility where service was rendered	If the service was rendered outside of the physician's office, enter that address here.
33	Physician's billing name, address, zip code, and phone	This information will be used to mail reimbursement. Be sure it is current. The physician's billing name is required; may be a practice or corporate name.

SSN, Social Security number; FECA, Federal Employee Compensation Act; EIN, employer ID number.

In the event of a work-related illness or injury, claims submitted to the group or individual health benefits plan will be returned with instructions to file with the workers' compensation administrator, who determines the validity of the claim and reimburses accordingly. Because your practice will likely be taking care of the patient for both routine medical care and work-related illness or injury, it is important to determine at the time services are rendered whether the illness or injury is work-related and, if so, to account and file for those services separately.

You are responsible for knowing your state's workers' compensation regulations and procedures. Consult your state's office for workers' compensation or your state's designated claims administrator of the workers' compensation program for specific information.

FILING CLAIMS

If the provider requires patients to make full payment at the time of the visit, the physician may still submit a claim on the patient's behalf; however, the patient may need to submit claims to the claims administrator for reimbursement. Most providers accept assignment of benefits, however. To do this, the patient must give written authorization for the claims administrator to reimburse the physician for billed charges. As a medical assistant, you may be responsible for obtaining all necessary claims information from the provider and the patient and then submitting a claim for payment to the claims administrator.

The patient's ID card is a source of information necessary for complete and accurate claims submission. Keep a copy of this card in the patient's file and be sure to update it at least yearly and preferably at each visit, since the patient's employment and eligibility may change.

In addition, a patient may be covered by more than one group plan. For example, a patient may be covered both on an employer's group plan and as a dependent on his or her spouse's group plan. The primary plan—the one that pays first—is the plan provided by the patient's employer. Any unpaid amount is then considered for payment by the spouse's group plan, which is considered secondary. This is called **coordination of benefits**.

Dependent children may be covered under one or two parents' plans. Unless the plans state otherwise, the plan of the parent whose birthday occurs first each calendar year (not necessarily the oldest parent) is the primary plan. This is known as the **birthday rule**. This rule is commonly used by benefit plans and claims administrators to coordinate the benefits of dependent children covered by two plans. If the parents are legally separated or divorced, however, the primary plan is the plan of the parent who has custody or, in some instances, is subject to a court order or divorce decree.

After establishing the primary plan and the claims submission destination, you prepare the claim for filing. The CMS-1500 was developed by the American Medical Association to standardize an acceptable claim form for different plans and different claims administrators. It is the most widely used method of filing a health claim (Fig. 16-3). The CMS-1500 is accepted by most claims administrators, including Blue Shield, Medicare, Medicaid, and TRICARE/CHAMPVA.

Most plans include a clause that excludes coverage for a stated period (usually 12 months) for a condition, called a **preexisting condition**, that existed before the plan's effective date. For example, a patient with a diagnosis of depression before the effective date of his or her plan would be covered for all other conditions from the effective date forward but would not be covered for services related to the diagnosis or treatment of depression for the preexisting exclusion period (in this example, 12 months).

Many pieces of information are necessary for timely and efficient claims processing. The insurance company or managed care plan cannot process claims with incomplete or inaccurate information and will return them to the provider for completion, correction, and resubmission. This lengthens the time the provider must wait for reimbursement, making accurate claims submission a critical aspect of your responsibilities. The most frequent causes for denial of a claim and the corrective actions that you can take are as follows:

1. The patient cannot be identified as a covered person. Confirm that coverage information on file is current, including insurance company and group number, and that the Social Security number is accurate.
2. Coding is deemed inappropriate for services provided. Review provided services and recode as necessary.
3. The patient is no longer covered by the plan. Bill the patient for the charges. The patient may provide confirmation of new coverage.
4. The data are incomplete. Complete the required data and resubmit the claim.
5. Services are not covered by the plan. Bill the patient for the charges unless there is a basis for an appeal.

Electronic Claims Submission

Although some practices continue to submit claims on paper through the mail and most claims administrators continue to accept this practice, most practices submit at least their

WHAT IF

The reason for a rejection or denial of a claim is not clear. What should you do?

If the reasons for denial of the claim are not clear, telephone the claims administrator and ask for clarification. Be sure to have the claim and papers with you when you make the telephone call.

LEGAL TIP

Keeping patient information confidential is a primary concern in all medical practices. You should not release any information about the patient to any party, including the claims administrator, without the written authorization of the patient or the patient's guardian. Obtain a written authorization to release information from each patient on his or her first visit to the practice. Keep this information in the patient's file. Any claims submitted by the physician's office must have "signature on file" on the claim form. With written authorization for the release of information, only such information as is pertinent to the claim and necessary for the processing of that claim should be released. Releasing any patient information without written consent is a breach of confidentiality.

Medicare and Medicaid claims electronically. As of October 2003, HIPAA requires nearly all, with very few exceptions, to be submitted electronically. The physician's office computer software includes the CMS-1500 format for convenient and automated claims filing. With a computer and a modem, health claims can be filed immediately, reducing the time for the reimbursement cycle. You will need to work closely with your practice's software vendor to ensure compatibility with the insurance companies' computer systems

Several regional and national clearinghouses receive health benefits claims and electronically direct them to the appropriate claims administrators. This system allows you to file all electronic claims through one clearinghouse rather than filing separately with each claims administrator.

The system requires that all fields on the electronic claim form be completed and in the required format. If the claim is incomplete or inaccurate, the system will not transmit the form. You can complete or correct the form online, allowing the form to be transmitted. Claims submitted electronically that do not meet the plan's criteria will be rejected by the clearinghouse and must be submitted by mail. In addition, claims that are particularly complicated or cumbersome, have attachments, or are otherwise unsuitable for electronic submission should be filed on paper with the claims administrator.

Explanation of Benefits

When the claims administrator settles a claim, that is, makes a payment, an **explanation of benefits (EOB)** is issued to both the provider and the patient (Fig. 16-4). The EOB tells how the payment was made, including deductible and coinsurance information. Some EOBs include informa-

tion for several claims on several patients that may have been processed during a particular period. You may be responsible for checking the EOB to be sure that all payments made to the physician are for the appropriate procedures and in the correct amounts.

POLICIES IN THE PRACTICE

Managed care contracts and negotiated services affect many practice policies. You must be knowledgeable and precise in administering practice policies, especially with regard to assignment of benefits and balance billing.

Assignment of benefits is a service the practice may provide. If assignment of benefits is accepted, the patient's signature must be on file, authorizing the claims administrator to reimburse the physician. Managed care plans require physicians to accept assignment, although many physicians do not accept assignment for non–managed care patients. If assignment is not accepted, the patient is responsible for paying all charges and filing a claim with the claims administrator for reimbursement directly to the patient.

Balance billing is prohibited by most managed care contracts. The physician cannot charge the patient the difference between the physician's usual charge and the allowable charge specified by the contract. For other types of plans, however, balance billing is not restricted, and the practice may bill the patient for any difference between the physician's charged fee and the amount allowable by the plan according to **usual, customary, and reasonable (UCR)** tables.

A few national firms provide UCR data to claims administrators who use that information to determine the maximum amount payable for any given service (the **plan maximum**). UCR data are calculated from surveys of the amount physicians charge for each service or procedure. That amount is calculated on a geographic basis to reflect regional variations in health care costs. Non–managed care plan physician reimbursements are based on a maximum allowable charge as specified in the UCR data. The physician may choose to bill the patient for the difference between the amount charged and the UCR amount.

LEGAL TIP

It is fraudulent to misrepresent or expand the services rendered on the coding of a claim so as to receive additional reimbursement. Unbundling procedures so as to receive a greater reimbursement is also fraudulent. **Unbundling** is the practice of submitting a claim with several separate procedure codes rather than the single code that represents the services performed. Most payers now have software that detects such practices and rejects the claim.

Explanation of Benefits

Employee Name: Joe Doe
SSN: 555-55-5555 (1)
Group No. 55555
Patient Name: Joe Doe

Date of Service: 6-15-2004
Provider: Dr. Jones
Provider TIN: 35-5555555

Date of Service (2)	Comment Code (3)	Amount of Charge (4)	Amount Allowed (5)	At (6)	Amount Paid (7)
6-15-2004	57	87.00	82.00	80%	65.60

Total (8)	65.60
Less Deductible (9)	25.00
Amount Paid (10)	40.60

Payable to: Dr. Jones
               Address

Comment Code:
57 - The amount charged exceeds Usual and Customary

Reading the EOB (Explanation of Benefits)

After the claim has been processed, an EOB will be issued. Although each payer has his or her own EOB format, this sample EOB illustrates the key points included in an EOB. The terms used may differ, and the formats differ widely.

(1) The top section typically includes the name of the employee and the Social Security number (SSN) or other identifying number, as well as the name of the patient, the group number, the date of service and provider name, and employer identification number (EIN) (Federal identification number assigned to the physician).

(2) The date of service is included and is shown as the date the service is actually rendered, not the date that was posted or billed.

(3) The Comment Code is a tool used on many EOBs to indicate a coded comment that is either on the bottom as exceeding "Usual and Customary." In this situation, the claim will be processed on the Usual and Customary amount. The difference between the amount charged ($87.00) and the amount allowed ($82.00) is $5.00. Unless the physician is contractually bound by an agreement with a managed care plan that forbids the practice of balance billing, that difference of $5.00 may be billed to the patient.

(4) Amount of Charge shows the amount that the physician's office billed for the service.

(5) Amount Allowed shows the amount of charge upon which the claim processing will be based (in this example, it is the amount of Usual and Customary).

(6) This indicates the percentage of co-insurance payable by the plan.

(7) Amount Paid shows the amount payable by the plan after co-insurance has been applied, but is not necessarily the amount that is actually paid (see #10).

(8) The Total shows the total submitted and payable after the claim has been processed.

(9) After all processing on the claim has been completed, any deductible is applied. In this example, Joe still had $25.00 to be applied to his annual deductible. Therefore, $25.00 is deducted from the amount paid and the actual reimbursement to the physician is $40.60. The amount applied to the deductible should be billed to the patient.

(10) The amount actually reimbursed.

FIGURE 16-4.

Chapter Summary

Most patients in the physician's office have some type of health care plan. Types of plans include group, individual, and government-sponsored health benefits, such as Medicare or Medicaid. Many physicians have contracts with managed care plans, such as HMOs and PPOs. Each type of plan has certain requirements regarding eligibility and claims submission, and you must be knowledgeable about those requirements. In particular, one of your primary duties is to file claims in a timely and accurate manner to ensure appropriate reimbursement for the physician. When filing claims, you must be careful to maintain patient confidentiality and to avoid fraud.

Critical Thinking Challenges

1. Jane and Joe are married, and both are employed and cover themselves and their two children on their health plans. Jane's birthday is July 23 and Joe's birthday is August 9. Joe is 2 years older than Jane. When claims are submitted for their two children, which spouse's plan is primary? Show which plan is primary and secondary for each family member.

	Primary	Secondary
Jane		
Joe		
Child 1		
Child 2		

2. The requirements for Medicaid vary from state to state. How do you determine the Medicaid requirements for your particular state? Locate the name, address, and telephone number of your state's resource.

Answers to Checkpoint Questions

1. With insured benefits, a monthly premium is paid by the employer or organization to an insurance company. The insurance company in turn is obligated to pay for any eligible health benefits. In contrast, self-funded benefits are provided to eligible employees or members by their employer or organization. Claims are processed by a professional claims administrator, such as a third-party administrator.

2. Persons enrolled in Social Security are automatically enrolled in Medicare Part A, which covers hospital services and expenses only, and Medicare Part B, which covers the physician's charges for inpatient or outpatient care as well as diagnostic services. Part B does not cover routine examinations, well care, routine immunizations, or cosmetic surgery. Part A is provided at no charge to Social Security recipients, and Part B caries a monthly fee. If Part B is not wanted, it must be declined.

3. Medicaid patients receive a new ID card each month.

4. The four elements of managed care programs are pre-certification of hospital admissions (often also called utilization management or **utilization review**—UM or UR), approved referrals, network, and assignment of benefits.

5. In a traditional insurance system, the individual, not the insurer, seeks medical services and thereby incurs the expense. An HMO promises to provide covered services rather than pay for them.

6. A primary difference between a HMO and a PPO is that patients with PPO coverage can see any physician of their choice and receive benefits; they simply have an incentive in the form of higher benefits when they see an in-network provider.

 ## Websites

Medicare for providers and recipients
    www.CMS.gov
Medicare for recipients
    www.Medicare.gov
Blue Cross Blue Shield
    www.bluecares.com
Local medical review policies
    www.LMRP.net
American Medical Association
    www.AMA-assn.org
All government agencies, federal and state
    www.firstgov.gov

17

Diagnostic Coding

CHAPTER OUTLINE

ROLE DELINEATION COMPONENTS

GENERAL: Legal Concepts
- Perform within legal and ethical boundaries

ADMINISTRATIVE: Administrative Procedures
- Perform basic administrative medical assisting functions

- Obtain reimbursement through accurate claims submission

ADMINISTRATIVE: Practice Finances
- Perform procedural and diagnostic coding

CHAPTER COMPETENCIES

LEARNING OBJECTIVES

Upon successfully completing this chapter, you will be able to:

1. Spell and define the key terms
2. Name and describe the coding system used to describe diseases, injuries, and other reasons for encounters with a medical provider
3. Give four examples of ways diagnostic coding is used
4. Describe the relationship between coding and reimbursement
5. Explain the format of the ICD-9-CM
6. List the steps in identifying a proper code
7. Name common errors in outpatient diagnostic coding

KEY TERMS

advance beneficiary notice
audits
conventions
cross-reference
E-codes
eponym

etiology
inpatient
International Classification of Diseases, Ninth Revision, Clinical Modification

late effects
main terms
medical necessity
outpatient

primary diagnosis
service
specificity
V-codes

CODING, AT ITS SIMPLEST, is the assignment of a number to a verbal statement or description. Medical coding is anything but simple. The ***International Classification of Diseases, Ninth Revision, Clinical Modification*** is a system for transforming verbal descriptions of disease, injuries, conditions, and procedures into numeric codes. It is essential that the physician and medical assistant work together to achieve accurate documentation, code assignment, and reporting of diagnoses and procedures. Use of standardized codes makes it easier for third-party payers to understand the reason for the patient's encounter with the health care provider and increases the likelihood of timely processing of claims and prompt payment when appropriate.

Coding is a way to standardize medical information for purposes such as collecting health care statistics, performing a medical care review, and indexing medical records. It is also used for health insurance claims processing (see Chapter 16). Because coding is the basis for reimbursement, it is imperative that you code patient visits accurately and precisely. Incorrect, insufficient, or incomplete coding on claims forms can lead to nonpayment for the physician as well as incorrect information in the insurance companies databases, which may effect the patient's insurability. For example, if a patient complaining of chest pain is coded as having "acute myocardial infarction" instead of "chest pain rule out myocardial infarction," that patient may be incorrectly labeled as having heart disease. The Current Procedural Terminology (CPT) codes, used to report services and procedures performed by health care providers, determine the amount paid (see Chapter 18), but the code assigned to the diagnosis or reason for the service or procedure proves the medical necessity for the services or procedures so that claims are paid. The third-party payer needs to know why the service was performed to assess **medical necessity**. Medical necessity means the procedure or service would have been performed by any reasonable physician under the same or similar circumstances. The ICD-9 diagnostic codes convey this information. Is a chest radiograph medically necessary for a patient who has gout? No, but it may be necessary for a patient with acute bronchitis. The diagnosis justifies the procedure.

Since Medicare considers certain procedures medically necessary only at certain intervals, having the patient sign an **advance beneficiary notice** (ABN) will ensure payment of treatments and procedures that will likely be denied by Medicare. An example is a Pap smear for a low-risk woman, which will be paid for once every 2 years. If the physician considers it *not* to be medically necessary, but the patient wants a Pap test, the patient will be responsible for payment and must sign an ABN.

Checkpoint Question

1. What is meant by medical necessity?

DIAGNOSTIC CODING

International Classification of Diseases, Ninth Revision, Clinical Modification (ICD-9-CM) is a statistical classification system based on the *International Classification of Diseases, Ninth Revision* (ICD-9), developed by the World Health Organization (WHO). The CM, which stands for clinical modification, addresses the intent of these codes to describe the clinical picture of the patient. These codes are much more precise than those needed for statistical grouping and trend analysis found in the ICD-9 and used in hospital coding.

The ICD-9-CM, which is now mandated by Health Insurance Portability and Accountability Act of 1996 (HIPAA), is the most current and comprehensive statistical classification of its kind. Containing more than 10,000 diagnostic codes and 1,000 procedure codes, it consists of three volumes:

- Volume 1: Tabular List of Diseases
- Volume 2: Alphabetic Index of Diseases
- Volume 3: Tabular List and Alphabetic Index of Procedures

The ICD-9-CM code books are available from several publishers, and although the presentation of the material may be different, the content must be the same. Depending on the publisher, these three volumes may be included within one book. In the physician's office, only Volumes 1 and 2 are used. Volume 3 is used by hospitals.

The diagnostic classification systems in Volumes 1 and 2 are maintained by a federal government agency, the National Center for Health Statistics (NCHS); the procedure classification (Volume 3) is maintained by the Centers for Medicare & Medicaid Services (CMS), the federal agency that regulates health care financing. All three volumes are updated regularly, with codes being added, revised, and sometimes deleted. Changes in the ICD-9-CM are published by NCHS and CMS with the approval of WHO. Both the American Health Information Management Association (AHIMA) and the American Hospital Association (AHA) advise and assist in keeping the classification system current.

Checkpoint Questions

2. What are the three volumes of the ICD-9-CM system?

3. What organization must approve any changes in the disease classification system?

Inpatient Versus Outpatient Coding

There is a big difference between coding medical claims in a hospital or other inpatient facility and coding for the physician in an outpatient medical practice. The systems and references used to assign codes to third-party claims is only one difference in the coding requirements and practices of the physician and the inpatient medical facility. Volumes 1 and 2 of the ICD-9 CM are used to report the diagnostic code that justifies physician services whether those services are provided in the office or in the hospital. Hospital coders use Volume 3 to report inpatient procedures, services, and supplies, as well as the reasons for the services.

The UB-92 (uniform bill) is used by institutions to report inpatient admissions and outpatient and emergency department services and procedures. These charges are for nursing services, building maintenance, and all costs associated with running the institution. These charges do not include physician services. The CMS-1500 (universal claim form) is used to report physician services, whether the physician sees the patient in the office, emergency department, hospital, or nursing home, because even though the physician may have been in the hospital, it is his **service** for which we are billing in the medical office.

The term **outpatient** is used to describe patients treated in the following places:

- Health care provider's office
- Hospital clinic
- Emergency department
- Hospital same-day surgery unit or ambulatory surgical center that releases the patient within 23 hours
- Observation status in a hospital (the patient is admitted for a short time for observation only, and the physician bills for his or her service during the stay)

The term **inpatient** refers to a patient who is admitted to the hospital for treatment with the expectation that the patient will remain in the hospital for 24 hours or more.

Hospital coders code only services provided by the hospital and hospital employees. Coders who are employed by the physician practice are concerned with the services provided by the physician no matter where the services are provided. For example, the hospital room, meals, and laboratory testing that a patient receives are billed and coded by the hospital billing department. The daily visits the physician makes to the patient are billed and coded by the physician's office.

Since the focus of this textbook is medical assisting, we concentrate on outpatient coding.

Checkpoint Question

4. Define the terms *inpatient* and *outpatient.*

ICD-9-CM: THE CODE BOOK

Coding books are available from several publishers, such as Ingenix and Medicode. The AMA (American Medical Association) Press also publishes coding books and training materials. The classification system is also available as part of a medical software package; one of these packages is CodeManager from the AMA. Although each publisher offers special features and helpful aids, the format remains the same. Some coders become comfortable with certain special features (i.e., AMA publications are spiral bound) and, since the content is the same, can choose among the various publications based on organization, illustrations, tabs, bullets, and color coding.

To become an expert medical coder, you need general knowledge of human anatomy and medical terminology. In addition to using a code book, you will need reference materials such as a medical dictionary and/or medical dictionary software.

To ensure accurate coding, update your ICD-9-CM coding books and software as needed. (Updates and addenda can be purchased from the publisher of your coding book.) You must update codes on superbills (preprinted bills listing a variety of procedures) or any other forms you use. Experts have estimated that millions of dollars in reimbursement have been lost because an incorrect code was taken from a standardized form that had not been updated. New codes are published each October, and most third-party payers require their use after January 1.

Checkpoint Question

5. How often is the ICD-9-CM updated?

Volume 1: Tabular List of Diseases

Volume 1 contains the classification of diseases (conditions) and injuries by code numbers. Figure 17-1 shows the table of contents from this volume. These 17 chapters cover groupings of diseases and injuries by **etiology** or cause (e.g., infectious diseases) and by anatomic system (e.g., digestive, respiratory). Each chapter has a heading or title (e.g., 16, Symptoms, Signs, and Ill-defined Conditions (780–799). Following the title in parentheses is the range of three-digit categories included in that chapter. In each chapter you will find subtitles in large type followed by a range of three-digit categories in parentheses (e.g., 16, Symptoms (780–789). These sections describe general disease. Three-digit codes followed by a title, the category codes, describe specific diseases (e.g., 780, general symptoms). The fourth digit further breaks down the category (e.g., 780.0, alteration of consciousness), and the fifth digit is the highest level of definition (e.g., 780.01, coma). Figure 17-2 is a sample page from the tabular list showing each level of classification.

Volume 1 is always used to code a diagnosis to its highest definition. This volume tells you how many digits are required to code a diagnosis correctly and to a level that most third-party payers will accept. Volume 1 also includes five appendices, outlined in Box 17-1.

Supplementary Classifications

Supplementary classifications in Volume 1 include V- and E-codes.

V-Codes. **V-codes**, which range from V01 to V82, provide a means of indexing the reason for hospital or physician office care for other than current or genuine illness, such as a history of illness, immunizations, or live-born infants according to type of birth. An example of a V-code is V10.04, used for a person with a personal history of a malignant neoplasm of the stomach. Because of this history, it would be

TABLE OF CONTENTS

F I G U R E   1 7 – 1 .   Table of contents from ICD-9-CM, Volume 1.

important for this patient to have regular checkups. You would not want to code the visit 230.2, neoplasm of the stomach, because that would imply the patient has the malignant neoplasm at this visit. The ICD-9-CM offers a variety of codes for HIV testing. The patient who is simply afraid carries one V-code, while the patient who has known exposure carries another. V-codes may be used alone if no disease diagnosis is appropriate or as the second or third code to help better explain the reason for the visit.

E-Codes. **E-codes**, which range from E800 to E999, are used to classify external causes of injuries and poisoning. Specificity is limited to the fourth digit level. E-codes are used in conjunction with codes in Chapters 1 to 17. They help to provide information of interest to industrial medicine, insurance underwriters, national safety programs, public health agencies, and others concerned with causes of injuries (e.g., auto accidents, accidents caused by heavy industrial machinery). These codes do not affect reimbursement.

✓5ᵗʰ **780.5 Sleep disturbances**

> **EXCLUDES** *that of nonorganic origin (307.40-307.49)*

780.50 Sleep disturbance, unspecified

780.51 Insomnia with sleep apnea

> DEF: Transient cessation of breathing disturbing sleep.

780.52 Other insomnia

> Insomnia NOS

> DEF: Inability to maintain adequate sleep cycle.

780.53 Hypersomnia with sleep apnea

> DEF: Autonomic response inhibited during sleep; causes insufficient oxygen intake, acidosis and pulmonary hypertension.

780.54 Other hypersomnia

> Hypersomnia NOS

> DEF: Prolonged sleep cycle.

780.55 Disruptions of 24-hour sleep-wake cycle

> Inversion of sleep rhythm
> Irregular sleep-wake rhythm NOS
> Non-24-hour sleep-wake rhythm

780.56 Dysfunctions associated with sleep stages or arousal from sleep

780.57 Other and unspecified sleep apnea

780.59 Other

✓4ᵗʰ **780 General symptoms**

✓5ᵗʰ **780.0 Alteration of consciousness**

> **EXCLUDES** *coma:*
> *diabetic (250.2-250.3)*
> *hepatic (572.2)*
> *originating in the perinatal period (779.2)*

780.01 Coma

> DEF: State of unconsciousness from which the patient cannot be awakened.

780.02 Transient alteration of awareness

> DEF: Temporary, recurring spells of reduced consciousness.

780.03 Persistent vegetative state

> DEF: Persistent wakefulness without consciousness due to nonfunctioning cerebral cortex.

780.09 Other

> Drowsiness   Stupor
> Semicoma   Unconsciousness
> Somnolence

780.1 Hallucinations

> Hallucinations: Hallucinations:
>   NOS   olfactory
>   auditory   tactile
>   gustatory

> **EXCLUDES** *those associated with mental disorders, as functional*
> *psychoses (295.0-298.9)*
> *organic brain syndromes (290.0-294.9, 310.0-310.9)*
> *visual hallucinations (368.16)*

> DEF: Perception of external stimulus in absence of stimulus; inability to distinguish between real and imagined.

✓5ᵗʰ **779.8 Other specified conditions originating in the perinatal period**

779.81 Neonatal bradycardia

> **EXCLUDES** *abnormality in fetal heart rate or rhythm*
> *complicating labor and delivery*
> *(763.81-763.83)*
> *bradycardia due to birth asphyxia (768.5-768.9)*

779.82 Neonatal tachycardia

> **EXCLUDES** *abnormality in fetal heart rate or rhythm*
> *complicating labor and delivery*
> *(763.81-763.83)*

779.89 Other specified conditions originating in the perinatal period

FIGURE 17-2.   Sample page from ICD-9-CM, Volume 1, showing categories, subheadings, and so on.

Box 17-1

ICD-9-CM APPENDICES

The following five appendices are found in Volume I
- Appendix A: Morphology of Neoplasms
    This appendix is used in conjunction with Chapter 2 in ICD-9-CM when coding neoplasms. It lists the five-digit alphanumeric codes used to identify the morphology of a neoplasm. For example, in the morphology code M8070/3, the 8070 indicates the morphology is squamous cell carcinoma. The /3 indicates that it is the primary site.
- Appendix B: Glossary of Mental Disorders
    Alphabetic list of mental disorders, including detailed descriptions of each disease.
- Appendix C: Classification of Drugs by American Hospital Formulary Service (AHFS) List Number and the ICD-9-CM Equivalents
    This appendix lists the AHFS list number (e.g., 24:04 for cardiac drugs) and the ICD9-CM code number for each one (e.g., 24.04 cardiac drugs would be equivalent to category 972.9, the ICD9-CM category "other and unspecified agents primarily affecting the cardiovascular system").
- Appendix D: Classification of Industrial Accidents by Agency
    This includes codes that can be used as a supplement to describe types of equipment or materials that may be responsible for an industrial accident or illness.
- Appendix E: List of Three-Digit Categories
    This is a list of all three-digit categories in ICD-9-CM.
    Appendices A through D are not recognized by most government programs, such as Medicare and Medicaid. As previously mentioned, ICD-9-CM has other uses, however, and you may find that you need the appendices to track such things as disorders treated.

Volume 2, Section 3, has a separate index to access E-codes, the Alphabetic Index to External Causes of Injury and Poisoning.

Checkpoint Question

6. List four reasons for using E-codes.

Volume 2: Alphabetic Index to Diseases

Volume 2, the alphabetic index to diseases, contains many diagnostic terms that do not appear in Volume 1. For example, itch, barbers, beard, and scalp are all listed under *Itch* in

Volume 2. In Volume 1 they are all listed under code 110.0. The index is arranged by condition. Always check all indentations in the index under the condition to ensure that you have the one most appropriate to the diagnosis you intend to code.

The alphabetic index is organized into three sections:

- Section 1, Alphabetic Index to Diseases and Injuries, is organized by **main terms** printed in boldface type. Section 1 is used for reporting the reason for patient encounters for most insurance claims. Following the main term is a code number, which refers you to the tabular listing (Volume 1). You must not accept this number as the correct code without a **cross-reference** or check of the tabular list. Never code directly from the alphabetic index. This could result in an incomplete or incorrect coding assignment. For example, if you have a patient with fluid overload and you look under fluid, it may seem logical to code the first code under fluid, which is abdomen, 789.5, but your patient is generally retaining fluid. If you use the alphabetic index only, you do not know that the correct code is 276.6, fluid overload, which excludes ascites, 789.5, and localized edema, 782.3. Box 17-2 lists several exceptions to the main term rule.
- Section 2, Table of Drugs and Chemicals, includes an extensive listing of drugs, chemical substances, and toxic agents. It also shows E-codes and American Hospital Formulary Service (AHFS) list numbers, which are in the table under the main term *drug*.
- Section 3, Alphabetic Index to External Cases of Injuries and Poisonings, leads you to codes that describe circumstances of injuries, accidents, and violence. These codes are not used for medical diagnoses. Main entries in this section usually are a type of accident or violence (e.g., assault, fall, collision). These codes can supplement the diagnostic code, but they should never be used alone or as principal diagnosis codes. E-codes

Box 17-2

EXCEPTIONS TO THE MAIN TERM RULE

Keep in mind the following exceptions to this rule:
1. Obstetric conditions may be found under the main terms *delivery*, *pregnancy*, and *puerperal*.
2. Complications of medical or surgical procedures can be found under *complication*.
3. Late effects are found under *late effect*.
4. V-codes are found under main entries such as *admissions*, *examination*, *history of observation*, *problem* (with), *status*, *vaccination*, *encounter for*, and *follow-up*.

Spanish Terminology

¿Qué son todo estos números?	What are all these numbers? Is that my bill?
No, estos números se utilizan para su seguro.	*No, these numbers are used for your insurance.*
Estos se llaman los números de codificación.	*These are called coding numbers.*

are frequently used with these codes. For example, a person who fractured a tibia in a fall off a sidewalk curb would be given a code from chapter 17, Volume 1, in the ICD-9-CM for the injury (e.g., fracture of tibia, closed, is 823.80), and an additional code, E880.0, indicates that the accident was a fall off a sidewalk curb.

Checkpoint Question

7. What are V-codes used for?

Volume 3: Inpatient Coding

Volume 3, the Tabular List and Alphabetic Index of Procedures, is used in inpatient facilities and is based on anatomy, not surgical specialty. There are no alphabetical characters in these procedure codes. The codes are two-digit categories with a maximum of two decimal digits where necessary. Most refer to surgical procedures, and the rest cover miscellaneous diagnostic and therapeutic procedures. An example of a procedure code is 31.61, larynx laceration suture. Volume 3 is used for inpatient coding only.

LOCATING THE APPROPRIATE CODE

Box 17-3 outlines CMS guidelines for diagnostic coding. These are explained next.

Using the ICD-9-CM Conventions

Figure 17-3 lists the conventions used in the ICD-9-CM indexes. **Conventions** are rules that apply to the assignment of the ICD-9 codes. They are found throughout both the Index to Diseases and the Tabular List and include general notes using specific terms, cross-references, abbreviations, punctuation marks, symbols, typeface, and format. They direct and guide the coder to the appropriate code and should be strictly adhered to. Each publisher uses these same conventions, and many add more to assist coders in providing the most complete and accurate reason for the encounter. For example, when you locate the word itch, you will find "see pruritus," the medical term for severe itching. This is a helpful tool for coders who are unfamiliar with medical terminology.

Box 17-3

CMS DIAGNOSTIC CODING GUIDELINES

CMS defines specific guidelines that provide the basic knowledge necessary to apply the correct ICD-9 codes. Although these guidelines were developed for use in submitting government claims, most insurance companies have also adopted them. Many variations exist among the private insurance companies; therefore, care must be taken in recognizing the different requirements for each third-party payer. Most coders operate on the assumption that the government regulations are the strictest, and following those guidelines will satisfy most third-party payers.

1. Identify each service and procedure, or supply with an ICD-9 code from 001.0 through V82.9 to describe the diagnosis, symptom, complaint, condition, or problem.
2. Identify services or visits for circumstances other than disease or injury, such as follow-up care after chemotherapy, with V-codes provided for this purpose.
3. Code the reason for the visit first and code any coexisting conditions that affect the treatment of the patient for that visit or procedure as supplementary information. Do not code a diagnosis that is no longer applicable.
4. Code to the highest degree of specificity. Carry the numeric code to the fourth or fifth digit when necessary.
5. Code a chronic diagnosis as often as it is applicable to the patient's treatment.
6. When only ancillary services are provided, list the appropriate V-code first and the problem second. For example, if a patient is receiving only physical therapy, list the V-code first, followed by the code for the condition on line 24E on the CMS-1500 form.
7. For ambulatory or outpatient surgical procedures, code the diagnosis applicable to the procedure. If the postoperative diagnosis is different from the preoperative diagnosis, use the postoperative diagnosis.

Conventions

Braces { }   These are used in the Tabular List to connect a series of terms to a common stem. Each term on the left of the brace is incomplete without one of the terms to the right of the bracket.

Brackets [ ]   Brackets enclose synonyms, alternate wording, or explanatory phrases

Colon :   A colon is used after an incomplete term that needs one or more of the modifiers that follow to make it assignable to a given category

Parentheses ( )   Parentheses enclose supplementary words that may be present or absent in the statement of a disease or procedure, without affecting the code number to which it is assigned.

NEC (not elsewhere classifiable)   Alerts the coder that the specified form of the condition is classified differently. Codes following NEC should be used only when the coder lacks the information necessary to code the term in a more specific category.

NOS (not otherwise specified)   The coder should continue to look for a more specific code

Note   Used to define terms and give coding instructions. Found most often with list of fifth digits.

"Includes"   Indicates separate terms as adjectives that further modify sites and conditions or to further define or give examples of the content of a certain category.

"Excludes"   A box with "excludes" in italics draws the reader's attention to instructions that direct the coder to the proper code. This convention is found in the Tabular List.

"See," "See Also," and "See Category"   Direct the coder to other terms or sections that should be considered. ALWAYS follow these instructions.

"Use additional code"   This directs the coder to add another code to further explain and give the third-party payer a better understanding of a diagnosis.

"Code First Underlying Disease"   This direction is used in the tabular list when a reason for an encounter results from another disorder. The coder is instructed to indicate the underlying disease that caused the current problem or symptom that brought the patient to the office.

Index to Disease Example

478.1   Other diseases of nasal cavity and sinuses

Abscess ⎫
Necrosis ⎬ Of nose (septum)
Ulcer ⎭

422.92   Septic myocarditis
      Myocarditis, acute or subacute:
        Pneumococcal
        Staphylococcal
      Use additional code to identify infectious organism [e.g., Staphylococcus 041.1]

See above example 478.1 (septum) may or may not be present in the diagnosis given.

Infection
    Streptococcal NEC 041.00
      Group
        A 041.01
        B 041.02

As soon as the bacterium is identified, code for specific infection.

At the time of the service, it has not been established whether a neoplasm is benign or secondary, for example. Remember, you are coding for a date of service with the information documented for that date of service.

	Allergic rhinitis (nonseasonal)
INCLUDES	477 Allergic rhinitis (seasonal)
	Hay fever
EXCLUDES	Allergic rhinitis with asthma (bronchial) (493.0)

Itch (see also Pruritus) 698.9

See 422.92 examples above.

362.72   Retinal dystrophy in other systemic disorders and syndromes
      Code first underlying disease, as:
        Bassen-Kornzweig syndrome (272.5)
        Refsum's disease (356.3)

FIGURE 17–3.   Conventions used in ICD-9.

Main Term

When trying to locate a diagnosis with more than one word, look first under the main term or condition. Often, a diagnosis may be an **eponym** (e.g., Ménière's disease or syndrome). These terms can be found under the main term *disease* or *syndrome*. In the diagnosis breast cyst, the main term is *cyst*. Find the condition, not the location. Remember the exceptions to the rules of using the main term.

Fourth and Fifth Digits

In many instances, a fourth digit has been added to a category to provide more detail, or **specificity**. These are subcat-

Box 17-4

STEPS IN LOCATING A DIAGNOSTIC CODE

1. Choose the main term within the diagnostic statement.
2. Locate the main term in Volume 2.
3. Refer to all notes and conventions under the main term.
4. Find the appropriate indented subordinate term.
5. Follow any relevant instructions, such as "see also."
6. Confirm the selected code by cross-referencing to Volume 1. Make sure you have added any fourth or fifth digits necessary.
7. Assign the code.

egory codes. Some codes also have a fifth digit because of the need to code to a higher specificity. For example, diabetes mellitus is category 250. It is necessary to use one of the fourth-digit subcategories to indicate the specific complications that may accompany the diabetes and then add a fifth digit to indicate whether the diabetes is insulin dependent or non–insulin dependent. Those codes requiring a fifth digit are identified in both Volumes 1 and 2. Incomplete coding here affects reimbursement and causes data errors. Figure 17-4 shows samples of fifth-digit classifications from the ICD-9-CM, Volumes 1 and 2. The code 807.1 tells the third-party payer that the patient was seen for an open fracture of a rib. The fifth digit is added to describe how many ribs. A patient who fractured two ribs would be assigned the code 807.12. This gives a more thorough picture of the patient's problem and enables the payer to determine whether the treatment is medically necessary.

Primary Codes

In outpatient coding, the **primary diagnosis** is simply the patient's chief complaint or the reason the patient sought medical attention today. It may be a routine follow-up visit, or there may be a new problem. The primary code is listed first on the CMS-1500 (Box 17-4).

When More Than One Code Is Used

In many cases, more than one code is used for a single patient visit. When patients have more than one diagnosis, it is necessary to convey an accurate picture of the patient's total condition. For example, an elderly patient may have the following diagnoses listed each time she visits the doctor: degenerative arthritis, type II diabetes mellitus, macular degeneration, hypertension, and pernicious anemia. If any of these conditions is related to or affects her treatment,

they should be listed as supplementary information. If she visits the doctor because she has influenza and her other diagnoses are not addressed at the visit, it is not necessary to list all the diagnoses given. The primary diagnosis is her reason for coming to the office (symptoms of influenza). But the fact that she is diabetic will affect her treatment and makes her visit medically necessary. Multiple codes should be sequenced with the proper service or procedure code on the proper line of the CMS-1500. Figure 17-5 shows the proper sequencing for another patient's CMS-1500. On line 1 of Section 24 on the CMS-1500 you place the code and charge for the visit. In Block 24E, the diagnosis code for the ankle injury appears first because that is what brought the patient to the office today. One Line 2 of 24A, the laboratory work is listed but is also referenced to the diagnosis on Line 21, Item 2, which is the proper code for the patient's diabetes; this is referenced to Item 2 on Line 24. If the patient did not have diabetes, the laboratory work would not be considered reasonable for a patient with an ankle injury. If this procedure were not followed, the laboratory work would be seen as medically unnecessary, and the physician would not be reimbursed.

Late Effects

Late effects are symptoms or conditions arising from an acute illness. The effects are present after treatment for the acute illness or injury has ended. Proper coding sequence requires that you list the code number identifying the residual or current condition first, with the code number identifying the cause or original illness or injury listed second. Key words used in the patient's medical records defining late effects include late, due to an old injury, due to a previous illness/injury, due to an illness or injury occurring a year or more ago, sequela of . . . , as a result of . . . , resulting from . . . , and so on. Patients who are status post cerebrovascular accident (CVA) may have residual effects from their original stroke, for example, and may have a diagnosis of left hemiparesis as a result of CVA 3 years ago. Figure 17-6 is a sample listing of a late effect from the ICD-9-CM.

LEGAL TIP

Remember that the ICD-9 codes placed on the CMA-1500 are confidential and should be protected as much as any other medical information. Forms left lying in common areas in the office may be seen by other patients. Keep printers and copies of these forms in a private place and share the diagnosis codes only with those who need the information to carry out their duties. Patients have the right to keep their diagnoses private.

INJURY AND POISONING   807–808.49

✓4ᵗʰ **807 Fracture of rib(s), sternum, larynx, and trachea**

The following fifth-digit subclassification is for use with codes 807.0-807.1:

0 **rib(s), unspecified**
1 **one rib**
2 **two ribs**
3 **three ribs**
4 **four ribs**
5 **five ribs**
6 **six ribs**
7 **seven ribs**
8 **eight or more ribs**
9 **multiple ribs, unspecified**

✓5ᵗʰ **807.0** **Rib(s), closed**   `MSP`

✓5ᵗʰ **807.1** **Rib(s), open**   `MSP`

807.2 **Sternum, closed**   `MSP`

DEF: Break in flat bone (breast bone) in anterior thorax.

807.3 **Sternum, open**   `MSP`

DEF: Break, with open wound, in flat bone in mid anterior thorax.

807.4 **Flail chest**   `MSP`

807.5 **Larynx and trachea, closed**   `MSP`
Hyoid bone   Trachea
Thyroid cartilage

A   **807.6** **Larynx and trachea, open**   `MSP`

Fracture — *continued*
multiple — *continued*
skull, specified or unspecified bones, or
face bone(s) with any other bone(s) —
continued

> *Note — Use the following fifth-digit*
> *subclassification with categories 800, 801,*
> *803, and 804:*
>
> 0   *unspecified state of consciousness*
> 1   *with no loss of consciousness*
> 2   *with brief [less than one hour] loss*
>   *of consciousness*
> 3   *with moderate [1-24 hours] loss of*
>   *consciousness*
> 4   *with prolonged [more than 24 hours]*
>   *loss of consciousness and return to*
>   *pre-existing conscious level*
> 5   *with prolonged [more than 24 hours]*
>   *loss of consciousness, without*
>   *return to pre-existing conscious level*
> *Use fifth-digit 5 to designate when a*
>   *patient is unconscious and dies*
>   *before regaining consciousness,*
>   *regardless of the duration of the*
>   *loss of consciousness*
> 6   *with loss of consciousness of*
>   *unspecified duration*
> 9   *with concussion, unspecified*

with
contusion, cerebral 804.1 `.5ᵗʰ`
epidural hemorrhage 804.2 `.5ᵗʰ`
extradural hemorrhage 804.2 `.5ᵗʰ`
hemorrhage (intracranial) NEC
804.8 `.5ᵗʰ`
intracranial injury NEC 804.4 `.5ᵗʰ`
laceration, cerebral 804.1 `.5ᵗʰ`
subarachnoid hemorrhage 804.2 `.5ᵗʰ`
B   subdural hemorrhage 804.2 `.5ᵗʰ`

F I G U R E   1 7 – 4 .   Samples of fifth-digit classifications from ICD-9-CM. (A) Volume 1. (B) Volume 2.

HEALTH INSURANCE CLAIM FORM

PLEASE DO NOT STAPLE IN THIS AREA

☐☐ PICA   PICA ☐☐

1. MEDICARE	MEDICAID	CHAMPUS	CHAMPVA	GROUP HEALTH PLAN	FECA BLK LUNG	OTHER	1a. INSURED'S I.D. NUMBER (FOR PROGRAM IN ITEM 1)
☒ (Medicare #)	☐ (Medicaid #)	☐ (Sponsor's SSN)	☐ (VA File #)	☐ (SSN or ID)	☐ (SSN)	☐ (ID)	000-00-0000A

2. PATIENT'S NAME (Last Name, First Name, Middle Initial)
Naomi A Dishman

3. PATIENT'S BIRTH DATE MM 04 DD 14 YY 24 SEX M ☐ F ☒

4. INSURED'S NAME (Last Name, First Name, Middle Initial)
Same

5. PATIENT'S ADDRESS (No., Street)
405 Carolina Ave

6. PATIENT RELATIONSHIP TO INSURED
Self ☐ Spouse ☐ Child ☐ Other ☐

7. INSURED'S ADDRESS (No., Street)

CITY Danville   STATE VA

8. PATIENT STATUS
Single ☐ Married ☒ Other ☐

CITY   STATE

ZIP CODE 24540   TELEPHONE (Include Area Code) (434) 555-5555

Employed ☐ Full-Time Student ☐ Part-Time Student ☐

ZIP CODE   TELEPHONE (INCLUDE AREA CODE) ( )

9. OTHER INSURED'S NAME (Last Name, First Name, Middle Initial)
NONE

10. IS PATIENT'S CONDITION RELATED TO:

11. INSURED'S POLICY GROUP OR FECA NUMBER

a. OTHER INSURED'S POLICY OR GROUP NUMBER

a. EMPLOYMENT? (CURRENT OR PREVIOUS)
☐ YES ☒ NO

a. INSURED'S DATE OF BIRTH MM DD YY SEX M ☐ F ☐

b. OTHER INSURED'S DATE OF BIRTH MM DD YY SEX M ☐ F ☐

b. AUTO ACCIDENT? PLACE (State)
☐ YES ☒ NO

b. EMPLOYER'S NAME OR SCHOOL NAME

c. EMPLOYER'S NAME OR SCHOOL NAME

c. OTHER ACCIDENT?
☒ YES ☐ NO

c. INSURANCE PLAN NAME OR PROGRAM NAME

d. INSURANCE PLAN NAME OR PROGRAM NAME

10d. RESERVED FOR LOCAL USE

d. IS THERE ANOTHER HEALTH BENEFIT PLAN?
☐ YES ☐ NO If yes, return to and complete item 9 a-d.

READ BACK OF FORM BEFORE COMPLETING & SIGNING THIS FORM.
12. PATIENT'S OR AUTHORIZED PERSON'S SIGNATURE I authorize the release of any medical or other information necessary to process this claim. I also request payment of government benefits either to myself or to the party who accepts assignment below.

SIGNED Signature of File   DATE 052803

13. INSURED'S OR AUTHORIZED PERSON'S SIGNATURE I authorize payment of medical benefits to the undersigned physician or supplier for services described below.

SIGNED

14. DATE OF CURRENT: MM 05 DD 28 YY 03 ILLNESS (First symptom) OR INJURY (Accident) OR PREGNANCY(LMP)

15. IF PATIENT HAS HAD SAME OR SIMILAR ILLNESS. GIVE FIRST DATE MM DD YY

16. DATES PATIENT UNABLE TO WORK IN CURRENT OCCUPATION FROM MM DD YY TO MM DD YY

17. NAME OF REFERRING PHYSICIAN OR OTHER SOURCE

17a. I.D. NUMBER OF REFERRING PHYSICIAN

18. HOSPITALIZATION DATES RELATED TO CURRENT SERVICES FROM MM DD YY TO MM DD YY

19. RESERVED FOR LOCAL USE

20. OUTSIDE LAB? ☐ YES ☐ NO $ CHARGES

21. DIAGNOSIS OR NATURE OF ILLNESS OR INJURY. (RELATE ITEMS 1,2,3 OR 4 TO ITEM 24E BY LINE)
1. 845.03
2. 250.00
3. ____.__
4. ____.__

22. MEDICAID RESUBMISSION CODE ORIGINAL REF. NO.

23. PRIOR AUTHORIZATION NUMBER

24. A. DATE(S) OF SERVICE From MM DD YY	To MM DD YY	B. Place of Service	C. Type of Service	D. PROCEDURES, SERVICES, OR SUPPLIES (Explain Unusual Circumstances) CPT/HCPCS	MODIFIER	E. DIAGNOSIS CODE	F. $ CHARGES	G. DAYS OR UNITS	H. EPSDT Family Plan	I. EMG	J. COB	K. RESERVED FOR LOCAL USE
05 28 03	05 28 03	11		99213		1	100 00	1				
05 28 03	05 28 03	11		82947		2	25 00	1				

25. FEDERAL TAX I.D. NUMBER SSN EIN
54-0000000 ☐ ☐

26. PATIENT'S ACCOUNT NO.
1234

27. ACCEPT ASSIGNMENT? (For govt. claims, see back)
☒ YES ☐ NO

28. TOTAL CHARGE $ 125 00

29. AMOUNT PAID $

30. BALANCE DUE $ 125 00

31. SIGNATURE OF PHYSICIAN OR SUPPLIER INCLUDING DEGREES OR CREDENTIALS (I certify that the statements on the reverse apply to this bill and are made a part thereof.)

SIGNED   DATE

32. NAME AND ADDRESS OF FACILITY WHERE SERVICES WERE RENDERED (If other than home or office)

33. PHYSICIAN'S, SUPPLIER'S BILLING NAME, ADDRESS, ZIP CODE & PHONE #
JOSEPH G NORTH, MD
1111 GRAYSON STREET
DANVILLE VA
PIN#   GRP#

(APPROVED BY AMA COUNCIL ON MEDICAL SERVICE 8/88)   **PLEASE PRINT OR TYPE**   APPROVED OMB-0938-0008 FORM CMS-1500 (12-90), FORM RRB-1500, APPROVED OMB-1215-0055 FORM OWCP-1500, APPROVED OMB-0720-0001 (CHAMPUS)

F I G U R E 1 7 – 5 .   Sample CMS-1500 claim form indicating proper sequencing.

LATE EFFECTS OF INJURIES, POISONINGS, TOXIC EFFECTS, AND OTHER EXTERNAL CAUSES (905-909)

Note: These categories are to be used to indicate conditions classifiable to 800-999 as the cause of late effects, which are themselves classified elsewhere. The "late effects" include those specified as such, or as sequelae, which may occur at any time after the acute injury.

✓4ᵗʰ **905 Late effects of musculoskeletal and connective tissue injuries**

    905.0 Late effect of fracture of skull and face bones
        Late effect of injury classifiable to 800-804

    905.1 Late effect of fracture of spine and trunk without mention of spinal cord lesion
        Late effect of injury classifiable to 805, 807-809

    905.2 Late effect of fracture of upper extremities
        Late effect of injury classifiable to 810-819

    905.3 Late effect of fracture of neck of femur
        Late effect of injury classifiable to 820

    905.4 Late effect of fracture of lower extremities
        Late effect of injury classifiable to 821-827

    905.5 Late effect of fracture of multiple and unspecified bones
        Late effect of injury classifiable to 828-829

    905.6 Late effect of dislocation
        Late effect of injury classifiable to 830-839

    905.7 Late effect of sprain and strain without mention of tendon injury
        Late effect of injury classifiable to 840-848, except tendon injury

    905.8 Late effect of tendon injury
        Late effect of tendon injury due to:
            open wound [injury classifiable to 880-884 with .2, 890-894 with .2]
            sprain and strain [injury classifiable to 840-848]

    905.9 Late effect of traumatic amputation
        Late effect of injury classifiable to 885-887, 895-897

A
        EXCLUDES *late amputation stump complication (997.60-997.69)*

Late

Late — *continued*
  effect(s) (of) — continued
    tuberculosis — *continued*
      genitourinary (conditions classifiable to 016) 137.2
      pulmonary (conditions classifiable to 010-012) 137.0
      specified organs NEC (conditions classifiable to 014, 017-018) 137.4
    viral encephalitis (conditions classifiable to 049.8, 049.9, 062-064) 139.0
    wound, open
      extremity (injury classifiable to 880-884 and 890-894, except .2) 906.1
      tendon (injury classifiable to 880-884 with .2 and 890-894 with.2) 905.8
      head, neck, and trunk (injury classifiable to 870-879) 906.0

B

FIGURE 17–6. Sample section of late effects in ICD-9-CM. (A) Volume 1. (B) Volume 2.

Coding Suspected Conditions

In the inpatient setting, coders list conditions after the patient's testing is complete. In other words, they are coding with complete information. In outpatient settings, however, the coder reports the reason for the patient visit as it occurs. When filing claims, the coder is limited by the information and documentation on hand at the time of the patient visit. If at the end of the visit the diagnosis is not confirmed, the physician may indicate "rule out," "suspected," or "probable." For example, a patient who comes in complaining of headache may be sent for magnetic resonance imaging (MRI) of the head because the physician suspects a serious disorder. On the patient's encounter form, the physician may list the diagnosis as "rule out brain tumor." It is not accurate to code the visit as brain tumor before it is confirmed by MRI. On this first visit to the physician's office, the reason for being seen is headache. The patient's symptom

WHAT IF

You need to code a condition described as acute, chronic, or both. What code should you use?

When a particular condition is described as both acute and chronic, code it according to the subentries in the alphabetic index (Volume 2) for the condition. If there are separate entries listed for acute, subacute, and chronic, use both codes. The first code listed should be for the acute condition, the reason the patient came to the office today. Respiratory and orthopedic conditions tend to be acute and chronic. That is, a patient with emphysema will always have underlying symptoms of progressive disease, but during the spring, pollen may aggravate the condition and cause acute breathing problems.

(headache) is the only confirmed reason for the encounter at this point. On the second visit to the doctor, the MRI has confirmed a glioma in the frontal lobe. For the second and all subsequent visits, glioma is coded as the reason for the encounter. Figure 17-2 shows a page from the ICD-9-CM that includes many of the symptom codes.

Checkpoint Question

8. Before a definitive diagnosis is made, what is coded?

Documentation Requirements

As discussed throughout this chapter, you should choose the code assigned to any given claim for a service or procedure based on the documentation available in the patient's record at the time of the service. An **audit** is conducted by the government, a managed care company, and a health care organization to determine compliance and to detect fraud. Remember, if it's not in the chart, it did not happen. Auditors verify the codes used based on information recorded in the chart on the date of service.

THE FUTURE OF DIAGNOSTIC CODING: *INTERNATIONAL CLASSIFICATION OF DISEASES, TENTH REVISION*

A new edition of the ICD, the *International Classification of Diseases, Tenth Revision* (ICD-10), is scheduled to be introduced sometime between 2003 and 2005. The WHO is responsible for revising the ICD to improve the quality of data input into clinical databases. The ICD-10-CM will include

more codes and will be used by every type of health care provider for all encounters, including hospice and home health care. The new codes are alphanumeric, but the format of the index is similar to the ICD-9-CM. Two new chapters relating to disorders of the eye and the ear are being added to the ICD-10. Computer software will be revised, and the ICD-9-CM code books will be obsolete.

Checkpoint Question

9. List two reasons for a chart audit.

CHAPTER SUMMARY

Medical outpatient diagnostic coding involves the use of numbers to describe diseases, injuries, and other reasons for seeking medical care. ICD-9-CM provides an index to report and track diseases. Diagnostic coding is linked to reimbursement because it assures that the physician's service or procedure was medically necessary. As a medical assistant, you must understand the format and guidelines for assigning a code or reason for each encounter, treatment, and/or service.

Critical Thinking Challenges

Tom Barksdale has been seen by the physician for controlled non–insulin-dependent type 2 diabetes mellitus for about 10 years. While being seen for a routine check of his blood sugar, he complains of numbness and tingling in his left lower leg and foot. An x-ray of both legs is performed, since poor circulation in the extremities can be a complication of diabetes. The x-ray confirms the diagnosis of peripheral neuropathy.

1. Which ICD-9 code should be listed with the office visit?
2. Which code indicates the reason for the x-ray?
3. Which code should be placed on the CMA-1500 first as the primary diagnosis or reason for the visit?

Answers:

1. 250.60
2. 337.1
3. 250.60

Answers to Checkpoint Questions

1. Medical necessity means a particular service or procedure is reasonable.
2. The three volumes of ICD-9-CM are Volume 1, the Tabular List of Diseases; Volume 2, the Alphabetic

Index of Diseases; and Volume 3, the Tabular List and Alphabetic Index of Procedures.

3. The World Health Organization must approve any changes in the ICD-9-CM system.

4. Inpatient refers to a patient who is admitted to the hospital for a stay anticipated to be longer than a day. An outpatient is one who is seen in the physician's office or for 1-day surgery and will stay in the inpatient facility for less than 24 hours.

5. ICD-9-CM is updated annually in October.

6. E-codes are used to provide information to (1) industry, (2) insurance underwriters, (3) national safety programs, and (4) public health agencies and others concerned with injuries and poisonings.

7. V-codes are used to report reasons for receiving services other than illness.

8. Before a definitive diagnosis is assigned to a patient, services must be coded with the patient's symptoms at the time he or she was seen.

9. Chart audits are conducted to assess compliance and to detect fraud.

 Websites

World Health Organization
www.who.int

Health and Human Services
www.hhs.gov

Centers for Medicare & Medicaid
www.cms.gov

American Health Information Management Association
www.ahima.org

American Hospital Association
www.aha.org

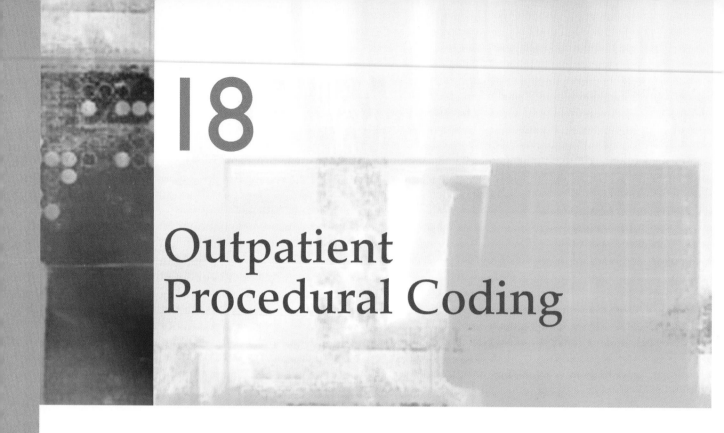

18

Outpatient Procedural Coding

CHAPTER OUTLINE

ROLE DELINEATION COMPONENTS

GENERAL: Legal Concepts
- Perform within legal and ethical boundaries

ADMINISTRATIVE: Administrative Procedures
- Perform basic administrative medical assisting functions.

- Obtain reimbursement through accurate claims submission.

ADMINISTRATIVE: Practice Finances
- Perform procedural and diagnostic coding.

CHAPTER COMPETENCIES

LEARNING OBJECTIVES

Upon successfully completing this chapter, you will be able to:
1. Spell and define the key terms
2. Explain the format of Current Procedural Terminology (CPT-4) and its use
3. Explain the Healthcare Common Procedure Coding System (HCPCS) and level 2 and 3 codes
4. Explain what diagnostic related groups (DRGs) are and how they are used to determine Medicare payments
5. Discuss the goals of resource-based relative value system (RBRVS)
6. Describe the relationship between coding and reimbursement

KEY TERMS

Current Procedural Terminology

descriptor

diagnostic related group

Healthcare Common Procedure Coding System

key component

modifiers

outlier

procedure

resource-based relative value scale

upcoding

As discussed in Chapter 17, coding is a way to standardize medical information for purposes such as collecting health care statistics, performing a medical care review, and indexing medical records. It is also used for health insurance claims processing (see Chapter 16 for more information). Because coding is linked to reimbursement, you must code accurately and precisely. Incorrect, insufficient, or incomplete coding on claims forms can lead to improper reimbursement for the physician as well as recording and possibly passing along inaccurate patient information.

PHYSICIAN'S CURRENT PROCEDURAL TERMINOLOGY

Physician's **Current Procedural Terminology** (CPT) is a comprehensive listing of medical terms and codes for the uniform coding of procedures and services provided by physicians. First published in 1966 by the American Medical Association (AMA), CPT initially focused mainly on surgical procedures, with a limited number of other codes to describe medical, radiology, laboratory, and pathology procedures. New editions were published in 1970, 1973, and 1977. The fourth edition, CPT-4, contains more than 7000 new codes. Although there has not been a major revision of the CPT since 1977, CPT-4 is updated annually, with the newest version available each December.

CPT-4 contains a listing of all current U. S. Food and Drug Administration–approved physicians' procedures and services. The AMA developed it in collaboration with various other health organizations. In the early 1980s, Congress decided to use CPT-4 to code all physicians' procedures and services for Medicare patients. The aim of CPT-4 was to establish a way in which interested parties would know what procedures and services had been provided to the patient without reading a lengthy report. For example, the CPT-4 allows insurance companies to:

- Communicate easily with one another
- Compare reimbursable amounts for procedures
- Speed claims processing

CPT-4 is a system of five-digit numeric codes and corresponding meanings, as illustrated in Figure 18-1, a sample page from the CPT-4 book.

Every code means something unique and is used only to describe a specific **procedure**, service, or medical supply provided by physicians to their patients. This is true for inpatients and outpatients. Codes and descriptions are updated, revised, or changed yearly. If your physician's office uses a superbill or preprinted routing slip that lists the procedures performed, you must update this form yearly and work with your software vendor to update your computer software. The CPT-4 code selected will be placed on the CMS-1500 universal claim form in Section 24, Box D, along with any modifiers used. Figure 18-2 is a sample universal claim form showing the proper placement of codes for consultation and chest radiography.

The CPT-4 book is divided into six major sections:

1. Evaluation and management
2. Anesthesia
3. Surgery
4. Radiology
5. Pathology and laboratory
6. Medicine

Reading Descriptors

When reading a code's **descriptor**, or description, you will read up to the semicolon and then look down for any indentations using the same words before the semicolon. For example, the code 25065 carries the following descriptor: Biopsy, soft tissue of forearm and/or wrist; superficial. The CPT code for a soft tissue biopsy of the forearm and/or wrist is 25065. If the tissue sample was taken from the superficial skin, 25065 is used. Look at the indented line that bears the code 25066. Because it is indented, you must look at the lines above to find the category. Then read up to the semicolon. The description of this code is Biopsy, soft tissue of forearm and/or wrist; deep superficial or intramuscular. Use of the indentation and the semicolon saves space and keeps the CPT books from becoming too long.

Guidelines

Each section begins with its own specific guidelines and a listing of specific procedures and services applicable in that field. The guidelines contain definitions, explanatory notes, a listing of the previously unlisted procedures found in that particular section, directions on how to file a special report, modifiers for use in that particular section, and definitions to assist the coder.

Unlisted Procedures and Special Reports

Occasionally, a physician will perform a service that is not listed in the CPT-4 book. CPT provides unlisted codes at the beginning of each section for use when an unusual, variable, or new procedure is done. When an unlisted code is used, however, you must submit a copy of the procedure report with the claim. This special report should include the following information:

1. Definition or description of the nature, extent, and need for the procedure
2. Time, effort, and equipment necessary to provide the service
3. Complexity of symptoms
4. Final diagnosis
5. Pertinent physical findings
6. Diagnostic and therapeutic procedures
7. Concurrent problems
8. Follow-up care

(27554 has been deleted. To report, see 27550, 27552, 27556, 27557, 27558)

27556 Open treatment of knee dislocation, with or without internal or external fixation; without primary ligamentous repair or augmentation/reconstruction

27557 with primary ligamentous repair

27558 with primary ligamentous repair, with augmentation/reconstruction

27560 Closed treatment of patellar dislocation; without anesthesia

(For recurrent dislocation, see 27420-27424)

27562 requiring anesthesia

(27564 has been deleted. To report, see 27560, 27562, 27566)

27566 Open treatment of patellar dislocation, with or without partial or total patellectomy

Manipulation

27570* Manipulation of knee joint under general anesthesia (includes application of traction or other fixation devices)

Arthrodesis

▲27580 Arthrodesis, knee, any techniques

Amputation

27590 Amputation, thigh, through femur, any level;

27591 immediate fitting technique including first cast

27592 open, circular (guillotine)

27594 secondary closure or scar revision

27596 re-amputation

27598 Disarticulation at knee

Other Procedures

27599 Unlisted procedure, femur or knee

Leg (Tibia and Fibula) and Ankle Joint

Incision

27600 Decompression fasciotomy, leg; anterior and/or lateral compartments only

27601 posterior compartment(s) only

27602 anterior and/or lateral, and posterior compartment(s)

(For incision and drainage procedures, superficial, see 10040-10160)

(For decompression fasciotomy with debridement, see 27892-27894)

27603 Incision and drainage, leg or ankle; deep abscess or hematoma

27604 infected bursa

▲27605* Tenotomy, percutaneous, Achilles tendon (separate procedure); local anesthesia

27606 general anesthesia

27607 Incision (eg, osteomyelitis or bone abscess) leg or ankle

(27608 has been deleted)

▲27610 Arthrotomy, ankle, including exploration, drainage, or removal or foreign body

(27611 has been deleted)

▲27612 Arthrotomy, posterior capsular release, ankle, with or without Achilles tendon lengthening

(See also 27685)

Excision

27613 Biopsy, soft tissue of leg or ankle area; superficial

▲27613 deep (subfascial or intramuscular)

(For needle biopsy of soft tissue, use 20206)

27615 Radical resection of tumor (eg, malignant neoplasm), soft tissue of leg or ankle area

FIGURE 18-1. Sample page from CPT 2003.

Evaluation and Management Codes

Evaluation and management (E/M) codes are five-digit numbers that begin with the number 9. These are the most frequently used codes. E/M codes describe various patient histories, examinations, and decisions physicians must make in evaluating and treating patients in various settings (e.g., office, outpatient, hospital). In essence, the E/M codes address what the physician does when interacting with the patient. For this reason, the physician's documentation must meet standards so the physician and coder (medical assistant) can decide which code to use for a specific patient–physician encounter.

To code the services described in the E/M section, you must be sure that the patient's medical record indicates that **key components** are present. Two of three key components are required for established patients and three of three for new patients. These components are the elements that make up the visit. All E/M codes contain the following components:

- History
- Physical examination
- Medical decision making
- Counseling
- Coordination of care

FIGURE 18-2. Sample insurance claim form for consultation and chest radiography.

- Nature of presenting problem
- Time

History, physical examination, and medical decision making are key components for a visit. The others are contributing elements.

Four classifications of histories and physical examinations are described in CPT-4. These include the following:

- Problem-focused
- Expanded problem-focused
- Detailed
- Comprehensive

Table 18-1 describes these classifications in greater detail. The provider must pick one of these based on information provided by the physician and documented in the patient's record.

The third key component, medical decision making, is defined in CPT-4 as one of the following:

- Straightforward
- Low complexity

Table 18-1 HISTORY AND PHYSICAL EXAMINATIONS

The physician or provider must select which history and physical examination code to use. You, however, should have a basic understanding of each category. It is important to note that there are separate codes for each category and separate codes for both new and established patients.

Type of History and Physical Examination	Patient Problems and Physician Time Required	Examples
Problem focused	Patient problems are self-limited and minor. Physician time: usually 10 minutes	• 9-month-old patient with diaper rash • 40-year-old patient with sunburn • 18-year-old patient with poison ivy • 60-year-old patient with a routine blood pressure check
Expanded problem focused	Patient problems are mild to moderate. Physician time: between 15–20 minutes	• 55-year-old patient with recurrent urinary tract infections • 16-year-old patient with chronic asthma presents with a cold • 76-year-old patient with osteoarthritis • 56-year-old patient with a stomach ulcer
Detailed	Patient problems are moderate to severe. Physician time: usually 30 minutes	• 18-year-old patient with first Pap smear and contraceptive education • 67-year-old patient with new onset of dysuria • 18-month-old patient with delayed motor skill development. • 34-year-old patient with diabetes requiring insulin dose changes
Comprehensive	Patient problems are moderate to severe. Physician time: usually 45 minutes	• 36-year-old patient with infertility • 8-year-old patient with new onset of diabetes • 65-year-old patient with history of left-sided weakness and confusion

• Moderate complexity
• High complexity

Medical decision making refers to the kinds of things the physician must do to establish a diagnosis for the patient (e.g., determine the management options available, the amount and complexity of the data to be reviewed, the risk of complications, or other problems, such as worsening of the illness or death). To qualify for a particular decision-making level, the physician must meet or exceed two of the three elements for an established patient and all three for a new patient.

Time spent with a patient (e.g., counseling or coordinating care) is sometimes the key component in determining E/M codes. When time spent with the patient is more than 50% of the typical time for the visit, time becomes the deciding factor in choosing an E/M code. For example, if a physician spends an additional 15 minutes counseling a patient in what would normally be only a 10-minute expanded problem-focused history and physical examination, the counseling was more than 50% of the typical 25-minute face-to-face time. The appropriate E/M code is one with a 25-minute time frame (10 minutes and an extra 15 minutes for counseling).

There are other special considerations regarding E/M codes. Initial hospital care codes can be used only by the admitting physician. All other physicians must use consultation codes for a first visit and then subsequent hospital care codes. Box 18-1 outlines the difference between a consultation and a referral. Emergency department service codes are to be used only when the service is rendered in a 24-hour hospital-based facility that specializes in providing treatment of unscheduled events.

Checkpoint Question

1. To code for a service in the E/M section, two of the three key components must be present for an established patient, and all three must be present for a new patient. What are the three key elements?

Anesthesia Codes

Anesthesia codes are five-digit codes that begin with 0. Anesthesia codes are divided by anatomic site and by specific type of procedure. For example, head, neck, and thorax

Box 18-1

IS IT A REFERRAL OR A CONSULTATION?

There are four subcategories of consultations: office, initial inpatient, follow-up inpatient, and confirmatory (in any setting). Each subcategory has specific reporting instructions. When a physician asks another provider to offer an opinion or advice regarding evaluation and management of a specific problem, the second provider becomes a consultant for the patient. The initial encounter is coded as a consultation, and the documentation must support the encounter. A letter should accompany the patient seeing a consulting physician, and the advising physician should send a letter back to the patient's primary physician outlining the findings. If the consulting physician takes over part or all of the patient's care, follow-up or subsequent visits are coded as regular subsequent visits. A confirmatory consultation is considered a second opinion, and the physician should offer only an opinion or advice. A confirmatory consultant does not take over the treatment of the patient. A referral is defined as passing on a patient to another physician. Referrals are coded as new patients, not consultations. Consider this scenario: A 17-year-old girl sees her family physician for recurrent sore throats. When the family physician realizes that the girl probably needs a tonsillectomy, the patient is *referred* to an otorhinolaryngologist for evaluation and possible surgery. The patient has been referred to the surgeon, who will take over that part of her care. When she has recovered from the procedure, she is discharged from the care of the surgeon and returns to her family physician for continued care.

In another example, a patient may be seen by an orthopedic surgeon for arthritis. When it is determined that the patient's problem may be rheumatoid arthritis, he may be sent to a rheumatologist for consultation. The rheumatologist advises the orthopedic surgeon on a treatment plan, but the orthopedic surgeon continues to see the patient and carries out that plan. Written communications between the two physicians are kept in the chart. The significant difference between a consultation and a referral is whether the patient's treatment is transferred to another physician for that problem.

are anatomic sites, and the codes in each section represent the specific procedure, such as plastic repair of cleft lip. Medical assistants in an anesthesiology practice code anesthesia procedures provided in the hospital setting, even though the office is an outpatient facility.

Two types of **modifiers** (letters or numbers added to a code to add detail to the code) are used in the anesthesia section. One type is the standard modifier that is found in all sections of CPT. The other type is the physical status modifier, a two-digit code beginning with the letter P and ending in a number from 1 to 6. These physical status modifiers indicate the patient's condition at the time of anesthesia and the corresponding complexity of services (e.g., P1 indicates a normal, healthy patient and P5 indicates a patient who is not expected to survive without the procedure).

Surgery Codes

Surgery codes begin with numbers 1 through 6. You need to be aware of the following elements, which are discussed in the guidelines of the surgery section.

Unstarred Codes

The CPT-4 codes in this section that do not have a star (*) refer to codes that include a surgical package. The code that follows identifies the surgical package including normal, uncomplicated follow-up care. The surgical package means that local infiltration, metacarpal, metatarsal, or digital block or topical anesthesia, the operation itself, and normal uncomplicated follow-up care are all included in the code that covers the operation itself.

If there is no star next to the code, it means that you cannot bill separately for preoperative and postoperative components.

The Centers for Medicare & Medicaid Services (CMS) has defined the surgical package for Medicare recipients somewhat differently. According to CPT-4, no complications or problems related to the surgery are included in the surgical package. If additional procedures are performed to correct or alleviate these problems, they should be coded separately. According to CMS, however, complications that do not require a revisit to the operating room are included in the price of surgery.

Some insurance carriers have a set number of follow-up days that is consistent for all unstarred surgical services. Check with your carrier to learn what these are so you can bill for the additional office, outpatient, or hospital visits.

Starred Codes

Codes with a star (*) are for the surgical service itself. The surgical package does not apply. You should code any preoperative anesthesia and postoperative components separately. Figure 18-1 includes several starred codes, for example, of repair—simple superficial wounds of scalp, neck, axilla, external genitalia, and so forth:

12001*—2.5 cm or less
12002*—2.6 cm to 7.5 cm
12004*—7.6 cm to 12.5 cm
12005—12.6 cm to 20.10 cm (notice no star)

If a patient came in for routine follow-up care of a scalp wound coded 12001, 12002, or 12004, the coder could also code for both office visits (99212). There is a corresponding fee for this service. If, however, the patient was returning for routine follow-up care for a wound repair that was originally coded 12005, the code 99024 (postoperative follow-up visit) could be used, but there is no charge for this because the service was already included in the surgical package. Remember, 12005 is not a starred procedure. Third-party payers have different rules about what constitutes a surgery package, so the coder must check with the relevant third-party payers.

Integumentary System

This section has codes for which a measurement is necessary. It is important that both the size of the defect and the size of the specimen be measured before they are sent to the laboratory. All excisions listed in the integumentary section include simple closure.

Repairs

CPT-4 defines three types of repairs: simple, intermediate, and complex. Repairs should be measured and recorded in centimeters to be coded appropriately.

Cast Reapplication

You cannot assign the same code for cast replacement as you did for the original cast application because the code for replacement does not include treatment of the fracture, as the original cast application code did; it, therefore, carries a lower reimbursement rate.

Multiple Procedures Furnished on the Same Day

Unless these are part of the overall service, they should be coded separately and placed on the claims form in order from major to minor.

Checkpoint Question

2. What items are included in a surgical package?

Radiology Codes

The radiology section of CPT-4 is divided into the following four subsections:

- Diagnostic radiology/diagnostic imaging
- Diagnostic ultrasound
- Radiation oncology
- Nuclear medicine

WHAT IF

You need help coding a chart. What should you do?

If you have a question about coding, never guess; find the correct answer. For example, you can ask colleagues, the office manager, or the physician. Insurance companies may have a help line. If you are a member of a professional health care organization, network with fellow members. The American Medical Association (AMA) publishes various books to assist in ICD and CPT coding. The AMA also has a magazine, *CPT Assistant*, that is written by CPT experts. It contains many articles designed to make coding easier. In addition, this magazine will keep you current with updates and changes. For further information on the *CPT Assistant* or other works the AMA publishes on coding, call 800-621-8335 or visit the website at **www.amapress.org.**

All radiology codes are five-digit numbers that begin with 7. They are generally arranged by anatomic site, from the top of the body to the bottom. Many radiology codes indicate the number of views for a particular study. Obviously, the facility must be reimbursed for film, developer, and the radiology technologist's time and service.

Some radiological tests require the administration of a contrast medium that enhances the image. The descriptors for such tests specify "with contrast" or "without contrast." "With contrast" refers to contrast medium that is given intravascularly. If the contrast medium is given orally or rectally, you use the code "without contrast."

If a physician performs the procedure and supervises and interprets a procedure (e.g., injects contrast medium and then supervises and interprets), two codes should be used. A written report in the patient's medical record is necessary for billing these codes. The code for the procedure can be found in the surgery, medicine, or radiology section, and the code for supervision and interpretation is found in the radiology section. If two physicians are participating (e.g., a surgeon and radiologist), the radiology portion is billed by the radiologist.

Pathology and Laboratory Codes

All codes in pathology and laboratory work are five-digit numbers that begin with 8. These codes are divided into sections for panels of tests, drug testing, consultations with pathologists, urinalysis, chemistry testing, antibody testing, cytopathology, and so on. The last part of the pathology and laboratory section includes services and procedures provided by a pathologist, including gross (can be seen by the naked eye) and microscopic examination of tissue removed in surgery. Each tissue specimen is submitted under a different identifying code for diagnosis by the pathologist. The codes represent the level of the physician's work. Post-mortem examination or autopsy is performed by a pathologist, and CPT-4 provides codes to report such examinations.

A subsection, automated multichannel tests, deserves a special note. When coding, check that the tests performed are included in the lists under this subsection. For example, the physician may perform the following three tests for a patient: bilirubin, direct; cholesterol; and blood urea nitrogen (BUN). To code this, you assign the code 80003, three clinical chemistry tests, because all of these tests are listed under the automated multichannel test subsection. If the tests performed were bilirubin, direct; cholesterol; and blood acetaldehyde, however, you would code 80002, two clinical chemistry tests, and 82000, blood acetaldehyde. That is because blood acetaldehyde was not on the list of clinical chemistry tests in the automated multichannel test subsections.

Medicine Codes

Like the E/M codes, medicine codes are five-digit numbers that begin with 9. Like the other five sections of the CPT-4, this section includes guidelines for appropriate coding.

Pay particular attention to the information related to the immunization injections subsection, which includes codes from 90701 to 90749. Typically, immunization injections are given when the patient comes to the physician's office for either a routine physical examination or for a minor problem, such as a sore throat. When the injection is given at the time of such a visit, use two codes: one for the service (usually an E/M code) and one for the immunization injection. For example, an established patient may come into the physician's office for a brief examination for a minor problem (e.g., controlled hypertension blood pressure check). The patient may be examined briefly by a nurse or medical assistant while the physician is in the office and may also be given an immunization for poliomyelitis. The coding for this is:

1. 99211, office and other outpatient visit for the evaluation and management of an established patient, which may not require the presence of a physician. Usually, the presenting problems are minimal. Typically, 5 minutes are spent performing or supervising services. (This code is generally used for examination by employees of the practice while a physician is in the office but not performing the examination.)
2. 90713, poliomyelitis vaccine.

For therapeutic or diagnostic injections (codes 90782–90799), you need to specify what was injected (90281–90399). For example, consider the code 90782, therapeutic injection of medication (specify); subcutaneous or intramuscular. This code is the same for a number of injectable therapeutic substances, making the additional, more specific code necessary. A code for administration should also be added (90471–90472). If a significant separately identifiable E/M service is performed, the appropriate E/M service code should be reported in addition to the injection code.

In Medicare claims, the cost of administering injections is included in the price of office and outpatient visits and other procedures furnished on the same day. Supplying the drug is a separate billable service, however, and should be assigned the appropriate code. (This may not be true of other carriers, so you need to check with them.)

Using the most specific codes for different injectable substances and supplies while keeping invoices to document actual cost helps verify charges submitted for these services.

The medicine section also includes cardiac diagnostic testing, such as electrocardiography and echocardiography. This section also lists the codes for performing cardiopulmonary resuscitation and dialysis treatment.

Checkpoint Question

3. A patient comes in for a tetanus booster, and the physician gives the booster and completes a routine physical examination. How many codes do you use for this visit?

CPT-4 Modifiers

CPT-4 provides a way to give additional information about a procedure through the use of additional numbers called modifiers.

There are several ways to write modifiers:

- Write the five-digit code with a hyphen followed by the two-digit modifier (e.g., 28702-22).
- Write the code without a hyphen separating it from the modifier (e.g., 2870222).
- Write the five-digit code that needs multiple modifiers with the first modifier as −99 (multiple modifiers), followed by the additional modifiers (e.g 28702-9922 . . .)

Of course, the modifier can never appear on the claim form by itself because it refers to the procedure and must be directly below it on the claim form (Fig. 18-2).

Box 18-2 provides a few examples of modifiers. A separate listing of available modifiers can be found in Appendix A of CPT-4. Check Appendix A first; then go to the appropriate section to verify that the modifier may be used with the specific CPT code. Failure to use an appropriate modifier causes database and billing errors.

Checkpoint Question

4. Where can a coder find a list of all CPT modifiers?

EXAMPLES OF CPT-4 MODIFIERS

Here are just a few examples of CPT-4 modifiers. A complete list can be found in Appendix A of CPT-4.

- *20 microsurgery or 09920:* This modifier signifies that the surgeon used an operating microscope to perform a procedure.
- *23 unusual anesthesia or 09923:* This modifier signifies that anesthesia was used in a procedure that normally would not require it.
- *26 professional component or 09926:* This modifier signifies that there are two components to the procedure, a professional and a technical one. For example, when a physician requests a radiograph, the radiology technologist takes the radiograph and the physician reads it. This modifier lets the insurance carrier know that the physician did not provide both service components.

HEALTHCARE COMMON PROCEDURE CODING SYSTEM

Because the AMA's CPT-4 codes do not include such items as ambulance service, wheelchairs, or injections, CMS designed another coding system based on the CPT-4. This system is referred to as the **Healthcare Common Procedure Coding System** or HCPCS.

The HCPCS uses codes contained in CPT-4 (now known as HCPCS Level 1) plus expanded codes developed by CMS and fiscal intermediaries to classify physician and nonphysician patient care services on the national level (now known as HCPCS Level 2). Level 2 HCPCS codes are most commonly referred to as the HCPCS codes, and Level 1 HCPCS codes are referred to as CPT. Since 1985, physicians have had to use the HCPCS to bill for services provided to Medicare patients either in the medical office or in the hospital. Since October 1986, physicians also have used the HCPCS to bill for services provided to Medicaid patients.

As of July 1, 1987, federal law requires hospitals to use the HCPCS to report outpatient surgery services to patients receiving health benefits sponsored by the federal government. By October 1, 1987, federal law had extended ambulatory surgical center (ASC) prospective payment methodology to hospital outpatient surgery payments. The purpose of this was twofold:

- To permit identification of ASC procedures so a blended payment rate could be applied to ambulatory surgery performed in the hospital outpatient department
- To provide a database for future payment amounts for all hospital outpatient services

The HCPCS includes three levels of codes, discussed in the following sections.

HCPCS Level 1 Codes

The HCPCS Level 1 codes are in CPT-4. This is a listing of terms and codes that provide a means to report physician procedures and services under both private and government-sponsored health insurance programs.

HCPCS Level 2 Codes: National Codes

The HCPCS Level 2 code listing comes out once a year in the *National Coding Manual*, which can be ordered from the American Hospital Association, American Medical Association, or other publishers of the CPT coding book. It includes codes for the following:

- Chemotherapeutic drugs
- Dental services
- Durable medical equipment
- Injections
- Ophthalmology services
- Orthotics
- Some pathology and laboratory and rehabilitation supplies
- Vision care

National codes are five-digit alphanumeric codes that begin with the letters A to V (e.g., L8100 is elastic support, elastic stocking, below knee, medium weight, each).

HCPCS Level 3 Codes: Local Codes

The HCPCS Level 3 codes were developed to address regional coding—the ability to code something performed or offered in one state that may or may not be performed or offered in another state. These codes, which are produced and made available through your state Medicare carrier, may vary from state to state. Local codes begin with letters W to Z. CMS takes full responsibility for the codes in the *National Coding Manual*, leaving local codes up to Medicare carriers in each state.

 Checkpoint Question

5. Where do you find codes for dental services?

REIMBURSEMENT

Diagnostic Related Groups

Diagnostic related groups (DRGs) are categories into which inpatients are placed according to the similarity of their diagnoses, treatment, and length of hospital stay. Initially, these categories were developed by Yale University researchers in the mid 1970s to aid the process of utilization review. Some 13,000 codes were run through a computer and grouped according to their clinical similarities (including similarities in resources used). Today, DRGs are used to determine reimbursement for Medicare patients' inpatient services. The fee attached to each DRG is based on the national average of all Medicare discharges and is adjusted for regional differences in hospital wages and updates. Hospitals are paid a set amount for each DRG regardless of actual costs for treating the patient. For example, if a hospital uses fewer resources to care for a patient and discharges that patient in less time, it may keep the difference between its actual cost and the DRG payment. Conversely, if the patient stays longer than usual and requires more services, the hospital absorbs the loss. A patient who has an unusually long stay or a complicated case is considered an **outlier**, and the hospital may be paid more than the standard DRG rate if the added expenses can be justified. The hospital coder uses ICD-9-CM codes to pick the appropriate DRG. The more information the hospital has prior to admission, the more accurate the coding; for example, for a patient admitted with chest pain, the hospital coder needs to know that the patient also has hypertension and diabetes.

You may be asked to schedule a patient for admission to the hospital. Assigning the correct ICD-9-CM code from the outpatient practice will influence the DRG to which the patient will be assigned. The hospital coder selects the proper DRG based on these factors:

- Principal diagnosis
- Surgeries
- Complications and comorbid conditions

Physicians can help with coding in the following ways:

- Record the appropriate documentation to identify each patient's problems, complaints, or other reasons for the encounter or visit.
- Work with the medical records or the office coding and billing staffs to determine the proper diagnosis to code, using terminology that includes specific diagnoses, symptoms, problems, or reasons for the encounter (ICD-9-CM codes describe all of these).

Resource-Based Relative Value Scale

As part of the 1989 Omnibus Budget Reconciliation Act (OBRA), the U. S. Congress stipulated that reimbursement to physicians for Medicare services is based on a fee schedule. This fee schedule sets a maximal fee for each service based on the **resource-based relative value scale** (RBRVS). The goal of RBRVS is to reduce Medicare Part B costs and to establish national standards for payment based on CPT-4 codes. (Remember, Part B Medicare covers physicians' services; Part A covers hospital expenses.)

Fee calculations are based on the following factors:

- Intensity of the service
- Time required
- Skills needed
- Overhead expenses
- Malpractice premiums

The particular fee is adjusted by a geographical practice cost index (GPCI), which reflects the difference in health care costs in different parts of the country. These determine the relative value unit (RVU). Finally, a national conversion factor is assigned yearly. The formula looks like this:, CPT code 99205 has an RVU of 4.58, and the national conversion factor is 36.7856. The Medicare allowed charge would be $168.48.

Checkpoint Question

6. Why are DRGs used?

FRAUD AND CODING

Billing for services not performed, using another patient's coverage to receive reimbursement, and falsifying records are examples of blatant fraud. The attorney general of the United States has jurisdiction over such cases, and in most states the Office of the Inspector General investigates reports of possible fraud. Less severe and undeliberate fraudulent practices also cause misuse of health care dollars, and CMS remains vigilant by conducting audits. Even though the physician you work for may already have been paid for a claim, the medical office may still be audited. As a federal program, Medicare has the same authority as the Internal Revenue Service to audit claims and may do so retroactively. This means that an audit can occur even a couple of years after payment has been received for claims. If the medical practice is found to be in error, the physician may be required to repay an amount owed plus interest. Even worse, such errors can jeopardize the physician's ability to participate in Medicare-funded programs. To avoid costly errors, be certain that you can justify your coding:

LEGAL TIP

When submitting Medicare or other insurance claims, do not bill for services the physician has not performed, and do not bill more for a service than it is worth. Billing high is called **upcoding**.

Millions of dollars have been budgeted to investigate fraud and abuse. Fiscal intermediaries (organizations under contract with the U. S. government to handle Medicare claims) randomly review and compare the documentation in the record and report their findings on the particular providers. Peer review organizations have been authorized by CMS to obtain medical records of Medicare beneficiaries for review.

- Keep adequate, accurate, and complete documentation in medical and billing records.
- Use the proper tools to code. Code books are updated yearly. Always use the most recent book.
- Follow the coding rules, becoming familiar with new rules and keeping up-to-date on any changes to existing ones. Medicare has regional updates, usually at no charge, and provides one of the best sources of changes.
- Work closely with the provider, and never code anything about which you are not sure.

CHAPTER SUMMARY

Medical coding involves the use of numbers to describe diseases, injuries, and procedures. It has several purposes, including indexing medical records, performing medical care reviews, deriving health statistics, and reimbursing physicians and hospitals for services. As a medical assistant, you are responsible for knowing the format and usage of CPT-4, the system used to report services and procedures by the physician. Accurate and thorough coding is essential to ensure appropriate reimbursement. You must assist the physician in making sure the proper documentation is available to substantiate the codes used on a claim. Because learning to code is an ongoing process, continuing education is vital. This can be accomplished by attending workshops in your geographic area or by joining a local association of coders, which may also sponsor coding clinics. Two such organizations are the American Academy of Professional Coders (AAPC) and the American Health Information Management Association (AHIMA). Other sources are local medical societies and your school. As in all other aspects of patient contact and care, coding of patients' records is covered by the Health Insurance Portability and Accountability Act of 1996 (HIPAA). Only those with a need to know should have access to patient records.

Critical Thinking Challenges

1. How would you handle a physician who you think overbills for procedures? To whom would you report this? How might you collect documentation of fraud?
2. Create a reminder card to be used when you are to assist with coding.
3. Assume you are working for a family practice physician. Identify three patient problems that you might encounter. Then use the CPT and ICD-9-CM coding books at your school library or the hospital library to find the correct codes.

Answers to Checkpoint Questions

1. The three key elements are history, physical examination, and medical decision making.
2. The surgical package consists of local infiltration, metacarpal, metatarsal, or digital blocks, topical anesthesia, the operation, and normal uncomplicated follow-up care.
3. There are two codes: one for the service and one for the immunization.
4. A list of all modifiers and their meanings is found in Appendix A of CPT-4.
5. Dental codes are found in the HCPCS Level 2 national codes.
6. DRGs are used to determine the reimbursement for Medicare patients' inpatient services.

 Websites

Coding Institute
    www.codinstitute.com
Compliant Billing Service
    www.compliantbilling.com
Medical Billing Association
    www.e-medbill.com

The Clinical Medical Assistant

Performing Clinical Duties

19

Medical Asepsis and Infection Control

CHAPTER OUTLINE

ROLE DELINEATION COMPONENTS

ADMINISTRATIVE: ADMINISTRATIVE PROCEDURES
- Perform basic administrative medical assisting functions

CLINICAL: FUNDAMENTAL PRINCIPLES
- Apply principles of aseptic technique and infection control
- Comply with quality assurance practices

CLINICAL: PATIENT CARE
- Prepare and maintain examination and treatment areas

GENERAL: PROFESSIONALISM
- Display a professional manner and image
- Demonstrate initiative and responsibility
- Work as a member of the health care team

GENERAL: COMMUNICATION SKILLS
- Recognize and respond effectively to verbal, nonverbal, and written communications

GENERAL: LEGAL CONCEPTS
- Perform within legal and ethical boundaries
- Document accurately
- Comply with federal and state health care legislation and regulations
- Comply with established risk management and safety procedures

GENERAL: INSTRUCTION
- Teach methods of health promotion and disease prevention

GENERAL: OPERATIONAL FUNCTIONS
- Perform inventory of supplies and equipment

CHAPTER COMPETENCIES

LEARNING OBJECTIVES
Upon successfully completing this chapter, you will be able to:
1. Spell and define key terms.
2. Describe conditions that promote the growth of microorganisms.
3. Explain the components of the infectious process cycle.
4. List the various ways microbes are transmitted.
5. Compare the effectiveness in reducing or destroying microorganisms using the four levels of infection control.
6. Describe the procedures for cleaning, handling, and disposing of biohazardous waste in the medical office.
7. Explain the concept of medical asepsis.
8. Discuss risk management procedures required by the Occupational Safety and Health Administration guidelines for the medical office.
9. List the required components of an exposure control plan.
10. Explain the importance of following Standard Precautions in the medical office.
11. Identify various personal protective equipment (PPE) items.
12. Describe circumstances when PPE items would be appropriately worn by the medical assistant.
13. Explain the facts pertaining to the transmission and prevention of the Hepatitis B virus and the Human Immunodeficiency Virus in the medical office.
14. Describe how to avoid becoming infected with the Hepatitis B and Human Immunodeficiency viruses.

PERFORMANCE OBJECTIVES
Upon successfully completing this chapter, you will be able to:
1. Perform a medical aseptic handwashing procedure (Procedure 19-1).
2. Remove and discard contaminated personal protective equipment appropriately (Procedure 19-2).
3. Clean and decontaminate biohazardous spills (Procedure 19-3).

KEY TERMS

aerobe	exposure control plan	OSHA	sanitation
anaerobe	exposure risk factors	pathogens	sanitization
asymptomatic	germicide	personal protective	standard precautions
bactericidal	immunization	equipment	sterilization
biohazard	infection	postexposure testing	transient flora
carrier	medical asepsis	resident flora	vector
disease	microorganisms	resistance	viable
disinfection	normal flora	spore	virulent

MANY PATIENTS ARE SEEN daily in the medical office for a variety of reasons, including physical examinations for employment, reassurance about a current health problem, and follow-up care for a chronic condition or surgical procedure. In addition, many patients request appointments because of illness. It is important for you to protect patients from each other with regard to contagious diseases and for you to protect yourself from acquiring the many microorganisms with which you will come into contact every day.

To prevent the spread of **disease** in the medical office, medical assistants must meet two goals. First, you must understand and practice **medical asepsis** at all times, using specific practices and procedures to prevent disease transmission. These practices and procedures also allow you to work with ill patients while reducing the chances that you will spread disease to other patients or become infected yourself. Second, you must teach the patients and their families about techniques to use at home to prevent the transmission of disease. Handwashing, the cornerstone of infection control, is discussed in this chapter and is emphasized in all subsequent chapters wherever contact with infectious material might be expected. In addition, this chapter describes how disease is transmitted and most important, how to prevent the spread of disease.

MICROORGANISMS, PATHOGENS, AND NORMAL FLORA

Microorganisms, living organisms that can be seen only with a microscope, are part of our normal environment. In addition to our physical environment, many microorganisms can be found on your skin and throughout your gastrointestinal, genitourinary, and respiratory systems, and some of these are required for good health. These microorganisms are normal and are referred to as **normal flora or resident flora**. Some microorganisms, however, are not part of the normal flora and may cause disease or **infection.** Disease-producing microorganisms are referred to as pathogens and are classified as bacteria, viruses, fungi, or protozoa. (See Chapter 42 for a more detailed discussion of microorganisms.)

When normal flora become too many in number or are transmitted to an area of the body in which they are not normally found, they are referred to as **transient flora**, which can become pathogens under the right conditions. For example, *Staphylococcus aureus*, a microorganism commonly found on the skin, may get into underlying tissue if the skin is broken. In this situation, the normal flora of the skin has become transient flora and may cause disease. Decreased **resistance** in the host is one condition that may allow transient flora to become pathogenic. Individuals who are elderly, receiving certain drugs to treat cancer, or under unusual stress may have a lowered resistance and be particularly susceptible to infections.

Although the body is protected by many nonspecific defenses against disease, infection or illness may occur if the natural barriers are overpowered or breached. These are some of the body's natural defenses that may prevent the invasion of pathogens into various body organs:

- Skin. As long as the skin is kept clean and remains intact or unbroken, *staphylococcal* (Staph) bacteria are not considered dangerous. Washing the skin frequently will flush away many of these bacteria along with any other microorganisms.
- Eyes. The eyelashes act as a barrier by trapping dust that may carry microorganisms before they have an opportunity to enter the eye. If any microorganisms do enter the eye, the enzyme lysozyme normally found in tears will destroy some microorganisms, including bacteria.
- Mouth. The greatest variety of microorganisms in the body is in the mouth. Saliva is slightly **bactericidal**, and good oral hygiene will remove or prevent the growth of many of the pathogens in the mouth.
- Gastrointestinal tract. Hydrochloric acid normally found in the stomach destroys most of the disease-producing pathogens that enter the gastrointestinal system. One bacterium, *Escherichia coli* (*E. coli*), is resident flora found in the large intestine and is necessary for digestion. It does not usually cause disease as long it remains within the gastrointestinal tract. *Helicobacter pylori* also resides in the digestive tracts of some individuals and may cause gastric ulcers.
- Respiratory tract. Hairs and cilia on the membrane lining of the nostrils are early defenses against airborne microorganisms. If these physical barriers do not stop an invasion, mucus from the membranes lining the respiratory tract should trap the microorganisms and facilitate their removal from the respiratory system as the person swallows, coughs, or sneezes.
- Genitourinary tract. The reproductive and urinary systems provide a less hospitable environment for microorganisms. The slightly acidic environment of these body systems reduces the ability of many microorganisms to survive. In addition, frequent urination flushes the urinary tract and removes many transient microorganisms.

While these systems have protective mechanisms to prevent infection, any of them may be overpowered by a particularly **virulent** organism. Transient flora are not usually pathogenic unless the person's defenses are compromised by a decrease in resistance.

Checkpoint Question

1. What are pathogenic microorganisms? How does the body prevent an invasion and subsequent infection naturally?

Conditions That Favor the Growth of Pathogens

All microorganisms require certain conditions to grow and reproduce. To reduce the number of microorganisms and potential pathogens in a clinical setting, you must eliminate as many of their life requirements as possible. These requirements include the following:

- Moisture. Few microorganisms can survive with little water or moisture. However, some microorganisms form **spores** and remain dormant until moisture is available.
- Nutrients. Microorganisms depend on their environment for nourishment. Surfaces (tables, counters, equipment) that are contaminated with organic matter (food products, body fluids, or tissue) promote the growth of microorganisms.
- Temperature. Although some microorganisms can survive even in freezing or boiling temperatures, those that thrive at a normal body temperature of 98.6°F are most likely to be pathogenic to humans. Many microorganisms that leave an infected person can survive for a while at room temperature; therefore, surfaces that are contaminated with dried organic material should be considered possibly pathogenic.
- Darkness. Many pathogenic bacteria are destroyed by bright light, including sunlight.
- Neutral pH. The pH of a solution refers to the measurement of its acid-base balance on a scale of 1 to 14,

with 7 being neutral. Many microorganisms are destroyed in an environment that is not neutral. The pH of blood, 7.35 to 7.45, is preferred by microorganisms that thrive in the human body.
- Oxygen. Microorganisms that need oxygen to survive are called **aerobes**. A few, however, do not require oxygen; these are called **anaerobes**. While most pathogens are aerobic, the microbes that cause tetanus and botulism are anaerobic.

If any one of these conditions is altered in any way, the growth and reproduction of the pathogen will be affected. Your role as a professional medical assistant in a medical office includes using this knowledge of microbial growth to inhibit the growth and reproduction of microorganisms in the office.

Checkpoint Question

2. Given the six conditions that favor the growth of pathogens, explain how you can alter the growth and reproduction of microorganisms by changing these factors.

The Infection Cycle

The infection cycle is often thought of as a series of specific links of a chain involving a causative agent or invading microorganism (FIG. 19-1). The first link in the chain is the reservoir host; this is the person who is infected with the

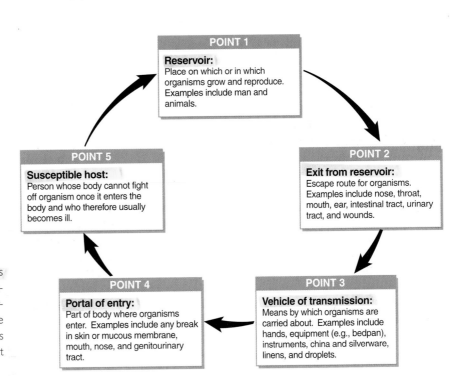

FIGURE 19-1. The infectious process cycle. Infections and infectious diseases are spread by starting from the reservoir (*point 1*) and moving in a circle to the susceptible host (*point 5*). Microorganisms can be controlled by interfering at any point in the cycle.

POINT 1
Reservoir: Place on which or in which organisms grow and reproduce. Examples include man and animals.

POINT 2
Exit from reservoir: Escape route for organisms. Examples include nose, throat, mouth, ear, intestinal tract, urinary tract, and wounds.

POINT 3
Vehicle of transmission: Means by which organisms are carried about. Examples include hands, equipment (e.g., bedpan), instruments, china and silverware, linens, and droplets.

POINT 4
Portal of entry: Part of body where organisms enter. Examples include any break in skin or mucous membrane, mouth, nose, and genitourinary tract.

POINT 5
Susceptible host: Person whose body cannot fight off organism once it enters the body and who therefore usually becomes ill.

microorganism. While this person may or may not show signs of infection, his or her body is serving as a source of nutrients and an incubator in which the pathogen can grow and reproduce. These persons are also called **carriers,** or **reservoirs, of disease.**

The reservoir host may transmit disease only when the pathogen has a means of exit. The second link in the chain is the manner in which the pathogen leaves the reservoir host. Means of exit include the mucous membranes of the nose and mouth, the openings of the gastrointestinal system (mouth or rectum), and an open wound.

In addition to the means of exit, the microbe must have a vehicle in which to leave the host. This next link in the chain, the **means of transmission, involves the vehicle that is used by the pathogen when it leaves the reservoir host and spreads through the environment.** Vehicles include mucus or air droplets from the oral or nasal cavities and direct contact between an unclean hand and another person or object. Sneezing and coughing without covering the nose and mouth are excellent methods of transmitting microorganisms into the environment and potential hosts.

The fourth link in the chain of the infectious process cycle is the portal of entry. This is the route by which the pathogen enters the next host. With inhalation of contaminated air droplets the respiratory system is the portal of entry. Another portal of entry is the gastrointestinal system: the pathogen enters the body in contaminated food or drink. Any break in the skin or mucous membranes can be a portal of entry for pathogenic microorganisms.

The final link in the infectious process cycle is the susceptible host (Box 19-1). This host is one to whom the pathogen is transmitted after leaving the reservoir host. If the conditions in the susceptible host are conducive to reproduction of the pathogen, the susceptible host becomes a reservoir host and the cycle repeats.

Checkpoint Question

3. How are the first and fifth links of the infection cycle related?

Modes of Transmission

In the third link of the infectious process cycle, the vehicle that spreads the microorganism is often called the mode of transmission. It is important for you to understand the mode of transmission used by various pathogens so that you can break this link in the infectious cycle and prevent the spread of disease.

Direct Transmission

Direct contact between the infected reservoir host and the susceptible host produces direct transmission. Direct transmission may occur when one touches contaminated blood or body fluids, shakes hands with someone who has

---

Box 19-1

THE SUSCEPTIBLE HOST

The susceptible host is unable to resist the invading pathogens for a variety of reasons:

- *Age.* As the body ages, defense mechanisms begin to lose their effectiveness. The immune system is no longer as active or as efficient as in youth. The immune system may also not be fully functional in the very young.
- *Existing disease.* The stress of an existing illness may deplete the immune system and allow microorganisms to cause illness in someone who might otherwise be able to fight it naturally.
- *Poor nutrition.* A diet deficient in nutrients such as proteins, carbohydrates, fats, vitamins, or minerals will not allow cells of the body to repair or reproduce as they are weakened by disease.
- *Poor hygiene.* Although multitudes of microbes exist on our skin, keeping the numbers down by practicing good hygiene will reduce the numbers of pathogens.

---

contaminated hands, inhales infected air droplets, or has intimate contact, such as kissing or sexual intercourse.

Indirect Transmission

Indirect transmission may occur through contact with a vehicle known as a vector. Vectors include contaminated food or water, disease-carrying insects, and inanimate objects such as soil, drinking glasses, wound drainage, and infected or improperly disinfected medical instruments. While visible blood and body fluids are obvious sources of infection, many infectious organisms remain **viable** for long periods on inanimate surfaces that are not visibly contaminated.

Sources of Transmission

Most reservoir hosts are humans, animals, and insects. Human hosts include people who are ill with an infectious disease, people who are carriers of an infectious disease, and people who are incubating an infectious disease but are not exhibiting symptoms. This last group can transmit disease even though they are ambulatory and **asymptomatic** (have no symptoms). Animal sources, which are less common, include infected dogs, cats, birds, cattle, rodents, and animals that live in the wild. Diseases that may be transmitted to humans from infected animals include anthrax and rabies.

In addition to flies and roaches, which carry many diseases, other insect sources feed on the blood of an infected reservoir

Table 19-1	COMMON COMMUNICABLE DISEASES
Disease	**Method of Transmission**
AIDS	Contact, or contact with contaminated sharps
Diphtheria	Airborne droplets, infected carriers
Rubella (German measles)	Airborne droplets, infected carriers
Influenza	Airborne droplets, infected carriers or direct contact with contaminated articles such as used tissues
Measles (rubeola)	Airborne droplets, infected carriers
Mumps	Airborne droplets, infected carriers or direct contact with materials contaminated with infected saliva
Mononucleosis	Airborne droplets or contact with infected saliva.
Pneumonia	Airborne droplets or direct contact with infected mucus
Tuberculosis	Airborne droplets, infected carriers
Tetanus	Direct contact with spores or contaminated animal feces
Rabies	Direct contact with saliva of infected animal such as an animal bite
Cholera	Ingestion of contaminated food or water.
Chicken pox (varicella)	Direct contact or droplets
Meningitis	Airborne droplets
Hepatitis B	Direct contact with infectious body fluid

host and then pass the disease to another victim or susceptible host. Ticks and mosquitoes may transmit diseases, including Lyme disease (ticks) and malaria (mosquitoes). TABLE 19-1 lists some common diseases and their methods of transmission.

Checkpoint Question

4. The medical office where you work has a policy of not opening screenless windows in examination rooms and the reception area. Why do you think this policy is or is not important?

PRINCIPLES OF INFECTION CONTROL

Most transmission of infectious disease in the medical office can be prevented by strict adherence to guidelines issued by the Occupational Safety and Heath Administration (OSHA) and the Centers for Disease Control and Prevention (CDC). While most medical assistants take extraordinary precautions when dealing with patients who are known carriers of infectious microorganisms, you may also treat an estimated five unknown carriers for each patient known to be infectious. Therefore, knowledge and use of effective infection control in relation to all patients is essential.

Medical Asepsis

Medical asepsis does not mean that an object or area is free from all microorganisms. It refers to practices that render an object or area free from pathogenic microorganisms. Commonly known as clean technique, medical asepsis prevents the transmission of microorganisms from one person or area to any other within the medical office (Box 19-2).

PATIENT EDUCATION

Basic Aseptic Technique

While performing procedures, take the opportunity to instruct your patients in basic aseptic techniques they can use at home to reduce the spread of disease.

- *Handwashing.* This routine aseptic technique is particularly important for patients and families in preventing the spread of disease. Instruct patients to wash their hands before and after eating meals, after sneezing, coughing, or blowing the nose, after using the bathroom, before and after changing a dressing, and after changing diapers.
- *Use tissue.* Explain to patients with respiratory symptoms that using a disposable tissue to cover the mouth and nose when coughing and sneezing decreases the potential to transmit the illness throughout the household. In addition, immediate and proper disposal of the used tissue is essential to prevent the spread of infection.
- *Changing bandages.* Patients and family members who change dressings on wounds should be instructed in the proper procedure for using sterile dressings and clean bandages. Always demonstrate the procedure for the patient and have the patient or family member return the demonstration to ensure their understanding.
- *Sanitation.* Explain the proper techniques for disposing of waste from members of the household with communicable diseases. If in doubt, consult the local public health department for guidelines.

Box 19-2.

GUIDELINES FOR MAINTAINING MEDICAL ASEPSIS

- Avoid touching your clothing with soiled linen, table paper, supplies, or instruments. Roll used table paper or linens inward with the clean surface outward.
- Always consider the floor to be contaminated. Any item dropped onto the floor must be considered dirty and be discarded or cleaned to its former level of asepsis before being used.
- Clean tables, counters, and other surfaces frequently and immediately after contamination. Clean areas are less likely than dirty ones to harbor microorganisms or encourage their growth.
- Always presume that blood and body fluids from any source are contaminated. Follow the guidelines published by OSHA and the CDC to protect yourself and to prevent the transmission of disease.

Handwashing is the MOST IMPORTANT medical aseptic technique to prevent the transmission of pathogens. The proper procedure for washing your hands is detailed in Procedure 19-1. Always wash your hands:

- Before and after every patient contact
- After coming into contact with any blood or body fluids
- After coming into contact with contaminated material
- After handling specimens
- After coughing, sneezing, or blowing your nose
- After using the restroom
- Before and after going to lunch, taking breaks, and leaving for the day

Because you should always assume that blood and body fluids are contaminated with pathogens, you should wear gloves when handling any specimens or when contact with contaminated material is anticipated. However, wearing gloves does not replace handwashing! In fact, your hands should be washed BEFORE you apply gloves and AFTER you remove them in all situations to prevent disease transmission.

Other medical aseptic techniques include general cleaning of the office, including the examination and treatment rooms, waiting or reception area, and clinical work areas. Floors are always considered contaminated, and dust and dirt are vehicles for transmission of microorganisms and should be regularly cleaned from all surfaces, including the floor. In addition, you should teach patients and their caregivers proper medical aseptic techniques for use in the home to prevent the spread of disease.

Checkpoint Question

5. Explain why wearing examination gloves does not replace handwashing.

Levels of Infection Control

Sterilization, the highest level of infection control, destroys all forms of microorganisms, including spores, on an inanimate surfaces. Sterilization methods include exposing the articles to various conditions, including steam under pressure in an autoclave; specific gases, such as ethylene oxide; dry heat ovens; and immersion in an approved chemical sterilizing agent (see Chapter 5 for a more complete discussion of sterilization techniques). Instruments or devices that penetrate the skin or come into contact with areas of the body considered sterile, such as the urinary bladder, must be sterilized using one of these methods. To save time, many medical offices use disposable sterile supplies and equipment to eliminate the need for manual sterilization (FIG. 19-2).

The next highest level of infection control is **disinfection**. Disinfectants or **germicides** inactivate virtually all recognized pathogenic microorganisms except spores on inanimate objects. There are three levels of disinfection, high, intermediate, and low. Each is described in more detail in the following section.

The lowest level of infection control is **sanitization**, which is cleaning any visible contaminants from the item using soap or detergent, water, and manual friction.

Sanitation

Most instruments, equipment, and supplies used in medical offices must be sanitized regularly according to the recom-

FIGURE 19-2. Equipment that must be sterile includes items that will penetrate the skin or come into contact with surgical incisions, such as surgical instruments. These items are disposable for one-time use only.

mendations of the manufacturer. Sanitation maintenance of a healthful, disease-free, and hazard-free environment. Sanitation often involves sanitization procedures that reduce the number of microorganisms on an inanimate object to a safe or relatively safe level. This is accomplished by thoroughly cleaning items such as instruments and equipment with warm, soapy water with mechanical action to remove organic matter and other residue. Cleaning or sanitizing must precede disinfection and sterilization.

Disinfection

Disinfectants, or germicides, inactivate virtually all recognized pathogenic microorganisms but not necessarily all microbial forms, including spores, on inanimate objects. These factors may affect disinfection:

- Prior cleaning of the object. Equipment and supplies that have been sanitized first are more effectively disinfected.
- The amount of organic material on the object. The more organic matter, such as blood or body tissues, on the item, the more disinfectant agent you must use.
- The type of microbial contamination. All blood and body fluids should be considered contaminated with blood-borne pathogens such as hepatitis B and HIV.
- The concentration of the **germicide** or chemical disinfectant that kills pathogens. Disinfectants diluted with water are relatively ineffective at killing microbes.
- The length of exposure to the germicide. The longer the disinfectant comes into contact with the contaminated object, the more thorough disinfection is likely to be.
- The shape or complexity of the object being disinfected. Objects that have rough edges, corners, or otherwise difficult-to-clean areas may require special techniques to disinfect all surfaces.
- The temperature of the process. Most disinfectants work adequately at room temperature.

Disinfection is categorized into three levels, high, intermediate, and low. High-level disinfection destroys most forms of microbial life except certain bacterial spores. This level of infection control, which is slightly less effective than sterilization, is commonly used to clean reusable instruments that come into contact with mucous membrane–lined body cavities that are not considered sterile, such as the vagina and the rectum. Methods of high-level disinfection include immersion in boiling water for 30 minutes (rarely used in the medical office) and immersion in an approved disinfecting chemical, such as glutaraldehyde or isopropyl alcohol for 45 minutes or according to the guidelines in the disinfectant label.

Intermediate-level disinfection destroys many viruses, fungi, and some bacteria, including *Mycobacterium tuberculosis* (*M. tuberculosis*), the bacterium that causes tuberculosis. However, intermediate disinfection does not kill bacterial spores. Intermediate disinfection is used for surfaces and instruments that come into contact with unbroken skin surfaces, including stethoscopes, blood pressure cuffs,

FIGURE 19-3. These products destroy many pathogenic microorganisms if used correctly.

and splints. Commercial chemical germicides that kill *M. tuberculosis* and solutions containing a 1:10 dilution of household bleach (2 oz of chlorine bleach per quart of tap water) are effective intermediate disinfectants.

Low-level disinfection destroys many bacteria and some viruses, but not *M. tuberculosis* or bacterial spores. This type of disinfection is adequate in the medical office for routine cleaning and removing surface debris when no visible blood or body fluids are on the items being disinfected. Disinfectants without tuberculocidal properties are used for low-level disinfection (FIG. 19-3). TABLE 19-2 describes disinfection methods, uses, and precautions of various chemicals.

 Checkpoint Question

6. What level of disinfection would you use to clean a reusable instrument that comes into contact with the vaginal mucosa, such as a vaginal speculum? Why?

OCCUPATIONAL SAFETY AND HEALTH ADMINISTRATION GUIDELINES FOR THE MEDICAL OFFICE

OSHA is the federal agency responsible for ensuring the safety of all workers, including those in health care. OSHA promulgates and enforces federal regulations that must be followed by all medical offices. The practices of individual offices regarding employees' health and safety must be put into either a policy and procedure manual or compiled separately as an infection control manual. Regardless of where the office policies are kept, however, they must be readily available to both employees of the medical office and OSHA representatives.

Table 19-2	DISINFECTION METHODS
Method	**Uses and Precautions**
Alcohol (70% isopropyl)	Used for noncritical items (countertops, glass thermometers, stethoscopes) Flammable Damages some rubber, plastic, and lenses
Chlorine (sodium hypochlorite or bleach)	Dilute 1:10 (1 part bleach to 10 parts water) Used for a broad spectrum of microbes Inexpensive and fast acting Corrosive, inactivated by organic matter, relatively unstable
Iodine or iodophors	Bacteriostatic agent Not to be used on instruments May cause staining
Phenols (tuberculocidal)	Used for environmental items and equipment Requires gloves and eye protection Can cause skin irritation and burns
Formaldehyde	Disinfectant and sterilant Regulated by OSHA Warnings must be marked on all containers and storage areas
Hydrogen peroxide	Stable and effective when used on inanimate objects. Attacks membrane lipids, DNA, and other essential cell components. Can damage plastic, rubber, and some metals.
Glutaraldehyde	Alkaline or acid Effective against bacteria, viruses, fungi, and some spores OSHA regulated; requires adequate ventilation, covered pans, gloves, masks Must display biohazard or chemical label.

DNA, deoxyribonucleic acid; OSHA, Occupational Safety and Health Administration.

Exposure Risk Factors and the Exposure Control Plan

Medical offices must provide clear instructions in the policy or infection control manual for preventing employee exposure and reducing the danger of exposure to biohazardous materials. The **exposure risk factor** for each worker by job description must be included in the written policy. It is based on the employee's risk of exposure to communicable disease. Administrative medical assistants have a low exposure risk and require only minimal protection to perform the duties associated with that position. However, clinical medical assistants have a higher exposure risk and require access to a variety of **personal protective equipment (PPE)**, such as gloves, goggles, and/or face shields, depending on the task at hand, and **immunization** against hepatitis B at no charge to the employee. The medical office must provide the appropriate equipment and supplies as outlined in this office policy according to OSHA.

Another written policy required by OSHA for offices with 10 or more employees is the **exposure control plan**. The medical office must have a written plan of action for all employees and visitors who may be exposed to **biohazardous** material despite all precautions. In the event of an exposure, you must first apply the principles of first aid and notify your immediate supervisor, office manager, or the office physician. The physician or supervisor should provide guidance

LEGAL TIP

BLOOD-BORNE PATHOGEN STANDARD TRAINING

According to OSHA, health care facilities, including physician offices, must provide training to newly hired employees who will be exposed to blood or other possibly infectious material while caring for patients. This training must be repeated yearly and include any new issues or policies recommended by OSHA, the CDC, the Department of Health and Human Services, or the U.S. Public Health Service. Items that must be included in the training:

- A description of blood-borne diseases, including the transmission and symptoms.
- Personal protective equipment available to the employee and the location of the PPE in the medical office.
- Information about the risks of contracting hepatitis B and about the HBV vaccine.
- The exposure control plan and postexposure procedures, including follow-up care in the event of an exposure.

regarding **postexposure testing** and follow-up procedures. Next you should complete and file an incident report (or exposure report) form explaining the circumstances surrounding the exposure. This report form not only documents the incident but also allows management to establish a policy to prevent this type of exposure in the future. In addition, the employer must record the exposure on an OSHA 300 log (FIG. 19-4) and report the exposure to OSHA if one or more of the following criteria are present:

- The work-related exposure resulted in loss of consciousness or necessitated a transfer to another job.
- The exposure resulted in a recommendation for medical treatment, such as vaccination or medication to prevent complications.
- The exposure resulted in the conversion of a negative blood test for a contagious disease into a positive blood test in the employee who was exposed.

Box 19-3 describes biohazard and safety equipment commonly used in medical offices.
Checkpoint Question

Checkpoint Question

7. Explain the difference between exposure risk factors and the exposure control plan.

Standard Precautions

Standard precautions are a set of procedures recognized by the CDC to reduce the chance of transmitting infectious microorganisms in any health care setting, including medical offices. By presuming that all blood and body fluids except perspiration are contaminated and by following these precautions, you can protect yourself and prevent the spread of disease. Specifically, these precautions pertain to contact with blood, all body fluids except sweat, damaged skin, and mucous membranes and require that you:

- Wash your hands with soap and water after touching blood, body fluids, secretions, and other contaminated items, whether you have worn gloves or not.
- An alcohol-based hand rub (foam, lotion, or gel) is acceptable to decontaminate the hands if the hands are not visibly dirty or contaminated.
- Wear clean nonsterile examination gloves when contact with blood, body fluids, secretions, mucous membranes, damaged skin, and contaminated items is anticipated.
- Change gloves between procedures on the same patient after exposure to potentially infective material.
- Wear equipment to protect your eyes, nose, and mouth and avoid soiling your clothes by wearing a disposable gown or apron when performing procedures that may splash or spray blood, body fluids, or secretions.

- Dispose of single-use items appropriately; do not disinfect, sterilize, and reuse.
- Take precautions to avoid injuries before, during, and after procedures in which needles, scalpels, or other sharp instruments have been used on a patient.
- Do not recap used needles or otherwise manipulate them by bending or breaking. If recapping is necessary to carry a used needle to a sharps container, use a one-handed scoop technique or a device for holding the needle sheath (see Chapter 26).
- Place used disposable syringes and needles and other sharps in a puncture-resistant container (sharps) as close as possible to the area of use.
- Use barrier devices (e.g., mouthpieces, resuscitation bags) as alternatives to mouth-to-mouth resuscitation (See Chapter 28).

Checkpoint Question

8. How will following standard precautions help to protect you against contracting an infection or communicable disease?

Personal Protective Equipment

In any area of the medical office where exposure to biohazardous materials might occur, PPE must be made available and used by all health care workers, including medical assistants. For instance:

- Gloves must be available and accessible throughout the office. If you or a patient is sensitive to the latex found in regular examination gloves, proper alternatives such as vinyl gloves must be available (Box 19-4).
- Disposable gowns, goggles, and face shields must be available in areas where splattering or splashing of airborne particles may occur (FIG. 19-5).
- You must wear gloves when performing any procedure that carries any risk of exposure, such as surgical procedures or drawing blood specimens, disposing of biohazardous waste, touching or handling surfaces that have been contaminated with biohazardous materials, or if there is any chance at all, no matter how remote, that you may come into contact with blood or body fluids.

Employers who do not make this equipment available are not in compliance with OSHA regulations and may face significant fines. However, employees are responsible for using the PPE correctly and appropriately and washing their hands frequently throughout the day. Remember: pathogens may be carried home to family members and to other persons who come into contact with you or the patient. When removing PPE after a procedure, remove all protective barriers before removing your gloves. Once you have removed all PPE, including your contaminated gloves (Procedure 19-2), always wash your hands.

OSHA's Form 300

Log of Work-Related Injuries and Illnesses

You must record information about every work-related death and about every work-related injury or illness that involves loss of consciousness, restricted work activity or job transfer, days away from work, or medical treatment beyond first aid. You must also record significant work-related injuries and illnesses that are diagnosed by a physician or licensed health care professional. You must also record work-related injuries and illnesses that meet any of the specific recording criteria listed in 29 CFR Part 1904.8 through 1904.12. Feel free to use two lines for a single case if you need to. You must complete an Injury and Illness Incident Report (OSHA Form 301) or equivalent form for each injury or illness recorded on this form. If you're not sure whether a case is recordable, call your local OSHA office for help.

Attention: This form contains information relating to employee health and must be used in a manner that protects the confidentiality of employees to the extent possible while the information is being used for occupational safety and health purposes.

Year 20____

U.S. Department of Labor
Occupational Safety and Health Administration

Form approved OMB no. 1218-0176

Establishment name _____

City _____ State _____

Identify the person

(A) Case no.	(B) Employee's name	(C) Job title (e.g., Welder)	(D) Date of injury or onset of illness

Describe the case

(E) Where the event occurred (e.g., Loading dock north end)	(F) Describe injury or illness, parts of body affected, and object/substance that directly injured or made person ill (e.g., Second degree burns on right forearm from acetylene torch)

Classify the case

Using these four categories, check ONLY the most serious result for each case:

Death (G)	Days away from work (H)	Remained at work Job transfer or restriction (I)	Remained at work Other recordable cases (J)

Enter the number of days the injured or ill worker was:

On job transfer or restriction (K)	Away from work (L)
___ days	___ days

Check the "injury" column or choose one type of illness:

(M)
(1) Injury
(2) Skin disorder
(3) Respiratory condition
(4) Poisoning
(5) All other illnesses

Page totals ▶

Be sure to transfer these totals to the Summary page (Form 300A) before you post it.

Page ___ of ___

Public reporting burden for this collection of information is estimated to average 14 minutes per response, including time to review the instructions, search and gather the data needed, and complete and review the collection of information. Persons are not required to respond to the collection of information unless it displays a currently valid OMB control number. If you have any comments about these estimates or any other aspects of this data collection, contact: US Department of Labor, OSHA Office of Statistics, Room N-3644, 200 Constitution Avenue, NW, Washington, DC 20210. Do not send the completed forms to this office.

FIGURE 19-4. The OSHA 300 log. (Courtesy of the U.S. Department of Labor.)

Box 19-3

BIOHAZARD AND SAFETY EQUIPMENT IN THE MEDICAL OFFICE

- *MSDS binder.* Material safety data sheets are forms prepared by the manufacturers of all chemical substances used in the medical office. The binder should contain sheets for all chemicals used in the office. Each sheet describes how to handle and dispose of the chemical and most important, the health hazards of the chemical and safety equipment needed when using it.
- *Biohazard waste containers.* Only waste contaminated with blood or body fluids or other potentially infectious material (OPIM) should be placed in biohazard waste containers. Sharps containers are used for disposal of items that have the potential to puncture or cut the skin.
- *Personal protective equipment.* Employers are required to provide PPE appropriate to the risk of exposure. For example, employees who may come into contact with blood, such as the clinical medical assistant giving an injection, need be protected only by wearing gloves. However, situations that may cause a splash or splatter of blood require full coverage of the skin, eyes, and clothing.
- *Eyewash basin.* Pressing the lever on the basin and turning on the faucets produces a stream of water that forces open the caps of the eyewash basin. To remove contaminants or chemicals from the eyes, lower your face into the stream and continue to wash the area until the eyes are clear or for the amount of time recommended on the MSDS.
- *Immunization.* Employers are required by OSHA to provide immunization against blood-borne pathogens if vaccines are available.

Checkpoint Question

9. What PPE should you wear when assisting the physician with a wound irrigation?

Handling Environmental Contamination

Although not all equipment or surfaces in the medical office must be sterile (free from all microorganisms), all equipment and areas must be clean. Sanitization is cleaning or washing equipment or surfaces by removing all visible soil. Any detergent or low-level disinfectant can be used to clean and disinfect areas such as floors, examination tables, cabinets, and countertops. Because you may be expected to perform cleaning tasks routinely or when these

WHAT IF

Your patient is offended that you are wearing gloves when drawing a blood specimen?

Sometimes patients become defensive and make statements to the effect that they are "disease free." If this happens to you, reassure the patient by saying that wearing gloves is a standard practice and is used for the protection of the patient also. Use this occasion to teach the patient about standard precautions and the importance of following these guidelines.

surfaces become soiled with visible blood or body fluids, you should understand how these procedures are correctly performed.

Any surface contaminated with biohazardous materials should be promptly cleaned using an approved germicide or a

Box 19-4

LATEX ALLERGY AND PREVENTION

The incidence among health care workers of allergic reactions to proteins in latex has increased in recent years. The proteins in latex, a product of the rubber tree that is used to make many products including examination gloves, may cause allergic reactions, especially with repeated exposure. The reactions can be mild (skin redness or rash, itching, or hives) or severe (difficulty breathing, coughing, or wheezing). Respiratory reactions often result when the powder in the gloves becomes airborne and is inhaled as the gloves are removed after use. To protect yourself from exposure and allergy to latex, the following guidelines may be useful:

- Use gloves that are not latex for tasks that do not involve contact or potential contact with blood or body fluids.
- When contact with blood or body fluids is possible, wear powder-free latex gloves. Powder-free gloves contain less protein than the powdered ones, reducing the risk of allergy.
- Avoid wearing oil-based lotions or hand creams before applying latex gloves. The oil in these products can break down the latex, releasing the proteins that cause the allergic reactions.
- Wash your hands thoroughly after removing latex gloves.
- Recognize the symptoms of latex allergy in yourself, your coworkers, and your patients.

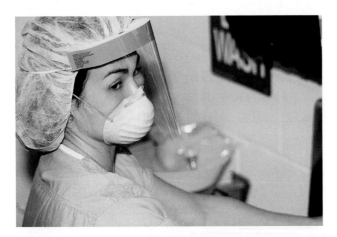

FIGURE 19-5. Personal protective equipment that must be provided for employees who may come into contact with contaminated materials includes gloves, goggles, face shields, and gowns or aprons to protect clothing.

FIGURE 19-6. A commercially prepared biohazard spill kit contains gloves, absorbent material, eye protection, and a biohazard bag for proper disposal. (Courtesy of Caltech Industries, Midland, MI)

dilute bleach solution. OSHA requires that spill kits or appropriate supplies be available, and commercial kits make cleaning contaminated surfaces relatively safe and easy. Commercial kits include clean gloves, eye protection if there is a risk of splashing, a gel to absorb the biohazardous material, a scoop, towels, and a biohazard waste container to discard all used items (FIG. 19-6). If your office does not purchase commercial kits, you should gather and store the following items together in the event that a biohazardous spill occurs:

- Eye protection, such as goggles
- Clean examination gloves
- Absorbent powder, crystals, or gel
- Paper towels
- A disposable scoop
- At least one biohazard waste bag
- A chemical disinfectant

In some cases, you may need a sharps container (FIG. 19-7) and spill control barriers. If there is a large amount of contamination on the floor, you should put on disposable shoe coverings to avoid transmitting microorganisms on your shoes. All gloves, paper towels, eye protection, and shoe coverings should be discarded in the biohazardous waste bags, which must be disposed of properly. Procedure 19-3 outlines the procedure for an area contaminated with blood or body fluids.

Although most medical offices use disposable patient gowns and drapes, some offices continue to use cloth. Hygienic storage of clean linens is recommended, and proper handling of soiled linens, disposable or not, is required. After applying clean examination gloves, handle soiled linen, including examination table paper, as little as possible by folding it carefully so that the most contaminated surface is turned inward to prevent contamination of the air. Contaminated linen should be placed in a biohazard bag in the examination room where the contamination occurred rather than carried through the hallways of the medical office. Some of-

fices using cloth linens contract with an outside company for the laundering. If linen materials are laundered at the office, use normal laundry cycles following the recommendations of the washer, detergent, and fabric.

 Checkpoint Question

10. How would you respond to an employee in the medical office who is unsure about how to clean up a spilled urine specimen? Is this biohazardous?

Disposing of Infectious Waste

Federal regulations from the Environmental Protection Agency (EPA) and OSHA set the policies and guidelines

FIGURE 19-7. All sharps should be disposed of properly by placing them in a plastic puncture-resistant sharps container like the one shown here. Note the biohazard symbol on the sharps container.

for disposing of hazardous materials, but individual states determine policies based on these guidelines. As a result, policies vary widely, and you should review your state and local regulations before making waste disposal decisions. Most medical offices are considered small generators of waste because they produce less than 50 pounds of waste each month. Facilities such as hospitals and large clinics that generate more than 50 pounds are considered large generators and must obtain a certificate of registration from the EPA and maintain a record of the quantity of waste and disposal procedures.

To remain compliant with any state and federal laws, facilities that are considered large generators of infectious waste and some smaller medical offices use an infectious waste service to dispose of biohazardous waste appropriately and safely. These services supply the office with appropriate waste containers and pick up filled containers regularly (Box 19-5). Once the filled containers are picked up by the waste service, the infectious waste is disposed of according to EPA and OSHA guidelines. The service maintains a tracking record listing the type of waste, its weight in pounds, and the disposal destination. When the waste has been destroyed, a tracking form documenting the disposal is sent to the medical office and should be retained in the office records for 3 years. This documentation must be provided to the EPA should an audit be performed to assess compliance. States impose stiff penalties, including fines and/or imprisonment, for violations of regulations involving biohazardous waste.

Because the fee charged by an infectious waste service is based on the type and amount of waste generated, you should follow these guidelines to help keep the cost down while maintaining safety:

- Use separate containers for each type of waste. Don't put bandages in sharps containers (puncture-resistant containers for needles or other sharp items) or paper towels used for routine handwashing in a biohazard bag.
- Fill sharps containers two-thirds full before disposing of them. Most containers have fill lines that must not be exceeded.
- Use only approved biohazard containers.
- When moving filled biohazard containers, secure the bag or top with a closure for that specific container.
- If the container is contaminated on the outside, wear clean examination gloves, secure it within another approved container, and wash your hands thoroughly afterward.
- Place biohazard waste for pick up by the service in a secure, designated area.

Checkpoint Question

11. After drawing a blood specimen from a patient, you notice that the tube of blood is leaking onto the examination table where you put it while finishing

TRIAGE

The following three situations occur at the same time in the office where you are employed:

A. You have just finished changing the dressing on a wound that is draining a moderate amount of blood. You still have your gloves on, but you need to document the procedure in the patient's medical record and instruct the patient regarding wound care.

B. As you are cleaning up the materials used to irrigate the wound, you spill the basin used to collect the irrigating solution and blood obtained from the procedure.

C. Another staff member knocks on the door of the examination room and informs you that you have a phone call.

How do you sort these tasks? What do you do first? Second? Third?

Tell the staff member in situation C that you cannot take a phone call now and ask him or her to take a message or refer the call to another medical assistant. The spill in situation B is a biohazardous spill and should be cleaned up and the area decontaminated immediately. You should be familiar with the policy and procedure of the medical office and clean the spill accordingly. Once the spill is cleaned and decontaminated, remove your gloves and wash your hands. Document the wound irrigation, dressing change, and patient education in situation A only after removing your gloves and washing your hands. To prevent the spread of microorganisms to the medical record, you should never handle the medical record while wearing contaminated gloves.

the procedure. How do you clean up the blood spill?

Hepatitis B and Human Immunodeficiency Viruses

One of the most persistent health care concerns in the medical office is the transmission of hepatitis B virus (HBV) and human immunodeficiency virus (HIV). Although HIV is the most visible public concern, HBV has been an occupational hazard for health care professionals for many years. HBV is more viable than HIV and may survive in a dried state on clinical equipment and counter surfaces at room temperature for more than a week. In this dried state, HBV may be passed through the medical setting by way of contact with

Box 19-5

PROPER WASTE DISPOSAL

Regular Waste Container

SA regular waste container.

A regular waste container should be used only for disposal of waste that is not biohazardous, such as paper, plastic, disposable tray wrappers, packaging material, unused gauze, and examination table paper. To prevent leakage and mess, liquids should be discarded in a sink or other washbasin, not in the plastic bag inside the waste can. NEVER discard sharps of any kind in plastic bags; these are not puncture resistant, and injury may result even with careful handling. Bags should not be filled to capacity. When the plastic bag is about two-thirds full, it should be removed from the waste can, the top edges brought together and secured by tying or with a twist tie. Remove the bag from the area and follow the office policy and procedure for disposal. Put a fresh plastic bag into the waste can.

A biohazard waste container.

Biohazard Waste Container

The biohazard waste container is reserved for the disposal of waste contaminated with blood or body fluids, including soiled dressings and bandages, soiled examination gloves, soiled examination table paper and cotton balls and applicators that have been used on or in the body.

contaminated hands, gloves, or other means of direct transmission. Fortunately, HBV can be contained by the proper use of standard precautions, and it can be killed easily by cleaning with a dilute bleach solution.

HBV and HIV are both transmitted through exposure to contaminated blood and body fluids. Accidental punctures with sharp objects contaminated with blood are one way to become infected, but the viruses may also enter the body through broken skin. Disorders of the skin, including dry cracked skin, dermatitis, eczema, and psoriasis, also allow entrance into the body if contact with contaminated surfaces or equipment occurs.

While there is no vaccine to prevent infection with HIV, employers whose workers, including clinical medical assistants, are at risk for HBV exposure are mandated by OSHA to provide the vaccine to prevent HBV at no cost to the employee. This vaccine is given in a series of three injections that normally produce immunity to the disease. It is recommended that a blood sample be drawn 6 months after the third injection of HBV vaccine to determine whether the person has developed immunity. The blood test can detect the presence, or titer, of antibodies against hepatitis B. The series is repeated if HBV immunity is not found, but the vaccine has been found to be very effective. The immunity may last as long as 10 years. Employees who choose not to receive the vaccine must sign a waiver or release form stating that they are aware of the risks associated with HBV. Individuals who contract hepatitis B may develop cirrhosis (destruction of the cells of the liver) and are at increased risk for developing liver cancer.

In the event of exposure to blood or body fluids infected with HBV, the postexposure plan should include an immediate blood test of the employee. Repeat blood titers should be obtained at specific intervals, usually 6 weeks, 3 months, 6 months, 9 months, and 1 year, as a comparison. If you have been immunized against HBV, usually no further treatment is required. However, if you waive the HBV series, hepatitis B immunoglobulin can be given by injection for immediate short-term protection, and the general series of three immunizations should be started.

The same schedule of evaluation is required after HIV exposure. Again, there is no vaccine to prevent HIV, but other HIV treatments for preventing transmission are being tested.

Checkpoint Question

12. Which virus is more of a threat to the clinical medical assistant: HIV or HBV? Why?

Procedure 19-1

Handwashing for Medical Asepsis

Purpose: To prevent the growth and spread of pathogen

Equipment: Liquid soap, disposable paper towels, an orangewood manicure stick, a waste can

Standard: This task should take 2 to 3 minutes.

Steps	Reason
1. Remove all rings and your wristwatch if it cannot be pushed up onto the forearm.	Rings and watches may harbor pathogens that may not be easily washed away. Ideally, rings should not be worn when working with material that may be infectious.
2. Stand close to the sink without touching it.	The sink is considered contaminated, and standing too close may contaminate your clothing.
3. Turn on the faucet and adjust the temperature of the water to warm.	Water that is too hot or too cold will crack or chap the skin on the hands, which will break the natural protective barrier that prevents infection.
4. Wet your hands and wrists under the warm running water, apply liquid soap, and work the soap into a lather by rubbing your palms together and rubbing the soap between your fingers at least 10 times.	This motion dislodges microorganisms from between the fingers and removes transient and some resident organisms.

Step 4. Wet hands and wrists.

(continues)

Procedure 19-1 *(continued)*

Handwashing for Medical Asepsis

Steps	Reason
5. Scrub the palm of one hand with the fingertips of the other hand to work the soap under the nails of that hand; then reverse the procedure and scrub the other hand. Also scrub each wrist. Step 5. Wash hands and wrists with firm rubbing and circular motions.	Friction helps remove microorganisms.
6. Rinse hands and wrists thoroughly under running warm water, holding hands lower than elbows; do not touch the inside of the sink. Step 6. Rinse hands thoroughly.	Holding the hands lower than the elbows and wrists allows microorganisms to flow off the hands and fingers rather than back up the arms.
7. Using the orangewood stick, clean under each nail on both hands.	Nails may harbor microorganisms. Metal files and pointed instruments may break the skin and make an opening for microorganisms. This may be done at the beginning of the day, before leaving for the day, or after coming into contact with potentially infectious material.

(continues)

Procedure 19-1 *(continued)*

Handwashing for Medical Asepsis

Steps	Reason
8. Reapply liquid soap and rewash hands and wrists.	Rewashing the hands after using the orangewood stick washes away any microorganisms that may have been removed with the orangewood stick.
9. Rinse hands thoroughly again while holding hands lower than wrists and elbows.	
10. Gently dry hands with a paper towel. Discard the paper towel and the used orangewood stick when finished.	Hands must be dried thoroughly and completely to prevent drying and cracking.

Step 10. Dry hands gently with a paper towel.

11. Use a dry paper towel to turn off the faucets and discard the paper towel.	Your hands are clean and should not touch the contaminated faucet handles.

Procedure 19-2

Removing Contaminated Gloves

Purpose: To remove contaminated gloves to prevent the spread of pathogenic microorganisms
Equipment: Clean examination gloves; biohazard waste container
Standards: This task should take 1 to 2 minutes.

Steps	Reason
1. Choose the appropriate size gloves for your hands and put them on.	Gloves should fit comfortably, not too loose and not too tight.
2. To remove gloves, grasp the glove of your nondominant hand *at the palm* and pull the glove away.	To avoid transferring contaminants to the wrist, be sure not to grasp the glove at the wrist.

Step 2. Grasp the palm of the glove on your nondominant gloved hand.

| 3. Slide your hand out of the glove, rolling the glove into the palm of the gloved dominant hand. | You should avoid touching either glove with your ungloved hand. |

Step 3A. Carefully remove the glove and avoid contaminating your bare skin.

continues

Procedure 19-2 *(continued)*

Removing Contaminated Gloves

Steps	Reason
Step 3B. Grasp the soiled glove with your gloved dominant hand.	
4. Holding the soiled glove in the palm of your gloved hand, slip your ungloved fingers under the cuff of the glove you are still wearing, being careful not to touch the outside of the glove.	Skin should touch skin but never the soiled part of the glove.
Step 4. Slip your free hand under the cuff of the remaining glove.	

continues

Procedure 19-2 *(continued)*

Removing Contaminated Gloves

Steps	Reason
5. Stretch the glove of the dominant hand up and away from your hand while turning it inside out, with the already removed glove balled up inside.	Turning it inside out ensures that the soiled surfaces of the gloves are enclosed.

Step 5. Remove the glove by turning it inside out over the previously removed glove.

Steps	Reason
6. Both gloves should now be removed, with the first glove inside the second glove and the second glove inside out.	
7. Discard both gloves as one unit into a biohazard waste receptacle.	
8. Wash your hands.	Wearing gloves is NOT a substitute for washing your hands!

Procedure 19-3

Cleaning Biohazardous Spills

Purpose:	To clean contaminated surfaces
Equipment:	Commercially prepared germicide OR 1:10 bleach solution, Gloves, Disposable towels, Chemical absorbent, Biohazardous waste bag, Protective eye wear (goggles or mask and face shield), Disposable shoe coverings. Disposable gown or apron made of plastic or other material that is impervious to soaking up contaminated fluids.
Standard:	This task should take 3 to 5 minutes.

Steps	Reason
1. Put on gloves. Wear protective eyewear, gown or apron, and shoe coverings if you anticipate any splashing.	A plastic gown or apron will protect your clothing from contaminants.
2. Apply chemical absorbent material to the spill as indicated by office policy. Clean up the spill with disposable paper towels, being careful not to splash.	
3. Dispose of paper towels and absorbent material in a biohazard waste bag.	The bag will alert anyone handling the waste that it contains biohazardous material.
4. Spray the area with commercial germicide or bleach solution and wipe with disposable paper towels. Discard towels in a biohazard bag.	
5. With your gloves on, remove the protective eyewear and discard or disinfect per office policy. Remove the gown or apron and shoe coverings and put in the biohazard bag if disposable or the biohazard laundry bag for reusable linens.	
6. Place the biohazard bag in an appropriate waste receptacle for removal according to your facility's policy.	
7. Remove your gloves and wash your hands thoroughly.	Wearing gloves does not replace proper hand washing.

CHAPTER SUMMARY

Following the principles of medical asepsis and infection control help ensure a safe environment for patients and health care providers in the medical office.

If you fail to follow these principles consistently, you will place yourself and others at risk for infection that may impair patients' recovery and affect health care workers' performance. Although avoiding contact with microorganisms in the environment is impossible, sanitation and disinfection will reduce the numbers of microorganisms and potential pathogens, making the environment clean and as disease free as possible. In addition, OSHA and the CDC issue regulations and standards for health care workers who work with blood and body fluids, and you must always follow them, including wearing PPE. In case of exposure, your office must have an exposure control plan and a postexposure plan to assist you in receiving appropriate medical attention and follow-up care.

Remember: Handwashing is the single most effective measure to prevent the spread of infection.

Critical Thinking Challenges

1. Review Table 19-1 on common communicable diseases. Create a patient education brochure that focuses on the spread of these diseases.
2. A patient who comes into your office has a leg wound that must be cared for at home. When asked about caring for the wound, he tells you that he knows how to do it, but you think he may be confused about the importance of using medical asepsis. How do you handle this situation?

Answers to Checkpoint Questions

1. Pathogenic microorganisms are microscopic organisms that cause disease. Natural ways that the body stops an invasion or destroys pathogens include tears (wash microbes away from the eyes and contain lysozyme, an effective disinfectant); hydrochloric acid in the stomach (produces a pH that kills many microbes that may get into the stomach); unbroken or intact skin (provides a barrier to invading microorganism); mucous membranes and cilia lining the respiratory tract (trap microorganisms that may be inhaled).

2. The conditions that favor the growth of microorganisms include moisture, nutrients, a warm temperature, darkness, a neutral or slightly alkaline pH, and oxygen. To prevent the growth of microbes, remove any moisture or sources of nutrition, use heat higher than 98.6°F, expose the area to light, or clean with acidic or alkaline chemicals.
3. The first link in the infection cycle (the reservoir host) provides nutrients and an incubation site for the pathogen. The fifth link (the susceptible host) allows the pathogen to enter and begin growing thus becoming the new reservoir host, repeating the cycle.
4. Opening screenless windows allows insects to come into the office. Insects may be reservoir hosts to certain diseases and contaminate items in the medical office.
5. Gloves are a barrier to prevent the skin from coming into contact with contaminated materials. However, once they are removed, standard precautions require that the hands be washed as an additional precaution.
6. Items or instruments that come into contact with unbroken mucous membranes in areas of the body that are not considered sterile (like the vagina) may be safely disinfected using a high-level disinfectant for the specified period.
7. Exposure risk factors are associated with specific jobs in terms of exposure to biohazardous or contaminated materials. The exposure control plan is a written document outlining the procedure that an employee or visitor should take to prevent contact with biohazardous material.
8. Following the standard precautions will help to protect you against contracting an infection or disease by preventing entrance of the pathogenic microorganisms into your body.
9. A wound irrigation requires wearing gloves and covering the eyes, nose, and mouth. This procedure has the potential to splash microorganisms into the environment.
10. Urine may be biohazardous and should be cleaned up by applying clean examination gloves, using paper towels or absorbent powder to absorb the urine, and placing all items used for cleaning up the spill into a biohazardous waste container. Once the urine is absorbed and discarded appropriately, the area or floor should be disinfected.
11. Again, all blood should be considered contaminated and should be cleaned up using the commercially prepared spill kit or with items assembled from the office. The broken blood tube should be placed in a sharps container, and once the blood has been wiped up, the table should be disinfected.
12. The virus that is actually more of a threat to the medical assistant is HBV. HBV may live in dried body secretions on an inanimate surface for up to 2 weeks. In

the "right" circumstances, contact with these dried secretions may cause infection in the exposed individual. Hepatitis B is a serious disease and may cause scarring and destruction of the liver tissue (leading to liver failure), an increased risk for developing liver cancer, and death.

 Websites

OSHA www.osha.gov

Latex allergy prevention http://www.cdc.gov/niosh/
    98-113.html

20

Medical History and Patient Assessment

CHAPTER OUTLINE

THE MEDICAL HISTORY
Methods of Collecting Information
Elements of the Medical History

CONDUCTING THE PATIENT INTERVIEW
Preparing for the Interview
Introducing Yourself
Barriers to Communication

ASSESSING THE PATIENT
Signs and Symptoms
Chief Complaint and Present Illness

ROLE DELINEATION

ADMINISTRATIVE: ADMINISTRATIVE PROCEDURES
- Perform basic administrative medical assisting functions

CLINICAL: PATIENT CARE
- Adhere to established patient screening procedures
- Obtain patient's history and vital signs

GENERAL: PROFESSIONALISM
- Display a professional manner and image
- Demonstrate initiative and responsibility

- Work as a member of the health care team
- Treat all patients with compassion and empathy

GENERAL: COMMUNICATION SKILLS
- Recognize and respect cultural diversity
- Adapt communications to individual's ability to understand
- Recognize and respond effectively to verbal, nonverbal, and written communications
- Use medical terminology appropriately

GENERAL: LEGAL CONCEPTS
- Perform within legal and ethical boundaries
- Prepare and maintain medical records
- Document accurately
- Implement and maintain federal and state health care legislation and regulations

GENERAL: INSTRUCTION
- Instruct individuals according to their needs
- Explain office policies and procedures

CHAPTER COMPETENCIES

LEARNING OBJECTIVES

Upon successfully completing this chapter, you will be able to:

1. Spell and define key terms.
2. Give examples of the type of information included in each section of the medical history.
3. Identify guidelines for conducting a patient interview.
4. Explain the difference between a sign and symptom and give examples of each.
5. Compare the chief complaint and present illness.
6. Discuss open-ended and closed-ended questions and explain when to use each type during the patient interview.

PERFORMANCE OBJECTIVES

Upon successfully completing this chapter, you will be able to:

1. Interview a patient using appropriate communication techniques (Procedures 20-1 and 20-2).
2. Correctly complete the various sections of the medical history form (Procedure 20-1).
3. Accurately document a chief complaint and present illness (Procedure 20-2).

KEY TERMS

(See glossary for definitions.)

assessment	demographic	HIPAA	over-the-counter
chief complaint	familial disorder	homeopathic medicine	signs
	hereditary traits	medical history	symptoms

To DIAGNOSE A PATIENT'S PRESENT ILLNESS, the physician needs the patient's past and current health information. As a professional medical assistant, you are often responsible for obtaining this information as part of the **medical history** and **assessment**. The medical history is a record containing information about a patient's past and present health status, the health status of related family members, and relevant information about a patient's social habits. Assessment begins with gathering information to determine the patient's problem or reason for seeking medical care. Typically, you ask standard questions and document the patient's responses during the assessment on preprinted forms or in a manner decided by the physician and outlined in the medical office policy and procedure manual.

THE MEDICAL HISTORY

Methods of Collecting Information

To complete the patient's medical history, you and the physician work cooperatively with the patient. In some medical practices, medical assistants gather initial patient information by interviewing the patient using a printed list of questions. Other medical offices ask the patient to fill out a standard form before or during the first appointment. Patients who receive the form in the mail are instructed to bring the completed document to the office at the initial visit. In either case, you must check the form for completeness, because the physician uses this information as the basis for more extensive questioning during the examination.

In other practices, the physician may prefer to complete the medical history form during the initial patient interview and examination. In this situation, you should be familiar with the form and ready to assist the physician if needed or asked to do so.

Elements of the Medical History

The medical history forms used by the office may vary with the practice specialty, but most forms are composed of these common elements: identifying data (database), past history (PH), review of systems (ROS), family history (FH), and social history. FIGURE 20-1 shows a medical history form. This information is confidential and protected by **HIPAA**, a federal law that protects the privacy of health information. No one except those directly involved in the patient's care may have access to it without the patient's permission.

These are the main elements of the medical history:

- Identifying database. The **demographic** information in this section, required for administrative purposes, always includes the patient's name, address, and phone number. It also includes the name, address, and phone number of the patient's employer and insurance carrier and the patient's health insurance policy number, social security number, marital status, gender, and race.
- Past history (PH). This section addresses the patient's prior health status and helps the physician plan appropriate care for any present illness. Information in this section typically includes allergies, immunizations,

TRIAGE

While working in the medical office, you begin the day by placing the following three patients into examination rooms:

Patient A, a new patient, arrives on time and was given the two-page medical history form to complete.

Patient B is an established patient who is scheduled to have his blood pressure checked today, since he started a new antihypertensive medication last month.

Patient C is a year-old baby who is scheduled to be seen today for a well-child check up and immunizations.

How would you sort these patients? Who should be seen first? Second? Third?

Patient B should be called back first, since he will probably take the least amount of time. Unless this patient's blood pressure is not responding to the antihypertensive medication or he has unanticipated problems, this type of visit is typically conducted in a timely manner as a convenience to the patient. Patient C should be seen next, since infant checkups usually require additional procedures that may require more time from the medical assistant and physician. Patient A should be given an adequate amount of time to complete the medical history forms, since this information will be necessary for the physician to understand the patient's current and future health problems. The patient should not be rushed to complete this paperwork. If necessary, you may call the patient back and assist with completion of the form, especially if the patient is having difficulty due to a physical disability, such as visual impairment, deformity, or trouble holding a pen or pencil because of arthritis.

childhood diseases, current and past medications, and previous illnesses, surgeries, and hospitalizations.

- Review of systems (ROS). A thorough review of each body system may elicit information that the patient forgot to mention earlier or thought was irrelevant. Specific questions, such as symptoms or known diseases, related to each system of the body are included in this section.
- Family history (FH). This section contains the health status of the patient's parents, siblings, and grandparents. This information is important because certain diseases or disorders have **familial** or **hereditary** tendencies. Familial diseases tend to occur often in a particular family, whereas hereditary diseases are transmitted from parent to offspring. If any immediate family member is deceased, the cause of death should be documented.

- Social history. The social history covers the patient's lifestyle, such as marital status, occupation, education, and hobbies. It may also include information about the patient's diet, use of alcohol or tobacco, and sexual history. This information may help the physician understand how present illness, including any treatment, may affect the lifestyle or how the lifestyle may affect the illness. The social history may also provide a guide for patient education, since some behaviors, such as tobacco use or a diet high in fat, may not yet be causing illness but can cause illness in the future.

Checkpoint Question

1. What is the difference between the past history and the family history?

CONDUCTING THE PATIENT INTERVIEW

Preparing for the Interview

As a medical assistant, your primary goal during a patient interview is to obtain accurate and pertinent information. To do this, you need to understand the basic components of communication and to use active listening skills. You should also use a variety of interviewing techniques, including reflecting, paraphrasing, asking for examples, asking questions, summarizing, and allowing silence. Communication also includes observation. Specifically, any objective or observable information concerning the patient's physical or mental status should be noted and documented in the patient's record as appropriate. Examples of observations about a patient's physical status include the general appearance (bruising or injury, pale or flushed skin). The mental or emotional condition of the patient includes observations such as lethargy, crying, tearfulness, and confusion. Judgments made about these observations should not be documented in the patient's record, because the terminology used (depressed, abused) may be diagnostic, which is out of the scope of training for the medical assistant. In the case of suspected abuse, you should document the observable information in medical record and alert the physician regarding your suspicions. Procedure 20-1 outlines the process for conducting a successful patient interview.

Before you start interviewing the patient, make sure you are familiar with the medical history form and any previous medical history provided by the patient. Shuffling papers while the patient is talking or asking questions out of order may distract the patient and disrupt the flow of the interview. If the patient is new to the medical practice, review the new patient questionnaire before beginning. Review the chart of any established patient and update information as indicated.

Professional Medical Associates – History Form

NAME: _____ DATE OF BIRTH: _____

What is the main reason for your visit to the doctor? _____

_____

Were you referred? _____ if so, by whom? _____

PAST MEDICAL HISTORY:

Are you allergic to any medication? _____

If so, list medications: _____

List current medications, dosage, and how many times a day you take them:

Medication	**Dose**	**Times A Day**

Alcohol Consumption: What type? _____ Amount _____ How Often? _____

History of Alcoholism? _____

When was your last TB or Tine test? _____

Have you ever had a positive test for tuberculosis? _____

When was your last Tetanus shot? _____

List all surgeries you have had in the past:

Date	**Type of Surgery**

List all past hospitalizations (not involving surgeries above):

Date	**Reason For Hospital Stay**

List all past problems with trauma (broken bones, lacerations, etc.):

_____

REVIEW OF SYSTEMS, PAST MEDICAL PROBLEMS:
If you have been told you have any of the problems listed below, or are having any of the problems listed below, please CIRCLE:

1. <u>GENERAL:</u> Weight loss, weight gain, fever, chills, night sweats, hot flashes, tire easily, problems with sleep, crying spells, history of cancer.

2. <u>SKIN:</u> Rash, sores that won't heal, moles that are new or changing, history of skin problems.

3. <u>HEENT:</u> Headache, eye problems, hearing problems, sinus problems, hay fever, dizziness, hoarseness, sores in your mouth that won't heal, dental problems.

   Do you chew tobacco or dip snuff? _____

4. <u>METABOLIC/ENDOCRINE:</u> Thyroid problems, diabetes or sugar problems, high cholesterol.

F I G U R E 2 0 - 1 .   A sample medical history form, front and back.

5. <u>RESPIRATORY:</u> Cough, wheezing, breathing problems, history of asthma, history of lung problems.

Do you smoke cigarettes or pipe? _____

How much? _____ For how long? _____

6. <u>BREAST (WOMEN):</u> Breast lumps, changes in nipples, nipple discharge, breast problems, family history of breast cancer. When was your last mammogram? _____

7. <u>CARDIOVASCULAR:</u> Heart murmur, rheumatic fever, high blood pressure, angina, heart problems, heart attack, abnormal heart rhythm, chest pain, palpitations, leg swelling, history of phlebitis or blood clots.

8. <u>GI:</u> Problems with appetite, swallowing, heartburn, nausea, vomiting, pain in the abdomen, constipation, diarrhea, blood in stool, history of ulcers, liver problems, hepatitis, jaundice, pancreas problems, gallbladder problems, or colon problems.

9. <u>REPRODUCTIVE (WOMEN):</u> Problems with irregular menstrual cycles, abnormal vaginal bleeding or discharge, history of sexually transmitted diseases, sexual problems.

AGE OF FIRST MENSES (PERIOD) _____ AGE OF MENOPAUSE _____

LAST PAP SMEAR _____ METHOD OF CONTRACEPTION _____

Obstetric History (Women)

NUMBER OF PREGNANCIES _____ PLEASE LIST AS FOLLOWS:

Delivery Date   Pregnancy Complications   Type Delivery   Baby's Weight

_____

_____

<u>MEN:</u> Problems with genital discharge, history of venereal diseases, sexual problems, prostate problems.

METHOD OF CONTRACEPTION _____

10. <u>UROLOGIC:</u> Problems with painful urination, urinary frequency, blood in urine, weak urinary stream, history of bladder or kidney infections, or kidney stones.

11. <u>MUSCULOSKELETAL:</u> Arthritis, back pain, cramps in legs.

12. <u>NEUROLOGIC:</u> Seizures, stroke, arm or leg weakness or numbness, black-out spells, memory or thinking problems, depression, anxiety, psychiatric problems.

13. <u>HEMATOLOGIC:</u> Anemia, bleeding problems, enlarged lymph nodes.

HAVE YOU EVER HAD A BLOOD TRANSFUSION? _____ DATE _____

FAMILY HISTORY:

List any medical problems that run in your family and which family members have these problems.

_____

_____

SOCIAL HISTORY:

MARITAL STATUS: _____

OCCUPATION: _____

EDUCATION: _____

HOBBIES: _____

WHAT DO YOU DO FOR ENJOYMENT? _____

FIGURE 20-1.   *(Continued)*

PATIENT EDUCATION

Genetic Diseases

The patient's family history can provide you with many teaching opportunities. If a patient indicates that previous members of his or her family had certain diseases, there may be a genetic link. A genetic disease is noted by a mark on the DNA (genetic material) for a specific illness or disease. The patient receives this mark from either or both parents. Some common examples include some forms of high blood pressure, diabetes, heart disease, obesity, and certain cancers. Examples of less common genetic disorders are Tay-Sachs disease, Marfan syndrome, and Huntington disease. Great strides have been made in genetic testing. This allows the patient to have the DNA examined for potential markers of diseases. For example, color blindness is a genetic disorder that can easily be seen on a DNA chain. Patients can have genetic testing done to see if they carry a particular disease marker. Genetic counseling may also be appropriate depending on the type of genetic disorder. Some insurance plans will pay for genetic testing and counseling. Advise the patient to contact his or her insurance company directly for specific coverage guidelines.

LEGAL TIP

You are responsible for ensuring that information in the patient's medical history is kept confidential. Legally and ethically, the patient has a right to privacy concerning his or her medical records, which includes storage in a secure place. Only health care providers directly involved in the patient's care should be allowed access to the records.

Introducing Yourself

Always begin the interview with new or established patients by identifying yourself, your title, and the purpose of the interview. For example, you might say, "Good morning, Mr. Frank. My name is Angela and I'm Dr. Martin's medical assistant. I would like to ask you a few questions that will help the doctor diagnose and treat you appropriately. Please be assured that your responses will be kept in strict confidence." Under no circumstance should you identify yourself as a nurse, since it is unethical and illegal to give the patient a false impression of your credentials.

The initial impression you make will be a lasting one, so be sure that your demeanor and words communicate genuine respect and concern. By developing professional rapport, you will gain the patient's confidence and trust in you, the physician, and the office staff. Some patients may be reluctant to share private information with you until a sense of trust has been established. This makes the professional role of the medical assistant as a caring and empathic health care worker even more important.

To safeguard confidential patient information and allow for open communication, conduct the interview in a private and comfortable place. Avoid public areas, such as the reception area, where distractions are likely and where others may hear the patient's answers. Interview the patient alone unless he or she wishes to have family members or significant others present (FIG. 20-2).

Barriers to Communication

As you begin speaking with the patient, you must assess any barriers to communication, such as unfamiliarity with English, hearing impairment, or cognitive impairment. Note the patient's verbal and nonverbal behavior during the interview and adjust your questioning if necessary. Avoid using highly technical or medical terminology when conversing with most patients. If the patient has impaired hearing or vision or difficulty understanding or speaking English, adjust your interviewing techniques to fit the patient's needs; however, remember that raising your voice is not necessary and will not improve communication or understanding with these patients. Instead, it is best to face the patient and maintain eye contact when speaking and use physical cues as appropriate.

FIGURE 20-2. Conduct the patient interview in a private office or examination room.

Spanish Terminology

¿Vive su padre?	Is your father living?
¿De qué murió?	What did he die of?
¿Vive su madre?	Is your mother living?
¿Tienen buena salud?	Are they in good health?
¿Algún familiar cercano ha muerto de un ataque al corazón?	Has anyone in your family died of a heart attack?

Checkpoint Question

2. Why is it important to review the medical history form before beginning the interview?

3. Why should you let the patient know that any information shared during the interview will be kept confidential?

ASSESSING THE PATIENT

Signs and Symptoms

During the interview, listen carefully as the patient describes current medical problems to identify **signs** and **symptoms**. Signs are objective information that can be observed or perceived by someone other than the patient. Signs include such things as rash, bleeding, coughing, and vital sign measurements. Signs may also be found during the physician's examination.

Symptoms, or subjective information, are indications of disease or changes in the body as sensed by the patient. Usually symptoms are not discernible by anyone other than the patient. They include complaints such as leg pain, headache, nausea, and dizziness. Observable signs that may indicate that a patient is having these symptoms include facial expressions, such as wincing during pain, holding onto rails or furniture for balance when walking, and gagging.

Chief Complaint and Present Illness

After recording the patient's medical history and reviewing the information for accuracy and clarity, you must find out exactly why the patient has come to see the physician for this appointment. Ask an open-ended question to encourage the patient to describe the chain of events leading to this visit. Open-ended questions allow the patient to answer with more than one or two words. For example, you might ask, "What is the reason for your appointment today?" or "Can you describe what has been going on?" Such questions require the patient to explain the visit by giving additional information. In contrast, answers to closed-ended questions usually necessitate only one or two words. Examples of closed-ended questions are "Do you have pain?" and "Are you able to sleep?" These questions can be answered with a simple yes or no and are not going to elicit responses that will useful to the physician attempting to make a diagnosis.

When open-ended questions are used to determine the reason for the visit, the patient's answer will reveal the **chief complaint** (CC). The CC, one statement describing the signs and symptoms that led the patient to seek medical care, is documented in the patient's medical record at each visit. Examples of a CC might include "I've had a headache for the past 3 days" or "Yesterday I lifted a heavy crate and hurt my back." You should document the CC on the progress report form in the patient's record, using the patient's own words in quotation marks whenever possible.

PATIENT EDUCATION

General Topics

While assessing a patient, you can also teach. Your teaching may include information about a specific disease or general care. For example, a diabetic patient may need instruction on glucose testing or diet control. General topics for all patients can include the following:

- Blood pressure management
- Stress management
- Diet or weight control tips
- The importance of exercise
- The effects of alcohol and tobacco
- Instructions for conducting breast or testicular self-examinations
- The importance of proper immunizations
- Cancer warning signs and prevention tips

PROGRESS NOTES

Name: _____

Date: _____ SS#: _____

Address: _____

Occupation: _____ Phone (home)_____ (work) _____

DOB: _____ Age: _____

Drug allergies: _____

DATE	TIME	REMARKS
7/6/XX	0800	cc: Pt. c/o "headache" and nasal congestion ×2 days. Denies fever, earache, sore throat, or nasal drainage.
		S. Stine, CMA

FIGURE 20-3. A progress note form.

WHAT IF

The patient appears highly anxious or intimidated about procedures that seem routine?

You can help put patients at ease by following these steps:

- Treat each patient as an individual with unique needs. Help elderly or disabled patients onto the examination table. If they are unsteady, keep them seated in a regular chair.
- When weighing patients, do not announce their weight aloud, since they may be embarrassed. Instead, ask them in the privacy of the examination room if they want to know their weight.
- Always offer a sheet or blanket to a patient who must change into an examination gown.
- When preparing a patient for a gynecologic examination, have her sit on the examination table until the physician is ready.
- If the physician is delayed, let the patient know. Explain generally the reason for the delay (e.g., an emergency) and let the patient know the approximate length of the delay.

The entry should include the date (day, month, and year) and the time of day. FIGURE 20-3 is an example of a progress report form used to document a patient's CC.

Once you have obtained the CC, continue to probe for more details to further define the patient's present illness (PI). The PI includes a chronological order of events, including dates of onset and any home remedies or other self-care activities, including **over-the-counter** and **homeopathic** medications. Over-the-counter medications are those that are available without prescriptions. They include natural drugs, such as herbs, vitamins, and some homeopathic agents. Homeopathic medications include small doses of agents that cause similar symptoms in healthy individuals and are given to a person who is ill to help cure the disease causing the symptoms. These questions could be used to obtain the PI:

- Chronology. How did this first begin?
- Location. Can you explain or show me exactly where the pain is?
- Severity. Can you describe the pain? Is the pain constant?
- Self-treatment. What medications have you taken for the pain? Do they help?
- Quality. Does anything that you do make the symptoms better? Worse?
- Duration. Have you had these symptoms before?

Avoid suggesting answers, such as "Is the pain sharp?" or "Is the pain worse when you walk?" Many patients will agree or answer positively because they think this must be the expected answer. In addition, don't coax patients by making suggestions of symptoms you might expect them to have based on the chief complaint. Some patients may agree to have the symptoms you describe if they feel that you are suggesting those that "should" be present.

After asking several open-ended questions, it may be appropriate to ask closed-ended questions to obtain specific data. For example, you might ask the patient, "How long have you had this pain?" This kind of question requires only a short answer, not a lengthy description.

Of course, not all patients visit the doctor because they are ill. Some appointments are for routine examinations or tests. In this case, the CC will include a statement about the reason for the visit (e.g., annual physical examination, employment examination); however, you should obtain any additional PI information as appropriate.

Checkpoint Question

4. Explain the difference between a sign and a symptom and give one example of each.

PATIENT EDUCATION

Preventive Medicine

While interviewing the patient about their chief complaint, you may have an opportunity to teach the patient about various topics. Emphasize to the patient that illnesses can often be treated easier and quicker if prompt medical attention is received. This is a very important point to stress to older patients with chronic medical problems such as diabetes. For example, a diabetic patient who presents with a small foot ulcer in its early stages may be able to be treated with medicated dressings. However, if the ulcer goes untreated and gets bigger, the patient may need surgery to clean the wound and may even require hospitalization for antibiotics. While interviewing the patient about their chief complaint, take the opportunity to stress the importance of preventative medicine.

Procedure 20-1

Interviewing the Patient to Obtain a Medical History

Purpose:	Complete the various sections of a medical history form while interviewing a patient.
Equipment:	Medical history form or questionnaire, black or blue pen.
Standard:	This task should take 10 minutes.

Steps	Reason
1. Gather the supplies.	You have everything you need before you begin.
2. Review the medical history form.	Be familiar with the order of the questions and the type of information required to allow for smooth communication with the patient.
3. Take the patient to a private and comfortable area of the office.	A private place prevents distractions and ensures confidentiality.
4. Sit across from the patient at eye level and maintain frequent eye contact.	Standing above the patient may be perceived as threatening and may result in poor communication.

(continues)

Procedure 20-1 (continued)

Interviewing the Patient to Obtain a Medical History

Steps	Steps
5. Introduce yourself and explain the purpose of the interview.	This helps to establish a professional rapport with the patient.
6. Using language the patient can understand, ask the appropriate questions and document the patient's responses. Be sure to determine the patient's CC and PI.	You must obtain accurate and complete data for the physician.
7. Listen actively by looking at the patient from time to time while he or she is speaking.	Patients can sense when the interviewer is not listening, so be sure that you show interest in what the patient is saying.
8. Regardless of the confidences shared by the patient, avoid projecting a judgmental attitude with words or actions.	Maintain professionalism and ensure the patient's trust.
9. If appropriate, explain to the patient what to expect during examinations or procedures at that visit.	Keeping the patient informed about his or her care may decrease anxiety.
10. Thank the patient for cooperating during the interview and offer to answer any questions.	Courtesy encourages the patient to have a positive attitude about the physician's office.

Charting Example

10/14/2005 11:00 a.m. CC: New patient checkup. Medical history form complete and in chart. Patient indicates no physical or health problems at this time. Family history of colon cancer and hypertension noted. E. _____ Parker, CMA

Procedure 20-2

Document a Chief Complaint and Present Illness

Purpose: Accurately record a CC and PI using open and closed questions while interviewing the patient.
Equipment: A cumulative problem list or progress notes form, black or blue ink pen
Standard: This procedure should take 10 minutes or less.

Steps	Reason
1. Gather supplies, including medical record containing cumulative problem list or progress note form.	You have everything you need before you start.
2. Review new or established patient's medical history form.	Be as familiar as possible with the patient to help you obtain a complete CC and PI.
3. Greet and identify the patient while escorting him or her to the examination room.	Greeting the patient by name helps develop professional rapport and eases patient's anxiety. Correctly identifying the patient may help to prevent errors.
4. Using open-ended questions, find out why the patient is seeking medical care; maintain eye contact.	Maintaining eye contact demonstrates that you are actively listening.
5. Determine the PI using open-ended and closed-ended questions.	Use closed-ended questions to obtain specific data only after the patient has responded to open-ended questions.
6. Document the CC and PI correctly on the cumulative problem list or progress report form.	Documentation should include the date, time, CC, PI, and your signature (first initial, last name, and title). Use only correct medical terminology and approved abbreviations.
7. Thank the patient for cooperating and explain that the physician will soon be in to examine the patient.	Courtesy encourages a positive attitude about the office. If you indicate a time frame in reference to the physician coming into the examination room, be honest.

Charting Example
09/15/2005 9:45 a.m. CC: Pt. c/o headache and nausea 3 × days. Has taken ibuprofen for the pain with "some relief." The pain is a "dull ache" in the frontal area of the head and face. No emesis. Face flushed, skin warm and dry. T 98.8°F, P 88, R 24, BP 190/110 (L) sitting S. _____ Vincer, CMA

CHAPTER SUMMARY

In every medical practice, a history is taken from each patient. As a professional medical assistant, you need to know the components of a standard medical history form. You may be required to obtain and document the information on the history form and to interview the patient to elicit the chief complaint and present illness. The physician relies on the information that you gather and document for diagnosing and treating patients, so it is essential that you question the patient carefully and document accurately.

Critical Thinking Challenges

1. Mrs. Smythe has always been impeccably groomed, articulate, and punctual for her monthly blood pressure checks. Today, she was 15 minutes late, her hair was not combed, she wore no makeup, and her clothes did not match. Are any of these observations worth noting on her chart?
2. After reviewing the following items, determine in which section of the medical history the information should be included and explain why. Identify any items that are irrelevant.
   - Sister died of breast cancer.
   - Son had chickenpox last year.
   - Patient has many allergies.
   - Father died of heart disease.
   - Mother is alive and well.
   - Brother works in real estate.
   - Patient smokes three packs of cigarettes a day.
   - Patient works in a cotton mill.
   - Patient is a runner and teaches aerobics.
   - Patient has recently lost 60 pounds.
   - Patient had an angioplasty last year.
3. Determine which of the following are signs and which are symptoms.
   - Nausea
   - Vomiting
   - Itching
   - Rash
   - Dizziness
   - Abdominal pain

- Pallor
- Tingling fingers and toes
- Ringing in the ears
- Fever
- Edema

4. Give open-ended questions for obtaining additional information from patients with the following complaints:
   - "I am tired; I don't sleep well at night."
   - "I have pain in the bottom of my foot when I walk."
   - "My stomach hurts and I threw up yesterday."
   - "I have indigestion every day."

Answers to Checkpoint Questions

1. The past history summarizes the patient's prior health status, and the family history summarizes the health status of the patient's parents, siblings, and grandparents.
2. You should be familiar with the medical history form before beginning the patient interview to promote smooth communication during the interview.
3. Yes, it is important to let the patient know that any information shared during the interview will be kept confidential. Understanding this enables patients to trust in the medical staff and encourages them to share important information that allows the physician to provide better care for the patient.
4. A sign is an objective (observable or measurable) indication of disease. An example of a sign is a patient's blood pressure or temperature reading or a laceration or rash. A symptom is a subjective indication of disease that is felt or noticed by the patient but not directly observable or measurable by the medical assistant or physician. Examples of symptoms include headache and nausea.

 Websites

The Health Insurance Portability and Accountability Act (HIPAA) www.cms.hhs.gov/hipaa
American Autoimmune Related Diseases Association www.aarda.org
March of Dimes www.marchofdimes.com
Genetic Alliance www.geneticalliance.org

21

Anthropometric Measurements and Vital Signs

ROLE DELINEATION

ADMINISTRATIVE: ADMINISTRATIVE
  PROCEDURES
  • Perform basic administrative functions.

CLINICAL: FUNDAMENTAL PRINCIPLES
  • Apply principles of aseptic technique and infection
    control.
  • Comply with quality assurance practices.

CLINICAL: PATIENT CARE
  • Adhere to established patient screening procedures.
  • Obtain patient's history and vital signs.
  • Prepare patient for examinations, procedures, and
    treatments.

GENERAL: PROFESSIONALISM
  • Display a professional manner and image.
  • Demonstrate initiative and responsibility.
  • Work as a member of the health care team.
  • Set priorities and perform multiple tasks.
  • Treat all patients with compassion and empathy.

GENERAL: COMMUNICATION SKILLS
  • Recognize and respect cultural diversity.
  • Adapt communications to individual's ability to
    understand.
  • Recognize and respond effectively to verbal,
    nonverbal, and written communications.
  • Use medical terminology appropriately.

GENERAL: LEGAL CONCEPTS
  • Perform within legal and ethical boundaries.
  • Document accurately.
  • Comply with established risk management and safety
    procedures.

GENERAL: INSTRUCTION
  • Instruct individuals according to their needs.
  • Teach methods of health promotion and disease
    prevention.

CHAPTER COMPETENCIES

LEARNING OBJECTIVES

Upon successfully completing this chapter, you will be able to:

1. Spell and define key terms.
2. Explain the procedures for measuring a patient's height and weight.
3. Identify and describe the types of thermometers.
4. Compare the procedures for measuring a patient's temperature using the oral, rectal, axillary, and tympanic methods.
5. List the fever process, including the stages of fever.
6. Describe the procedure for measuring a patient's pulse and respiratory rates.
7. Identify the various sites on the body used for palpating a pulse.
8. Define Korotkoff sounds and the five phases of blood pressure.
9. Identify factors that may influence the blood pressure.
10. Explain the factors to consider when choosing the correct blood pressure cuff size.

PERFORMANCE OBJECTIVES

Upon successfully completing this chapter, you will be able to:

1. Measure and record a patient's weight (Procedure 21-1).
2. Measure and record a patient's height (Procedure 21-2).
3. Measure and record a patient's oral temperature using a glass mercury thermometer (Procedure 21-3).
4. Measure and record a patient's rectal temperature using a glass mercury thermometer (Procedure 21-4).
5. Measure and record a patient's axillary temperature using a glass mercury thermometer (Procedure 21-5).
6. Measure and record a patient's temperature using an electronic thermometer (Procedure 21-6).
7. Measure and record a patient's temperature using a tympanic thermometer (Procedure 21-7).
8. Measure and record a patient's radial pulse (Procedure 21-8).
9. Measure and record a patient's respirations (Procedure 21-9).
10. Measure and record a patient's blood pressure (Procedure 21-10).

KEY TERMS

afebrile
aneroid
anthropometric
baseline
calibrated
cardiac cycle

cardinal signs
diastole
diaphoresis
febrile
hyperpyrexia
hypertension

intermittent
palpation
postural hypotension
pyrexia
relapsing fever
remittent fever

sphygmomanometer
sustained fever
systole
tympanic thermometer

VITAL SIGNS, also known as **cardinal signs**, are measurements of bodily functions essential to maintaining life processes. Vital signs frequently measured and recorded by the medical assistant include the temperature (T), pulse rate (P), respiratory rate (R), and blood pressure (BP). In addition, medical assistants take **anthropometric** measurements, or the height and weight, of patients and document them in the medical record. This information is essential for the physician to diagnose, treat, and prevent many disorders.

Measurements taken at the first visit are recorded as **baseline** data and are used as reference points for comparison during subsequent visits. After the first office visit, the height is usually not taken; however, the vital signs and weight are taken and recorded for each adult patient at each visit to the medical office.

ANTHROPOMETRIC MEASUREMENTS

Weight

An accurate weight is always required for pregnant patients, infants, children, and the elderly. In addition, weight monitoring may be required if the patient has been prescribed medications that must be carefully calculated according to body weight or for a patient who is attempting to gain or lose weight.

Since most medical practices have only one scale, placement of the scale is important. Many patients are uncomfortable if they are weighed in a place that is not private. Types of scales used to measure weight include balance beam scales, digital scales, and dial scales (FIG. 21-1). Weight may be measured in pounds or kilograms, depending upon the preference of the physician and the type of scale in the medical office. Procedure 21-1 describes how to measure and record a patient's weight.

Height

Height can be measured using the movable ruler on the back of most balance beam scales. Some offices use a graph ruler mounted on a wall (FIG. 21-2), but more accurate measures can be made with a parallel bar moved down against the top of the patient's head. Height is measured in inches or centimeters, depending upon the physician's preference. Procedure 21-2 describes how to measure an adult patient's height. Refer to Chapter 39 for the procedure for measuring the height and weight of infants and children.

Checkpoint Question

1. Why is it important to measure vital signs accurately at every patient visit?

VITAL SIGNS

Temperature

Body temperature reflects a balance between heat produced and heat lost by the body (FIG. 21-3). Heat is produced during normal internal physical and chemical processes called metabolism and through muscle movement. Heat is normally lost through several processes, including respiration,

FIGURE 21-1. The three types of scales used in medical offices include the digital, dial, and balance scales.

FIGURE 21-2. A wall-mounted device to measure height and the sliding bar on the balance scale.

elimination, and conduction through the skin (TABLE 21-1). Normally, the body maintains a constant internal temperature of around 98.6° Fahrenheit (F) or 37.0° Celsius (C) (centigrade). A patient whose temperature is within normal limits is said to be **afebrile**, while a patient with a temperature above normal is considered **febrile** (has a fever).

Thermometers are used to measure body temperature using either the Fahrenheit or Celsius scale. Box 21-1 compares temperatures taken a variety of ways in Celsius and in Fahrenheit. Since glass thermometers used in the medical office may be marked in either scale, you should be able to convert from one scale to another (see Appendix VI). The patient's temperature can be measured using the oral, rectal, axillary, or **tympanic** method. The oral method is most commonly used, but use of the tympanic thermometer is increasing; if used accurately, it gives a reading that is comparable to the oral temperature. A reading of 98.6°F orally is considered a normal average for body temperature rectal or axillary and readings will vary slightly. Rectal temperatures are generally 1°F higher than the oral temperature because of the vascularity and tightly closed environment of the rectum. Axillary temperatures are usually 1°F lower because of lower vascularity and difficulty in keeping the axilla tightly closed. When recording the body temperature, you must indicate the temperature reading and the method used to obtain it, such as oral, rectal, axillary, or tympanical. A rectal temperature reading of 101°F is equivalent to 100°F

orally, and an axillary reading of 101°F is equivalent to 102°F orally.

Checkpoint Question

2. How does an oral temperature measurement differ from a rectal measurement? Why?

Fever Processes

Although a patient's temperature is influenced by heat lost or produced by the body, it is regulated by the hypothalamus in the brain. When the hypothalamus senses that the body is too warm, it initiates peripheral vasodilation to carry core heat to the body surface via the blood and increases perspiration to cool the body by evaporation. If the temperature registers too low, vasoconstriction to conserve heat and shivering to generate more heat will usually maintain a fairly normal core temperature. Temperature elevations and variations are often a *sign* of disease but are not a disease in themselves. These factors may cause the temperature to vary:

- *Age.* Children usually have a higher metabolism and therefore a higher body temperature than adults. The elderly, with a slower metabolism, usually have lower readings than younger adults. Temperatures of both the very young and the elderly are easily affected by the environment.
- *Gender.* Women usually have a slightly higher temperature than men, especially at the time of ovulation.
- *Exercise.* Activity causes the body to burn more calories for energy, which raises the body temperature.
- *Time of day.* The body temperature is usually lowest in the early morning, before physical activity has begun.
- *Emotions.* Temperature tends to rise during times of stress and fall with depression.
- *Illness.* High or low body temperatures may result from a disease process.

FIGURE 21-3. Factors affecting the balance between heat loss and heat production.

Table 21-1.   MECHANISMS OF HEAT TRANSFER

Mechanism	Definition	Example
Radiation	Diffusion or dissemination of heat by electro-magnetic waves	The body gives off waves of heat from uncovered surfaces.
Convection	Dissemination of heat by motion between areas of unequal density	An oscillating fan blows cool air across the surface of a warm body.
Evaporation	Conversion of liquid to vapor	Body fluid (perspiration and insensible loss) evaporates from the skin.
Conduction	Transfer of heat during direct contact between two objects.	The body transfers heat to an ice pack, melting the ice.

Mechanisms of heat transfer.

Adapted with permission from Taylor C, Lillis C, Le Mone P. Fundamentals of Nursing, 2nd ed. 388. Philadelphia: Lippincott, 1993; 388.

Stages of Fever

An elevated temperature, or fever, usually results from a disease process, such as a bacterial or viral infection. Body temperature may also rise during intense exercise, anxiety, or dehydration unrelated to a disease process, but these elevations are not considered fevers. **Pyrexia** refers to a fever of 102°F or higher rectally or 101°F or higher orally. An extremely high temperature, 105° to 106°F, is **hyperpyrexia** and is considered dangerous, since the intense internal body heat may damage or destroy cells of the brain and other vital organs. The fever process has several clearly defined stages:

1. The *onset* may be abrupt or gradual.
2. The *course* may range from a day or so to several weeks. Fever may be **sustained** (constant), **remittent** (fluctuating), **intermittent** (occurring at intervals), or **relapsing**, (returning after an extended period of normal readings). TABLE 21-2 describes and illustrates these courses of fever.
3. The *resolution*, or return to normal, may occur as either a *crisis* (abrupt return to normal), or *lysis* (gradual return to normal).

Checkpoint Question

3. Explain why the body temperature of a young child may be different from that of an adult.

Types of Thermometers

Glass Mercury Thermometers. Oral, rectal, and axillary temperatures have traditionally been measured using the mercury glass thermometer. This thermometer consists of

Box 21-1

TEMPERATURE COMPARISONS

	Fahrenheit	Celsius
Oral	98.6	37.0
Rectal	99.6	37.6
Axillary	97.6	36.4
Tympanic	98.6	37.0

a glass tube divided into two major parts. The bulb end is filled with mercury and may have a round or a slender tip. Glass thermometers have different shapes for oral and rectal use. Rectal thermometers have a rounded, or stubbed, end and are usually color coded red on the opposite flat end of the thermometer. Thermometers with a long, slender bulb are used for axillary or oral temperatures and are color-coded blue (FIG. 21-4). When the glass thermometer is placed in position for a specified period, body heat expands the mercury, which rises up the glass column and remains there until it is physically shaken back into the bulb.

PATIENT EDUCATION

Fever

When instructing patients about fever, explain that temperature elevations are usually a natural response to disease and that efforts to bring the temperature back to normal may be counterproductive. However, if the patient is uncomfortable or the temperature is abnormally high, it should be brought down to about 101°F, and the body's natural defenses may still be able to destroy the pathogen without extreme discomfort to the patient.

After consulting with the physician, instruct all patients regarding the following comfort measures:

- Drink clear fluids as tolerated to rehydrate body tissues if nausea and vomiting are not present.
- Keep clothing and bedding clean and dry, especially after **diaphoresis** (sweating).
- Avoid becoming chilled. Chills cause shivering, which raises the body temperature.
- Rest and eat a light diet as tolerated.
- Use antipyretics to keep comfortable, but do not give aspirin products to children under 18 years of age. Aspirin has been associated with Reye's syndrome, a potentially fatal disorder, following cases of viral illnesses and varicella zoster (chickenpox).

Table 21-2.	VARIATIONS IN FEVER PATTERNS
Type of Fever	**Description**
Sustained	Remains elevated, with very little fluctuation.
Remittent	Fluctuates several degrees but never reaches normal.
Intermittent	Cycles frequently between periods of normal or subnormal temperatures and spikes of fever.
Relapsing	Recurs after a brief but sustained period of normal temperature.

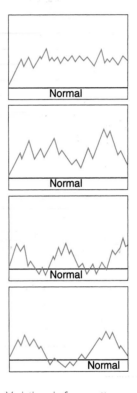

Variations in fever patterns.

Adapted with permission from Timby BK. Fundamental Skills and Concepts in Patient Care, 6th ed. Philadelphia: Lippincott-Raven, 1996.

The long stem of the Fahrenheit thermometer is calibrated with lines designating temperature in even degrees: 94°, 96°, 98°, 100°, and so on. Uneven numbers are marked only with a longer line. Between these longer lines, four smaller lines designate temperature in 0.2° increments. The thermometer is read by noting the level of the mercury in the glass column. For example, if the level of the mercury falls on the second smaller line past the large line marked 100, the reading is 100.4°F. Celsius thermometers are marked for each degree (35°, 36°, 37°, and so on), with 10 markings between the whole numbers (FIG. 21-5). If the mercury falls on the third small line past the line marked 37, the temperature reading is recorded as 37.3°C.

FIGURE 21-4. Glass mercury thermometers. **Front.** Slender bulb, oral. **Center.** Rounded bulb, red tip, rectal. **Back.** Blue tip, oral.

Before using an electronic thermometer, place it in a disposable clear plastic sheath (FIG. 21-6). When you take the thermometer from the patient, remove the sheath by pulling the thermometer out, which turns the sheath inside out and traps the saliva inside it. Dispose of the sheath in a biohazard container and sanitize and disinfect the thermometer according to the office policy. Usually, washing the thermometers with warm—not hot—soapy water and soaking in a solution of alcohol is sufficient. The procedures for measuring oral, rectal, and axillary temperatures using glass mercury thermometers are described in Procedures 21-3 to 21-5.

Electronic Thermometers. Electronic thermometers are portable battery-operated units with interchangeable probes (FIG. 21-7). The base unit of the thermometer is battery operated, and the interchangeable probes are color-coded blue for oral or axillary and red for rectal. When the probe is properly positioned, the temperature is sensed and a digital readout shows in the window of the handheld base. Electronic thermometers are usually kept in a charging unit between uses to ensure that the batteries are operative at all times. The

procedure for taking and recording an oral temperature using an electronic thermometer is described in Procedure 21-6.

Tympanic Thermometers. Another type of thermometer used in medical offices today is the tympanic, or aural, thermometer. This device is usually battery powered. The end is fitted with a disposable cover that is inserted into the ear much like an otoscope (FIG. 21-8). With the end of the thermometer in place, a button is pressed and infrared light bounces off the tympanic membrane, or eardrum. When correctly positioned, the sensor in the thermometer determines the temperature of the blood in the tympanic membrane. The temperature reading is displayed on the unit's digital screen within 2 seconds. This device is considered highly reliable for temperature measurement. Procedure 21-7 describes the complete process for obtaining a body temperature with a tympanic thermometer.

Centigrade

Rectal

Oral

Fahreneit

Rectal

Oral

FIGURE 21-5. The two glass thermometers on the top are calibrated in the Celsius (centigrade) scale, and the two on the bottom use the Fahrenheit scale. Note the blunt bulb on the rectal thermometers and the long thin bulb on the oral thermometers.

FIGURE 21-6. (A and B) An electronic thermometer is placed in a disposable sheath before use.

WHAT IF

You have been assigned to disinfect the glass mercury thermometers used in your medical office?

Although glass thermometers are always placed in a disposable sheath before use, the thermometer should be sanitized and disinfected after each use. The procedure should be outlined in the office policy and procedure manual, but the following steps can be used as a guide:

- Wearing gloves, wash the thermometer with cool or tepid soapy water. Do not use hot water, since too much heat may break the thermometer.
- After rinsing with cool water, dry the thermometer to avoid diluting your disinfecting solution.
- Pour a disinfecting soaking solution (70% alcohol is commonly used) into a tray or container with a lid. The lid will prevent the soaking solution from evaporating.
- Soak the thermometers for a prescribed period, usually 3 to 4 hours, before rinsing, drying, and storing.

FIGURE 21-8. The tympanic thermometer in use.

 Checkpoint Question

4. Why is a tympanic membrane temperature more accurate than an axillary temperature?

Disposable Thermometers. Single-use disposable thermometers are fairly accurate but are not considered as reliable as electronic, tympanic, or glass thermometers. These thermometers register quickly by indicating color changes on a strip. They are not reliable for definitive measurement, but they are acceptable for screening in settings such as day care centers and schools (FIG. 21-9). Other disposable thermometers are available for pediatric use in the form of sucking devices, or pacifiers, but these are not used in the medical office setting.

Pulse

As the heart beats, blood is forced through the arteries, expanding them. With relaxation of the heart, the arteries relax also. This expansion and relaxation of the arteries can be felt at various points on the body where you can press an artery against a bone or other underlying firm surface. These areas are known as pulse points. With **palpation**, each expansion of the artery can be felt and is counted as one heartbeat. A pulse in specific arteries supplying blood to the extremities also indicates that oxygenated blood is flowing to that extremity.

The heartbeat can be palpated (felt) or auscultated (heard) at several pulse points. The arteries most commonly used are the carotid, apical, brachial, radial, femoral, popliteal, posterior tibial, and dorsalis pedis (FIG. 21-10). Palpation of the

FIGURE 21-7. Two types of electronic thermometers and probes.

FIGURE 21-9. Disposable paper thermometer. The dots change color to indicate the body temperature.

FIGURE 21-10. Sites for palpation of peripheral pulses.

FIGURE 21-11. Measuring a radial pulse. (Reprinted with permission from Bickely LS. Bates' Guide to Physical Examination and History Taking, 8th ed. Philadelphia: Lippincott Williams & Wilkins, 2003.)

pulse is performed by placing the index and middle fingers, the middle and ring fingers, or all three fingers over a pulse point (FIG. 21-11). The thumb is not used to palpate a pulse. The apical pulse is auscultated using a stethoscope with the bell placed over the apex of the heart (FIG. 21-12), and a Doppler unit is used to amplify the sound of peripheral pulses that are difficult to palpate.

Pulse Characteristics

While palpating the pulse, you also assess the rate, rhythm, and volume as the artery wall expands with each heartbeat. The *rate* is the number of heartbeats in 1 minute. This number can be determined by palpating the pulse and

Table 21-3. VARIATIONS IN PULSE RATE BY AGE	
Age Minute	Beats p
Birth to 1 year	110–170
1–10 years	90–110
10–16 years	80–95
16 years to midlife	70–80
Elderly adult	55–70

counting each heartbeat while watching the second hand of your watch either for 30 seconds and then multiplying that number by 2 or for 1 minute. In healthy adults, the average pulse rate is 60 to 100 beats per minute. At other ages, there is a large variance of pulse rates as shown in TABLE 21-3.

The *rhythm* is the interval between each heartbeat or the pattern of beats. Normally, this pattern is regular, with each heartbeat occurring at a regular, consistent rate. An irregular rhythm should be counted for 1 full minute to determine the rate, and the irregular rhythm should be documented with the pulse rate.

Volume, the strength or force of the heartbeat, can be described as soft, bounding, weak, thready, strong, or full. Usually the volume of the pulse is recorded only if it is weak, thready, or bounding.

Factors Affecting Pulse Rates

Many factors affect the force, speed, and rhythm of the heart. Young children and infants have a much faster heart rate than adults. A conditioned athlete may have a normal heart rate below 60 beats per minute. Older adults may have a

FIGURE 21-12. Measuring an apical pulse. (Reprinted with permission from Bickely LS. Bates' Guide to Physical Examination and History Taking, 8th ed. Philadelphia: Lippincott Williams & Wilkins, 2003.)

Table 21-4. FACTORS AFFECTING PULSE RATES

Factor	Effect
Time of day	The pulse is usually lower early in the morning than later in the day.
Gender	Women have a slightly higher pulse rate than men.
Body type and size	Tall, thin people usually have a lower pulse rate than shorter, stockier people.
Exercise	The heart rate increases with the need for increased cardiac output (the amount of blood ejected from either ventricle in one minute).
Stress or emotions	Anger, fear, excitement, and stress will raise the pulse; depression will lower it.
Fever	The increased need for cell metabolism in the presence of fever raises the cardiac output to supply oxygen and nutrients; the pulse may rise as much as 10 beats/minute per degree of fever.
Medications	Many medications raise or lower the pulse as a desired effect or an undesirable side effect.
Blood volume	Loss of blood volume to hemorrhage or dehydration will increase the need for cellular metabolism and will increase the cardiac output to supply the need.

faster heart rate, as the myocardium compensates for decreased efficiency. Other factors that affect pulse rates are listed in TABLE 21-4.

The radial artery is most often used to determine pulse rate because it is convenient for both the medical assistant and the patient (Procedure 21-8). If the radial pulse is irregular or hard to palpate, the apical pulse is the site of choice (FIG. 21-13). Peripheral pulses that are difficult to palpate may also be auscultated with a Doppler unit (FIG. 21-14), a small battery-powered or electric device that consists of a main box with control switches, a probe, and an earpiece unit that plugs into the main box and resembles the earpieces to a stethoscope. The earpiece may be detached so the sounds can be heard by everyone in the room if desired. Follow these steps to use a Doppler device:

1. Apply a coupling or transmission gel on the pulse point before placing the end of the probe, or transducer, on the area. This gel creates an airtight seal between the probe and the skin and facilitates transmission of the sound.

2. With the machine on, hold the probe at a 90° angle with light pressure to ensure contact. Move the probe as necessary in small circles in the gel until you hear the pulse (Fig. 21-14). When contact with the artery is made, the Doppler will emit a loud pumping sound with each heartbeat. Adjust the volume control on the Doppler unit as necessary.

3. After assessing the rate and rhythm of the pulse, clean the patient's skin and the probe with a tissue or soft cloth. Do not clean the probe with water or alcohol, as this may damage the transducer.

Checkpoint Question

5. What characteristics of a patient's pulse should be assessed, and how should they be recorded in the medical record?

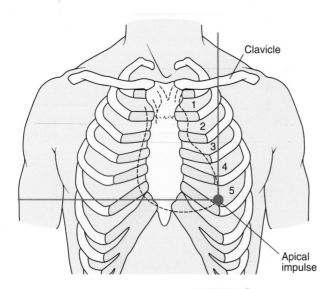

FIGURE 21-13. Finding the apical pulse.

FIGURE 21-14. The dorsalis pedis pulse being auscultated using a Doppler device.

TRIAGE

While working in a medical office, you have just taken these three patients' vital signs:

A. A 52-year-old woman complaining of dyspnea. Her respiratory rate is 38, her pulse is 112 and irregular, and her blood pressure is 150/86.

B. A 43-year-old man with a pulse of 54 and blood pressure of 98/52. He denies any shortness of breath, chest pain, or dizziness.

C. A 65-year-old man who had open-heart surgery 2 weeks ago. He states that yellow drainage is coming from the surgical wound on his chest. His temperature is 101.8°F orally, his blood pressure is 118/62, and his pulse is 118 and regular.

How do you sort these patients? Who should be seen first? Second? Third?

Patient A should be seen first. The physician should immediately see any patient complaining of trouble breathing. Her respiratory and pulse rates are faster than normal for an adult. Patient C should be seen second because of his temperature and pulse rate. Patient B should be seen last. A pulse rate of 52 and blood pressure of 98/52 are low, but the patient is not complaining of any symptoms. If he is physically fit, his vital signs may normally be lower than average. If he were complaining of dizziness or feeling faint, he would need to be seen sooner.

Respiration

Respiration is the exchange of gases between the atmosphere and the blood in the body. With respiration, the body expels carbon dioxide (CO_2) and takes in oxygen (O_2). External respiration is inhalation and exhalation, during which air travels through the respiratory tract to the alveoli so that oxygen can be absorbed into the bloodstream. Internal respiration is the exchange of gases between the blood and the tissue cells. Respiration is controlled by the respiratory center in the brainstem and by feedback from chemosensors in the carotid arteries that monitor the CO_2 content in the blood.

As the patient breathes in (inspiration), oxygen flows into the lungs and the diaphragm contracts and flattens out, lifting and expanding the rib cage. During expiration, air in the lungs flows out of the chest cavity as the diaphragm relaxes, moves upward into a dome-like shape, and allows the rib cage to contract. Each respiration is counted as one full inspiration and one full expiration.

Observing the rise and fall of the chest to count respira-

tions is usually performed as a part of the pulse measurement. Generally you should not make the patient aware that you are counting respirations, because patients often change the voluntary action of breathing if they are aware that they are being watched. Respirations can be counted for a full minute or for 30 seconds with the number multiplied by 2. When appropriate, a stethoscope may be used to auscultate respirations.

Respiration Characteristics

The characteristics of respirations include rate, rhythm, and depth. *Rate* is the number of respirations occurring in 1 minute. *Rhythm* is time, or spacing, between each respiration. This pattern is equal and regular in patients with normal respirations. Any abnormal rhythm is described as irregular and recorded as such in the patient's record after the rate.

Depth is the volume of air being inhaled and exhaled. When a person is at rest, the depth should be regular and consistent. There are normally no noticeable sounds other than the regular exchange of air. Respirations that are abnormally deep or shallow are documented in addition to the rate. Abnormal sounds during inspiration or expiration are usually a sign of a disease process. These abnormal sounds are usually recorded as crackles (wet or dry sounds) or wheezes (high-pitched sounds) heard during inspiration or expiration.

Factors Affecting Respiration

In healthy adults, the average respiratory rate is 14 to 20 breaths per minute. TABLE 21-5 shows the normal variations in respiratory rates according to age. Patients with an elevated body temperature usually also have increased pulse and respiratory rates. A respiratory rate that is much faster than average is called tachypnea, and a respiratory rate that is slower than usual is referred to bradypnea. Further descriptions of abnormal or unusual respirations include the following:

dyspnea difficult or labored breathing.
apnea no respiration.
hyperpnea abnormally deep, gasping breaths.
hyperventilation a respiratory rate that greatly exceeds the body's oxygen demand.

Table 21-5. VARIATIONS IN RESPIRATION RANGES BY AGE	
Age	**Respirations per Minute**
Infant	20 +
Child	18–20
Adult	12–20

hypopnea   shallow respirations.
orthopnea   inability to breathe lying down; the patient
usually has to sit upright to breathe.

Procedure 21-9 lists the steps for counting and recording
respirations.

Checkpoint Question

6. What happens within the chest cavity when the
diaphragm contracts?

Blood Pressure

Blood pressure is a measurement of the pressure of the
blood in an artery as it is forced against the arterial
walls. Pressure is measured in the contraction and relaxation phases of the cardiac cycle, or heartbeat. When the
heart contracts, it forces blood from the atria and ventricles
in the phase known as **systole**. This highest pressure level
during contraction is recorded as the systolic pressure and
is heard as the first sound in taking blood pressure (Procedure 21-10).

As the heart pauses briefly to rest and refill, the arterial
pressure drops. This phase is known as **diastole**, and the
pressure is recorded as the diastolic pressure. Systolic and diastolic pressure result from the two parts of the **cardiac cycle**, the period from the beginning of one heartbeat to the beginning of the next. When measured using a stethoscope and
sphygmomanometer, or blood pressure cuff, these two
pressures constitute the blood pressure and are written as a
fraction, with the systolic pressure over the diastolic pressure. The normal adult systolic blood pressure is 100 to 140,
and the normal diastolic pressure is 60 to 90, with an average
adult blood pressure of 120/80. A lower pressure may be
normal for athletes with exceptionally well-conditioned cardiovascular systems. Blood pressure that drops suddenly
when the patient stands from a sitting or lying position is
postural hypotension, or orthostatic hypotension; it may
cause symptoms including vertigo. Some patients with postural hypotension may faint. Extra precautions should be
taken when assessing patients going from lying down to sitting or standing.

Two basic types of sphygmomanometers are used to
measure blood pressure: the **aneroid**, which has a circular
dial for the readings, and the mercury, which has a mer-

F I G U R E   2 1 - 1 5 .   A mercurcury column sphygmomanometer and an aneroid sphygmomanometer.

cury-filled glass tube for the readings (FIG. 21-15). Although only one type actually contains mercury, both
types are calibrated and measure blood pressure in millimeters of mercury (mm Hg). A blood pressure of 120/80
indicates the force needed to raise a column of mercury to
the 120 calibration mark on the glass tube during diastole
and 80 during diastole. The elasticity of the person's arterial walls, the strength of the heart muscle, and the quantity
and viscosity (thickness) of the blood all affect the blood
pressure.

The sphygmomanometer is attached to a cuff by a rubber
tube. A second rubber tube is attached to a hand pump with
a screw valve. This device is used to pump air into the rubber bladder in the cuff. When the screw valve is turned
clockwise, the bladder in the cuff around the patient's arm is
inflated by multiple compressions of the pump. As the bladder inflates, the pressure created against the artery at some
point prohibits blood from passing through the vessel. When
the screw valve is slowly opened by turning it counterclock-
wise, the blood pressure can be determined by listening carefully with the stethoscope placed on the artery to the sounds
produced as the blood begins to flow through the vessel. Procedure 21-10 describes the steps for correctly obtaining a patient's blood pressure using the radial artery.

Spanish Terminology

Voy a tomar su pulso radial.	I am going to take your radial pulse.
Voy a tomar su presión de sangre.	I am going to take your blood pressure.
Voy a tomar la temperatura.	I am going to take your temperature.
Fiebre?	Fever?

Checkpoint Question

7. What happens to the heart during systole? Diastole?

Korotkoff Sounds

Korotkoff sounds can be classified into five phases of sounds heard while auscultating the blood pressure as described by the Russian neurologist Nicolai Korotkoff. Only the sounds heard during phase I (represented by the first sound heard) and phase V (represented by the last sound heard) are recorded as blood pressure. You may hear other Korotkoff sounds during the procedure, but it is not necessary to record them. Table 21-6 describes the five phases of Korotkoff sounds that may be heard when auscultating blood pressure.

Pulse Pressure

The difference between the systolic and diastolic readings is known as the pulse pressure. For example, with the average adult blood pressure of 120/80, the difference between the numbers 120 and 80 is 40. The average normal range for pulse pressure is 30 to 50 mm Hg. Generally the pulse pressure should be no more than one-third of the systolic reading. If the pulse pressure is more or less than these parameters, the physician should be notified.

PATIENT EDUCATION

Hypertension

After taking a patient's blood pressure, tell the patient what the reading was. Patients with high blood pressure should be encouraged to keep a personal log of their blood pressure readings. Teach the patient about the risks and possible complications of not controlling their blood pressure. Emphasize the importance of taking prescribed antihypertensive medications every day as directed. Emphasize that the patient should never stop taking blood pressure medication without the doctor's permission, even if the blood pressure seems to be under control: the readings may be under control because of the medication. Teach patients how to take their blood pressure at home. Patients should be warned that freestanding blood pressure machines in pharmacies and supermarkets are to be used only as a screening device. These machines are not always calibrated properly or calibrated on a regular basis. The readings may not be accurate.

Phase	Sounds
I	Faint tapping heard as the cuff deflates (systolic blood pressure)
II	Soft swishing
III	Rhythmic, sharp, distinct tapping
IV	Soft tapping that becomes faint
V	Last sound (diastolic blood pressure)

Table 21-6. FIVE PHASES OF BLOOD PRESSURE

Auscultatory Gap

Patients with a history of **hypertension**, or elevated blood pressure, may have an auscultatory gap heard during phase II of the Korotkoff sounds. An auscultatory gap is the loss of any sounds for a drop of up to 30 mm Hg (sometimes more) during the release of air from the blood pressure cuff after the first sound is heard. If the last sound heard at the beginning of the gap is recorded as the diastolic blood pressure, the documented blood pressure is inaccurate and may result in misdiagnosis and treatment of a condition that the patient does not have. As a result, it is important for you to listen and watch carefully as the dial or column of mercury falls until you are certain that you have heard the last sound, or diastolic pressure.

Factors Influencing Blood Pressure

Atherosclerosis and arteriosclerosis are two disease processes that greatly influence blood pressure. These diseases affect the size and elasticity of the artery lumen. The general health of the patient is also a major factor. General health includes dietary habits, alcohol and tobacco use, the amount and type of exercise, previous heart conditions such as myocardial infarctions, and family history of cardiac disease. These other factors normally affect blood pressure:

- *Age.* As the body ages, vessels begin to lose elasticity and more force is needed to expand the arterial wall. The buildup of atherosclerotic patches inside the artery also increases the force needed for blood flow.
- *Activity.* Exercise raises the blood pressure temporarily, and inactivity or rest usually lowers the pressure.
- *Stress.* The sympathetic nervous system stimulates the release of the hormone epinephrine, which raises the pressure in the fight or flight response.
- *Body position.* Blood pressure normally falls when a person lies supine.
- *Medications.* Some medications lower the pressure, and others may cause an elevation.

Because so many variables can affect a patient's blood pressure, a diagnosis of hypertension is usually not made by the physician unless a pattern of three or four elevated pressures are documented over time.

WHAT IF

A patient has a dialysis shunt (a surgically made venous access port that allows a patient with little or no kidney function to be connected to a dialysis machine) in his left arm? Should you use that arm to take his blood pressure?

No! Taking blood pressure in that arm might permanently damage the shunt, and the patient would not be able to receive dialysis until another shunt was prepared by a surgeon. A patient who has had a mastectomy should also not have a blood pressure taken in the arm on the affected side, since the lymphatic circulation in that extremity is impaired. The patient with a dialysis shunt or mastectomy should have the medical record clearly marked indicating that no blood pressure or blood draws are to be performed on the designated arm. Most patients are aware of the importance of not taking blood pressure or specimens from the affected arm and will alert you before you mistakenly perform the procedure.

Blood Pressure Cuff Size

Before beginning to take a patient's blood pressure, assess the size of the patient's arm and choose the correct size accordingly. The width of the cuff should be 40% to 50% of the circumference of the arm. To determine the correct size, hold the narrow edge of the cuff at the midpoint of the upper arm. Wrap the width, not the length, around the arm. The cuff width should reach not quite halfway around the arm (Fig. 21-16). Varying widths of cuffs are

FIGURE 21-16.   Choosing the right blood pressure cuff.

FIGURE 21-17.   Three sizes of blood pressure cuffs (from left): a large cuff for obese adults, a normal adult cuff, and a pediatric cuff.

available from about 1 inch for infants to 8 inches for obese adults (Fig. 21-17). The blood pressure measurement may be inaccurate by as much as 30 mm Hg if the cuff size is incorrect. Box 21-2 lists causes of errors in blood pressure readings.

 Checkpoint Question

8. How are the pulse pressure and the auscultatory gap different?

Box 21-2

CAUSES OF ERRORS IN BLOOD PRESSURE READINGS

- Wrapping the cuff improperly
- Failing to keep the patient's arm at the level of the heart while taking the blood pressure
- Failing to support the patient's arm on a stable surface while taking the blood pressure
- Recording the auscultatory gap for the diastolic pressure
- Failing to maintain the gauge at eye level
- Applying the cuff around the patient's clothing and attempting to listen through the clothing
- Allowing the cuff to deflate too rapidly or too slowly
- Failing to wait 1 to 2 minutes before rechecking using the same arm
- Improper size of cuff

Measuring Weight

Purpose:	Accurately measure and record a patient's weight.
Equipment:	Calibrated balance beam scale, digital scale, or dial scale; paper towel.
Standard:	This procedure should take 5 minutes.

Steps	Reason
1. Wash your hands.	Handwashing before contact with patients aids in infection control.
2. Ensure that the scale is properly balanced at zero.	This helps prevent an error in measurement.
3. Greet and identify the patient. Explain the procedure.	Identifying the patient prevents errors, and explaining the procedure promotes cooperation.
4. Escort the patient to the scale and place a paper towel on the scale.	Since the patient will be standing in bare feet or stockings, the paper towel minimizes microorganism transmission.
5. Have the patient remove shoes and heavy outerwear and put down purse.	Unnecessary items must be removed to get an accurate reading.
6. Assist patient onto scale facing forward, standing on paper towel, without touching or holding on to anything if possible while watching for difficulties with balance.	Some patients may feel unsteady as the plate of the scale settles.
7. Weigh the patient: A. *Balance beam scale:* Slide counterweights on bottom and top bars (start with heavier bars) from zero to approximate weight. Each counterweight should rest securely in notch with indicator mark at proper calibration. To obtain measurement, balance bar must hang freely at exact midpoint. To calculate weight, add top reading to bottom one. (Example: If heavier counterweight reads 100 and lighter one reads 16 plus three small lines, record weight as 116.75 lb.). B. *Digital scale:* Read and record weight displayed on digital screen. C. *Dial scale:* Indicator arrow rests at patient's weight. Read this number directly above the dial.	Reading at an angle would result in an incorrect measurement.
8. Return the bars on the top and bottom to zero.	A balance beam scale should be returned to zero after each use.
9. Assist the patient from the scale if necessary and discard the paper towel.	Patients may lose balance and fall when stepping down from the scale; they should be observed and assisted as necessary. The paper towel may be left in place if the height is going to be obtained.
10. Record the patient's weight.	If the weight and height are measured at the same time, they are recorded together.

Charting Example
12/22/2005 2:00 P.M. Wt. 155# _____ J. Briten, CMA

Procedure 21-2

Measuring Height

Purpose: Accurately measure and record a patient's height.

Equipment: A scale with a ruler.

Standards: This procedure should take less than 5 minutes.

Steps	Purpose
1. Wash your hands if this procedure is not done at the same time as the weight.	Typically, height is obtained with weight; your hands are already washed.
2. Have the patient remove shoes and stand straight and erect on the scale, heels together, eyes straight ahead. (Patient may face the ruler, but a better measurement is made with the patient's back to the ruler).	The posture of the patient must be erect for an accurate measurement.
3. With measuring bar perpendicular to the ruler, slowly lower it until it firmly touches the patient's head. Press lightly if the patient's hair is full or high.	Hair that is full should not be included in the height measurement.

(continues)

Procedure 21-2 *(continued)*

Measuring Height

Steps	Purpose

Step 3. Measure where the bar slides out of the scale (or point of movement). This measure read 63 inches, or 5 feet 3 inches.

4. Read the measurement at the point of movement on the ruler. If measurements are in inches, convert to feet and inches (e.g., if the bar reads 65 plus two smaller lines, read it at 65.5. Since 12 inches equals 1 foot, the patient is 5 feet 5.5 inches tall).	
5. Assist the patient from the scale if necessary; watch for signs of difficulty with balance.	
6. Record the weight and height measurements in the medical record.	

Charting Example
10/14/2005 9:15 A.M. Ht. 5 feet 5.5 inches; Wt. 136.25 lb._____ Y. Torres, CMA

Measuring Oral Temperature Using a Glass Mercury Thermometer

Purpose	Accurately measure and record a patient's oral temperature using a glass mercury thermometer.
Equipment:	Glass mercury oral thermometer; tissues or cotton balls; disposable plastic sheath; gloves; biohazard container; cool, soapy water; disinfectant solution
Standard:	This procedure should take 10 minutes

Steps	Reason
1. Wash your hands and assemble the necessary supplies.	Handwashing aids infection control.
2. Dry the thermometer if it has been stored in a disinfectant solution by wiping it from the bulb and going up the stem with a tissue or cotton ball.	Removing the wet disinfectant allows the thermometer to slip easily into the sheath.
3. Carefully check the thermometer for chips or cracks.	A chipped or cracked thermometer could injure the patient.
4. Check the reading by holding the stem horizontally at eye level and turning it slowly.	It is easiest to see the mercury in the column in this position.
5. If the reading is above 94°F, shake down the thermometer by securely grasping it at the end of the stem with your thumb and forefinger and snapping your wrist several times. Avoid hitting the thermometer against anything while snapping your wrist.	The reading must begin below 94°F to provide an accurate temperature reading. The reading will never decrease in the thermometer unless the mercury is physically forced into the bulb
6. Insert the thermometer into the plastic sheath.	Follow the package instructions for placing the thermometer correctly in the sheath.
7. Greet and identify the patient. Explain the procedure and ask about any eating, drinking of hot or cold fluids, gum chewing, or smoking within the past 15 minutes.	Eating, drinking, gum chewing, or smoking may alter the oral reading. If the patient has done any of these within 15 minutes, wait 15 minutes or select another route.
8. Place the thermometer under the patient's tongue to either side of the frenulum.	This is the area of highest vascularity and will give the most accurate reading.
9. Tell the patient to keep the mouth and lips closed but not to bite down on the thermometer.	Keeping the mouth and lips closed prevents air from entering the mouth and causing an inaccurate reading. Biting down on the thermometer may break it.
10. Leave the thermometer in place for 3 to 5 minutes. *Note*: The patient's pulse, respirations, and blood pressure may be taken during this time (See Procedures 21-8 to 21-10).	The thermometer may be left in place for 3 minutes if there is no evidence of fever and the patient is compliant. It should be left in place for 5 minutes if the patient is febrile or noncompliant (talks or opens mouth frequently).
11. At the appropriate time, remove the thermometer from the patient's mouth while wearing gloves. Remove the sheath by holding the very edge of the sheath with your thumb and forefinger and pulling down from the open edge over the length of the thermometer to the bulb. Discard the sheath into a biohazard container.	

(continues)

Procedure 21-3 *(continued)*

Measuring Oral Temperature Using a Glass Mercury Thermometer

Steps	Reason
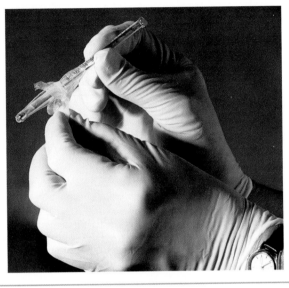 Step 11. Remove the sheath by grasping the end nearest the tip and inverting the plastic toward the bulb. The soiled area should now be inside the sheath.	
12. Hold the thermometer horizontal at eye level and note the level of mercury that has risen into the column.	
13. Sanitize and disinfect the thermometer according to the office policy and wash your hands.	Wash the thermometer with cool or tepid soapy water, rinse with cool water, and dry well. Place the thermometer in a disinfectant solution, such as 70% isopropyl alcohol, according to office policy.
Step 13. Store clean thermometers in a covered instrument tray padded with gauze to prevent chipping or cracking of the glass.	
14. Record the patient's temperature.	Procedures are considered not done if they are not recorded. The vital signs (temperature, pulse, respirations, and blood pressure) are usually recorded together.

Measuring a Rectal Temperature

Purpose: Accurately measure and record a rectal temperature using a glass mercury thermometer.

Equipment: Glass mercury rectal thermometer; tissues or cotton balls; disposable plastic sheath; surgical lubricant; biohazard container; cool, soapy water; disinfectant solution; gloves.

Standard: This procedure should take 5 minutes.

Steps	Reason
1. Wash your hands and assemble the necessary supplies.	Handwashing aids infection control.
2. Dry the thermometer if it has been stored in a disinfectant solution by wiping it from the bulb up the stem with a tissue or cotton ball.	Removing the wet disinfectant allows the thermometer to slip easily into the sheath.
3. Carefully check the thermometer for chips or cracks.	A chipped or cracked thermometer may injure the patient.
4. Check the reading in the thermometer by holding the stem horizontally at eye level and turning it slowly to see the mercury column.	It is easiest to see the mercury in the column in this position.
5. If the reading is above 94°F, shake down the thermometer by securely grasping it at the end of the stem with your thumb and forefinger and snapping your wrist several times. Avoid hitting the thermometer against anything while snapping your wrist.	The mercury must begin below 94°F to get an accurate temperature reading.
6. Insert the thermometer into the plastic sheath.	Follow the package instructions.
7. Spread lubricant onto a tissue and then from the tissue onto the sheath of the thermometer.	When using a tube of lubricant, avoid cross-contamination by not applying lubricant directly to the thermometer. A lubricant should always be used for rectal insertion to prevent patient discomfort.
8. Greet and identify the patient and explain the procedure.	

Step 9. The patient in a side-lying position draped appropriately. (Reprinted with permission from LifeART. Philadelphia: Lippincott Williams & Wilkins, 2004.)

Procedure 21-4 *(continued)*

Measuring a Rectal Temperature

Steps	Reason
9. Ensure the patient's privacy by placing the patient in a side-lying position facing the examination room door and draping appropriately.	If the examination room door is opened, a patient facing the door is less likely to be exposed. The side-lying position facilitates exposure of the anus.
10. Apply gloves and visualize the anus by lifting the top buttock with your nondominant hand.	Never insert the thermometer without first having a clear view of the anus.
11. Gently insert the thermometer past the sphincter muscle about 1.5 inches for an adult, 1 inch for a child, and 0.5 inch for an infant.	Inserting the thermometer at these depths helps prevent perforating the anal canal.
12. Release the upper buttock and hold the thermometer in place with your dominant hand for 3 minutes. Replace the drape without moving the dominant hand.	The thermometer will not stay in place if it is not held. Replacing the drape will ensure the patient's privacy.
13. After 3 minutes, remove the thermometer and sheath. Discard the sheath into a biohazard container.	The lubricant or sheath may obscure the mercury column and should be removed before you read the thermometer.
14. Note the reading with the thermometer horizontal at eye level.	
15. Give the patient a tissue to wipe away excess lubricant and assist with dressing if necessary.	
16. Sanitize and disinfect the thermometer according to the office policy.	
17. Remove your gloves and wash your hands.	This prevents the spread of microorganisms.
18. Record the procedure and mark the letter R next to the reading, indicating that the temperature was taken rectally.	Temperatures are presumed to have been taken orally unless otherwise noted in the medical record. The vital signs (temperature, pulse, respirations, and blood pressure) are usually recorded together.

Note: Infants and very small children may be held in your lap or over your knees for this procedure. Hold the thermometer and the buttocks with your dominant hand while securing the child with your nondominant hand. If the child moves, the thermometer and your hand will move together, avoiding injury to the anal canal.

Charting Example

09/11/2005 8:30 A.M. T 100.2° (R) _____ J. Barth, CMA

Measuring an Axillary Temperature

Purpose:	Accurately measure and record an axillary temperature using a glass mercury thermometer.
Equipment:	Glass mercury (oral or rectal) thermometer; tissues or cotton balls; disposable plastic sheath; biohazard container; cool, soapy water; disinfectant solution.
Standard:	This procedure should take 15 minutes.

Steps	Reason
1. Wash your hands and assemble the necessary supplies.	Handwashing aids infection control.
2. Dry the thermometer if it has been stored in a disinfectant solution by wiping it from the bulb up the stem with a tissue or cotton ball.	Removing the wet disinfectant allows the thermometer to slip easily into the sheath.
3. Carefully check the thermometer for chips or cracks.	A chipped or cracked thermometer may injure the patient.
4. Check the reading in the thermometer by holding the stem horizontally at eye level and turning it slowly to see the mercury column.	It is easiest to see the mercury in the column in this position.
5. If the reading is above 94°F, shake down the thermometer by securely grasping it at the end of the stem with your thumb and forefinger and snapping your wrist several times. Avoid hitting the thermometer against anything while snapping your wrist.	The mercury must begin below 94°F to get an accurate temperature reading.
6. Insert the thermometer into the plastic sheath.	Follow the package instructions.
7. Expose the patient's axilla without exposing more of the chest or upper body than is necessary.	The patient's privacy must be protected at all times.
8. Place the bulb of the thermometer deep in the axilla and bring the patient's arm down, crossing the forearm over the chest. Drape the patient as appropriate for privacy.	This position offers the best skin contact with the thermometer and maintains a closed environment.

Step 8. With the thermometer in the axilla, the arm should be down and the forearm should be crossed across the chest.

(continues)

Procedure 21-5 *(continued)*

Measuring an Axillary Temperature

Steps	Reason
9. Leave the thermometer in place for 10 minutes.	Axillary temperatures take longer than oral or rectal ones. Since the thermometer is secure in the axilla, it is not necessary to hold it in place unless the patient does not understand to leave the arm down.
10. At the appropriate time, remove the thermometer from the patient's axilla and remove the sheath by holding the very edge of the sheath with your thumb and forefinger, pulling down from the open edge over the length of the thermometer to the bulb. Discard the sheath into a biohazard container.	
11. Hold the thermometer horizontal at eye level and note the level of mercury that has risen into the column.	
12. Sanitize and disinfect the thermometer according to the office policy.	
13. Wash your hands.	This prevents the spread of microorganisms.
14. Record the procedure and mark a letter A next to the reading, indicating that the reading is axillary.	Temperatures are presumed to have been taken orally unless otherwise noted in the medical record. The vital signs (temperature, pulse, respirations, and blood pressure) are usually recorded together.

Charting Example
02/01/2005 3:45 P.M. T 97.8°F (A) _____ B. DeMarcus, CMA

Procedure 21-6

Measuring Temperature Using an Electronic Thermometer

Purpose: Accurately measure and record a patient's temperature using an electronic thermometer.

Equipment: Electronic thermometer with oral or rectal probe, lubricant and gloves for rectal temperatures, disposable probe cover, biohazard container.

Standard: This task should take 5 minutes.

Steps	Reason
1. Wash your hands and assemble the necessary supplies.	Handwashing aids infection control.
2. Greet and identify the patient and explain the procedure.	Identifying the patient prevents errors.
3. Choose the most appropriate method (oral, axillary, or rectal) and attach the appropriate probe to the battery-powered unit.	
4. Insert the probe into a probe cover. Covers are usually carried with the unit in a specially fitted box attached to the back of the unit.	All probes fit into one size probe cover. If using the last probe cover, be sure to attach a new box of covers to the unit to be ready for the next patient.
5. Position the thermometer appropriately for the method.	If measuring the temperature rectally, be sure to apply lubricant to the probe cover and hold the probe in place.
6. Wait for the electronic unit to beep when it senses no signs of the temperature rising further. This usually occurs within 20 to 30 seconds.	
7. After the beep, remove the probe and note the reading on the digital display screen on the unit.	
8. Discard the probe cover in a biohazard container by depressing a button, usually on the end of the probe. Most units automatically shut off when the probe is reinserted into the unit.	Always note the temperature reading before replacing the probe in the slot on the unit.
9. Remove your gloves if any, wash your hands, and record the procedure.	Record the temperature exactly as if taken with a glass mercury thermometer. Be sure to indicate a rectal or axillary reading by recording an R or A next to the reading in the documentation. The vital signs (temperature, pulse, respirations, and blood pressure) are usually recorded together.
10. Return the unit and probe to the charging base.	Although the unit is battery powered, it should be kept in the charging base so that the battery is always adequately charged.

Charting Example
11/28/2005 10:15 A.M. T 101°(O) _____ D. Snap, CMA

Procedure 21-7

Measuring Temperature Using a Tympanic Thermometer

Purpose: Accurately measure and record a patient's temperature using a tympanic thermometer.

Equipment: Tympanic thermometer, disposable probe covers, biohazard container.

Standard: This task should take 5 minutes.

Steps	Reason
1. Wash your hands and assemble the necessary supplies.	Handwashing aids infection control.
2. Greet and identify the patient and explain the procedure.	Identifying the patient prevents errors.
3. Insert the ear probe into a probe cover.	Always put a clean probe cover on the ear probe before inserting it.
4. Place the end of the ear probe in the patient's ear canal with your dominant hand while straightening out the ear canal with your nondominant hand.	Straighten the ear canal of most patients by pulling the top posterior part of the outer ear up and back. For children under 3 years of age, pull the outer ear down and back.
5. With the ear probe properly placed in the ear canal, press the button on the thermometer. The reading will be displayed on the digital display screen in about 2 seconds.	
6. Remove the probe and note the reading. Discard the probe cover in a biohazard container.	The probe covers are for one use only.
7. Wash your hands and record the procedure.	Record the temperature as if using a glass mercury thermometer. Be sure to indicate that the tympanic temperature was taken. The vital signs (temperature, pulse, respirations, and blood pressure) are usually recorded together.
8. Return the unit and probe to the charging base.	The unit should be kept in the charging base so that the battery is always adequately charged.

Charting Example

04/13/2005 2:00 P.M. T 99.4°tympanic _____ M. Smythe, CMA

Procedure 21-8

Measuring the Radial Pulse

Purpose: Accurately measure and record a patient's radial pulse.

Equipment: A watch with a sweep second hand.

Standard: This procedure should take 3 to 5 minutes.

Steps	Reason
1. Wash your hands.	Handwashing aids infection control.
2. Greet and identify the patient and explain the procedure.	In most cases, the pulse is taken at the same time as the other vital signs.
3. Position the patient with the arm relaxed and supported either on the lap of the patient or on a table.	If the arm is not supported or the patient is uncomfortable, the pulse may be difficult to find and the count may be affected.
4. With the index, middle, and ring fingers of your dominant hand, press with your fingertips firmly enough to feel the pulse but gently enough not to obliterate it.	Do not use your thumb; it has a pulse of its own that may be confused with the patient's. You may place your thumb on the opposite side of the patient's wrist to steady your hand.
5. If the pulse is regular, count it for 30 seconds, watching the second hand of your watch. Multiply the number of pulsations by 2, since the pulse is always recorded as beats per minute. If the pulse is irregular, count it for a full 60 seconds.	Counting an irregular pulse for less than 60 seconds may give an inaccurate measurement.
6. Record the rate in the patient's medical record with the other vital signs. Also, note the rhythm if irregular and the volume if thready or bounding.	Procedures are considered not to have been done if they are not recorded. The vital signs (temperature, pulse, respirations, and blood pressure) are usually recorded together.

Charting Example

06/12/2005 11:30 A.M. Pulse 78 and irregular _____ E. Kramer, CMA

Procedure 21-9

Measuring Respirations

Purpose: Accurately measure and record a patient's respirations.

Equipment: A watch with a sweeping second hand.

Standard: This procedure should take 3 to 5 minutes.

Steps	Reason
1. Wash your hands	Handwashing aids infection control.
2. Greet and identify the patient and explain the procedure.	In most cases, the respirations are counted at the same time as the other pulse.
3. After counting the radial pulse and still watching your second hand, count a complete rise and fall of the chest as one respiration. *Note:* Some patients have abdominal movement rather than chest movement during respirations. Observe carefully for the easiest area to assess for the most accurate reading.	A patient who is aware that you are observing respirations may alter the breathing pattern. It is best to begin counting respirations immediately after counting the pulse without informing the patient.
4. If the breathing pattern is regular, count the respiratory rate for 30 seconds and multiply by 2. If the pattern is irregular, count for a full 60 seconds.	Counting an irregular respiratory pattern for less than 60 seconds may give an inaccurate measurement.
5. Record the respiratory rate in the patient's medical record with the other vital signs. Also, note the rhythm if irregular along with any unusual or abnormal sounds, such as wheezing.	Procedures are considered not to have been done if they are not recorded. The vital signs (temperature, pulse, respirations, and blood pressure) are usually recorded together.

Charting Example

09/15/2005 8:45 A.M. Resp 16 _____ J. Thompson, CMA

Procedure 21-10

Measuring Blood Pressure

Purpose:	Accurately measure and record a patient's blood pressure.
Equipment:	Sphygmomanometer, Stethoscope
Standard:	This procedure should take 5 minutes.

Steps	Purpose
1. Wash your hands and assemble your equipment.	Handwashing aids infection control.
2. Greet and identify the patient and explain the procedure.	Identifying the patient prevents errors, and explaining the procedure eases anxiety.
3. Position the patient with the arm to be used supported with the forearm on the lap or a table and slightly flexed, with the palm upward. The upper arm should be level with the patient's heart.	Positioning the arm with the palm upward facilitates finding and palpating the brachial artery. If the upper arm is higher or lower than the heart, an inaccurate reading may result.
4. Expose the patient's arm.	Any clothing over the area may obscure the sounds. If the sleeve is pulled up, it may become tight and act as a tourniquet, decreasing the flow of blood and causing an inaccurate blood pressure reading.
5. Palpate the brachial pulse in the antecubital area and center the deflated cuff directly over the brachial artery. The lower edge of the cuff should be 1 to 2 inches above the antecubital area.	If the cuff is placed too low, it may interfere with the placement of the stethoscope and cause noises that obscure the Korotkoff sounds.
6. Wrap the cuff smoothly and snugly around the arm and secure with the Velcro edges.	
7. With the air pump in your dominant hand and the valve between your thumb and forefinger, turn the screw clockwise to tighten. Do not tighten it to the point that it will be difficult to release.	The cuff will not inflate with the valve open. If the valve is too tightly closed, it will be difficult to loosen with one hand after the cuff is inflated.

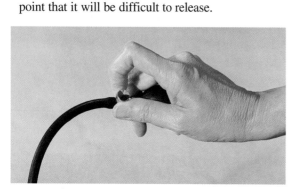

Step 7. Holding the bulb and the screw valve properly allows you to inflate and deflate the cuff easily.

(continues)

Procedure 21-10 *(continued)*

Measuring Blood Pressure

Steps	Reason
8. While palpating the brachial pulse with your nondominant hand, inflate the cuff and note the point or number on the dial or mercury column at which you no longer feel the brachial pulse.	The dial or mercury column should be at eye level. Noting this number gives you a reference point for reinflating the cuff when taking the blood pressure.

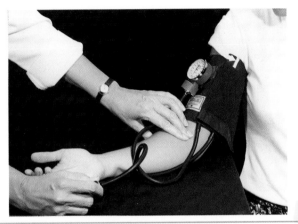

Step 8. Palpate the brachial pulse before auscultating the blood pressure.

Steps	Reason
9. Deflate the cuff by turning the valve counterclockwise. Wait at least 30 seconds before reinflating the cuff.	Always wait at least 30 seconds after deflating the cuff to allow circulation to return to the extremity.
10. Place the stethoscope earpieces in your ears with the openings pointed slightly forward. Stand about 3 feet from the manometer with the gauge at eye level. The stethoscope tubing should hang freely without touching or rubbing against any part of the cuff.	With the earpieces pointing forward in the ears, the openings follow the natural opening of the ear canal. The manometer should be at eye level to decrease any chance of error when it is read. If the stethoscope rubs against other objects, environmental sounds may obscure the Korotkoff sounds.
11. Place the diaphragm of the stethoscope against the brachial artery and hold it in place with your nondominant hand without pressing too hard.	If not pressed firmly enough, you may not hear the sounds. Pressing too firmly may obliterate the pulse.

Step 11. Hold the stethoscope diaphragm firmly against the brachial artery.

(continues)

Procedure 21-10 *(continued)*

Measuring Blood Pressure

Steps	Reason
12. With your dominant hand, turn the screw on the valve just enough to close the valve; inflate the cuff. Pump the valve bulb to about 30 mm Hg above the number noted during step 8.	Inflating more than 30 mm Hg above baseline is uncomfortable for the patient and unnecessary; inflating less may produce an inaccurate systolic reading.
13. Once the cuff is appropriately inflated, turn the valve counterclockwise to release the air at about 2 to 4 mm Hg per second.	Releasing the air too fast will cause missed beats, and releasing it too slowly will interfere with circulation.
14. Listening carefully, note the point on the gauge at which you hear the first clear tapping sound. This is the systolic sound, or Korotkoff I.	Aneroid and mercury measurements are always made as even numbers because of the way the manometer is calibrated.

Step 14A. The meniscus on the mercury column in this example reads 120 mm Hg.

Step 14B. The gauge on the aneroid manometer reads 80 mm Hg.

15. Maintaining control of the valve screw, continue to listen and deflate the cuff. When you hear the last sound, note the reading and quickly deflate the cuff. *Note:* Never immediately reinflate the cuff if you are unsure of the reading. Totally deflate the cuff and wait 1 to 2 minutes before repeating the procedure.	The last sound heard is Korotkoff V and is recorded as the bottom number or diastolic blood pressure.
16. Remove the cuff and press the air from the bladder of the cuff.	

(continues)

Procedure 21-10 *(continued)*

Measuring Blood Pressure

Steps	Reason
17. If this is the first recording or a new patient, the physician may also want a reading in the other arm or in another position.	Blood pressure varies in some patients between the arms or in different positions such as lying or standing.
18. Put the equipment away and wash your hands.	
19. Record the reading with the systolic over the diastolic, noting which arm was used (120/80 LA). Also record the patient's position if other than sitting.	Procedures are considered not done if they are not recorded. The vital signs (temperature, pulse, respirations, and blood pressure) are usually recorded together.

Charting Example
11/08/2005 3:30 P.M. T 98.6°O, P 78, R 16, BP 130/90 (LA) sitting, 110/78 (LA) standing _____Y. Torres, CMA

CHAPTER SUMMARY

Anthropometric measurements include height and weight. Vital signs include temperature (T), pulse (P), respirations (R), and blood pressure (BP). When a patient first visits the medical office, these measurements are recorded as a baseline and used as a comparison for data collected at subsequent visits. These measurements, which provide important data for the physician to use in diagnosing and treating illnesses, are very frequently performed by medical assistants.

Critical Thinking Challenges

1. You are asked to teach a patient, Mr. Stone, how to take his blood pressure at home once in the morning and once at night and record these readings for 1 month. Create a brochure for patients that explains the procedure in understandable terms and design a sheet that Mr. Stone can use easily to record these readings.
2. Ms. Black arrived late for her appointment, frantic and explaining that she had car trouble on the way to the office, could not find a parking place, and just locked her keys inside her car. How do you expect these events to affect her vital signs? Explain why.
3. What size cuff do you choose for Mrs. Cooper, an elderly woman who is 5 feet 3 inches tall and weighs approximately 90 pounds? Why?
4. An elderly woman with osteoporosis requests that her height be taken and recorded today, since she "feels shorter." Do you explain that the office policy requires measuring height only at the first visit and give her the previously recorded measurements, or do you comply with her request?

Answers to Checkpoint Questions

1. Accurately measuring vital signs assists the physician in diagnosing and treating various disorders.
2. Rectal temperature measurements are usually 1° higher than oral measurements because of the vascularity and tightly closed environment of the rectum.
3. A child's body temperature may be slightly higher than an adult's because of the faster metabolism in a child.
4. Tympanic thermometers measure the temperature of the blood in the eardrum. The ear canal is a closed environment with the probe in place, providing a rapid, noninvasive, and accurate reading when performed correctly.
5. Measuring a patient's pulse entails assessing and recording the rate (number of heartbeats in 1 minute), rhythm (regular or irregular), and volume (thready, bounding).
6. Contraction of the diaphragm causes negative pressure in the lungs, which respond by filling with inhaled air.
7. During systole, the heart contracts and forces blood out and through the arteries. In diastole, the heart relaxes and fills with blood.
8. The pulse pressure is the difference between the systolic and diastolic blood pressures, and the auscultatory gap is an abrupt but temporary end to the tapping sound heard when auscultating the blood pressure.

 Websites

National Reye's Syndrome Foundation
    www.reyessyndrome.org
American Society of Hypertension www.ash-us.org
American Lung Association www.lungusa.org

22

Assisting With the Physical Examination

CHAPTER OUTLINE

ROLE DELINEATION

ADMINISTRATIVE: ADMINISTRATIVE PROCEDURES
- Perform basic administrative medical assisting functions

CLINICAL: FUNDAMENTAL PRINCIPLES
- Apply principles of aseptic technique and infection control
- Comply with quality assurance practices

CLINICAL: PATIENT CARE
- Obtain patient's history and vital signs
- Prepare and maintain examination and treatment areas
- Prepare patient for examinations, procedures, and treatments
- Assist with examinations, procedures, and treatments
- Coordinate patient care information with other health care providers

GENERAL: PROFESSIONALISM
- Display a professional manner and image
- Demonstrate initiative and responsibility
- Work as a member of the health care team
- Set priorities and perform multiple tasks
- Treat all patients with compassion and empathy

GENERAL: COMMUNICATION SKILLS
- Recognize and respect cultural diversity
- Adapt communications to individual's ability to understand
- Recognize and respond effectively to verbal, nonverbal, and written communications
- Serve as a liaison

GENERAL: LEGAL CONCEPTS
- Perform within legal and ethical boundaries
- Prepare and maintain medical records
- Document accurately
- Implement and maintain federal and state health care legislation and regulations

GENERAL: INSTRUCTION
- Instruct individuals according to their needs
- Explain office policies and procedures
- Teach methods of health promotion and disease prevention

CHAPTER COMPETENCIES

LEARNING OBJECTIVES
Upon successfully completing this chapter, you will be able to:
1. Spell and define key terms.
2. Identify and state the use of the basic and specialized instruments and supplies used in the physical examination.
3. Describe the four methods used to examine the patient.
4. List the basic sequence of the physical examination.
5. State your responsibilities before, during, and after the physical examination.

PERFORMANCE OBJECTIVES
Upon successfully completing this chapter, you will be able to:
1. Assist the physician with a patient's physical examination (Procedure 22-1).

KEY TERMS

applicator	diagnosis	nasal septum	range of motion (ROM)
asymmetry	extraocular	occult	rectovaginal
auscultation	gait	palpation	sclera
Babinski reflex	hernia	Papanicolaou (Pap) test or	speculum
baseline	inguinal	smear	symmetry
bimanual	inspection	percussion	transillumination
bruit	lubricant	peripheral	tympanic membrane
cerumen	manipulation	PERRLA	

THE PURPOSE of the complete physical examination is to assess the patient's general state of health and detect signs and symptoms of disease. New patients usually receive a complete physical examination, which gives the physician **baseline** information about the patient. This baseline information is valuable for future comparison and can aid the physician in **diagnosis** (identifying a disease or condition). Routine examinations are performed thereafter at regular intervals to help maintain the patient's health and prevent disease.

The three basic components of patient assessment are the medical history, the physical examination, and any laboratory and diagnostic tests requested by the physician. Once the data from these three components are collected and evaluated, the physician will make a judgment about the patient's condition and devise a plan of care. As a medical assistant, you are responsible for assisting with taking the medical history, preparing the patient for the examination, and assisting the physician during the examination. In addition, you may collect specimens for diagnostic testing. During the examination, you must anticipate the needs of the physician and patient and be prepared to assist as necessary.

BASIC INSTRUMENTS AND SUPPLIES

Instruments used during the physical examination enable the examiner to see, hear, or feel areas of the body being assessed. In most cases, it is the physician who uses these instruments, but you must be familiar with instruments and supplies. These instruments should be kept in a special

FIGURE 22-1. Common supplies used in the adult physical examination: tape measure, gloves, tongue depressors, and cotton-tipped applicators.

FIGURE 22-2. A reflex hammer.

tray or drawer in a convenient location in each examination room. The exact equipment used varies among medical offices according to physicians' preferences and the specialty. Supplies that should be available in the examination room include a tape measure, gloves, tongue depressors, and cotton-tipped **applicators** (FIG. 22-1). The purpose of the most common instruments used in the physical examination are described in the following sections.

Percussion Hammer

The percussion hammer is used to test neurologic reflexes. Also called a reflex hammer, this instrument has a stainless steel handle and a hard rubber head (FIG. 22-2). The head is used to test reflexes by striking the tendons of the ankle, knee, wrist, and elbow. The tip of the handle may be used to stroke the sole of the foot to assess **Babinski's reflex**. Some hammers have a brush and needle in the handle specifically used to test sensory perception.

Tuning Fork

The tuning fork is used to test hearing. It is a stainless steel instrument with a handle at one end and two prongs at the other end (FIG. 22-3). The examiner strikes the prongs

FIGURE 22-3. A tuning fork.

FIGURE 22-4. A nasal speculum. (Courtesy of Katena Products, Denville, NJ.)

against his or her hand, which causes them to vibrate and produce a humming sound. While vibrating, the handle is placed against a bony area of the skull near one of the ears and the patient is asked to describe what, if anything, is heard in that ear. Depending upon the results of this hearing test, the physician may order additional auditory tests.

Nasal Speculum

The nasal speculum is a stainless steel instrument that is inserted into the nostril to assist in the visual inspection of the lining of the nose, nasal membranes, and septum. The tip of the instrument is inserted into the nose and the handles squeezed, opening the end and allowing for visualization (FIG. 22-4). Nasal specula are also available in a disposable form.

Otoscope and Audioscope

The otoscope permits visualization of the ear canal and tympanic membrane. The **tympanic membrane**, or eardrum, is a thin, oval membrane between the outer and middle ear that transmits sound vibrations to the inner ear. The otoscope has a stainless steel handle at one end and a head with a light, a magnifying lens, and a cone-shaped hollow speculum at the other end. A portable otoscope has batteries in the handle to operate the light in the head; other otoscopes are part of a unit attached to the wall and plugged into an electrical outlet (FIG. 22-5). In both types, the hollow speculum is covered with a disposable speculum cover before it is placed in the ear canal. An otoscope with a specialized nasal speculum tip may be used to examine the nose.

The audioscope is used to screen patients for hearing loss. Although it looks like an otoscope, the audioscope's handle has a variety of indicators and selection buttons that can be used to adjust its tones. The examiner places the tip of the audioscope in the patient's ear and asks the patient to respond to each of the tones that is produced. The results are recorded in the patient's medical record.

Ophthalmoscope

The ophthalmoscope is used to examine the interior structures of the eyes. Like the otoscope, it may have a stainless steel handle that contains batteries or may be mounted on the wall (FIG. 22-6). The head of the ophthalmoscope also has a light source, magnifying lens, and opening through which to view the eye. Portable units may have

A

B

FIGURE 22-5. (A) A portable otoscope. (Reprinted with permission from Taylor C, Lillis C, LeMone P. Fundamentals of Nursing: The Art and Science of Nursing Care, 4th ed. Philadelphia: Lippincott Williams & Wilkins, 2001.) (B) Wall-mounted examination instruments. From left: sphygmomanometer with cuff, ophthalmoscope, otoscope, and dispenser for disposable otoscope speculum covers. (Courtesy of Welch Allyn, Skaneatels Falls, NY.)

FIGURE 22-6. A portable ophthalmoscope. (Reprinted with permission from Taylor C, Lillis C, LeMone P. Fundamentals of Nursing: The Art and Science of Nursing Care, 4th ed. Philadelphia: Lippincott Williams & Wilkins, 2001.)

a common base handle with various otoscope or ophthalmoscope tips that can be attached for different examinations.

Examination Light and Gooseneck Lamp

Some offices are equipped with an adjustable overhead examination light for better visualization during the examination. The gooseneck lamp is a floor lamp with a movable stand that bends at the neck for use when the overhead lighting is not adequate (FIG. 22-7). You have the responsibility to make sure all examination lights are in proper working order and to direct the light toward the area of the body as indicated by the physician.

FIGURE 22-8. A stethoscope. (Reprinted with permission from Nettina SM. The Lippincott Manual of Nursing Practice, 7th ed. Philadelphia: Lippincott Williams & Wilkins, 2001.)

Stethoscope

The stethoscope is used for listening to body sounds. The bell or diaphragm is at one end and is placed on the patient's body. This end is connected to two earpieces by flexible rubber or vinyl tubing (FIG. 22-8). The two earpieces have plastic or rubber tips that must be adjusted and directed outward before being placed in the examiner's ears. The stethoscope is used to listen to the sounds of the heart, lungs, and intestines. It is also used for taking blood pressure.

Penlight or Flashlight

A penlight or flashlight provides additional light to a specific area during the examination. The penlight is the shape and size of a ballpoint pen and is easily carried in the examiner's pocket (FIG. 22-9). A common flashlight may be used if a penlight is not available. The penlight is often used to examine the eyes, nose, and throat.

FIGURE 22-7. An examination light.

FIGURE 22-9. A penlight.

Checkpoint Question

1. Which instruments are used to test the ears and hearing?

INSTRUMENTS AND SUPPLIES USED IN SPECIALIZED EXAMINATIONS

In addition to the basic instruments described previously, specialized equipment may be used during the physical examination. This chapter introduces the specialized examinations and equipment. A more detailed description of specialty examinations is provided in **Unit 2**.

Head Light or Mirror

An ear, nose, and throat specialist (otorhinolaryngologist) may wear a headlight or head mirror during the examination of these structures. This instrument consists of a light or mirror attached to a headband that fits over the examiner's head (FIG. 22-10). A head light provides direct light on the area being examined; the mirror reflects light from the examination light into the area.

Laryngeal Mirror and Laryngoscope

The laryngeal mirror is a stainless steel instrument with a long, slender handle and a small, round mirror (FIG. 22-11). It is used to examine areas of the patient's throat and larynx that may not be directly visible.

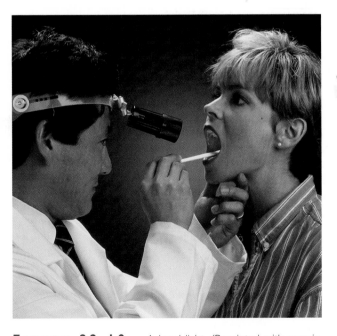

FIGURE 22-10. A head light. (Reprinted with permission from Willis MC. Medical Terminology: A Programmed Learning Approach to the Language of Health Care. Baltimore: Lippincott Williams & Wilkins, 2002.)

FIGURE 22-11. A laryngeal mirror. (Reprinted with permission from Anatomical Chart Company.)

The laryngoscope handle is similar to the battery handle of an otoscope or ophthalmoscope, but the head allows attachment of curved or straight laryngoscope stainless steel blades and a small light source (FIG. 22-12). The examiner places the blade in the patient's throat to visualize the larynx or vocal cords, which cannot be seen by simply looking down the patient's throat.

Vaginal Speculum

The general physical examination of female patients may include a pelvic examination and **Papanicolaou** (Pap) smear. This is a simple test in which cells obtained from the cervix or vagina are examined microscopically for abnormalities including cancer. To obtain the cells for a Pap smear, or to visually examine internal female reproductive structures,

FIGURE 22-12. A laryngoscope handle and blades (straight and curved).

FIGURE 22-13. Vaginal specula.

the vaginal speculum is inserted into the vagina to expand the opening (FIG. 22-13). This instrument is made of stainless steel or disposable plastic.

To obtain vaginal or cervical cells, the physician may use the Ayre spatula or cervical scraper (FIG. 22-14). This scraper is about 6 inches long and made of plastic or wood. One tip has an irregular shape that is placed in the cervical opening and rotated to collect the specimen; the other end is rounded and may be used to collect cells from the vaginal cul-de-sac. A histobrush may also be used to obtain cells for a Pap smear; it is made of nylon or plastic with soft bristles at one end. The collected cells are transferred to either a glass slide or a liquid preservative and sent to a

FIGURE 22-14. Cotton-tipped applicator (*left*), Ayre spatula (*center*), and histobrush (*right*). Cotton-tipped applicators of this size are frequently used to remove excess vaginal secretions or to apply medications during the gynecological examination.

WHAT IF

The physician is performing a genital and pelvic examination of a disabled female patient and she cannot assume the lithotomy position?

Both genital and rectal examinations may be performed in the dorsal recumbent or Sims position for patients (such as the elderly or disabled) who cannot comfortably assume the usual positions, including the lithotomy position.

laboratory for analysis. Chapter 38 has additional information about the gynecological examination and the role of the medical assistant.

Lubricant

Lubricant is a water-soluble gel used to reduce friction and provide easy insertion of an instrument in the physical examination. After cells are obtained for a Pap smear, lubricant may also be used for a **bimanual** examination, in which one gloved, lubricated hand is inserted into the vagina while the other hand is placed on the abdomen. This examination allows the examiner to palpate internal structures of the pelvic cavity. Lubricant may also be used for rectal examinations.

Anoscope, Proctoscope, and Sigmoidoscope

The instruments used for examination of the rectum and colon vary in length as appropriate for the structure to be examined. The anoscope is a short stainless steel or plastic speculum that is inserted into the rectum to inspect the anal canal. An obturator with a rounded tip extends beyond the anoscope to allow the instrument to be easily inserted into the rectum (FIG. 22-15). After the anoscope is inserted, the obturator is removed for visualization of the internal lining of the rectum.

FIGURE 22-15. The anoscope with the obturator. (Courtesy of Welch Allyn.)

FIGURE 22-16. A flexible sigmoidoscope. (Courtesy of Olympus.)

The proctoscope is another type of speculum that is used to visualize the rectum and the anus. It is longer than the anoscope and allows the examiner to inspect more areas of the rectum. While it also consists of an obturator that is removed after the instrument is inserted, a fiberoptic light handle and magnifying lens are attached. The tubular part of the scope is marked in centimeters so that the depth of abnormalities in the anal canal can be noted.

A longer instrument used to visualize the rectum and the sigmoid colon is the sigmoidoscope. This instrument consists of a tube with an obturator, fiberoptic light handle, and magnifying lens (FIG. 22-16). It may be rigid and made of stainless steel, or it may be flexible. The advantages of the flexible sigmoidoscope include a smaller diameter, greater depth during the examination, better visualization of the intestinal mucosa, and less discomfort for the patient.

During all rectal examinations, you need a suction machine, cotton-tipped applicators, glass microscope slides, specimen containers, and laboratory request slips available. Tissue or stool specimens obtained during any rectal procedure must be properly preserved and protected for transport to the laboratory for analysis. More information regarding examinations of the colon is found in Chapter 34.

 Checkpoint Question

2. What are the uses of the anoscope, proctoscope, and sigmoidoscope? What is the function of an obturator?

EXAMINATION TECHNIQUES

While performing the physical examination, the physician uses four basic techniques to gather information. These include **inspection**, **palpation**, **percussion**, and **auscultation**. Each technique is described in more detail in the following sections.

Inspection

Inspection is looking at areas of the body to observe physical features. The examiner inspects the patient's general appearance, including movements, skin and membrane color, contour, and **symmetry** or **asymmetry**, which is equality or inequality in size and shape. Inspection is done both with the naked eye and with instruments, using either room lighting or a special light source. In some cases, inspection includes use of the sense of smell to note any unusual odors of the breath (such as a fruity smell in a diabetic patient) or foul odors from infected wounds or lesions.

Palpation

Palpation is touching or moving body areas with the fingers or hands. The examiner palpates the body to determine pulse characteristics and the presence of growths, swelling, tenderness, or pain. Organs can be palpated to assess their size, shape, and location. Skin temperature, mois-

Spanish Terminology

Voy a examinarle.	I am going to examine you.
Voy a reviser sus orejas.	I am going to check your ears.
Voy a reviser su boca.	I am going to check your nose.
Saque la lengua.	Stick out your tongue.
Voy a reviser su piel.	I am going to examine your skin.
Voy a reviser su abdomen (vientre).	I am going to examine your abdomen.
Voy a reviser su espalda.	I am going to examine your back.

ture, texture, and elasticity may also be assessed by palpation. Palpation performed with both hands is called bimanual palpation; if the fingers are used, it is called a digital examination. **Manipulation** is the passive movement of the joints to determine the extent of movement or **range of motion**.

Percussion

Percussion is tapping or striking the body with the hand or an instrument to produce sounds. Direct percussion is performed by striking the body with a finger. Indirect percussion is done by placing a finger on the area and then striking this finger with a finger of the other hand while listening to the sounds and feeling the vibrations. This allows the examiner to determine the position, size, and density of air or fluid within a body cavity or organ.

Auscultation

Auscultation is listening to the sounds of the body. This examination method uses a stethoscope or the ear placed directly on the patient's body. Areas of the body that can be auscultated include the heart, lungs, abdomen, and blood vessels. In the abdominal examination, auscultation is performed before palpation and percussion, which can affect normal bowel sounds.

Checkpoint Question

3. Which of the examination techniques requires the use of the hands and fingers to feel organs or structures?

RESPONSIBILITIES OF THE MEDICAL ASSISTANT

Room Preparation

Medical assistants are usually responsible for preparing the examination rooms, equipment, and supplies in the clinical area. The examination room should be clean, well lighted, well ventilated, and at a comfortable temperature for the patient. The examination table is decontaminated with an appropriate disinfectant between patients, and the paper on the table is removed and replaced with clean paper. At the beginning of each day, you are responsible for checking each examination room for adequate supplies and equipment, including the working condition of equipment. Batteries in otoscopes, ophthalmoscopes, and laryngoscopes are to be checked daily and replaced as needed.

Patient Preparation

Once the examination room is ready, you will call the patient back by name from the waiting room and escort him or her to the treatment room. It is important that you develop rap-

port with your patients and practice good interpersonal skills. This helps put your patients at ease and increases their confidence in you and the physician. Your goal is to create a positive, supportive, caring, and friendly atmosphere. Treat each patient as an individual and speak clearly with a confident tone of voice as you explain any procedures.

Before the physician sees the patient, it may be your responsibility to obtain and record the patient's history, chief complaint, and vital signs. If a urine specimen is needed, explain how to obtain the specimen, direct the patient to the bathroom, and explain what to do with the specimen.

Once in the examination room, give the patient instructions for disrobing and putting on the examination gown. Depending on the type of examination to be performed, the patient may wear the gown with the opening in the front or in the back. Leave the room while the patient undresses unless the patient needs help. Then ask the patient to sit on the examination table, helping if needed, and cover the legs with a drape. Place the chart outside the examining room door and notify the physician that the patient is ready.

Assisting the Physician

During the physical examination, you may assist the physician by handing him or her instruments or supplies and directing the light appropriately. For legal reasons, you may be required to remain in the room when a male examiner examines a female patient or when a female examiner examines a male patient. Procedure 22-1 describes the steps for assisting the physician with the physical examination.

Depending on the examination and the physical condition of the patient, you may also assist the patient into

TRIAGE

While working in a family practice, you have to complete these three tasks:

A. A patient was just discharged and the examination room has to be restocked and cleaned.

B. The physician states that she is ready to perform a gynecological examination and needs your assistance.

C. A suture tray has to be set up for a 3-year-old with a facial laceration.

How do you sort these tasks? What do you do first? Second? Third?

First assist the physician with the examination. When possible, limit the waiting time for female patients to have their gynecological examination. Next, set up the suture tray. Third, clean and restock the examination room.

appropriate positions and adjust the drape to expose only the body area being examined (FIG. 22-17). Be supportive and offer reassurance to the patient during the examination. Always assess the patient's facial expression and level of anxiety by noting verbal and nonverbal behavior during the examination. TABLE 22-1 lists standard examination positions, the body parts usually examined in these positions, and the instruments needed by the physician for these examinations.

Postexamination Duties

After the physical examination, you should perform any follow-up treatments and procedures as necessary or as ordered by the physician. Always offer the patient help returning to a sitting position after the examination. Ask the patient to

dress, and leave the room unless the patient needs your assistance. Tell the patient what to do after getting dressed. In many offices, the patient gets dressed and remains in the examining room until the medical assistant gives further instructions; in other offices, patients are told to go to the front desk to schedule future appointments or receive further instructions or prescriptions. In either situation, you are responsible for reinforcing any instructions given by the physician and providing appropriate patient education. Unless the patient was advised to wait in the examination room for instructions after dressing, escort the patient to the front desk for scheduling future appointments and addressing billing issues. Check the medical record to be sure that all data have been accurately documented before releasing the record to the billing department.

FIGURE 22-17. Patient examination positions. (A) The erect or standing position. The patient stands erect facing forward with the arms at the sides. (B) The sitting position. The patient sits erect at the end of the examination table with the feet supported on a footrest or stool. (C) The supine position. The patient lies on the back with arms at the sides. A pillow may be placed under the head for comfort. (D) The dorsal recumbent position. The patient is supine with the legs separated, knees bent, and feet flat on the table. (E) The lithotomy position, similar to the dorsal recumbent position but with the patient's feet in stirrups rather than flat on the table. The stirrups should be level with each other and about 1 foot out from the edge of the table. The patient's feet are moved into or out of the stirrups at the same time to prevent back strain. (F) The Sims position. The patient lies on the left side with the left arm and shoulder behind the body, right leg and arm sharply flexed on the table, and left knee slightly flexed. (G) The prone position. The patient lies on the abdomen with the head supported and turned to one side. The arms may be under the head or by the sides, whichever is more comfortable. (H) Knee-chest position. The patient kneels on the table with the arms and chest on the table, hips in the air, and back straight. (I) Fowler's position. The patient is half-sitting with the head of the examination table elevated 80 to 90°. (J) Semi-Fowler position. The patient is in a half-sitting position with the head of the table elevated 30 to 45° and the knees slightly bent.

Table 22-1	EXAMINATION POSITIONS AND THEIR USES	
Position	**Body Parts**	**Instruments Needed**
Sitting	General appearance	
	Head, neck	Stethoscope
	Eyes	Ophthalmoscope, penlight
	Ears	Otoscope, tuning fork
	Nose	Nasal speculum, penlight, substances to smell
	Sinuses	Penlight
	Mouth	Glove, tongue blade, penlight
	Throat	Glove, tongue blade, penlight, laryngeal mirror, laryngoscope
	Axilla, arms	
	Chest	Stethoscope
	Breasts	
	Upper back	Stethoscope
	Reflexes	Percussion hammer
Supine	Chest	Stethoscope
	Abdomen	Stethoscope
	Breasts	
Lithotomy, dorsal recumbent, Sims	Female genitalia and internal organs	Gloves, vaginal speculum, Ayre spatula, histobrush, lubricant
	Female rectum	Glove, lubricant, fecal occult blood test
Standing, dorsal recumbent, Sims	Male genitalia and hernia	Gloves
	Male rectum	Gloves, lubricant, fecal occult blood test
	Prostate	Glove, lubricant
	Legs	Percussion hammer
	Spine, posture, gait, coordination, balance, strength, flexibility	
Prone	Back, spine, legs	
Knee-chest	Rectum	Glove, lubricant, anoscope, proctoscope, or sigmoidoscope, fecal occult blood test
	Female genitalia	Glove, lubricant, vaginal speculum, Ayre spatula, histobrush
	Prostate	Glove, lubricant
Fowler's	Head, neck, chest	Stethoscope

Clean all reusable equipment, and properly dispose of any disposable supplies or equipment used during the examination. Cover the examination table with clean paper and prepare the room for the next patient.

Checkpoint Question

4. What are your four basic responsibilities in the performance of the physical examination?

PHYSICAL EXAMINATION FORMAT

The physical examination of the patient begins with the patient seated on the examining table with a drape sheet over the lap and covering the legs. The physician usually progresses through the examination in an orderly, methodical sequence. The patient's general appearance, behavior, speech, posture, nutritional status, hair distribution, and skin are observed throughout the examination. These next sections describe the areas of the body examined, including normal and abnormal findings.

Head and Neck

The patient's skull, scalp, hair, and face are inspected and palpated for size, shape, and symmetry. The examiner looks for nodules, masses, and local trauma. The patient may be asked to roll the head in all directions to assess range of motion and to check for any limitations of movement. The trachea and lymph nodes on the anterior neck are palpated for size and symmetry. The thyroid gland, also on the anterior neck, is palpated for size and symmetry. The patient may be asked to swallow to facilitate palpating this gland. The carotid arteries are palpated and auscultated on both sides of the neck to check for any **bruit** (abnormal sound) caused by abnormal blockage.

Eyes and Ears

Usually you perform the visual acuity test before the physician's examination (see Chapter 31). The physician also inspects the **sclera**, or fibrous tissue covering the eye, for normal color. The pupils are inspected with a light to see if they are equal in size, round, and normally reactive to light and accommodation (adjustment). **Normal pupil reaction is recorded as PERRLA, which means the pupils are *equal*, *round*, and *reactive* to *light* and *accommodation*.** Eye movement is assessed by asking the patient to follow the examiner's fingers. Normal movement may be documented as "EOM intact," which means **extraocular** (outside the eye) movement intact. **Peripheral** vision, or side vision while looking straight ahead, may also be assessed. Using the ophthalmoscope, the physician visualizes the interior of the eye and evaluates the condition of the retina and any pathology of the interlobular blood vessels.

The ears are inspected and palpated for size, symmetry, lesions, and nodules. The otoscope is used to examine the interior of the ear canal, including any **cerumen**, or ear wax. The tympanic membrane is checked for color and intact or broken condition. **Normally the tympanic membrane is pearly gray and concave (FIG. 22-18).** However, infection may cause discoloration, and fluids behind the eardrum may cause the membrane to bulge outward. Auditory acuity is tested with the tuning fork or the audioscope (see Chapter 31).

FIGURE 22-18. A normal tympanic membrane. (Reprinted with permission from Moore KL, Dalley AF. Clinically Oriented Anatomy, 4th ed. Baltimore: Lippincott Williams & Wilkins, 1999.)

PATIENT EDUCATION

The Sense of Taste and Smell

When obtaining the medical history, ask the patient whether he or she has had any problems with tasting or smelling. A sudden loss in the ability to taste or smell can be the result of medication, sinus infection, and certain types of tumor. Lack of taste sensation can be a result of normal aging. Normally, the tongue is covered with small bumps called papillae. Each papilla holds about 100 taste buds that allow sweet, salty, sour, and bitter tastes to be identified. The average adult has about 10,000 taste buds. The cells that make up the taste buds are replaced about every 2 weeks. Scientists estimate that by 80 years of age, most people have lost 60 to 80% of their taste buds, and unfortunately, the remaining taste buds are less sensitive than earlier in life. Sweet and salty taste buds tend to be the most affected.

Nose and Sinuses

The external nose is palpated for abnormalities and inspected using a nasal speculum and light. The position of the **nasal septum** is noted for any deviation to the right or left. Each nostril is inspected for color of the mucosa, discharge, lesions, obstructions, polyps, swelling, or tenderness. The sense of smell may be assessed by having the patient close the eyes and identify a common substance such as alcohol, lemon, strawberry, or peppermint.

The paranasal sinuses are also inspected and palpated. With the technique of **transillumination** to visualize the sinuses, the room is darkened and a penlight or flashlight placed against the upper cheek or periorbital ridge.

Mouth and Throat

The physician inspects the mucous membranes of the mouth, gums, teeth, tongue, tonsils, and throat using clean gloves, a light source, and a tongue blade. A laryngeal mirror may also be used. The examiner assesses general dental hygiene and salivary gland function and looks for any abnormalities in the oral cavity, including color, ulcerations, and nodules.

Checkpoint Question

5. What is the tympanic membrane and how does infection affect its appearance?

Chest, Breasts, and Abdomen

The anterior chest is examined with the gown removed to the waist. The physician observes the general appearance and symmetry of the chest and breast area, the respiratory rate and pattern, and any obvious masses or swelling. Palpation includes the axillary lymph nodes and the area over the heart. Underlying structures may also be percussed. Using a stethoscope, the examiner auscultates the lungs for abnormal sounds, at which time the patient may be asked to take deep breaths. The heart sounds and apical pulse are also assessed.

Inspection and palpation of the posterior chest include the muscles of the back and spine. This is followed by percussion of the back to assess lung fields. With a stethoscope the examiner listens to posterior lung sounds, again with the patient asked to take deep breaths.

The breasts may be palpated in both male and female patients. The supine position is preferred for palpation of the breasts because the breast tissue flattens out, making any abnormalities easier to feel. The tissue subject to breast examination includes not only the breast and nipple, but the tissue extending up to the clavicle, under the axilla, and down to the bottom of the rib cage.

After the breasts are examined, the drape is lowered to expose the abdomen to the pubic area. The patient's chest is draped or gowned to just below the breasts. The abdomen is inspected for contour, symmetry, and pulsations from the aorta, a large artery that extends from the heart down the center of the thoracic and abdominal cavities. The examiner uses the stethoscope to auscultate the bowel sounds. Percussion may be used to determine the outlines of the abdominal organs, and palpation is used to assess any organ enlargement, masses, pain, or tenderness.

The lower abdomen and groin are palpated to assess enlargement of **inguinal** lymph nodes and detect any **hernia.** A hernia is protrusion of an organ, such as the intestines, through a weakened muscle wall. The femoral arteries, which pass through each groin, may also be palpated and auscultated.

Checkpoint Question

6. Why is the patient supine for palpation of the breasts?

Genitalia and Rectum

The physician puts on clean gloves to examine the external male genitalia and then the rectum. The genitalia are inspected to note symmetry, lesions, swelling, masses, and hair distribution. The scrotal contents may be visualized using transillumination in a darkened room. In addition, the scrotum is palpated for testicular size, contour, and consistency. The male patient is then asked to stand and bear down as if having a bowel movement while the examiner places a gloved index finger upward along the side of the scrotum in the inguinal ring to assess for a hernia.

The physician asks the patient either to bend over the examination table or to assume the Sims position to inspect the anus for lesions and hemorrhoids. The examiner inserts a gloved and lubricated finger into the rectum to palpate the rectal sphincter muscle and prostate gland for size, consistency, and any masses. An **occult** blood (hidden blood) stool test may be obtained on any stool obtained from the gloved finger. (Chapter 34 describes the procedure for processing the occult blood stool specimen.)

The female genitalia and rectum are usually examined with the patient in the lithotomy position and with one corner of the drape extending over the genitalia and the other corner covering the patient's chest. A gooseneck lamp is adjusted to direct light on the vaginal area, and the external genitalia are inspected for lesions, edema, cysts, discharge, and hair distribution. With clean gloves, the examiner inserts the vaginal speculum and inspects the condition of the vaginal mucosa and cervix. A Pap smear sample from the cervix is obtained and the speculum removed. At this time, the examiner performs a bimanual examination to palpate the internal reproductive organs for size, contour, consistency, and any masses. Two fingers of the gloved dominant hand are inserted into the vagina while the gloved nondominant hand is placed on the lower abdomen to compress the internal organs. (See Chapter 38 for a complete description of the procedure for assisting with a gynecological examination.)

Sometimes a **rectovaginal** examination is necessary to palpate the posterior uterus and vaginal wall. The examiner places a gloved index finger in the vagina and the middle finger in the rectum at the same time. The rectum is usually inspected and palpated for lesions, hemorrhoids, and sphincter tone. A stool specimen may be obtained from the gloved finger to test for occult blood.

Legs

The legs are inspected and the peripheral pulse sites palpated with the patient supine. The patient stands, with assistance if needed, and the peripheral pulse sites may be palpated again and legs observed for varicose veins.

Reflexes

The examiner uses the percussion hammer to test the patient's reflexes by striking the biceps, triceps, patellar, Achilles, and plantar tendons. The patient is usually sitting when these reflexes are checked but may move to supine for checking the plantar reflexes.

Posture, Gait, Coordination, Balance, and Strength

The general posture of the patient and the spine may be inspected with the patient standing. The patient may be asked to walk and perform other movements so that **gait** and coordination can be observed. A balance test may be done by having the patient stand with the feet together and eyes closed. Range of motion and strength of arms and legs are assessed.

Checkpoint Question

7. What is the function of the rectovaginal and bimanual pelvic examinations?

GENERAL HEALTH GUIDELINES AND CHECKUPS

Physicians vary as to how often they recommend a complete physical examination. For patients aged 20 to 40 years, physical examinations are scheduled about every 1 to 3 years. Annual examinations are typically performed on patients over age 40 unless a medical condition requires more frequent visits.

For women, the first Pap smear is recommended at age 18 to 20 and then annually thereafter. A breast examination by a physician is recommended every 3 years for women aged 20 to 40 to detect lumps and thickenings that could be malignancies, but breast self-examinations should be performed monthly to allow the patient to detect and report any abnormalities in breast tissue between visits to the physician (see Chapter 38). As with most cancers, early detection of breast cancer is the key to survival. A baseline mammogram is recommended for those aged 35 and 40, every 2 years from 40 to 50 years of age, and then annually after 50. If the patient is at risk for developing breast cancer, the physician may recommend mammograms earlier and more often.

All patients should have a baseline electrocardiogram (ECG) at age 40 and follow-up ECGs as necessary. A rectal examination and fecal occult blood are recommended annually beginning at age 40. At age 50, a proctoscopic examination (colonoscopy) is recommended and if the results are negative, every 3 to 5 years thereafter.

Adult immunizations are generally recommended as follows:

- Tetanus booster every 10 years, or sooner if the patient has an open wound.
- One injection of pneumonia vaccine (Pneumovax) at age 60 to 65 years.
- After age 65, an annual flu shot (influenza A and B) should be given.

PATIENT EDUCATION

The Body's Warning Signals

Teach patients the CAUTION acronym to recognize these early warning signs of cancer:

C Change in bowel or bladder habits
A A sore that does not heal
U Unusual bleeding or discharge
T Thickening, lumps, or changes in the shape of the breasts or testicles
I Indigestion or difficulty swallowing
O Obvious change in a wart or mole
N Nagging cough or hoarseness of the voice

Frequent, severe headaches and persistent abdominal pain are other signals that should not be ignored. Instruct patients not to overlook the following signs in their children:

- Continual crying for no obvious reason
- Unexplained nausea and vomiting
- General failure to thrive
- Spontaneous bleeding or bleeding that does not stop in the normal amount of time
- Bumps, lumps, masses, or swelling anywhere on the body
- Frequent stumbling for no apparent reason

- Some doctors also recommend a series of three hepatitis B injections for any adult patient who has not received this immunization.

You should take every opportunity to educate patients regarding the signs and symptoms that may signal health problems and when to call the physician.

Checkpoint Question

8. Why are monthly self breast examinations important for women aged 20 to 40 years?

Procedure 22-1

Assisting with the Adult Physical Examination

Purpose: Prepare the room and patient for the general physical examination, assist the physician during the examination, assist the patient as needed after the examination, and clean up the examination room, supplies, and equipment.

Equipment: A variety of instruments and supplies, including the stethoscope, ophthalmoscope, otoscope, penlight, tuning fork, nasal speculum, tongue blade, percussion hammer, gloves, and patient gown and draping supplies.

Standard: This procedure should take 15 minutes.

Steps	Reason
1. Wash your hands.	Hand washing aids in infection control.
2. Prepare the examination room and assemble the equipment.	A clean room that is free of contamination prevents transfer of microorganisms.
3. Greet the patient by name and escort him or her to the examining room.	Identifying the patient by name prevents errors.
4. Explain the procedure.	Explaining the procedure reduces anxiety and may help to ensure compliance.
5. Obtain and record the medical history and chief complaint.	
6. Take and record the vital signs, height, weight, and visual acuity.	The vital signs and other measurements give the physician an overall picture of the patient's health.
7. If the physician requires it, instruct the patient to obtain a urine specimen and escort him or her to the bathroom.	Even if a urine specimen is not part of the physical examination, an empty bladder makes abdominal and/or pelvic examinations more comfortable.
8. Once the patient has returned from the bathroom, instruct him or her in disrobing and how to put on the gown (open in the front or the back). Leave the room unless the patient needs assistance.	The gown must open in the direction that provides accessibility for the examination. Elderly and disabled persons may need help disrobing and putting on the gown.
9. Help the patient sit on the edge of the examination table and cover the lap and legs with a drape.	The sitting position is often the first position used by the physician.
10. Place the medical record outside the examination room and notify the physician that the patient is ready.	Alerting the physician helps prevent delays.
11. Assist the physician by handing him or her the instruments as needed and positioning the patient appropriately.	Anticipating the physician's needs promotes efficiency and saves time.
A. Begin by handing the physician the instruments necessary for examining the following: • Head and neck • Eyes • Ears • Nose • Sinuses	 Stethoscope Ophthalmoscope, penlight Otoscope, tuning fork, audioscope Penlight, nasal speculum Penlight

(continues)

Procedure 22-1 *(continued)*

Assisting with the Adult Physical Examination

Steps	Reason
• Mouth	Tongue blade, penlight. Hand over the tongue blade holding it in the middle. When it is returned to you, grasp it in the middle again so that you do not touch the end that was in the patient's mouth.
• Throat	Glove, tongue blade, laryngeal mirror, penlight
B. Help the patient drop the gown to the waist for examination of the chest and upper back. Hand the physician the stethoscope.	Only the parts of the body being examined should be exposed. Always preserve patients' privacy and keep them covered as much as possible.
C. Help the patient pull the gown up and remove the drape from the legs so that the physician can test the reflexes. Hand the physician the reflex hammer.	
D. Help the patient to lie supine, opening the gown at the top to expose the chest again. Place the drape to cover the waist, abdomen, and legs. Hand the physician the stethoscope.	
E. Cover the patient's chest and lower the drape to expose the abdomen. Hand the physician the stethoscope.	
F. Assist with the genital and rectal examinations. Hand the patient tissues following these examinations.	Tissues may be used to wipe off excess lubricant.

For females

- Assist the patient to the lithotomy position and drape appropriately.
- For examination of the genitalia and internal reproductive organs, provide a glove, lubricant, speculum, microscope slides or prep solution, and spatula or brush.
- For the rectal examination, provide a glove, lubricant, and fecal occult blood test slide.

For males

- Help the patient stand and have him bend over the examination table for a rectal and prostate examination.
- For a hernia examination, provide a glove.
- For a rectal examination, provide a glove, lubricant, and fecal occult blood test slide.
- For a prostate examination, provide a glove and lubricant.

G. With the patient standing, the physician can assess the legs, gait, coordination, and balance.

(continues)

Assisting with the Adult Physical Examination

Steps	Reason
15. Help the patient sit at the edge of the examination table.	The physician often discusses findings with the patient at this time and may provide instructions.
16. Perform any follow-up procedures or treatments.	
17. Leave the room while the patient dresses unless the patient needs assistance.	Leaving the room provides privacy for the patient.
18. Return to the examination room when the patient has dressed to answer any questions, reinforce instructions, and provide patient education.	Compliance depends on full understanding of the treatment plan. Patient education is the responsibility of all health care workers, including the medical assistant.
19. Escort the patient to the front desk.	You can clarify appointment scheduling or billing issues.
20. Properly clean or dispose of all used equipment and supplies. Clean the room with a disinfectant and prepare for the next patient.	All instruments, supplies, and equipment that came into direct contact with the patient must be appropriately decontaminated or disposed of.
21. Wash your hands and record any instructions from the physician. Also note any specimens and indicate the results of the test or the laboratory where the specimens are being sent for testing.	Procedures and instructions are considered not to have been done if they are not recorded.

Charting Example

01/19/2005 1:30 p.m. CC: Annual physical examination complete per Dr. Smith. ECG done; results given to Dr. Smith. Blood drawn and sent to Acme lab for a CBC, electrolytes, and liver panel. Pt. instructed to return to office in 2 weeks to discuss results of laboratory tests. Pt. given written and verbal instructions regarding an 1800-calorie low-sodium diet to follow as ordered per Dr. Smith. Pt. verbalized understanding. _____ J. Bohr, CMA

CHAPTER SUMMARY

Your role as a medical assistant during the physical examination is to assist both the physician and the patient. Efficiency, accuracy, and attention to detail are crucial as you assist the physician and anticipate what will be needed in the examination. Assessing the patient's needs, developing a good interpersonal relationship, and providing support to the patient are important to help the patient have a pleasant office visit.

Critical Thinking Challenges

1. During the physical examination, the physician asks the patient to walk across the room. What can be determined about the patient's health from observing the patient's gait?
2. After the physical examination, a patient asks you, "Why did the physician hit my chest with his fingers while listening?" How do you explain to the patient what the doctor was doing?
3. Why is it possible for the physician to assess vascular health by checking the interior eye with the ophthalmoscope?
4. How can you anticipate what instruments or supplies the physician may need during the physical examination? Why is this important?

Answers to Checkpoint Questions

1. The tuning fork and audioscope are used to test hearing. The otoscope is used to assess the internal structures of the ear.
2. The anoscope is the shortest and is used to inspect the anal canal. The proctoscope is longer than the anoscope and is used to visualize the rectum and the anus. The sigmoidoscope is the longest of the three and is used to inspect the rectum and sigmoid colon.
3. The examination technique that requires the use of the hands or fingers is palpation.
4. The clinical medical assistant is responsible for preparing the examination room, preparing the patient, assisting the physician, and cleaning the examination room and equipment after the examination.
5. The tympanic membrane, also called the eardrum, is a thin membrane between the outer and middle ear that transmits sound waves to the inner ear. Normally it is a pearly gray and concave. However, in the presence of an infection and fluid behind it, it may be discolored and bulge outward.
6. When the patient is supine, the breast tissue flattens out, making it easier for the examiner to feel any abnormalities.
7. The rectovaginal examination is done to palpate the posterior uterus and vaginal wall.
8. Monthly self breast examinations are important in women aged 20 to 40 to detect abnormal lumps or thickenings that may be malignancies. Cancers are most likely to be cured if detected and treated early.

WWW.GO Websites

American Academy of Family Physicians www.aafp.org

familydoctor.org from the American Academy of Family Physicians www.familydoctor.org

American College of Physicians—Internal Medicine www.acponline.org

CDC Screen for Life: National Colorectal Cancer Action Campaign www.cdc.gov/cancer/screenforlife/

American Cancer Society www.cancer.org

National Breast Cancer Foundation www.nationalbreast-cancer.org

23

Surgical Instruments and Sterilization

CHAPTER OUTLINE

PRINCIPLES AND PRACTICES
  OF STERILE ASEPSIS
Sterilization

SURGICAL INSTRUMENTS
  Forceps
  Scissors
  Scalpels and Blades
  Towel Clamps
  Probes and Directors
  Retractors

CARE AND HANDLING OF
  SURGICAL INSTRUMENTS

STORAGE AND RECORD
  KEEPING

MAINTAINING SURGICAL
  SUPPLIES

ROLE DELINEATION

ADMINISTRATIVE: ADMINISTRATIVE PROCEDURES
- Perform basic administrative medical assisting functions

CLINICAL: FUNDAMENTAL PRINCIPLES
- Apply principles of aseptic technique and infection control
- Comply with quality assurance practices

CLINICAL: PATIENT CARE
- Prepare and maintain examination and treatment areas

GENERAL: PROFESSIONALISM
- Display a professional manner and image
- Demonstrate initiative and responsibility
- Work as a member of the health care team
- Set priorities and perform multiple tasks

GENERAL: LEGAL CONCEPTS
- Perform within legal and ethical boundaries
- Comply with established risk management and safety procedures

GENERAL: OPERATIONAL FUNCTIONS
- Perform routine maintenance of administrative and clinical equipment

CHAPTER COMPETENCIES

LEARNING OBJECTIVES
Upon successfully completing this chapter, you will be able to:
1. Spell and define key terms.
2. Describe several methods of sterilization.
3. Categorize surgical instruments based on use and identify each by its characteristics.
4. Identify surgical instruments specific to designated specialties.
5. State the difference between reusable and disposable instruments.
6. Explain the procedure for storing supplies, instruments, and equipment.
7. Describe the necessity and procedure for maintaining documents and records of maintenance for instruments and equipment.

PERFORMANCE OBJECTIVES
Upon successfully completing this chapter, you will be able to:
1. Sanitize equipment and instruments (Procedure 23-1)
2. Properly wrap instruments in preparation for sterilization in an autoclave (Procedure 23-2)
3. Operate an autoclave while observing for pressure, time, and temperature determined by the items being sterilized (Procedure 23-3)

KEY TERMS

autoclave	hemostat	ratchet	scissors
disinfection	needle holder	sanitation	serration
ethylene oxide	obturator	sanitize	sound
forceps	OSHA	scalpel	sterilization

THE GOAL OF SURGICAL ASEPSIS is to free an item or area from all microorganisms, both pathogens and others (see Chapter 19). The practice of surgical asepsis, also known as sterile technique, should be used during any office surgical procedure, when handling sterile instruments to be used for incisions and excisions into body tissue, and when changing wound dressings. Surgical asepsis prevents microorganisms from entering the patient's environment; medical asepsis prevents microbes from spreading to or from patients.

In a medical office, your responsibilities may include assisting with minor surgical procedures while maintaining surgical asepsis. To manage this responsibility, you must do the following:

- Become familiar with many types of surgical instruments
- Understand the principles and practices of surgical asepsis
- Understand and use **disinfection** and **sterilization** techniques
- Use equipment designed for sterilization, treatment, and diagnostic purposes
- Maintain accurate records and inventory of purchases related to surgical equipment and supplies

The physician expects you to understand sterile technique and to be able to maintain sterility throughout procedures. Any break in sterile technique, no matter how small, can lead to infection the body cannot fight. Even small infections can delay the patient's recovery and are physically, mentally, and financially costly to the patient.

PRINCIPLES AND PRACTICES OF SURGICAL ASEPSIS

As a medical assistant, you are responsible for preventing infection in accordance with the principles and practices of asepsis as it relates to items used during minor office surgical procedures. Surgical asepsis requires the absence of microorganisms, infection, and infectious material on instruments, equipment, and supplies. Disinfection, or medical asepsis, is different from sterilization (TABLE 23-1). By becoming familiar with the manufacturer's recommendations for processing instruments according to the purposes for which the items will be used, you will be able to determine the appropriate level of asepsis.

TRIAGE

While you are working in a medical office, these three situations arise:

A. You have to sanitize instruments soaking in detergent that were used earlier in the day during a minor surgical procedure.

B. A 45-year-old woman who just had a mole removed needs postoperative instructions before discharge, and the treatment room where the procedure was done is in need of cleaning for the next patient.

C. A load in the autoclave that ran earlier is finished. The sterilized packs have to be put away.

How do you sort these tasks? What do you do first? Second? Third?

The patient in situation B should be taken care of first. You should take time to explain any postoperative instructions and follow-up care clearly as indicated by the physician. Once the patient is discharged, the treatment room should be cleaned and any used surgical equipment discarded appropriately or prepared for sanitation according to appropriate standard precautions. The next task includes sanitizing the soaking instruments, rinsing each of them thoroughly, and allowing them to dry completely. While they are drying, the autoclave load from earlier can be put away. At that point, the clean instruments can be wrapped and placed in the autoclave for sterilization.

Table 23-1	COMPARISON OF MEDICAL AND SURGICAL ASEPSIS	
	Medical Asepsis	**Surgical Asepsis**
Definition	Destroys microorganisms after they leave the body	Destroys microorganisms before they enter the body
Purpose	Prevents transmission of microbes from one person to another	Prevents entry of microbes into the body in invasive procedures
When used	During contact with a body part that is not normally sterile	During contact with a normally sterile part of the body
Differences in handwashing technique	Hands and wrists are washed for 1 to 2 minutes	Hands and forearms are washed for 5–10 minutes with a brush

Sterilization

While **sanitation** and disinfection are adequate for maintaining medical asepsis in the medical office, these practices are not sufficient to process instruments and equipment used during sterile procedures (see Chapter 19). Objects requiring surgical asepsis must be **sanitized** first and sterilized by either a physical or chemical process. Procedure 23-1 describes the procedure for sanitizing instruments in preparation for sterilization. Sterilization is the complete elimination or destruction of all forms of microbial life, including spore forms. Steam under pressure, dry heat, **ethylene oxide** gas, and liquid chemicals are principle sterilizing agents. Although in medical offices steam under pressure is the most frequently used method of sterilization, the method depends on the nature of the material to be sterilized and the type of microorganism to be destroyed. TABLE 23-2 describes the various methods of sterilization and the temperatures and time of exposure if applicable.

Checkpoint Question

1. How do sanitization, disinfection, and sterilization differ?

Sterilization Equipment

Several types of sterilization equipment are used in clinics and medical offices. As a clinical medical assistant, it is your responsibility to do the following:

- Become familiar with the uses and operation of each piece of equipment

Table 23-2 STERILIZATION METHODS	
Methods	**Concentration or Level**
Heat	
Moist heat (steam under pressure)	250°F or 121°C for 30 min
Boiling	212°F or 100°C for ≥ 30 min
Dry heat	340°F or 171°C for 1 hour
	320°F or 160°C for 2 hours
Liquids	
Glutaraldehyde	Follow manufacturer's recommendations or OSHA requirements and guidelines
Formaldehyde	Follow manufacturer's recommendations or OSHA requirements and guidelines
Gas	
Ethylene oxide	450–500mg/L 50°C

OSHA, Occupational Safety and Health Administration.

- Schedule periodic preventive maintenance or servicing of the equipment
- Maintain adequate supplies for general operational needs

The Autoclave

The most frequently used piece of equipment for sterilizing instruments today is the autoclave (FIG. 23-1). The autoclave has two chambers: an outer one where pressure builds and an inner one where the sterilization occurs. Distilled water is added to a reservoir, where it is converted to steam as the preset temperature is reached. The steam is forced into the inner chamber, increasing the pressure and raising the temperature of the steam to 250°F or higher, well above the ordinary boiling temperature of water (212°F or 100°C). The pressure has no effect on sterilization other than to increase the temperature of the steam. The high temperature allows for destruction of all microorganisms, including viruses and spores.

An air exhaust vent on the bottom of the autoclave allows the air in the chamber to be pushed out and replaced by the pressurized steam. When no air is present, the chamber seals and the temperature gauge begins to rise. Most automatic autoclaves can be set to vent, time, turn off, and exhaust at preset times and levels. Older models may require that the steps be advanced manually. All manufacturers provide instructions for operating the machine and recommendations for the times necessary to sterilize different types of loads. These instructions should be posted in a prominent place near the machine.

Sterilization is required for surgical instruments and equipment that will come into contact with internal body tissues or cavities that are considered sterile. The autoclave is commonly used to sterilize minor surgical instruments, surgical storage trays and containers, and some surgical equipment, such as bowls for holding sterile solutions. Instruments or equipment subject to damage by water should not be sterilized in the autoclave. These items can be sterilized with gas. Items that are not subject to water damage but may be destroyed by heat can be cold-sterilized or soaked for a prescribed amount of time in a liquid such as glutaraldehyde or formaldehyde. Always follow the manufacturer's recommendations for sterilizing instruments or equipment and for using any chemical products for sterilization. Procedure 23-2 describes preparation of instruments for sterilization in the autoclave.

Checkpoint Question

2. What is an autoclave, and how does it work?

Sterilization Indicators

Tape applied to the outside of the material used to wrap instruments or supplies for the autoclave indicates that the items have been exposed to steam, but the tape cannot ensure the sterility

A   **B**

F I G U R E 2 3 - 1 .   (A) An autoclave that may be found in the medical office; note the clearly marked dials and gauges. (B) The interior of the autoclave.

of the contents (Box 23-1 and FIGURE 23-2). Sterilization indicators placed inside the packs register that the proper pressure and temperature were attained for the required time to allow steam to penetrate the inner parts of the pack (FIG. 23-3). Improper wrapping, loading, or operation of the autoclave may prevent the indicator from registering properly.

Types of indicators include those that change colors at high temperatures. Specially designed tubes containing wax pellets are also used to indicate that the required temperature was reached, as evidenced by the melted wax. Although most types of sterilization indicators work well, the best method for determining effectiveness of sterilization is the culture test. Strips impregnated with heat-resistant spores are wrapped and placed in the center of the autoclave between the packages in a designated load, such as the first load of the day. The strips are removed from their packets and placed in a broth culture to be incubated according to the instructions of the manufacturer. At the end of the incubation period, the culture is compared to a control to determine that all spores have been killed. If sterilization was not achieved, the load must be reprocessed.

 Checkpoint Question

3. What is the difference between a sterilization indicator and autoclave tape?

Loading the Autoclave

Load the autoclave loosely to allow steam to circulate. If too many items are packed into the autoclave, steam will not penetrate the items in the center. Place empty wrapped containers or bowls on their sides with the lids wrapped separately. If containers are upright in the autoclave, air, which is heavier than steam, will settle into the interior of the container and keep steam from circulating to the inner surfaces. Place all packs on their sides to allow for the maximum steam circulation and penetration.

 Checkpoint Question

4. Why is the loading of the autoclave important? How would you load it?

Operating the Autoclave

All components of autoclaving—temperature, pressure, steam, and time—must be correct for the items to reach sterility. Follow the instruction manual carefully. All machines use the same principles, but operation varies. Become familiar with the function of the machine in your facility. Instructions may be covered in plastic or laminated and posted beside the machine for easy reference.

The autoclave has a reservoir tank that should be filled with distilled water only. Tap water contains chemicals and minerals that would coat the interior chamber, clog the exhaust valves, and hinder the overall operation of the autoclave. When filling the internal chamber of the autoclave with dis-

---

Box 23-1

AUTOCLAVE INDICATOR TAPE

Autoclave tape is designed to change color in the presence of heat and steam. In extreme instances the tape may change appearance when stored too close to heat sources. Most tapes have imprinted lines that darken after exposure, but sterilization of the package contents is not ensured by a color change on the autoclave tape. Proper sterilization can be assumed only if accompanying sterilization indicators have registered that all elements of the sterilization process (time and temperature) have been achieved.

FIGURE 23-2. The stripes on autoclave indicator tape change color, indicating that the pack has been exposed to steam.

tilled water from the reservoir, be sure the water level is at the fill line. If too much water is added to the chamber, the steam will be saturated and may not be efficient, and too little water will not produce the required amount of steam. Procedure 23-3 outlines the general steps for operating an autoclave.

The temperature, pressure, and time required vary with the items being sterilized. In most cases, 250°F at 15 pounds of pressure for 20 to 30 minutes will be sufficient, but you should follow the manufacturer's instructions for the load content. Solid or metal loads take slightly less time than soft, bulky loads. The timer should not be set until the proper temperature has been attained. Some microorganisms, such as spores, are killed only if exposed to high enough temperature for a specific amount of time.

When the items have been in the autoclave at the right temperature for enough time, the timer will sound, indicating that the cycle is finished. Be sure to vent the autoclave to allow the pressure to drop safely. After the pressure has dropped to a safe level, open the door of the autoclave slightly to allow the temperature to drop and the load to cool and dry. Newer autoclaves vent automatically. Do not handle or remove items from the autoclave until they are dry, because bacteria from your hands would be drawn through the moist coverings and contaminate the items inside the wrapping. Once the items are dry, remove the packages and store them in a clean, dry, dust-free area. Packs that are sterilized on site in the autoclave are considered sterile for 30 days and must be sterilized again after this period. Always store recently autoclaved items toward the back of the cabinet, rotating the previously autoclaved items to the front. In addition, you are responsible for performing maintenance on the autoclave at regular intervals. Post a schedule for this maintenance near the machine; allow for cleaning the lint trap, washing out the interior of the chamber with a cloth or soft brush, and checking the function of all components. This schedule can remind and document the service with space for initialing or signing after the maintenance has been done.

 Checkpoint Question

5. Why is it important to set the timer on the autoclave during a cycle only after the correct temperature has been reached?

SURGICAL INSTRUMENTS

You must be able to identify surgical instruments according to their design and function. A surgical instrument is a tool or device designed to perform a specific function, such as cutting, dissecting, grasping, holding, retracting, or suturing. Surgical instruments are designed to perform specific tasks based on their shape; they may be curved, straight, sharp, blunt, serrated, toothed, or smooth. Many are made of stainless steel and are reusable; others are disposable. It is your responsibility to know the proper use and care of the surgical instruments in your clinical setting.

Most instruments used in office procedures can be identified by carefully examining the instrument. The most widely used surgical instruments are **forceps, scissors, scalpels,** and clamps. TABLE 23-3 shows the most commonly used instruments and equipment by specialty.

Forceps

Forceps are surgical instruments used to grasp, handle, compress, pull, or join tissue, equipment, or supplies. The types of forceps include the following:

- **hemostat clamp** A surgical instrument with slender jaws used for grasping blood vessels and establishing hemostasis.
- **Kelly clamp** A curved or straight forceps or hemostat; those with long handles are widely used in gynecological procedures.
- **sterilizer forceps** Used to transfer sterile supplies,

FIGURE 23-3. Sterilization indicators and autoclave indicator tape. Gas indicator tape (*left*) and steam indicator tape (*right*).

Table 23-3	COMMONLY USED INSTRUMENTS AND EQUIPMENT BY SPECIALTY	
	Instruments	**Use**
Obstetrics, gynecology	Vaginal speculum	Open vagina to view vaginal walls, cervical os; perform procedures; sized; may be reusable metal or disposable plastic
	Tenaculum	Grasping and holding tissue with hooklike tips
	Uterine **sounds**	Assess depth of uterus; graduated in inches or centimeters
	Uterine dilator	Widens cervical os; usually 3–18 mm
	Curet	Blunt or sharp; for scraping endometrium
	Biopsy forceps	Secure pieces of tissue for microscopic study

Gynecology instruments. (A) Graves vaginal speculum. (B) Pederson vaginal speculum. (C) Duplay tenaculum forceps. (D) Schroeder tenaculum forceps. (E) Sims uterine sound. (F) Simpson uterine sound, malleable. (G) Hand uterine dilator. (H) Hegar uterine dilator. (I) Thomas uterine curets. (J) Sims uterine curets.

Orthopedics	Cast saw	Remove cast
	Cutters or spreaders	

Orthopedic instruments. (A) Oscillating plaster saw. (B) Stille plaster shears. (C) Hennig plaster spreader.

Table 23-3 (CONTINUED)

	Instruments	Use
Urology	Urethral sounds	Explore bladder depth, direction; dilate urethral meatus in stenosis; sized Fr 8–26
	Prostate biopsy	Removes tissue for microscopic study

A

B

Urology instruments. (A) Otis-Dittel urethral sound. (B) Dittel urethral sound.

	Instruments	Use
Proctology	Anoscopes, proctoscopes	Visualize lower intestinal tract; most have **obturator** for ease of insertion
	Sigmoidoscope	Visualize lower sigmoid colon; rigid or flexible, with fiberoptic light; some have suction device
	Punch biopsy	Remove small piece of tissue via small circular hole
	Alligator biopsy	Jaws grasp and excise tissue

A

B

C

Proctology instruments. (A) Ives rectal speculum (Fansler). (B) Pratt rectal speculum. (C) Hirschman anoscope.

	Instruments	Use
Otology, rhinology	Nasal or ear forceps	Insert or remove materials from nose or ear canal
	Nasal speculum	Opens, extends nostrils for visualization of nasal passages
	Curet	Remove cerumen from deep ear canal

A

B

C

D

Otology and rhinology. (A) Wilde ear forceps. (B) Lucae bayonet forceps. (C) Buck ear curet. (D) Vienna nasal speculum.

(continues)

Table 23-3 (CONTINUED)

	Instruments	Use
Ophthalmology	Eye loop, lid retractor Tonometer	Hold eyelids open for removal of foreign bodies Measure intraocular pressure to diagnose glaucoma

A   Desmarres lid retractor

Bailey foreign body remover   B

C   Schiotz tonometer

Ophthalmology. (A) Desmarres lid retractor. (B) Bailey foreign body remover. (C) Schiotz tonometer.

Dermatology	Punch biopsy	Removes small circular sections of skin for microscopic studies; sized 2–8 mm, disposable or reusable
	Comedone extractor	Remove blackheads, open pustules

A   06–4120   06–4121   06–4122   B

Dermatology instruments. (A) Keyes cutaneous punch. (B) Schamberg comedone extractor.

Fr, French.

equipment, and other surgical instruments to a sterile field. May also be called sterile transfer forceps.

- **needle holder** Used to hold and pass a needle through tissue during suturing.
- **spring or thumb forceps** Used for grasping tissue for dissection or suturing, such as tissue forceps and splinter forceps.

A variety of forceps can be seen in FIGURE 23-4. All forceps are available in many sizes, with or without **serrations** or teeth, with curved or straight blades, and with ring tips, blunt tips, or sharp tips. Many have **ratchets** in the handles to hold the tips tightly together; these are notched mechanisms that click into position to maintain tension. Some have spring handles that are compressed between the thumb and index finger to grasp objects.

Physicians use a variety of forceps. You should study the names and purposes of each type to assist the physician when a specific instrument is requested.

Scissors

Scissors are sharp instruments composed of two opposing cutting blades held together by a central pin at the pivot. Scissors are used for dissecting superficial, deep, or delicate tissues and for cutting sutures and bandages. Scissors have blade points that are blunt, sharp, or both, depending on the use of the instrument. The types of scissors include the following:

- **straight scissors** cut deep or delicate tissue and sutures
- **curved scissors** dissect superficial and delicate tissues
- **suture scissors** cut sutures; straight top blade and curved-out, or hooked, blunt bottom blade to fit under, lift, and grasp sutures for snipping.
- **bandage scissors** remove bandages; flattened blunt tip on the bottom longer blade safely fits under bandages; most common type is the Lister bandage scissors.

FIGURE 23-5 shows various types of scissors.

FIGURE 23-4. (A) Rochester-Pean forceps. (B) Rochester-Ochsner forceps. (C) Adson forceps. (D) Bozeman forceps. (E) Crile hemostat. (F) Kelly hemostat. (G) Halsted mosquito hemostat. (H) Allis forceps. (I) Babcock forceps. (J) DeBakey forceps. (K) Allis tissue forceps. (L) Duplay tenaculum forceps. (M) Crile-Wood needle holder. (N) Ballenger sponge forceps. (O) Fine-point splinter forceps. (P) Adson dressing forceps. (Q) Potts-Smith dressing forceps. (Courtesy of Sklar Instruments, West Chester, PA).

FIGURE 23-5. (A) Straight-blade operating scissors. *Left to right:* S/S, S/B, B/B. (B) Curved-blade operating scissors. *Left to right:* S/S, S/B, B/B. (C) Spencer stitch scissors. (D) Suture scissors. (E) Lister bandage scissors. S/S, sharp/sharp; S/B, sharp/blunt; B/B, blunt/blunt. (Courtesy of Sklar Instruments, West Chester, PA).

FIGURE 23-6. (A) Scalpel handles. (B) Surgical blades. (C) Complete sterile disposable scalpel. (Courtesy of Sklar Instruments, West Chester, PA).

Scalpels and Blades

A scalpel is a small surgical knife with a straight handle and a straight or curved blade. A reusable steel scalpel handle can hold different blades for different surgical procedures. Straight or pointed blades are used for incision and drainage procedures, while curved blades are used to excise tissue. Reusable handles are used only with disposable blades. Many offices use disposable handles and blades packaged as one sterile unit. FIGURE 23-6 shows various scalpels and blades.

FIGURE 23-7. (A) Backhaus towel clamp. (B) Jones cross-action towel clamp. (Courtesy of Sklar Instruments, West Chester, PA).

FIGURE 23-8. (A). Director and tongue tie. (B) Double-ended probe. (C) Probe with eye. (Courtesy of Sklar Instruments, West Chester, PA).

Towel Clamps

Towel clamps are used to maintain the integrity of the sterile field by holding the sterile drapes in place, allowing exposure of the operative site (FIG. 23-7). A sterile field is a specific area that is considered free of all microorganisms.

Probes and Directors

Before entering a cavity or site for a procedure, the physician may first probe the depth and direction of the operative area. A probe shows the angle and depth of the operative area, and a director guides the knife or instrument once the procedure has begun (FIG. 23-8).

Retractors

Retractors hold open layers of tissue, exposing the areas beneath. They may be plain or toothed; the toothed retractor may be sharp or blunt. Retractors may be designed to be held by an assistant or screwed open to be self-retaining. FIGURE 23-9 shows several types of retractors.

 Checkpoint Question

6. What types of instruments are used to remove tissue during a biopsy?

CARE AND HANDLING OF SURGICAL INSTRUMENTS

To ensure that surgical instruments always function properly, follow these guidelines:

1. Do not toss or drop instruments into a basin or sink. Surgical instruments are delicate, and the blade or

FIGURE 23-9. (A) Volkman retractor. (B) Lahey retractor. (C) Senn retractor. (Courtesy of Sklar Instruments, West Chester, PA).

tip is easily damaged by improper handling. Should you drop an instrument accidentally, carefully inspect it for damage. Damaged instruments can usually be repaired and should not be discarded unless repair is not feasible.

2. Avoid stacking instruments in a pile. They may tangle and be damaged when separated.

3. Always store sharp instruments separately to prevent dulling or damaging the sharp edges and to prevent accidental injury. Disposable scalpel blades should be removed from reusable handles and placed in puncture-proof sharps biohazard containers. If a disposable scalpel is used, the whole unit is discarded into the sharps container. Syringes with needles attached and suture needles should also be discarded in a sharps container, never in the trash or with other instruments for processing. Delicate instruments, such as scissors or tissue forceps or those with lenses, are kept separate to be sanitized and sterilized appropriately.

4. Keep ratcheted instruments open when not in use to avoid damage to the ratchet mechanism.

5. Rinse gross contamination from instruments as soon as possible to prevent drying and hardening, which makes cleaning more difficult. Always wear gloves and follow OSHA standards to prevent contact with possibly infected blood or body fluids.

6. Check instruments before sterilization to ensure that they are in good working order and identify instruments in need of repair.
   A. Blades or points should be free of bends and nicks.
   B. Tips should close evenly and tightly.
   C. Instruments with box locks should move freely but should not be too loose.
   D. Instruments with spring handles should have enough tension to grasp objects tightly.

E. Scissors should close in a smooth, even manner with no nicks or snags. (Scissors may be checked by cutting through gauze or cotton to be sure there are no rough areas).

F. Screws should be flush with the instrument surface. They should be freely workable but not loose.

WHAT IF

While pouring a liquid sterilization solution such as glutaraldehyde into a container, the chemical spills?

OSHA and state regulations have defined a specific law to protect you from hazardous materials. The law, The Right to Know, requires that all companies, including medical offices, using hazardous materials have material safety data sheets (MSDS) available to their employees. MSDS are prepared by the chemical manufacturer and clearly state how to handle and dispose of the chemical. These forms also include a list of possible health hazards to workers and identify the safety equipment needed for using the chemical. Never handle any type of chemical spill without first reading the MSDS. You are required to add to the MSDS binder any MSDS that accompany any supplies or equipment containing hazardous materials. This notebook should be placed in a stationary area where it can be easily consulted in case of an emergency involving hazardous materials.

7. Use instruments only for the purpose for which they were designed. For instance, never use surgical scissors to cut paper or open packages, because this may damage the cutting edges.

8. Sanitize instruments before they are sterilized so that sterilization will work effectively.

Checkpoint Question

7. Why should you avoid dropping surgical instruments, and what should you do if one drops accidentally?

STORAGE AND RECORD KEEPING

When using and maintaining sterile instruments, equipment and supplies, staff are responsible for correctly storing these items, keeping accurate records of warranties and maintenance agreements and keeping reordering information on hand. You should be familiar with the manufacturer's recommendations for each instrument or piece of equipment. Most offices have specific storage or supply areas for keeping sterile and other instruments and equipment. This area should be kept clean and dust free and should be close to the area of need. Clean and sterile supplies and equipment must be separated from soiled items and waste.

Medical assistants are also responsible for keeping accurate records of sterilized items and equipment. Information that must be recorded includes maintenance records and load or sterilization records. These records should include the following:

- Date and time of the sterilization cycle
- General description of the load
- Exposure time and temperature
- Name or initials of the operator
- Results of the sterilization indicator
- Expiration date of the load (usually 30 days)

The maintenance records include service provided by the manufacturer's representative and daily or recommended maintenance to keep the equipment in optimum working condition.

Checkpoint Question

8. What six items should be included on a sterilization record?

MAINTAINING SURGICAL SUPPLIES

As a clinical medical assistant, you should keep an up-to-date master list of all supplies including purchases and replacements. Generally, one person is responsible for maintaining inventory, keeping maintenance schedules, and placing orders. If too many staff are involved, these tasks may be overlooked or efforts may be duplicated. Instruction manuals for all equipment should be kept on file and consulted when ordering supplies for replacement or maintenance. Equipment records for each item should include the following:

- Date of purchase
- Model and serial numbers of the equipment
- Time of recommended service
- Date service was requested
- Name of the person requesting the service
- Reason for the service request
- Description of the service performed and any parts replaced
- Name of the person performing the service and the date the work was completed
- Signature and title of the person who acknowledged completion of the work

Warranties and guarantees should be kept with the equipment records, along with the name of the manufacturer's contact person. A tickler file should be kept to remind the staff of the need for manufacturer service and concurrent or periodic maintenance by the staff.

Parts and supplies for items that are vital to the operation of the facility should always be kept on hand. The shelf life of the item, the storage space available, and the time required to order and receive an item should be considered when deciding what items to keep in inventory. If a piece of equipment cannot function without all of its components or if some of those components have a short life, replacements must be readily available. For example, an ophthalmoscope without a light is virtually useless.

Procedure 23-1

Sanitizing Equipment for Disinfection or Sterilization

Purpose: Properly sanitize instruments in preparation for disinfection or sterilization.

Equipment: Instruments or equipment to be sanitized, gloves, eye protection, impervious gown, soap and water, small handheld scrub brush.

Standard: This procedure should take 10 minutes.

Steps	Reason
1. Put on gloves, gown, and eye protection.	These devices protect against splattering and prevent contamination of your clothes.
2. Take any removable sections apart. If cleaning is not possible immediately, soak the instrument or equipment to prevent their sticking together.	
3. Check for operation and integrity of the equipment. Defective equipment should be repaired or discarded appropriately according to office policy.	
4. Rinse the instrument with cool water.	Hot water cooks proteins on, making the contaminants more difficult to remove.
5. After the initial rinse, force streams of soapy water through any tubular or grooved instruments to clean the inside as well as the outside.	
6. Use a hot, soapy solution to dissolve fats or lubricants on the surface. Use the soaking solution indicated by office policy.	
7. After soaking for 5 to 10 minutes, use friction with a soft brush or gauze to wipe down the instrument and loosen transient microorganisms. Abrasive materials should not be used on delicate instruments and equipment. Brushes work well on grooves and joints. Open and close the jaws of scissors or forceps several times to ensure that all material has been removed.	
8. Rinse well.	Proper rinsing removes soap or detergent residue and any remaining microorganisms.
9. Dry well before autoclaving or soaking in disinfectant.	Excess moisture decreases the effectiveness of the autoclave by delaying drying, and it dilutes the disinfectant.
10. Any items (brushes, gauze, solution) used in sanitation are considered grossly contaminated and must be properly disinfected or discarded.	

Procedure 23-2

Wrapping Instruments for Sterilization in an Autoclave

Purpose:	Properly prepare and wrap instruments for sterilization in the autoclave.
Equipment:	Instruments or equipment to be sterilized, wrapping material, autoclave tape, sterilization indicator, black or blue ink pen.
Standard:	This procedure should take 10 minutes.

Steps	Reason
1. Assemble the equipment and supplies. Check the instruments being wrapped for working order.	Any instruments found to be defective, broken, or otherwise needing repair should not be wrapped or autoclaved.
2. Be sure that the wrapping material has these properties: • Permeable to steam but not contaminants • Resists tearing and puncturing during normal handling • Allows for easy opening to prevent contamination of the contents • Maintains sterility of the contents during storage	The wrap may be double layers of cotton muslin, special paper, or appropriately sized instrument pouches.

A

B

Step 2. Autoclave pouches are convenient and come in a variety of sizes.

Steps	Reason
3. Tear off one or two pieces of autoclave tape. On one piece, indicate in ink the contents of the pack or the name of the instrument that will be wrapped, the date, and your initials.	After the item is wrapped, the contents cannot be seen. Also, dating the package allows the user to determine the quality of the contents based on the amount of time (usually 30 days) that sterilized contents are considered sterile.

(continues)

Procedure 23-2 *(continued)*

Wrapping Instruments for Sterilization in an Autoclave

Steps	Purpose
4. When using autoclave wrapping material made of cotton muslin or special paper, begin by laying the material diagonally on a flat, clean, dry surface. Place the instrument in the center of the wrapping material with the ratchets or handles open. Include a sterilization indicator.	The ratchets should be left open during autoclaving to allow steam to penetrate and sterilize all surfaces.

Step 4. The ratchets are open.

Steps	Purpose
5. Fold the first flap at the bottom of the diagonal wrap up and fold back the corner making a tab.	Making a tab allows for easier opening of the pack without contaminating the contents.

Step 5. Make a tab with the corner.

(continues)

Wrapping Instruments for Sterilization in an Autoclave

Steps	Purpose
6. Fold the left corner of the wrap, then the right, each making a tab for opening the package. Secure the package with autoclave tape. 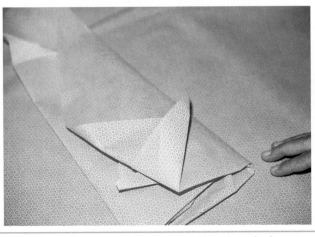	Step 6. The bottom, left, and right corners of the wrap are folded.
7. Fold the top corner down, making the tab tucked under the material. **A** **B**	Step 7. **(A)** The top corner is folded down. **(B)** Secure the wrapped instrument package with autoclave tape.

Procedure 23-3

Operating an Autoclave

Purpose: Safely sterilize instruments or equipment using an autoclave.

Equipment: Sanitized and wrapped instruments or equipment, distilled water, autoclave operating manual

Standard: This procedure should take 1 hour.

Steps	Reason
1. Assemble the equipment, including the wrapped articles and the sterilization indicator in each package according to office policy.	Some offices want a separately wrapped indicator autoclaved with the load for checking that the procedure was performed properly without opening a pack.
2. Check the water level of the autoclave reservoir and add more if needed.	Use only distilled water in the reservoir tank.
3. Add water to the internal chamber of the autoclave to the fill line.	Too little water makes too little steam; too much water may cause saturated steam, extending drying time, and may wick microorganisms into the damp packages.
4. Load the autoclave:	
A. Place trays and packs on their sides 1 to 3 inches apart.	Air circulation is not possible if items are tightly packed. Vertical placement forces out heavier air rather than pooling in the containers.
B. Put containers on their side with the lid off.	Air can circulate in containers on their side with the lid off.
C. In mixed loads, place hard objects on the bottom shelf and softer packs on the top racks.	Hard objects may form condensation that will drip onto softer items and wet them.
5. Read the instructions and close to the machine. Most machines follow the same protocol:	

5. Read the instructions and close to the machine. Most machines follow the same protocol:

   A. Close the door and secure or lock it.

   B. Turn the machine on.

   C. When the temperature gauge reaches the point required for the contents of the load (usually 250°F), set the timer. Many autoclaves can be programmed for the required time.

   D. When the timer indicates that the cycle is over, vent the chamber.

   E. After releasing the pressure to a safe level, crack the door of the autoclave to allow additional drying. Most loads dry in 5–20 min. Hard items dry faster than soft ones.

(continues)

Procedure 23-3   (continued)

Operating an Autoclave

Steps	Reason
6. When the load has cooled, remove the items.	
7. Check the separately wrapped sterilization indicator, if used, for proper sterilization.	If the indicator registers that the load was properly processed, the items in the additional packs are considered sterile; if not, the items should be considered not sterile and the load must be reprocessed.
8. Store the items in a clean, dry, dust-free area for 30 days.	After 30 days, reprocessing is necessary. The pack need not be rewrapped, but the autoclave tape should be replaced with new tape with the current date.
9. Clean the autoclave per manufacturer's suggestions, usually by scrubbing the interior chamber with a mild detergent and a soft brush. Attention to the exhaust valve will prevent lint from occluding the outlet. Rinse the machine thoroughly and allow it to dry.	Always follow the manufacturer's recommendations for cleaning the autoclave.

CHAPTER SUMMARY

Most areas of the medical office require medical asepsis to maintain cleanliness and prevent the spread of infection to the patients and staff. However, when body tissues need repair or must be opened surgically, sterile technique or surgical asepsis is required. You are responsible for maintaining surgical asepsis, which necessitates that you understand the principles and practices of medical and surgical asepsis, know disinfection and sterilization techniques, use equipment to sterilize and disinfect, and keep accurate records and adequate supplies on hand. In addition, your responsibilities include being familiar with instruments used in office surgical procedures, the content of the next chapter.

Critical Thinking Challenges

1. As the clinical medical assistant at Dr. Will's office, you have been asked to orient new employees to various aspects of the practice and develop an orientation booklet for all staff members. Design a booklet that contains the following information:

   • A basic explanation of the surgical equipment commonly used in the practice

   • The procedures for sanitizing, disinfecting, and sterilizing instruments
   • The operating instructions for the autoclave

2. Create a record that can be used to document sterilization using the autoclave.
3. Research the various types of commercial cold chemical sterilization solutions. Design a step-by-step procedure for using the solution to disinfect and sterilize. Note any hazards or safety precautions that should be followed when working with the chemical.

Answers to Checkpoint Questions

1. Sanitation is maintenance of a healthful, disease-free environment by removing organic matter and other residue. Disinfection is destruction of pathogenic microorganisms but not their spores. Sterilization destroys all microorganisms and their spores on an item or instrument.
2. An autoclave is a steam pressure chamber for sterilizing medical instruments or supplies. Distilled water is converted to steam, and as the pressure increases, the temperature of the steam increases to allow for destruction of microorganisms and their spores.
3. Autoclave tape is used on the outside of a wrapped instrument or pack to identify the contents of the pack,

the date the item was autoclaved, and the initials of the person who wrapped the pack. After exposure to steam, dark brown or black stripes will appear on the tape, acknowledging that the pack has been processed in the autoclave or exposed to steam. Sterilization indicators are placed inside the pack to indicate sterility of the contents.

4. Load the autoclave loosely; do not try to pack too many items in at once, because the steam cannot penetrate to items in the center of a crowded chamber. Place empty containers on their sides with the lids off and place all packs on their sides to allow for maximum steam circulation and penetration.

5. The time indicated for sterilization should be started only after the appropriate temperature has been reached, since the temperature and time are both important for destruction of microorganisms and their spores. Items that have been exposed to the high temperature for less time than indicated by the manufacturer of the autoclave may not be sterile.

6. The physician may use forceps to remove tissue for biopsy.

7. Because surgical instruments are delicate, improper handling may easily damage sharp blades or pointed tips. If you do drop an instrument, inspect it carefully for damage. Many instruments are expensive, but damaged instruments can usually be repaired.

8. The six items to include on a sterilization record are (1) date and time of the cycle, (2) a general description of the load, (3) time and temperature, (4) name or initials of the operator, (5) results of the sterilization indicator, and (6) load expiration date.

 Websites

Medical Resources New and Reconditioned Equipment: Midmark and Ritter Autoclaves
www.medicalresources.com

Amsco autoclaves and sterilizers: Alfa Medical
www.sterilizers.com

Sklar surgical instruments www.sklarcorp.com

Glutaraldehyde occupational hazards
www.cdc.gov/niosh/2001-115.html

Glutaraldehyde guidelines for safe use and handling in health care facilities
www.state.nj.us/health/eoh/survweb/glutar.pdf

Occupational Safety and Health Administration
www.governmentguide.com

24

Assisting With Minor Office Surgery

ROLE DELINEATION

ADMINISTRATIVE: ADMINISTRATIVE
PROCEDURES
- Perform basic administrative medical assisting
functions
- Understand and adhere to managed care policies and
procedures

CLINICAL: FUNDAMENTAL PRINCIPLES
- Apply principles of aseptic technique and infection
control
- Comply with quality assurance practices

CLINICAL: DIAGNOSTIC ORDERS
- Collect and process specimens

CLINICAL: PATIENT CARE
- Adhere to established patient screening procedures
- Prepare and maintain examination and treatment areas
- Prepare patient for examinations, procedures, and
treatments
- Recognize and respond to emergencies
- Coordinate patient care information with other
health care providers

GENERAL: PROFESSIONALISM

- Display a professional manner and image
- Demonstrate initiative and responsibility
- Work as a member of the health care team
- Set priorities and perform multiple tasks
- Adapt to change
- Treat all patients with compassion and empathy

GENERAL: COMMUNICATION SKILLS

- Recognize and respect cultural diversity
- Adapt communications to individual's ability to understand
- Recognize and respond effectively to verbal, nonverbal, and written communications
- Use medical terminology appropriately
- Serve as a liaison

GENERAL: LEGAL CONCEPTS

- Perform within legal and ethical boundaries
- Prepare and maintain medical records
- Document accurately
- Comply with established risk management and safety procedures

GENERAL: INSTRUCTION

- Instruct individuals according to their needs
- Explain office policies and procedures
- Teach methods of health promotion and disease prevention

GENERAL: OPERATIONAL FUNCTIONS

- Perform routine maintenance of administrative and clinical equipment

CHAPTER COMPETENCIES

LEARNING OBJECTIVES

Upon successfully completing this chapter, you will be able to:

1. Spell and define key terms.
2. List your responsibilities before, during, and after minor office surgery.
3. Identify the guidelines for preparing and maintaining sterility of the field and surgical equipment during a minor office procedure.
4. State your responsibility in relation to informed consent and patient preparation.
5. Describe the types of needles and sutures and the uses of each.
6. Explain the purpose of local anesthetics and list three commonly used in the medical office.
7. Describe the various methods of skin closure used in the medical office.
8. Explain your responsibility during surgical specimen collection.
9. Describe the guidelines for applying a sterile dressing.
10. List the types of laser surgery and electrosurgery used in the medical office and explain the precautions for each.

PERFORMANCE OBJECTIVES

Upon successfully completing this chapter, you will be able to:

1. Open sterile surgical packs (Procedure 24-1).
2. Use sterile transfer forceps (Procedure 24-2).
3. Add sterile solution to a sterile field (Procedure 24-3).
4. Perform skin preparation and hair removal (Procedure 24-4).
5. Apply sterile gloves (Procedure 24-5).
6. Apply a sterile dressing (Procedure 24-6).
7. Change an existing sterile dressing (Procedure 24-7).
8. Assist with excisional surgery (Procedure 24-8).
9. Assist with incision and drainage (Procedure 24-9).
10. Remove sutures (Procedure 24-10).
11. Remove staples (Procedure 24-11).

KEY TERMS

approximate	coagulate	fulgurate	purulent
atraumatic	dehiscence	keratosis	swaged needle
bandage	dressing	lentigines	traumatic
cautery	electrode	preservative	

As a clinical medical assistant, you will have many responsibilities when minor surgery is performed in the physician's office. These include the following:

1. Reinforcing the physician's instructions to the patient regarding preparation for surgery, including at-home skin preparation as directed, fasting from food or fluids, bowel preparation, and other preparations that may be ordered.
2. Identifying the patient and gathering the proper equipment and supplies before the physician is ready to do the procedure.
3. Obtaining and witnessing the informed consent document if instructed to do so by the physician.
4. Preparing the treatment room, instruments, supplies, and equipment.
5. Assisting the physician during the procedure.
6. Applying a **dressing** and **bandage** to the surgical wound.
7. Instructing the patient about postoperative wound care, including observing the wound for changes that indicate infection or problems with healing.
8. Assisting the patient as needed before, during, and after the procedure.
9. Assisting with postoperative instructions such as prescriptions, medications, and scheduling return visits.
10. Removing and caring for instruments, equipment, and supplies, including properly disposing of disposable items, sharps, and contaminated or unused supplies.
11. Preparing the room for the next patient.

Although the types of surgery performed in the medical office vary with the type of medical specialty, the procedure for preparing the patient and setting up the supplies and equipment will require the same process, known as sterile technique. Procedures performed in many general practice offices include suture insertion and removal, incision and drainage, and sebaceous cystectomy. Some gynecological procedures and urinary procedures also require sterile technique.

PREPARING AND MAINTAINING A STERILE FIELD

Minor office surgery involves procedures that penetrate the body's normally intact surface. Whenever a patient has an open wound, surgical asepsis must be maintained to prevent pathogens from entering the body tissues and causing an infection. Follow the guidelines listed below to maintain sterility before and during a sterile procedure:

1. Do not let sterile packages get damp or wet. Microorganisms can be drawn into the package by wicking, or absorption of the liquid along with the pathogens in it. If a package sterilized in the medical office gets moist, it must be repackaged in a clean, dry wrapper and sterilized again. Damp or wet disposable packages must be discarded.

2. Always face a sterile field to ensure that the area has not been contaminated. If you must leave the area or work with your back to the sterile field, the field must be covered with a sterile drape using sterile technique.
3. Hold all sterile items above waist level. When sterile items are not in your field of vision, you must presume that they have become contaminated.
4. Place sterile items in the middle of the sterile field. A 1-inch border around the field is considered contaminated.
5. Do not spill any liquids, even sterile liquids, onto the sterile field. Remember, the surface below the field is not sterile, and moisture will allow microorganisms to be wicked up into the surgical field.
6. Do not cough, sneeze, or talk over the sterile field. Microorganisms from the respiratory tract can contaminate the field.
7. Never reach over the sterile field. Dust or lint from clothing can contaminate the sterile field.
8. Do not pass soiled supplies, such as gauze or instruments, over the sterile field.
9. If you know or suspect that the sterile field has been contaminated, alert the physician. Sterility must be reestablished before the procedure can continue.

Sterile Surgical Packs

Preparing the treatment or examination room for a surgical procedure is usually the responsibility of the medical assistant. Many medical offices keep a box with index cards or a loose-leaf binder listing the surgical procedures that are commonly performed in the office, including the items needed for setup. Some medical offices prepackage sterile setups in a suitable wrapper and prepare them in the office by autoclave sterilization (Fig. 24-1). These setups are labeled according to the type of procedure (e.g., lesion removal, suture setup) and contain the general instruments for that procedure. Some basic supplies (e.g., gauze sponges,

FIGURE 24-1. A wrapped sterile surgical pack.

cotton balls, and towels) may also be included before autoclaving.

To reduce the time and effort of sterilizing packs on site, many offices use commercially packaged disposable surgical packs. Disposable surgical packs have become increasingly popular because they are convenient and come with an almost infinite variety of contents. They may contain one sterile article (such as a 4 × 4 sterile dressing) or a complete sterile surgical setup. Many of the supplies are packaged in peel-apart wrappers with two loose flaps that can be pulled apart and the sterile items dropped carefully onto the operative field. The insides of the wrappers may be opened out and used as sterile field. Some packages are enclosed in plastic and wrapped inside a barrier material that can be used as a sterile field.

Directions for opening are clearly marked on the outside of sterile packs and should be read carefully before opening. If the surgical pack is opened improperly, the contents will be contaminated and cannot be used. Commercially prepared sterile packs are generally more expensive than packages prepared at the medical office, so care must be taken to avoid waste. Labels on commercially prepared packs list the contents in the pack item by item; site-prepared packs usually only state the type of setup. You should check the expiration date on the package; if the pack has expired, it must not be used, since sterility is in question. Procedure 24-1 describes the steps for opening sterile surgical packs.

As discussed in Chapter 23, a sterilization indicator should be put inside each surgical package to show that it has been properly sterilized. Tapes, strips, and packaging with indicator stripes or dots on the outside of the packs do not guarantee sterility. In the autoclave, sterility is achieved only by the right combination of temperature, pressure, steam, and time. In addition, improperly packing the autoclave can impede steam penetration to the articles. Therefore, sterilization indicators should be packaged within each pack and must be checked before beginning the surgical procedure. When you open a package of sterile objects, the procedure is the same whether the items are sterilized at the office or commercially prepared. For all sterile packs or supplies, keep in mind that:

1. Clean hands are used to open the sterile items or packages. The unsterile area is the outside surface of the outside wrapper.
2. The sterile area includes the inside surface of the outside wrapper, the inside wrapper if any, and the contents of the package. These areas or items must not come into contact with any surface, including the hands, or they are considered contaminated and must be replaced.
3. Items are considered contaminated and should be repackaged and sterilized again:
   A. When moisture is present on the pack
   B. If the items are dropped outside the sterile field
   C. If the date on the outside of the package is beyond 30 days for site-prepared packages or the

posted expiration date on commercially prepared packages
   D. If the sterilization indicator inside the pack has not changed color
   E. If the wrapper is torn, damaged, or wet
   F. When any area is known or thought to have been touched by a contaminated item.

Checkpoint Question

1. What are the nine guidelines that must be followed to maintain a sterile field?

Sterile Transfer Forceps

Setting up the sterile field requires clean hands and careful technique to avoid contaminating the contents inside the sterile area or field. In the event that sterile items must be manipulated or placed on the sterile field, sterile transfer forceps or sterile gloved hands must be used, since the hands can never be sterilized. The tips of the forceps and the articles being transferred must both remain sterile (FIG. 24-2). The handles, however, are considered medically aseptic, not sterile, because these are touched by the bare hands of the person using them. Sterile transfer forceps are stored in a dry sterile container, in a wrapped sterile package, or in a sterile solution in a closed container system, such as the Bard Parker, which helps protect the tips of the forceps from contamination. In a closed dry container system, the forceps and container must be sanitized and autoclaved daily. In a closed sterile solution system, the forceps and the container are sterilized at least every day, and fresh sterilization solution is added daily. Only one forceps should be stored in a container to decrease the chance of contamination. After using the sterile transfer forceps without contaminating, place the forceps back in the container for use throughout the procedure or in other procedures scheduled that day. Follow office policy for sterilizing the forceps. Proper use of sterile transfer forceps requires that certain guidelines be followed (Procedure 24-2).

FIGURE 24-2. Sterile transfer forceps may be used to add or move items on the sterile field.

Adding Peel-back Packages and Pouring Sterile Solutions

Procedure packages are frequently prepared with supplies (e.g., cotton balls and gauze squares) to eliminate the need to add more at the time of setup. However, patient assessment at the time of surgery may suggest the need for additional items. These small supplies are usually provided commercially in peel-apart packages. These packages may contain small or single items to be added to the surgical field. The package has an upper edge with two flaps that are used to open the package in a manner that maintains the sterility of the contents. The package is properly opened by using both hands with the thumbs just inside the tops of the edges. The flaps are separated using a slow, outward motion of the thumbs and flaps (FIG. 24-3). Keep in mind that the inside of

F I G U R E   2 4 - 4 .   The physician may use forceps to remove small supplies from peel-back packages.

the sealed package and the contents are sterile but will be contaminated if touched by anything that is not sterile, such as your fingers, or if talking, coughing, or sneezing occurs as you open it. There are three ways to add the contents of peel-back packages to the sterile field:

1. *Sterile transfer forceps.* Peel the edges apart with a rolling motion as described earlier. Holding down the two edges, lift the contents up and away with the forceps (FIG. 24-4).
2. *Sterile gloved hand.* This method requires two persons, usually the medical assistant, who opens the package, and the physician, who removes the contents with a sterile gloved hand. You must carefully hold the edges to avoid contaminating the physician's gloves (FIG. 24-5).
3. *Flip of the contents onto a sterile field.* To do this, you step back from the sterile field to prevent your hands and the outer wrapper, which is not sterile, from crossing it. Pull the edges down and away from the package contents and carefully toss or flip the item onto the middle of the sterile field without touching the 1-inch border around the sterile field. This 1-inch area is considered not sterile.

In most cases, items in presterilized peel-back envelopes cannot be sterilized after being opened and must be discarded even if not used. Because such items are relatively expensive, they should not be opened unnecessarily. A supply of items that might be needed during the procedure should be placed conveniently close to the area and added only if needed.

Whether site prepared or commercially prepared, trays are not processed or stored with liquids in open containers. Solutions must be added as needed at the time of setup. Some procedures require sterile water or saline, while others

A

B

F I G U R E   2 4 - 3 .   (A) Open sterile packets by grasping the edges and rolling the thumbs outward. (B) Opening the packet properly forms a sterile field.

FIGURE 24-5. Sterile gloved hands may be used to remove sterile items.

require an antiseptic solution, such as Betadine. These will be poured into sterile containers added to the sterile field with sterile transfer forceps (Procedure 24-3).

Checkpoint Question

2. What are three ways that contents of peel-back packages can be added to the sterile field?

PREPARING THE PATIENT FOR MINOR OFFICE SURGERY

Patient Instructions and Consent

Many of the minor surgical procedures that are performed in the medical office require a full explanation of the procedure and informed consent (FIG. 24-6). Either the patient agrees and the procedure is performed or the patient refuses and the procedure is not done. The informed consent document must state the procedure, its purpose and expected results along with possible side effects, risks, and complications. Although the physician is responsible for informing the patient of the details of the procedure and any risks involved, the patient may ask questions, including how long the procedure will last, what preparations will be needed, or whether fasting will be necessary. You may answer these questions after verifying the information with the physician.

It is always a good practice to give specific written instructions to the patient for any preparations to be made before arriving at the office so that the procedure can be done on schedule and with no preventable risk to the patient. The physician may prescribe medication for the patient to take at home before the procedure. As with any patient instructions, you should notify the physician if the patient seems confused or does not understand the instructions. Encourage the patient to call the office if questions arise later. Of course, the instructions should be documented in the medical record.

Positioning and Draping

Before positioning the patient for a minor surgical procedure, ask the patient to void; this helps prevent discomfort during the procedure. Offer to help the patient remove whatever clothing is necessary to expose the operative site. Expose only the area necessary for the procedure to ensure the patient's privacy. An air-conditioned office may be uncomfortably cool for patients. You may provide additional sheets or a blanket for comfort.

Assist the patient to assume a comfortable position on the examining table that offers exposure of and access to the operative site. Provide pillows for comfort and support. Do not make patients maintain uncomfortable positions, such as the lithotomy or knee-chest, while waiting for the physician. Position the patient only when the physician is ready to begin the procedure. At the end of the procedure, assist the patient from the table, allowing as much time as needed. Often patients who did not need help removing clothing will require help dressing following minor office surgery. Be aware of this and assist as necessary.

The type of procedure and the patient's position determine the type of drapes used to expose the operative site and cover the patient. Disposable paper drapes are most commonly used in the medical office. They come in many sizes and shapes, each suited for specific uses. Paper drapes can be used alone, in combination, or with separate drape sheets and towels. Fenestrated drapes have an opening to expose the operative site while covering adjacent areas. Fenestrated drapes may be small, such as those used for suture insertion, or large, such as those used to cover the legs and lower abdomen but expose the perineal area. Some sterile drapes are combined with adhesive-backed clear plastic, which sticks to the patient's skin and eliminates the need for towel clamps.

LEGAL TIP

Informed Consent
In today's litigious society, physicians routinely obtain signed informed consent forms even for minor office procedures. Printed forms are available, or the office may have its own form. Such forms may be used for procedures requiring legal witnessed signatures. Other more generic ones have blank spaces to add information relevant to the procedure to be performed. All forms should have spaces for the date and signatures of the patient, physician, and witness or witnesses. The medical assistant is not responsible for informing the patient but often witnesses the signing of the document by the patient. It is the physician's legal responsibility to inform the patient before the consent form is signed by the patient or legal guardian.

SPECIAL CONSENT TO OPERATION OR OTHER PROCEDURE(S)

PATIENT _____   PATIENT NUMBER _____

DATE _____   TIME _____

1.   I HEREBY AUTHORIZE DOCTOR _____ AND/OR SUCH ASSIS-
     TANTS AS MAY BE SELECTED BY HIM, TO PERFORM THE FOLLOWING PROCEDURE(S):
     _____

     ON _____
             (NAME OF PATIENT OR MYSELF)

2.   THE PROCEDURE(S) LISTED ABOVE HAVE BEEN EXPLAINED TO ME BY DR.
     AND I UNDERSTAND THE NATURE AND THE CONSEQUENCES OF THE PROCEDURE(S).

3.   I RECOGNIZE THAT, DURING THE COURSE OF THE OPERATION, UNFORESEEN CONDI-
     TIONS MAY NECESSITATE ADDITIONAL OR DIFFERENT PROCEDURES THAN THOSE SET
     FORTH. I FURTHER AUTHORIZE AND REQUEST THAT THE ABOVE NAMED SURGEON, HIS
     ASSISTANTS, OR HIS DESIGNEES PERFORM SUCH PROCEDURES AS ARE IN HIS PRO-
     FESSIONAL JUDGMENT NECESSARY AND DESIRABLE, INCLUDING, BUT NOT LIMITED TO,
     PROCEDURES INVOLVING PATHOLOGY AND RADIOLOGY. THE AUTHORITY GRANTED
     UNDER THIS PARAGRAPH SHALL EXTEND TO REMEDYING CONDITIONS NOT KNOWN TO
     DR. _____ AT THE TIME THE OPERATION IS COMMENCED.

4.   I AM AWARE THAT THE PRACTICE OF MEDICINE AND SURGERY IS NOT AN EXACT SCI-
     ENCE AND I ACKNOWLEDGE THAT NO GUARANTEES HAVE BEEN MADE TO ME AS TO THE
     RESULTS OF THE OPERATION OR PROCEDURE.

5.   TISSUE REMOVED DURING SURGERY SHALL BE SENT TO PATHOLOGY TO BE EXAMINED
     AND DISPOSED OF IN ACCORDANCE WITH THE RULES AND REGULATIONS OF THE MED-
     ICAL STAFF OF THE SURGERY CENTER.

Procedure has been discussed with patient. (Surgeon's Signature) _____   SIGNATURE OF PATIENT _____

PATIENT IS UNABLE TO SIGN BECAUSE   ❏ HE (SHE) IS A MINOR _____ YEARS OF AGE

                                      ❏ OTHER (SPECIFY) _____

WITNESS _____   PERSON AUTHORIZED TO SIGN FOR PATIENT _____

                        RELATIONSHIP OF ABOVE TO PATIENT _____

FIGURE 24-6. Sample consent form.

Sterile drapes are applied by picking up the drape on the 1-inch border (no gloves needed), lifting over the surgical area without contaminating the drape, and laying the drape on the patient from farthest away to closest (FIG. 24-7). This ensures that you do not reach over the drape after it is placed on the patient.

When removing contaminated drapes from the patient following a procedure, put on clean examination gloves and carefully roll the items away from the body, keeping the contaminated areas innermost. This helps to surround the dirtier areas of the sheet with the cleaner area and helps prevent contaminating your clothing. Because the sheets, towels, or drapes may be contaminated with blood or other body fluids, follow standard precautions (see Chapter 19).

Preparing the Patient's Skin

The goal of preoperative skin preparation is to remove as many microorganisms as possible from the skin to decrease the chance of wound contamination. Skin preparation may be simply applying an antiseptic solution to the area or may include removing gross contaminants and hair from the operative area. Hair can be removed with depilatory creams but often requires shaving the skin (Procedure 24-4).

FIGURE 24-7. Applying a sterile drape

Checkpoint Question

3. What is a fenestrated drape?

ASSISTING THE PHYSICIAN

Local Anesthetics

When office surgery of any kind is performed, the site is first anesthetized (numbed) with a local anesthetic to minimize the pain and discomfort felt by the patient. Occasionally, when a wound contains embedded debris that must be removed prior to repair, the local anesthetic will be injected before preparing the wound site to facilitate wound cleaning. Lidocaine (Xylocaine) and lidocaine with epinephrine (0.5–2%) are two of the many local anesthetics commonly used in medical offices. Others are lidocaine (Baylocaine), mepivacaine (Carbocaine), and bupivacaine (Marcaine). Epinephrine is added to local anesthetics to cause vasoconstriction and to slow absorption by the body and lengthen the anesthetic's effectiveness. It may be used when the physician anticipates a long procedure, but anesthesia with epinephrine should never be used on the tips of the fingers, toes, nose, or penis, since the vasoconstriction may cause death of tissue in these areas.

Two methods may be used to administer local anesthesia. In one method, you draw the anesthetic for the physician into a syringe, keeping the vial beside the syringe for the physician's approval. In this case, the anesthetic is usually given to the patient before the physician puts on sterile gloves, since the outside of the syringe and needle unit are not sterile.

The second method is used if the physician puts on sterile gloves before administering the anesthetic. In this case, a sterile syringe and needle are included on the sterile field setup. When the physician is ready to administer the anesthetic, you show the physician the label on the vial, clean the rubber stopper of the vial with an alcohol swab, and hold the vial while the physician draws the required amount into the syringe (FIG. 24-8). There are many methods of holding the vial securely while the physician withdraws the medication. You and the physician together develop a method to maintain surgical asepsis.

Wound Closure

Many types of wounds require closure to ensure rapid healing with minimal scarring. This is accomplished by bringing the edges of the wound as close together as possible in their original position (approximation). Sutures are used to close wounds and incisions and to bring tissue layers into close approximation. Skin closures are performed after cyst or tissue sample removal, to close lacerations, or anytime skin surfaces require assistance for healing. Supplies used to suture skin include needles and suture material. Skin staples are sometimes used to close large incisions over areas where **dehiscence** can occur, such as the knee, hip, or abdomen, but these are not usually inserted in the medical office.

Needles and Sutures

Needles used in minor office surgery are chosen for the type of surgery to be performed. Needles are classified thus:

- By shape, curved or straight
- By point, tapered or cutting
- By eye, **atraumatic** (swaged) or **traumatic** (with an eye)

FIGURE 24-8. Hold the vial containing the anesthetic downward, supporting that wrist with the other hand.

Spanish Terminology

Es alergico a la Novocaina u otros tipos de anesthesia?	Are you allergic to Novocaine or other anesthetics?
Debe firmar esta formulario.	You need to sign this form.
Usted tiene tres puntos.	You have three stitches.
Le duelen los puntos?	Do your stitches hurt?
Vuelva a la oficina el lunes.	Return to the office on Monday.

Round straight needles are called domestic needles, and straight cutting needles are called Keith needles. Curved needles used in surgical procedures are usually clamped in a needle holder before being handed to or used by the physician. Straight needles are not clamped in a needle holder but are handed to the physician with the point up. Straight needles are rarely used in medical offices.

Cutting needles are used on tough tissues, such as skin. Round or tapered (noncutting) needles are used on subcutaneous tissue, peritoneum, and muscle. Atraumatic, or **swaged, needles** have suture material that has been mechanically attached to the needle by the manufacturer and do not require threading. These are called atraumatic because they cause less trauma than threaded ones as they pass through the tissues. Unlike atraumatic or swaged needles, threaded needles have an eye with a double thickness of suture that must be pulled through tissues. The double thickness of this suture makes a larger and therefore more traumatic opening in the tissues than a swaged suture.

In medical offices curved swaged needles are used far more often than any other type. Swaged needles are selected for a procedure according to the size and length of the suture material and the attached needle gauge clearly marked on the packaging material. When a suture must be threaded through an eyed needle, both needle gauge and suture size must be selected. The physician usually selects the suture and needle, but you should know your physician's preferences and anticipate needs whenever possible. Sutures, needles, and suture–needle combinations are contained in peel-apart packages that are sterile on the inside so that they can be added to the sterile field (FIG. 24-9). This may be done by sterile transfer forceps, a sterile gloved hand, or by carefully flipping them onto the sterile field.

Sutures come in various gauges (diameters) and lengths. Very thick sutures are numbered 1 to 5, with 5 being the thickest. Sutures smaller than size 1 are expressed with added zeros. Small sutures, which become progressively smaller, range from 1-0 to 10-0 or smaller (i.e., 1-0, 2-0, 3-0, and so forth). A very fine 10-0 suture, which is about the diameter of a human hair, is generally used in microsurgery. When a fine suture is needed, such as on the face and neck, 23-0 and 24-0 sutures are commonly used. A very fine suture decreases scarring and gives a better cosmetic result.

Sutures also come in absorbable and nonabsorbable forms. **Absorbable sutures, or catgut (made from the intestines of sheep or cattle), are readily broken down in the body and usually do not have to be removed.** The two forms of absorbable gut suture are chromic, which is chemically treated to delay absorption for several days, and plain, which is not treated and is more quickly absorbed. Absorbable sutures are used most frequently in hospitals during surgery on deep tissues.

Nonabsorbable sutures are available in a great variety of brands, sizes, lengths, and swaged needles; they are the most versatile. **Nonabsorbable sutures either remain in the body permanently or are removed after healing.** Nonabsorbable sutures are used on the skin, intestines, or bone; to ligate larger vessels; and to attach heart valves and various artificial and natural grafts. Nonabsorbable sutures are made of fibers such as silk, nylon, Dacron, or cotton or stainless steel wire.

FIGURE 24-9. Suture material and needles are supplied in see-through packages with the size of the suture material and the type of needle listed on the packet. The inside of the packet is sterile.

Skin Staples

Another form of nonabsorbable suture is the metal skin clip or staple. These are commonly made of stainless steel, but some very specialized types are made of sterling silver for use in neurosurgery and other procedures. When nonabsorbable sutures or staples are used to close skin wounds, they must be removed when the wound has healed completely. Depending on the location of the skin wound, nonabsorbable sutures or staples remain in place for varying lengths of time: the head and neck may require 3 to 5 days, whereas the arms and legs may require 7 to 10 days.

A

 Checkpoint Question

4. How do swaged needles differ from threaded ones?

Adhesive Skin Closures

Adhesive skin closures are used to approximate the edges of a small wound if sutures are not needed. They are appropriate where there is little tension on the skin edges. The strips are placed transversely across the line of the wound to bring the wound edges in close approximation (FIG. 24-10). In most instances, the strips are left in place until they fall off. However, in some cases, the physician may want them removed or replaced if soiled with drainage. When removing these strips, carefully lift the edges distal to the wound and pull gently toward the wound. Never pull the strips away from the wound as tension on the wound site may disrupt the healing process.

B

F I G U R E 2 4 - 1 0 . Adhesive skin closures. (A) These lightweight lengths of porous tape are used for closing small wounds. (B) Strips are placed transversely across a wound.

Specimen Collection

Many minor office surgical procedures yield specimens that must be sent to a laboratory to be examined by a pathologist. Specimens include samples of tissue, wound exudate, foreign bodies, and so on. The medical assistant must choose the proper container with the appropriate **preservative** (substance that delays decomposition) for the type of procedure being performed. The laboratory where the specimen is sent usually provides the appropriate containers with preservative, and you should have a stock of them on hand. Hold the open container steady to avoid touching the sides as the physician drops the specimen into the preservative (FIG. 24-11).

You are responsible for attaching a label to the specimen container with the patient's name and the date written clearly on the label, and you must complete a laboratory request form to send with the specimen. These forms require information such as the patient's name, age, sex, identification number or social security number, date, type of specimen, type of examination, and the physician's name or laboratory

contract number. Specimens obtained during a minor surgical procedure must be transported to the pathology laboratory as quickly as possible.

Electrosurgery

Electrosurgery uses high-frequency alternating electric current to destroy or cut and remove tissue. It is used to **coagulate**, or clot, small bleeding vessels. Electrosurgery is considered an alternative to traditional office surgery and is rapidly gaining favor for many procedures. An advantage of electrical surgery is the cautery produced by the electricity that seals small bleeding vessels and coagulates nearby cells to reduce bleeding and loss of cell fluid. Electrosurgical units use disposable **electrodes** with tips of various sizes and shapes to deliver the desired amount of electric current to the tissues (FIG. 24-12). The following procedures are considered electrosurgery:

- *Fulguration* destroys tissue with controlled electric sparks. As the physician holds the electrode tip 1 to 2 mm from the site, a series of sparks destroys the superficial cells at the site.

FIGURE 24-11. Tissue samples are placed in the preservative by the physician.

FIGURE 24-12. A disposable electrosurgical unit. The blade is designed either to cut or to cauterize.

- *Electrodesiccation* dries and separates tissue with an electric current. The electrode is placed directly on the site.
- *Electrocautery* causes quick coagulation of small blood vessels with the heat created by the electric current. Electrocautery is commonly referred to as electrocoagulation.
- *Electrosection* is used for incision or excision of tissue. Bleeding is minimal with this type of procedure, but more damage can occur to surrounding tissues.

Medical offices frequently use electrosurgery to remove moles, cysts, warts, and certain types of skin and cervical cancers. Electrosurgical equipment includes various elec-

trode tips, such as blades, needles, loops, and balls, each with specific uses.

During electrosurgery, your responsibilities are to ensure the safety and comfort of the patient and to pass the electrode to the physician as needed. As with all instruments, the electrode must be passed in its functional position. The electrode is handed to the physician with the tip down.

Because electric current is delivered to the tip by the electrosurgical machine, great care should be exercised to prevent injuries. Although the physician activates the device, it is possible to cause injury to the patient, physician, or yourself by careless handling of the device. Take care to ground the patient before electrosurgery. Metal conducts electricity and can cause serious burns. When assisting with electrosurgery, follow these safety measures:

- Ensure that all working parts are in good repair. The electrical current is carefully regulated; if the machine is defective, serious injury to the patient may occur.
- Ensure that all metal is removed from the patient. The patient must be asked about any metal implants or a cardiac pacemaker. Metal conducts electricity and can cause burns. Metal implants may become very hot, and pacemakers may malfunction during the procedure.
- Ensure that the patient is grounded with a pad supplied by the manufacturer. Attach it to the patient at a site recommended by the manufacturer (some recommend placing the pad far from the operative site; others suggest placing it near the site). Improper placement can result in injury.
- Place the grounding pad firmly and completely against the patient's skin. Apply a conducting gel to the pad and to the patient's skin, or use an adhesive-backed pad to facilitate conduction through the grounding pad. Areas of skin against the pad that are not well connected will result in hot spots and may burn the patient.

Although disposable tips are usually used today, reusable tips are still used in some offices. Reusable tips are disinfected and processed in the autoclave according to the manufac-

TRIAGE

The physician has just performed a needle biopsy for a lesion on Mr. Smith's lower back. You have to do these three tasks:

A. Label the specimen and complete the laboratory requisition form.

B. Apply a dressing to Mr. Smith's lower back.

C. Help Mr. Smith get dressed and into a wheelchair.

How do you sort these tasks? What do you do first? Second? Third?

The correct order is A, B, C. All specimens must be immediately labeled. Incorrectly labeled specimens or poorly completed requisition forms may result in the laboratory not being able to test the specimen. It is appropriate to apply a dressing to the wound and then assist the patient to get dressed and into a wheelchair.

turer's directions. Reusable tips may be polished with steel wool if they become dull. Disposable tips should be discarded after use. Electrosurgical machines should be inspected periodically to ensure proper working order. The operating manual states the periodic maintenance to be performed by office staff and routine inspections to be performed by trained technicians. Surfaces should be kept clean and dry; machines should be kept covered when not in use.

Checkpoint Question

5. Which type of electrosurgery is used for incision or excision of tissue?

Laser Surgery

Lasers are devices that focus high-intensity light in a narrow beam to create extreme heat and energy. In medicine, lasers can be used to cut tissue and coagulate small bleeding vessels. There are many types of lasers, each with fairly specific applications in medicine. These are the most common types of lasers encountered in the medical office:

- Argon laser, used for coagulation
- Carbon dioxide laser, used for cutting tissue
- ND: YAG, used for coagulation and to separate warts and moles from surrounding tissues

Light from the laser is not usually visible. Colored filters are used to illuminate the laser's target, enabling the physician to direct the laser beam to the affected area. As with other electronic devices, attention to care and handling of the laser helps ensure that it is in good working order when it is needed. It is important to read and follow the manufacturer's recommended maintenance procedures as described in the instruction manual.

Everyone who is in the room, including the patient, during the laser procedure is required to wear goggles for eye protection. Health care workers are recommended to complete a training program before assisting with laser procedures to ensure that safety precautions are followed.

Checkpoint Question

6. What is one important safety feature worth noting when assisting with a laser procedure?

POSTSURGICAL PROCEDURES

Sterile Dressings

Sterile dressings are items such as 4×4 inch absorbent gauze sponges and nonadhering dressings that have been processed for use on open wounds. Sterile dressings are generally prepackaged in small numbers but may come in bulk containers. They are manufactured in various sizes and shapes, each for a specific use and chosen according to the size of the wound and the amount of drainage.

Dressings should be handled with sterile technique. A sterile dressing may be secured by various bandages (sling, cravat, roller, tubular gauze) to hold the dressing in place, protect the injured part, or restrict movement. Chapter 29 describes bandaging techniques. Procedure 24-5 describes putting on sterile gloves, Procedure 24-6 explains applying a sterile dressing to a surgical wound, and Procedure 24-7 explains changing an existing dressing on a wound.

A sterile dressing is considered contaminated if it is damp or outdated, if its wrapper is damaged, or if it is improperly removed from its wrapper. Sterile dressings are used directly over a wound for the following:

1. To cover and protect from contamination
2. To absorb drainage such as blood, serum, or pus
3. To exert pressure on an open wound to control bleeding
4. To hide disfigurement during healing
5. To hold medications against a wound to facilitate healing

When you remove a sterile dressing or change an existing one, always wear clean examination gloves and carefully observe for any drainage or exudates, noting this in the patient's chart. The terminology for describing wound drainage is outlined in Box 24-1. Immediately following the closure of a wound, it is normal to see serous or serosanguinous drainage in scant or moderate amounts, depending on the extent of the wound or incision. **Purulent** drainage, or drainage with color other than pink, is a sign of infection. Notify the physician when the wound is uncovered so that it can be examined and a decision made regarding how well healing is progressing. Box 24-2 describes the types and phases of wound healing.

Box 24-1

WOUND DRAINAGE

When observing wound drainage, be sure to note:

Color
- Serous (clear)
- Sanguinous (blood tinged)
- Serosanguinous (pinkish or clear and red mixed)
- Purulent (white, green, or yellow-tinged drainage; usually accompanied by an unpleasant odor characteristic of infection)

Amount
- Copious (large amount)
- Medium (moderate amount)
- Scant (small amount)

The amount can also be quantified by indicating the size of the drainage (e.g., 2-inch diameter, entire 4×4 dressing saturated) or the size of the dressing.

B o x   2 4 - 2

THE HEALING PROCESS

Types of Wound Healing

Healing by Primary Intention: This simplest form of healing occurs in wounds whose edges are closely approximated, allowing the entrance of little or no bacteria to complicate the process. The edges of the wound lie closely together, new cells form quickly to bind the site, and capillaries expand themselves across the tissue break to restore circulation to the tissues. Scarring is usually minimal.

Healing by Secondary Intention: Granulation of tissue is present in the wound and the edges of the wound join indirectly. Because the skin edges are not closely approximated, additional new cells are required to fill spaces in the lesion. Capillaries may not be able to reach across the gap to restore full circulation. Nerves may not rejoin, which results in diminished nerve stimulus through the area. A large scab forms to protect the area while healing

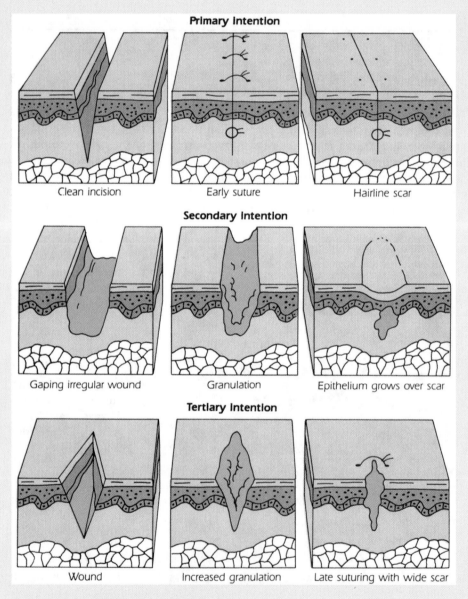

Types of wound healing. (*Top*) Primary intention. *Left to right*: Clean incision; early suture; hairline scar. (*Center*) Secondary intention. *Left to right*: Gaping irregular wound; granulation epithelium grows over scar. (*Bottom*) Tertiary intention. *Left to right*: Wound; increased granulation; late suturing with wide scar.

Box 24-2 (continued)

goes on below it. Scarring is more severe than with primary intention healing.

Healing by Tertiary Intention: The wound initially is left open if there is the possibility that the wound may already be contaminated with microorganisms and closing it would only trap the microorganisms, increasing the potential for an infection. The wound is left open to fill in with granular tissue. There is considerable scar formation.

Phases of Wound Healing

Phase I (inflammatory, lag, or exudative phase): This phase usually lasts from 1 to 4 days. The body attempts to heal itself by increasing the circulation to the part and by beginning to reroute or repair the supplying vessels. The increased circulation brings with it more white blood cells to mount a defense against pathogens. Serum and red blood cells brought by the additional blood form a gluelike fibrin to plug the wound. As the fibrin dries, it pulls the edges of the wound closer together and forms a scab. Signs that this phase is working are edema from the tissue fluid, warmth from the extra blood, redness from the vasodilation, and pain from the pressure on the nerve endings caused by the edema.

*Phase II (proliferative, healing, or granulation phase):*This phase may last from several days to several weeks. The]vessels continue to repair themselves and may reroute if damage is severe. The scab from phase I continues to dry and to pull the edges of the wound as closely together as possible.

Phase III (remodeling, maturation, or scarring phase): This phase may take from weeks to years, depending upon the severity of the wound. Fibroblasts build scar tissue to guard the area.

PATIENT EDUCATION

Postoperative Instructions

After any surgical procedure, the patient should receive written and verbal discharge instructions, including how to care for the postoperative wound, taking prescribed medications correctly, and returning to the office for follow-up visits, dressing changes, and suture removal as ordered by the physician. The patient should be informed of the signs and symptoms of infection and should be instructed to report the following conditions:

- Excessive bleeding from the wound (additional teaching should include how to stop any excessive bleeding by applying direct pressure or elevating the body area).
- Redness, red streaks, or excessive swelling around the surgical site.
- Fever.

Tell the patient to call the office if these symptoms arise. In addition, you will tell the patient:

- When to return to the office to have the dressing or bandage changed or how and when to change the bandage or dressing at home.
- The need for follow-up visits. Have the patient schedule the appointment or appointments before leaving and provide an appointment card for each appointment.
- After speaking with the physician, tell the patient when he or she can take a shower or bath and whether the surgical wound can get wet. (Whether the wound may get wet depends on location and depth of the wound and the surgeon's preference.)
- If a specimen was taken for a pathology test, tell the patient when the results will be available.
- Answer any questions about postoperative experience and always encourage patients to call the office at any time if a problem or concern arises.

A,B

B

FIGURE 24-13. Clean a wound outward from the site following any of the numbered patterns shown here.

 Checkpoint Question

7. What is the difference between a dressing and a bandage?

Cleaning the Examination Table and Operative Area

In preparation for the next patient, all used equipment must be discarded properly or transported to the equipment room for sanitizing before sterilization. The examination room must be cleaned as part of the procedure. Remove papers and sheets in a rolling movement so outside surfaces cover the interior of the bundle. Do not let table covers and sheets come into contact with your clothing. Discard the sheets and covers appropriately. After applying gloves, wipe down the examination table, surgical stand, sink, counter, and other surfaces used during the procedure with an approved disinfectant or dilute bleach solution and allow them to dry. Replace the table sheet paper for the next patient.

COMMONLY PERFORMED OFFICE SURGICAL PROCEDURES

Two of the most frequently performed minor surgeries in the general medical office are excision of skin lesions (moles, **lentigines**, **keratoses**, and skin tags) and incision and drainage of abscesses. Follow standard precautions when assisting with these surgical procedures.

Excision of a Lesion

Physicians may excise lesions with electrocautery, laser, **cryosurgery**, or standard surgical equipment. Procedure 24-8 describes the steps for assisting the physician during the excision of a skin lesion using standard equipment. Some lesions are desiccated or **fulgurated**; however, many lesions are sent to pathology for diagnosis after excision.

Incision and Drainage

An abscess is a local collection of pus in a cavity surrounded by inflamed tissue. It results from the body's response to an infectious process when pathogens have entered through a break in the skin. Abscesses may be referred to as boils, furuncles (one lesion), or carbuncles (several lesions grouped closely together) and are very painful. The site must be incised and the infected material drained before healing can take place (Procedure 24-9).

ASSISTING WITH SUTURE AND STAPLE REMOVAL

In many instances you will be required to remove sutures from a wound. **Patients should understand that they might feel a pulling sensation during suture removal but should not feel pain.** First, cleanse the area with an antiseptic solution. Either wearing sterile gloves or using sterile transfer forceps with clean hands (Procedure 24-2), clean the

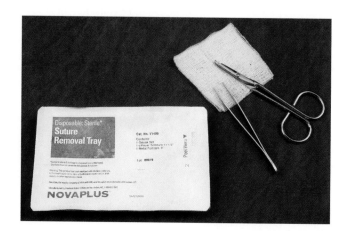

FIGURE 24-14. A disposable suture removal kit.

area in a circular motion away from the wound or in straight wipes away from the suture line (FIG. 24-13). The wipe is discarded after each sweep and a new one is used for the next sweep across the area. Either a sterile disposable suture removal kit, which contains all of the equipment needed for suture removal (FIG. 24-14), or sterile reusable equipment may be used (Procedure 24-10).

Following hospital surgery, some incisions are closed with metal staples rather than sutures. Patients often leave the hospital before the staples can be removed safely and return later to the physician's office to have them removed. Frequently it will be your responsibility to remove the staples. Most offices use staple removal kits similar to the kits supplied for suture removal. Included in the staple removal kit is a special instrument for removing the staples instead of suture scissors. Procedure 24-11 describes the process for removing staples.

WHAT IF

You accidentally cut your finger while cleaning up after a minor office surgical procedure?

Remove your gloves and immediately wash your hands with an antiseptic solution. Then have the physician evaluate the wound. The physician may suggest that you perform a surgical scrub or irrigate the wound, and antibiotics may be prescribed. The patient should be asked for permission to take a blood sample to test for hepatitis B, hepatitis C, and HIV. State laws vary regarding the legality of health care workers demanding a blood sample for testing. After blood from the patient is examined for the hepatitis B surface antigen, you may be given hepatitis B immunoglobulin (HBIG) and/or hepatitis B vaccine. You should consider obtaining the vaccine for hepatitis now. Many states require that health care workers be immunized at their employer's expense. Finally, be sure to notify your supervisor of any work-related injury so that it may be appropriately documented. The Needlestick Safety and Prevention Act requires that a sharps injury log be maintained and that it include the type and brand of device involved in the incident, the area in which the incident occurred, and a description of the incident. The name of the employee should not be recorded in the injury log. Preventing accidental exposure to contaminated blood or body fluids requires being alert and working without distractions.

Procedure 24-1

Opening Sterile Packs

Purpose: Open sterile packages without contaminating the contents.
Equipment: Surgical pack, surgical or Mayo stand.
Standard: This procedure should take 10 minutes.

Steps	Reason
1. Verify the procedure to be performed and remove the appropriate tray or item from the storage area. Check the label for contents and expiration date. Check the package for tears and moisture.	Packages that have passed the expiration date should not be used. Moist or torn areas contaminate the contents of the package.
2. Place the package, with the label facing up, on a clean, dry, flat surface such as a Mayo or surgical stand. Wash your hands.	Although the field will be protected by a barrier undersurface, microorganisms must be kept at a minimum by using an area as free of pathogens as possible. The surgical stand makes it easy to move the field for the physician's convenience. Your hands should be clean for this procedure.
3. Without tearing the wrapper, carefully remove the sealing tape. With commercial packages, carefully remove the outer protective wrapper.	Many disposable packages are wrapped in clear plastic film that will become the sterile field when properly opened. Packages prepared in the office are sealed with autoclave tape, which should clearly indicate that the package has been through the autoclave.
4. Loosen the first flap of the folded wrapper by pulling it up, out and away; let it fall over the far side of the table or stand.	This prevents you from having to reach across the sterile field again.

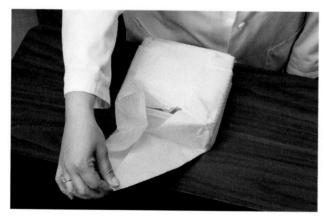

Step 4. Open the first flap away from you.

(continues)

Procedure 24-1 (continued)

Opening Sterile Packs

Steps	Reason
5. Open the side flaps in a similar manner, using your left hand for the left flap and your right hand for the right flap. Touch only the unsterile outer surface; do not touch the sterile inner surface.	This method minimizes your movement over the sterile areas of the package.

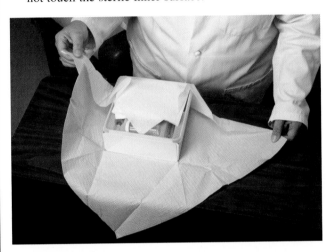

Step 5. Open the side flaps.

6. Pull the remaining flap down and toward you by grasping the outside surface only. The outer surface of the wrapper is now against the surgical stand; the sterile inside of the wrapper forms the sterile field.

Step 6. Pull the remaining flap down and toward you.

(continues)

Opening Sterile Packs

Steps	Reason
7. Repeat steps 4 to 6 for packages with a second or inside wrapper. This wrapper also provides a sterile field upon which to work. The field is now ready for the procedure to begin.	
8. If you must leave the area after opening the field, cover the tray and its contents with a sterile drape. Without leaving or turning your back on the sterile setup area, open the sterile drape and carefully lift it out of the package by the edges without contaminating it. Carefully lay the drape over the sterile field, working from your body out so that your arms do not cross the uncovered sterile field but do cross the drape that has been placed over the tray.	

Procedure 24-2

Using Sterile Transfer Forceps

Purpose: Use sterile transfer forceps without contamination during a sterile setup.

Equipment: Sterile transfer forceps in a container with sterilization solution, sterile field, sterile items to be transferred.

Standard: This procedure should take 10 minutes.

Steps	Reason
1. Slowly lift the forceps straight up and out of the container without touching the outside of the container or its inside above the level of the solution.	The area above the soaking solution and the rim are considered not sterile.
2. Hold the forceps with the tips down at all times.	This prevents the solution from running toward the unsterile handles and then back to the grasping blades and tips, which would contaminate them.
3. Keep the forceps above waist level.	This prevents accidental and unnoticed contamination.
4. With the forceps, pick up the articles to be transferred and drop them onto the sterile field, but do not let the forceps come into contact with the sterile field.	The forceps may be moist from the soaking solution, which may wick microorganisms from the surface below onto the sterile field. *Note*: Transfer forceps that have been wrapped and autoclaved may be placed with tips on the sterile field and handles extending beyond the 1-inch border that is considered contaminated. Doing this allows you to move objects around the field for the physician's convenience.
5. Carefully place the forceps back in the sterilization solution.	The sterilization solution in the forceps container keeps the tips of the forceps sterile for future use. The solution should be changed at least daily or according to office policy.

Procedure 24-3

Adding Sterile Solution

Purpose: Pour a sterile solution into a container on the sterile field without contamination.

Equipment: Sterile setup, container of sterile solution, sterile bowl or cup.

Standard: This procedure should take 10 minutes.

Steps	Reason
1. As with any drug or medication, identify the correct solution by carefully reading the label. If necessary, use the sterile transfer forceps and place the sterile bowl or cup on the sterile field.	The label should be checked three times to prevent errors: when taking the container from the shelf, before pouring the solution, and when returning the container to the shelf.
2. Check the expiration date on the label; do not use the solution if it is out of date, if the label cannot be read, or if the solution appears abnormal. Sterile water and saline bottles must be dated when opened and must be discarded if not used within 48 hours.	Out-of-date solutions may have changed chemically or deteriorated and are not considered sterile.
3. If you are adding medication, such as lidocaine, to the solution, show the medication label to the physician now.	This allows for verification of the contents.
4. Remove the cap or stopper. Hold the cap with your fingertips, the cap opening down to prevent contamination of the inside of the cap. If you must put the cap down, place it on a side table (not the sterile field) with the open end up. If you are pouring the entire contents onto the sterile field, discard the cap. Retain the bottle to keep track of the amount added to the field and for charting later. It can then be discarded.	If the cap becomes contaminated and is returned to the bottle, the contents are considered contaminated. Placing the cap on a surface with the opening up prevents contamination of the interior of the cap.

(continues)

Procedure 24-3   *(continued)*

Adding Sterile Solution

Steps	Reason
5. Grasp the container with the label against the palm of your hand (known as palming the label).	If solution runs down the side of the bottle in this position, it will not obscure the label.
6. Pour a small amount of the solution into a separate container or waste receptacle.	The lip of the bottle is considered contaminated; pouring off this small amount cleanses the lip.
7. Without reaching across the sterile field, carefully and slowly pour the desired amount of solution into the sterile container from not less than 4 inches and not more than 6 inches above the container. The bottle of solution should never touch the sterile container or tray, as this will cause contamination.	Pouring the solution slowly reduces the chance of splashing and overfilling. Solution poured too fast or from an improper height may splash. Touching the container to objects on the sterile field contaminates the field. If the solution splashes onto the field, wicking will cause contamination from the surface below.

Step 7. Hold the cap facing downward to prevent contamination of the inside.

Steps	Reason
8. After pouring the desired amount of solution into the sterile container, recheck the label for the contents and expiration date and replace the cap carefully, without touching the bottle rim with any unsterile surface of the cap.	This ensures accuracy. Careful replacement of the cap ensures that the contents remain sterile.
9. Return the solution to its proper storage area or discard the container after checking the label again.	This ensures accuracy.

Procedure 24-4

Performing Hair Removal and Skin Preparation

Purpose: Prepare the skin by removing any hair and applying an antiseptic solution before a surgical procedure.

Equipment: Nonsterile gloves; shave cream, lotion, or soap; new disposable razor; gauze or cotton balls; warm water; antiseptic; sponge forceps.

Standard: This procedure should take 10 minutes.

Steps	Reason
1. Wash your hands.	Handwashing aids infection control.
2. Assemble the equipment.	This ensures that all supplies are available. A new razor must be used for each patient to prevent the transmission of pathogens and to ensure the closest possible shave.
3. Greet and identify the patient. Explain the procedure and answer any questions.	This prevents errors in treatment, helps gain compliance, and eases anxiety.
4. Put on gloves.	Standard precautions must be observed when contact with blood or body fluids is possible.
5. Prepare the patient's skin. A. For shaving, apply shaving cream or soapy lather to the area. Pull the skin taut and shave by pulling the razor across the skin in the direction of hair growth. Repeat this procedure until all hair is removed from the operative area. Rinse and thoroughly pat the shaved area dry with a gauze square. B. If the patient's skin is not to be shaved, wash and rinse with soap and water and dry the skin thoroughly.	Shaving cream or soapy lather on the skin reduces friction and helps prevent scratching. Shaving in the direction of hair growth gives the closest shave while reducing the chance of nicking the skin. Rinsing removes soap residue and hair from the shaved area. Pat dry rather than rub to prevent abrasions. Using gauze squares for drying picks up stray hairs that might have been left behind during rinsing.
6. Apply antiseptic solution of the physician's choice to the skin surrounding the operative area using sterile gauze sponges, sterile cotton balls, or antiseptic wipes. Holding the gauze or cotton ball in the sterile sponge forceps, wipe the skin in circular motions starting at the operative site and working outward. Discard each sponge after a complete sweep has been made. If the area is large or circles are not appropriate, the sponge may be wiped straight outward from the operative site, then discarded and the procedure repeated until the entire area has been thoroughly cleaned. At no time should a wipe that has passed over the skin be returned to the cleaned area or to the antiseptic solution.	Discarding sponges after each stroke prevents contamination of the wound by microorganisms brought back to the area from the surrounding skin.

(continues)

Procedure 24-4   *(continued)*

Performing Hair Removal and Skin Preparation

Steps	Reason
7. Holding dry sterile gauze sponges in the sponge forceps, thoroughly pat the area dry. In some instances, the area may be allowed to air dry.	Moist skin may moisten the sterile drapes, causing wicking and contaminating the site.
8. Instruct the patient not to touch or cover the prepared area.	This avoids contaminating the operative site, which would require repeating the procedure.
9. Inform the physician that the patient is ready for the procedure. Drape the prepared area with a sterile drape if the physician will be delayed for more than 10 or 15 minutes.	

Procedure 24-5

Applying Sterile Gloves

Purpose:	Apply prepackaged sterile gloves without contamination.
Equipment:	One package of sterile gloves in the appropriate size.
Standard:	This procedure should take 5 minutes.

Steps	Reason
1. Remove rings and other jewelry.	Rings may pierce the gloves and contaminate the procedure.
2. Wash your hands.	Wearing gloves is not a substitute for handwashing but must be done in addition to it.
3. Place the prepackaged gloves on a clean, dry, flat surface with the cuffed end toward you.	Sterile gloves are packaged for ease of application in this fashion.

A. Pull the outer wrapping apart to expose the sterile inner wrap.

Step 3A. Pull the outer wrapping apart to expose the sterile inner wrap.

B. With the cuffs toward you, fold back the inner wrap to expose the gloves.

(continues)

Procedure 24-5   *(continued)*

Applying Sterile Gloves

Steps

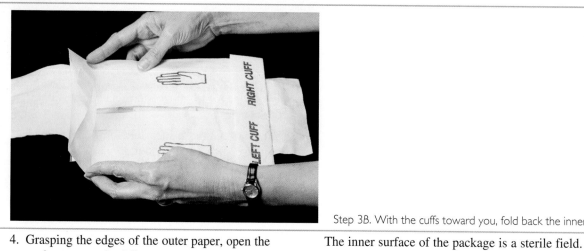

Step 3B. With the cuffs toward you, fold back the inner wrap.

4. Grasping the edges of the outer paper, open the package out to its fullest.

The inner surface of the package is a sterile field.

Step 4. (A and B) Grasp the edges and open the package.

(continues)

Procedure 24-5   *(continued)*

Applying Sterile Gloves

Steps	**Reason**
5. Using your nondominant hand, pick up the dominant hand glove by grasping the folded edge of the cuff, lifting it up and away from the paper. The folded edge of the cuff is contaminated as soon as it is touched with the ungloved hand. Be very careful not to touch the outside surface of the sterile glove with your ungloved hand.	Lift it up and away to avoid letting the fingers of the glove brush an unsterile surface.

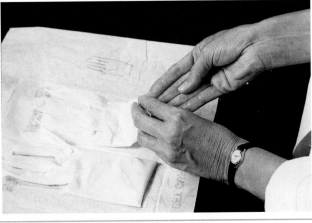

Step 5. Using your nondominant hand, lift the cuff of the glove for the dominant hand, touching only the inner surface of the cuff. Curl your thumb inward as you insert your hand.

Steps	**Reason**
6. Curl your fingers and thumb together and insert them into the glove. Then straighten your fingers and pull the glove on with your nondominant hand still grasping the cuff.	This prevents accidental touching of the outside surface of the glove.
7. Unfold the cuff by pinching the inside surface that will be against your wrist and pulling it toward the wrist.	This ensures that only the unsterile portions are touched by the hands.

Step 7. Pull the glove snugly into place, touching only the inside surface of the cuff.

(continues)

Procedure 24-5 *(continued)*

Applying Sterile Gloves

Steps	Reason
8. Place the fingers of your gloved hand under the cuff of the remaining glove, lift the glove up and away from the wrapper, and slide your ungloved hand carefully into the glove with your fingers and thumb curled together.	This prevents the sterile glove from accidentally touching an unsterile surface and ensures that the fingers will not brush the sterile surface of the glove.

Step 8. With your thumb curled, slip the gloved dominant hand into the cuff of the remaining glove.

Steps	Reason
9. Straighten your fingers and pull the glove up and over your wrist by carefully unfolding the cuff.	At all times, sterile must touch sterile only. Folding the cuffs out to their fullest allows the greatest area of sterility.

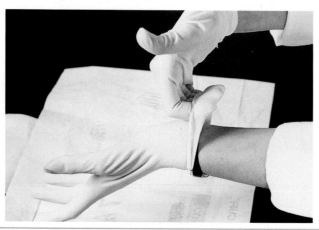

Step 9. Unfold the cuff and pull the glove on snugly.

Steps	Reason
10. Settle the gloves comfortably onto your fingers by lacing your fingers together and adjusting the tension over your hands.	The gloves should fit snugly without wrinkles or areas that bind the fingers.

(continues)

Procedure 24-5 (continued)

Applying Sterile Gloves

Steps	Reason
Step 10. Adjust the fingers for a comfortable fit.	
11. Remove contaminated sterile gloves exactly as you would remove contaminated nonsterile gloves and discard them appropriately.	If removed correctly, one glove will be balled into the other with no opportunity to touch the soiled area of either glove.

Procedure 24-6

Applying a Sterile Dressing

Purpose: Using sterile dressings and sterile technique, apply a sterile dressing to a surgical wound without contamination.

Equipment: Sterile gloves, sterile gauze dressings, scissors, bandage tape, any medication to be applied to the dressing if ordered by the physician.

Standard: This procedure should take 10 minutes.

Steps	Reason
1. Wash your hands.	Handwashing aids infection control.
2. Assemble the equipment and supplies.	This ensures that all of the supplies are available before beginning the procedure.
3. Greet and identify the patient. Ask about any tape allergies before selecting tape. With the size of the dressing in mind, cut or tear lengths of tape to secure the dressing. Set the tape aside in a convenient place.	Patients must be identified to prevent errors in treatment. Some patients are sensitive to certain tape adhesives. Many types of hypoallergenic tape are available. Having tape cut and prepared saves time and may prevent the dressing from slipping while tape is cut after the dressing is applied.

(continues)

Procedure 24-6   (continued)

Applying a Sterile Dressing

Steps	Reason
4. Explain the procedure and instruct the patient to remain still during the procedure and to avoid coughing, sneezing, and talking until the procedure is complete.	Unexpected movements by the patient may result in contamination of the sterile supplies and the wound. Talking, coughing, and sneezing release droplets of moisture containing microorganisms from the respiratory tract that may contaminate the sterile field and the wound.
5. Open the dressing pack to create a sterile field, leaving the sterile dressing on the inside of the opened package. Observe the principles of surgical asepsis. Many packets are designed to be peeled apart.	Sterile technique ensures sterility of the dressing after it is open. Packages of dressings are sterile on the inside; if opened properly, the inner surface may be used as a sterile field.

Step 5. Open the sterile dressing pack or packs.

6. To maintain sterility:	Using sterile technique prevents contamination of the dressings and wound.
A. If sterile gloves are to be used, open the appropriate package of gloves. Using sterile technique, put on the gloves. Before touching any sterile items.	
B. If using sterile transfer forceps to apply the dressing (the no-touch method), use sterile technique to arrange the dressing on the wound, and do not touch the dressing or the site with the hands.	

A

B

Step 6. (A) Using sterile gloves. (B) Using sterile transfer forceps.

(continues)

Procedure 24-6 *(continued)*

Applying a Sterile Dressing

Steps	Reason
7. Apply to the sterile dressing that will directly cover the wound any topical medication ordered by the physician, being careful not to touch the end of the medication bottle or tube to the dressing.	The outside end of the medication bottle or tube may not be sterile.
8. Using the already opened sterile dressings and sterile technique, apply the number of dressings necessary to cover and protect the wound. Sterile dressings must be carefully placed on the wound and not allowed to drag over the skin.	If the dressing is dragged over the skin, it will be contaminated by microorganisms from the surrounding skin and may cause infection.
9. Apply the previously cut lengths of tape over the dressing to secure it, but avoid overuse of tape. When the wound is completely covered, you may remove your gloves or keep them on while you tape the dressing. Discard the gloves in the proper receptacle.	Tape is used only to keep the dressing in place. It should allow observation of any bleeding or drainage. Too much tape can cause perspiration that will dampen the dressing and compromise sterility. Tape should not obstruct blood circulation. Excessive tape also must later be removed, which may hurt. A bandage may be applied over the dressing to hold it in place, add support, or immobilize the area.
10. When the patient is to change dressings at home, provide appropriate instructions. Dressings should be kept clean and dry and changed when wet or soiled. Otherwise, dressings should be changed as instructed by the physician. Make sure patients understand the signs of infection, such as redness, swelling, pain, or undue warmth at the site, and instruct them to call the office at once if these appear. Also say what to do in case of excessive bleeding or drainage and how to manage any drains.	Microorganisms may be transported to the wound by capillary action if the dressing is wet or soiled.
11. Wearing clean examination gloves, properly dispose of or care for equipment and supplies. Disposable articles contaminated with wound drainage or blood go into a biohazard container. Clean the work area, remove your gloves, and wash your hands.	Follow standard precautions.
12. Return reusable supplies (unopened sterile gloves or dressings, tape) to their appropriate storage areas; all others should be discarded correctly.	Unopened supplies should be returned to the appropriate storage areas for reuse. Discarding uncontaminated reusables is wasteful.
13. Record the procedure.	Procedures are considered not to have been done if they are not recorded in the patient's record.

Charting Example

10/14/2005 4:45 P.M. DSD applied to surgical wound (L) anterior forearm. No bleeding from incision, edges well approximated with 4 sutures intact. Pt. given verbal and written instructions on dressing change and wound care at home. To RTO in 5 days for suture removal. _____ L. Hicks, CMA

Procedure 24-7

Changing an Existing Dressing

Purpose: Carefully remove an existing dressing from a wound and cover it with a sterile dressing using sterile technique.

Equipment: Sterile gloves, nonsterile gloves, sterile dressing, prepackaged skin antiseptic swabs or sterile antiseptic solution in a sterile basin and sterile cotton balls or gauze, tape, approved biohazard containers.

Standard: This procedure should take 10 minutes.

Steps	Reason
1. Wash your hands.	Handwashing aids infection control.
2. Assemble the equipment and supplies.	This ensures that all supplies are available before you begin the procedure.
3. Greet and identify the patient. Explain the procedure and answer any questions.	This prevents errors in treatment, helps gain compliance, and eases anxiety.
4. Prepare a sterile field, including opening sterile dressings. If using a sterile container and solution, open the package containing the sterile basin and use the inside of the wrapper as the sterile field for the basin. Flip the sterile gauze or cotton balls into the basin and appropriately pour in the antiseptic solution. If using prepackaged antiseptic swabs, carefully open an adequate number for the size of the wound and set them aside without contaminating them.	
5. Instruct the patient not to talk, cough, sneeze, laugh, or move during the procedure.	Respiratory droplets may contaminate the sterile field. Movement may cause accidental contamination of the field.
6. Wearing clean gloves, carefully remove the tape from the wound dressing by pulling it toward the wound. Remove the old dressing. *Note:* If the dressing is difficult to remove because of dried blood, it may be soaked with sterile water or saline for a few minutes to loosen it. Gently pull the edges of the dressing toward the center. Never pull on a dressing that does not come off easily. If this procedure does not sufficiently loosen the dressing or causes undue discomfort to the patient, immediately notify the physician.	Tape pulled away from the direction of the wound may pull the healing edges of the wound apart.
7. Discard the soiled dressing into a biohazard container. Do not pass it over the sterile field.	The dressing will be soiled with blood and body fluids and must be considered hazardous. Dressings passed over the sterile field will shed microorganisms and contaminate the area.

(continues)

Procedure 24-7 (continued)

Changing an Existing Dressing

Steps	Reason
8. Inspect the wound for degree of healing, amount and type of drainage, appearance of wound edges, and so on.	The wound is inspected now because wound cleaning removes most exudate. Make a mental note for charting when the procedure is complete.
9. Observing medical asepsis, remove and discard your gloves. The physician may want to inspect the wound before you remove exudate or drainage to determine whether healing is proceeding as expected. If a culture is ordered, the specimen must be taken before the wound is cleaned to ensure the most reliable findings.	
10. Using proper technique, put on sterile gloves. Clean the wound with the antiseptic solution ordered by the physician. Clean in a straight motion with the cotton or gauze or the prepackaged antiseptic swab. Discard the wipe (cotton ball, swab) after each stroke and use a fresh sterile one to continue. Never return the wipe to the antiseptic solution or to the skin after one sweep across the area.	The wound must be cleaned before fresh dressings are applied. Returning the wipe to the wound area or solution brings microorganisms from the surrounding skin to the open lesion.
11. Remove your gloves and wash your hands.	Your hands must be washed before you apply the sterile dressing with sterile gloves or sterile transfer forceps.
12. Change the dressing using the procedure for sterile dressing application and using sterile gloves or sterile transfer forceps (Procedure 24-6).	
13. Record the procedure.	Procedures are considered not to have been done if they are not recorded.

Charting Example

11/23/2005 11:30 A.M. Wound to (R) lower leg changed, small amount of yellow purulent drainage noted—Dr. Blake aware. Wound culture for C&S obtained and sent to Acme laboratory. Wound cleansed with Betadine as ordered; DSD reapplied. Moderate amount of redness and swelling at wound site; edges well approximated. Instructed to RTO in 2 days for C&S results and dressing change. _____ B. Lamont, CMA

Procedure 24-8

Assisting with Excisional Surgery

Purpose: Prepare for and assist with excisional surgery while maintaining sterile technique.

Equipment: *At the side:* Sterile gloves, local anesthetic, antiseptic wipes, adhesive tape, specimen container with completed laboratory request, *On the field:* Basin for solutions, gauze sponges and cotton balls, antiseptic solution, sterile drape, dissecting scissors, disposable scalpel, blade of physician's choice, mosquito forceps, tissue forceps, needle holder, suture and needle of physician's choice.

Standard: This procedure should take 15 minutes.

Steps	Reason
1. Wash your hands.	Handwashing aids in infection control.
2. Assemble the equipment.	This ensures that all supplies are available.
3. Greet and identify the patient. Explain the procedure and answer any questions.	This prevents errors in treatment, helps gain compliance, and eases anxiety.
4. Set up a sterile field on a surgical stand with the at-the-side equipment close at hand. Cover the field with a sterile drape until the physician arrives.	
5. Position the patient appropriately.	The required position depends on the location of the lesion.
6. Put on sterile gloves or use sterile transfer forceps and cleanse the patient's skin as described in Procedure 24-4. Some physicians prefer to do this themselves after gloving, using supplies on the field. The physician's preference always takes precedence over any outlined procedure.	The antiseptic discourages the entrance of microorganisms into the wound. After cleansing the skin, remove the gloves, if used, and wash the hands.
7. The physician will perform the procedure; you may be asked to assist. This usually involves adding supplies as needed, watching closely for opportunities to assist the physician, and comforting the patient.	It is not necessary for you to wear sterile gloves during the procedure unless the physician requires you to handle sterile instruments or supplies.
8. If the lesion is to be referred to pathology for analysis, you will be required to assist with collecting the specimen in an appropriate container.	Always follow standard precautions, wearing examination gloves when handling specimens. Have the container ready to receive the specimen.
9. At the end of the procedure, wash your hands and dress the wound using sterile technique (Procedure 24-6).	*The wound must be covered to protect the incision from contamination.*
10. Thank the patient and give appropriate instructions for care of the operative site, changing the dressing, postoperative medications, and follow-up visits as ordered by the physician.	Courtesy encourages the patient to have a positive attitude about the physician's office.

(continues)

Procedure 24-8 *(continued)*

Assisting with Excisional Surgery

Steps	Reason
11. Wearing gloves, clean the examining room in preparation for the next patient. Discard all used disposables in appropriate biohazard containers. Return unused items to their proper places. Remove your gloves and wash your hands.	Standard precautions must be followed.
12. Record the procedure.	Procedures are considered not to have been done if they are not recorded. Documentation of the procedure requires postoperative vital signs, care of the wound, instructions on postoperative care, and processing any specimens.

Charting Example

09/19/2005 8:45 A.M. Mole to posterior (L) shoulder removed per Dr. Snider. Specimen sent to Acme lab. T 98.4 (O) P 96 R20 BP 134/78 (R) sitting. 4 × 4 DSD applied to surgical incision; minimal sanguinous drainage noted. Pt. given verbal and written instructions on wound care, postop antibiotics, pain medication, and follow-up visits. Verbalized understanding. To RTO ×2 days for drsg change. _____ B. Cole, CMA

Procedure 24-9

Assisting with Incision and Drainage (I & D)

Purpose: Prepare for and assist with an incision and drainage procedure while maintaining sterile technique.

Equipment: *At the side:* sterile gloves, local anesthetic, antiseptic wipes, adhesive tape, sterile dressings, packing gauze, culture tube if the wound may be cultured.

              On the field: basin for solutions, gauze sponges and cotton balls, antiseptic solution, sterile drape, syringes and needles for local anesthetic, commercial I & D sterile setup OR scalpel, dissecting scissors, hemostats, tissue forceps, 4 × 4 gauze sponges, probe (optional).

Standard: This procedure should take 15 minutes.

The steps for this procedure are similar to those in Procedure 24-8. Specifically, you are expected to prepare the surgical field and the patient's surgical area as instructed or preferred by the physician. After the procedure, the wound must be covered to avoid further contamination and to absorb drainage. The exudate is a hazardous body fluid requiring standard precautions. Although a culture and sensitivity may be ordered on the drainage from the infected area, no other specimen is usually collected.

Charting Example

04/15/2005 11:30 A.M. Postop VS T 100.4 (O) P 88 R 24 BP 128/88 (R) sitting. 4 × 4 DSD applied to surgical wound on (L) posterior neck. Given verbal and written instructions on wound care, dressing changes, and follow-up. Verbalized understanding. _____ E. Black, CMA

Procedure 24-10

Removing Sutures

Purpose:	Using aseptic technique, remove sutures from a wound.
Equipment:	Skin antiseptic, sterile gloves, prepackaged suture removal kit OR thumb forceps, suture scissors, gauze.
Standard:	This procedure should take 10 minutes.

Steps	Reason
1. Wash your hands and apply clean examination gloves.	Handwashing aids infection control.
2. Assemble the equipment.	This ensures that all supplies are available.
3. Greet and identify the patient. Explain the procedure and answer any questions.	This prevents errors in treatment, helps gain compliance, and eases anxiety.
4. If dressings have not been removed, remove them and properly dispose of them in the biohazard container. Remove your gloves and wash your hands if a soiled dressing was removed.	
5. Put on clean examination gloves and cleanse the wound with an antiseptic, such as Betadine, using a new antiseptic gauze for each swipe down the wound and removing any old drainage or blood.	The wound must be as free of pathogens as possible before removal of the sutures to prevent contamination of the wound.
6. Open the suture removal packet using sterile asepsis or set up a field for on-site sterile equipment. Put on sterile gloves.	Suture removal is a sterile procedure.
7. The knots will be tied so that one tail of the knot is very close to the surface of the skin; the other will be closer to the area of suture that is looped over the incision. A. With the thumb forceps, grasp the end of the knot closest to the skin and lift it slightly and gently up from the skin.	

(continues)

Removing Sutures

Steps	**Reason**
B. Cut the suture below the knot as close to the skin as possible.	Cutting below the knot and close to the skin frees the knot at an area that has not been exposed to the outside surface of the body. The only part of the suture that will pull through the tissues will be the suture that was under the skin surface.
C. Use the thumb forceps to pull the suture out of the skin with a smooth, continuous motion at a slight angle in the direction of the wound.	This prevents tension on the healing tissue.

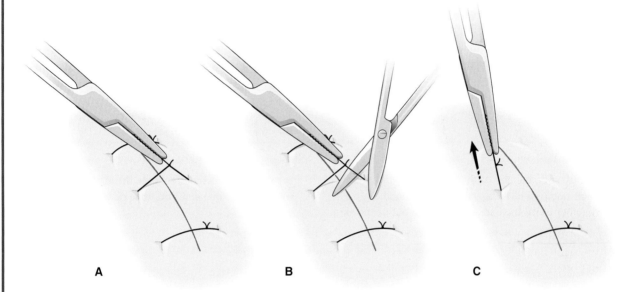

A   B   C

Step 7. (A) With the hemostat or thumb forceps, lift the stitch up and away from the skin. This permits the blades of the scissors to slide under the stitch. (B) Cut the stitch near the skin. (C) Using the forceps, pull the freed stitch up and out.

8. Place the suture on the gauze sponge. Repeat the procedure for each suture to be removed.	This helps in counting the number removed; if six sutures were inserted and are now to be removed, there should be six sutures on the gauze sponge at the end of the procedure.
9. Clean the site with an antiseptic solution, and if the physician has so indicated, cover it with a sterile dressing.	Some wounds still need to be protected; some have healed well enough to be left uncovered.
10. Thank the patient and properly dispose of the equipment and supplies. Clean the work area, remove your gloves, and wash your hands.	Standard precautions must be followed. Courtesy encourages a positive attitude about the physician's office.
11. Record the procedure, including the time, location of sutures, number removed, and condition of the wound.	Procedures are considered not to have been done if they are not recorded.

Charting Example

06/26/2005 3:30 P.M. ×6 sutures removed from (L) ring finger. Wound well approximated, no drainage. _____ J. Rose, RMA

Removing Staples

Purpose:	Using aseptic technique, remove staples from a wound.
Equipment:	Antiseptic solution or wipes, gauze squares, sponge forceps, prepackaged sterile staple removal instrument, examination gloves, sterile gloves.
Standard:	This procedure should take 10 minutes.

Steps	Reason
1. Wash your hands.	Handwashing aids infection control.
2. Assemble the equipment.	This ensures that all supplies are available.
3. Greet and identify the patient. Explain the procedure and answer any questions.	This prevents errors in treatment, helps gain compliance, and eases anxiety.
4. If the dressing is still in place, put on clean examination gloves and remove it. Dispose of the dressing in a biohazard container.	The dressing is contaminated and must be handled with standard precautions. Remove gloves and wash your hands.
5. Clean the incision with antiseptic solution. Pat dry with sterile gauze sponges.	The incision must be cleaned before removing the staples to avoid infection. If exudate is present, the staples may not be easy to see.
6. Put on sterile gloves.	Staple removal is a sterile procedure.
7. Gently slide the end of the staple remover under each staple to be removed. Press the handles together to lift the ends of the staple out of the skin.	The remover is designed to open the staple so that the ends will lift free and minimize discomfort.

Step 7. Slide the end of the staple remover under each staple. Press the handles together to lift the ends of the staple out of the skin.

Steps	Reason
8. Place each staple on a gauze square as it is removed.	This helps in counting the staples at the end of the procedure.
9. When all staples are removed, gently clean the incision as instructed for all procedures. Pat dry and dress the site if ordered to do so by the physician.	The area should be cleaned and dried before any new dressing is applied to avoid wicking microorganisms. Healing may be far enough along to allow the wound to remain uncovered.
10. Thank the patient and properly care for or dispose of all equipment and supplies. Clean the work area, remove your gloves, and wash your hands.	Standard precautions must be followed.

(continues)

Procedure 24-11 *(continued)*

Removing Staples

Steps	Reason
11. Record the procedure.	Procedures are not considered to have been done if they are not recorded.

Charting Example

3/17/2005 10:30 A.M. ×15 staples removed from (L) knee incision; edges well approximated, no redness or drainage noted. Wound left open to air as ordered by Dr. Perez. _____ B. Daniels, CMA

CHAPTER SUMMARY

With the spiraling costs of health care, many procedures that were once performed only in hospitals are now being performed in medical offices. As a medical assistant, you will be required to become more proficient in minor surgical procedures as offices change to meet the needs of the patients. Continuing education, research, and on-the-job training will keep you current on the changes in the field of surgery and in the new equipment that is used during minor office surgical procedures. However, no matter how technical or sophisticated the surgical procedure or equipment, you must not forget the feelings of apprehension many patients have. While it is your responsibility to prepare the treatment room and assist the physician, you are also obligated to instruct the patient accurately on any presurgical preparations, obtain third-party authorization if necessary, reassure the patient during the procedure, and give the patient accurate information about postsurgical care as ordered by the physician. Of course, after the procedure you must also disinfect the examination room and prepare it for future patients.

Critical Thinking Challenges

1. Dr. Brown has just informed Mrs. Levine that she should return tomorrow for office surgery. While you are alone with the patient, Mrs. Levine begins to cry and expresses great concern about the procedure. What should you do?
2. Refer to an anatomy book and review the anatomy of a hair follicle. Why are skin nicks more likely if the hair is shaved in the opposite direction of its natural growth?
3. Why is it preferable for infected wounds to heal with delayed or unclosed surface edges?
4. Prepare a patient education sheet outlining postoperative wound care.

Answers to Checkpoint Questions

1. To maintain a sterile field, you must keep sterile packages dry, face the sterile field, keep sterile items above waist level, keep items in the middle of the field, avoid spills, not cough or sneeze near the field, never reach over the field, not pass contaminated items over the field, and alert the physician if the field becomes contaminated.
2. Contents of a peel-back package can be added to the sterile field with sterile forceps or a sterile gloved hand or by flipping them onto the field.
3. A fenestrated drape has an opening to expose the treatment site while covering adjacent areas.
4. Swaged (atraumatic) needles have the appropriate size suture material attached by the manufacturer. Threaded needles have an eye with a double thickness of suture that must be pulled through the tissues.
5. Electrosection is the type of electrosurgery used for incision or excision of tissue.
6. When assisting with laser procedures, everyone present must protect their eyes by wearing goggles.
7. Dressings are used to cover and protect a wound, absorb drainage, exert pressure, hide disfigurement, and hold medications against the skin. Bandages are placed over dressings to hold the dressing in place, protect the injured part, or restrict movement.

 Websites

American Society of Plastic Surgeons
www.plasticsurgery.org
American Society for Dermatologic Surgery
www.asds-net.org
Center for Laser Surgery www.lasersurgery.com

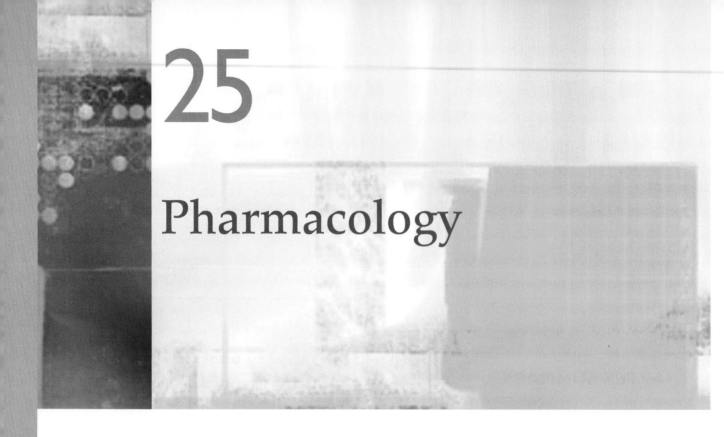

25

Pharmacology

CHAPTER OUTLINE

MEDICATION NAMES

LEGAL REGULATIONS
Food and Drug Administration
Drug Enforcement Agency

SOURCES OF DRUGS

DRUG ACTIONS AND
INTERACTIONS
Pharmacodynamics
Pharmacokinetics
Drug Interactions
Side Effects and Allergies

SOURCES OF INFORMATION

PRESCRIPTIONS

ROLE DELINEATION

CLINICAL: FUNDAMENTAL PRINCIPLES
- Apply principles of aseptic technique and infection control

CLINICAL: PATIENT CARE
- Assist with examinations, procedures, and treatments
- Prepare and administer medications and immunizations
- Maintain medication and immunization records

GENERAL: COMMUNICATION SKILLS
- Recognize and respond effectively to verbal, nonverbal, and written communications
- Use medical terminology appropriately

GENERAL: LEGAL CONCEPTS
- Perform within legal and ethical boundaries
- Document accurately
- Implement and maintain federal and state health care legislation and regulations
- Comply with established risk management and safety procedures

GENERAL: OPERATIONAL FUNCTIONS
- Perform inventory of supplies and equipment

CHAPTER COMPETENCIES

LEARNING OBJECTIVES

Upon successfully completing this chapter, you will be able to:

1. Spell and define key terms.
2. Identify chemical, trade, and generic drug names.
3. Name the regulations and branches of government that impact prescription medications and controlled substances.
4. Explain the various drug actions and interactions including pharmacodynamics and pharmacokinetics.
5. Describe the difference between medication side effects and allergies.
6. Name the sources for locating information on pharmacology.

KEY TERM LIST

allergy	contraindication	pharmacodynamics	synergism
anaphylaxis	drug	pharmacokinetics	trade name
antagonism	generic name	pharmacology	
chemical name	interaction	potentiation	

As A CLINICAL MEDICAL ASSISTANT, you may be responsible for administering medications under the supervision of the physician. It is important that you acquire knowledge of medications, their uses and potential abuses, range of dosages, methods of administration, and adverse effects. **Pharmacology** is the term given to the study of drugs, their actions, dosages, and side effects. A **drug** is a chemical substance that affects body function or functions. Medications are available in many forms and are administered in various ways to produce therapeutic effects.

MEDICATION NAMES

Most medications have a **chemical name**, a **generic name,** and a **trade name** (Box 25-1). The chemical name is the first name given to any medication. It identifies the chemical components of the drug. The generic name is assigned to the medication during research and development. When the drug is available for commercial use and distribution by the original manufacturer, it is given a brand, or trade, name. The trade name is registered by the U.S. Patent Office and has the official trademark symbol (TM) after its name. After the patent expires, any other company that manufactures the medication may assign its own trade name to the generic equivalent. The first letter of a trade name is always capitalized; generic names begin with lowercase letters.

Drugs can be classified according to their actions and effects on the body. TABLE 25-1 lists some commonly used drugs, prescription and nonprescription, and their classifications.

 Checkpoint Question

1. What is the difference between a drug's chemical name and trade name?

LEGAL REGULATIONS

Food and Drug Administration

Consumers in the United States are protected by federal regulations regarding the production, prescribing, or dispensing of medications. In 1906, the Pure Food and Drug Act was passed. After being amended in 1938, it required that the safety of a drug be proved before distribution to the public. The amended law was renamed the Federal Food, Drug, and Cosmetic Act. In 1952, the Durham-Humphrey Amendment banned many drugs from being dispensed without a prescription. The Kefauver-Harris Amendment of 1962 required testing of prescription and nonprescription medications for effectiveness before their release for sale. The Food and Drug Administration (FDA) was established to regulate the manufacture and distribution of drugs and food products and to ensure accuracy in the ingredients listed on the labels of food and drug products.

Drug Enforcement Agency

In 1970, the Controlled Substances Act was passed to regulate the manufacture and distribution of drugs whose use may result in dependency or abuse. This act also requires that anyone who manufactures, prescribes, administers, or dispenses controlled substances register with the United States Attorney General under the Bureau of Narcotics and Dangerous Drugs (BNDD). The Drug Enforcement Agency (DEA) is a branch of the Department of Justice (DOJ) and is designated to exercise strong regulatory control over all drugs listed by the BNDD. This authority extends to prescribing, refilling, and storing controlled substances in the medical office. The DEA is concerned with controlled

Table 25-1   CLASSIFICATIONS OF DRUGS

Therapeutic Classification	Effect, Action, Uses	Common Examples
Adrenergic blocking agents	Affect alpha receptors of adrenergic nerves	Metoprolol tartrate (Lopressor); propranolol hydrochloride (Inderal)
Adrenergic agents	Mimic activity of sympathetic nervous system	Epinephrine (Adrenaline); ephedrine sulfate
Analgesics	Relieve pain	Aspirin, acetaminophen (Tylenol), codeine
Antacids	Neutralize or reduce acidity of stomach	Magnesia (Milk of Magnesia); calcium carbonate (Tums)
Anthelmintics	Kill parasitic worms	Piperazine citrate, mebendazole (Vermox)
Antianginal agents	Promote vasodilation	Nitroglycerine, diltiazem hydrochloride (Cardizem)
Antianxiety agents	Act on subcortical brain to relieve symptoms of anxiety	Alprazolam (Xanax); chlordiazepoxide (Librium); diazepam (Valium)
Antiarrhythmics	Reduce or prevent irregular cardiac rhythms	Procainamide hydrochloride (Pronestyl); esmolol(Brevibloc)
Antibiotics	Interrupt or interfere with growth of or destroy microorganisms	Penicillin, ampicillin, lop cefaclor, tetracycline
Anticoagulants and thrombolytics	Prevent or dissolve blood clots	Heparin sodium, coumadin, streptokinase (Streptase)
Anticonvulsants	Reduce excitability of brain	Phenobarbital, phenytoin (Dilantin)
Antidepressants	Prevent or reduce symptoms of psychological depression	Amitriptyline hydrochloride (Elavil); fluoxetine hydrochloride (Prozac)
Antidiarrheals	Decrease intestinal peristalsis	Loperamide hydrochloride (Imodium A-D)
Antiemetic agents	Prevent nausea, vomiting	Dimenhydrinate (Dramamine); promethazine hydrochloride (Phenergan)
Antifungals	Destroy or retard growth of fungi	Ketoconazole (Nizoral), miconazole nitrate (Monistat 3 or 7)
Antihistamines	Counteract effects of histamine on organs and structures	Chlorpheniramine maleate (Chlor-Trimeton); diphenhydramine hydrochloride (Benadryl)
Antihypertensives	Increase size of arteries	Methyldopate hydrochloride (Aldomet), prazosin (Minipress)
Antiinflammatory agents	Reduce irritation and swelling of tissues	Aspirin, ibuprofen (Motrin); naproxen (Naprosyn)
Antineoplastic agents	Slow tumor growth	Cyclophosphamide (Cytoxan)
Antipsychotics	Exact mechanism not understood; used to treat psychoses	Chlorpromazine (Thorazine), haloperidol (Haldol)
Antipyretics	Decrease body temperature	Aspirin, acetaminophen (Tylenol)
Antitussives, mucolytics, expectorants	Relieve cough, loosen respiratory secretions, aid removal of thick secretions	Codeine sulfate, Benylin, Entex

(continued)

Table 25-1 *(Continued)*

Therapeutic Classification	Effect, Action, Uses	Common Examples
Antivirals	Inhibit viral replication	Acyclovir (Zovirax), AZT
Bronchodilators	Dilate bronchi	Albuterol sulfate (Ventolin), Alupent
Cardiotonics	Increase force of myocardium	Digoxin (Lanoxin), Primacor
Cholinergic blockers	Affect autonomic nervous system	Atropine sulfate, scopolamine hydrobromide
Cholinergics	Mimic activity of parasympathetic nervous system	Neostigmine (Prostigmin), pilocarpine hydrochloride
Decongestants	Reduce swelling of nasal passages	Pseudoephedrine hydrochloride (Sudafed)
Diuretics	Increase secretion of urine by kidneys	Furosemide (Lasix), chlorothiazide (Diuril)
Emetics	Promote vomiting	Ipecacuanha (Ipecac syrup)
Histamine H_2 antagonists	Inhibit action of histamine at H_2 receptor cells of stomach	Cimetidine (Tagamet), ranitidine (Zantac)
Hormones, female	Prevent symptoms of menopause	Estradiol (Estraderm), medroxyprogesterone acetate (Provera)
Hormones, male	Therapy for testosterone deficiency	Androgen (Testamone)
Immunological agents	Stimulate immune response to protect against disease	Vaccines against pneumococcus, influenza virus; diphtheria and tetanus toxoid
Insulin, oral hypoglycemics	Control diabetes	NPH, ultralente insulin; tolbutamide (Orinase), glipizide (Glucotrol)
Sedatives, hypnotics	Sedatives relax and calm; hypnotics induce sleep	Butabarbital sodium, Restoril
Stimulants	Increase activity of central nervous system	Doxapram hydrochloride (Dopram), amphetamine sulfate
Thyroid, antithyroid agents	Alter amount of thyroid hormone produced	Levothyroxine sodium (T4) (Levothroid)

Summarized from Scherer JC, Roach SS. Introductory Clinical Pharmacology, 5th ed. Philadelphia: Lippincott-Raven, 1996.

Box 25-1

EXAMPLE OF A DRUG'S NAMES

Chemical name	7-chloro-1,3-dihydro-1-methyl-5-phenyl-2H-1,4-Benzodiaxepin-2-one
Trade name	Valium
Generic name	Diazepam

substances only; medications not subject to abuse are not regulated by this agency.

As a medical assistant, you may be responsible for maintaining or reminding the physician about professional records and licensure, including registration with the DEA. When the physician registers with the U.S. Attorney General under the BNDD, a registration number (DEA number) is issued. Physicians are registered for 3 years after application and acceptance. The DEA does not take responsibility if the physician's registration expires. The registration retires with the physician; it does not stay with the medical office.

The DEA is also responsible for revising the list of drugs in the Schedule of Controlled Substances (TABLE 25-2). These substances have been identified as having a potential for abuse and dependency. Drug dependence, sometimes referred to as addiction, can be either psychological, physical, or both. A patient who has developed physical dependence on a drug will have mild to severe physiological symptoms that gradually decrease in intensity after the drug is stopped. Patients who are psychologically dependent have acquired a need for the feeling brought on by the drug. Patients who are prescribed controlled substances must be monitored closely for signs of physical or psychological dependence.

Controlled substances in Schedule II are received from suppliers using a Federal Triplicate Order Form DEA 222. Schedules III to V do not require triplicate forms, but invoices for receipts of the substances must be maintained for 2 years. As controlled substances are received, they are listed on a special inventory form in the office (FIG. 25-1). Their receipt should be signed by two employees. Every time a controlled substance leaves the medical office inventory, the drug name, patient, dose, date, ordering physician, and employee who handled the procedure must be recorded. These inventory forms must be kept for 2 years. Controlled substances kept in the medical office must be locked in a safe or in a secure locked box. The number of persons with access to the keys or cabinet should be limited. If drugs are lost or stolen, the local law enforcement agency must be notified immediately.

If controlled substances are prescribed and not administered at the office, some states require only that the information be recorded in the patient's chart; others require a separate file of prescription copies of controlled substances. Law enforcement officials recommend that the DEA number not be preprinted on the prescription. Officials at regional DEA offices are available to answer any questions regarding the drugs under its control. As a medical assistant, you should make sure the physician's office is on the DEA's periodic mailing list to keep abreast of changes.

Checkpoint Question

2. What information must be documented when a controlled substance is administered in the medical office?

SOURCES OF DRUGS

Drugs are available from numerous natural sources, such as plants, minerals, and animals. They may also be synthetic (prepared in the laboratory by artificial means). TABLE 25-3 lists a number of commonly prescribed drugs and their sources.

DRUG ACTIONS AND INTERACTIONS

Pharmacodynamics

Pharmacodynamics is the study of the ways drugs act on the body, including the actions on specific cells, tissues, and organs. All drugs cause cellular change (drug action) and some degree of physiological change (drug effect). An action of a local drug, such as an ointment or lotion applied to the skin, is limited to the area where it is administered. A drug administered for a systemic effect is absorbed into the blood and carried to the organ or tissue on which it will act. An example of this is antibiotic therapy for a urinary tract infection. The antibiotic tablets are taken orally, but once they are absorbed, the action takes place in the urinary bladder, where the drug destroys any microorganisms. A systemic effect can be produced by administering drugs orally (by mouth), sublingually (under the tongue), rectally, by injection, transdermally (through the skin), or by inhalation (through the lungs). A number of factors can influence a drug's action in the body (Box 25-2).

Pharmacokinetics

Pharmacokinetics is the study of the action of drugs within the body based on the route of administration, rate of absorption, duration of action, and elimination from the body. Specifically, the processes included in pharmacokinetics include absorption (getting the drug into the bloodstream), distribution (movement of the drug from the bloodstream into the cells and tissues), metabolism (the physical and chemical breakdown of drugs by the body, including the liver), and excretion (byproducts sent to the kidneys to be removed from the body). In the presence of hepatic disease, the liver may not be able to break down the drug properly, and the patient

Table 25-2 CONTROLLED SUBSTANCES

Schedule	Description	Examples
I	Highest potential for abuse; no accepted medicinal use in U.S.; no accepted safety standards, although some are used in carefully controlled research projects	Opium, marijuana, lysergic acid diethylamide (LSD), peyote, mescaline
II	High potential for abuse; accepted medicinal use in U.S. but with severe restrictions. Abuse can lead to psychological or physiologic dependence. Require written prescription; prescription cannot be refilled or called in to pharmacy by medical office. Only in extreme emergencies may physician call in prescription; handwritten prescription must be presented to pharmacist within 72 hours.	Morphine, codeine, cocaine, secobarbital (Seconal), amphetamines, hydromorphone (Dilaudid), methylphenidate (Ritalin)
III	Limited potential for psychological or physiological dependence. Prescription may be called in to pharmacy by physician and refilled up to 6 times in 6 months.	Paregoric, acetaminophen (Tylenol) with codeine, Fiorinal
IV	Lower potential for abuse than those in schedules II and III; can be called into pharmacy by medical office employee; may be refilled up to 5 times in 6 months.	Chlordiazepoxide (Librium), diazepam (Valium), propoxyphene (Darvon), phenobarbital
V	Lower potential for abuse than those in schedules I to IV.	Buprenorphine (Buprenex), Codeine in cough preparations

Five schedules, or categories, of controlled substances were established by the Bureau of Narcotics and Dangerous Drugs. Medications in the five schedules may be revised periodically after review.

FIGURE 25-1. Controlled substances inventory form.

Table 25-3   COMMON DRUGS AND THEIR SOURCES

Source	Drug	Use
Plants		
Cinchona bark	Quinidine	Antiarrhythmic
Purple foxglove	Digitalis	Cardiotonic
Opium poppy	Paregoric	Antidiarrheal
	Morphine	Analgesic
	Codeine	Antitussive, analgesic
Minerals		
Magnesium	Milk of Magnesia	Antacid, laxative
Silver	Silver nitrate	Placed in eyes of newborns to kill *Neisseria gonorrhoeae*;
Chemical		
		cautery of lesions
Gold	Solganal	Arthritis treatment
Animal proteins		
Pork, beef pancreas	Insulin	Antidiabetic hormone
Pork, beef stomach acids	Pepsin	Digestive hormone
Animal thyroid glands	Thyroid, USP	Hypothyroidism
Synthetics		
	Demerol	Analgesic
	Lomotil	Antidiarrheal
	Gantrisin	Sulfonamide
Semisynthetics		
Escherichia coli	Humulin	Antidiabetic hormone
Bacteria, altered DNA molecules		

LEGAL TIP

If you suspect that a physician or any other health care professional is illegally diverting controlled substances, you have a legal and ethical responsibility to report this suspicion. Gather and document evidence and the reasons you suspect diversion of substances. You should have a clear and compelling case to present to the proper authorities, usually the local police. In addition, if a physician is involved, report this evidence to the Drug Enforcement Agency and the American Medical Association (AMA). You should also notify the state medical society. If the suspected health care worker is not a physician, report it to the appropriate supervisor or superior. Most states have programs to assist health care professionals in obtaining appropriate psychological help to deal with addiction or dependency issues. In most instances, you will remain anonymous.

WHAT IF

Bob Sandler, a 38-year-old accountant, was first seen in the office 2 weeks ago for a back injury that occurred after doing some home repair work the previous weekend. At the initial visit, the physician prescribed an opioid pain medication and a muscle relaxant. Today, Mr. Sandler tells you that his medications were stolen and he would like a refill for both. What if both drugs had a high potential for abuse and were often purchased illegally on the street? Would you suspect that the patient was selling his medication? How could you be sure that this was not occurring?

While the medical assistant must be an advocate for the patient, he or she must also be vigilant about the possibility of drug abuse in the patient population and the community at large. It is imperative that the medical assistant gather as much information as possible about "lost" or "stolen" medications and report any illegal activities to the proper authorities. Patients whose medications with a high potential for abuse have been stolen will want to report the theft to the police. Some physicians want to see a police report before issuing another prescription.

Drug Interactions

When two or more drugs are taken simultaneously, one drug may increase, decrease, or cancel the effects of the other. These interactions may occur with prescribed drugs, over-the-counter medications, herbal or other natural supplements, and alcohol consumption. These **interactions** must always be taken into account when prescribing, administering, obtaining a medication history, or educating a patient about taking medications. Types of interactions include **synergism** (two drugs working together), **antagonism** (an effect in which one drug decreases the effect of another), and **potentiation** (occurs when one drug prolongs or multiplies the effect of another drug). Physicians prescribing two or more drugs may be using these drug interactions to cause a desired effect. An example of this is use of a muscle relaxant and a pain medication to reduce the pain associated with an injury to a muscle or muscle group. However some drug interactions produce undesirable effects. For example, antacids taken to relieve symptoms of indigestion may prevent absorption of antibiotics, such as tetracycline (antagonism), while sedatives and barbiturates taken together can cause central nervous system depression (synergism). TABLE 25-4 lists other important drug-related terms you should know.

PATIENT EDUCATION

Food–Drug Interaction

Many medications interact with food. Some medications are best absorbed when taken on an empty stomach. Two such medications are the antibiotics ampicillin and nafcillin (Unipen). Other medications should be taken with food to decrease the potential for stomach upset. These include ibuprofen (Motrin, an analgesic and anti-inflammatory); amoxicillin, an antibiotic; and verapamil (Calan, a heart medication). Certain medications interact with specific types of food. For example, green leafy vegetables can interact with coumadin, an anticoagulant, and make the patient's bleeding time increase. Also, grapefruit juice interacts with atorvastatin (Lipitor), a medication used to lower blood cholesterol levels, to reduce its efficacy. It is important for patients to know about any food–drug interaction that may affect them. Information about food and drug interactions can be found in most pharmacology books. You will need to learn as much as you can about the medications that are commonly prescribed by the physician with whom you are working.

Box 25-2

FACTORS INFLUENCING DRUG ACTION

Age	Elderly people have slow metabolic processes. Age-related kidney and liver dysfunctions also extend breakdown and excretion times, so it is necessary to monitor the cumulative effects of drugs in the elderly. Children may have a more immediate response to drugs and therefore must be assessed frequently.
Weight	Many dosages are calculated and administered according to the patient's weight. As a general rule, the larger the patient, the greater the dose; however, individual sensitivity should be taken into consideration.
Sex	Women's reactions to certain drugs may be different from those of men because of the ratio of fat to body mass or fluctuating hormone levels.
Existing pathology	If the body is compromised by a disease process, absorption, distribution, metabolism, and excretion may be altered.
Tolerance	Some medications given over a long period cause the body to become resistant to their effects, requiring larger doses to achieve the desired response.

Medical assistants should administer medications only under the direct order of a physician. In no circumstance should the dosage be adjusted or altered unless the assistant is specifically instructed to do so by the physician, since this constitutes illegally practicing medicine.

may undergo toxic effects caused by an accumulation of the drug in the liver or the bloodstream. In this situation, the drug may be noted as **contraindicated** by the manufacturer, or not recommended for use, in patients with a history of liver disease. Some drugs reach the kidneys relatively unchanged; these drugs can be detected in the urine during excretion, when the waste products of drug metabolism are eliminated from the body. However, if the kidneys are compromised by disease, medication may not be properly eliminated, adding to the danger of a cumulative, or building, effect and possible toxicity or poisoning.

WHAT IF

Mrs. Jones calls your office and asks that her prescription for digoxin be refilled. As you are talking with her, you pull her chart to record the call. While reviewing her chart, you notice that she has not had a digoxin blood level drawn as planned by the physician's schedule. How do you handle this situation?

Because digoxin may cause a toxic cumulative effect, it is important that patients taking this drug have their blood level monitored regularly. Explain to Mrs. Jones that you will check with the physician and call her back. You should note your conversation in Mrs. Jones's medical record, then put the chart on the physician's desk or discuss it personally at a convenient time. When the physician has made a decision, call Mrs. Jones with instructions for the drug's renewal and her course of action.

Side Effects and Allergies

When gathering a patient's medical history, you must always ask about allergies of any sort, particularly allergies to medications. A drug **allergy** is a reaction such as hives, dyspnea, or wheezing. In addition, the allergic reaction **anaphylaxis** can be life threatening. Allergic reactions can be immediate or delayed 2 hours or longer, depending on the route of administration; however, many allergic reactions occur within minutes if the medication is administered by injection. The medical assistant must interview the patient carefully about symptoms of allergies and note in the medical record medications that produce true allergic symptoms. Drug allergies should always be noted prominently on the front of the patient's medical record and on each page of the medica-

tion record. Because of the possibility of an anaphylactic reaction, patients should never be given medications that they have had an allergic reaction to in the past. You should always check the chart and ask the patient before administering any medications in the medical office as an additional safety measure.

Many patients state that they have an allergy to certain medications when in fact the reaction was **side effects**. Side effects are reactions to medications that are predictable (as noted by the manufacturer of the medication) and that occur in some patients who take the medication. For example, some medications may cause nausea unless taken with food, and in this case, nausea may be listed by the manufacturer as a side effect. Other medications may cause drowsiness or dryness of the mouth. While side effects are often annoying, they are not life threatening and should not be noted on the patient's allergy list.

If a patient is receiving allergy medications or any medication that has a high incidence of allergic reactions (e.g., penicillin), the patient should wait for 20 to 30 minutes and be rechecked before leaving the office. Some offices require all patients receiving injections to wait for a specific amount of time (15 to 20 minutes) before leaving the office. Always follow the policies of the medical office with regard to administering medications.

Checkpoint Question

3. How does synergism differ from antagonism?

SOURCES OF INFORMATION

The *Physician's Desk Reference* (PDR) is widely used as a reference for drugs in current use. It is intended for physicians, but since the medical assistant must know about various medications administered in the office, the *PDR* is a valuable resource for anyone, including the medical assistant, to use before administering medications. This resource is clearly written to identify a drug's chemical name, brand name or names, and generic name. It also lists the properties,

Table 25-4	DRUG-RELATED TERMS
Term	**Meaning**
Therapeutic classification	States the purpose for the drug's use (e.g., cardiotonic, anti-infective, antiarrhythmic)
Teratogenic category	Level of risk to fetal or maternal health, from category A to D, with increasing danger at each level. Category X drugs should never be given during pregnancy.
Indications	Diseases and conditions for which the particular drug is prescribed.
Contraindications	Conditions or instances for which the particular drug should not be used.
Adverse reaction	Undesirable side effects of a particular drug.
Hypersensitivity	Excessive reaction; also known as drug allergy. Body must build this response; first exposures may or may not indicate that a problem is developing.
Idiosyncratic reaction	Abnormal or unexpected reaction to a drug peculiar to the individual patient; not technically an allergy.

Spanish Terminology

Tome la medicina con jogo.	Take the medicine with juice.
Tome la medicina antes de las comidas.	Take the medicine before meals.
Tome la medicina después de las comidas.	Take the medicine after meals.
Tiene alergias?	Do you have any allergies?

indications, side effects, contraindications, dosages, and so on. One section of the PDR contains pictures of various medications. This book is sometimes distributed to physicians free of charge; however, it is also available for use in libraries and for purchase in bookstores.

The *United States Pharmacopeia Dispensing Information* (USPDI) consists of two paperback volumes providing drug information for the health care provider. It defines drug sources, chemistry, physical properties, tests for identity, storage, and dosage. The USPDI does not contain photographs of the medications and must be purchased by the physician.

The *American Hospital Formulary Service* (AHFS), distributed to practicing physicians, contains concise information arranged according to drug classifications. The *Compendium of Drug Therapy* is published annually and is also distributed to physicians. It includes photographs of the drugs and phone numbers of major pharmaceutical companies and poison control centers.

PRESCRIPTIONS

Medications may be administered (given in the office), dispensed (a supply given for later use), or prescribed (a written order to be filled by a pharmacist). You may be permitted to complete the prescription form and obtain the physician's signature if directed to do so by the physician. An established protocol and traditional form must be followed when filling out prescriptions:

Line 1. *Date.* Prescriptions must be filled within 6 months of the date of issuance.

Line 2. *Patient's name and address.* The pharmacist needs this information to fill the prescription.

Line 3. *Superscription.* The symbol Rx is found at the top left of the blank prescription pad. Literally it means recipe, or "take thou."

Line 4. *Inscription.* This includes the name of the medication, the desired form (e.g., liquid, tablet, capsule), and the strength (e.g., 250 mg, 500 mL).

Line 4. *Subscription.* This states the amount to be dispensed (e.g., 60 tablets, 120 mL).

Line 5. *Signature.* This section notes any instructions for taking the medication (e.g., with meals, three times a day, four times a day).

Line 6. *Refills.* The number of times a prescription can be refilled should be indicated on the prescription, generally no more than 5 times within 6 months. If no refills are indicated, the word none should be circled or 0 should be written in.

Line 7. *Physician's signature.* The physician is responsible for prescriptions written in his or her office and should check and sign all prescriptions.

Line 8. *Generic.* Some physicians and insurance companies allow generic substitutes for some medications but not others. Note on the prescription whether generic substitutions can be made. If the physician does not want a specific medication substituted with a generic drug, "DAW" can be written on the prescription which means "dispense as written."

All prescribed medications must be documented in full in the patient's record (FIG. 25-2). Prescriptions that are

DATE	TIME	ORDERS
7/5/xx	1000	Prescription for ampicillin 250 mg, p.o., qid X 7 days as ordered by Dr. Smith
		Sally Smith, CMA

FIGURE 25-2. Documentation of a prescribed medication in a patient record.

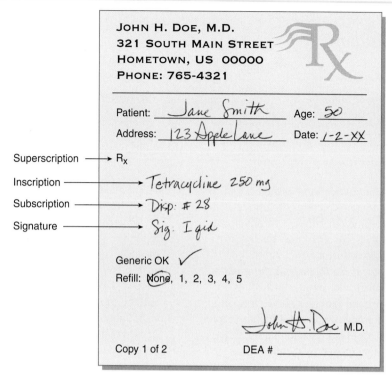

JOHN H. DOE, M.D.
321 SOUTH MAIN STREET
HOMETOWN, US 00000
PHONE: 765-4321

Patient: _Jane Smith_   Age: _50_
Address: _123 Apple Lane_   Date: _1-2-XX_

Superscription ———▶ R$_X$

Inscription ——————▶ _Tetracycline 250 mg_

Subscription —————▶ _Disp: # 28_

Signature ——————▶ _Sig: I qid_

Generic OK ✓
Refill: None, 1, 2, 3, 4, 5

John H. Doe M.D.

Copy 1 of 2   DEA # _____

FIGURE 25-3. Prescription form.

TRIAGE

Three patients have called the office asking you for prescription refills. It is 10 in the morning. What is the correct priority order for looking at the patient's medical record and calling the pharmacy for a refill?

A. A 52-year-old patient says she went to take her methyldopa (Aldomet) this morning but was out of it. She takes it every morning at 9 for her blood pressure.

B. A mother says her 3-year-old son spilled the bottle of ampicillin on the floor. The next dose is due at 2 this afternoon.

C. A 66-year-old patient says she is out of her sleeping pills. She wants a refill for temazepam (Restoril).

How do you sort these patients? Which prescription should be called in to the pharmacy first? Second? Third?

Important: Before calling any medication refill into the pharmacy, you must look at the patient's medical record and be sure there are refill orders on the chart. Also, you must follow your office's policy on prescription refills.

Patient A should be done first; it is important that blood pressure medications be taken at the same time every day. Patient B is next so that the 2 P.M. dose is not missed. Patient C's prescription should be handled last of these three.

called or faxed to the pharmacist must also be documented. The chart is a legal document and may be called into court in the event of legal action. If the medication order is not recorded, it will be presumed that the medication was never ordered. FIGURE 25-3 shows a sample prescription form.

Checkpoint Question

4. What does the superscription on the prescription indicate and how does it differ from the subscription?

CHAPTER SUMMARY

Medications are administered, dispensed, or prescribed to patients to produce therapeutic effects. They are available in many forms and can be administered in various ways. Some medications, called controlled substances, may result in dependency and abuse. These drugs are strictly regulated by the federal government. As a medical assistant, you will need to keep current on the legal regulations concerning the manufacture, sale, and prescribing of medications. You must also understand the actions, effects, and interactions of drugs to carry out a physician's medication orders.

Critical Thinking Challenges

1. What type of information regarding medications do patients need to know? Is there anything they do not need to know?
2. Using a drug reference book such as the PDR, look up a medication that you have taken. What are the medication's trade and generic names? Are there any side effects or contraindications? Explain what you learned about this medication that you did not already know.

Answers to Checkpoint Questions

1. A drug's chemical name identifies the chemical components of the drug; the trade name is the name under which the manufacturer distributes the drug commercially.
2. When a controlled substance is administered, you must document the drug name, patient, dose, date, ordering physician, and your name as the employee who administered the drug.
3. Synergism refers to an interaction between two drugs or other substances in which the action of one is enhanced by the other. Antagonism is an interaction in which one drug or substance decreases the effects of another.
4. The superscription indicates the medication name, desired form, and strength. The subscription indicates the amount of medication to dispense.

 Websites

www.fda.gov/medwatch
www.pdr.net
www.emedguides.com
http://medlineplus/gov/
http://nccam.nih.gov

26

Preparing and Administering Medications

CHAPTER OUTLINE

ROLE DELINEATION

CLINICAL: FUNDAMENTAL PRINCIPLES
- Apply principles of aseptic technique and infection control

CLINICAL: PATIENT CARE
- Prepare patient for examinations, procedures, and treatments
- Assist with examinations, procedures, and treatments

- Prepare and administer medications and immunizations
- Maintain medication and immunization records
- Coordinate patient care information with other health care providers
- Initiate intravenous medications and administer intravenous medications with appropriate training as permitted by state law

GENERAL: PROFESSIONALISM
- Display a professional manner and image
- Work as a member of the health care team
- Treat all patients with compassion and empathy

GENERAL: COMMUNICATION SKILLS
- Recognize and respect cultural diversity
- Adapt communications to individual's ability to understand
- Recognize and respond effectively to verbal, nonverbal, and written communications
- Use medical terminology appropriately
- Serve as a liaison

GENERAL: LEGAL CONCEPTS
- Perform within legal and ethical boundaries
- Document accurately
- Implement and maintain federal and state health care legislation and regulations
- Comply with established risk management and safety procedures

GENERAL: INSTRUCTION
- Instruct individuals according to their needs

CHAPTER COMPETENCIES

LEARNING OBJECTIVES
Upon successfully completing this chapter, you will be able to:
1. Spell and define the key terms.
2. List the safety guidelines for medication administration.
3. Explain the difference between the oral and parenteral routes of medication administration.
4. Describe the parts of a syringe and needle and name the parts that must be kept sterile.
5. Compare the types of injections (intradermal, subcutaneous, and intramuscular) and locate the sites and anatomical landmarks used to determine where each may be administered safely.
6. List the various needle lengths, gauges, and preferred sites for each type of injection.
7. Explain and demonstrate how to calculate adult and child dosages.
8. Identify and list the rights used for medication administration.
9. Discuss when the Z-track method for administering an intramuscular injection is indicated.

10. Describe the procedure for reading an intradermal tuberculosis screening test and explain what is meant by a positive result.
11. Explain the principles for calculating an intravenous fluid rate.

PERFORMANCE OBJECTIVES
Upon successfully completing this chapter, you will be able to:
1. Administer oral medications (Procedure 26-1).
2. Prepare an injection (Procedure 26-2).
3. Administer an intradermal injection (Procedure 26-3).
4. Administer a subcutaneous injection (Procedure 26-4).
5. Administer an intramuscular injection (Procedure 26-5)
6. Administer an intramuscular injection using the Z-track method (Procedure 26-6).
7. Apply transdermal medications (Procedure 26-7).
8. Prepare an intravenous line for medication administration (Procedure 26-8).

KEY TERMS

ampule	diluent	metric system	sublingual medication
apothecary system of measurement	gauge	nebulizer	topical medication
	induration	ophthalmic medication	vial
buccal medication	infiltration	otic medication	
contraindication	Mantoux	parenteral medication	

MEDICATION ADMINISTRATION BASICS

Before administering any medications in the medical office, you should be familiar with the medication ordered by the physician and the procedures necessary to administer the drug accurately and safely. As a clinical medical assistant, you must look up any drugs you are not familiar with to determine the drug classification, the usual dosage, and the route of administration. In addition, you should be thoroughly familiar with the terminology, abbreviations, symbols, and signs used in prescribing, administering, and documenting medications. The abbreviations listed in TABLE 26-1 are most commonly used and should be memorized.

Safety Guidelines

To ensure safety when administering medications, follow these guidelines:

1. Know the policies of your office regarding the administration of medications.
2. Give only the medications that the physician has ordered in writing. Do not accept verbal orders.
3. Check with the physician if you have any doubt about a medication or an order.
4. Avoid conversation and other distractions while preparing and administering medications. It is important to remain attentive during this task.
5. Work in a quiet, well-lighted area.
6. Check the label when taking the medication from the shelf, when preparing it, and when replacing it on the shelf or disposing of the empty container. This is known as the three checks for safe administration.
7. Place the order and the medication side by side to compare for accuracy.
8. Check the strength of the medication (e.g., 250 versus 500 mg) and the route of administration.
9. Read labels carefully. Do not scan labels or medication orders.
10. Check the patient's medical record for allergies to the actual medication or its components before administering.
11. Check the medication's expiration date.
12. Be alert for color changes, precipitation, odor, or any indication that the medication's properties have changed. If the medication has changed in consistency, color, or odor, discard it appropriately.
13. Measure exactly. There should be no bubbles in liquid medication.
14. Have sharps containers as close to the area of use as possible.
15. Put on gloves for all procedures that might result in contact with blood or body fluids.
16. Stay with the patient while he or she takes oral medication. Watch for any reaction and record the patient's response.
17. Never return a medication to the container after it is poured or removed.
18. Never recap, bend, or break a used needle.
19. Never give a medication poured or drawn up by someone else.
20. Never leave the medication cabinet unlocked when not in use.
21. Never give keys for the medication cabinet to an unauthorized person. Limit access to the medication cabinet by limiting access to the cabinet keys.

Checkpoint Question

1. When are the three checks for safe medication administration performed?

Seven Rights for Correct Medication Administration

Medication errors should not occur during careful preparation or administration. By observing the seven rights during medication administration, you will eliminate the potential for many errors (Box 26-1). The seven rights include the following:

1. Right patient. Ask the patient to state his or her name. Some patients will answer to any name, so simply saying the name is not assurance that you have the correct patient.
2. Right time. Most medications ordered to be given in the office are to be given before the patient leaves. Some patients may have to be told when the next dose is due.
3. Right dose. Check doses carefully. Many medications come in various strengths.
4. Right route. Some medications are prepared for administration by a variety of routes. Is it oral, **parenteral**, **otic**, **ophthalmic**, or **topical**?
5. Right drug. Many medication names are very much alike; for instance Orinase and Ornade may be confused if you are not careful. Always look up unfamiliar medications in a drug reference book such as the *Physicians Desk Reference* (PDR).
6. Right technique. Check how the medication is to be given, such as orally and with or without food. Intramuscular, subcutaneous, and intradermal injections should be given only after carefully choosing a site and with the correct procedure.
7. Right documentation. The medical record is a legal document. Make sure that the medication is documented after it is administered (not before) and that you have documented it in the correct medical record. All medications given in the medical office must be documented immediately with the name of the medication, the dose, route, and site (if injected) and signed by the medical assistant. The patient's response should be charted as well when appropriate.

Table 26-1 ABBREVIATIONS

Abbreviation	Meaning	Abbreviation	Meaning
aa	of each	NS	normal saline
ac	before meals	OD	right eye
ad lib	as desired	OS	left eye
AM, am, A.M.	morning	OU	both eyes
amp	ampule	os	mouth
amt	amount	oz	ounce
aq	aqueous	p	after
bid	twice a day	pc	after meals
c̄	with	pm, PM	afternoon or evening
cap	capsule	po, PO	by mouth
cc	cubic centimeter	prn, PRN	whenever necessary
DC, disc, d/c	discontinue	pt	pint
disp	dispense	q	every
dl, dL	deciliter	qd	every day
dr	dram	qh	every hour
DW	distilled water	q2h	every 2 hours
elix	elixir	q3h	every 3 hours
et	and	qid	four times a day
ext	extract	qod	every other day
fl, fld	fluid	qs	quantity sufficient
g, gm	gram	qt	quart
gr	grain	R	right, rectal
gt(t)	drop(s)	Rx	take, prescribe
h, hr	hour	s̄	without
hs, HS	hour of sleep	SC, subcu, subq, S/Q, SQ	subcutaneously
Id, ID	intradermal	Sig	label
IM	intramuscular	SL	sublingual
IV	intravenous	sol	solution
Kg	kilogram	SOS	once if necessary
L, l	liter	sp	spirits
lb	pound	ss	one-half
m, min	minim	stat, STAT	immediately
mcg, μg	microgram	supp	suppository
mEq	milliequivalent	syr	syrup
ml, mL	milliliter	tab	tablet
n	normal	T, tb, tbs, tbsp	tablespoon
NaCl	sodium chloride	t, tsp	teaspoon
NKA	no known allergies	tid	three times a day
noc	night	tinc	tincture
NPO	nothing by mouth	ung	ointment

MEDICATION ERRORS

Even if you are extremely careful, you may make an error when administering a medication. It is imperative that you report the error to the physician and that intervention measures start immediately. The error and all corrective actions must be documented thoroughly in the patient's medical record. An incident report should be filed in the medical office as verification that all possible precautions were taken for the patient.

Systems of Measurement

The most common system of measurement used in the medical office is the **metric system**; however, the **apothecary system of measurement** is still used by some physicians. The household system of measurement is most often used by patients, but this system should be avoided in the medical setting, since the measurements are not as accurate as in the metric system (Box 26-2). While working in the clinical setting, you may find it necessary to convert from one system to another. In addition, you may be required to calculate a dose in one system of measurement using mathematical equations. It is necessary to master the elements of the systems of measurement before attempting to calculate dosages.

Metric, Household, and Apothecary Systems

The metric system is used in the United States and throughout the world. Because it is based on multiples of 10, decimals, not fractions, are used. In the metric system, the base unit of *length* is the *meter* (m). The base unit of *weight* is the *gram* (g or gm). Liter (L or l) is used to measure fluid volume. Prefixes used in the metric system show a fraction or multiple of the base. These prefixes are often used:

- Micro- (0.000001)
- Milli- (0.001)
- Centi- (0.01)
- Deci- (0.1)
- Kilo- (1000.0)

For example, using the base unit of a gram, fractional measurements are as follows:

- Microgram (mcg, μg), one-millionth of a gram (×0.000001)
- Milligram (mg), one-thousandth of a gram (×0.001)
- Kilogram (kg), 1000 grams (×1000.0)

Decagrams and centigrams are not used in medication administration.

With the base unit of a liter (1 L = approximately 1.06

quarts), fractional measurements are in milliliters (ml, mL), measures are rarely used in medication administration. Also, 1 cubic centimeter (cc), a solid, is equivalent to 1 mL and therefore, the measures are used interchangeably at times.

The apothecary system is used less frequently now than in the past and is gradually being replaced by the metric system. In the apothecary system, liquid measurements include drop (gt) or drops (gtt), minim (min, m), fluid dram (fl dr), fluidounce (fl oz), pint (pt), quart (qt), and gallon (gal). Measurements for solid weights include grain (gr), dram (dr), ounce (oz), and pound (lb). Roman numerals are used for smaller numbers, and fractions may be used when necessary. Decimals are never used in the apothecary system.

The household system of measurement includes measures such as the teaspoon (tsp), tablespoon (tbsp), ounce (oz), cup (c), pint (pt), quart (qt), and pound (lb). While this system is not used in the medical office for calculating doses, patients may need to be instructed on the proper household measurement for taking medications ordered in the metric system (e.g., 5 mL is equivalent to 1 tsp). TABLE 26-2 lists commonly used equivalents in the metric, apothecary, and household systems of measurement.

Checkpoint Question

2. What are three systems of measurement, and which one should be avoided? Why?

Converting Between Systems of Measurement

Apothecary or Household to Metric. To convert from one system to another system, use the following rules:

- To change grains (apothecary system) to grams (metric system), divide the number of grains ordered by 15. Example: gr 30 ÷ 15 = 2 g.

HOUSEHOLD MEASURES

Household measurements include cups, medicine droppers, teaspoons (tsp), and tablespoons (tbsp). These are some of the approximate equivalents to household measurements:

1 tsp = 1 fluid dram = 5 mL
1 tbsp = 0.5 fluidounce = 4 fluid drams = 15 mL
2 tbsp = 1 fluidounce = 30 mL

Caution patients who will be using household measurements to avoid using table flatware and regular cups. Standard measuring spoons and cups are more accurate.

Table 26-2	MOST COMMONLY USED APPROXIMATE EQUIVALENTS	
Metric	**Apothecary**	**Household**
0.06 g	gr i	
0.06 mL	min i	1 drop
1.0 g	gr xv	
1.0 mL	min xv	0.2 tsp
5.0 mL	1 dr	1 tsp
15 mL	0.5 oz	1 tbsp
30 mL	1 oz	2 tbsp
500 mL	16 oz	1 pt
1000 mL	32 oz	1 qt

There are many discrepancies among these approximate equivalents. For example, 30 mL is the accepted equivalent for 1 oz, but 29.57 mL is the exact equivalent. Such discrepancies are inevitable when equivalencies between the two systems are not exact. The discrepancies are within a 10% margin of error, which usually is acceptable in pharmacology. Reprinted with permission from Taylor C, Lillis C, Le Mone P. Fundamentals of Nursing: The Art and Science of Nursing Care, ed 2. Philadelphia: Lippincott, 1993;1347.

- To change grains (apothecary system) to milligrams (metric system), multiply the grains by 60. Use this rule with less than 1 grain. Example: gr 1/4 × 60 = 15 mg.
- To change ounces (household) to milliliters (metric system), multiply the ounces by 30. Example: 4 oz × 30 = 120 mL.
- To change milliliters (metric system) to fluidounces (household system), divide the milliliters by 30. Example: 150 mL ÷ 30 = 50 oz.
- To change kilograms (metric system) to pounds (household system), multiply the kilograms by 2.2. Example: 50 kg × 2.2 = 110.0 lb.
- To change pounds to kilograms (metric system), divide the pounds (household system) by 2.2. Example: 44 lb ÷ 2.2 = 20 kg.

Metric to Metric. In the metric system, it is sometimes necessary to convert measurements using the same unit of measure. For example, the physician may order 0.5 g of medication and the medication label reads 500 mg. To convert within the metric system, use the following rules:

- To change grams to milligrams, multiply grams by 1000 or move the decimal point three places to the right. Example: 0.5 g × 1000 = 500 mg
- To change milligrams to grams, divide the milligrams by 1000 or move the decimal point three places to the left. Example: 500 mg ÷ 1000 = 0.5 g.
- To change milligrams to micrograms, multiply the milligrams by 1000 or move the decimal three places to the right. Example: 5 mg × 1000 = 5000 µg.
- To change micrograms to milligrams, divide the micrograms by 1000 or move the decimal three places to the left. Example: 500 µg ÷ 1000 = 0.5 mg.

- To change liters to milliliters, multiply the liters by 1000 or move the decimal three places to the right. Example: 0.01 L × 1000 = 10 mL.
- To change milliliters to liters, divide the milliliters by 1000 or move the decimal three places to the left. Example: 100 mL ÷ 1000 = 0.1 L.

There is no conversion necessary when changing cubic centimeters to milliliters; they are approximately the same.

Calculating Adult Dosages

Administration of medication is an exact science; errors in calculation can kill the patient. Although the physician will order the amount of medication to be administered to the patient, you may have to calculate the amount of medication to withdraw into a syringe or pour into a medicine cup. There are two methods by which doses are most frequently calculated for adults: the ratio method and the formula method. Measurements must be in the same system (preferably metric) and unit before a calculation can be made. For example, if the medication is ordered in the apothecary or household system but is packaged in the metric system, you must first convert the order (apothecary or household) to the metric system. If the medication is ordered in grams but is packaged in milligrams, the ordered dose must be converted to milligrams before any calculations can be made. When using the metric system, be careful to keep the decimal point in the correct place during calculations and be sure to convert fractions to decimals.

Ratio and Proportion. When using the ratio method to calculate doses, you must use the amount of medication ordered and the information on the medication label to create a ratio. Once the ratio has been determined, the proportion, or relationship between the two ratios, can be calculated to give you the amount of medication to administer. To calculate a dose using the ratio and proportion method, set up the problem thus:

$$\text{Dose on hand : Known quantity}$$
$$= \text{Dose desired : Unknown quantity}$$

Example 1. The physician orders erythromycin 250 mg. The label on the package reads erythromycin 100 mg/mL. The equation can be written thus:

$$100 \text{ mg} : 1 \text{ mL} = 250 \text{ mg} : X$$
Multiply the extremes (first and fourth terms) = 100X
Multiply the means (second and third terms) = 250
Write the proportion as follows: 100X = 250
Divide both sides of the equal sign by 100 to solve for X.
$$250 ÷ 100 = 2.5$$

Therefore, you withdraw and administer 2.5 mL of erythromycin for the patient to receive the 250 mg ordered by the physician. *Note*: When you document the medication after administration, the amount given is the amount ordered by the physician, not the amount drawn up.

Example 2. The physician orders phenobarbital 25 mg. On hand are 12.5-mg tablets. State the equation:

$$12.5 \text{ mg} : 1 \text{ tablet} = 25 \text{ mg} : X$$
$$\text{Multiply the extremes} = 12.5X$$
$$\text{Multiply the means} = 25 \text{ mg}$$
$$25 = 12.5X$$
$$\text{Divide both sides by } 12.5$$
$$25 \div 12.5 = 2 \text{ tablets}$$

In this example, you administer two tablets of phenobarbital to the patient and record that 25 mg was given.

The Formula Method. The formula method is written thus:

$$(\text{Desired} \div \text{On hand}) \times \text{Quantity} = \text{Dose}$$

Example 1. The physician orders ampicillin 0.5 g. On hand you have ampicillin 250 mg capsules. How much ampicillin should be administered? Remember, both doses must be in the same unit of measure. Convert grams to milligrams: multiply the grams by 1000 or move the decimal point three places to the right. The answer is 0.5 g equals 500 mg. With this information, you may set up your problem thus:

$$500 \text{ mg (desired)} \div 250 \text{ mg (on hand)}$$
$$\times 1 \text{ (quantity)} = 2 \times 1 = 2$$

In this example, you administer two capsules and chart that 0.5 g or 500 mg was given to the patient.

Example 2. The physician orders 0.35 g of a medication and you have on hand a liquid of 700 mg/mL. How many milliliters do you prepare to administer? Remember, measurements must be in equivalent units, so 0.35 g must be changed to milligrams.

$$(350 \text{ mg} \div 700 \text{ mg}) \times 1 \text{ mL} = 0.5 \text{ mL} = 0.5 \text{ mL}$$

Checkpoint Question

3. Before calculating doses, what must be done with the measurements?

Calculating Pediatric Doses

Several formulas are used to calculate children's doses. One method uses body surface area (BSA) and requires a scale known as a nomogram (FIG 26-1). The BSA method is considered to be the most accurate method for children up to 12 years of age and for adults who are below normal percentiles for body weight. The nomogram chart estimates the BSA in square meters according to the patient's height and weight. A straight line is drawn from the patient's height in inches or centimeters (column 1) to the patient's weight in kilograms or pounds (column 3). The line intersects on the BSA column (column 2) to give the BSA of the

Height		Surface Area	Weight	
Feet	Centimeters	Square Meters	Pounds	Kilograms

FIGURE 26-1. Nomogram for estimating surface area of infants and young children. To determine the surface area of the patient, draw a straight line between the point representing the height on the left vertical scale and the point representing the weight on the right vertical scale. The point at which this line intersects the middle vertical scale indicates the patient's surface area in square meters.

Spanish Terminology

Tome la medicina cuatro veces al día.	Take the medicine four times a day.
Tome la medicina tres veces al día.	Take the medication three times a day.
Esta medicina quita (alivia) el dolor.	This medication is a pain killer.
Que medicinas toma?	What medications do you take?

child (FIG. 26-2). After obtaining the BSA estimate, the following formula is used to calculate the dosage:

$$(\text{BSA} \times \text{adult dose}) \div 1.7 = \text{child's dose}$$

Other rules for calculating pediatric doses include Young's rule, Clark's rule, and Fried's rule. Young's rule is used to calculate doses for children aged 12 months to 12 years. This method requires that you determine the age of the child in years and divide by the age of the child in years plus 12. This number is multiplied by the adult dose.

$$\text{Pediatric dose} = \frac{\text{child's age in years}}{\text{child's age in years} + 12} \times \text{adult dose}$$

Clark's rule is more accurate than Young's rule because it allows for variations in body size and weight for different ages. Using Clark's rule, the weight of the child is divided by 150 (presumed weight of average adult) and multiplied by the average adult dose to determine the pediatric dose.

$$\text{Pediatric dose} = \frac{\text{child's weight in pounds}}{150 \text{ pounds}} \times \text{adult dose}$$

Fried's rule, used for calculating doses for infants less than 2 years of age, bases the dose on the age of the child in months. In this case, 150 used in calculations is the age in

WHAT IF

A child arrives at the medical office in cardiac arrest? How does the physician have time to calculate the dose for the child's body weight?

In such a situation, the physician does not have the time to perform the calculations and instead may rely on a printed graph that lists precalculated emergency drug doses. Also, some hospital emergency departments have computer software that will automatically calculate and print a list of pediatric emergency medications and their doses.

months of a 12.5-year-old child, presuming that a child of that age would be eligible for an adult dose. Using Fried's rule, the child's age in months is divided by 150, then multiplied by the average adult dose.

$$\text{Pediatric dose} = \frac{\text{child's age in months}}{150 \text{ months}} \times \text{adult dose}$$

Many medications that require careful calibration are dosed per kilogram of body weight. Instructions for calculation are included in the package insert that comes with the medication. For instance, the insert may state, "Adults and children over 25 kg (55 lb), give 500 mg. Children less than 25 kg, give 25 mg/kg." If the child to whom this medication is to be given weighs 20 lb, this weight must be converted to kilograms. If 1 kg is 2.2 lb, this child weighs 9 kg. The equation for calculating the child's dosage is as follows:

$$25 \text{ mg} \times 9 \text{ kg} = 225 \text{ mg}$$

Checkpoint Question

4. What is the most accurate method used to calculate a pediatric dose?

ROUTES OF MEDICATION ADMINISTRATION

Medication can be administered in many ways and is chosen by the physician after considering many factors. Sometimes the route is chosen because of cost, safety, or the speed by which the drug will be absorbed into the body. Certain drugs may be administered by only one route, while others may be administered in a variety of ways. Some drugs may be toxic if given by a certain route, some may be effective only if given by a specific route, and sometimes absorption will occur only through one particular route.

Height		Surface Area	Weight	
Feet	Centimeters	Square Meters	Pounds	Kilograms

FIGURE 26-2. Using the nomogram, the child who is 32 inches tall and weighs 40 pounds has a BSA of 0.6 m².

Oral, Sublingual, and Buccal Routes

Of all of the medication routes, the oral route is most preferred by patients and is the easiest to administer. However, medications taken orally, or by mouth, are usually slow to take effect, and this route cannot be used for unconscious patients, those with nausea and vomiting, or those who are ordered to take nothing by mouth. Drugs given orally may be administered as tablets, capsules, pills, or liquids (Procedure 26-1). Most are absorbed through the walls of the gastrointestinal tract. Drugs given orally in the medical office usually come in unit dose packs that contain the amount of the drug for a single dose. These may be left by pharmaceutical sales representatives to be given as samples to patients (FIG 26-3). Unit dose packages are labeled with the trade name, generic name, precautions, instructions for storage, and an expiration date. TABLE 26-3 lists common solid and liquid forms of oral medications.

The physician may also order medications to be taken sublingually or buccally. Medication taken sublingually is placed under the patient's tongue; it must not be swallowed. The drug is dissolved by the saliva in the mouth and is absorbed directly into the bloodstream through the oral mucosa covering the sublingual vessels. Caution the patient not to eat or drink until the medication has totally dissolved.

Medication given by the buccal route is placed in the pouch between the cheek and gum at the side of the

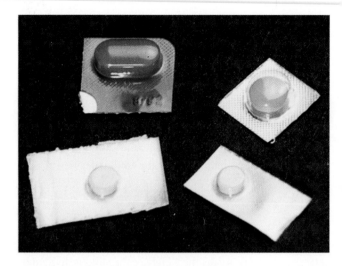

FIGURE 26-3. Unit dose packages.

mouth. Buccal absorption of medication occurs through the vascular oral mucosa. Few medications are manufactured for this route. The patient must not eat or drink until the medication is completely absorbed.

Checkpoint Question

5. What are the disadvantages of the oral route for medication administration?

Table 26-3 FORMS OF ORAL MEDICATIONS	
Form	**Description**
Solids	
Buffered caplet	Medication with added agent to decrease or counteract acidity to prevent gastric irritation.
Capsule	Powdered or granulated; in a gelatin sheath designed to dissolve in gastric enzymes or high in small intestine.
Enteric coated tablet	Compressed dry; coated to withstand gastric acidity and dissolve in intestines; may be destroyed by gastric enzymes or damaging to gastric mucosa. Never crush or break enteric coated tablets.
Gelcap	Oil-based medication in a soft gelatin capsule.
Lozenge	Firm, compressed form, usually for local effect in mouth or throat. Caution patients to let lozenges dissolve slowly and avoid drinking fluids after using lozenge.
Powder	Finely ground form; may be difficult for some patients to swallow.
Spansule, or time-release capsule	Gelatin capsule filled with medication that will dissolve over time rather than all at once. Never open a time-release capsule unless recommended by manufacturer.
Tablet	Medication shaped and colored for easy identification. Tablets usually dissolve high in the GI tract; may be broken in half only if scored for that purpose.
Liquids	
Elixir	Medication dissolved in alcohol and flavored; less sweet than syrups, usually preferred by adults. Not appropriate for alcoholics or diabetics.
Emulsion	Medication combined with water and oil; must be thoroughly shaken to disperse medication evenly.
Extract	Highly concentrated form made by evaporating volatile plant oils; may be administered as drops; usually given in a liquid to disguise strong taste.
Gel	Medication suspended in thin gelatin or paste.
Suspension	Particles dissolved in liquid; must be shaken well before use.
Syrup	Very sweet form frequently used for children; usually flavored in addition to having a high sugar content.

INJECTIONS: MAINTAINING STERILITY

The following parts of a hypodermic setup must be kept sterile:
- Syringe tip
- Inside of barrel
- Shaft of plunger
- Needle

Parenteral Administration

If a patient cannot take medications orally, if the drug cannot be absorbed through the gastrointestinal system, or if rapid absorption of the drug is desired, the parenteral route is used. Parenteral administration refers not only to injections but to all ways drugs are administered other than via the gastrointestinal tract. Administration by injection is the most efficient method of parenteral drug administration, but it can also be the most hazardous. While the effects may be quite rapid, the medication cannot be retrieved once injected, and because the skin is broken, it is possible for infection to develop if strict aseptic technique is not followed (Box 26-3).

Equipment for Injections

Ampules, Vials, Cartridges. Medications used for injections are supplied in **ampules**, **vials**, and cartridges (FIG 26-4). Ampules are small glass containers that must be broken at the neck so that the solution can be aspirated into the syringe. When the ampule is opened, all medication in it must be either used or discarded. It must not be saved for later use, since once the ampule is broken, sterility cannot be maintained.

Vials are glass or plastic containers sealed at the top by a rubber stopper. They may be single-dose or multiple-dose containers. The contents of vials may be in solution or in powder, which requires reconstitution with a specific amount and type of **diluent** (diluting agent), usually sterile water or saline. Certain drugs, such as phenytoin (Dilantin), require a special diluent supplied by the manufacturer. When a powdered drug is reconstituted in a multiple-dose vial, the following must be written on the label:

1. Date of reconstitution
2. Initials of the person who reconstituted the drug
3. Diluent used

To reconstitute dry medication, withdraw the diluent using aseptic technique, add the diluent to the vial containing the powder, and roll the bottle between your palms to dissolve the medication completely. Shaking the vial may cause unnecessary bubbles. When the powder has completely dis-solved, calculate the dose based on the amount of diluent added to the powder. The instructions from the manufacturer of the drug usually indicate how much diluent to add to the powder and the resulting concentration of the mixture necessary for calculating dosages. You should always check the vial label or manufacturer's instructions before adding the diluent to determine the resulting dosage.

Vials intended for multiple doses may hold up to 50 mL and may be used repeatedly by inserting a needle through the self-sealing rubber stopper to remove a portion of the solution. Unit dose vials usually contain 1 to 2 mL, and all of the solution is removed for a single injection.

Prefilled syringes contain a premeasured amount of medication in a disposable cartridge with a needle attached. The prefilled cartridge and needle are placed in a holder for administration (FIG 26-5). Examples of prefilled cartridges and holders are the Tubex and the Carpuject. After a prefilled cartridge and holder are used, only the used cartridge should be discarded in a sharps biohazard container. The holder is reusable.

Needles and Syringes. The choice of needle and syringe used for an injection depends on the type of injection and the size of the patient. The 3-mL hypodermic syringe is the type most commonly used for injections. In the medical office syringes designed to hold 5 mL or more are usually used for irrigation only, not for injections. All syringes consist of a plunger, body or barrel, flange, and tip (FIG. 26-6). Types of syringes used for parenteral administration include tuberculin, or 1 mL, syringes and insulin syringes that are calibrated in units and are used for insulin only.

Needle lengths vary from 0.375 inch to 1.5 inch for standard injections. **Gauge** refers to the diameter of the needle lumen. Needle gauge varies from 18 (large) to 30 (small); the higher the number, the smaller the gauge. Medical supply companies package hypodermic needles separately in color-coded packages (FIG. 26-7) or in color-coded envelopes with the syringe attached. The sizes are also written on the pack-

FIGURE 26-4. Ampules, vials, prefilled cartridges, and holders.

F I G U R E   2 6 - 5 .   Prefilled syringes. (A) Prefilled medication cartridges and injector devices. (B) Inserting the cartridge into the injector device. (C) Ready for injection.

F I G U R E   2 6 - 6 .   Parts of a needle and syringe. (Reprinted with permission from Cohen BJ. Medical Terminology: An Illustrated Guide. Philadelphia: Lippincott Williams & Wilkins, 2003.)

in minims (m). The tuberculin (TB) syringe is narrow and has a total capacity of 1 mL; 100 calibration lines mark it. Each line represents 0.01 mL. Every tenth line is longer than the others to indicate 0.1 mL. TB syringes are used for newborn and pediatric doses, for intradermal skin tests, and any time small amounts of medication are to be given (FIG. 26-8).

F I G U R E   2 6 - 7 .   Needles. (A) Different gauges and lengths. (B) Parts of a needle.

age. Choose the package with a needle length and gauge appropriate for the route of the injection. For example, an intramuscular injection for an adult requires a needle length of 1.5 inches, depending on the size of the patient and the fat to muscle ratio. The needle gauge varies from 20 to 25 depending on the thickness of the medication to be administered. **Thick medications, such as penicillin and hormones, are difficult to draw into a syringe using a small-gauge needle, such as a 25 or 27, and equally difficult to inject into the patient.** Subcutaneous injections are generally given using a short, small-gauge needle: 25 gauge 0.625 inch, or 23 gauge, 0.5 inch.

All hypodermic syringes are marked with 10 calibrations per milliliter on one side of the syringe. Each small line represents 0.1 mL. The other side of the syringe may be marked

F I G U R E 2 6 - 8 . Syringes. *Top to bottom:* 10 mL, 3 mL, tuberculin or 1 mL, insulin, and low-dose insulin.

The insulin syringe is used strictly for administering insulin subcutaneously to diabetic patients. It has a total capacity of 1 mL; however, the 1-mL volume is marked as 100 units (U) to represent the strength of 100 U insulin per milliliter when full. Each group of 10 U is divided by five small lines, and each line represents 2 U. Most of the insulin used today is U-100, which means that it has 100 U of insulin in each milliliter. The insulin syringe must be marked U-100 to match the insulin used. Procedure 26-2 describes the steps required for preparing an injection.

Checkpoint Question

6. What are ampules and vials, and how do they differ?

Types of Injections

Intradermal injections. Intradermal medications are administered into the dermal layer of the skin by inserting the needle at a 10° to 15° angle, almost parallel to the skin surface (FIG. 26-9). When an intradermal injection is administered correctly, the needle tip and lumen are slightly visible under the skin, and a small bubble, known as a wheal, is raised in the skin. Recommended sites for intradermal injections include the anterior forearm and the back. Intradermal injections are used exclusively to administer skin tests for tuberculosis screening, the **Mantoux** test, and allergy testing. Procedure 26-3 describes the steps for giving an intradermal injection.

The tine test is another skin test used for routine screening of tuberculosis, but it is not considered as diagnostic as the Mantoux test. Both methods use purified protein derivative (PPD) from a live tuberculin bacillus culture to test for the presence of tuberculin antibodies. The tine applicator contains small tines impregnated with PPD. After cleansing the forearm, press the tine applicator firmly into the intradermal

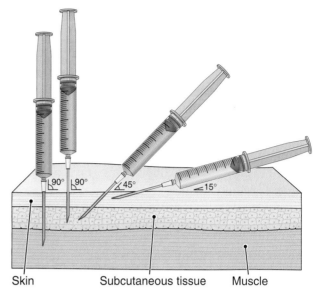

Skin   Subcutaneous tissue   Muscle

■ Intramuscular injection
■ Subcutaneous injection
□ Intradermal injection

F I G U R E 2 6 - 9 . Angles of insertion for intramuscular, subcutaneous, and intradermal injections. (Reprinted with permission from Cohen BJ. Medical Terminology: An Illustrated Guide. Philadelphia: Lippincott Williams & Wilkins, 2003.)

layer of the skin (FIG. 26-10). A positive tine test is usually followed by a Mantoux test. Both the tine test and the Mantoux test must be read within 48 to 72 hours. **A positive Mantoux reaction has induration, a hard raised area over the injection site, larger than 10 mm. This positive reaction indicates the possibility of exposure to tuberculosis; however, it does not indicate that the patient has active tuberculosis** (see Chapter 32). A complete medical history and further testing by sputum culture and radiography are required for a definitive diagnosis. Redness over the intradermal injection site should not be considered induration. An induration of less than 10 mm in a patient with no known

F I G U R E 2 6 - 1 0 . Administering the tine test for tuberculosis screening.

risk factors, such as previous tuberculosis or HIV infection, is considered negative.

Subcutaneous Injections. Subcutaneous (SQ or SC) injections are given into the fatty layer of tissue below the skin by positioning the needle and syringe at a 45° angle to the skin (see Fig. 26-9). **The subcutaneous route is chosen for drugs that should not be absorbed as rapidly as through the intramuscular or intravenous (IV) route.** Common sites include the upper arm, thigh, back, and abdomen. Procedure 26-4 describes the steps for administering a subcutaneous injection.

Intramuscular Injections. Intramuscular (IM) injections are given by positioning the needle and syringe at a 90° angle to the skin (see Fig. 26-9). **Absorption of IM medications is fairly rapid because of the rich vascularity of muscle.** If slower absorption is desired, the medication is mixed with an oil base rather than saline or water to prolong absorption time. A 1- to 1.5-inch needle is required to administer an intramuscular injection to an adult. The length of the needle depends on the muscle chosen for injection and the size of the patient.

Recommended sites for IM injections include the deltoid (FIG. 26-11), dorsogluteal (FIG. 26-12), ventrogluteal (FIG. 26-13), and vastus lateralis (FIG. 26-14) muscles. The rectus

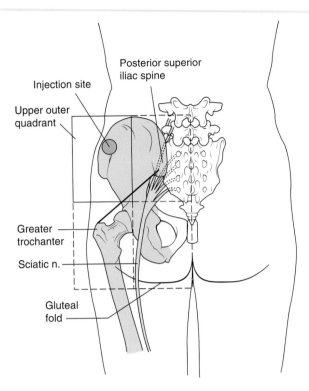

FIGURE 26-12. The dorsogluteal site for intramuscular injection is lateral and slightly superior to the midpoint of a line drawn from the trochanter to the posterior superior iliac spine. Correct identification of this site minimizes the possibility of accidentally damaging the sciatic nerve.

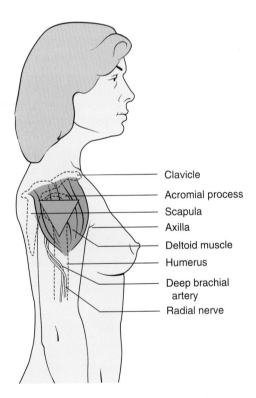

FIGURE 26-11. The deltoid muscle for intramuscular injection is located by palpating the lower edge of the acromial process. At the midpoint, in line with the axilla on the lateral aspect of the upper arm, a triangle is formed. Medications are administered within this triangle.

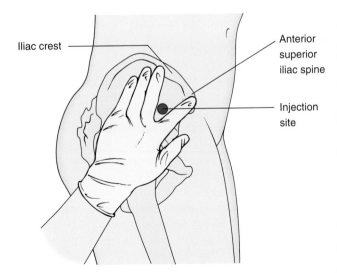

FIGURE 26-13. The ventrogluteal site is located by placing the palm on the greater trochanter and the index finger toward the anterior superior iliac spine. The middle finger is then spread posteriorly away from the index finger as far as possible. A V or triangle is formed by this maneuver. The injection is made in the middle of the triangle.

the line of injection. An example of a medication that should be administered using this technique is iron dextran, used to treat iron deficiency anemia. The Z-track method prevents leakage by sealing off the layers of skin along the route of the needle (FIG. 26-16). If the medication is extremely caustic, directions may include changing the needle after drawing up the solution. An additional precaution may include drawing up to 0.5 mL of air into the syringe after the medication has been aspirated into the syringe. When the medication is injected at a 90° angle, the additional air rises to the top of the syringe and is injected after the medication. This clears the needle and the path of the injection (FIG. 26-17). Procedure 26-6 describes the steps for administering an intramuscular injection using the Z-track method.

Checkpoint Question

7. Name the types of injections and the possible sites for each type.

Other Medication Routes

Rectal Administration. Rectal medications are packaged in the form of suppositories or liquids administered as a retention enema (FIG. 26-18). They can provide a local effect or be absorbed through the rectal mucosa for a systemic effect.

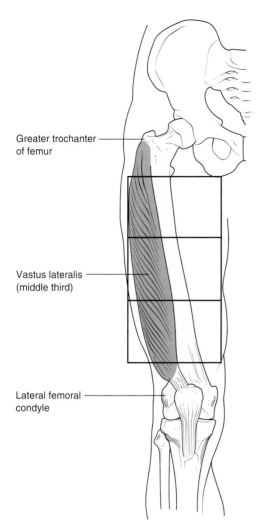

FIGURE 26-14. The vastus lateralis site for intramuscular injections is identified by dividing the thigh into thirds horizontally and vertically. The injection is given in the outer middle third.

femoris (FIG. 26-15) can also be used when the other sites are **contraindicated**. It is recommended that no more than 1 mL be injected into the deltoid muscle and no more than 3 mL into the other muscles in an adult. Children less than 2 years of age should never receive injections in the gluteal muscle, since this muscle is not well developed until the child is walking. The muscle chosen for the injection depends on the preference of the medical assistant, the patient, and the amount of medication to be administered. Also, some pharmaceutical companies recommend a specific site for injection, and the medical assistant should use this site as indicated. Gold sodium thiomalate, a medication used to treat arthritis, is an example of a medication that has specific guidelines for administration set forth by the manufacturer. Procedure 26-5 describes the steps for administering an intramuscular injection.

Z-track Method of Intramuscular Injection. This method is used for IM administration of medications that may irritate or damage the tissues if allowed to leak back along

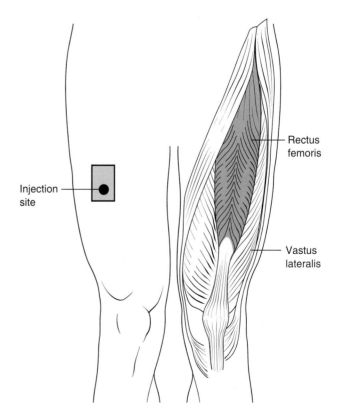

FIGURE 26-15. The rectus femoris site for intramuscular injections is used only when other sites are contraindicated.

FIGURE 26-16. The Z-track is used to administer medications that are irritating to subcutaneous tissue. The skin is pulled to one side, the needle is inserted, and the solution is injected after careful aspiration. When the needle is withdrawn and the displaced tissue is allowed to return to its normal position, the solution is prevented from escaping from the muscle tissue.

Rectal medications may be used for patients who are NPO (allowed nothing by mouth) or who have nausea and vomiting, but they are never used for patients who have diarrhea. Suppositories have a cocoa butter or glycerin base that melts at body temperature. They should be stored in the refrigerator to prevent melting. Rectal medications are rarely administered in the medical office, but you may be required to instruct the patient in the proper technique for administration at home. Both retention enemas and rectal suppositories should be retained by the patient for about 20 to 30 minutes before elimination.

Vaginal Administration. Vaginal medications include creams, tablets, cocoa butter–based suppositories, and solutions for douches. Examples include hormonal creams and antibiotic or antifungal preparations (FIG.

26-19). **Very few medications other than those for local effects are prescribed for the vaginal route.** Instruct the patient to remain lying for a while after the insertion of vaginal medications. For comfort, the patient may have to wear a light pad to absorb any drainage.

Transdermal Administration. Dermal medications, which are applied to the skin, include topical creams, lotions, ointments, and transdermal medications. **Topical medications (creams, ointments, sprays, and lotions) produce local effects, while transdermal medications produce systemic effects.** Medication administered transdermally is delivered to the body by absorption through the skin. Delivery is slow and maintains a steady, stable level of medication. You should never cut a transdermal patch, since doing so alters the rate of absorption. Dermal patches are placed on the skin, usually on the chest or back, upper arm, or behind the ear (for medications that prevent motion sickness). Procedure 26-7 describes the steps for applying transdermal medications.

Air above medication

Medication

Air lock

FIGURE 26-17. An air bubble added to the syringe after the medication has been accurately measured helps to expel solution that is trapped in the shaft of the needle when the injection is given. It also helps to trap the injected solution in the intramuscular tissue.

TRIAGE

While you are working in a medical office setting, the following three situations arise:

A. A 50-year-old man is complaining of dyspnea, and the doctor has ordered a nebulizer treatment.

B. A 65-year-old woman needs her first dose of an antibiotic.

C. A 47-year-old woman slipped on the ice in the parking lot and is having moderate pain in the right ankle. The doctor has ordered a pain medication injection.

How do you sort these patients? Whom do you see first? Second? Third?

Patient A should be treated first; any patient with chest pain or shortness of breath should be treated as a number 1 priority. Patient C should be medicated for pain control. Last, patient B should be given the antibiotic. Remember, you must closely monitor this patient for 30 minutes for signs of an allergic reaction. All three of these patients need to be closely evaluated after receiving their medications. Ask yourself, is the patient breathing better? Is the pain better? Communicate your findings with the physician.

FIGURE 26-18. (A) Rectal suppositories. (B) Rectal suppositories should be placed well beyond the internal sphincter.

Inhalation. Inhalation is administration of medication, water vapor, or gas by inspiration of the substance into the lungs. Medication administered by inhalation is absorbed quickly through the alveolar walls into the capillaries, but a disease condition may make absorption difficult to predict. Patients with chronic pulmonary disease or disorder may self-administer certain medications with a handheld **nebulizer** or inhaler, both producing a fine spray of medicated mist that is inhaled directly into the lungs (see Chapter 32).

Intravenous Route. With the IV route, a sterile solution of a drug is injected through a catheter into a vein by venipuncture. **IV medication has the quickest action because it enters the bloodstream immediately.** Only drugs intended for IV administration should be given by this route. In most cases, the physician administers IV medications, but some ambulatory care centers expect medical assistants to be proficient at setting up the equipment and fluids for an IV, performing the venipuncture, and regulating the IV fluids as directed by the physician. The equipment necessary for starting an IV includes the fluids (determined by the physician), the IV catheter (angiocatheter), and the tubing and valve that connect the fluids to the catheter and regulate the flow of fluids into the patient (FIG. 26-20).

Once the IV line is started, the fluids are administered through the vein either to replace fluids lost by the patient or to administer medications through special ports on the tubing. Examples of fluids that come prepackaged for use in IV therapy are Ringer's lactate (RL), dextrose 5% and water (D_5W), 0.9% normal saline, 0.45% normal saline, or a combination (D_5NS, D_5RL). The physician chooses the type and amount of fluid to be administered. An administration set (tubing) is used, with one end (the end with the drip chamber) inserted into the IV fluid bag and the other end into the IV catheter af-

PATIENT EDUCATION

Administering Rectal Medications at Home

Some medications have to be administered rectally. You should teach the patient or family member to perform this procedure if the medication is to be taken at home. Here are some key points to discuss:

- Gloves should be worn.
- A small amount of a lubricant should be added to the suppository for easy insertion. The lubricant maybe supplied with the suppository, or it can be purchased separately at the pharmacy.
- Advise the patient to remain lying on the bed for about 15 minutes after the suppository is inserted.
- The suppository should be inserted past the anal sphincter.

A

B

FIGURE 26-19. (A) Vaginal suppository and applicator. (B) Insertion of vaginal cream using applicator.

ter it is in the vein (Procedure 26-8). After securing the IV catheter and attaching the administration set tubing, adjust the flow of fluids by adjusting the roller clamp and carefully watching the fluids drip into the drip chamber. Carefully count the drops per minute so you can adjust the flow of fluids to the exact rate desired. The amount of fluid to be administered is ordered by the physician in terms of milliliters per hour (e.g., 125 mL/hour). Using this physician order, determine how fast to run the solution following this procedure:

- Determine the drop factor (number of drops needed to deliver 1 mL of fluid) as noted on the administration set tubing package (Macrodrop systems deliver 10 or 20 drops per milliliter, and microdrip systems deliver 60 drops per milliliter.)
- The physician order will include the type of fluid (e.g., RL, D_5W), the amount (e.g., 125 mL), and the time frame (e.g., per hour).
- Use the following formula to calculate the number of drops per minute necessary to deliver the amount of fluid:

- Drops per minute = volume in milliliters ÷ time in minutes × drop factor (gtt/min)
- Example: physician order reads Ringers lactate 100 mL/hour. Administration set delivers 10 gtt/mL.
- 100 ÷ 60 = 1.67 (volume ÷ time in minutes)
- 1.67 × 10 gtt = 17 gtt/min (16.7 rounded up to nearest tenth = 17)
- Regulate the roller clamp so that 17 drops per minute flow into the drip chamber to deliver 100 mL/hour.

If the physician would like the patient to have an IV line but not necessarily the fluids, a to-keep-open (TKO) or keep-vein-open (KVO) rate will be ordered. The flow of fluids into the vein to prevent clotting may be 15 to 30 mL/hour as determined by the physician. The same formula is used to calculate this rate (rate = volume ÷ time × drop factor).

The medical assistant must be vigilant about watching the IV fluids and the site of venipuncture. **Infiltration** occurs when IV fluid infuses into the tissues surrounding the vein, usually because the catheter has been dislodged. Carefully securing the IV catheter and the administration tubing usually prevents this. In case of infiltration, stop the flow of fluids, remove the catheter, and notify the physician. Infiltration is characterized by the following:

- Swelling and pain at the IV site
- A slow or absent flow rate into the drip chamber of the administration set with the roller clamp open
- No blood return or backup into the tubing when the fluid bag is below the level of the heart

If the physician orders that the IV be reinserted, you must use either the other arm or a site above the level of infiltration. Procedure 26-8 outlines the steps for insertion of an IV line.

FIGURE 26-20. IV equipment, including the fluid, tubing, and needle or catheter.

Procedure 26-1

Administering Oral Medications

Purpose: Accurately administer oral medications.

Equipment: Physician's order, oral medication, disposable calibrated cup, glass of water, patient's medical record.

Standard: This procedure should take 5 minutes.

Steps	Reason
1. Wash your hands.	Handwashing aids infection control.
2. Review the physician's medication order and select the correct medication. Compare the label to the physician's instructions. Note the expiration date. Check the label three times: when taking it from the shelf, while pouring, and when returning it to the shelf.	Carefully dispensing medications helps prevent errors. Outdated medication should not be administered but should be discarded appropriately.
3. Calculate the correct dose if necessary.	
4. If using a multidose container, remove the cap from the container, touching only the outside of the lid. Single, or unit dose, medications come individually wrapped in packages that may be opened by pushing the medication through the foil backing or peeling back a tab on one corner.	The inside of the lid of a multidose bottle will be contaminated if touched.
5. According to your calculations and the label, remove the correct dose of medication. A. For solid medications i. Pour the capsule or tablet into the bottle cap to prevent contamination.	

Step 5.A.i. Pour the tablet into the bottle cap.

(continues)

Procedure 26-1   (continued)

Administering Oral Medications

Steps	Reason

ii. Transfer the medication to a disposable cup.

Step 5.A.ii. Transfer the medication to a disposable cup.

B. For liquid medications

   i. Open the bottle and put the lid on a flat surface with the open end up to prevent contamination of the inside of the cap.

   ii. Palm the label to prevent liquids from dripping onto the label and possibly damaging it or making it illegible.

Step 5.B.ii. Palm the label of the container when pouring liquids.

   iii. With the opposite hand, place your thumbnail at the correct calibration on the cup. Holding the cup at eye level, pour the proper amount of medication into the cup, using your thumbnail as a guide.

(continues)

Procedure 26-1 *(continued)*

Administering Oral Medications

Steps	Reason
6. Greet and identify the patient. Explain the procedure. Ask the patient about medication allergies that may not be noted on the chart.	Identifying the patient prevents errors. Explaining the procedure helps ease anxiety and may improve compliance. The medical record should be checked for allergies, but the patient should also be asked, since allergies may not have been noted.
7. Give the patient a glass of water to wash down the medication unless contraindicated and administer the medication by handing the patient the disposable cup containing the medication.	Water helps the patient swallow the medication, but water is contraindicated for medications intended for a local effect (such as cough syrup or lozenges) and for buccal or sublingual medications.
8. Remain with the patient to be sure that all of the medication is swallowed. Observe any unusual reactions and report them to the physician and enter in the medical record.	You cannot assume that the patient swallowed the medication unless you observe it.
9. Thank the patient and give any appropriate instructions.	
10. Wash your hands.	
11. Record the procedure in the patient's medical record, noting the date, time, name of medication, dose administered, route of administration, and your name.	Procedures are considered not to have been done if they are not recorded.

Charting Example

12/14/2003 8:45 A.M. Ampicillin 125 mg PO given to patient—NKA. _____ T. Jones, CMA

Procedure 26-2

Preparing Injections

Purpose:	Accurately prepare a medication by injection.
Equipment:	Physician's order, medication for injection, ampule or vial, antiseptic wipes, needle and syringe of appropriate size, small gauze pad, biohazard sharps container, patient's medical record.
Standard:	This procedure should take 5 minutes.

Steps	Reason
1. Wash your hands.	Handwashing aids infection control.
2. Review the medication order and select the correct medication. Compare the label to the physician's instructions. Note the expiration date. Check the label three times: when taking it from the shelf, while drawing it up into the syringe, and when returning to the shelf.	Carefully dispensing medications helps prevent errors. Outdated medication should not be administered to a patient but should be discarded appropriately.
3. Calculate the correct dose if necessary.	
4. Choose the needle and syringe according to the route of administration, type of medication, and size of the patient.	
5. Open the needle and syringe package. Assemble if necessary. Make sure the needle is firmly attached to the syringe by grasping the needle at the hub and turning it clockwise onto the syringe.	Needles and syringes often are preassembled, or they may be purchased separately. A needle that is not firmly attached may be detached during the procedure

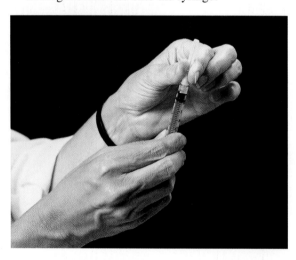

Step 5. Grasp the needle at the hub and turn it clockwise.

(continues)

Procedure 26-2 (continued)

Preparing Injections

Steps	Reason
6. Withdraw the correct amount of medication	

A. From an ampule

i. With the fingertips of one hand, tap the stem of the ampule lightly to remove any medication in or above the narrow neck.

ii. Wrap a piece of gauze around the ampule neck to protect your fingers from broken glass. Grasp the gauze and ampule firmly with the fingers. Snap the stem off the ampule with a quick downward movement of the gauze. Be sure to aim the break away from your face. Dispose of the ampule top in a biohazard sharps container to prevent injury.

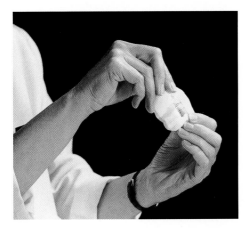

Step 6.A.ii. Grasp the gauze and ampule firmly.

iii. After removing the needle guard, insert the needle lumen below the level of the medication. Withdraw the medication by pulling back on the plunger of the syringe without letting the needle touch the contaminated edge of the broken ampule. Withdraw the desired amount of medication and dispose of the ampule in a biohazard sharps container.

iv. Remove any air bubbles by holding the syringe with the needle up and gently tap the barrel of the syringe until the air bubbles rise to the top. Draw back on the plunger to add a small amount of air, then gently push the plunger forward to eject the air out of the syringe. Be careful not to eject any medication if the required dosage has been drawn up.

(continues)

Procedure 26-2   (continued)

Preparing Injections

Steps	Reason

B. From a vial

    i. Using the antiseptic wipe, cleanse the rubber stopper of the vial to avoid introducing bacteria into the medication.

Step 6.B.i. Clean the rubber stopper with an antiseptic wipe.

    ii. Remove the needle guard and pull back on the plunger to fill the syringe with an amount of air equal to the amount of medication to be removed from the vial.

Step 6.B.ii. Pull back on the plunger, sucking air into the syringe.

(continues)

Procedure 26-2 *(continued)*

Preparing Injections

Steps	Reason

iii. Insert the needle into the vial through the center of the cleansed vial top. Inject the air from the syringe into the vial above the level of the medication to avoid producing foam or bubbles in the medication. Injecting an equal amount of air into the vial will prevent a vacuum from forming in the vial, which would make withdrawal of the medication difficult.

Step 6.B.iii. Insert the needle through the rubber stopper.

iv. With the needle inside the vial, invert the vial, holding the syringe at eye level. Aspirate, or withdraw, the desired amount of medication into the syringe.

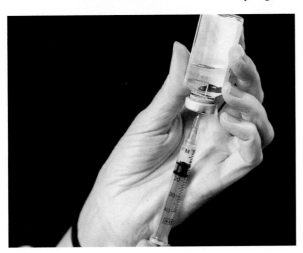

Step 6.B.iv. Invert the vial.

(continues)

Procedure 26-2   *(continued)*

Preparing Injections

Steps	Reason

v. Displace any air bubbles in the syringe by gently tapping the barrel of the syringe with the fingertips. Remove the air by pushing the plunger slowly and forcing the air into the vial.

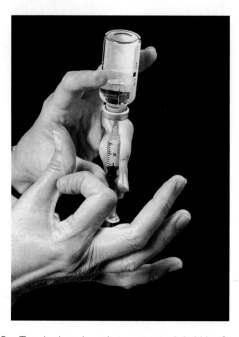

Step 6.B.v. Tap the barrel gently to remove air bubbles from the medication.

Steps	Reason
7. Carefully recap the needle by placing the needle guard on a hard, flat surface and without contaminating the needle, insert the needle into the cap and scoop up the cap with one hand.	Recapping the needle protects the sterility of the needle until the medication can be administered. Recapping with two hands should be avoided to prevent needle sticks, especially after giving an injection.

Administering an Intradermal Injection

Purpose:	Accurately prepare and administer a medication by intradermal injection.
Equipment:	Physician's order, medication for injection, ampule or vial, antiseptic wipes, needle and syringe of appropriate size, small gauze pad, biohazard sharps container, clean examination gloves, patient's medical record
Standard:	This procedure should take 10 minutes.

Steps	Reason
1. Wash your hands.	Handwashing aids infection control.
2. Review the order and select the correct medication. Compare the label to the physician's instructions. Note the expiration date. Check the label three times: when taking it from the shelf, while drawing it up into the syringe, and when returning to the shelf.	Carefully dispensing medications helps prevent errors. Outdated medication should not be administered to a patient but should be discarded appropriately.
3. Prepare the injection according to the steps in Procedure 26-2.	
4. Greet and identify the patient. Explain the procedure and ask the patient about medication allergies that may not be noted on the medical record.	Correctly identifying the patient prevents errors.
5. Select the appropriate site for the injection. Recommended sites are the anterior forearm and the middle of the back.	
6. Prepare the site by cleansing with an antiseptic wipe using a circular motion starting at the anticipated injection site and working toward the outside. Do not touch the site after cleaning.	The site must be prepared by first removing microorganisms from the area. Wiping in a circular motion will carry the microorganisms away from the site.
7. Put on gloves.	Standard precautions must be followed for protection against exposure to blood.
8. Remove the needle guard. Using your nondominant hand, pull the patient's skin taut.	Stretching the skin allows the needle to enter the skin with little resistance and secures the patient against movement.

Step 8. Insert the needle at a 10 to 15° angle.

(continues)

Procedure 26-3   *(continued)*

Administering an Intradermal Injection

Steps	Reason
9. With the bevel of the needle facing upward, insert the needle at a 10–15° angle into the upper layer of the skin. When the bevel of the needle is under the skin, stop inserting the needle. The needle will be slightly visible below the surface of the skin. It is not necessary to aspirate when performing an intradermal injection.	The needle should be inserted almost parallel to the skin to ensure that penetration occurs within the dermal layer. The bevel of the needle facing up will allow the wheal to form. If the bevel faces down, no wheal will form.
10. Inject the medication slowly by depressing the plunger. A wheal will form as the medication enters the dermal layer of the skin. Hold the syringe steady for proper administration.	Moving the needle once it has penetrated the skin will cause discomfort to the patient.
11. Remove the needle from the skin at the angle of insertion. Do not use an antiseptic wipe or gauze pad when withdrawing the needle. Do not press or massage the site. Do not apply an adhesive bandage.	Pressure on the wheal may press the medication into the tissues or out of the injection site. Any redness or swelling produced by applying an adhesive bandage could result in an inaccurate reading of the test.
12. Do not recap the needle. Dispose of the needle and syringe in an approved biohazard sharps container. The sharps container should be placed where you have easy access to it after the injection is given.	Discarding the needle and syringe without recapping helps reduce the risk of an accidental needle stick.
13. Remove your gloves and wash your hands.	
14. Depending upon the type of skin test administered, the length of time required for the body tissues to react, and the policies of the medical office, perform one of the following: A. Read the test results. Inspect and palpate the site for the presence and amount of induration. B. Tell the patient when to return (date and time) to the office to have the results read. C. Instruct the patient to read the results at home. Make sure the patient understands the instructions. Have the patient repeat the instructions if necessary.	
15. Document the procedure, site, and results. Document any instructions to the patient.	Procedures are considered not to have been done if they are not recorded.

Charting Example

05/04/2004 10:35 A.M. Mantoux test, 0.1 mL PPD ID to (L) anterior forearm. Pt. given verbal and written instructions to RTO in 48–72 hours for reading the results—verbalized understanding. _____ P. King, CMA

Procedure 26-4

Administering a Subcutaneous Injection

Purpose: Accurately prepare and administer a medication by subcutaneous injection.

Equipment: Physician's order, medication for injection, ampule or vial, antiseptic wipes, needle and syringe of appropriate size, small gauze pad, biohazard sharps container, clean examination gloves, adhesive bandage, patient's medical record

Standard: This procedure should take 10 minutes.

Steps	Reason
1. Wash your hands.	Handwashing aids infection control.
2. Review the medication order and select the correct medication. Compare the label to the physician's instructions. Note the expiration date. Check the label three times: when taking it from the shelf, while drawing it up into the syringe, and when returning to the shelf.	Carefully dispensing medications helps prevent errors. Outdated medication should not be administered to a patient and should be discarded appropriately.
3. Prepare the injection according to the steps in Procedure 26-2.	
4. Greet and identify the patient. Explain the procedure and ask the patient about medication allergies that may not be noted on the medical record.	Correctly identifying the patient prevents errors.
5. Select the appropriate site for the injection. Recommended sites include the upper arm, thigh, back, and abdomen.	
6. Prepare the site by cleansing with an antiseptic wipe using a circular motion starting at the anticipated injection site and working outward. Do not touch the site after cleaning.	The site must be prepared by first removing microorganisms from the area. Wiping in a circular motion will carry the microorganisms away from the site.
7. Put on gloves.	Standard precautions must be followed for protection against exposure to blood.
8. Remove the needle guard. Using your nondominant hand, hold the skin surrounding the injection site in a cushion fashion.	Holding the skin up and away from the underlying muscle will ensure entrance into the subcutaneous tissues. Proper technique will help ensure that the subcutaneous tissue, not the muscle, is entered.
9. With a firm motion, insert the needle into the tissue at a 45° angle to the skin surface. Hold the barrel between the thumb and the index finger of the dominant hand and insert the needle completely to the hub.	A quick, firm motion is less painful to the patient. Full insertion ensures that the medication is inserted into the proper tissue.
10. Remove your nondominant hand from the skin.	

(continues)

Procedure 26-4 *(continued)*

Administering a Subcutaneous Injection

Steps	Reason
11. Holding the syringe steady, pull back on the syringe gently. If blood appears in the hub or the syringe, a blood vessel has been entered. If this occurs, do not inject the medication. Remove the needle and prepare a new injection.	If medication intended for subcutaneous administration is administered into a blood vessel, the medication can be absorbed too quickly, producing undesirable results.
12. Inject the medication slowly by depressing the plunger.	If medication is injected too rapidly, pressure will cause discomfort and possibly tissue damage.
13. Place a gauze pad over the injection site and remove the needle at the angle at which it was inserted. Gently massage the injection site with the gauze pad with one hand while discarding the needle and syringe into the sharps container with the other hand. Do not recap the used needle. Apply an adhesive bandage if needed.	Discarding the needle and syringe without recapping helps reduce the risk of an accidental needle stick. Massaging helps to distribute the medication so that it can be more completely absorbed.
14. Remove your gloves and wash your hands.	
15. An injection given for allergy desensitization requires that the patient remain in the office for at least 30 minutes for observation of any reaction. If any patient has any unusual reaction after any injection, notify the physician immediately.	
16. Document the procedure, site, and results. Document any instructions to the patient.	Procedures are considered not to have been done if they are not recorded.

Charting Example

03/04/2004 9:30 A.M. FBS 180. Regular insulin 5 units SQ (R) anterior thigh. _____ Collins, RMA

Administering an Intramuscular Injection

Purpose: Accurately prepare and administer a medication by intramuscular injection.

Equipment: Physician's order, medication for injection, ampule or vial, antiseptic wipes, needle and syringe of appropriate size, small gauze pad, biohazard sharps container, clean examination gloves, adhesive bandage, patient's medical record.

Standard: This procedure should take 10 minutes.

Steps	Reason
1. Wash your hands.	Handwashing aids infection control.
2. Review the order and select the correct medication. Compare the label to the physician's instructions. Note the expiration date. Check the label three times: when taking it from the shelf, while drawing it up into the syringe, and when returning to the shelf.	Carefully dispensing medications helps prevent errors. Outdated medication should not be administered to a patient but should be discarded appropriately.
3. Prepare the injection according to the steps in Procedure 26-2.	
4. Greet and identify the patient. Explain the procedure and ask the patient about medication allergies that might not be noted on the medical record.	Correctly identifying the patient prevents errors.
5. Select the appropriate site for the injection. Recommended sites include the deltoid, vastus lateralis, dorsogluteal, and ventrogluteal areas; however, the site should be chosen according to the medication, age, and size of the patient.	Skill and accuracy are crucial when locating intramuscular injection sites, since major blood and nerve vessels may lie near the muscles.
6. Prepare the site by cleansing with an antiseptic wipe using a circular motion starting at the anticipated injection site and working toward the outside. Do not touch the site after cleaning.	The site must be prepared by first removing microorganisms from the area. Wiping in a circular motion will carry the microorganisms away from the site.
7. Put on gloves.	Standard precautions must be followed for protection against exposure to blood.
8. Remove the needle guard. Using your nondominant hand, hold the skin surrounding the injection site either taut with the thumb and index fingers or by grasping the muscle in a small person with little body fat.	Holding the skin taut in an average or overweight adult will allow for easier insertion of the needle. Bunching the muscle produces a deeper mass in a very thin person.
9. While holding the syringe like a dart, use a quick, firm motion to insert the needle into the tissue at a 90° angle to the surface. Hold the barrel between the thumb and index finger of the dominant hand and insert the needle completely to the hub.	A quick, firm motion is least painful to the patient. Full insertion at 90° ensures that the medication is inserted into the proper muscle tissue.

(continues)

Procedure 26-5   *(continued)*

Administering an Intramuscular Injection

Steps	Reason
10. Remove your nondominant hand from the skin and gently pull back on the plunger while holding the syringe steady. If blood appears in the hub or the syringe, a blood vessel has been entered. If this occurs, do not inject the medication. Remove the needle and prepare a new injection.	If medication intended for intramuscular administration is administered into a blood vessel, the medication can be absorbed too quickly, producing undesirable results.
11. Inject the medication slowly by depressing the plunger.	If medication is injected too rapidly, pressure will cause patient discomfort and possibly tissue damage.
12. Place a gauze pad over the injection site and remove the needle at the angle at which it was inserted. Gently massage the injection site with the gauze pad with one hand while discarding the needle and syringe into the sharps container with the other hand. Do not recap the used needle. Apply an adhesive bandage if needed.	Discarding the needle and syringe without recapping helps reduce the risk of an accidental needle stick. Massaging helps to distribute the medication into the tissues so that it can be more completely absorbed.
13. Remove your gloves and wash your hands.	
14. Observe the patient for any unusual reactions. If any patient has any unusual reaction after any injection, notify the physician immediately.	
15. Document the procedure, site, and results. If instructions were given to the patient, document these also.	Procedures are considered not to have been done if they are not recorded.

Charting Example

05/06/2004 2:00 P.M. Solu-Medrol 20 mg IM (L) DG. _____ O. Campbell, CMA

Procedure 26-6

Administering an Intramuscular Injection Using the Z-Track Method

Purpose: Accurately prepare and administer a medication by Z-track intramuscular injection.

Equipment: Physician's order, medication for injection, ampule or vial, antiseptic wipes, needle and syringe of appropriate size, small gauze pad, biohazard sharps container, clean examination gloves, adhesive bandage, patient's medical record.

Standard: This procedure should take 10 minutes.

Steps	Reason
1. Follow steps 1–7 as described in Procedure 26-5. Note: The ventrogluteal, vastus lateralis, and dorsogluteal sites work well for the Z-track method; the deltoid does not.	
2. Remove the needle guard. Rather than pulling the skin taut or grasping the tissue as you would for an intramuscular injection, pull the top layer of skin to the side and hold it with the nondominant hand throughout the injection.	
3. While holding the syringe like a dart, use a quick, firm motion to insert the needle into the tissue at a 90 degree angle to the skin surface. Hold the barrel between the thumb and the index finger of the dominant hand and insert the needle completely to the hub.	A quick, firm motion is less painful to the patient. Full insertion at 90° ensures that the medication is inserted into the proper muscle tissue.
4. Aspirate by withdrawing the plunger slightly. If no blood appears, push the plunger in slowly and steadily. Count to 10 before withdrawing the needle.	If medication intended for intramuscular administration is administered into a blood vessel, the medication can be absorbed too quickly, producing undesirable results. Counting to 10 before removing the needle allows time for the tissues to begin absorbing the medication.
5. Place a gauze pad over the injection site and remove the needle at the same angle at which it was inserted while releasing the skin. Do not massage the area. Discard the needle and syringe into the sharps container. Apply an adhesive bandage if needed.	Discarding the needle and syringe without recapping helps reduce the risk of an accidental needle stick.
6. Remove your gloves and wash your hands.	
7. Observe the patient for any unusual reactions. If any patient experiences any unusual reaction after any injection, notify the physician immediately.	
8. Document the procedure, the site, and the results. If instructions were given to the patient, document these also.	Procedures are considered not to have been done if they are not recorded.

Charting Example

07/11/2004 3:30 P.M. Imferon 25 mg IM Z-track (R) DG. _____ E. Edwards, CMA

Procedure 26-7

Applying Transdermal Medications

Purpose: Accurately prepare and administer a transdermal medication.

Equipment: Physician's order, Medication, Clean examination gloves, Patient medical record

Standard: This procedure should take 5 minutes.

Steps	Reason
1. Wash your hands.	Handwashing aids infection control.
2. Review the order and select the correct medication. Compare the label to the physician's instructions. Note the expiration date. Check the label three times: when taking it from the shelf, while drawing it up into the syringe, and when returning to the shelf.	Carefully dispensing medications helps prevent errors. Outdated medication should not be administered to a patient but should be discarded appropriately.
3. Greet and identify the patient. Explain the procedure and ask the patient about medication allergies that might not be noted on the medical record.	Correctly identifying the patient prevents errors.
4. Select the appropriate site and perform any necessary skin preparation. The usual sites are the upper arm, chest or back, and behind the ear. These sites should be rotated. Ensure that the skin is clean, dry, and free from any irritation. Do not shave areas with excessive hair; trim the hair close with scissors.	Shaving may abrade the skin and cause the medication to be absorbed too rapidly.
5. If there is a transdermal patch already in place, remove it carefully while wearing gloves. Discard the patch in the trash. Inspect the site for irritation.	Touching the medication with bare hands may cause it to be absorbed into your skin, causing undesirable reactions.
6. Open the medication package by pulling the two sides apart. Do not touch the area of medication.	
7. Apply the medicated patch to the patient's skin following the manufacturer's directions. Press the adhesive edges down firmly all around, starting at the center and pressing outward. If the edges to not stick, fasten with tape.	Starting at the center eliminates air spaces that may prevent contact with the skin.
8. Wash your hands.	
9. Document the procedure and the site of the new patch in the medical record.	Procedures are considered not to have been done if they are not recorded.

Charting Example

09/06/2004 8:30 A.M. Transdermal nitroglycerine 0.2 mg/hr patch to left anterior chest. _____ R. Evans, RMA

Procedure 26-8

Obtaining and Preparing an Intravenous Site

Purpose: Accurately start a peripheral IV line.

Equipment: Physician's order, including the type of fluid to be used and the rate; IV solution; infusion administration set; IV pole; blank labels; appropriate sized IV catheter; antiseptic wipes; tourniquet; small gauze pad; biohazard sharps container; clean examination gloves; bandage tape; adhesive bandage; patient medical record; IV catheter (Angiocath)

Standard: This procedure should take 15 minutes.

Steps	Reason
1. Wash your hands.	Handwashing aids infection control.
2. Review the physician's order and select the correct catheter, solution, and administration set. Compare the label on the infusion solution and administration set with the physician's order. Note the expiration dates on the infusion solution and the administration set.	Carefully checking the order and the solution helps prevent errors. Outdated solutions or equipment should not be used but should be discarded appropriately.
3. Prepare the solution by attaching a label to the solution indicating the date, time and name of the patient and hanging the solution on an IV pole. Remove the administration set from the package and close the roller clamp.	Although there may be other clamps on the administration set, close only the roller clamp, since this is the primary clamp that will be used to adjust the flow rate.
4. Remove the end of the administration set by removing the cover on the spike (above the drip chamber). Remove the cover from the infusion port on the bottom of the bag) and insert the spike end of the administration set into the IV fluid.	Maintain sterility of the end of administration set and the port on the infusion solution bag at all times.

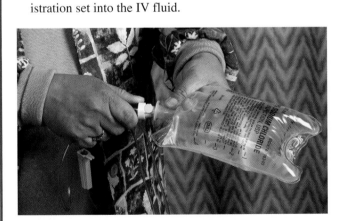

Step 4. The spike on the administration set tubing will be inserted completely into the port on the IV solution bag.

5. Fill the drip chamber on the administration set by squeezing the drip chamber until it is about half full.	Do not fill the drip chamber completely. You must observe the flow of drops into this chamber to determine the rate.

(continued)

Obtaining and Preparing an Intravenous Site

Steps	Reason

Step 5. Fill the drip chamber about half full.

Steps	Reason
6. Open the roller clamp and allow fluid to flow from the drip chamber through the length of the tubing, displacing any air. Do not remove the cover protecting the end of the tubing. Close the roller clamp when the fluid has filled the tubing and no air is noted. Drape the filled tubing over the IV pole and perform a venipuncture.	If there are any defects in the tubing (e.g., leaks), discard and obtain a new administration set.
7. Greet and identify the patient. Explain the procedure and ask the patient about medication allergies that may not be noted on the medical record.	Correctly identifying the patient prevents errors.
8. Prepare the IV start equipment by tearing or cutting 2 or 3 strips of tape to be used to secure the IV catheter after insertion. Inspect each arm for the best available vein.	After inserting the IV, you will not be able to let go of the catheter to tear or cut tape without the danger of the catheter falling out or being pulled out by the weight of the tubing.
9. Wearing gloves, apply the tourniquet 1 to 2 inches above the intended venipuncture site. The tourniquet should be snug but not too tight. Ask the patient to open and close the fist of the selected arm to distend the veins.	Standard precautions must be followed for protection against exposure to blood. Making a fist raises the vessels out of the underlying tissues and muscles.

(continued)

Procedure 26-8 *(continued)*

Obtaining and Preparing an Intravenous Site

Steps	Reason

Step 9. Pull the tourniquet snugly around the arm.

10. Secure the tourniquet with a half-bow. Make sure the ends of the tourniquet extend upward to avoid contaminating the venipuncture site.

11. Select a vein by palpating with your gloved index finger to trace the path of the vein and judge its depth. Release the tourniquet after palpating the vein if it has been left on for more than 1 minute.

12. Prepare the site by cleansing with an antiseptic wipe using a circular motion starting at the anticipated venipuncture site and working outward. Do not touch the site after cleaning.

Step 12. Prepare the venipuncture site by working outward from the center.

13. Place the end of the administration set tubing on the examination table for easy access after venipuncture. Anchor the vein to be punctured by placing the thumb of the nondominant hand below the intended site and holding the skin taut.

(continued)

Obtaining and Preparing an Intravenous Site

Steps	Reason
14. Remove the needle cover from the IV catheter. Using the nondominant hand to hold the catheter by the flash chamber, not the hub of the needle, with the dominant hand insert the needle and catheter unit directly into the top of the vein with the bevel of the needle up at a 15 to 20° angle for superficial veins. Watch for a blood flashback into the flash chamber.	Holding the catheter by the hub may prevent you from seeing problems during insertion of the catheter. A blood flashback indicates that the needle, not necessarily the catheter, has been correctly inserted into the vein. A pop may be felt when the vein has been entered.
15. When the blood flashback is observed, lower the angle of the needle until flush with the skin and slowly advance the needle and catheter unit about 0.25 inch.	Step 15. After the needle and catheter unit has been inserted into the vein, slowly advance the unit about 1/4 of an inch and stop.
16. Once the needle and catheter unit have been inserted slightly into the lumen of the vein, hold the flash chamber of the needle steady with the nondominant hand while sliding the catheter (using the catheter hub) off of the needle and into the vein with the dominant hand. The catheter should be advanced into the vein up to the hub.	
17. With the needle partly occluding the catheter, release the tourniquet. Remove the needle and discard into a biohazard sharps container. Connect the end of the administration tubing to the end of the IV catheter that has been inserted into the vein. Open the roller clamp and adjust the flow according to the physician's order.	A sterile 2 × 2 gauze may be placed under the catheter hub to absorb blood that will flow back out of the catheter after the needle has been completely removed before the tubing is attached.
18. Secure the hub of the IV catheter with tape by placing one small strip, sticky side up, under the catheter and crossing one end over the hub; stick it to the skin on the opposite side of the catheter. Cross the other end of the tape in the same fashion and stick it to the skin on the opposite side of the hub. A transparent membrane adhesive dressing can be applied over the entire hub and insertion site.	Avoid placing tape directly over the insertion site so that signs of infection or other problems can be observed readily.

(continued)

Obtaining and Preparing an Intravenous Site

Steps	Reason

Step 18. (A) Tape the catheter in place carefully. (B) Apply an adhesive dressing over the entire hub and insertion site.

Steps	Reason
19. Make a small loop with the administration set tubing near the IV insertion site and secure with tape.	This will prevent the catheter from being pulled if the tubing should be pulled or tugged.
20. Remove your gloves, wash your hands, and document the procedure in the medical record, indicating the size of the IV catheter and the location, type of infusion, and rate.	Procedures are considered not to have been done if they are not recorded.

Charting Example

05/11/2004 11:45 A.M. IV started with #22 Angiocath, (L) anterior forearm, 1000 mL RL solution at TKO rate.
_____ J. Partin, CMA

CHAPTER SUMMARY

The administration of medication is one of the most challenging and exacting procedures performed in the medical office. Few other procedures require such intense concentration and attention to detail or include such potential for danger to the patient. You will be asked to practice interpersonal skills such as tact and diplomacy to make these procedures acceptable to the patient and to allay the anxiety felt by almost all patients during the administration of medications.

Critical Thinking Challenges

1. Create a chart that you can carry with you to convert among the metric, apothecary, and household systems of measurement.

2. Design a brochure that will teach patients about taking oral medications.
3. You are giving an intramuscular injection. After inserting the needle, you aspirate by pulling back slightly on the plunger. As you do this, blood appears in the syringe. What has happened? What should you do?
4. After calculating a dose for an IM medication, you determine that 2 mL of medication must be administered. The patient insists that the injection be given in the arm. Is this appropriate? Why or why not?

Answers to Checkpoint Questions

1. The three checks are performed when the medication is taken from the shelf, when it is poured, and when it is put back on the shelf.
2. The three systems used to measure medications are the metric, apothecary, and household systems. Household measurements, which patients often use, should be avoided because they are inaccurate.

3. To calculate doses, you must ensure that the measurements are in the same system and in the same unit of measurement.
4. The most accurate method used to calculate a child's dose is by the body surface area (BSA) using the nomogram.
5. Oral medication typically takes effect slowly. Also, the oral route cannot be used for patients who are unconscious, have nausea and vomiting, or are NPO.
6. Ampules and vials are medication containers. An ampule is a glass container with a narrow neck that must be broken to obtain the medication. A vial is a glass or plastic container sealed with a rubber stopper. Vials may contain medication in either wet or dry form.
7. Types of injections include intradermal, subcutaneous, and intramuscular. Sites for intradermal injections include the anterior forearm and the back. Sites for subcutaneous injections include the upper arm, thigh, back, and abdomen. Sites for intramuscular injections include the deltoid, ventrogluteal, and vastus lateralis muscles.

 Websites

Medwatch www.fda.gov/medwatch
Physicians Desk Reference www.pdr.net
eMedguides www.emedguides.com
National Center for Complementary and Alternative Medicine http://medlineplus/gov/ http://nccam.nih.gov

27

Diagnostic Imaging

CHAPTER OUTLINE

ROLE DELINEATION

ADMINISTRATIVE: ADMINISTRATIVE PROCEDURES
- Perform basic administrative medical assisting functions
- Schedule inpatient and outpatient admissions and procedures

CLINICAL: FUNDAMENTAL PRINCIPLES
- Apply principles of aseptic technique and infection control
- Comply with quality assurance practices
- Screen and follow up patient test results

CLINICAL: PATIENT CARE
- Prepare patient for examinations, procedures, and treatments
- Coordinate patient care information with other health care providers

GENERAL: PROFESSIONALISM
- Display a professional manner and image
- Work as a member of the health care team
- Set priorities and perform multiple tasks

GENERAL: COMMUNICATION
- Recognize and respect cultural diversity
- Adapt communications to individual's ability to understand
- Recognize and respond effectively to verbal, nonverbal, and written communications
- Use medical terminology appropriately
- Serve as a liaison

GENERAL: LEGAL CONCEPTS
- Perform within legal and ethical boundaries
- Document accurately

- Implement and maintain federal and state health care legislation and regulations
- Comply with established risk management and safety procedures
- Recognize professional credentialing criteria

GENERAL: INSTRUCTION
- Instruct individuals according to their needs

CHAPTER COMPETENCIES

LEARNING OBJECTIVES
Upon successfully completing this chapter, you will be able to:
1. Spell and define the key terms.
2. Explain the theory and function of x-rays and x-ray machines.
3. State the principles of radiography and radiation therapy.
4. Describe routine and contrast media, computed tomography, sonography, magnetic resonance

imaging, nuclear medicine, and mammographic examinations.
5. Discuss the legal and ethical considerations in radiology.
6. Explain the role of the medical assistant in radiological procedures.

KEY TERM LIST

cassette	nuclear medicine	radiolucent	tomography
contrast medium	radiograph	radionuclide	ultrasound
film	radiography	radiopaque	x-rays
fluoroscopy	radiologist	teleradiology	
magnetic resonance imaging	radiology		

PRINCIPLES OF RADIOLOGY

The discovery of **x-rays** in the late nineteenth century forever changed the practice of medicine. Routine x-ray imaging, computed tomography (CT), sonography, **magnetic resonance** imaging, and **nuclear medicine** are now commonly used diagnostic and therapeutic procedures. Advances in radiation therapy continue to be at the forefront of the treatment for cancer.

Radiology continues to evolve through technological changes that provide ever-increasing diagnostic information to physicians. As the technology advances, the need to teach patients becomes even more important. Medical assistants are often directly involved in preparing patients for outpatient radiographic procedures, performing basic radi-

ographic procedures in the medical office, and assisting in the general educational process.

X-rays and X-ray Machines

X-rays are high-energy waves that cannot be seen, heard, felt, tasted, or smelled and that can penetrate fairly dense objects, such as the human body. This penetrating ability is what allows x-rays to be powerful diagnostic and therapeutic tools. Diagnostically, these penetrating waves create two-dimensional shadowlike images on **film** that is similar to photographic film. Unprocessed film must be protected from light and kept in a special holder called a **cassette** before use. Once the film inside the cassette has been exposed to x-rays, the cassette is placed in a special machine that removes the film and processes it. The processed film containing a visible image is called a **radiograph** (FIG. 27-1). The process by which these films are produced is called **radiography**.

Electricity of extremely high voltage in the x-ray tube produces x-rays. The x-rays leave the tube in one primary direction as a beam, through a device used to control the size of the beam. The light that shines on the patient is not part of the beam but is a positioning aid that illuminates the area covered by the beam. A patient may hear noises coming from the tube area during an exposure, but these are made by the equipment, not the x-rays.

Today, x-ray machines are sophisticated and technologically advanced. Many are designed to work with computers to produce digital images of the body. Fluoroscopic units can reveal motion within the body. Most permanently installed radiographic units include a special table, some of which can be electronically rotated from the horizontal to the vertical (FIG. 27-2). In this situation, the radiographic film is placed in a cassette that slides into a slot or opening on the table.

Images are formed on the x-ray film as the rays either pass through or are absorbed by the tissues of the body. **Radiolucent** tissues, such as air in the lungs, permit the passage of x-rays, while **radiopaque** tissues, such as bone, do not permit the passage of x-rays. Because bone is dense and absorbs much of the radiation beam, these structures appear white on a radiograph. Air is not dense and does not absorb much radiation. Therefore, air in a structure shows up dark on a radiograph. Other body tissues, such as muscle, fat, and fluid, show as varying shades of gray because of the way each tissue absorbs the x-rays. Physicians who

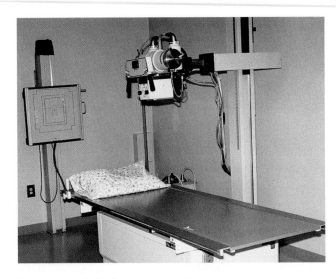

FIGURE 27-2.   Permanently installed radiographic unit.

specialize in interpreting the images on the processed film are **radiologists**.

Outpatient X-rays

The medical community is making a conscious effort to have as much treatment as possible done on an outpatient basis, and so some medical offices have on-site x-ray equipment. Outpatient diagnostic imaging centers have also been created to offer these services. Some companies specialize in providing minimal x-ray services to patients in long-term care facilities or the patients' homes.

In some states, you may be permitted to take and process simple images such as bone or chest radiographs. The training for medical assistants varies, but most curricula include a formal course in the theory of radiography and a written examination offered by the state radiographic association for the general operator. In other states, only licensed radiographers may take and process radiographs. You should be familiar with your state laws and comply with any regulations.

Checkpoint Question

1. What are x-rays?

Patient Positioning

The x-ray exposure on film is a two-dimensional image. Because the human body is a three-dimensional structure, x-ray examinations usually require a minimum of two exposures taken at 90° to each other. For instance, a chest radiographic examination requires one exposure from the back and another from the side (FIG. 27-3). Other examinations necessitate three or more exposures at different an-

FIGURE 27-1.   A radiograph of the chest.

Anteroposterior projection

Posteroanterior projection

Right lateral projection

Left lateral projection

Left posterior oblique projection

Right posterior oblique projection

Left anterior oblique projection

Right anterior oblique projection

FIGURE 27-3. Standard positions for x-ray examinations.

gles. These different angles of exposure are the basis for standard positioning for x-ray examinations (Box 27-1).

Examination Sequencing

Most radiographic procedures can be performed in any order of convenience, but certain procedures must follow certain sequences in specific situations. For example, patients with gallbladder symptoms may go through a series of procedures, progressing from the simple noninvasive oral cholecystogram (an x-ray of the gallbladder after the inges-

tion of a **contrast medium** orally) to the more complex operative cholangiogram (x-ray of the bile ducts after injection with a contrast medium during a surgical procedure).

Another example is barium studies, the name given to examinations performed after administration of barium sulfate. A patient with gastrointestinal (GI) symptoms may undergo a series of barium studies to assist the physician in diagnosis. Because of the nature of the barium studies and the length of time required to eliminate the barium from the digestive tract, barium enemas are usually scheduled after upper GI examinations. If an endoscopic study, such formed. If an upper GI examination, commonly referred to as an upper GI or barium swallow, is performed first, it may be several days before all of the barium is out of the patient's system. Any residual barium in the GI tract can obscure vital structures in subsequent procedures, preventing them from contributing diagnostic information. The proper sequencing of scheduling the barium enema first and the upper GI last will usually provide diagnostic information in a shorter time.

Checkpoint Question

2. Why is it important to schedule a barium enema before an upper GI or barium swallow?

Radiation Safety

Of primary concern to all radiation workers and patients is the proper and safe use of radiant energy. The hazards of radiation have been known for many decades, and warnings about x-ray radiation are usually posted in appropriate areas (FIG. 27-4). X-rays have the potential to cause cellular or genetic damage to the body, and the results of this damage may not manifest for several years after exposure. The adverse effects are most extreme for rapidly reproducing cells. Pregnant women, children, and reproductive organs of adults are at the highest risk because of their rapid cell division and growth.

Radiation safety procedures for patients include the following:

1. Minimizing exposure amounts.
2. Avoiding unnecessary examinations.
3. Limiting the area of the body exposed.
4. Shielding sensitive body parts, such as the gonads and the thyroid gland.
5. Evaluating the pregnancy status of female patients before performing examinations.

TRIAGE

While working in a medical office setting, the physician has asked you to call the hospital and schedule Mrs. Roberts for these three tests. What is the correct order for scheduling these tests to be performed?

A. Fiberoptic endoscopic procedure

B. Barium enema

C. Upper GI series

The correct order is fiberoptic endoscopy, upper GI, and finally the barium enema. It is important that procedures be scheduled correctly to ensure optimal results.

as an esophagogastroscopy, is ordered, it is imperative that these be scheduled before any procedure involving barium to avoid having the barium obstruct or interfere with the visualization of internal structures.

The barium study that requires filling only the large intestine with barium is the barium enema. Because this procedure involves the last part of the GI tract, this barium can be eliminated fairly quickly so that other examinations can be per-

FIGURE 27-4. A posted x-ray warning sign.

Safety procedures for clinical staff working around x-ray equipment include the following:

1. Limiting the amount of time exposed to x-rays.
2. Staying as far away from the x-rays as possible during exposure, preferably standing behind a barrier such as a wall lined with lead.
3. Using available shielding for protection, such as lead aprons and gloves (FIG. 27-5).
4. Avoiding holding patients during exposures. For children requiring assistance, a parent wearing a lead apron may be recruited during the procedure.
5. Wearing individual dosimeters, small devices that contain radiographic film clipped to the outside of the uniform, to record the amount of radiation, if any, to

FIGURE 27-6. The dosimeter records the amount of radiation to which a worker has been exposed.

which the worker has been exposed (FIG. 27-6). These badges are provided by the employer and are obtained from companies that specifically monitor any radiation exposure of individual health care providers.
6. Ensuring proper working condition of the equipment by scheduling routine maintenance.

For both patients and medical assistants working around radiation, these concerns can be summed up in what is called the ALARA concept: doing whatever is necessary to keep radiation exposure *as low as reasonably achievable.*

DIAGNOSTIC PROCEDURES

Routine radiographic examinations require little or no preparation of the patient and are the most commonly performed examinations. These procedures are most read-

FIGURE 27-5. Proper protection includes a lead-lined apron, goggles, and gloves. (Courtesy of Protech, Palm Beach Gardens, FL.)

Spanish Terminology

Tiene que estar en ayunas antes de la prueba.	You must not eat or drink anything before the test.
Debe comer una comida ligera la noche antes de la prueba.	You may eat a light supper the night before the test.
Debe seguir estas instrucciónes al pie de la letra.	You must follow these directions exactly.
Tengo que tomarle una placa.	I have to take an x-ray.

ily accepted by the patient and are named for the part of the body involved in the radiographic procedure (TABLE 27-1). These studies are performed for viewing primarily bone structure or abnormalities.

Mammography

Mammography, x-ray examination of the breast, is used as a screening tool for breast cancer (Box 27-2). Each breast is compressed in a specialized device to even the thickness, allowing for an optimal diagnostic image. Needle localization studies using the information gained from the mammogram allow the physician to withdraw small amounts of cells from suspicious areas in a minimally invasive procedure. Mammography has become a vital adjunct to biopsy (FIG. 27-7).

Contrast Medium Examinations

Within the abdomen, many structures having similar radiation absorption rates are superimposed on each other. This makes differentiating structures difficult. The use of a radiopaque contrast medium helps differentiate between body structures by artificially changing the absorption rate of a particular structure. For example, barium sulfate absorbs radiation and shows white on a radiograph (FIG. 27-8). There are many contrast media for various applications. Iodinated compounds are used in many areas of the body, including the kidneys and blood vessels and some CT scans. Patients who may have an intestinal perforation may be given an iodinated contrast medium instead of barium because that material spilling into the peritoneum is much less troublesome to the patient than barium would be.

Radiographic examinations using contrast media are performed to evaluate not only a structure but also its function. For example, patients having excretory urography have a contrast medium injected, and the anatomical structure of each kidney is evaluated as the medium passes through the urinary tract. Contrast media may be introduced into the body in several ways, including by mouth, intravenously, or through a catheter, depending on the material and area of the body being examined. Of particular concern to patients is the preparation they must undergo before some contrast examinations, especially barium studies. Prepara-

---

TABLE 27-1	ROUTINE RADIOGRAPHIC EXAMINATIONS BY BODY REGION
Region	**Patient Preparation**
Trunk	Disrobing of the area: chest, ribs, sternum, shoulder, scapula, clavicle, abdomen, hip, pelvis, sternoclavicular, acromioclavicular, sacroiliac joints
Extremities	Removing jewelry or clothing that might obscure parts of interest: fingers, thumb, hand, wrist, forearm, elbow, humerus, toes, foot, os calcis, ankle, lower leg, knee, patella, femur
Spine	Disrobing of the appropriate area: cervical, thoracic, or lumbar spine; sacrum; coccyx
Head	Removing eyewear, false eyes, false teeth, earrings, hairpins, hairpieces: skull, sinuses, nasal bones, facial bones and orbits, optic foramen, mandible, temporomandibular joints, mastoid and petrous portion, zygomatic arch

---

Box 27-2

AMERICAN CANCER SOCIETY GUIDELINES FOR MAMMOGRAPHY SCREENING

- Mammography for women who do not have symptoms, such as palpable breast masses or masses found on prior radiological examination.
  - If you are 40–49 years of age, every 1–2 years
  - If you are 50 years of age or over, every year
- Screening mammogram by age 40

FIGURE 27-7. A patient being positioned for a mammography (Lorad M-IV mammography machine).

tion of the patient for a barium study might include the following:

- Liquid diet only for the evening meal on the day before the examination.
- Laxatives the day preceding the examination to help clean the intestinal tract.
- Nothing by mouth (NPO) after midnight the day before the examination. This usually includes no gum chewing or cigarette smoking, because both activities in-

FIGURE 27-8. A radiograph of the large intestine filled with barium. The barium makes the large intestine show up as white on the radiograph.

WHAT IF

A patient has been scheduled for a barium study and asks you why she may not drink water before the test?

As a medical assistant, you must understand the reason for fasting and reinforce to the patient the importance of following all instructions carefully. The patient may not understand the consequences of not following instructions, including having to repeat the test or procedure.

crease gastric secretions that may interfere with the ability of the contrast medium to coat the wall of the intestine.

This general preparation applies to any contrast examination of the abdominal structures. Although this type of radiographic procedure is not performed in the medical office, you must ensure that the patient has proper instructions for preparing for the procedure and is notified of the scheduled time and facility. If patients are not properly prepared for contrast studies, they may have to be rescheduled for another time and day and must undertake the preparations again. Explaining the importance of the preparation can be one of the most important contributions you can make to the patient's care in contrast examinations.

Checkpoint Question

3. How do contrast media help in differentiating between body structures?

Fluoroscopy

Fluoroscopy, or fluoro studies, use x-rays to observe movement within the body. The movement may be of a contrast medium, such as barium sulfate through the digestive tract or iodinated compounds showing the beating of the heart or blood flow through specific blood vessels. Fluoroscopy is also used as an aid to other types of treatments, such as reducing fractures and implanting devices such as pacemakers.

Computed Tomography

Tomography is a procedure in which the x-ray tube and film move in relation to one another during the exposure, blurring out all structures except those in the focal plane. **CT uses a combination of x-rays from a tube circling the patient and analyzed by computers to create cross-sectional im-**

FIGURE 27-9. A computed tomography scanner. (Courtesy of Philips Medical Systems).

ages of the body. CT may be done with or without contrast medium. In addition, some CT units can create three-dimensional images, so that organs can be viewed from all angles (FIG. 27-9).

Sonography

Ultrasound, or sonography, uses high-frequency sound waves, not x-rays, to create cross-sectional still or real-time (motion) images of the body, usually with the help of a computer. This application is often used to demonstrate heart function or abdominal or pelvic structures. It is commonly used in prenatal testing to visualize the developing fetus. Many obstetricians routinely schedule at least one sonogram before the fourth month of pregnancy (FIG. 27-10).

FIGURE 27-10. A sonogram showing a fetus 9 weeks after a patient's last monthly period.

Magnetic Resonance Imaging

Magnetic resonance imaging (MRI) uses a combination of high-intensity magnetic fields, radio waves, and computer analysis to create cross-sectional images of the body. MRI does not use x-rays. The image depends on the chemical makeup of the body. MRI is commonly used for a variety of studies, including the central nervous system and joint structure. Some MRI studies are performed with contrast. Typically, the patient must be prepared for a long procedure snugly enclosed in a machine that makes numerous knocking and whirring noises. Some facilities use open MRI, which does not make a patient feel as claustrophobic as closed MRI (FIG. 27-11). Patients with fear of enclosed places may require a mild sedative before closed MRI.

 Checkpoint Question

4. How does fluoroscopy differ from CT and sonography?

Nuclear Medicine

Nuclear medicine entails the injection of small amounts of **radionuclides**, radioactive materials with short life spans, designed to concentrate in specific areas of the body. Sophisticated computer cameras detect the radiation and create an image. This technique is commonly used to study the thyroid, brain, lungs, liver, spleen, kidney, bone, and breast. These examinations are commonly called scans.

A sophisticated nuclear medicine study, *positron emission tomography (PET)*, uses specialized equipment to produce detailed sectional images of the body's physiological processes. Another procedure, *single photon emission computed tomography (SPECT)*, is a nuclear study that produces sectional images of the body as detectors move around the patient. Both of these procedures are useful in the early di-

FIGURE 27-11. An open MRI machine.

PATIENT EDUCATION

Advancement in Surgical Procedures

Patients often become confused, saying things like, "My mother was in the hospital for 2 weeks following her cholecystectomy, and the doctor says I will be in only 2 days. Why?" Many surgical procedures are done with the interventional radiology. In the 1960s, a patient would be admitted to the hospital for weeks following gallbladder surgery. The surgery required a long incision and often resulted in significant pain for the patient. In the 1980s the incision became smaller and hospital admission averaged 1 week. Today, the gallstones are removed with a laparoscope guided by an interventional radiologist. The procedure, laparoscopy, is quicker, and patients have a smaller wound and a shorter hospital stay, often only a day. Another major advance is treating abdominal aortic aneurysms with a similar procedure, resulting in shorter hospital admissions and less pain. You need to stay abreast of these advances so that you can be informed and reassure patients and their families about new procedures.

agnosis of physiological and cellular abnormalities such as those associated with cancerous tumors.

INTERVENTIONAL RADIOLOGICAL PROCEDURES

Interventional radiological techniques are designed to treat specific disease conditions. For some patients, these therapeutic techniques are so effective that there is no need for surgery. Some interventional procedures may be lifesaving. These are some types:

- *Percutaneous transluminal coronary angioplasty (PTCA)*, also known as balloon angioplasty, is used to enlarge the lumen of a coronary artery with a balloon-tipped catheter. Using fluoroscopy, the catheter is placed at a point of partial occlusion or stenosis. The balloon is then briefly inflated, compressing the plaque against the sides of the vessel. After the balloon is deflated, the catheter is removed and the lumen of the vessel remains larger, allowing for improved blood flow through the blood vessel. Balloon angioplasties may be performed in almost any blood vessel.
- *Laser angioplasties* use laser beams to remove deposits in vessels using fluoroscopy.
- *Vascular stents* (plastic or wire tubes) may be inserted into the stenosed, or constricted, area of a vessel to

maintain its patency. Fluoroscopy is used to guide placement of the stent.
- *Embolizations* artificially stop active bleeding from a blood vessel or reduce blood flow to a diseased area of an organ.

Checkpoint Question

5. How can PTCA save lives?

RADIATION THERAPY

A major force in the fight against cancer for many years has been radiation therapy. The use of high-energy radiation to destroy cancer cells may not only prolong the lives of many patients but also save lives. Used in conjunction with surgery, chemotherapy, or both, radiation is possibly the best-known treatment for cancer. Because the radiation is intense enough to destroy cancer cells, it may also damage adjacent normal cells. Therefore, treatments must be planned carefully and precisely by a radiologist, a physician who specializes in radiology.

Treatment consists of a precise, carefully planned regimen of therapy, including the frequency and amount of radiation to be used and the number of exposures during a given period. The area of the body to be exposed must be defined exactly so that each treatment is identical. The therapy consists of placing the patient in a position described by the treatment plan and having the exact amount of radiation administered by a radiology technician. Usually the patient has little to do but lie still.

The patient's prognosis varies with the situation. Most patients have some side effects, which may include hair loss, weight loss, loss of appetite, skin changes, and digestive system disturbances. Once the treatment plan is carried out, most of the side effects disappear.

THE MEDICAL ASSISTANT'S ROLE IN RADIOLOGICAL PROCEDURES

Because professional medical assistants have a variety of responsibilities in patient care, they often are in an ideal position to help alleviate patients' anxiety regarding radiology. Anxiety may be relieved by giving patients information about examinations they do not understand, by making patients feel comfortable enough to ask questions, and by answering questions in terms the patient can understand.

Patient Education

Some patients who have experience with the medical system have learned to overcome their anxieties and to find answers to their questions. No matter how much they have been through before, however, there is always something new or something they do not understand that makes them feel they have lost control of their situation. Being sensitive to patients' feelings is one of the greatest talents anyone in medicine can possess and should be an important part of your training and personality.

Unfortunately, many patients must undergo procedures they do not understand and do not know enough about to be able to ask relevant questions. Many feel like spectators rather than participants in their own care. Medical assistants can affect a patient's emotional response to a radiological procedure by explaining what to expect in simple, everyday language, not technical medical terms (FIG. 27-12). The technical aspects of radiology make it difficult for patients to understand. The key to success in explaining these procedures to patients is simplicity, leaving the details to the physician.

As noted earlier, explaining the preparations for examinations and their importance is vital to the success of many procedures. Equally important may be an explanation of what to do after the procedure. A barium enema, for instance, can lead to constipation if the patient does not drink enough fluids after the examination. This simple direction can save the patient much distress.

Assisting With Examinations

As a medical assistant, you may be expected to assist with radiological examinations thus:

- Tell the patient what clothing to remove or assist with clothing removal as needed.
- Help the patient take the position for the procedure, emphasizing the importance of remaining still and following breathing directions.
- Perform specific radiological procedures, such as bone or chest radiography, as permitted by your state's laws and your education and training.
- Place film in an automatic processor and reload new film into the cassette.
- Distribute or file radiographs and reports appropriately.

FIGURE 27-12. The medical assistant explains radiological procedures so they are easy to understand.

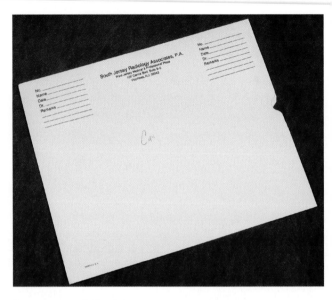

FIGURE 27-13. An x-ray envelope used for storing processed radiographs.

Handling and Storing Radiographic Films

Advancing technology and the need for quality control have led to automated processing and developing of film to eliminate human error. Automated processing machines produce a film usually in less than 2 minutes. Because processors vary by manufacturer, you need to be proficient in the operation of your particular facility's equipment.

Unexposed film must be protected from moisture, heat, and light by storage in a cool, dry place, preferably in a lead-lined box. Film packets, exposed or unexposed, must be opened in a darkroom using only the darkroom light for illumination. The film is placed in a cassette for use in any area outside the darkroom. Intensifying screens in the cassette are used to reduce the amount of exposure required. Special sleeves or envelopes of various sizes are available for storing the film that has been labeled with the name of the patient (FIG. 27-13). Film must be protected and stored in a cool, dry area.

Checkpoint Question

6. How can the medical assistant help with radiological examinations?

TRANSFER OF RADIOGRAPHIC INFORMATION

Radiographic images obtained on site for use by the physician remain part of the patient's permanent record. Digital images can be saved on a computer diskette or compact disk. In many cases, however, radiographic studies are performed at one site for consultation or referral at another site. X-ray films belong to the site where the study was performed.

The examining physician or radiologist generally writes a summary of the examination to the referring physician. You may need the patient's permission to have the summary of findings sent to the office physician.

With a short-term referral, the examining physician usually returns the films to the referring physician. Patients who have ongoing concerns or who change physicians may request the information contained in their records after submitting written consent. In addition, the patient may obtain copies of the original radiographs if necessary.

Teleradiology

The use of computed imaging and information systems, **teleradiology**, is providing new benefits in medicine. Many institutions use a picture archiving and communication system (PACS) in which computers store and transmit images. Digital images from CT, for instance, can be transmitted via telephone lines to distant locations. This allows consultation with experts on a difficult case within a matter of minutes. Previously unavailable expertise can be brought to rural areas for greatly improved patient care. The result is improved patient care over large geographic areas, not just in specific locations. The term teleradiology is often used to describe this radiology over a great distance.

CHAPTER SUMMARY

Radiology is continually evolving as a tool to diagnose and treat disease. As a medical assistant, you must understand the common types of diagnostic and therapeutic radiological procedures. You may also be responsible for teaching patients about these procedures in general and about any particular preparations required. When assisting the physician, always follow radiation safety precautions carefully for the protection of yourself and your patient.

Critical Thinking Challenges

1. A mother of a 6-year old child voices concerns about the dangers of x-rays. How do you address her fears?
2. Summarize the key points of radiation safety; then write a policy booklet for new employees. Create a poster highlighting the most important points of radiation safety to hang in the staff lounge.

3. Constipation is a common problem among patients who have barium studies. How can patient education diminish this problem? Develop a brief instruction sheet to give to these patients.

Answers to Checkpoint Questions

1. X-rays are high-energy waves that travel at the speed of light. X-rays can penetrate fairly dense objects, such as the human body. They cannot be seen, heard, felt, tasted, or smelled.
2. Barium enemas fill only the large intestine with barium. Because the large intestine is the last part of the GI tract, this barium can be eliminated quickly. If an upper GI examination is performed first, it may be days before barium can be eliminated, which may delay other examinations.
3. Contrast media help differentiate between body structures by artificially changing the absorption rate of a particular structure so that it can be seen clearly instead of blending in with adjacent structures. For example, barium sulfate absorbs radiation and shows up as white areas on a radiograph.
4. Fluoroscopy uses x-rays to show movement within the body. CT uses x-rays and a computer to create cross-sectional images of the body. Sonography uses high-frequency sound waves to create cross-sectional still or real-time (motion) images of the body.
5. PTCA can save a patient's life by reopening the lumen of a coronary artery to allow sufficient blood flow and oxygen to keep the heart muscle alive.
6. Medical assistants can help with radiological examinations by providing instruction to patients, positioning patients, handling x-ray film, and distributing or filing radiographs and reports. In some states, the medical assistant may take simple x-rays.

 Websites

Radiology Info: The radiology information resource for patients http://www.radiologyinfo.org
Virtual hospital: A digital library of health information http://www.vh.org
American Society of Radiological Technologists http://www.asrt.org

28

Medical Office Emergencies

CHAPTER OUTLINE

ROLE DELINEATION

ADMINISTRATIVE: ADMINISTRATIVE PROCEDURES
- Perform basic administrative functions

CLINICAL: FUNDAMENTAL PRINCIPLES
- Apply principles of aseptic technique and infection control
- Comply with quality assurance practices

CLINICAL: PATIENT CARE
- Adhere to established patient screening procedures
- Obtain patient history and vital signs
- Recognize and respond to emergencies
- Coordinate patient care information with other health care providers

GENERAL: PROFESSIONALISM
- Display a professional manner and image
- Demonstrate initiative and responsibility
- Work as a member of the health care team
- Set priorities and perform multiple tasks
- Adapt to change
- Enhance skills through continuing education

GENERAL: COMMUNICATION SKILLS
- Adapt communications to individual's ability to understand
- Recognize and respond effectively to verbal, nonverbal, and written communications
- Use medical terminology appropriately
- Serve as a liaison

GENERAL: LEGAL CONCEPTS
- Perform within legal and ethical boundaries
- Document accurately
- Comply with established risk management and safety procedures

CHAPTER COMPETENCIES

LEARNING OBJECTIVES
Upon successfully completing this chapter, you will be able to:

1. Spell and define the key terms.
2. Describe the role of the medical assistant in an emergency before the ambulance arrives.
3. Identify the five types of shock and the management of each.
4. Describe how burns are classified and managed.
5. Explain the management of allergic reactions.
6. Describe the management of poisoning and the role of the poison control center.
7. List the three types of hyperthermic emergencies and the treatment for each type.
8. Discuss the treatment of hypothermia.
9. Describe the role of the medical assistant in managing psychiatric emergencies.

KEY TERMS

allergen	heat cramps	infarction	septic shock
anaphylactic shock	heat stroke	ischemia	shock
cardiogenic shock	hematoma	melena	splint
contusion	hyperthermia	neurogenic shock	superficial burn
ecchymosis	hypothermia	partial-thickness burn	
full-thickness burn	hypovolemic shock	seizure	

MEDICAL OFFICE EMERGENCY PROCEDURES

Emergency medical care is the immediate care given to sick or injured persons. When properly performed, it can mean the difference between life and death, rapid recovery and long hospitalization, temporary disability and permanent disability. Emergency medical care in the medical office entails identifying the emergency, delivering basic first aid, and furnishing temporary assistance or basic life support until a rescue squad and advanced life support can be obtained.

An emergency can occur anywhere and to anyone. For example, a patient who is being seen for a routine examination may have a heart attack, collapse, and require immediate cardiopulmonary resuscitation (CPR). A diabetic patient or coworker may lapse into a diabetic coma. A patient may fall down a flight of stairs and receive trauma to the head or limbs. In a life-threatening situation, the well-prepared medical assistant can obtain important information and perform lifesaving procedures before the ambulance or rescue squad arrives, increasing the patient's chance for survival. Medical assistants should be certified in CPR and removing foreign body airway obstructions. Effective January 1, 2005, the American Association of Medical Assistants will require certified medical assistants who are renewing their credentials to demonstrate proof of current CPR certification. This training may be provided by the American Red Cross, American Heart Association, American Safety and Health Institute, or National Safety Council. You should contact one of these agencies for specific information regarding training and certification. This chapter is not meant to provide a comprehensive study of all aspects of emergency care; it briefly reviews the information in such a training course.

Emergency Action Plan

Every medical office should have an emergency action plan, including the following:

- The local emergency rescue service telephone number (usually 911)
- Location of the nearest hospital emergency department
- Telephone number of the local or regional poison control center
- Procedures for various emergencies
- List of office personnel who are trained in CPR
- Location and list of contents of the emergency medical kit or crash cart

Whether confronted with a cardiac emergency or psychiatric crisis, medical assistants must be able to coordinate multiple ongoing events while rendering patient care. Contributing to the complexity of a medical emergency are such factors as panicky family members, the arrival of emergency personnel, and possibly language barriers. You must be able to remain calm in these situations while reacting competently and professionally.

Emergency Medical Kit

Proper equipment and supplies should be readily available in a medical emergency. Although the office's equipment and supplies vary with the medical specialty, emergency equipment and supplies are fairly standard. This equipment should be kept in a designated location that is accessible to all staff. Standard supplies for a medical emergency kit are listed in Box 28-1. Although items used

---

Box 28-1

EMERGENCY MEDICAL KIT AND EQUIPMENT

These are standard supplies that can be used to make up an emergency medical kit:
- Activated charcoal
- Adhesive strip bandages, assorted sizes
- Adhesive tape, 1 and 2 inch rolls
- Alcohol (70%)
- Alcohol wipes
- Antimicrobial skin ointment
- Chemical ice pack
- Cotton balls
- Cotton swabs
- Disposable gloves, latex
- Elastic bandages, 2- and 3-inch widths
- Gauze pads, 2 × 2 and 4 × 4 inch widths
- Roller, self-adhesive gauze, 2- and 4-inch widths
- Safety pins, various sizes
- Scissors
- Syrup of ipecac
- Thermometer
- Triangular bandage
- Tweezers
    In addition to these contents, the following equipment should be available:
- Blood pressure cuff (pediatric and adult)
- Stethoscope
- Bag-valve mask device with assorted size masks
- Flashlight or penlight
- Portable oxygen tank with regulator
- Oxygen masks
- Suction unit and catheters
    Additional equipment if available:
- Various sizes of endotracheal tubes
- Laryngoscope handle and various sizes of blades
- Automatic external defibrillator
- Intravenous supplies (catheters, administration set tubing, assorted solutions)
- Emergency drugs including atropine, epinephrine, and sodium bicarbonate

during an emergency should be replaced as soon as possible, a medical assistant or other staff member, such as a nurse, should check the contents of the emergency kit or crash cart regularly, perhaps weekly, to verify that contents are available and that no item has gone beyond the expiration date. If so, the expired items should be replaced immediately.

The Emergency Medical Services System

The initial element of any emergency medical services (EMS) system is citizen access. The availability of rapid, systematic intervention by personnel specifically trained in providing emergency care is an integral part of the EMS system. Most communities have a 911 system to report emergencies and summon help by telephone. The communications operator at the local EMS station will answer the call, take the information, and alert the EMS, fire, or police department as needed. In communities without a 911 system, emergency calls are usually made directly to the local ambulance, fire, or police department. You should know the emergency system used in your community. Emergency phone numbers should be prominently displayed by all telephones in the medical office.

Some communities have an enhanced 911 system that automatically identifies the caller's telephone number and location. If the telephone is disconnected or the caller loses consciousness, the communications operator can still send emergency personnel to the scene. In the medical office, an emergency requiring notification of the EMS includes situations that are life threatening or have the potential to become life threatening, such as the symptoms of a heart attack, **shock**, or severe breathing difficulties. In each of these cases, the medical assistant provides immediate care to the patient, including CPR if necessary, while directing another staff member to notify the physician. During assessment of the emergency by the physician, the medical assistant should continue to provide first aid or be prepared to assist the physician in administering first aid while another staff member notifies the EMS. The staff member who calls EMS should be able to describe the emergency to the communications operator. The operator will then know what level of emergency personnel and rescue equipment to send. Excellent communication skills and cooperation between health care team members is essential during a medical office emergency.

Documentation in the medical record is an important responsibility in all patient care, including emergency care. EMS personnel depend on accurate and complete information regarding the patient's symptoms, the nature of the emergency, and any treatment performed prior to their arrival. This information should be placed in the patient's record in chronological order as events occurred or treatments were performed. Any vital signs taken during the emergency should also be recorded. Emergencies that in-

volve visitors or staff must also be documented, and in this case, a blank paper or progress note page will be sufficient to record the details and outline the care provided. Information should include but not be limited to the following:

1. Basic identification, including name, age, address, and location of the patient's emergency contact if known.
2. The chief complaint if known.
3. Times of events, beginning with recognition of the emergency, management techniques, and changes in patient's condition.
4. The patient's vital signs.
5. Specific emergency management rendered in the office, such as CPR, bandaging, splinting, and medications administered before and after the emergency.
6. Observations of the patient's condition, including any slurred speech, lethargy, confusion, and so on.
7. Any medical history, allergies, or current medications if known.

When the EMS personnel arrive, assist them as necessary. Let them examine the patient and take over the emergency care. You can also help by removing any obstacles to removal of the patient by stretcher and keeping family members in the reception area or a private room.

Checkpoint Question

1. What should you attempt to document before the ambulance arrives in an emergency?

PATIENT ASSESSMENT

The two primary objectives in assessment of the patient are to identify and correct any life-threatening problems and provide necessary care. Each step of the assessment must be managed effectively before proceeding to the next. For example, airway, breathing, and circulation must be intact before you take a history. In addition, survey the scene quickly to identify hazards or clues to the patient's condition. For example, an elderly person found at the bottom of a stairway will likely have head or neck injuries and should be treated in such a way as to avoid moving the head, neck, or spinal column. Emesis found near a person that resembles coffee grounds may be a clue to bleeding in the gastrointestinal system that may result from peptic ulcer disease and hemorrhage.

Recognizing the Emergency

When providing emergency care, do not assume that the obvious injuries are the only ones. Less noticeable or internal injuries may also have occurred during an accident. You should look for the causes of the injury, which may provide a clue to the extent of physical damage. For example, the elderly patient who fell downstairs may have a noticeable bump on the forehead; this is obvious, but perhaps the patient has an injury in the cervical spine that is not as readily noticeable. In the case of an injury to the head or back when spinal fracture is possible, be especially careful not to move the victim any more than necessary and avoid rough handling.

The Primary Assessment

Once you are at the victim's side, an initial survey of the patient is the first step in emergency care. This is a rapid evaluation, usually done in less than 45 seconds. The purpose of the primary assessment is to identify and correct any life-threatening problems. Quickly assess the following aspects of the patient:

- Responsiveness
- Airway
- Breathing
- Circulation

Checking for responsiveness means noting whether the patient is conscious or unconscious. If the patient is unconscious, attempt to awaken the patient by speaking and touching the shoulder. If no response occurs, assess the patient's airway by using the head tilt–chin lift method. Patients who may have neck injuries should have the airway opened using the jaw thrust method to avoid further injury to the spinal cord (FIGS. 28-1 and 28-2). An unconscious patient who is supine is likely to have a partial or total airway obstruction caused by the tongue falling back into the oropharynx, producing snoring respirations or total airway obstruction. Opening the patient's airway may be necessary to allow adequate respirations.

Once the airway is open, evaluate the patient's breathing by watching for movement of the chest up or down while listening and feeling over the mouth and nose for signs of adequate ventilation. If the patient is not breathing, artificial respiration must be started immediately. A face mask with a one-way valve or a bag–valve–mask device is recommended when performing rescue breathing and should be used if available (FIG. 28-3). Respirations that are too fast, too slow, or irregular also require medical intervention. Immedi-

FIGURE 28-1. The head tilt–chin lift technique for opening the airway. The head is tilted backward with one hand (*down arrow*) while the fingers of the other hand lift the chin forward (*up arrow*).

ate intervention for these conditions may include breathing into a mask or paper bag for respirations that are too fast (hyperventilation) or administering oxygen as directed by the physician. Any obvious noises, such as stridor or wheezes, are noted and reported to the physician (see Chapter 32).

Evaluate circulation in adults and children by checking the carotid pulse (FIG. 28-4). The brachial pulse is used to evaluate circulation in infants. If no pulse is found, begin cardiopulmonary resuscitation immediately (FIG. 28-5). Some medical offices may have an automatic external defibrillator (AED) as part of the emergency medical kit (FIG. 28-6). Although these devices should not be used on infants, adults and children with life-threatening heart rhythms have an increased chance of survival if defibrillated quickly and appropriately. Training to use the AED is included in most CPR classes today.

FIGURE 28-2. The jaw thrust technique for opening the airway. The hands are placed on either side of the head. The fingers of both hands grasp behind the angle of the jaw, bringing it up (*arrow*).

FIGURE 28-3. Using the bag–valve–mask, begin rescue breathing if no breathing is noted in the primary survey.

FIGURE 28-5. Chest compressions should be started if no signs of circulation, including a pulse, are present.

Also check for any hemorrhage, and if it is found, control the bleeding quickly. If a pulse is present or becomes palpable during CPR, note the rate and quality frequently. Evaluate perfusion, or blood flow through the tissues, by checking the temperature and moisture of the skin.

Checkpoint Question

2. What is the purpose of the primary assessment?

The Secondary Assessment

After conducting a primary assessment and assessing that the patient's airway, breathing, and circulation are adequate, a secondary assessment can be performed. The secondary assessment includes asking the patient questions to obtain additional information and performing a more thorough physical evaluation to find less obvious problems than those noted in the primary assessment. To gain an accurate impression during the secondary assessment, the following four areas are assessed:

1. General appearance. The patient's skin color and moisture, facial expression, posture, motor activity, speech, and state of alertness provide important clues about the mental and physical condition. Check for a medical bracelet or necklace. Medicine bottles in a pocket or purse can also be helpful.

Level of consciousness. By the time you have completed the primary survey and noted the patient's general appearance, the level of consciousness may be apparent. A decrease in oxygen to the cells of the brain, neurological damage from a cerebrovascular accident (stroke), and intracranial swelling are just some of the conditions that

FIGURE 28-4. Check for circulation by palpating the carotid pulse.

FIGURE 28-6. The automatic external defibrillator can be used to defibrillate a life-threatening heart rhythm.

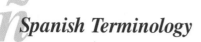

Spanish Terminology

Tiene dolor?	Do you have pain?
Tiene dificultad para respirar?	Are you having any problem breathing?
Cuando ocurrio el accidente?	When did the accident happen?
Calmese, por favor. La ambulancia esta en camino.	Calm down. The ambulance is on the way.

may alter a patient's level of consciousness. The AVPU system uses a common language to describe the patient's level of consciousness:

- A, *A*wake and alert
- V, responds to *v*oice
- P, responds only to *p*ain
- U = *U*nresponsive or unconscious

2. Vital signs. After noting the general appearance and determining the level of consciousness, assess the vital signs, including the pulse and respiratory rates and blood pressure. Assessment of temperature is important for patients who have altered skin temperature or have been exposed to environmental temperature extremes. Patients with a history of infection, chills, or fever and children with **seizures** should always have their temperature taken.

3. Skin. An initial evaluation of the temperature and moisture of skin should have been noted during the primary survey. A more thorough look should now be taken. Skin is normally dry and somewhat warm. Moist, cool skin may indicate poor blood flow to the tissues and possibly shock. The color of the skin should be noted as an indication of the circulation near the surface of the body and oxygenation of the tissues. TABLE 28-1 summarizes abnormal skin colors and the possible causes or conditions.

The Physical Examination

A head-to-toe survey that includes examination of the head and neck, chest and back, abdomen, and extremities in this sequence should be done only after completing the primary and secondary surveys. Although the physician usually performs this examination, you must be prepared to assist as needed while continuing to reassure the patient.

Head and Neck. If a cervical spine injury is suspected, immediately immobilize the spine and avoid manipulating the neck during examination of the head. Inspect the

Table 28-1	ABNORMAL SKIN COLORS AND THEIR CAUSES	
Color	**Possible Cause**	**Possible Conditions**
Pink	Vasodilation	Heat illness
	Increased blood flow	Hot environment
		Exertion
		Fever
		Alcohol consumption
White, pale	Decreased blood flow	Shock, fainting
	Decreased red blood cells	Anemia
	Vasoconstriction	Cold exposure
Blue	Inadequate oxygenation	Airway obstruction
		Congestive heart
failure		
		Chronic bronchitis
Yellow	Increased bilirubin	Liver disease
	Retention of urinary elements	Renal disease

Reprinted with permission from Jones SA, Weigel A, White RD, et al. Advanced Emergency Care for Paramedic Practice. Philadelphia: Lippincott, 1992:116.

face for edema, bruising, bleeding, and drainage from the nose or ears. Examine the mouth for loose teeth and dentures. The condition and severity of a neurological injury or patient with altered consciousness can be assessed by checking the pupils with a flashlight or penlight. The pupils should be checked for several characteristics:

- Equality in size
- Dilation bilaterally in darkness or dim light
- Rapid constriction to light in both eyes
- Equal reaction to light

To evaluate the pupils for these qualities, shade both eyes from the light and use a flashlight or small penlight at an angle 6 to 8 inches from each eye. The conscious patient should not look directly into the light. Report the findings to the physician.

Chest and Back. The anterior chest is evaluated to some degree when the patient's respiratory status is evaluated. A further inspection of the chest should be done after removing clothing from a patient with trauma or abnormal vital signs. Patients with cardiac or respiratory complaints should also have their chest more thoroughly evaluated. Palpation of the chest and back may reveal the possibility of rib fractures.

Abdomen. The abdomen of all patients is evaluated, but it is particularly important for those with GI symptoms or suspicion of blood or fluid loss as seen in vaginal bleeding, vomiting, or **melena** (blood in the stool). The abdomen is inspected for scars, bruises, and masses. A distended abdomen may indicate hemorrhage in the abdominal cavity.

Arms and Legs. An examination of the arms and legs is the last step of the head-to-toe survey. Inspect the arms and legs for swelling, deformity, and tenderness. Also note any tremors in the hands. To determine the neurological status of the arms and legs, assess strength, movement, range of motion, and sensation, including comparing one side of the body with the other. Muscle strength in the upper extremities is checked by having the patient squeeze both of your hands at the same time. Leg strength may be determined by having the patient push each foot against your hand, again at the same time, while noting any weakness in one side or the other. Assess sensation by using a safety pin or other tool to determine the patient's response to pain. Throughout the examination, you must note the comparison of both sides, including any weakness or decreased sensation in one side or the other. Again, the physician will most likely be performing this examination, but you must be prepared to assist as needed.

Checkpoint Question

3. What diagnostic signs are evaluated in the secondary assessment?

TYPES OF EMERGENCIES

Shock

Shock is lack of oxygen to the individual cells of the body, including the brain, as a result of a decrease in blood pressure. Although the cause of the low blood pressure varies, the body initially adjusts for any type of shock by increasing the strength of the heart contractions and the heart rate while constricting the blood vessels throughout the body. As shock progresses, the body has more difficulty trying to adjust, and eventually tissues and body organs have such severe damage that the shock becomes irreversible and death ensues. Box 28-2 describes the signs and symptoms of shock.

Types of Shock

Hypovolemic shock is caused by loss of blood or other body fluids. If the cause is blood loss, it is hemorrhagic shock. Dehydration caused by diarrhea, vomiting, or profuse sweating can also lead to hypovolemic shock.

Cardiogenic shock is an extreme form of heart failure that occurs when the function of the left ventricle is so compromised that the heart can no longer adequately pump blood to body tissues. This type of shock may follow death of cardiac tissue during a myocardial infarction (heart attack).

TRIAGE

While working in a medical office setting, the following three patients arrive at the same time:

A. A 4-month-old child arrives with his mother. Mother says the child has had vomiting and diarrhea for 2 days and adds, "He is so sleepy and hard to arouse."

B. A 76-year-old man arrives in the office and says, "I was bitten by a spider on my right hand yesterday. My hand is now swollen and hot."

C. A 48-year-old man comes in and says, "I burned my hand on a cup of coffee about 1 hour ago." He is complaining of pain. You notice the hand is red and has two small blisters on the palm.

How do you sort these patients? Whom do you see first? Second? Third?

See patient A first. Anytime there is change in anyone's mental status, it should be treated as a priority. This child may be dehydrated and headed for hypovolemic shock. Patient C should be seen next. Last, see the man with a spider bite.

SIGNS AND SYMPTOMS OF SHOCK

- Low blood pressure
- Restlessness or signs of fear
- Thirst
- Nausea
- Cool, clammy skin
- Pale skin with cyanosis (bluish color) at the lips and earlobes
- Rapid and weak pulse

Neurogenic shock is caused by a dysfunction of the nervous system following a spinal cord injury. Normally, the diameter of all blood vessels is controlled by the involuntary nervous system and smooth muscles surrounding the vessels. After a spinal cord injury, the nervous system loses control of the diameter of the blood vessels, and vasodilation ensues. Once the blood vessels are dilated, there is not enough blood in the general circulation, so that blood pressure falls and shock ensues.

Anaphylactic shock is an acute general allergic reaction within minutes to hours after the body has been exposed to an offending foreign substance. You must carefully observe patients for this type of shock after giving medications and during allergy testing (see later section on anaphylaxis).

Septic shock is caused by a general infection of the bloodstream in which the patient appears seriously ill. It may be associated with an infection such as pneumonia or meningitis or it may occur without an apparent source of infection, especially in infants and children. Initially, a fever is present, but the body temperature falls, a clinical sign suggestive of sepsis.

Management of the Patient in Shock

Shock can be the result of many types of medical crisis or trauma. After performing the primary and secondary assessments, observe the following list of general guidelines for managing a patient in shock:

1. Observe the patient for and maintain an open airway and adequate breathing.
2. Control bleeding.
3. Administer oxygen as directed by the physician.
4. Immobilize the patient if spinal injuries may be present.
5. Splint fractures.
6. Prevent loss of body heat by covering the patient with a blanket, especially if the patient is cold.
7. Assist the physician with starting an intravenous line as ordered.
8. Elevate the feet and legs of a patient with low systemic blood pressure.

9. Transport the patient to the closest hospital as soon as possible by notifying the EMS.

Checkpoint Question

4. What does *shock* mean?

Bleeding

Soft tissue injuries involve the skin and/or underlying musculature. An open injury to these tissues is a wound. Box 28-3 describes common soft-tissue injuries and wounds.

When a blunt object strikes the body, it may crush the tissue beneath the skin. Although the skin does not always break, severe damage to tissue and blood vessels may cause

TYPES OF SOFT TISSUE INJURIES

- **Abrasion**, the least serious type of open wound, is little more than a scratch on the surface of the skin. All abrasions, regardless of size, are painful because of the nerve endings involved.
- **Laceration** results from snagging or tearing of tissues that leaves a freely bleeding jagged wound. Skin may be partly or completely torn away, and the laceration may contain foreign matter that can lead to infection. A wound caused by a broken bottle or a piece of jagged metal is a laceration.
- **Major arterial laceration** can cause significant bleeding if the sharp or jagged instrument cuts the wall of a blood vessel, especially an artery. Uncontrolled major arterial bleeding can result in shock and death.
- **Puncture wounds** can result from sharp, narrow objects like knives, nails, and ice picks. Punctures also can be caused by high-velocity penetrating objects, such as bullets. A special case of the puncture wound is the *impaled object wound*, in which the instrument that caused the injury remains in the wound. The object can be anything—a stick, arrow, piece of glass, knife, steel rod—that penetrates any part of the body.
- **Avulsion** is a flap of skin torn loose; it may either remain hanging or tear off altogether. Avulsions usually bleed profusely. Most patients who present with an avulsion work with machinery. Home accidents with lawn mowers and power tools are common causes of avulsion.
- **Amputation** is caused by the ripping, tearing force of industrial and automobile accidents, often great enough to tear away or crush limbs from the body.

WHAT IF

You encounter a person bleeding on the street and you do not have any personal protective equipment with you?

If the person is conscious, instruct him or her to cover the wound and apply pressure with a hand or piece of cloth. You can also make a large, bulky dressing with a piece of clothing and hold it on the area that is bleeding, avoiding direct contact with the victim's blood. In many cases it is up to you to decide whether or not to participate in a street emergency. However, some states have specific laws that require health care professionals to render emergency care.

bleeding within a confined area. This is called a closed wound. Types of closed wounds include **contusions**, **hematomas**, and crush injuries. A contusion is a bruise or collection of blood under the skin or in damaged tissue. The site may swell immediately or 24 to 48 hours later. As blood accumulates in the area, a characteristic black and blue mark, called **ecchymosis**, is seen.

A blood clot that forms at the injury site, generally when large areas of tissue are damaged, is a hematoma. As much as a liter of blood can be lost in the soft tissue when a large bone is fractured. Crush injuries are usually caused by extreme external forces that crush both tissue and bone. Even though the skin remains intact, underlying organs may be severely damaged. Regardless of the type of swelling in a closed wound, the treatment includes the application of ice to reduce and prevent additional swelling to the area (see Chapter 30).

In an open wound, the skin is broken and the patient is susceptible to external hemorrhage and wound contamination. An open wound may be the only surface evidence of a more serious injury, such as a fracture. Open wounds include abrasions, lacerations, major arterial lacerations, puncture wounds, avulsions, amputations, and impalements. When managing any patient with an open wound, follow standard precautions to protect yourself against disease transmission and to protect the patient from further contamination.

Management of Bleeding and Soft Tissue Injuries

Management of open soft tissue injuries includes controlling bleeding by applying direct pressure and elevating the wound above the level of the heart if possible. Sterile gauze should be used to cover the wound. Manage-

ment of an amputated body part includes controlling the bleeding but also preserving the severed part for possible reattachment later. To preserve the severed body part:

- Place the severed part in a plastic bag.
- Place this bag in a second plastic bag. This second bag will provide added protection against moisture loss.
- Place both sealed bags in a container of ice or ice water, but do not use dry ice.

An impaled object should not be removed but requires careful immobilization of the patient and the injured area of the body. Because any motion of the impaled object can cause additional damage to the surface wound and underlying tissue, you must stabilize the object without removing it by placing gauze pads around the object and securing with tape. The immobilized impaled object can be carefully removed after transportation to the hospital.

Burns

The four major sources of burn injury are thermal, electrical, chemical, and radiation. *Thermal burns*, also called heat burns, result from contact with hot liquids, solids, superheated gases, or flame. *Electrical burns* are caused by contact with low- or high-voltage electricity. Lightning injuries are also considered electrical burns. *Chemical burns* result when wet or dry corrosive substances come into contact with the skin or mucous membranes. The amount of injury with a chemical burn depends on the concentration and quantity of the chemical agent and the length of time it is in contact with the skin. *Radiation burns* are similar to thermal burns and can occur from overexposure to ultraviolet light or from any extreme exposure to radiation.

Classification of Burn Injuries

Classification of burn injuries depends on the depth, or tissue layers involved. Factors that determine the depth of the burn include the agent causing the burn, the temperature, and the length of time exposed. Burns are classified according to the depth of injury: superficial (first degree), partial thickness (second degree), or full thickness (third degree). TABLE 28-2 describes the characteristics of burns according to depth.

Calculation of Body Surface Area

The extent of body surface area (BSA) injured by the burn is most commonly estimated by a method called the rule of nines. This method calculates the percentage of total body surface of individual sections of the body. With the rule of nines for an adult, 9% of the skin is estimated to cover the head and another 9% for each arm, including front and back (FIG. 28-7). Twice as much, or 18%, of the total skin area covers the front of the trunk, another 18%

Table 28-2   CHARACTERISTICS OF BURNS ACCORDING TO DEPTH

Depth, Causes	Skin Involvement	Symptoms	Wound Appearance	Recuperative Course
Superficial (first degree)				
Sunburn, low intensity, flash	Epidermis	Tingling, hyperesthesia, pain soothed by cooling	Reddened; blanches with pressure; little or no edema	Complete recovery within a week; some peeling
Partial thickness (second degree)				
Scalds, flash flame	Epidermis, dermis	Pain, hyperesthesia, sensitivity to cold air	Blistered, mottled red base; Broken epidermis; Weeping surface; Edema	Recovery in 2–3 weeks; some scarring, depigmentation; infection may convert to third degree
Full thickness (third degree)				
Flame, long exposure to hot liquids, electric current	Epidermis, dermis, sometimes subcutaneous tissue	Pain free; shock; hematuria, possible entrance, exit wounds if electrical	Dry, pale white, leathery, or charred; broken skin with fat exposed; edema	Eschar sloughs; grafting needed, scarring, loss of contour function; loss of digits or extremity possible

Reprinted with permission from Smeltzer SC, Bare BG. Brunner and Suddarth's Textbook of Medical–Surgical Nursing, ed 8. Philadelphia: Lippincott-Raven, 1996; 1550.

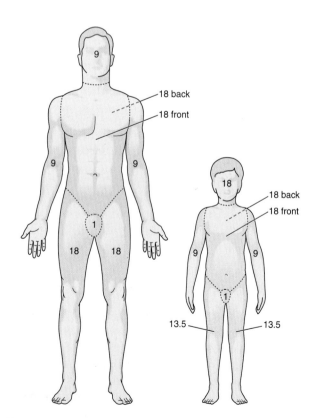

FIGURE 28-7.   The rule of nines.

for the back of the trunk, and 18% for each lower extremity. The area around the genitals is the additional 1% of the BSA. In infants and children, the percentages are the same except that the head is 18% and each lower extremity is 13.5% of the total BSA.

Management of the Burn Victim

Follow these guidelines for managing burn patients in the medical office:

1. If necessary, eliminate the source of the burn.
2. Have someone notify the physician and call EMS.
3. Assess the patient's airway, breathing, and circulation. Begin CPR if necessary.
4. Remove all jewelry and clothing as necessary to evaluate the extent of the burn.
5. Wrap the patient in a clean, dry sheet.
6. Administer oxygen as instructed by the physician.
7. Treat the patient for shock and accompanying low blood pressure.
8. Assist with the necessary procedures for transporting the patient to the hospital.

 Checkpoint Question

5. What are the four major sources of burn injuries?

Musculoskeletal Injuries

Injuries to muscles, bones, and joints are some of the most common problems encountered in providing emergency care. The seriousness varies widely, from simple injuries, such as a fractured finger, to major or life-threatening conditions, such as open fracture to the femur, which can cause severe bleeding. Injuries to muscles, tendons, and ligaments occur when a joint or muscle is torn or stretched beyond its normal limits. Fractures and dislocations are usually associated with external forces, although some arise from disease, such as bone degeneration.

Management of Musculoskeletal Injuries

It is often difficult to distinguish between strains, sprains, fractures, and dislocations in an emergency. Therefore, in most cases assume the area is fractured and immobilize it accordingly. Proper splinting includes immobilizing the joint above and below the fracture site. Splinting helps prevent further injury to soft tissues, blood vessels, and nerves from sharp bone fragments and relieves pain by stopping motion at the fracture site. As soon as possible, apply ice to the injured area to reduce the swelling that commonly occurs with this type of injury, but never attempt to reduce, or put back into place, a dislocated area.

Types of Splints

Any device used to immobilize a sprain, strain, fracture, or dislocated limb is a **splint**. Splinting material may be soft or rigid and can be improvised from almost any object that can provide stability. Commercial types include traction, air, wire ladder, and padded board splints. Regardless of the type of splint, you must examine the extremity for signs of impaired circulation. To check the circulation of an extremity:

- Observe the skin color and nail beds of the affected extremity. A pale or cyanotic color indicates that the circulation is impeded.
- Locate a pulse in the artery distal to the affected extremity. A weak or absent pulse also indicates that circulation is decreased to the area.
- Watch for increased swelling of the extremity. While this may not indicate that the circulation is impaired, the swelling itself can reduce circulation.

If the circulation is impaired with the splint in place, it must be removed or loosened immediately to provide for adequate blood flow or tissue **ischemia** (decrease in oxygen) and **infarction** (death) may occur.

Cardiovascular Emergencies

Cardiovascular disease accounts for nearly 1 million deaths each year in the United States. The most common problem is coronary artery disease. Approximately two-thirds of sudden deaths from coronary artery disease occur out of the hospital, and most occur within 2 hours of the onset of symptoms. As coronary artery disease progresses, less and less oxygen can get to the cardiac muscle, which leads to tissue ischemia and eventual infarction of the cardiac tissue. The early symptoms of a myocardial infarction (heart attack) include the following:

- Chest pain not relieved by rest
- A complaint of pressure in the chest or upper back
- Nausea or indigestion
- Chest pain that radiates up into the neck and jaw or down one arm
- Anxiety

Early treatment, including basic life support, early defibrillation, and advanced life support can prevent many of these deaths. If cardiopulmonary resuscitation is initiated promptly and the patient is rapidly and successfully defibrillated, the patient's survival chances improve. As noted earlier, an automatic external defibrillator, or AED, may be available in your medical office and should be used as soon as possible after it is determined that the victim does not have a pulse. When applied to the patient's chest, the AED will analyze the rhythm and advise the operator to shock, or defibrillate, the patient by simply pressing a button.

Neurological Emergencies

A seizure is caused by an abnormal discharge of electrical activity in the brain. During a seizure, erratic muscle movements, strange sensations, and a complete loss of consciousness can occur. A seizure is not a disease but a manifestation or symptom of an underlying disorder. Epilepsy, head injury, and drug toxicity can cause seizures. A thorough patient history is important when assessing these patients. It should include the following:

- Information about previous seizure disorders
- Frequency of seizures if recurrent
- Prescribed medications
- Any history of head trauma
- Alcohol or drug abuse
- Recent fever
- Stiff neck (as seen in meningitis)
- A history of heart disease, diabetes, or stroke.

In managing a patient having a seizure, you must give priority to assessing the patient's responsiveness, airway, breathing, and circulation. In certain types of seizures, the patient loses consciousness and therefore cannot protect the airway. During the seizure the muscles of the body, including those of the face, will contract tightly. If you attempt to force an object between the teeth to prevent the patient from biting the tongue, the result will most likely be injury to you or the patient. Frequently, patients vomit during the seizure and lose bowel or bladder control. Particular attention and care are necessary to clear and maintain the airway without causing injury to yourself or the patient. Assisting the patient into the recovery position (on one side) will help secretions such as blood or vomit drain from the mouth. Secretions may be removed from the mouth using a suction machine if available.

After gaining control of the airway, perhaps the most important thing you can do for a patient during a seizure is protect the patient from injury. If the patient lost consciousness and fell at the beginning of the seizure, care will be necessary to protect the neck and cervical spine until immobilization can occur.

Allergic and Anaphylactic Reactions

A severe allergic reaction called anaphylaxis causes most emergency department visits related to allergies. An allergic reaction is a generalized reaction that can occur within minutes to hours after the body has been exposed to a substance recognized by the immune system as foreign and to which it is oversensitive. The systemic signs and symptoms of anaphylaxis are more severe than for a simple allergic reaction, but repeated exposure to a substance that produces allergic reactions may ultimately lead to an anaphylactic reaction and should be avoided.

PATIENT EDUCATION

Choking

A common misconception is that only children choke. The reality is that each year many adults choke to death. Here are some important teaching tips for people aged 20 to 70:

- Chew your food. Focus on eating. Do not eat and drive a car at the same time.
- Avoid excessive alcohol consumption, especially while eating.
- Laugher and talking increase your chance of choking. Do not talk with food in your mouth.

Here are some important teaching points for older people:

- Be sure dentures fit snugly. Go for an annual dental evaluation.
- As we age, our saliva glands produce less saliva. Saliva is needed to dissolve food into small pieces and also helps with swallowing. Therefore, pay special attention while you eat. Older patients need to chew food longer and take smaller bites.

Common Allergens

An **allergen** is a substance that gives rise to hypersensitivity or allergy. The allergen may be a drug, insect venom, food, or pollen and may be injected, ingested, inhaled, or absorbed through the skin or mucous membranes. A person may have symptoms within seconds after exposure to an allergen, or the reaction may be delayed for several hours. You must ask every patient about allergies at every visit and indicate them on the front of the patient's chart and the medication record. Check the patient's medical record and ask about allergies *before* administering any medications in the office; this is essential to prevent allergic reactions or anaphylaxis in patients with known hypersensitivity.

Although the exact incidence of anaphylactic reactions is difficult to pinpoint, it is estimated that 1% to 2% of patients who receive penicillin in the United States have some form of allergy to the drug and that 1 in 50,000 injections of penicillin results in death from anaphylaxis. However, you must be alert to the signs and symptoms of allergic reactions after administering any medication, not just penicillin. Patients with moderate to severe allergy symptoms often receive frequent injections of specific allergens to reduce the symptoms associated with allergies. These patients should be monitored especially closely for anaphylaxis, and they should not be permitted to leave the office for a prescribed amount of time, often 20 to 30 minutes after the injection. When documenting that an injection was given, you should also note the condition of the patient upon discharge.

Signs and Symptoms

The initial signs and symptoms of an allergic reaction may include severe itching, a feeling of warmth, tightness in the throat or chest, or a rash. The primary rule for any exposure is that the sooner the symptoms occur after the exposure, the more severe the reaction is likely to be. Be observant and ready to treat any patient who has these symptoms, since airway obstruction, cardiovascular collapse, and shock can occur if the situation worsens. Since the primary cause of death in an anaphylactic reaction is swelling of the tissues in the airway, leading to airway obstruction, observe the patient closely for signs of airway involvement, including wheezing, shortness of breath, and coughing. Choking or tightness in the neck and throat may signal this danger. Tachycardia, hypotension, pale skin, dryness of the mouth, diaphoresis (profuse sweating), and other signs of shock may also be present.

Management of Allergic and Anaphylactic Reactions

The patient having a severe allergic reaction will often be anxious. Some allergic reactions are mild, without respiratory problems or signs of shock. These simple reactions can be managed by administering oxygen or medications such as antihistamines to relieve symptoms as directed by the physician. If respiratory involvement occurs without signs of shock, the physician may order that epinephrine (1:1000) be given subcutaneously. The patient with a severe anaphylactic reaction who is in shock needs more aggressive therapy, including additional medications, an intravenous line, and monitoring of the cardiac rhythm. The primary goal when treating a patient having an anaphylactic reaction is restoring respiratory and circulatory function. The following steps are required for managing allergic reactions, including anaphylaxis:

- Do not leave the patient, but have another staff member request that the physician immediately evaluate the patient and bring the emergency kit or cart, including oxygen.
- Assist the patient to a supine position.
- Assess the patient's respiratory and circulatory status by obtaining the blood pressure, pulse, and respiratory rates.
- Observe the skin color and warmth.
- If the patient complains of being cold or is shivering, cover with a blanket.
- Upon the direction of the physician, start an intravenous line and administer oxygen and other medications as ordered.
- Document vital signs and any medications and treatments.
- Communicate relevant information to the EMS personnel, including copies of the progress notes or medication record as needed.

 Checkpoint Question

6. What is the primary cause of death in anaphylaxis?

Poisoning

The likelihood that one will be exposed to toxins in the home or workplace is increasing. Over-the-counter and prescription medications are common in homes. Household chemicals are an additional hazard and are often designed to have a pleasant odor and color. Industrial chemicals offer another possibility of poisoning. These chemicals may affect a single victim or many victims in the event of a hazardous materials incident. Most toxic exposures occur in the home, and almost 50% occur in children aged 1 to 3 years. While about 90% of reported poisonings are accidental, intentional exposures usually affect adolescents and adults, and they tend to have a higher death rate. Fortunately, deaths from drug overdoses and poisoning are rare, but you must know how to respond if a patient comes to the office or telephones with a possible poisoning.

Poison Control Center

The American Association of Poison Control Centers (AAPCC) has established standards and regional poison control centers throughout the country. These centers are staffed by physicians, nurses, and pharmacists. When information about a poisoning or drug overdose is not readily available, the poison control center is a valuable resource, and the phone number should be posted near all phones in the medical office. The professionals at the poison control center can usually evaluate a potential or known toxic exposure, instruct the caller in the use of syrup of ipecac to induce vomiting if indicated, and check on the patient's progress by follow-up telephone calls.

Management of Poisoning Emergencies

Exactly how and when a poison control center is consulted should be part of the medical office's protocol. Few toxic substances have specific antidotes, so the management of the poisoning is aimed at treating the signs and symptoms and assessing the involved organ systems. The patient may go to the medical office after the poisoning, or more commonly, the patient or caregiver telephones the office requesting information. In either situation, you must obtain the following information *before* making the call to poison control:

- The nature of the poisoning (ingested, inhaled, skin exposure)
- The age and weight of the victim
- The name of the substance
- An estimate of the amount of poison
- When the exposure occurred
- The patient's present signs and symptoms

Once the poison control center has been notified and instructions given, you must be prepared to treat the patient as directed and notify the EMS to transport the patient to the hospital. Never give a patient syrup of ipecac or otherwise induce vomiting unless directed to do so by the professionals at the poison control center.

Heat- and Cold-Related Emergencies

Environmental temperature is one of the many variables to which the body normally adjusts, maintaining equilibrium. Human beings depend on the ability to control core body temperature within a range of several degrees. Measured rectally, this core temperature is 37.6°C (99.6°F). The peripheral temperature is usually lower (98.6°F orally). Several conditions can disrupt the normal heat-regulating mechanisms of the body. These are divided into two main categories: **hyperthermia** and **hypothermia**.

Hyperthermia

Hyperthermia is the general condition of excessive body heat. Correct management depends on assessment of the underlying cause. The first type of hyperthermia includes **heat cramps**: muscle cramping that follows a period of heavy exertion and profuse sweating in a hot environment. While sweat is primarily water, it also contains the electrolyte sodium, which is needed for muscle function. Heavy sweating, which is a normal compensatory mechanism to cool the body, will result in a sodium deficit, which compromises muscle function and produces muscle cramps. A patient with heat cramps often complains of cramping in the calves of the legs and in the abdomen. Cramping may also occur in the hands, arms, and feet. Mental status and blood pressure usually remain normal, although an increased pulse rate is common.

Heat cramps signal the need for cooling and rest. In uncomplicated cases, the patient is encouraged to take fluids by mouth, but nausea may make intravenous infusion necessary. If the patient is able to take fluids by mouth, give a commercial electrolyte solution such as Gatorade, or salt can be added to water or fruit juice at 1 teaspoon per pint. Cramps can sometimes be prevented entirely with similar oral intake before physical exertion and every 20 minutes during exercise. Salt tablets are not recommended because they may cause nausea.

Heat exhaustion results most often from physical exertion in a hot environment without adequate fluid replacement. Body temperature usually remains normal or slightly above normal. Patients have central nervous system symptoms such as headache, fatigue, dizziness, or syncope (fainting). Although the skin is typically moist and the pulse rate is high, skin color, blood pressure, and respiratory rate vary with the degree to which the body is able to hold off the distress. Patients in late stages of heat exhaustion have pale skin, low blood pressure, and rapid respiration.

Heat stroke is a true emergency. The body is no longer able to compensate for the rapid rise in body temperature (past 105°F) and may undergo brain damage or death. Heat stroke victims can deteriorate quickly to coma, and many patients have seizures. The skin is classically hot, flushed, and dry. Vital signs are elevated initially but may drop, with ensuing cardiopulmonary arrest. Heat stroke demands rapid cooling of the body. After alerting the physician, follow office policy for the management of hyperthermia and heat stroke, which will include these steps:

- Move the patient to a cool area.
- Remove clothing that may be holding in the heat.
- Place cool, wet cloths or a wet sheet on the core surface areas of the body where the ability to cool the central blood is the greatest: the scalp, neck, axilla, and groin.
- Administer oxygen as directed by the physician and apply a cardiac monitor.
- Notify the EMS for transportation to the hospital.

Hypothermia

The body's core temperature can drop several degrees without loss of normal body function. The body usually tolerates a 3° to 4°F drop in temperature without symptoms; hypothermia is an abnormally low body temperature, below 35°C (95°F). Internal metabolic factors and significant heat loss to the external environment can lead to hypothermia. Very cold air and immersion in cold water can cause a rapid drop in core temperature. These are the signs and symptoms of hypothermia:

- Cool, pale skin
- Lethargy and mental confusion
- Shallow, slow respirations
- Slow, faint pulse rate

Basic management of hypothermia includes handling the patient gently, removing wet clothing, and covering the patient to prevent further cooling. If there is evidence of rewarming (skin warm, respirations approaching normal, no shivering) and the patient is alert and able to swallow, give warm fluids by mouth. Avoid drinks that constrict peripheral blood vessels, such as those that contain caffeine (coffee and tea). Fluids that cause dilation of the blood vessels, such as alcohol, should also be avoided. Warm beverages with sugar, such as hot chocolate, can be given to begin replacement of the fuel that the body needs to restore normal heat production. No fluids should be given by mouth to patients who have a diminished or changing level of consciousness.

Frostbite

Windy subfreezing weather creates the greatest risk for **frostbite**. Small body parts with a high ratio of surface area to tissue mass (fingers, toes, ears, and nose) are most vulnerable to frostbite, although larger areas of the extremities are also vulnerable during profound cooling. Exposure to cold can cause tissues to freeze, and the frozen cells die.

The type and duration of contact are the two most important factors in determining the extent of frostbite injury. Touching cold fabric, for example, is not nearly as dangerous as coming into direct contact with cold metal, particularly if the skin is wet or even damp. The combination of wind and cold is dangerous. *Superficial frostbite* appears as firm and waxy gray or yellow skin in an area that loses sensation after hurting or tingling. Prolonged exposure can lead to blistering and eventually *deep frostbite*, which most often affects the hands and feet. No warning symptoms appear after the initial loss of feeling. Freezing progresses painlessly once the nerve endings are numb. Skin becomes inelastic and the entire area feels hard to the touch. Deep frostbite results in tissue death, and the affected tissue must be removed surgically or amputated.

Superficial frostbite can be managed by warming the affected part with another body surface, for example placing an ungloved hand over the nose or ears. Management for more than superficial frostbite is rapid rewarming after any systemwide hypothermia has been corrected. Deep frostbite should be managed only in the hospital to prevent further damage to the tissue. After notifying the EMS, you may be asked to do the following as directed by the physician:

- Immerse the frozen tissue in lukewarm water (41°C, 105°F) until the area becomes pliable and the color and sensation return.
- Do not apply dry heat.
- Do not massage the area; massage may cause further tissue damage.
- Avoid breaking any blisters that may form.

If rewarming is not attempted, bandage the frostbitten part with dry sterile dressings while waiting for the EMS to transport the patient to the hospital. Frostbitten tissue is similar to burned tissue in that it is vulnerable to infection. Take care to keep the affected part as clean as possible. All frostbite victims should be assessed for hypothermia. Clothing offers good protection against weather only if it is loose enough to avoid restricting circulation. Tight gloves, cuffs, boots, and straps add to the danger.

Behavioral and Psychiatric Emergencies

Psychological distress may be mild, moderate, or severe. The degree of intensity determines the type and amount of intervention necessary. A psychiatric emergency is different from an emotional crisis, and you must know how to differentiate between the two. A psychiatric emergency is any situation in which the patient's moods, thoughts, or actions are so disordered or disturbed that harm or death may result for the patient or others if no intervention occurs. An emotional crisis, on the other hand, is a situation with much less intensity. While it may be distressing to the patient, in most cases it is not likely to end in danger, harm, or death without immediate intervention. However, if neglected entirely, an emotional crisis may escalate to a full psychiatric emergency.

A true behavioral emergency, like a medical emergency, carries a serious threat. Urgent behavioral situations usually require some form of professional psychological evaluation and intervention and require transportation to the hospital. The following guidelines are useful for handling a psychiatric emergency:

- Notify the physician and the EMS as directed.
- Offer reassurance and general support to the patient and any caregivers or family members who may be present.
- Accurately document information, including vital signs and the patient's behavior.

CHAPTER SUMMARY

Medical assisting requires interpersonal skills and the ability to communicate clearly, but it is equally important for you to recognize the need for immediate medical intervention when faced with an emergency. If you are prepared with the appropriate knowledge and training to deal with emergencies, you can provide first aid and life support measures that can mean the difference between life and death. In addition, being prepared will lend you confidence in administering first aid and life support, which will reassure your patient, family members, and other members of the health care team.

Critical Thinking Challenges

1. When an emergency occurs, the patient's family members may become anxious and emotionally distraught. How can you help to calm an anxious family member?
2. Reread the "What If" question in this chapter. Analyze how you would respond to such a situation.
3. Investigate the Good Samaritan law in your state.

Answers to Checkpoint Questions

1. Before the ambulance arrives, you should document basic identification, the chief complaint, times that specific events occurred, vital signs, techniques used to treat the patient, and any observations.
2. The purpose of the primary assessment is to identify and correct any life-threatening problems.
3. The diagnostic signs of the secondary assessment are general appearance, level of consciousness, vital signs, and skin appearance.
4. Shock is defined as lack of oxygen to individual cells resulting from low blood pressure.
5. The four major types of burn injuries are thermal, electrical, chemical, and radiation.
6. The primary cause of death from anaphylaxis is airway obstruction.

 Websites

American Association of Poison Control Centers
www.aapcc.org
American Heart Association www.americanheart.org
American Red Cross www.redcross.org
American Safety and Health Institute
www.ashinstitute.com
National Safety Council www.nsc.org

Clinical Duties
Related to Medical
Specialties

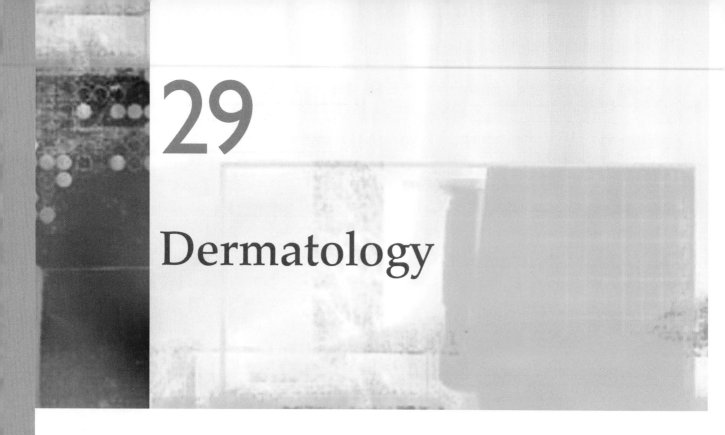

29

Dermatology

CHAPTER OUTLINE

COMMON DISORDERS OF THE INTEGUMENTARY SYSTEM
Skin Infections
Inflammatory Reactions
Disorders of Wound Healing
Disorders Caused by Pressure
Alopecia
Disorders of Pigmentation
Skin Cancers

DIAGNOSTIC PROCEDURES
Physical Examination of the Skin
Wound Cultures
Skin Biopsy
Urine Melanin
Wood's Light Analysis

BANDAGING
Types of Bandages
Bandage Application Guidelines

ROLE DELINEATION

CLINICAL: FUNDAMENTAL PRINCIPLES
- Apply principles of aseptic technique and infection control
- Screen and follow up patient test results

CLINICAL: DIAGNOSTIC ORDERS
- Collect and process specimens
- Perform diagnostic tests

CLINICAL: PATIENT CARE
- Adhere to established patient screening procedures
- Obtain patient history and vital signs
- Prepare and maintain examination and treatment areas
- Prepare patient for examinations, procedures, and treatments
- Assist with examinations, procedures, and treatments
- Coordinate patient care information with other health care providers

GENERAL: PROFESSIONALISM

- Display a professional manner and image
- Demonstrate initiative and responsibility
- Work as a member of the health care team
- Set priorities and perform multiple tasks
- Adapt to change
- Treat all patients with compassion and empathy

GENERAL: COMMUNICATION SKILLS

- Recognize and respect cultural diversity
- Adapt communications to individual's ability to understand
- Recognize and respond effectively to verbal, nonverbal, and written communications
- Use medical terminology appropriately
- Serve as a liaison

GENERAL: LEGAL CONCEPTS

- Perform within legal and ethical boundaries
- Prepare and maintain medical records
- Document accurately
- Comply with established risk management and safety procedures

GENERAL: INSTRUCTION

- Instruct individuals according to their needs
- Teach methods of health promotion and disease prevention

CHAPTER COMPETENCIES

LEARNING OBJECTIVES

Upon successfully completing this chapter, you will be able to:

1. Spell and define the key terms.
2. Describe common skin disorders.
3. Explain common diagnostic procedures.
4. Prepare the patient for examination of the integument.
5. Assist the physician with examination of the integument.
6. Explain the difference between bandages and dressings and give the purpose of each.
7. Identify the guidelines for applying bandages.

PERFORMANCE OBJECTIVES

Upon successfully completing this chapter, you will be able to:

1. Apply a warm or cold compress. (Procedure 29-1)
2. Assist with therapeutic soaks. (Procedure 29-2)
3. Apply a tubular gauze bandage. (Procedure 29-3)

KEY TERMS

alopecia	dermatophytosis	impetigo	psoriasis
abscess	dressing	macule	pustule
bandage	eczema	malignant tumor	seborrhea
benign tumor	erythema	neoplasm	*Staphylococcus*
bulla	exudate	nodule	*Streptococcus*
carbuncle	fissure	papilloma	urticaria
cellulitis	folliculitis	papilloma virus	verruca
comedo	furuncle	papule	vesicle
cyst	herpes simplex	pediculosis	wheal
dermatitis	herpes zoster	pruritus	Wood's light

COMMON DISORDERS OF THE INTEGUMENTARY SYSTEM

The skin, or integument, is the largest organ of the body. Clear skin glowing with health indicates a good general state of wellness; pallor, cyanosis, or dry, scaly skin indicates poor general health. Although it has many functions, including maintaining homeostasis, one of the most important functions of the integumentary system is to protect the underlying tissues and organs from the external environment. FIGURE 29-1 shows a cross-section of the normal anatomy of the skin and accessory structures. Unbroken skin provides a protective barrier that prevents the entrance of microorganisms and is the body's first line of defense against infection. In addition, the skin protects the body from mechanical injury, damaging substances, and the ultraviolet rays of the sun. The study of the skin is dermatology, and a physician who specializes in disorders of the skin is a dermatologist. The general practice physician may diagnose diseases of the integumentary system or may refer patients to the dermatologist.

Checkpoint Question

1. How does the integument help to prevent infection?

Skin Infections

Many integumentary disorders are manifested by lesions or abnormalities in skin tissue (FIG. 29-2). These lesions may be primary or secondary to primary lesions. When working with a patient who may have a skin infection, you should always wear protective equipment, such as examination gloves, since the drainage from any lesions may be infective.

Bacterial Infections

Impetigo. **Impetigo** is a contagious bacterial infection of the skin that is common in young children. It may be caused by **Staphylococcus** or **Streptococcus** microorganisms. Lesions appear on exposed areas, such as the face and neck. Terms used to describe many skin lesions, not just those seen in a patient with impetigo, include the following:

macule   small, flat skin discoloration (Fig. 29-2*A*).
vesicle   small fluid-filled sac (Fig. 29-2*D*).
bulla   large fluid-filled sac (Fig. 29-2*E*).
pustule   pus-filled sac (Fig. 29-2*F*).

Initially, impetigo may appear as an area of **erythema**; however, patches of vesicles that produce honey-colored drainage and crusts follow the redness (Fig. 29-2*K*). These vesicles leave red areas when the crusts are removed.

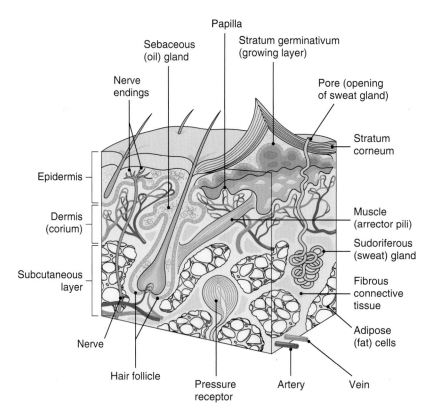

FIGURE 29–1.   Cross-section of the skin. (Reprinted with permission from Cohen BJ, Wood DL. Memmler's The Human Body in Health and Disease. Philadelphia: Lippincott Williams & Wilkins, 2000.)

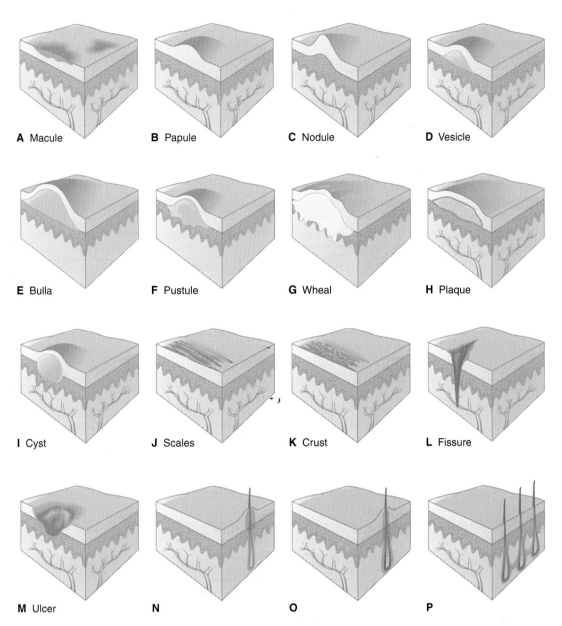

A Macule **B** Papule **C** Nodule **D** Vesicle

E Bulla **F** Pustule **G** Wheal **H** Plaque

I Cyst **J** Scales **K** Crust **L** Fissure

M Ulcer **N** **O** **P**

FIGURE 29–2. Skin lesions. _Primary lesions:_ (A) Macule. Flat, circumscribed discoloration. (B) Papule. Palpable elevated solid lesion smaller than 1 cm; colors vary. (C) Nodule. Raised solid lesion larger than 1 cm. (D) Vesicle. Small elevation filled with clear fluid. (E) Bulla. Vesicle or blister larger than 1 cm. (F) Pustule. Lesion containing pus. (G) Wheal. Transient elevation of the skin caused by edema of the dermis and surrounding capillary dilation. (H) Plaque. Elevated solid lesion on skin or mucosa; larger than 1 cm. (I) Cyst. Tumor that contains semisolid or liquid material. _Secondary lesions:_ (J) Scales. Heaped-up horny layer of dead epidermis. (K) Crust. Covering formed from serum, blood, or pus drying on the skin. (L) Fissures. Cracks in the skin. (M) Ulcer. Lesion formed by local destruction of the epidermis and part of the underlying dermis. _Other lesions:_ (N) Superficial folliculitis. Local infection of a hair follicle. (O) Furuncle. Acute inflammation deep within hair follicle. (P) Carbuncle. Infection involving subcutaneous tissues around several hair follicles.

Treatment is washing the area 2 or 3 times a day and applying a topical antibiotic as ordered by the physician. Oral antibiotics may also be prescribed for severe cases. Scratching must be discouraged to prevent the spread of the infection, and patients must be instructed to wash towels, washcloths, and bed linens daily. Individuals at risk for developing impetigo are those in poor health, those with conditions such as anemia or malnutrition, and those with poor hygiene; however, any person handling contaminated laundry or otherwise exposed to the infectious material should be encouraged to practice frequent medical asepsis such as handwashing.

Folliculitis. **Folliculitis** is a superficial infection of a hair follicle (Fig. 29-2N). It is characterized by itching, burning, and the formation of a **pustule**. Treatment is aimed at promoting drainage and healing. Saline soaks or compresses (Procedures 29-1 and 29-2) may be ordered for 15 minutes twice a day followed by application of an anti-infective ointment or cream and a dressing to absorb any drainage. If folliculitis is left untreated, it may lead to the formation of an **abscess**. An abscess is formed when a small sac of pus, or purulent material, accumulates at the site of inflammation. The causative agent of these infections is often *Staphylococcus.*

Furuncle. A **furuncle**, more commonly known as a boil, is a deep-seated infection of a hair follicle or gland (Fig. 29-2O). Friction and pressure at the site may contribute to its formation. A hard, painful **nodule** forms (Fig. 29-2C), enlarges for several days, then erupts, with pus oozing from the site. The cause of the infection is often *Staphylococcus.* Treatment of a furuncle includes application of moist heat to assist in ripening it, or bringing it to a head, and antibiotic therapy. Often a minor surgical procedure known as incision and drainage is performed to remove the purulent material and facilitate healing.

Carbuncle. A **carbuncle** consists of infection in an interconnected group of hair follicles or several furuncles joined together in a mass (Fig. 29-2P). The subcutaneous tissue in the surrounding area is also involved, and *Staphylococcus* is often responsible. Carbuncles are hard, round, extremely painful swellings that enlarge over several days to a week. Eventually they soften and erupt, discharging pus from several sites. When the skin sloughs away, a scarred cavity remains. The patient often has a fever. Treatment of a carbuncle is with systemic antibiotics, moist heat (Procedures 29-1 and 29-2), and incision and drainage once the lesion has matured. A topical anti-infective agent and loose bandages are also applied to the area. The site may require a wick, or sterile gauze packing, to remain in the cavity for several days to facilitate healing.

Cellulitis. When an existing wound is infected and the infection spreads to the surrounding connective tissue, **celluli-** tis results. The skin becomes hot, red, and edematous. If it is not treated, the underlying tissue may be destroyed or develop an **abscess**. A systemic anti-infective, such as an antibiotic, usually provides rapid and successful treatment.

Checkpoint Question

2. Which three bacterial infections develop in the hair follicles? Briefly describe each.

Viral Skin Infections

Herpes Simplex. Herpes simplex infections produce lesions commonly known as cold sores or fever blisters. The lesions, which appear on the lips, mouth, face, and nose, are small vesicles grouped on a red base. They eventually erupt, leaving a painful ulcer and then a crust. The infection may be precipitated by other infections, such as upper respiratory infections, or by menstruation, fatigue, trauma, stress, or exposure to the sun.

The causative agent is herpes simplex virus I (HSVI). (Herpes simplex II is responsible for the sexually transmitted disease known as genital herpes.) Typically, HSV1 infections are recurrent, and no effective treatment eliminates or controls the disease. During an outbreak, the lesions appear and demonstrate the characteristics noted earlier and should be considered infectious. Antiviral drugs, such as valacyclovir or acyclovir, have been shown to decrease the severity of the outbreaks in some people, but do not offer a cure. Treatment is aimed at relieving discomfort with topical anesthetic ointment to relieve the pain until the lesions heal, usually in 5 to 7 days.

Herpes Zoster. **Herpes zoster**, or shingles, is caused by the same virus that causes chickenpox. It is believed that after an initial infection with the varicella virus, the virus lies dormant in the nervous system for years. Herpes zoster usually occurs in adults and may become active in times of physical or emotional stress. When reactivated, the virus spreads down a nerve to the skin, causing redness, swelling, and pain. After about 48 hours, a band of lesions develops. They begin as **papules**, small, red solid elevations on the skin (Fig. 29-2B). Shingles commonly appear on the face, back, and chest and are frequently unilateral. These lesions progress to vesicles and pustules, then dry crusts, and may last for 2 to 5 weeks. Scarring and alterations in pigmentation are common. Pain often remains after the lesions have disappeared, in some cases for several months.

The treatment of a herpes zoster breakout includes an opioid analgesic for the discomfort or nerve block for severe pain. Locally, calamine lotion may be used for itching. The area must be protected from air and the irritation of clothing. Acyclovir is sometimes used to alleviate the severity of the disease.

Verruca. A **verruca** is a wart, or squamous cell **papilloma** (benign skin tumor) that appears as a rough, raised lesion with a pitted surface. Warts may occur singly or in groups and may be found anywhere on the skin or mucous membranes. They commonly appear on the fingers, hands, or feet and may vary in size, shape, and appearance. The causative agents include **papillomaviruses,** and the treatment is removal. Removing a wart may be achieved with keratolytic agents, which cause softening and shedding of the skin; liquid nitrogen, which freezes and destroys the affected tissue; podophyllum resin, a caustic agent found in many over-the-counter wart medications; laser therapy, which removes the affected tissue using radiation of the visible infrared spectrum of light; or surgery. They may also disappear spontaneously.

Checkpoint Question

3. Which viral skin infection is linked to a common childhood disorder? Explain.

Fungal Skin Infections

Fungal infection of the skin (**dermatophytosis**) is caused by a group of molds called dermatophytes. There are several types of dermatophytes, but the treatment is similar. The group of fungal diseases called tinea is collectively known as ringworm; its members are named according to the area of the body infected. All tinea infections are considered contagious.

Tinea Capitis. Tinea capitis affects the scalp. It is contagious and appears most frequently in children. It is characterized by round gray scale patches (dried skin flakes) and areas of **alopecia** (baldness). There are usually no symptoms except light itching.

Tinea Corporis. Tinea corporis (also known as tinea circinata) manifests on hairless portions of the body. It is characterized by itchy red rings that are clear in the center with a scaly border (Fig. 29-2*J*). It is frequently found on the face and arms but may also be found on the trunk.

Tinea Cruris. Tinea cruris, known in lay terms as jock itch, is found on the skin in the groin area and the gluteal folds. The lesions, which cause marked itching, are red macules with clear centers and scaly borders.

Tinea Pedis. Tinea pedis, or athlete's foot, is characterized by itching, burning, and stinging between the toes and on the soles of the feet. The lesions may appear as red, weepy vesicles, as chronic dry scales, or as **fissures** (cracklike lesions) between the toes (Fig. 29-2*L*).

Tinea Unguium. Also known as onychomycosis, tinea unguium causes thickening, discoloration, and crumbling of the nails, most often the toenails. It is difficult to cure and often requires months of local antifungal preparations. In severe cases, an oral antifungal medication, griseofulvin, is prescribed.

Tinea Versicolor. Tinea versicolor, also known as pityriasis versicolor, is a fungal infection; however, it is not caused by dermatophytes. It is not known exactly what sort of fungus is the causative agent. The disease causes a multicolor rash, generally over the upper trunk. It is most common in young people in warm weather, and it is chronic. Its lesions vary from macular to raised, round, or oval, from darkly pigmented to depigmented and are slightly scaly. There are usually no symptoms. Diagnosis of tinea versicolor is determined with a **Wood's light**, an ultraviolet light used in a darkened room to show abnormalities in the skin as fluorescent. Treatment includes the use of selenium sulfide for 7 days along with topical antifungal cream or lotion.

Treatment of Tinea Infections. All of the tinea infections are treated with topical antifungal powders, creams, or shampoos. Antifungal medications such as griseofulvin may be prescribed orally for severe cases. Inflamed lesions may be treated with wet compresses or soaks. General measures for treating fungal infections and preventing the spread of infection is to keep the area clean and dry, because fungi thrive in moist conditions. Clothing should be loose fitting and laundered daily. Socks and underclothing should be changed frequently, and clothing should not be shared with others. Shower shoes should be worn in public showers and pools, since these areas are usually wet, providing an optimum environment for the fungus to grow on floors and be transmitted directly to the feet.

Checkpoint Question

4. What is the difference between tinea capitis and tinea pedis?

Parasitic Skin Infections

Scabies. Scabies is a contagious skin disorder caused by the itch mite *Sarcoptes scabiei*. It is spread by direct contact and produces small vesicles or pustules between the fingers, at the inner wrist, elbows, axillae, waist, and groin. The itching caused by the mite is worst at night, when the female burrows under the epidermis to lay her eggs.

Treatment for scabies is aimed at disinfestation. For adults, an antiparasitic such as 1% lindane cream is applied from the neck down at bedtime. One application of 5% permethrin, or Elimite, cream is effective and is the drug of choice for children. All bedding and clothing for the entire family should be laundered daily until the infestation is resolved.

Pediculosis. **Pediculosis** is an infestation of the skin with a parasite known commonly as lice. *Three types of the louse* Pediculus humanus infest the body: the scalp (*pediculosis capitis*, by *P. humanis var. capitis*), the body (*pediculosis corporis* by *P. humanis var. corporis* or *var. vestimenti*), the eyelashes or eyelids (*pediculosis palpebrarum*, also by *P. capitis*), and the pubic hairs (*pediculosis pubis*). Wherever they are found, itching is intense and the skin often becomes secondarily infected from scratching. Lice feed on human blood and lay eggs (nits) on body hair or clothing fibers. Nits may be seen on hair shafts close to the skin or in seams of clothing.

Pediculosis is common among populations with overcrowding, such as head lice in schools, and poor hygiene. The infestation is transmitted through physical contact with an infested person, by sitting on an infested toilet seat, or by sharing a comb, brush, clothing, or bedding that is infested. Benzene hexachloride creams, lotions, or shampoos are used for all types of pediculosis. All clothing and linen must be dry cleaned or washed in hot water and ironed. Sealing items in plastic bags for 30 days or heating them to 140°F will kill lice on items that cannot be laundered.

Inflammatory Reactions

Eczema

Eczema is an inflammatory skin disorder usually involving only the epidermal layer of the skin. It is more common in children than adults and is characterized by itching and lesions that generally begin as red patches, proceed to weepy vesicles, and end up as dry scaly crusts. They appear on the face, neck, bends of the knees and elbows, and the upper trunk. It is not clear why some patients develop this disorder, which is chronic and may have periods of remission and exacerbation. Possible causes of eczema depend on the individual and may include the following:

- Food allergies to fish, eggs, and milk products
- Medication or chemical allergies
- Sensitivity to irritating soaps, household cleaning products, deodorants, and perfumes
- Inhalants such as pollen, dust, or animal dander
- Poor circulation to a body part
- Ultraviolet rays

Treatment is removing the cause and promoting healing of the lesions. The causative agent should be avoided if it is known. The patient should maintain good hydration and keep the skin well moistened with emollients. A humid environment is recommended. Warm, not hot, baths should be taken daily with a nondrying soap. The skin should be dried immediately and scratchy clothing should be avoided.

Exudative lesions are treated with soaks, baths, or wet dressings for 10 to 30 minutes 3 or 4 times daily. Domeboro, Aveeno, or bicarbonate is good for these purposes. In addition, the physician may order the following treatments:

- Topical corticosteroid lotion, cream, or ointment to be used twice a day.
- Bandages at night to protect against scratching.
- Antihistamines for severe **pruritus** (itching).
- For scales, a topical steroid ointment. Systemic corticosteroids, such as prednisone, may be ordered in severe cases.

Seborrheic Dermatitis

Seborrheic **dermatitis** (skin inflammation), also known as **seborrhea**, is an overproduction of sebum. It is a chronic disorder resulting in greasy yellow scales primarily on the scalp, where it is called seborrheic dandruff. Underlying redness and pruritus may be present. The eyelids, face, chest, back, umbilicus, and body folds may also be affected. It is thought that seborrhea is caused by a genetic predisposition and a combination of hormones, nutrition, infection, or stress. It is treated with shampoo and topical corticosteroid lotion.

Urticaria

Urticaria, or hives, is an acute inflammatory reaction of the dermis. It begins with itching, followed by erythema and swelling. The **wheals** (Fig. 29-2*G*) have a pale center with a red edge. They resemble a mosquito bite and appear in clusters anywhere on the body. Hives are self-limiting, lasting from a few days to a few weeks. The most common causes include contact with these substances:

- Foods, including shellfish, strawberries, tomatoes, citrus fruits, eggs, and chocolate
- Inhalants, including feathers or animal dander
- Chemicals, cosmetics, and medications
- Sunlight
- Insect bites or stings
- Heat, cold, or pressure on the skin
- Infection
- Stress

Treatment of urticaria is reduction of the inflammatory response. The cause should be avoided if known. Antihistamines are usually given to reduce itching and swelling, and a short course of prednisone is sometimes ordered. Starch or Aveeno baths twice a day may be ordered to make the patient more comfortable. Epinephrine is given if the symptoms of urticaria develop rapidly and are associated with dyspnea. These symptoms are indicative of anaphylaxis, a severe life-threatening emergency (see Chapter 28).

Spanish Terminology

El sarpullido es picante.	The rash is itchy.
¿Cuán largo ha tenido usted ese lunar?	How long have you had that mole?
He tenido este lunar durante 5 años.	I have had this mole for 5 years.
Esta ampolla es dolorosa.	This blister is painful.

Acne Vulgaris

Acne vulgaris is an inflammatory disease of the sebaceous glands. Its cause is not known in all cases, and it may occur in any adult, but it commonly occurs during adolescence as a result of the increase in hormone production. It is characterized by pimples, **comedones** (blackheads), **cysts** (fluid-filled sacs beneath the skin) (Fig. 29-2*I*), and scarring. The lesions may occur on the face, neck, upper chest, back, and shoulders. Overactive sebaceous glands produce excessive sebum that gets trapped in a follicle, producing a dark substance that results in a blackhead. Leukocytes accumulate, producing pus.

Treatment for acne includes a regimen of tretinoin (Retin-A), benzoyl peroxide, and tetracycline. Sunlamp treatments are sometimes used to dry the lesions.

Psoriasis

Psoriasis is a chronic inflammatory skin disorder characterized by bright red plaques (Fig. 29-2*H*) covered with dry, silvery scales. Although the cause is unknown, it is a chronic disorder and often difficult to treat. Psoriasis is usually found on the scalp, elbows, knees, base of the spine, palms, soles, and around the nails. There are usually no vesicles, and itching varies from mild to severe. Exacerbations are common during cold weather, stress, and pregnancy. Treatment includes tar preparations and topical steroid cream or ointment. Exposure to ultraviolet light 3 times a week may also be prescribed.

Checkpoint Question

5. What is urticaria, and which layer of the skin does it affect?

Disorders of Wound Healing

Keloids

Keloids, an overproduction of scar tissue, occur as a complication of wound healing. The scar tissue forms as a result of excessive collagen accumulation. A raised nodule forms and does not resolve with time. The cause is unknown. It occurs most frequently in young women, especially during pregnancy, and is particularly common in African Americans. The most common sites are the neck and shoulders. Injections of cortisone are sometimes effective in treating keloids.

Disorders Caused by Pressure

Callus and Corn

A callus, sometimes called a callosity, is a raised painless thickening of the epidermis. It is caused by pressure or friction on the hands and feet. A corn is a hard, raised thickening of the stratum corneum on the toes. It results from chronic friction and pressure, especially from poorly fitting shoes. The pressure compresses the dermis, making it thin and tender and causing pain and inflammation. Soft corns can form between the toes.

The treatment for calluses and corns begins with relieving the pressure. Shoes should be made of soft leather and fit properly. Liners may be inserted in shoes to relieve pressure. Bandages and corn pads also help correct the problem. Sometimes the physician recommends surgical intervention or use of a keratolytic agent to cause chemical peeling.

Decubitus Ulcers

Decubitus ulcers are also called pressure sores and are caused by prolonged pressure to an area of the body, usually over a bony prominence (Fig. 29-2*M*). The pressure impairs blood supply, oxygen, and nutrition to the area, which results in an ulcerative lesion and eventual tissue death. The most common sites are over the sacrum and hips, but these ulcers may also occur on the back of the head, ears, elbows, heels, and ankles. They are most common in aged, debilitated, and immobilized patients. Bedridden and wheelchair-bound patients are at risk for developing decubiti unless they are repositioned frequently, every 2 hours, to relieve pressure. Special mattresses, pads, and pillows are useful in preventing pressure sores.

Decubitus ulcers are graded, or staged, according to the degree of tissue involvement (TABLE 29-1). Treatment consists of topical antibiotic powder and adhesive absorbent bandages and dressings. Deep infections may require systemic antibiotics and possibly surgical debridement.

Stage	Description
TABLE 29-1	**STAGING OR GRADING FOR DECUBITUS ULCERS**
I	Red skin does not return to normal when massaged or when pressure is relieved.
II	Skin is blistered, peeling, or cracked superficially.
III	Skin is broken, with loss of full thickness; subcutaneous tissue may be damaged; serous or bloody drainage may be present.
IV	Deep, craterlike ulcer shows destruction of subcutaneous tissue; fascia, connective tissue, bone, or muscle exposed and may be damaged.

Intertrigo

Intertrigo is a disorder of skin breakdown that occurs in the body folds of obese persons. The combination of heat, moisture, and friction of the skin against itself in these areas causes the skin to break down. Humid climates and poor hygiene often aggravate the condition. Erythema and skin fissures result, and the affected area itches, stings, and burns.

Treatment for intertrigo is proper hygiene and an attempt to keep the area clean and dry. Talcum powder or cornstarch is often recommended. Antibacterial or antifungal lotion or powder is necessary if secondary infection is present.

Alopecia

Alopecia, or baldness, may be the result of physical trauma, systemic disease, bacteria or fungal infection, chemotherapy, excessive radiation, hormonal imbalance, or genetic predisposition. Baldness caused by scarring and inherited male pattern baldness are permanent and cannot be reversed; however, the drug minoxidil may be recommended by the physician to stimulate hair growth in male pattern baldness. For other causes of baldness, treatment of the underlying disorder often results in new hair growth.

Disorders of Pigmentation

Albinism

Albinism is a genetically determined condition of partial or total absence of the pigment melanin in the skin, hair, and eyes. The skin is pale, the hair is white, and the irises of the eyes appear pink. The skin will not tan and is prone to sunburn. Because no pigment is present to protect the underlying eye structures from the ultraviolet rays of the sun, eye problems may develop as a result of this disorder. Albinism has no treatment.

Vitiligo

Vitiligo is a progressive chronic destruction of melanocytes, cells in the epidermis that produce melanin, a skin pigment. This disorder is thought to be an autoimmune disorder in patients with an inherited predisposition. The depigmented areas occur as white patches that sometimes have a hyperpigmented border. It usually occurs in exposed areas of the skin.

There is no effective treatment for vitiligo. Patients are advised to protect the areas from the sun because they are prone to sunburn in the absence of melanin. Waterproof cosmetics may be used to cover the area.

Leukoderma

Leukoderma is a permanent local loss of skin pigment that results from damage caused by skin trauma. It is particularly common in African Americans. Causes of leukoderma include contact with caustic chemicals and the sequela of burn or infection.

Nevus

A nevus, also known as a birthmark or mole, is a congenital pigmented skin blemish. It is usually circumscribed and may involve the epidermis, connective tissue, nerves, or blood vessels. Nevi are usually **benign**, not cancerous, but may become **malignant** (cancerous). Patients should be cautioned to watch for changes in the color, size, and texture of any nevus. Bleeding and itching should also be reported (Box 29-1).

WHAT IF

An elderly patient comes into the office with multiple decubitus ulcers? What should you do?

The elderly are always at risk for developing skin ulcerations; however, the physician must assess the situation to determine whether the patient is receiving adequate care at home. Patients who arrive in the medical office with multiple ulcers in different stages of healing may be abused or neglected. Elder abuse is less often identified, but some experts believe it is as common as child abuse. If you suspect elder abuse, contact your local department of social services. The investigation may substantiate the abuse (requiring referral to law enforcement) or may identify ways to alleviate the situation (caregiver education, respite care) without removing the patient from home. In some states the law requires reporting elder abuse. The physician who fails to do so can be fined or be subject to other penalties.

Box 29-1

ON THE LOOKOUT FOR MALIGNANT MELANOMA

Most melanomas are pigmented, elevated skin lesions; they frequently develop in a new or existing mole. About 54,200 new melanomas were diagnosed in the United States during 2003, and about 7,600 people will die of melanomas. The key to treatment of this potentially deadly cancer is early detection of changes in size, color, shape, elevation, texture, or consistency of any pigmented area, old or new, or in any spot or bump (see illustrations). Being familiar with what is normal for you makes you more likely to notice what is abnormal.

The eventual outcome of melanoma is governed by how deeply it has invaded the skin, which also determines how aggressively the cancer will be treated. A cancer prevention message first used in Australia and currently being promoted in the United States is "Slip! Slop! Slap! Wrap!" which may help individuals to remember Slip on a shirt! Slop on sunscreen! Slap on a hat! And put on wrap-around sunglasses to protect your eyes and the skin around them.

Mole Patrol

Mole inspection is simpler if you keep in mind the American Cancer Society's ABCD rule for distinguishing a normal mole or other skin blemish from and abnormal one:

Asymmetry. Half of the mole does not match the other.
Border. The edges are irregular: ragged, notched, or blurred.
Color. The color is not uniform but may be differing shades of tan, brown, or black, sometimes with patches of red, white, or blue.
Diameter. The mole is larger than a pencil eraser— about 6 mm, or a quarter of an inch—or is growing.

Reprinted with permission from *Harvard Medical Letter*, June 1991, p. 4, American Cancer Society.

Checkpoint Question

6. What are four disorders of pigmentation? Briefly describe them.

Skin Cancers

Basal Cell Carcinoma

Basal cell carcinoma is a slow-growing cancer that appears most commonly on exposed areas of the body, usually the face, but may also occur on the shoulders or chest. The lesion has a waxy appearance with a depressed center and a rolled edge where blood vessels may be apparent. Metastasis (spreading to other areas of the body) almost never occurs, but if left untreated, the lesions will grow locally and may ulcerate and damage surrounding tissues (FIG. 29-3). The most common treatment for basal cell carcinoma is surgical removal, and this may be done in the physician's or dermatologist's office. Radiation therapy and cryosurgery, or removal using a cold agent such as liquid nitrogen, are alternative treatments.

Squamous Cell Carcinoma

Squamous cell carcinoma is slightly less common than basal cell carcinoma. It may occur in any squamous (scaly) epithelial area of the body, such as the lungs, cervix, or anus, but is most frequently found on the skin (FIG. 29-4). Squamous cell carcinoma is a slow-growing, malignant **neoplasm** (tumor). The lesions are firm, red, horny or prickly, and painless, and they range widely in size. Those on exposed areas are thought to result from exposure to the sun. Other areas not normally exposed, such as mucous membranes, are thought to be affected as the result of frequent irritation. Treatment is the same as for basal cell carcinoma. Although basal cell carcinoma is not generally metastatic, squamous cell carcinoma will spread readily through underlying and surrounding tissues.

Malignant Melanoma

Malignant melanoma is a cancer of the skin that forms from melanocytes. Lesions vary from macules to nodules and often have an irregular border and a variety of colors

FIGURE 29-3. Basal cell carcinoma. (Reprinted with permission from Goodheart HP. Goodheart's Photoguide of Common Skin Disorders. Philadelphia: Lippincott Williams & Wilkins, 2003.)

FIGURE 29-4. Squamous cell carcinoma. (Reprinted with permission from Goodheart HP, Goodheart's Photoguide of Common Skin Disorders. Philadelphia: Lippincott Williams & Wilkins, 2003.)

Box 29-2

EFFECTS OF SUNLIGHT ON THE SKIN

Exposure to the sun's ultraviolet rays is the major cause of skin cancers. In addition, ultraviolet rays cause sunburn and premature aging of the skin. Primary prevention of skin cancer consists of limiting exposure to ultraviolet light by wearing proper clothing and using sunscreen. Exposure to the sun is not recommended during the five peak hours of the day, from 10:00 A.M to 3:00 P.M. A sunscreen with at least a 15 SPF (sun protective factor) is considered good protection in blocking ultraviolet rays. Most sunscreens contain PABA (aminobenzoic acid), which causes allergy in many people. However, a number of PABA-free sunscreens are available. The use of sunlamps and tanning beds should be avoided.

(FIG. 29-5). Mixtures of white, blue, purple, and red are the most common. The tumor grows both in radius and in depth into the dermis. In about 30% to 35% of cases, it grows in a preexisting nevus.

Malignant melanoma, which is thought to be caused by excessive exposure to sunlight, is the leading cause of death due to skin disease. It is the ninth most common cancer. The incidence is 1 in 105 individuals in the United States. Those at highest risk for developing the disease have blond or red hair, fair skin, blue eyes, and a tendency to sunburn and spend a lot of time out of doors (Box 29-2).

Treatment of malignant melanoma is surgical removal after a biopsy, possibly including removal of lymph tissue. The patient's prognosis depends on the depth of the tumor.

Tumors over 1.5 mm often metastasize to the lymph nodes, liver, lungs, and brain and are often fatal (Box 29-1).

Checkpoint Question

7. Which is more likely to metastasize, basal cell or squamous cell carcinoma?

DIAGNOSTIC PROCEDURES

Physical Examination of the Skin

Examination of the skin is performed mostly by inspection. Many lesions can be diagnosed by the characteristic size, shape, and distribution on the skin. However, laboratory

A   B

FIGURE 29-5. Malignant melanoma. (*Left*) Superficial melanoma. (*Right*) Nodular melanoma.

studies may be necessary to confirm a diagnosis. As the medical assistant, you may assemble the equipment as directed by the physician, verify that an informed consent has been obtained for surgical procedures, and properly direct specimens to the appropriate laboratories. Observe standard precautions when handling any specimens, including those obtained from the skin.

Before the examination, prepare the examination room and the patient. Use a gown and draping appropriate to the patient's symptoms and area to be examined. During the examination, aid the physician by ensuring that the lighting is adequate and directed properly, assisting in obtaining wound cultures, maintaining asepsis, and applying topical medications, sterile dressings, and bandages. Protect skin lesions from further infection by using medical or surgical asepsis as indicated.

After the dermatological examination, reinforce the patient's instructions about caring for the skin condition at home, such as:

- Keeping bandages clean and dry
- Returning to the office to have sutures or staples removed
- How long to avoid getting the area wet
- Applying topical medications

Clean and disinfect the examination room according to the office policy.

Wound Cultures

Obtain a wound culture by getting a sample of wound **exudate** (drainage) using a sterile swab, applying the specimen to a growth medium, and allowing the microorganisms to grow. A sample of the propagated culture is placed on a slide in the laboratory and observed under a microscope to diagnose bacterial or fungal infection. In the medical office, you will obtain wound cultures by following these steps:

1. Wash your hands and put on gloves.
2. If a dressing is present, remove it and dispose of it in a biohazard container. Assess the wound for signs of infection by observing the color, odor, and amount of exudate.
3. Obtain a wound collection device that contains the sterile swab for collecting the specimen and a culture medium for transporting to the laboratory.
4. Open and remove the sterile culture tube and insert the cotton-tipped applicator end of the swab into the exudate, being sure to saturate the swab with drainage (FIG. 29-6). Place the swab back in the culture tube and crush the ampule of transport medium (FIG. 29-7). Label the culture tube, fill out a laboratory requisition slip, and send it to the laboratory according to the office and laboratory policies.
5. Clean the wound and apply a sterile dressing using sterile technique.
6. Remove your gloves, wash your hands, and document the procedure.

FIGURE 29-6. Insert culture swab into the wound to obtain a sample.

FIGURE 29–7.   Crush ampule of medium.

Skin Biopsy

The purpose of a skin biopsy is to remove a small piece of tissue from a lesion so that it may be examined under a microscope to determine whether it is a benign or malignant growth. A local anesthetic is injected by the physician and sterile asepsis is used throughout the procedure (see Chapter 6). The three types of skin biopsy performed by the physician are excision, punch, and shave. In an excision biopsy, the entire lesion is removed for evaluation. When a punch biopsy is done, a small section is removed from the center of the lesion. A shave biopsy cuts the lesion off just above the skin line. The sample of tissue is sent to the laboratory for analysis.

Urine Melanin

Melanin is not normally present in the urine unless the patient has malignant melanoma. A urine test to detect the presence of melanin is done with a random sample of urine from the patient. The specimen is sent to the laboratory, allowed to sit for 24 hours, and then examined under a microscope for the presence of melanin.

Wood's Light Analysis

Wood's light is an ultraviolet light that is used to detect fungal and bacterial infections, scabies, and alterations in pigment. When it is directed 4 to 5 inches from the patient's skin in a darkened room, certain abnormalities in the skin and hair appear as fluorescent colors that can be diagnosed by the physician and treated accordingly.

Checkpoint Question

7. Why is a skin biopsy performed?

BANDAGING

Bandages are strips of woven materials, typically absorbent, that are used for many purposes:

1. Applying pressure to control bleeding
2. Holding a **dressing** in place
3. Protecting dressings and wounds from contamination
4. Immobilizing an injured part of the body
5. Supporting an injured part of the body

Types of Bandages

- *Roller bandages* are soft woven materials packaged in a roll. Roller bandages are available in various lengths and widths from 1 inch to 6 or more inches.

TRIAGE

While working in a medical office setting, the following three situations are occurring:

A. The physician has asked you to apply a tubular gauze dressing to a 47-year-old woman with a finger injury.

B. The receptionist has asked you to come to the waiting room to see a patient who just arrived in the office complaining of urticaria and shortness of breath. The receptionist tells you that the patient is allergic to bees and was stung by a bee about 20 minutes ago.

C. An 80-year-old woman is ready to be discharged but needs to be taught how to do a therapeutic soak for a foot ulcer. She has diabetes.

How do you sort these patients? Whom do you see first? Second? Third?

Patient B should be taken directly to an examination room and seen first. She is most likely having an allergic reaction to a bee sting *and may develop anaphylaxis*. Patient A should be seen next. Applying a dressing should take only a few minutes. Patient C should be seen last. Teaching a patient a new skill requires time and attention to detail. You should demonstrate and then have the patient return the demonstration.

The bandage size used depends on the part being bandaged and the desired thickness of the completed bandage. Most bandages are made of a porous, lightweight material and are either sterile or clean. Gauze bandages conform easily to angular surfaces of the body. A crepelike stretchy gauze is made to adjust to various body contours and resists unrolling much better than plain roller gauze. Kling and Conform are two frequently used brands.

- *Elastic bandages,* such as the Ace brand, are special bandage rolls with elastic woven throughout the fabric. They are generally brownish tan. Unlike other types of roller gauze, elastic bandages can be given to the patient to take home to be washed and reused many times. Because of the elastic fibers, great care must be exercised when applying the bandage to prevent compromising circulation and still give support to the injured part. Elastic bandages should be applied without wrinkling in concentric or overlapping layers. Bandages should fit snugly but not too tightly. Adjust the bandage if it seems too loose or if the patient says it is uncomfortable or tight. Some elastic bandages have an adhesive backing, which helps keep the layers in place and provides a secure, snug, and comfortable fit. **To avoid applying it too tightly, never stretch or pull on the elastic bandage during application.** Ask the patient how tight the bandage feels as it is being applied and instruct the patient on signs of impaired circulation by checking the extremity distal to the bandage for these indications:

  A. Increased swelling or pain
  B. Pale skin
  C. Cool skin compared to the other extremity

- *Tubular gauze bandages* are used to enclose rounded body parts. The bandage resembles a hollow tube and is very stretchy. It is used to enclose fingers, toes, arms, and legs and even the head and trunk. Tubular gauze bandages are available in various widths from 0.672 inch to 7 inches to fit any part of the body. Tubular gauze is applied using a metal or plastic tubular framelike applicator. The applicator is available in various sizes and should be slightly larger than the body part to be covered. This enables the gauze to slide easily over the body part. Applicators are marked according to a size number that corresponds to different sizes of tubular gauze. Procedure 29-3 describes the specific steps for applying a tubular gauze bandage.

Bandage Application Guidelines

When properly applied, bandages should feel comfortably snug and should be fastened securely enough to remain in place until removed. Bandages can be fastened with safety pins, adhesive tape, or clips. You gain the patient's confidence when you apply a bandage that is comfortable and neat looking and that stays in place. Patients become understandably upset when bandages fall off during normal activities. These are general guidelines for applying bandages:

1. Observe the principles of medical asepsis, including handwashing to prevent the transfer of pathogens. Surgical asepsis is not necessary. The bandage may be used to cover a sterile dressing or may be used alone if there is no open wound.
2. Keep the area to be bandaged and the bandage itself dry and clean, because moisture may wick bacteria into the wound. A moist bandage encourages the growth of pathogens and is uncomfortable for the patient.
3. Never place a bandage directly over an open wound. Apply a sterile dressing first and cover it with a bandage for protection. The bandage should extend approximately 1 to 2 inches beyond the edge of the dressing.
4. Never allow skin surfaces of two body parts to touch each other under a bandage. Wound healing may cause opposing surfaces to adhere and result in scar tissue formation. For example, burned fingers must be dressed separately but may be bandaged together.
5. Pad joints and any bony prominence to help prevent skin irritation caused by the bandage rubbing against the skin over a bony area.
6. Bandage the affected part in the normal position: joints should be slightly flexed to avoid muscle strain, discomfort, and pain. Muscle spasms may occur if the part is made to assume an unnatural position.
7. Apply bandages beginning at the distal part and extending to the proximal part of the body. Bandage turns that extend distal to proximal aid in return of venous blood to the heart and help make the bandage more secure.
8. Always talk with the patient during the bandaging. If the patient complains that it is too tight or too loose, adjust the bandage. Instruct the patient to do the same at home. The bandage should fit snugly, but if it is too tight, it may impair circulation. If it is too loose, it may fall off.
9. When bandaging hands and feet, leave the fingers and toes exposed whenever possible to make it easier to check for circulatory impairment. If the skin feels cold or looks pale, the nail beds look cyanotic, or the patient complains of swelling, numbness, or tingling of the toes or fingers, remove the bandage immediately and reapply it correctly.

FIGURE 29-8 illustrates various techniques for wrapping bandages.

FIGURE 29–8. The six basic techniques for wrapping a roller bandage. (A) A *circular turn* is used to anchor and secure a bandage when it is started and ended. Hold the free end of the rolled material in one hand and wrap it about the area and back to the starting point. (B) A *spiral turn* partly overlaps a previous turn. The overlapping varies from half to three-fourths of the width of the bandage. Spiral turns are used to wrap a cylindrical part of the body like the arms and legs. (C) A *spiral reverse turn* is a modification of a spiral turn. The roll is reversed halfway through the turn. This works well on tapered body parts, such as the forearm and wrist. (D) A *figure-of-8 turn* is best used when an area spanning a joint, like the elbow or knee, requires bandaging. It is made by making oblique turns that alternately ascend and descend, simulating the number 8. (E) A *spica turn* is a variation of the figure-of-8 turn. It differs in that the wrap includes a portion of the trunk or chest. (F) The *recurrent turn* is made by passing the roll back and forth over the tip of a body part. Once several recurrent turns have been made, the bandage is anchored by completing the application with another basic turn like the figure-of-8. A recurrent turn is especially beneficial when wrapping the stump of an amputated limb.

Procedure 29-1

Applying a Warm or Cold Compress

Purpose: Apply warm or cold compresses according to a physician's order.

Equipment: Warm compresses: appropriate solution (water with possible antiseptic if ordered), warmed to 110°F or recommended temperature; bath thermometer; absorbent material (cloths, gauze); waterproof barriers; hot water bottle (optional); clean or sterile basin; gloves. Cold compresses: appropriate solution; ice bag or cold pack; absorbent material (cloths, gauze); waterproof barriers; gloves.

Standard: This procedure should take 40 minutes, depending on the physician's order.

Steps	Reason
1. Wash your hands and put on gloves.	Handwashing aids infection control.
2. Check the physician's order and assemble the equipment and supplies.	
3. Pour the appropriate solution into the basin. For hot compresses, check the temperature of the warmed solution.	The solution must not be hot enough to injure the patient.
4. Greet and identify the patient. Explain the procedure.	Identifying the patient prevents errors in treatment. Explaining the procedure helps ease anxiety and ensure compliance.
5. Ask patient to remove clothing as appropriate and to put on a gown. Drape as appropriate.	Privacy must always be provided.
6. Protect the examination table with waterproof barrier.	Wet surfaces are uncomfortable for the patient and may cause chilling.
7. Place absorbent material or gauze in the prepared solution. Wring out excess moisture.	Compresses should be moist but not dripping; avoid wetting the patient.
8. Lightly place the compress on the patient's skin and ask about the temperature for comfort. Observe the skin for changes in color.	Always ask the patient whether the temperature of the compress is causing pain or discomfort.

Step 8. Gently touch the wet compress to the affected area.

(continues)

Procedure 29-1   (continued)

Applying a Warm or Cold Compress

Steps	Reason
9. Gently arrange the compress over the area and contour the material to the area. Insulate the compress with plastic or other waterproof barrier.	Unless the material is against the skin, temperature will not be transferred to the area of concern. Insulating the area with the waterproof barrier will retard temperature loss and avoid getting the rest of the patient wet.
10. Check the compress frequently for moisture and temperature. Hot water bottles or ice packs may be used to maintain the temperature. Rewet absorbent material as needed.	The temperature should stay fairly constant. If the material dries, benefits will be lost.
11. After the prescribed amount of time, usually 20–30 minutes, remove the compress, discard disposable materials, and disinfect reusable equipment.	Equipment should be available for the next use. Cross-contamination must be avoided.
12. Remove your gloves and wash your hands.	
13. Document the procedure, including duration of treatment, type of solution, temperature of solution if a warm compress was used, skin color after treatment, assessment of the area, and the patient's response.	Procedures are considered not to have been done if they are not recorded.

Note: If compress is being applied to an area with an open lesion, sterile technique is required.

Note: Warm compresses will speed suppuration to increase healing. Cold compresses will slow bleeding and decrease inflamation.

Charting Example
10/16/2004 10:45 A.M. Hot compress applied to left ankle ×20 min. Skin pink after treatment; no broken areas noted on the skin. _____ B. Barth, CMA

Procedure 29-2

Assisting With Therapeutic Soaks

Purpose: Perform a therapeutic soak as directed by the physician.

Equipment: Clean or sterile basin or container to contain the body part comfortably, solution and/or medication, dry towels, bath thermometer, gloves.

Standard: This procedure should take 15 minutes.

Steps	Reason
1. Wash your hands and apply your gloves.	Handwashing aids infection control.
2. Assemble the equipment and supplies, including a basin or container of the appropriate size. Pad surfaces of container.	If the container is uncomfortably small, soaking the body area will be difficult and may cause muscle spasms. Surfaces should be padded for comfort.
3. Fill the container with solution and check the temperature with a bath thermometer. The temperature should be below 110°F to avoid blood pressure changes caused by vasodilation.	Assessing the temperature will prevent burning or injuring tissues.
4. Greet and identify the patient. Explain the procedure.	Identifying the patient prevents errors in treatment. Explaining the procedure helps ease anxiety and ensure compliance.
5. Slowly lower the area to be soaked into the container and check the patient's reaction. Arrange the part comfortably. Check for pressure areas and pad the edges as needed for comfort.	Immersing the part too quickly can shock the patient. If the patient is not comfortable, muscle spasms or strain may result.

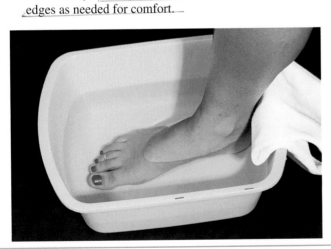

Step 5. The basin should be large enough to immerse the entire body area. Pad the edge for comfort.

6. While soaking, check the temperature of the solution every 5–10 minutes. If additional water or solution must be added to maintain the temperature, remove some of the solution and then add warmed solution while holding your hand between the patient and the stream of the solution being poured. Mix or swirl the soak to ensure constant, even temperature.	The proper temperature must be maintained for maximum benefit. Avoid pouring the solution or water directly against the patient's skin.

(continues)

Procedure 29-2   *(continued)*

Assisting With Therapeutic Soaks

Steps	Reason
 Step 6. Shield the patient's skin when adding warm water to the soak.	
7. Soak for the prescribed amount of time, <u>usually 15–20 minutes</u>. Remove the part from the solution and carefully dry the area with a towel.	The area may be sensitive to brisk rubbing but must be dried to prevent chilling the patient or causing discomfort.
8. Properly care for the equipment; appropriately dispose of single-use supplies.	
9. Document the procedure, including duration of treatment, type and temperature of solution, skin color after treatment, assessment of the area, including the condition of any lesions, and the patient's response.	Procedures are considered not to have been done if they are not recorded.

Charting Example

4/19/2004 12:20 P.M. Soaked left great toe in Betadine solution ×15 min. Mod. amount of tan drainage from ingrown toenail during soaking. _____ J. Brighton, RMA

Procedure 29-3

Applying a Tubular Gauze Bandage

Purpose: Apply tubular gauze bandage to a digit or extremity.

Equipment: Tubular gauze, applicator, tape, scissors.

Standard: This procedure should take 15 minutes.

Steps	Reason
1. Wash your hands and assemble the equipment.	Handwashing aids infection control.
2. Greet and identify the patient. Explain the procedure.	This prevents error in treatment, helps gain the patient's compliance, and eases anxiety.
3. Choose the appropriate size tubular gauze applicator and gauze width according to the size of the area to be covered. Manufacturers of tubular gauze supply charts with suggestions for the appropriate size for various body parts.	The applicator and gauze should slip easily over the body part. Choose an applicator slightly larger than the part to be covered. The gauze designed to fit the chosen applicator will provide a secure fit.
4. Select and cut or tear adhesive tape in lengths to secure the gauze ends.	Tape ensures that the gauze will not slip off. Having it at hand before beginning the procedure saves time and effort.
5. Place the gauze bandage on the applicator in the following manner:	

    A. Be sure the applicator is upright (open end up) and placed on a flat surface.

    B. Pull a sufficient length of gauze from the stock box; do not cut it yet.

    C. Open the end of the length of gauze and slide it over the upper end of the applicator; estimate and push the amount of gauze that will be needed for this procedure onto the applicator.

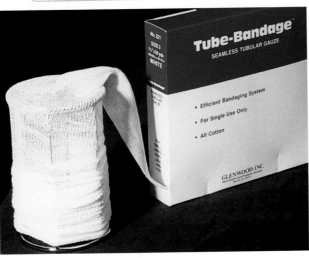

Step 5C. Place the applicator upright and slide the end of the gauze over the applicator.

    D. Cut the gauze when the required amount of gauze has been transferred to the applicator.

(continues)

Procedure 29-3   *(continued)*

Applying a Tubular Gauze Bandage

Steps	**Reason**
6. Place the applicator over the distal end of the affected part (finger, hand, toe, leg) and begin to apply the gauze by pulling it over the applicator onto the skin. Hold it in place as you move to step 7.	The applicator should begin distally and work proximally.
7. Slide the applicator up to the proximal end of the affected part. Holding the gauze at the proximal end of the affected part, pull the applicator and gauze toward the distal end.	This keeps the bandage from slipping. If the bandage is not held in place at the early stages of application, it may not completely cover the part.

Step 7. Hold the gauze at the proximal end of the affected part and pull the applicator toward the distal end.

8. Continue to hold the gauze in place at the proximal end. Pull the applicator 1–2 inches past the end of the affected part if the part is to be completely covered. Sometimes the gauze need not extend beyond a limb but covers only the area around the wound.	The bandage will be secured at the distal end if the part is to be completely covered. If the distal portion of the limb is not to be covered, the bandage must extend at least 1 inch beyond the wound site to ensure adequate coverage.

Step 8. Pull the applicator 1 to 2 inches past the affected area.

9. Turn the applicator one full turn to anchor the bandage.	The bandage will be securely held in place by the twist.

(continues)

Procedure 29-3 (continued)

Applying a Tubular Gauze Bandage

Steps	Reason
10. Move the applicator toward the proximal part as before.	

Step 10. Move the applicator toward the proximal part.

Steps	Reason
11. Move the applicator forward about 1 inch beyond the original starting point. Anchor the bandage again by turning it as before.	Anchoring provides a secure fit.

Step 11. Move the applicator forward about 1 inch beyond the starting point.

Steps	Reason
12. Repeat the procedure until the desired coverage is obtained. The final layer should end at the proximal part of the affected area. Any extra length of gauze can be cut from the applicator. Remove the applicator.	The part should be adequately covered to protect the wound.
13. Secure the bandage in place with adhesive tape or cut the gauze into two tails and tie them at the base of the tear. Tie the two tails around the closest proximal joint. Use the adhesive tape sparingly to secure the end if not using a tie.	The bandage must be securely fastened to keep it in place until it is changed.

(continues)

Procedure 29-3   (continued)

Applying a Tubular Gauze Bandage

Steps	Reason
 Step 13. Secure the bandage with adhesive tape.	
14. Properly care for or dispose of equipment and supplies. Clean the work area. Wash your hands.	Standard precautions must be followed.
15. Record the procedure.	Procedures are considered not to have been done if they are not recorded.

Charting Example
02/08/2004 9:15 A.M. Sterile dressign change to right index finger; tubular bandage applied and secured over dressing.
_____ T. Matthews, CMA

CHAPTER SUMMARY

As the largest and certainly the most visible organ of the body, the skin with its accessories offers the first glimpse into the total state of health. Assessment of the integument is the first step of any physical examination. Although the dermatologist will treat patients with a variety of integumentary system disorders, the medical assistant in other medical offices will be exposed to many examples of integumentary diseases and disorders listed in this chapter and must learn to assist the physician in correctly identifying the forms of skin lesions.

Critical Thinking Challenges

1. Sunlight or ultraviolet rays are needed to convert vitamin D necessary for calcium and phosphorous absorption. Why is it important that children be exposed to sunlight regularly during their growing years?

2. Why do molds and fungi thrive in a public shower or pool? Consider the factors needed for microorganisms to thrive.
3. Why is hot water contraindicated in cases of eczema?

Answers to Checkpoint Questions

1. Intact skin helps prevent invasion by microorganisms into underlying tissue.
2. Folliculitis, furuncle, and carbuncle are bacterial skin infections that develop in the hair follicles. Folliculitis is infection of one hair follicle. A furuncle is an infection deep within the hair follicle. A carbuncle is an infection of subcutaneous tissue around several hair follicles.
3. Herpes zoster, also known as shingles, is caused by varicella virus, the virus that causes chickenpox. This virus can lie dormant for many years after the initial exposure. When reactivated, the virus spreads down a nerve to the skin, resulting in redness, swelling, pain, and eventual development of lesions.

4. Tinea capitis is a fungal infection that affects the scalp; tinea pedis is a fungal infection that affects the feet and is also known as athlete's foot.

5. Urticaria, also known as hives, is an acute inflammatory reaction of the dermis; it is characterized by itching and the development of wheals.

6. Four pigmentation disorders are albinism (partial or total absence of pigment in the skin, hair, and eyes), vitiligo (chronic destruction of melanocytes), leukoderma (local loss of pigment), and nevus (pigmented skin blemish).

7. Squamous cell carcinoma will spread through underlying and surrounding tissue.

8. A skin biopsy is used to examine a lesion for benign and malignant cells.

 Websites

American Cancer Society www.cancer.org
American Academy of Dermatology www.aad.org
American Board of Dermatology www.abderm.org
American Society of Dermatology www.asd.org
Dermatology Image Atlas, Johns Hopkins University
   http://dermatlas.med.jhmi.edu

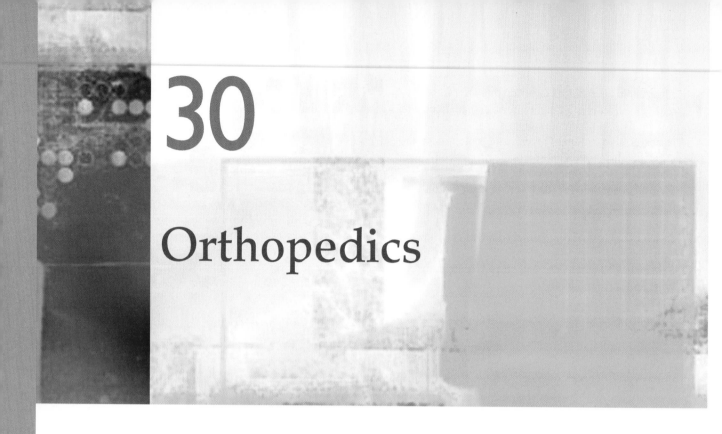

30

Orthopedics

CHAPTER OUTLINE

ROLE DELINEATION

ADMINISTRATIVE: ADMINISTRATIVE PROCEDURES

- Perform basic administrative medical assisting functions
- Schedule inpatient and outpatient admissions and procedures

CLINICAL: FUNDAMENTAL PRINCIPLES

- Apply principles of aseptic technique and infection control
- Screen and follow up patient test results

CLINICAL: PATIENT CARE

- Adhere to established patient screening procedures
- Prepare patient for examinations, procedures, and treatments
- Assist with examinations, procedures, and treatments
- Coordinate patient care information with other health care providers

GENERAL: PROFESSIONALISM

- Display a professional manner and image
- Work as a member of the health care team
- Set priorities and perform multiple tasks
- Treat all patients with compassion and empathy

GENERAL: COMMUNICATION SKILLS

- Recognize and respect cultural diversity
- Adapt communications to individual's ability to understand
- Recognize and respond effectively to verbal, nonverbal, and written communications
- Use medical terminology appropriately
- Serve as a liaison

GENERAL: LEGAL CONCEPTS

- Perform within legal and ethical boundaries
- Document accurately
- Comply with established risk management and safety procedures

GENERAL: INSTRUCTION

- Instruct individuals according to their needs

CHAPTER COMPETENCIES

LEARNING OBJECTIVES

Upon successfully completing this chapter, you will be able to:

1. Spell and define the key terms.
2. List and describe disorders of the musculoskeletal system.
3. Compare the different types of fractures.
4. Identify and explain diagnostic procedures of the musculoskeletal system.
5. Describe the various types of ambulatory aids.
6. Discuss the role of the medical assistant in caring for the patient with a musculoskeletal system disorder.

PERFORMANCE OBJECTIVES

Upon successfully completing this chapter, you will be able to:

1. Apply a triangular arm sling (Procedure 30-1)
2. Apply cold packs (Procedure 30-2).
3. Use a hot water bottle or commercial hot pack (Procedure 30-3).
4. Measure a patient for axillary crutches (Procedure 30-4).
5. Instruct a patient in various crutch gaits (Procedure 30-5).

KEY TERMS

ankylosing spondylitis	callus	goniometer	phonophoresis
arthrogram	contracture	iontophoresis	prosthesis
arthroscopy	contusion	kyphosis	reduction
arthroplasty	electromyography	lordosis	scoliosis
bursae	embolus		

THE MUSCULOSKELETAL SYSTEM AND COMMON DISORDERS

Muscles allow movement of the body through contraction and relaxation. Bones support the body and respond to the contractions and relaxations (FIG. 30-1). Because the two systems depend on each other to function, they are often referred to as a single system—the musculoskeletal system. Within this system are joints, areas where two or more bones are held together by connective tissue and cartilage. The integrity of the entire system is required for normal body support and movement (FIG. 30-2).

When there is a problem with the musculoskeletal system, orthopedists and physical therapists often provide appropriate treatment and rehabilitation. However, medical assistants working in other specialties, such as family practice, also care for patients with musculoskeletal disorders. The most common disorders of the musculoskeletal system are sprains, dislocations, fractures, joint disruptions, and degeneration. The musculoskeletal system reacts to injury or disease with pain (Box 30-1), swelling, inflammation, deformity, and/or limitation of range and function.

Sprains and Strains

Injury to a joint capsule and its supporting ligaments is called a sprain, and injury to a muscle and its supporting tendons is called a strain. Damage to a muscle, ligament, or tendon may result in joint instability. If the ligament is completely torn, it cannot efficiently stabilize the joint. Common symptoms are inflammation and pain. Applying ice at the time of injury helps reduce swelling and pain. For mild sprains, treatment includes exercise to prevent joint stiffness and muscle atrophy. Therapeutic devices and compression wraps reduce swelling. Moderate sprains must be treated with care to prevent further injury, because the ligaments are weakened and healing may take 6 to 8 weeks. Severe sprains often require surgery, and the recovery may take longer than 8 weeks.

In the spine, a sprain to the facet joint (the area between vertebrae) can cause pain not only at the point of difficulty but also radiating into an extremity (radicular pain) as a result of impingement on the nerve root that passes close to the joint. For example, an injury to the facet joint between vertebrae of the lower back often causes pain in the back and radiating down one leg or the other. An injury to the anterior cruciate ligament in the knee greatly compromises the joint's stability. The knee becomes swollen, painful, and unstable and has limited motion. Complete tears in the ligaments of the knee require surgery and extensive rehabilitation. An injury to the Achilles tendon in the lower posterior leg is extremely painful and limits the ability to walk. A tear in this tendon requires surgery followed by immobilization.

Dislocations

Dislocation of a joint, also called a luxation, occurs when the end of the bone is displaced from its articular surface. It can be caused by trauma or disease, or it may be congenital. Common sites of dislocations include the shoulders, elbows, fingers, hips, and ankles. A subluxation is a partial dislocation in which the bone is pulled out of the socket but all joint structures maintain their proper relationships. Partial dislocations can result from weakness, decreased muscle tone, gravity, or neurological deficit. The muscles bear most of the responsibility for preventing subluxation. Common symptoms of dislocations include pain, pressure, limited movement, and deformity. Numbness and loss of a pulse in the affected extremity can also occur. Treatment includes realigning the bones and immobilization of the joint. The patient may have to do exercises to strengthen supporting muscles to avoid recurrences.

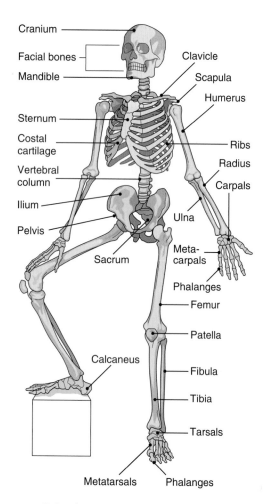

FIGURE 30–1.   The axial skeleton is shown in yellow; the appendicular skeleton is shown in blue. (Reprinted with permission from Cohen BJ, Wood DL. Memmler's The Human Body in Health and Disease. Philadelphia: Lippincott Williams & Wilkins, 2000.)

Labels in figure: Cranium, Facial bones, Mandible, Sternum, Costal cartilage, Vertebral column, Ilium, Pelvis, Sacrum, Calcaneus, Metatarsals, Clavicle, Scapula, Humerus, Ribs, Radius, Carpals, Ulna, Metacarpals, Phalanges, Femur, Patella, Fibula, Tibia, Tarsals, Phalanges

Checkpoint Question

1. How does a luxation differ from a subluxation?

Flexion/extension

Pronation/supination

Abduction/adduction

Circumduction

dorsiflexion/plantar flexion

Rotation

Inversion/eversion

FIGURE 30-2. Normal range of motion of selected joints. (Reprinted with permission from Cohen BJ, Wood DL. Memmler's The Human Body in Health and Disease. Philadelphia: Lippincott Williams & Wilkins, 2000.)

Box 30-1

RELIEVING MUSCULOSKELETAL PAIN

Rest or immobilization or both may be needed to relieve pain in acute soft tissue strains, sprains, and inflammations. Because painful movement may cause further damage to the injured tissue, restriction of movement may also be required. This can be accomplished by rest and by the use of a cast, brace, sling, splint, collar, elastic wrap, or corset. If weight bearing is painful or inadvisable because of fracture or musculoskeletal pathology, an ambulatory aid (e.g., cane, walker, or crutches) may be used.

The use of hot moist packs, a heating pad, or warm baths can help increase circulation, relax spasms, and ease sore muscles. Ice packs help prevent swelling, decrease inflammation, and reduce contusions, which may follow a direct blow on a muscle.

With contusions, the capillaries (small blood vessels) rupture and bleed into the tissue. Swelling and inflammation may result. Reduction of the bleeding is crucial; it is accomplished by applying cold packs and a pressure bandage. Immobilization to prevent further injury is also important. Within a few days, pain-free exercises and heat applications should be introduced to begin healing.

Generally, movement should begin as soon as possible after a soft tissue injury to maintain a healthy joint and resilient muscles. Gently active or passive movement in the pain-free range, mild joint immobilization, traction, or exercise can be effective in maintaining normal range, function, and strength.

Fractures

A fracture is a break or disruption in a bone. The causes of fractures include falls, other trauma, disease, tumors, and unusual stress. There are many types of fractures, each with its own set of problems (TABLE 30-1). However, all fractures have one symptom in common: pain. Other manifestations may include swelling, hemorrhage, lack of movement or unusual movement, **contusions**, and deformity of the body part involved.

Treatment is **reduction** (realigning the bones) by placing the broken ends into proper alignment. Casting, splinting, wrapping, and taping are means of maintaining and immobilizing a closed reduction while the bone heals. If it is not pos-

Table 30-1 TYPES OF FRACTURES

Type	Description
Simple or closed	Does not protrude through the skin; usually treated with closed reduction.
Compound or open	Broken end protrudes through skin; infection a major concern; surgery often required.
Spiral	Occurs with torsion or twisting injuries; appears to be **S**-shaped on radiographs.
Impacted	One bone segment driven into another.
Greenstick	Common injury in children; partial or incomplete break in which only one side of a bone is broken, like a green stick.
Transverse	At right angles to axis of bone; generally caused by excessive bending force or direct hit on bone.
Oblique	Slanted across axis of bone.
Comminuted	Bone is fragmented, usually by much direct force; difficult to reduce because many pieces of bone must be held in proper alignment; more complicated to treat if articular surface is involved, so surgery usually required. Severe soft tissue damage common because of the force necessary to cause the fracture.
Compression	Damage from application of strong force against both ends, such as a fall; vertebrae susceptible to compression fractures, especially in elderly.
Depressed	Fracture of flat bones (usually skull), causing fragment to be driven below surface of bone.
Avulsion	Caused by strong force applied to bone by sharp twisting, pulling motion of attached ligaments or tendons resulting in a tearing away of bone fragments.
Pathological	Usually result of disease process such as osteoporosis (brittle bones), **Paget's disease** (a chronic skeletal disease in the elderly with bowing of the long bones), bone cysts, tumors, or cancer.

Closed

Open

Greenstick

Comminuted

A

Types of fractures.

(continued)

Table 30-1 *(Continued)*

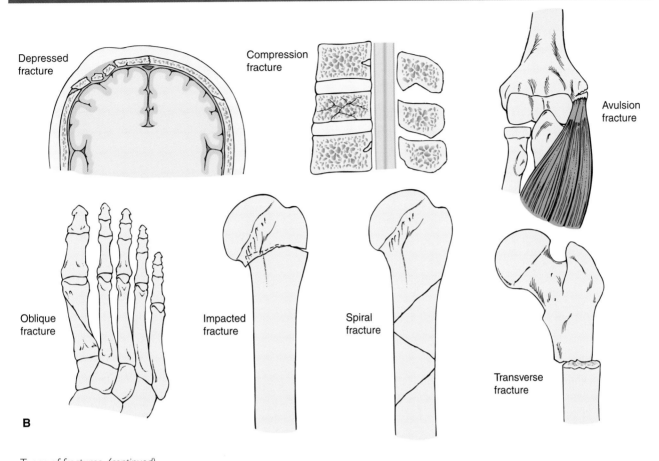

Depressed fracture

Compression fracture

Avulsion fracture

Oblique fracture

Impacted fracture

Spiral fracture

Transverse fracture

B

Types of fractures. *(continued)*

sible to obtain proper alignment by a closed reduction, surgery is required; this open reduction may require the insertion of pins, a plate, or other hardware to maintain alignment of the bones. Fractures in the shoulder are serious because the immobilization necessary for healing may cause scar tissue (adhesions) to form in the capsule, resulting in a severe loss of motion and function. These patients require extensive physical therapy to regain complete use of the involved arm.

Casts

Fractures must be immobilized to facilitate healing of the bone in the proper alignment. In most instances, both proximal and distal joints are included in the cast to ensure that movement is restricted. Box 30-2 describes various types of casts. The casting material is either plaster or fiberglass. Traditional plaster casts are bandages impregnated with calcium sulfate crystals and are supplied as rolls of material in widths appropriate to a variety of sites. After water is added to the dry rolls of bandage and the wet material is applied to the extremity, a chemical reaction generates heat that may be uncomfortable to the patient for a short time, usually less than 30 minutes. This chemical reaction is nec-

essary to produce a rigid dressing when dry. The bandage will mold smoothly to the casting site as it is applied.

A plaster cast is rather soft until it is fully dry, which can take as long as 72 hours. Patients must be cautioned not to exert pressure on the drying cast so as to avoid pressure sores from indentations. Plaster casts must be kept dry at all times.

Because of its lighter weight, water resistance, and durability, fiberglass is rapidly becoming the material of choice for casting. The polyurethane additives harden in minutes, eliminating the extended drying time. After the cast has set, the material will not soften when wet but must be dried to prevent skin lesions. The fabric has a more open weave than plaster, which helps maintain skin integrity.

Assisting With Plaster or Fiberglass Cast Application. After positioning the patient comfortably before the procedure begins, drape the patient to expose only the part to be casted, avoiding unnecessary exposure and protecting other skin areas from the casting material. The part to be casted should be clean and dry; apply a bandage or dressing to any lesions before casting. Assemble the following items:

- Tubular soft fabric stocking material large enough to encircle the limb

PATIENT EDUCATION

Helping Elderly Patients Avoid Hip Fractures

Older patients are particularly likely to fall and fracture bones. One of the most common broken bones is the head of the femur. These fractures take a long time to heal and often result in the patient being admitted to a skilled nursing facility for rehabilitation. It is important to teach older patients fall prevention techniques. Here are some important tips:

- Always wear shoes with good, solid tie strings.
- Be sure that lighting is adequate, both inside the home and outside.
- Remove scatter rugs inside the home.
- Place grab bars throughout the home.

Advise the patient that one-floor living is best, and teach the patient ways to reorganize the home to avoid climbing stairs.

- Roller padding, also called sheet wadding
- Casting material
- Bucket of cool or tepid water
- Plaster or cast knife (FIG. 30-3)
- Utility gloves

WHAT IF

Your patient has a cervical fracture?

Fractures to the cervical spine can be life threatening or seriously disabling. There are seven cervical vertebrae. Fractures to the first cervical vertebra (C-1), the most superior vertebra, tend to be fatal unless immediately and aggressively treated by emergency services personnel before transport to a trauma center. Fractures to the second and third cervical vertebrae (C-2 and C-3) often result in permanent or long-term respiratory dependency. Vertebrae fractures of the fourth to seventh cervical vertebrae (C-4 to C-7) will result in various levels of paralysis and motor impairment. If you suspect a patient has a cervical fracture or other vertebral fracture, keep the patient still and call for emergency personnel. Never move the patient unless the patient is in immediate danger. The ambulance technicians will properly immobilize the patient for transport to the hospital, where radiographic tests will diagnose the extent of the injury.

Box 30-2

TYPES OF CASTS

- *Short arm cast* extends from below the elbow to mid palm.
- *Long arm cast* extends from the axilla to mid palm. The elbow is usually at a 90°angle.
- *Short leg cast* extends from below the knee to the toes; the foot is in a natural position.
- *Long leg cast* extends from the upper thigh to the toes; the knee is slightly flexed and the foot is in a natural position.
- *Walking cast* may be either short leg or long leg; the cast is extra strong to bear weight and may include a walking heel.
- *Body cast* encircles the trunk, usually from the axilla to the hip.
- *Spica cast* encircles part of the trunk and one or two extremities.

The limb is covered first with the soft knitted tubular material with extra fabric above and below the projected casting length to allow for a padded fold at each end. The soft roller padding is applied in fairly thick layers over bony prominences (FIG. 30-4). The physician wraps the limb from distal to proximal with the soaked casting material. You may be responsible for soaking the material until bubbles no longer form around the rolls. The rolls should be pressed, not wrung, until they are wet through but not dripping. Wear utility gloves to protect your hands from the material. When

FIGURE 30-3.   Plaster or cast knife. (Courtesy of Sklar Instruments, West Chester, PA).

FIGURE 30–4. Applying a roller bandage.

the site is adequately covered, rough edges are trimmed with the plaster knife and the knitted fabric is folded back to form cuffs at each end. The skin outside the cast is cleansed of casting material to avoid discomfort and skin breakdown.

Because the unsupported weight of an arm cast may put undue stress and strain on the shoulder muscles, a sling is ordered to relieve and redistribute the weight. Slings are also used when casting is not necessary but the arm must be immobilized to facilitate healing. Procedure 30-1 describes the steps for applying a sling.

Plaster or Fiberglass Cast Removal Cuts are made in the cast through its length on opposite sides, dividing it into halves. An electric oscillating circular saw known as a cast cutter is used (FIG. 30-5). Assure the patient that this will not cut the skin. Wear safety goggles to protect your eyes from flying particles and caution the patient also. The cast will be split apart with a cast spreader and the padding will be cut with utility scissors. The patient should be warned that the skin will be pale and dry and the muscle will be weak and shrunken from disuse. Also explain that the skin may be sensitive to touch and temperature. Creams and lotions help alleviate the dryness, and physical therapy and exercise will restore the muscle tone.

Healing of Fractures

The most important criterion for successful healing of a fracture is an adequate blood supply. The blood secretes an important gluelike substance known as **callus**, which is deposited around the break. Callus holds the ends of the bones together; with time, the callus turns to bone. The bone cells mold the callus and smooth the fracture site to close to its original size. Immobilization of the fracture site allows successful molding and reshaping.

If the blood supply is inadequate to the healing bone or tissue, union may be delayed or absent. If damage is sufficient or if severe trauma, disease, tumor, or complications are involved, amputation may be necessary. Amputation is a drastic measure that is performed only when all other avenues are exhausted. A **prosthesis** enables the amputee to resume functional activities such as walking, grasping, and holding. The elderly heal slowly. Prosthetic joint replacement may be necessary if bone restructuring is inadequate (Box 30-3).

A potentially life-threatening complication of a fracture is a fat **embolus**. This type of embolus results from the release of fat droplets from the yellow marrow of the long bones. If the embolus lodges in the coronary or pulmonary vessels or in a large vessel in the brain, it can block the vessel, causing an infarction and death.

 Checkpoint Question

2. What is the difference between an open and closed reduction?

LEGAL TIP

A cast that is applied improperly can lead to nerve and vascular damage, resulting in permanent loss of function to the extremity. (In extreme situations, a surgical amputation may be required.) To ensure proper care and to avoid lawsuits, it is essential that distal extremity circulation be assessed and documented before and after reductions and casting.

FIGURE 30–5. A cast cutter and saw. (Courtesy of M-PACT Worldwide, Eudora, KS)

Box 30-3

BONE HEALING IN THE ELDERLY

A fractured femur in the elderly raises special concerns. Bone-repairing osteoblasts are less able to use calcium to restructure bone tissue at any site in the elderly, but the neck of the femur, the most common fracture site, is especially vulnerable to delayed or imperfect healing because the blood supply is poor. Fractures through this area, involving the femoral head or neck or just inferior to the greater trochanter, may require hip arthroplasty or total hip replacement.

Most hip joint replacement prostheses are metal or polyethylene molded to conform to the joints they are designed to replace. Total hip replacement, usually used for degenerative joint disease or rheumatoid arthritis, replaces the head and neck of the femur and the acetabular surface. Knee replacement replaces both the head of the tibia and the distal epiphysis of the femur.

Early repair and return to mobility prevent contractures and atrophy of the supporting muscles. Postoperative walking prevents many of the complications associated with prolonged confinement in the elderly, such as pathological fractures, static pneumonia, and renal calculi.

Acetabular (pelvic) component

Femoral (distal) component

Femoral (proximal) component

Tibial component

Hip and knee replacement.

Bursitis

Bursae, small padlike sacs filled with a clear synovial fluid, surround some joints in areas of excessive friction, such as under tendons and over bony prominences. Their primary purposes are to reduce friction between moving parts and to prevent damage. The subdeltoid bursa in the shoulder between the deltoid muscle and the joint capsule is the most common site of bursitis, an inflammation of the bursa. Other frequent sites include the olecranon process at the elbow, the trochanter at the hip, the prepatellar bursae at the knee, and the heel.

The most common symptom of bursitis is pain during range-of-motion movement (Fig. 30-2). In subdeltoid bursitis, pain occurs in the midrange of abduction but not at the beginning or end of the range. Pain occurs in the shoulder and arm when the inflamed bursa is pinched between the head of the humerus and the clavicle during abduction.

Treatment for bursitis usually consists of antiinflammatory medications, rest, heat or cold applications, ultrasound to promote healing, and activities within the pain-free range. Physical therapy for range-of-motion exercises may also be ordered by the physician.

Arthritis

Osteoarthritis, or degenerative joint disease, is caused by wear and tear on the weight-bearing joints. As the articular cartilage degenerates, the ends of the bones enlarge, causing an intrusion of bone into the joint cavity. The patient has pain and restricted movement in the affected joint. Treatment of osteoarthritis includes administration of antiinflammatory medications and intra-articular corticosteroid injections to control the pain and inflammation. Patients may also require the use of an ambulatory aid such as a cane, walker, or crutches to decrease joint stress.

Rheumatoid arthritis is a systemic autoimmune disease that attacks the synovial membrane lining of the joint. Ultimately it leads to inflammation, pain, stiffness, and crippling deformities. It usually begins in non–weight-bearing joints such as the fingers but eventually may affect many joints, including the hands, wrists, elbows, feet, ankles, knees, and neck.

Marie-Strumpell disease, or **ankylosing spondylitis**, is rheumatoid arthritis of the spine. It is characterized by extreme forward flexion of the spine and tightness in the hip flexors. Rheumatoid arthritis in children is known as Still's disease.

The treatment for rheumatoid arthritis is similar to the treatment for osteoarthritis: anti-inflammatory medications orally and corticosteroid or gold injections into the affected joint, heat and cold applications, and protection of painful joints with splints or braces. In severe cases, the joint may be surgically replaced with an artificial one.

Checkpoint Question

3. How does osteoarthritis differ from rheumatoid arthritis?

Tendonitis

Muscles are attached to bones by tendons, which aid the body's mobility and stability. Tendonitis is inflammation of these structures. This disorder usually occurs after strains, sprains, overuse, or overstretching of the tissue. Although pain does not occur with passive movement, active movement is painful, and resistance to movement is intensely painful because the tissue must contract during active and resisted movement. Local tenderness is usual. The most common site of tendonitis is at the supraspinatus tendon in the shoulder, one of the rotator cuff muscles. Palpation over the tendon will elicit exquisite pain. Sometimes tendonitis is caused by calcium deposits, and this type is calcific tendonitis.

The treatment for tendonitis consists of oral anti-inflammatory medications, rest, heat or cold applications, ultrasound, **iontophoresis** (electrical transfer of ions), massage, and transverse friction massage (deep massage across the fibers of the tendons). Usually the patient is referred to a licensed massage therapist is for the massage or transverse friction massage.

Fibromyalgia

Fibromyalgia causes multiple often nonspecific symptoms including widespread pain in specific body areas, muscular stiffness, fatigue, and difficulty sleeping. This disorder varies from person to person, and the symptoms can be intermittent, making diagnosis difficult. Although the exact cause of this disorder is not known, some evidence suggests abnormalities in the immune system, perhaps resulting from a viral infection. Although it does not lead to other serious diseases, fibromyalgia tends to be chronic and is diagnosed by ruling out all other diseases and disorders with similar symptoms.

Treatment for fibromyalgia is based on relieving the symptoms with nonsteroidal anti-inflammatory medications, exercise, rest, and personal counseling as indicated for clinical depression that often accompanies this disorder because it is chronic.

SPINE DISORDERS

The vertebral column (FIG. 30-6) is made up of 33 vertebrae and numerous joints. The cervical, thoracic, and lumbar vertebrae are separated from each other by 23 intervertebral discs; the vertebrae of the sacrum and coccyx are fused, with no discs separating the bones. These vertebrae and their discs absorb and transmit the shock of running, walking, and jumping and keep the spine flexible for a high degree of mobility. Many strong ligaments and structures support and protect the spine, including the anterior and posterior longitudinal ligaments and the four natural curves in the spine. However, back injuries are common and are a leading cause of work-related injury among health care professionals. Box 30-4 offers some suggestions for avoiding back strain, and patients can use these general guidelines as well.

Abnormal Spinal Curvatures

Exaggerated or abnormal curvatures of the spine affect the posture and the alignment of the shoulders and hips. An abnormally deep lumbar curve is **lordosis**, or swayback. Abnormal thoracic curvature, particularly the upper portion, is called **kyphosis**, or hunchback. A side-to-side or lateral curvature is called **scoliosis**; it is commonly screened for in school children, especially girls, and if severe enough, surgically corrected during adolescence (FIG. 30-7).

Treatment of abnormal spinal curvatures entails the use of bracing to straighten the curve to a normal position. Transcutaneous muscle stimulation devices cause the muscles on one side to contract and draw the spine into its proper position. When necessary, orthopedic surgery is performed to straighten the spinal column.

Herniated Intervertebral Disc

The lumbar spine is one of the most frequently injured parts of the body because it absorbs the body's full weight and the weight of anything that is carried. Because most of the movement in the lumbar spine occurs at the L-4 to L-5 and L-5 to S-1 segments, most herniated discs are seen at these levels, but injury can occur in any disc in the spine.

A disc herniates when its soft center, known as the nucleus, ruptures through its tough outer layer to protrude

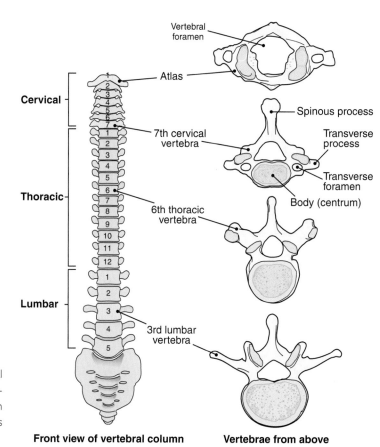

FIGURE 30-6. (*Left*) Front view of the vertebral column. (*Right*) Vertebrae from above. (Reprinted with permission from Cohen BJ, Wood DL. Memmler's The Human Body in Health and Disease. Philadelphia: Lippincott Williams & Wilkins, 2000.)

Front view of vertebral column   Vertebrae from above

AVOIDING BACK STRAIN

You can prevent back strain by using good body mechanics.

- When lifting a heavy object, keep the object close to your body. Never lift an object with extended arms.
- Never lift and twist at the same time. Lift the object, then reposition your feet by pivoting or taking two steps to turn.
- Bend your knees, not your back, when lifting.
- Ask for assistance from coworkers when you must lift or move obese patients or heavy objects.
- Maintain proper posture at all times; slouching causes muscle strain.

If you do sustain an injury at work, inform your supervisor immediately and document what happened. Complete an incident report in accordance with the facility's policy.

---

into the spinal canal, sometimes pressing on the spinal cord. It is usually caused by severe trauma, degenerative change, or strenuous strain. Common symptoms include severe back pain, numbness in one or both extremities, spasms, weakness, and limitation of movement. Flexion radiates pain into the extremities, and extension is restricted and causes pain at the spinal segment. Having the patient raise one leg from the supine position (known as the straight leg raise test) indicates whether the back pain is from a disc. A positive sign includes back pain with the leg at 45° to 60°. A flattened lumbar curve and a lateral shift of the spine are fairly common. Radiography may show a narrowed disc space.

Because bone strength throughout the body is diminished during confinement or inactivity, total bed rest is no longer a common treatment for most musculoskeletal disorders, including herniated discs, although pain limits activity. The treatment for herniated discs may include physical therapy for traction, massage, and mild extension exercises. While most disc herniations and bulges can be treated successfully without surgery, severe, unremitting pain, numbness, and progressive weakness of an extremity are indications for surgery to remove the injured disc.

Checkpoint Question

4. What are three abnormal curvatures of the spine? Briefly describe each.

DISORDERS OF THE UPPER EXTREMITIES

The structures of the upper extremity include the shoulder, elbow, wrist, and hand. Movement of the shoulder occurs

in a ball-and-socket joint, which is the most mobile joint in the body. The elbow, a hinge joint, is made up of the articulation of the humerus with the radius (lateral) and the ulna (medial) and allows movement in one direction only.

The complex structure of the wrist allows for a variety of movements, including flexion, extension, ulnar deviation, radial deviation, and circumduction. However, the most intricate and specialized movements of the musculoskeletal system occur in the hand. The thumb, the first digit, accounts for 50% of hand function. The muscles that control the precision movements and fine motor activities of the hand are known as intrinsic muscles because they have both of their attachments, origin (the end of the muscle that stays relatively stationary or fixed) and insertion (the more movable end of the muscle), in the hand.

Rotator Cuff Injury

The rotator cuff is formed by the tendons of four muscles that hold the joint surfaces together during joint motion. Injury to the rotator cuff muscles in the shoulder can cause severe pain, weakness, and loss of function. Surgical intervention for rotator cuff injury is often necessary because the tendons do not heal quickly on their own. An extended period of postoperative rehabilitation and physical therapy is usually needed to increase range of motion and strength and to regain the use of the shoulder. Professional athletes, particularly baseball pitchers, are prone to rotator cuff injuries.

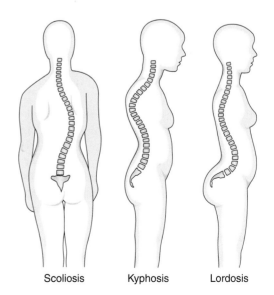

Scoliosis   Kyphosis   Lordosis

FIGURE 30-7. Abnormalities of the spinal curves. (Reprinted with permission from Cohen BJ, Wood DL. Memmler's The Human Body in Health and Disease. Philadelphia: Lippincott Williams & Wilkins, 2000.)

PATIENT EDUCATION

Posture and Back Pain

Poor posture can lead to back pain, and pain and injury can lead to poor posture. Also, as people age, natural changes in the body may affect posture. For example, the discs become less resilient and give in to forces such as gravity and body weight. Muscles lose flexibility, and the spine degenerates. In addition, a sedentary lifestyle causes weakness and shortening in some muscles and overstretching in others. The most common posture faults are the forward head posture and rounded shoulders.

In patients with poor posture, the bones are not aligned properly, and the muscles, joints, and ligaments become strained and stressed. Weak, tight, and inflexible muscles cannot support the back's natural curves. Years of poor posture can affect the position and function of the vital organs.

Maintaining good posture—or correcting poor posture—can help reduce a bulging disc or relieve the biomechanical stress caused by poor skeletal alignment, greatly aiding musculoskeletal system functioning.

Adhesive Capsulitis, or Frozen Shoulder

Frozen shoulder, a shortening of the muscles and joint structures known as a **contracture**, affects the entire shoulder joint and its capsule. It usually results from a fracture or disease process that prevents movement; however, anything that causes pain or restricts motion (e.g., tendonitis, bursitis, nerve damage, stroke, sprain, or strain) can lead to a frozen shoulder. Contractures develop when the joint is immobilized, allowing the collagen fibers to stick to each other and thereby limiting the movement in the joint. Adhesions and additional collagen are produced in response to injury, which results in a painful, tight, and constricted capsule. The shoulder movements most restricted are abduction and external rotation (Fig. 30-2). Because full active range of motion is not possible, weakness and atrophy ensue.

Treatment consists of administration of anti-inflammatory medications and heat or cold applications. The physician may also prescribe physical therapy to include ultrasound, mobilization or manipulation, and stretching exercises. Recovery is slow and typically painful. Contractures in the joints are often preventable with proper management and by moving the joint through a full range of motion each day.

Lateral Epicondylitis, or Tennis Elbow

Lateral epicondylitis, often called tennis elbow, is a common elbow injury, a sprain or strain of the tendons of origin of the wrist and finger extensor muscles. Symptoms include extreme pain with extension of the wrist, such as when trying to lift a cup or glass. Resistance to wrist extension and supination are the diagnostic tests for tennis elbow, because both movements greatly increase the pain.

Treatment consists of ice applications, **phonophoresis** (ultrasound with cortisone) or iontophoresis, avoiding movements that cause the pain, use of a forearm strap just distal to the elbow to take the pressure off the tendon, transverse friction massage, and gentle passive exercise to maintain mobility. In prolonged, extreme cases, surgery may be indicated.

Carpal Tunnel Syndrome

A repetitive motion injury, carpal tunnel syndrome occurs when the carpal bones and transverse carpal ligaments compress the median nerve at the wrist. Symptoms include numbness in the thumb and index and middle fingers and pain and weakness in the affected hand and wrist. Often pain awakens the patient at night. Patients who are diagnosed with carpal tunnel syndrome should be questioned regarding their work environment. This syndrome is common among typists, computer operators, assembly line workers, and those performing other jobs that demand frequent and repetitive grasping, twisting, and flexion to the wrist.

Diagnostic tests for carpal tunnel syndrome include Phalen's test, in which holding the wrist in flexion reproduces the symptoms; Tinel's test, in which the wrist is held in hyperextension and the transverse carpal ligament is thumped, causing tingling in the hand and fingers; and nerve conduction tests.

Treatment of carpal tunnel syndrome can be conservative, with anti-inflammatory medications and immobilization of the wrist with a brace or splint. If surgical intervention is necessary, it consists of release of the transverse carpal ligament.

Dupuytren Contracture

Dupuytren contracture results in flexion deformities of the fingers, most often the ring and little fingers. It is caused by contractures of the fascia in the palm of the hand due to the proliferation or overgrowth of fibrous tissue. As the fibrous tissue grows thicker, function is lost because the fingers cannot be straightened. Dupuytren contracture is easily diagnosed by inspection and palpation. Surgery is often required to release the contractures. Although no medications are available to treat this disorder, corticosteroid injections may temporarily improve function in the hand. Stretching of the tight structures in the early stages may slow the progression.

DISORDERS OF THE LOWER EXTREMITIES

The musculoskeletal structures of the lower extremities include the hip, knee, ankle, and feet. The hip, a ball-and-socket joint, is important for weight bearing and walking. The acetabulum, the socket of the hip joint, is deep enough to hold most of the femoral head and is surrounded by three strong ligaments.

The largest joint in the body, however, is the knee. Locking the knee into extension allows one to stand for long periods without using the muscles. An integral part of the knee is the patella, which lies inside the quadriceps tendon and protects the hinge joint. Two important sets of ligaments, the collateral and cruciate ligaments, stabilize the knee. The knee is often injured, because it is supported entirely by muscles and ligaments and because it is one of the most stressed joints, lying as it does between the two longest bones in the body.

Chondromalacia Patellae

Chondromalacia patellae is a degenerative disorder affecting the cartilage that covers the back of the patella, or kneecap. It usually occurs in young women and in athletes who perform activities that stress the knee, such as running, jumping, and bicycling. A common complaint is pain when walking down stairs or getting out of a chair. Rest, physical therapy, bracing or taping the knee, anti-inflammatory medications, ice therapy, and exercises to strengthen the quadriceps muscles can help to relieve the symptoms. If these treatments are not effective, an endoscope may be used to examine the joint and surrounding tissue for further problems (**arthroscopy**) (FIG. 30-8). In severe and chronic cases, a surgical procedure, **arthroplasty**, may be performed to repair or remove damaged cartilage.

Plantar Fasciitis

Plantar fasciitis is the most frequent cause of pain in the bottom of the foot. It is caused by inflammation of the plantar fascia ligament, which stretches across the bottom of the foot. Although the cause of plantar fasciitis is not always known, repetitive activities that stress the plantar fascia ligament, such as running and walking for extended periods on hard surfaces may cause it. Factors that may aggravate it include wearing improperly fitted shoes and being overweight. Diagnosis includes a history of pain in the foot and heel when getting out of bed or after sitting for long periods. Deep palpation over the plantar (sole) surface of the heel bone will elicit pain. Radiography of the foot may be ordered to identify stress fractures, bone cysts, or heel spurs; however, ligaments do not show up clearly on radiographs, which are not routinely ordered to diagnose plantar fasciitis.

Treatment of choice is a foot orthotic device (splint or heel pad) to support the arch and distribute the weight evenly. Physical therapy to stretch the ligament, ice therapy, massage, ultrasound, and nonsteroidal anti-inflammatory medications may also relieve the pain. Chronic planter fasciitis may necessitate wearing a night splint, which holds the affected foot at a 90°angle, preventing shortening and tightening of the plantar fascia during the night. Surgery is rarely done because of the high incidence of recurrence.

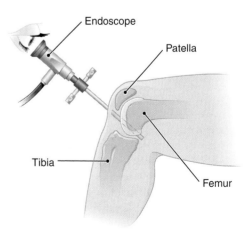

FIGURE 30–8. An arthroscopic examination of the knee. (Reprinted with permission from Cohen BJ. Medical Terminology: An Illustrated Guide. Philadelphia: Lippincott Williams & Wilkins, 2003.)

Gout

Gout, a metabolic disease of overproduction of uric acid, is a form of arthritis caused by the deposit of uric acid crystals into a joint, usually in the great toe. Although the cause of gout is unknown, the patient may have a history of injury to the joint, obesity, and a high-protein diet, especially a diet high in purines (alcoholic beverages, turkey, sardines, trout, bacon, and organ meats). The patient with gout complains of a painful, hot, inflamed joint; symptoms worsen unless treated. Periods of remission and exacerbation may occur. Gout may become chronic and can lead to multiple joint involvement with chronic pain, degeneration, and deformity. Symptoms are relieved by taking nonsteroidal anti-inflammatory medications and by avoidance of purine-rich foods and alcohol. Medication to prevent uric acid formation or foster its excretion from the body may also be prescribed.

Muscular Dystrophy

The congenital disorders collectively known as muscular dystrophy are characterized by varying degrees of progressive wasting of skeletal muscles. There is no neurological involvement, but the skeletal muscles waste and weaken. Some forms of the disease affect the heart and other organs. The most common type of muscular dystrophy, Duchenne, is apparent in males in early childhood and is usually fatal by young adulthood as respiratory and cardiac muscles fail. Several forms, such as facioscapulohumeral and limb girdle dystrophy, progress slowly from a childhood onset and result in varying degrees of disability. Duchenne, facioscapulohumeral, and limb girdle dystrophies are genetically transmitted.

Diagnosis of muscular dystrophy is based on family and patient history. The characteristic signs are frequently the most obvious diagnostic indicators of the disease. They include muscle weakness, clumsiness, frequent falling, and muscle spasms. **Electromyography** and muscle biopsy are used to rule out nervous system involvement. There is no known cure for any form of muscular dystrophy; however, exercise, physical therapy, and the use of splints or braces can relieve the symptoms. As mobility decreases, the use of a cane, walker, or wheelchair may be useful in maintaining independence.

Osteoporosis

Porous bones, or osteoporosis, is a condition in which the bones are deficient in calcium and phosphorus, making them brittle and vulnerable to fractures. The cause may be dietary, with general deficiencies in calcium, vitamin D, or phosphorus, or it may be primary progressive inability to metabolize calcium brought on by estrogen deficiency in elderly women or sedentary lifestyle, alcoholism, liver disorder, or rheumatoid arthritis.

There are few signs of osteoporosis other than a gradual loss of stature or height, progressive kyphosis (or dowager's

hump), and spontaneous, nontraumatic fractures. Diagnosis includes bone scan, densitometry (a test that measures the density of the bones), thyroid and parathyroid studies, and serum calcium and phosphorus determinations. Treatment is preventing fractures by increasing appropriate levels of exercise to strengthen the bones. Hormone therapy with estrogen or a combination of estrogen and progesterone may be prescribed for postmenopausal women to prevent loss of minerals from the bones that occurs with the natural decrease in these hormones during menopause. Calcium and vitamin D supplements are beneficial to arrest the progression but will not cure the underlying degenerative factors once osteoporosis has begun.

Bone Tumors

Bone tissue is rarely the primary site for malignancies but is frequently a site of metastasis. Primary osteosarcomas occur most often in young men, although they may occur at any age in either sex. Osteogenic sarcomas originate in the bony tissue, while nonosseous tumors seed to the bones from other sites. Ewing sarcoma, originating in the marrow and invading the shaft of the long bones, is common in young adults, especially adolescent boys.

TRIAGE

While working in a medical office setting, the following three situations are occurring:

A. You need to teach a 78-year-old patient to use a walker.

B. A 47-year-old woman just arrived in the office complaining of pain in her left wrist. She fell in the parking lot. You have been instructed to apply a cold pack to her wrist.

C. A 12-year-old patient needs a sling applied to her right arm.

How do you sort these patients? Whom do you see first? Second? Third?

Patient B should be attended first. A cold pack should be applied to the injured wrist as soon as possible to help control the swelling and decrease the pain. Patient C should be seen next. Applying a sling will take less time than teaching patient A to use the walker. Teaching an older patient may take extra time, skill demonstration, and return demonstration. In addition, a detailed patient education instruction pamphlet about the use of the walker should be given to the patient and explained

Spanish Terminology

Voy a ponerle una tabilla en la pierna.	I am going to put a splint on the leg.
Voy a examiner la pierna.	I am going to examine your leg.
Doble las rodillas, no la espalda.	Bend your knees, not your back.
Le duelen las articulaciónes?	Do you have pain in your joints?

There is no known cause of malignant skeletal tumors, but one hypothesis is that rapid development of bone tissue during growth spurts is a predisposing factor. Bone pain is the most common early sign. The pain is most intense at night, is usually dull and centered at the site, and is not relieved by resting the body part. Depending on the site, the mass may be palpable through the skin and muscles. Biopsy is the definitive diagnostic test after bone scans suggest the need. Surgical treatment includes excision of the tumor, including a large margin of surrounding bone structure and nearby lymph nodes, or amputation if the tumor is in an extremity. Chemotherapy and radiation are usually indicated also.

COMMON DIAGNOSTIC PROCEDURES

Physical Examination

The physician's evaluation of the musculoskeletal system usually includes an assessment of structure and function, movement, and pain. An important part of the evaluation is the history, which includes the patient's description of the events and circumstances that led to the decision to seek medical help.

The physician observes the patient's overall physical state by noting how the patient walks, sits, stands, and moves. Concentrating on the area of concern, the physician evaluates the problem by visual inspection, palpation, and diagnostic tests. Pain and limited or compromised functions are warning signals. Strength also affects function and is a part of any musculoskeletal evaluation. Other important considerations are skin color, temperature, tone, and tenderness; abnormal findings may indicate underlying disease.

Diagnostic Studies

The most frequently used tools for detecting disorders of the musculoskeletal system are radiology and diagnostic imaging, which are used to diagnose fractures, dislocations, and degeneration or diseases of the bones and joints. Other radiographic studies include **arthrograms**, x-ray studies of the joints that may show joint disease, and myelograms, which help detect intervertebral disc conditions. A bone scan analyzes bone growth, density, tumors, and other pathology.

Computed tomography (CT) and magnetic resonance imaging (MRI) may reveal soft tissue disease, such as tumor, metastatic lesions, and ruptured or bulging discs. Electromyography and nerve conduction velocity tests measure the health and fitness of the nerves as they relate to conduction of nerve impulses and muscle function.

Goniometry is measurement of the amount of movement available in a joint by a protractorlike device called a **goniometer** (FIG. 30-9). A bone or muscle biopsy is also a valuable diagnostic tool. It allows intense examination of the tissue under a microscope to determine cell damage, neoplasms (tumor or growth), or other types of diseases.

 Checkpoint Question

5. What 10 procedures can be used to diagnose musculoskeletal disorders?

FIGURE 30–9. A goniometer. (Reprinted with permission from Weber J, Kelley J. Health Assessment in Nursing. Philadelphia: Lippincott Williams & Wilkins, 2003.)

Table 30-2	Heat and Cold Treatments: Types and Purposes	
Dry Heat	**Moist Heat**	**Purposes**
Hot water bottle	Compresses	Relieve muscle spasms or tension; relieve pain; hasten healing by increasing blood flow to an area; provide local or systemic warming
Heating pad	Warm soaks	
Thermal pad		
Disposable heat pack		
Heat lamp		
Dry Cold	**Moist Cold**	**Purposes**
Ice bag	Compresses	Limit initial edema by decreasing capillary permeability (caution: cold retards edema by decreasing blood flow to the area); decrease bleeding or hemorrhage; decrease inflammation; relieve pain by numbing nerve pathways; provide local or systemic cooling
Ice collar	Cold soaks	
Disposable ice pack		

THE ROLE OF THE MEDICAL ASSISTANT

Warm and Cold Applications

Because of the time necessary for warm or cold applications, these procedures are not often done in the office. However, your responsibility may include instructing the patient in administering the treatments at home. Patients should understand the purpose of the procedure, how to perform it, the expected results, and any precautions or danger signs. TABLE 30-2 discusses the types of heat and cold applications and the purposes of each. Procedure 30-2 describes the steps for applying a cold pack, and Procedure 30-3 describes a hot pack application.

Precautions

When exposed to cool or warm temperatures, the body quickly adapts. For example, the water in a swimming pool feels cool at first, but after a short while, the body becomes used to the temperature and it no longer feels cool. The body has adapted. Using this reasoning, patients should be instructed that the benefits of heat or cold therapy are continuing even though they may not be able to feel the initial temperature change.

The body responds to extremes of temperature for extended periods by exerting an opposite effect called the rebound phenomenon. For example, heat applied to an area will cause dilation of the blood vessels, or vasodilation. However, if heat is applied beyond 30 minutes, vasoconstriction will occur as the body attempts to compensate for the heat. Therefore, applications left on longer than recommended by the physician will have an opposite effect to the one intended.

Some areas of the body, those with thin skin and few nerve receptors, such as the abdomen, are more sensitive to heat than areas such as the palms of the hands. When applying heat, remember that the very young, the elderly, the

confused or disoriented patient, and patients with circulatory disorders or diabetes are particularly subject to burns. Box 30-5 provides additional guidelines for the proper use of heat and cold.

Generally, the temperature should be kept within the following guidelines:

- Warm: tepid, 95–98°F, to very warm, 115°F
- Cold: neutral, 93/95°F, to very cold, 50°F

Box 30-5

PROPER USE OF HEAT AND COLD: WHEN NOT TO USE HEAT OR COLD AND WHY

Do not use heat:
- Within 24 hours after an injury, because it may increase bleeding
- For noninflammatory edema, because increased capillary permeability will allow additional tissue fluid to build up
- In cases of acute inflammation, because increased blood supply will increase the inflammatory process
- In the presence of malignancies, because cell metabolism will be enhanced
- Over the pregnant uterus
- On areas of erythema or vesicles, because it will compound the existing problem
- Over metallic implants, because it will cause discomfort

Do not use cold:
- On open wounds, because decreased blood supply will delay healing

In the presence of already impaired circulation, because it will further impair circulation

Box 30-6

SAFETY TIPS FOR USING WALKING AIDS

Remind the patient to:

- Check the rubber tips frequently and replace worn tips immediately. (Most ambulatory aids require rubber tips, although some walkers have rollers.)
- Check screws and bolts frequently; tighten as needed.
- Remove scatter rugs and small pieces of furniture that may cause falls.
- Use caution on wet surfaces to avoid falling.
- To avoid damage to the axillary nerve, do not place the axillary bars against the axilla.
- Avoid back and neck strain by standing straight and looking ahead.

Checkpoint Question

6. How does the body respond to prolonged exposure to temperature extremes?

Ambulatory Assist Devices

Patients may lose their ability to move normally because of an accident or injury, disease process, neurological or muscular defect, or degeneration. Patients who require assistance to maintain mobility may use crutches, a cane, a walker, or a wheelchair. Medical assistants often are responsible for teaching patients how to use these ambulatory aids safely (Box 30-6).

Crutches

Crutches may be either wooden or tubular aluminum. The most common form is the axillary crutch, which extends from just under the patient's axillae to the floor, with hand grips to distribute weight to the palms. Axillary crutches may be prescribed for short-term conditions when the patient cannot bear weight on one extremity. The Lofstrand or Canadian crutch is usually aluminum and reaches just to the forearms, with a metal cuff to maintain its position on the arms and a covered hand grip to distribute the weight (FIG. 30-10). Lofstrand crutches allow the patient to release and use the hands without losing the crutches. These work well for patients who will need crutches for a long period or who have poor coordination. Procedures 30-4 and 30-5 explain the steps necessary for measuring and fitting a patient with axillary crutches and teaching a patient the proper gait techniques.

PATIENT EDUCATION

Tips for Crutch Walking

To go up stairs:

- Stand close to the bottom step.
- With the body's weight supported on the hands, step up on the first step with the unaffected leg.
- Bring the affected side and the crutches up to the step at the same time.
- Resume balance before proceeding to the next step.
- *Remember:* The good side goes up first!

To descend stairs:

- Stand close to the edge of the top step.
- Bend from the hips and knees to adjust to the height of the lower step. Do not lean forward (leaning forward may cause a fall).
- Carefully lower the crutches and the affected leg to the next step before moving the other extremity.
- Next, lower the unaffected leg to the lower step and regain balance.
- *Remember:* The affected foot goes down first!

To sit:

- Back up to the chair until you feel its edge on the back of your legs.
- Move both crutches to the hand on the affected side and reach back for the chair with the hand on the unaffected side.
- Lower yourself slowly into the chair.

A   B

FIGURE 30-10. Types of crutches. (**A**) Axillary crutches. (**B**) Lofstrand, or Canadian, or forearm crutches.

FIGURE 30–11. Three types of canes. (**A**) Single-ended canes with half-circle handles are recommended for patients requiring minimal support. (**B**) Single-ended canes with straight handles are recommended for patients with hand weakness. (**C**) Three- or four-prong canes are recommended for patients with poor balance.

Canes

A cane is used when the patient needs extra support and stability but requires only a small measure of assistance with weight bearing. The standard cane may be used when the patient needs very slight assistance. The tripod (three legs) or quad cane (four legs) is useful when the patient needs greater stability (FIG. 30-11). Tripod and quad canes can stand alone when patients need to use their hands or have other support. They tend to be bulkier and heavier than standard canes, but because they offer greater stability and safety, they are good for patients who need more support than the standard cane affords.

To measure for proper cane length, have the patient stand erect. The cane should be level with the patient's greater trochanter, and the patient's elbow should be bent at a 30° angle. To walk with a cane, the patient should:

1. Position the cane on the unaffected side about 4 to 6 inches to the side and about 2 inches ahead of the foot.
2. Advance the cane and the affected leg together.

3. Bring the unaffected leg forward to a position just ahead of the cane.
4. Repeat the steps.

Walkers

A walker is a comfortable aid for the elderly and others with conditions that cause weakness or poor coordination. A walker is a lightweight aluminum frame shaped like three sides of a rectangle; however, because walkers are somewhat bulky, maneuvering in close quarters can be difficult. The walker frame should be level with the patient's hip, and the patient's elbow should be bent at about a 30° angle (FIG. 30-12). To use a walker:

1. Stand erect and move the walker ahead about 6 inches.
2. Using an easy walking gait with hands on the walker grips, step into the walker.
3. Move the walker ahead again.
4. Repeat the steps.

 Checkpoint Question

7. On which side of the body is the cane positioned?

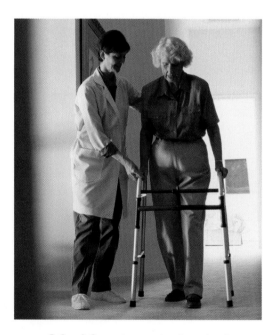

FIGURE 30–12. A properly adjusted walker.

Procedure 30-1

Applying a Triangular Arm Sling

Purpose: Correctly apply a triangular arm sling.

Equipment: A canvas triangular arm sling, 2 safety pins.

Standard: This procedure should take 10 minutes.

Steps	Reason
1. Wash your hands.	Handwashing aids infection control.
2. Assemble the equipment and supplies. Greet and identify the patient and explain the procedure.	Identifying the patient prevents errors in treatment. Explaining the procedure helps ease anxiety and ensure compliance.
3. Position the affected limb with the hand at slightly less than a 90°angle so that the fingers are a bit higher than the elbow.	This position helps reduce swelling of the hand and fingers.
4. Place the triangle with the uppermost corner at the shoulder on the unaffected side (extend the corner across the nape of the neck), the middle corner at the elbow of the affected side, and the third corner pointing at the foot of the unaffected side.	
5. Bring up the third corner to meet the upper corner at the side of the neck, *never* at the back of the neck.	A knot at the back of the neck will be uncomfortable for the patient.
6. Tie or pin the sling at the knot. Secure the elbow by fitting any extra fabric neatly around the limb and pinning.	
7. Check the patient's comfort and distal extremity circulation.	
8. Document the appliance in the patient's chart.	Procedures are considered not to have been done if they are not recorded.

(continues)

Procedure 30-1   *(continued)*

Applying a Triangular Arm Sling

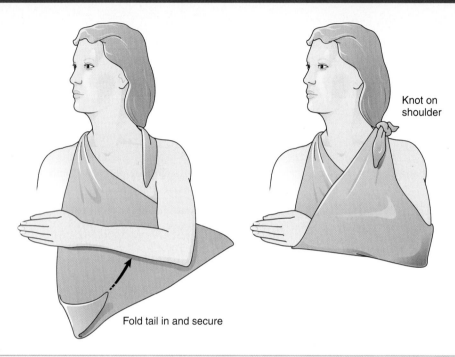

Knot on shoulder

Fold tail in and secure

Note: Fitted canvas slings with buckles or Velcro are also available.

Charting Example

10/28/2004 11:15 A.M. Triangular arm sling applied to (R) arm as orderd. Fingers to (R) hand warm and pink, no swelling. To return to office in 4 days. _____ T. Burton, RMA

Handwritten notes (on overlaid paper):
Ex. 8-6
216 - 217
Nov. 20
ERTSS
for RedCross
Electronic requirement
for Medicare. ? Check to

Procedu

Appl

Purpose:	
Equipment:	...the physician's order.
	...sable cold pack, small towel or cover for ice pack, gauze
Standard:	

Steps	**Reason**
1. Wash y	Handwashing aids infection control.
2. Assemb ice bag read th	Avoid wetting and chilling the patient. Small bits of ice help the bag to conform to the patient's contours better than large pieces.
3. Fill a r flat on contain	If the bag is too full of ice or air, it will not conform easily to the patient's contours.
4. If usin	
5. Cover	The cover will absorb condensation and make the procedure more comfortable for the patient.
6. Greet and identify the patient. Explain the procedure.	Identifying the patient prevents errors in treatment. Explaining the procedure helps ease anxiety and ensures compliance.
7. After assessing the skin for color and warmth, place the covered ice pack on the area.	The area must be assessed for the documentation before treatment begins. The cold pack should not come into direct contact with the skin.
8. Secure the ice pack with gauze or tape.	It should lie securely against the patient's skin for the greatest benefit. Pins may puncture the ice bag.
9. Apply the treatment for the prescribed amount of time, no longer than 30 minutes.	Longer than the prescribed time or 30 minutes may cause an adverse rebound effect, causing increased blood flow and swelling.
10. During the treatment, assess the skin under the pack frequently for mottling, pallor, or redness. Remove the ice pack at once if these appear.	These signs indicate an adverse reaction and should be reported to the physician immediately after removing the ice pack.
11. Properly care for or dispose of equipment and supplies. Wash your hands.	If the equipment is reusable, it should be prepared for the next patient by disinfecting according to office policy. If it is disposable, discard it appropriately.
12. Document the procedure, site of the application, results including the condition of the skin after the treatment, and the patient's response.	Procedures are considered not to have been done if they are not recorded.

Charting Example

11/22/2004 10:45 A.M. Ice bag applied to (L) anterior thigh as ordered ×20 minutes. Skin before treatment swollen, with large contusion noted, no break in skin. After treatment, area pale and cool to touch, swelling decreased. Verbal and written instructions given for application qid at home; pt. verbalized understanding. _____ B.Barry, CMA

Procedure 30-3

Use a Hot Water Bottle or Commercial Hot Pack

Purpose: Apply a hot pack appropriately according to the physician's order.

Equipment: A hot water bottle or commercial hot pack, towel or other suitable covering for the hot pack.

Standard: This procedure should take 30 minutes.

Steps	Reason
1. Wash your hands.	Handwashing aids infection control.
2. Assemble equipment and supplies, checking the hot water bottle for leaks.	Checking for leaks avoids wetting the patient.
3. Fill the hot water bottle about two-thirds full with warm (110°F) water; place the bottle on a flat surface with the opening up and press out the excess air.	Excess air will prevent the bottle from conforming to the patient's contours.

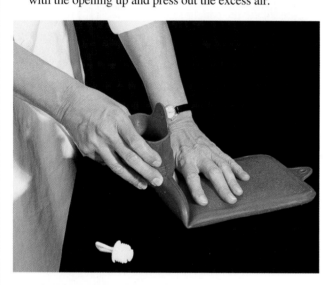

Step 3. Express air from the bottle before capping.

Steps	Reason
4. If using a commercial hot pack, follow the manufacturer's directions for activating it.	
5. Wrap and secure the pack or bottle before placing it on the patient's skin.	Covering the bag will increase the patient's comfort and prevent burning the skin.

(continues)

Procedure 30-3   *(continued)*

Use a Hot Water Bottle or Commercial Hot Pack

Steps	Reason
Step 5. Wrap and secure the bag before placing on the patient's skin.	
6. Greet and identify the patient. Explain the procedure.	Identifying the patient prevents errors in treatment.
7. After assessing the color of the skin where the treatment is to be applied, place the covered hot pack on the area.	The area must be assessed for documentation before the treatment begins. The hot pack should not touch the skin. Heat therapy should be used cautiously in patients with circulatory disorders, diabetics, and the elderly.
8. Secure the hot pack with gauze or tape.	It should be securely against the patient's skin for the greatest benefit. Pins may puncture the hot pack.
9. Apply the treatment for the prescribed amount of time, but no longer than 30 minutes.	Longer than the prescribed time or 30 minutes may cause an adverse rebound effect and decreased blood flow to the area.
10. During the treatment, assess the skin every 10 minutes for pallor (rebound), excessive redness (pack too hot), swelling (tissue damage). If you see any of these signs, immediately remove the hot pack.	These signs indicate an adverse reaction and should be reported to the physician immediately after you remove the hot pack.
11. Properly care for or dispose of equipment and supplies. Wash your hands.	Reusable equipment should be disinfected for the next patient. Disposables should be discarded appropriately.
12. Document the procedure, site of the application, results including condition of the skin after treatment, and the patient's response.	Procedures are considered not to have been done if they are not recorded.

Charting Example
7/11/2004 3:00 P.M. Hot pack to left shoulder posterior upper back ×30 minutes as ordered. Skin pink before treatment, slightly reddened after treatment. Pt. stated pain in upper back and shoulder relieved. Oral and written instructions given for applications at home qid, verbalized understanding. _____ S. Rose, CMA

Measure a Patient for Axillary Crutches

Purpose: Accurately measure a patient for axillary crutches.

Equipment: Axillary crutches with tips, pads for the axillae, and hand rests as needed; tools to tighten bolts.

Standard: This procedure should take 10 minutes.

Steps	Reason
1. Wash your hands.	Handwashing aids infection control.
2. Assemble the equipment, including crutches of the correct size.	Axillary crutches must always be fitted to the height of the patient.
3. Greet and identify the patient.	This helps avoid errors in treatment.
4. Ensure that the patient is wearing low-heeled shoes with safety soles.	Low-heeled shoes with good soles assist with adjusting the crutches to the patient's height and help prevent falls. While using the crutches, patients should wear shoes with the same heel height to avoid an improper crutch fit.
5. Have the patient stand erect. Support the patient as needed.	
6. While standing erect, have the patient hold the crutches naturally with the tips about 2 inches in front of and 4–6 inches to the sides of the feet. This is called the tripod position, and all crutch gaits start from this position.	
7. Using the tools as needed, adjust the central support in the base so that the axillary bar is about 2 finger-breadths below the patient's axillae. Tighten the bolts for safety at the proper height.	If the axillary bar presses on the axillae, nerve damage may occur. If it is too low, the crutches will be difficult to manage and will cause poor posture and back strain.

A

Step 7A. Adjust the crutches to the patient's height by removing the wing nut and bolt and moving the extension.

(continues)

Measure a Patient for Axillary Crutches

Steps	Reason

B

Step 7B. Tighten the bolt securely.

8. Adjust the hand grips by raising or lowering the bar so that the patient's elbow is at a 30-degree angle when the bar is gripped. Tighten bolts for safety.

Hand grips that are too high or too low will compromise safety and may cause nerve pressure.

A

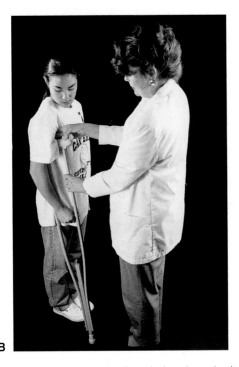

B

Step 8A. Adjust the hand grips by raising or lowering along the shaft of the crutch.

Step 8B. Crutches are properly adjusted when the patient's elbow is at a 30-degree angle and two fingers can be inserted under the axillae on top of the crutch axillary bar.

(continues)

Procedure 30-4   *(continued)*

Measure a Patient for Axillary Crutches

Steps	Reason
9. If needed, pad axillary bars and hand grips with soft material, such as large gauze pads or small towels and secure with tape to prevent friction.	If padding is used on the axillary bars, make sure the padding is not touching the axilla; this is to avoid pressure and damage to the axillary nerve.
10. Wash your hands and record the procedure.	Procedures are considered not to have been done if they are not recorded.

Charting Example

3/17/2005 4:40 P.M. Pt. measured for axillary crutches as ordered; no pressure to axilla; elbows at 30°angle. Given oral and written instructions on using crutches safely and the three-point and swing-through gaits. Demonstrated both procedures without difficulty. Verbalized understanding of instructions. Reinforced physician order for no weight bearing with (L) leg ×3 days, to return to office in 4 days. _____ B. Daye, RMA

Procedure 30-5

Instruct a Patient in Various Crutch Gaits

Purpose: Properly instruct a patient in various gaits using axillary crutches.

Equipment: Axillary crutches measured appropriately for a patient.

Standard: This procedure should take 10 minutes.

Steps	Reason
1. Wash your hands.	Handwashing aids infection control.
2. Have the patient stand up from a chair, holding both crutches on the affected side, then sliding to the edge of the chair. The patient pushes down on the chair arm on the unaffected side, then pushes to stand. With one crutch in each hand, he or she rests on the crutches until balance is restored.	
3. Assist the patient to the tripod position.	To ensure safety and proper balance, crutches should be in this position before proceeding with any gait.
4. Depending upon the patient's weight-bearing ability, coordination, and general state of health, instruct the patient in one or more of the following gaits: A. Three-point gait, most commonly used for crutch training. For use when only one leg can bear weight or only partial weight bearing is allowed on the affected leg. Used by amputees, those with injury to one leg, and leg or foot surgery patients. Requires coordination and upper body strength.	

(continues)

Procedure 30-5 (continued)

Instruct a Patient in Various Crutch Gaits

Crutch gaits.

(continues)

Procedure 30-5   *(continued)*

Instruct a Patient in Various Crutch Gaits

Steps	Reason
i. Move both crutches forward with the unaffected leg bearing weight.	
ii. Supporting weight on hand grips, bring unaffected leg past crutches.	
iii. Repeat.	
B. Two-point gait requires partial weight bearing, good coordination. Two points are raised and two points always on the floor.	
i. Move right crutch and left foot forward.	
ii. As these points rest, move right foot and left crutch forward.	
iii. Repeat.	
C. Four-point gait, slowest and safest of the gaits. At least three points are on the ground at all times. The affected leg must bear partial weight. For patients with degenerative diseases, spasticity, poor coordination.	
i. Move right crutch forward.	
ii. Move left foot just ahead of left crutch.	
iii. Move left crutch forward.	
iv. Move right foot just ahead of right crutch.	
v. Repeat.	
D. Swing-through gait	
i. Move both crutches forward.	
ii. With weight on hands, swing body ahead of crutches, both legs leaving the floor together.	
iii. Move crutches ahead.	
iv. Repeat.	
E. Swing-to gait	
i. Move both crutches forward.	
ii. With weight on hands, swing body even with crutches, both legs leaving the floor.	
iii. Move crutches ahead.	
iv. Repeat.	
5. Wash your hands and record the procedure.	Procedures are considered not to have been done if they are not recorded.

Charting Example
See example for Procedure 30-4.

CHAPTER SUMMARY

The musculoskeletal system provides support and protection for vital organs and allows movement and mobility. The skeleton is the frame on which muscles are attached, and the bones are held together at the joints, which provide stability and flexibility. Muscles enable the body to stand upright, to move, and to perform specific and detailed functions requiring strength and dexterity. The integrity of the entire musculoskeletal system allows for safe, pain-free, normal movement. This chapter discusses various disorders that may affect the musculoskeletal system, including the cause when known, the diagnosis, and treatments that may be prescribed. Although the orthopedic physician specializes in the diagnosis and treatment of these conditions, you should expect to see patients with disorders of the musculoskeletal system in various medical offices, including pediatrics and family practice.

Critical Thinking Challenges

1. Create a patient education brochure for the use of ambulatory aids. Be sure to include a brief description of the purpose of each aid along with the procedure steps.
2. The youth baseball league playoffs are coming to your town, and you are asked to staff the first aid station. What kinds of orthopedic injuries do you expect to see, and why? Develop a list of the first aid supplies that you want to have available and explain the reasons for your selections.

Answers to Checkpoint Questions

1. Luxation is a complete dislocation; subluxation is a partial dislocation.
2. An open reduction includes surgery; a closed reduction does not.

3. Osteoarthritis is a degenerative joint disease caused by wear and tear on the weight-bearing joints in which the articular cartilage degenerates and the ends of the bones enlarge. Rheumatoid arthritis is a systemic autoimmune disease that attacks the synovium of the joint, ultimately leading to inflammation, pain, stiffness, and crippling deformities. It usually begins in the non–weight-bearing joints but eventually affects most of the joints of the appendicular skeleton.
4. Abnormal spinal curvatures include scoliosis (lateral curve), kyphosis (hunchback), and lordosis (swayback).
5. The 10 procedures that can be used to diagnose musculoskeletal disorders are physical examination, computed tomography, magnetic resonance imaging, electromyography, nerve conduction velocity, goniometry, arthrography, myelography, bone scan, and radiography.
6. After long exposure to temperature extremes, the body exerts the opposite effect. For example, heat applications lasting longer than 30 minutes will cause vasoconstriction rather than the intended vasodilation. This is called the rebound phenomenon, or rebound effect.
7. The cane is positioned on the unaffected side of the body.

 Websites

Virtual Hospital: A digital library of health information
http://www.vh.org
MedicineNet http://www.medicinenet.com
Medlineplus Health Information http://www.medlineplus.gov
Arthritis Foundation http://www.arthritis.org
Muscular Dystrophy Association http://www.mdausa.org
What you need to know about orthopedics http://www.orthopedics.about.com

31

Ophthalmology and Otolaryngology

CHAPTER OUTLINE

ROLE DELINEATION

ADMINISTRATIVE: ADMINISTRATIVE
  PROCEDURES
- Perform basic administrative medical assisting functions
- Understand and adhere to managed care policies and procedures

CLINICAL: FUNDAMENTAL PRINCIPLES
- Apply principles of aseptic technique and infection control
- Comply with quality assurance practices
- Screen and follow up patients' test results

CLINICAL: DIAGNOSTIC ORDERS
- Collect and process specimens
- Perform diagnostic tests

CLINICAL: PATIENT CARE
- Adhere to established patient screening procedures
- Prepare and maintain examination and treatment areas
- Prepare patients for examinations, procedures, and treatments
- Assist with examinations, procedures, and treatments
- Prepare and administer medications and immunizations
- Coordinate patient's health care information with other health care providers

GENERAL: PROFESSIONALISM
- Display a professional manner and image
- Demonstrate initiative and responsibility
- Work as a member of the health care team
- Set priorities and perform multiple tasks
- Adapt to change
- Treat all patients with compassion and empathy

GENERAL: COMMUNICATION SKILLS
- Recognize and respect cultural diversity
- Adapt communications to individual's ability to understand
- Recognize and respond effectively to verbal, nonverbal, and written communications
- Use medical terminology appropriately
- Serve as a liaison

GENERAL: LEGAL CONCEPTS
- Perform within legal and ethical boundaries
- Prepare and maintain medical records
- Document accurately
- Comply with established risk management and safety procedures

GENERAL: INSTRUCTION
- Instruct individuals according to their needs
- Teach methods of health promotion and disease prevention

GENERAL: OPERATIONAL FUNCTIONS
- Perform routine maintenance of administrative and clinical equipment

CHAPTER COMPETENCIES

LEARNING OBJECTIVES
Upon successfully completing this chapter, you will be able to:
1. Spell and define the key terms.
2. List and define disorders associated with the eye, ear, nose, and throat.
3. Identify diagnostic procedures commonly performed on the eye, ear, nose, and throat.
4. Describe patient education procedures associated with the eye, ear, nose, and throat.

PERFORMANCE OBJECTIVES
Upon successfully completing this chapter, you will be able to:
1. Measure distance visual acuity with a Snellen chart (Procedure 31-1)
2. Measure color perception with an Ishihara color plate book (Procedure 31-2)
3. Instill eye medication (Procedure 31-3)
4. Irrigate the eye (Procedure 31-4)
5. Administer an audiometric hearing test (Procedure 31-5)
6. Irrigate the ear (Procedure 31-6)
7. Instill ear medication (Procedure 31-7)
8. Instill nasal medication (Procedure 31-8)
9. Take a sample for a throat culture (Procedure 31-9)

KEY TERMS

astigmatism	myopia	otolaryngologist	retinal degeneration
cerumen	myringotomy	otoscope	tinnitus
decibel (db)	ophthalmologist	presbycusis	tonometry
fluorescein angiography	ophthalmoscope	presbyopia	upper respiratory infection
hyperopia	optician	refraction	(URI)
intraocular pressure	optometrist		

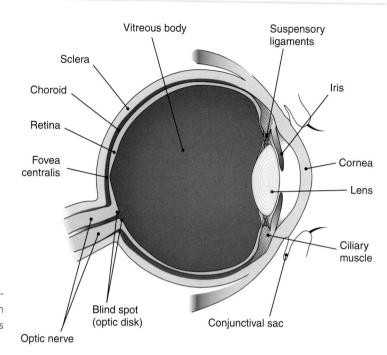

FIGURE 31–1. The eye. (Reprinted with permission from Cohen BJ, Wood DL. Memmler's The Human Body in Health and Disease. Philadelphia: Lippincott Williams & Wilkins, 2000.)

Medical assistants working for **ophthalmologists**, who specialize in disorders of the eyes, or **otolaryngologists**, who specialize in disorders of the ears, nose, and throat—also known as ENT physicians, are expected to perform basic procedures associated with these body systems. Medical assistants working in general family practice and pediatric offices also encounter patients with eye or ear disorders and are expected to perform basic procedures associated with the eyes, ears, nose, and throat in these settings as well. This chapter describes the various disorders, diagnostic tests, and treatment modalities that are included in the eye, ear, nose, or throat examination.

COMMON DISORDERS OF THE EYE

Light waves are reflected off of all objects and are transmitted through various structures of the eye including the cornea, lens, and retina (FIG. 31-1). These impulses are transmitted via the optic nerve to the occipital lobe of the cerebral cortex in the brain. When the rays of light are bent, or refracted, by the curvature of the cornea and lens, the occiput recognizes whether the objects are in or out of focus. If the objects are out of focus to the occiput, impulses are sent to change the shape of the lens or the position of the extrinsic muscles to sharpen the image.

While the eye is a complex, highly developed organ, any of its many components may malfunction or become infected or diseased. The most common eye disorders that you may encounter in a medical office are described in the following sections. In addition, Box 31-1 describes guidelines for assisting sight-impaired patients in a medical office.

Cataract

A cataract is an opacity, or clouding, of the lens that leads to decreased visual acuity. Most commonly, cataracts are bilateral and seen in the elderly. A rare condition in infancy can result from maternal exposure to the rubella virus. This condition is known as congenital cataracts. Occasionally, trauma to the lens or chemical toxicity causes clouding of the lens.

Box 31-1

ASSISTING SIGHT-IMPAIRED PATIENTS

Follow these tips to assist a sight-impaired patient:
- Ask patients how you can help, and follow their requests and suggestions. Many sight-impaired patients know best what they need.
- When escorting the patient, offer your arm. Tell the patient the approximate length of the hallway and advise the patient of any turns, such as, "It should be about 20 steps and then we'll take a right." Avoid stairs if possible, but if you must assist a sight-impaired patient up or down stairs, advise the person of the number of steps. Many patients prefer to hold the railings for balance.
- If the patient has a guide dog, do not approach the dog without first speaking to the patient and receiving approval.
- If the patient needs extensive teaching on a particular subject, suggest using a tape recorder to record the instructions.

The symptoms include gradual blurring and loss of vision over months as the clouding of the lens slowly progresses. The observer may see a milky opacity at the pupil rather than the normal black opening. An examination with an **ophthalmoscope** reveals the white area behind the pupil if the cataract has not advanced to the point where it can be seen unassisted.

The treatment for cataracts is surgical removal of the opaque lens. This surgery is beneficial in 95% of patients and is usually an outpatient procedure. After the cloudy lens has been removed, an intraocular lens is implanted or the patient's vision is corrected by contact lenses or special glasses.

Sty, or Hordeolum

A sty, or hordeolum, is an infection of any of the lacrimal glands of the eyelids, causing redness, swelling, and pain. The causative infectious organism is often *Staphylococcus aureus*, a microorganism commonly found on the skin. Warm compresses will hasten suppuration of the infection, and topical antibiotic drops or ointments attack the microorganism. You may be responsible for teaching the patient the procedure for applying warm compresses and instilling ophthalmic drops or ointment.

Conjunctivitis

Conjunctivitis, an infection of the mucous membrane covering the sclera and cornea (conjunctiva) of the eye, is caused by several species of bacteria or viruses. Additional causes of conjunctivitis include allergens or irritants without an infectious process. Many pathogens cause unilateral conjunctivitis, but allergic conjunctivitis is almost always bilateral.

Signs and symptoms of conjunctivitis include tearing and occasionally exudates and pain. Bacterial and viral conjunctivitis, or pink eye, is highly contagious and can rapidly spread through schools and day care centers. It is spread by contact when an infectious child rubs the eyes, handles objects such as toys or books, and spreads the infection to the next child who comes into contact with the contaminated object. The infected child should not go to school or day care until the infection is treated and has been resolved. Good hygiene, including handwashing, helps prevent the spread of infectious conjunctivitis. Antibiotic ophthalmic drops or ointment are prescribed by the physician if the cause of the conjunctivitis is bacterial. To prevent the spread of conjunctivitis, you should instruct the patient to do the following:

- Avoid rubbing the eyes to prevent spreading the infection to the other eye or to other people
- Discard all eye makeup that may be infectious
- Wash all towels, washcloths, and pillowcases after use

 Checkpoint Question

1. What is the difference between a sty and conjunctivitis?

Corneal Ulcer

A corneal ulcer is erosion of the surface of the cornea, leaving scar tissue that may lead to visual disturbances or blindness. Corneal ulcers are caused by several types of bacteria, fungi, viruses, and protozoa or by trauma, allergen, or toxin. Signs and symptoms include tearing, pain on blinking, and sensitivity to light. A visual examination with a penlight shows an irregular corneal surface. A fluorescein dye is administered by placing a strip gently in the sulcus of the eye; this stains the perimeter of the ulcer to confirm the diagnosis. Treatment includes rest and antibiotic therapy.

Retinopathy

Retinopathy is a general term for disease or disorder affecting the retina. A decrease in the blood supply to the highly vascular retina will cause **retinal degeneration**, pathological changes in cell structure that impair or destroy the retina's function. The causes include atherosclerosis that impedes blood flow to the retina, the microcirculatory changes associated with diabetes (diabetic retinopathy), and vascular changes resulting from long-term hypertension. Depending on the cause, the patient's loss of vision may be sudden or gradual. Loss of vision may be preceded by small intraocular hemorrhages, night blindness, or loss of the central visual field. If small vessels rupture and scar, they may pull against the retina and cause retinal detachment that results in blindness. Diagnosis is made by a thorough eye examination and **fluorescein angiography**. This procedure is injection of fluorescent dye into one of the veins of the arms and photographing the blood vessels of the eye as the dye moves through it. The treatment of retinopathy is based on treating the underlying cause. Although some forms of retinopathy respond well to treatment, others progress to full blindness.

Glaucoma

Glaucoma describes a group of disorders that result in increased intraocular pressure, or pressure within the eye. As aqueous humor is formed in the posterior chamber just in front of the lens it flows through the pupil to the anterior chamber just behind the cornea. It eventually filters into the canal of Schlemm. Any pathology that impedes the outflow of aqueous humor (genetics, vasoconstriction) will increase the pressure, either very gradually or quite suddenly. The gradual form of glaucoma (open-angle glaucoma) may present with mild or no pain, visualizing halos around lights, and loss of peripheral vision. Most adult glaucoma patients have this type of glaucoma. Angle-closure glaucoma, an acute and sudden blockage, is characterized by severe eye pain, blurred vision, headache, nausea, and vomiting. Blindness may result within days of the onset of acute glaucoma unless the condition is diagnosed and treated quickly.

Treatment for chronic glaucoma includes medication, often a diuretic, to decrease intraocular pressure by slowing

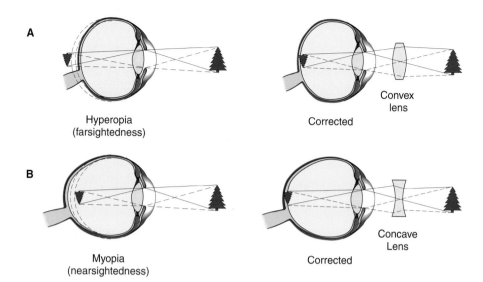

A
Hyperopia
(farsightedness)

Convex
lens
Corrected

B
Myopia
(nearsightedness)

Concave
Lens
Corrected

F I G U R E   3 1 – 2 .   (A) The hypertropic eye with convex corrective lens. (B) The myopic eye with concave corrective lens. (Reprinted with permission from Cohen B J, Wood D L. Memmler's The Human Body in Health and Disease. Philadelphia: Lippincott Williams & Wilkins, 2000.)

the formation of aqueous humor within the eyes or by improving the flow. Acute glaucoma may necessitate an iridectomy, or removal of part of the iris, to increase the outflow of the humor. Frequent eye examinations, including **tonometry**, may detect glaucoma and facilitate treatment before visual deficiencies and blindness result.

Refractive Errors

Errors of **refraction** are the most common of all eye problems. The primary types of refractive errors are **hyperopia**, **myopia**, **astigmatism**, and **presbyopia**. Hyperopia, also known as farsightedness, occurs in an eyeball that is too short from front to back to allow the lines of vision to reflect distinctly on the fovea centralis. The person with hyperopia cannot focus on objects near the face.

Myopia, also known as nearsightedness, results when the eyeball is too long. The lines of vision converge before they reach the fovea centralis and begin to diverge again at the fovea. Objects must be near the face for the image to be focused far back on the retina.

Astigmatism is unfocused refraction of light rays on the retina. It results from lens or corneal irregularities. If the cornea is not smooth, images refracted through it will not project sharply onto the retina; the effect is much like peering through wavy glass.

Presbyopia is vision change resulting from loss of lens elasticity with age. The lens normally adjusts to refract light from near or far. As a person ages, the ciliary bodies that hold and adjust the lens and the lens itself lose elasticity and no longer accommodate near vision; far vision may be unaffected. Symptoms usually begin gradually around age 40. Most adults are affected to some degree by age 50.

All refractive errors are treated with either corrective lenses or reshaping the lens with laser surgery (FIG. 31-2). An **optometrist** is a trained specialist who measures errors of refraction and prescribes lenses. An **optician** is a trained specialist who grinds lenses to fulfill corrective prescriptions written by either an optometrist or an ophthalmologist, a medical doctor who treats eye disorders or performs surgical corrections.

 Checkpoint Question

2. What are four common refractive errors? Briefly explain each.

Strabismus

Strabismus is a misalignment of eye movements, usually caused by muscle incoordination. Although most newborns are born with some degree of strabismus, coordination improves as the infant grows and the eye muscles strengthen. However, the strabismus does not resolve in some cases and requires medical intervention. Strabismus may take any of these forms:

- Esotropic, also known as cross eyes or convergent eyes
- Exotropic, also known as wall eyes or divergent eyes
- Hypotropic, deviation downward
- Hypertropic, deviation upward
- Concomitant, with both eyes moving together
- Nonconcomitant, with the two eyes moving independently

Treatment may require only patching, or covering, the unaffected eye to force the affected eye's muscles to strengthen.

In some cases, surgery is required to correct the deviant muscle or muscles.

Color Deficit

Color deficit is an absence of or a defect in color perception. Red, green, or blue perception may be impaired or absent. The term *color deficient* or *color deficit* is commonly used rather than referring to the disorder as color blindness.

This disorder is usually inherited on the X chromosome and affects more men than women. Occasionally color deficit results from damage to the cones by medications or other substances that are toxic to the color-receptive nerve cells. Color deficit has no cure or correction.

DIAGNOSTIC STUDIES OF THE EYE

In most medical offices the basic examination equipment includes the **ophthalmoscope**, a lighted instrument used to examine the inner surfaces of the eye (FIG. 31-3). In many instances, visually examining the interior structures of the eyes can alert the physician to a number of vascular and hypertensive conditions, since the blood vessels of the eye and the inner structures such as the retina are easily viewed.

Visual Acuity Testing

Visual acuity, or clearness, is commonly assessed in the medical office using the Snellen eye chart. These charts are hung 20 feet from the patient at eye level in an area with good lighting and few distractions (Procedure 31-1). Normal vision (20/20) means the patient can see at 20 feet what the normal eye sees at 20 feet. The figures on the charts—letters, numbers, a series of E's, or common symbols—are progressively smaller to test levels of perception (FIG. 31-4). For patients who cannot read or who do not speak English, the E chart may be used. A patient who can see only the line (letters or E's) on the chart at the 20/40 level has visual acuity at 20 feet equivalent to what a person with normal vision can see at 40 feet. The patient should wear any corrective lenses for the test unless the physician requests that the examination be done without them. Each eye is tested separately with the opposite eye covered but not closed.

The picture chart is used for children. If a child is to be tested, first spend a few moments familiarizing the child with the objects on the chart. For example, if the picture is of a dog and the child has never seen one, the illustration may not be recognized as a dog. If necessary, enlist a parent or coworker to help with the eye cover.

 Checkpoint Question

3. When is the E chart used to test visual acuity?

Color Deficit Testing

The Ishihara method is used to test for color deficits (Procedure 31-2). It consists of 14 color plates with many 4-colored dots forming a number, a letter, or a pattern of contrasting color in arrangement of dots (FIG. 31-5). Patients with deficient color perception are unable to see the design, numbers, or letters on plates 1 to 11, depending on the color deficiency. Although there is no cure or treatment for color deficits, knowledge of the deficit may help the patient with regard to coordinating clothing or choosing colors for decorating.

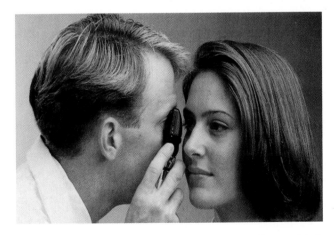

F I G U R E   3 1 – 3 . Examination of the eye with an ophthalmoscope. (Reprinted with permission from Willis MC. Medical Terminology: A Programmed Learning Approach to the Language of Health Care. Baltimore: Lippincott Williams & Wilkins, 2002.)

FIGURE 31–4. Snellen charts used to assess distant vision. The charts in the center and at far right are used for young children and illiterate adults.

Tonometry and Gonioscopy

Using a tonometer, the physician measures the intraocular pressure or tension in the eye. The anterior eye is anesthetized with eye drops, and the instrument is moved against the cornea to measure the pressure required to produce an indentation or to flatten a small area of the cornea. This test is an important part of the eye examination to diagnose glaucoma. Although it is not routinely performed at the general practice medical office, tonometry is painless and done regularly at the ophthalmologist's or optometrist's office.

Gonioscopy, also performed at the ophthalmologist's or optometrist's office, is use of a special instrument (gonioscope) to measure the angle of the anterior chamber between the iris and the cornea. This test is useful to the physician in determining the cause of the increased intraocular pressure.

FIGURE 31–5. Ishihara color plate. (Courtesy of B. Proud. Copyright.)

THERAPEUTIC PROCEDURES FOR THE EYE

Instilling Eye Medications

Medical assistants frequently have the responsibility of instilling ophthalmic medications and teaching patients about the procedure for home use. Instillations are used to treat infection or irritation, to dilate the pupil for retinal examination, and to apply anesthetic for treatment or testing (Proce-

TRIAGE

You have these three tasks:

A. A patient needs an eye examination as part of a physical examination for employment.

B. A patient came into the office complaining of "something in my left eye" after clearing some brush and weeds in a garden. After the physician examines the patient, you are instructed to irrigate the left eye to remove the debris.

C. A pharmacist telephones with a question about a patient's prescription for glaucoma medication.

How do you sort these tasks? What do you do first? Second? Third?

After asking the receptionist to take a message from the pharmacist, take care of patient B. Debris in the eye can scratch the cornea and result in further damage and discomfort for the patient and should be removed as soon as possible. Next, complete and record the eye examination for patient A's physical examination. Once these situations are resolved, call the pharmacist and answer any questions, clarify concerns, or refer the matter to the physician.

dure 31-3). Eye irrigations may also be ordered by the physician, usually to remove foreign bodies. Procedure 31-4 describes the steps for an eye irrigation.

COMMON DISORDERS OF THE EAR

The ear is divided into three sections: the external ear, the middle ear, and the inner ear (FIG. 31-6). When sound waves hit the tympanic membrane, the vibrations pass through structures in the middle and inner ear. The auditory, or eustachian, tube connects the middle ear with the nasopharynx, and during swallowing, pressure is equalized in the middle ear. This equalization through the eustachian tube prevents pressure from building up in the middle ear and rupturing the tympanic membrane.

Patients who have problems with the ear or hearing are often referred to an otolaryngologist. Medical assistants in general practices also encounter patients with various disorders of the ears, because pain and hearing loss are a frequent outcome of certain diseases and can occur at any age.

Ceruminosis

Ceruminosis, or impacted earwax, is a frequent reason for diminished hearing. **Cerumen** is usually soft and moist and leaks out in such small amounts that it is unnoticed. Occasionally, the cerumen becomes hard and dry or excessive

---

Box 31-2

ASSISTING HEARING-IMPAIRED PATIENTS

Follow these tips to assist a hearing-impaired patient:
- Speak normally; do not yell or raise your voice. Doing so will not facilitate the hearing capabilities of the patient.
- Get the patient's attention before speaking and make sure he or she can see your lips while you talk.
- Speak clearly, but remember that the patient is hearing impaired, not mentally challenged.
- If the patient is deaf and requires an interpreter, speak to the patient, not the interpreter.

---

hair in the ear holds the wax in the ear canal, causing it to build up against the tympanic membrane.

The presenting symptoms may be a gradual hearing loss or **tinnitus**, an extraneous noise heard in one or both ears. An examination of the ear canal with an **otoscope** shows the obvious reason. The wax may be softened by warm ear drops or hydrogen peroxide and removed by an ear curet or by gently washing with an irrigating device using water at room temperature.

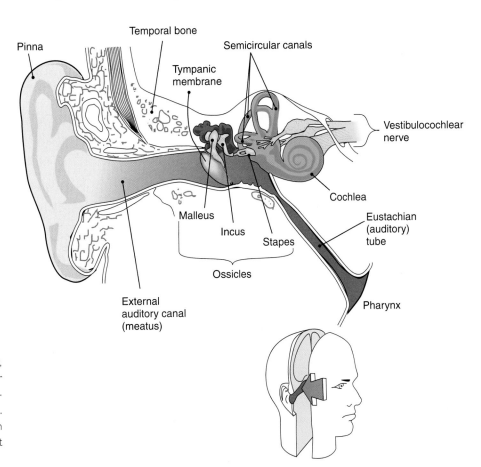

FIGURE 31–6. The ear, showing the outer, middle, and inner subdivisions. (Reprinted with permission from Cohen BJ, Wood DL. Memmler's The Human Body in Health and Disease. Philadelphia: Lippincott Williams & Wilkins, 2000.)

WHAT IF

Your patient asks you if a hearing aid could help her?

Hearing aids help many people, but they do not fully restore the ability to hear. The purpose of the aid is to amplify sound waves. Not all patients with hearing loss are good candidates for hearing aids. For example, patients who have permanent nerve damage generally do not have significant improvement with standard hearing aids.

The two basic types of aids are bone conduction receivers, which sit behind the ear and press against the skull, and air conduction receivers, which fit into the auditory canal. The size and type of hearing aid depends on the patient's specific condition and need. Binaural (both ears) aids are available and often can be fitted into eyeglasses for inconspicuous appearance.

Patients must understand that a hearing aid will improve their hearing, not correct it. Teach patients about maintenance requirements so they can keep the device in good working condition and explain how to adjust the volume control. Have the patient speak to the physician with any concerns about purchasing and using a hearing aid.

Conductive and Perceptual Hearing Loss

Conductive and perceptual hearing loss are the two categories of hearing impairment. In conductive loss, sound waves are not appropriately transmitted to the level of the cochlea. In perceptual, or sensorineural, loss, transmission from the oval window to the receptors in the brain is impaired. Many patients present with both, a condition called mixed deafness.

Causes of hearing loss include heredity, infection, trauma, ototoxic drug, some neurological diseases, exposure to loud noises, and **presbycusis**. Presbycusis usually results from a hardening of the joints between the ossicles (three small bones in the middle ear), which occurs with aging.

Diagnosis of hearing loss of any type is done by testing the hearing using an audiometer (FIG. 31-7) in the medical office. Treatment is aimed at addressing the underlying cause of the hearing loss if possible. A stapedectomy may be performed for otosclerosis, with a replacement for the impaired joint. Cochlear implants are gaining favor for those whose hearing loss is caused by impairment in the cochlear receptors. Conductive hearing loss can be treated successfully in most instances with hearing aids; perceptual loss is far more difficult to correct.

Checkpoint Question

4. What is the difference between conductive and perceptual hearing loss?

Ménière's Disease

Ménière's disease, a degenerative condition of unknown cause, affects the inner ear and upsets the body's ability to maintain equilibrium in addition to causing loss of hearing. The symptoms include vertigo, sensorineural hearing loss, and tinnitus. Severe symptoms may lead to nausea and vomiting. Periods of remission are followed by exacerbation. Although there is no cure, many of the symptoms can be treated with palliative medication. If the symptoms persist or increase and become incapacitating, it may be necessary to destroy the organs of the inner ear. The result of this drastic measure is immediate relief of symptoms, but the patient is irreversibly deaf.

Otitis Externa

Also known as swimmer's ear, otitis externa is an inflammation or infection of the external ear. It is common in summer and is caused by any number of pathogens that grow in the warm, moist ear canal. The presenting symptoms include pain on movement of any adjoining structures around the ear, jaw, and auricle. Otoscopy reveals a red, swollen ear canal. Debris (pus or excessive cerumen) must be gently washed from the area (see Procedure 31-6). Otitis externa is best treated by an antibiotic, either topical or systemic, warm compresses, and medication to relieve pain.

Applying an alcohol solution after swimming can help prevent this problem. Encourage patients who are prone to otitis externa to wear earplugs while swimming and to avoid using objects such as swabs or hairpins to clean inside the ear canal.

FIGURE 31–7. The audiometer.

PATIENT EDUCATION

Otological Disorders

Teach patients to recognize symptoms of otological disorders (hearing loss, pain, drainage) and to report them promptly to the physician. Proper attention at the early stage of an infection or injury can often prevent serious or irreversible damage.

Instruct patients that it is acceptable to clean the external ear with a cotton-tipped applicator but that they should not to put the applicator inside the ear canal. This drives cerumen deeper into the ear and creates more impaction than may already be present.

Tell children not to put small objects such as beans, peas, or small parts of toys in their ears, because they may become lodged and removal may require surgery. Caution parents to complete all antibiotic treatment for children's ear infections even though the symptoms subside. The infection may linger after the patient is asymptomatic. Ear recheck appointments should be kept as scheduled to ensure that the child is free of infection.

Otitis Media

Otitis media, an inflammation or infection of the middle ear, is frequently caused by an upper respiratory infection. Pathogens responsible for pharyngitis, nasopharyngitis, and the common cold frequently travel through the warm, moist eustachian tube to the middle ear. As the infection increases, the mucous membranes of the eustachian tubes swell, closing off the opening to the middle ear. With no way to drain, fluid builds up as a response to the infection and causes pain and pressure on the flexible tympanic membrane. If pressure is sufficient, the membrane may tear or perforate spontaneously to relieve the pressure. This disorder is common in infants and children because of the relatively horizontal position of the eustachian tube between the nasopharynx and middle ear.

Symptoms include severe pain, fever of varying degrees, and mild to moderate hearing loss. Infants may be fussy and tug at their ears. Any elevation in a child's temperature should be a warning to check for otitis media. Diagnosis is usually made by otoscopy, which may reveal a reddened, bulging tympanic membrane. Bubbles can sometimes be seen behind the thin membrane. Treatment is an antibiotic for bacterial infection and an analgesic for pain relief. A decongestant may reduce some of the swelling. In severe chronic cases, a **myringotomy** (surgical incision into the tympanic membrane) may be performed to relieve pressure. Tubes may be inserted through the tympanic membrane and

remain for several months to equalize the pressure if the problem persists.

Children have very short, almost horizontal eustachian tubes, which can be problematic if microorganisms from the nasopharynx are forced into the middle ear by coughing. The problem is compounded for children who are put to bed with a bottle of milk or formula. The milk acts as a hospitable medium for bacteria.

Otosclerosis

Otosclerosis is a disorder of the ossicles of the inner ear, especially the stapes bone. This disorder, thought to be hereditary, results from ossification or hardening of the bones causing loss of hearing of low tones. The treatment for otosclerosis is hearing aids or microsurgical implantation of a stapedial prosthesis to replace the sclerotic joint and allow movement of the bones.

DIAGNOSTIC STUDIES OF THE EAR

Visual Examination

Using an otoscope, the physician can view the auditory canal and eardrum. Disposable otoscopes are available; reusable otoscopes use disposable speculum covers that are changed between patients (FIG. 31-8). Some reusable otoscopes use the same base as an ophthalmoscope.

Audiometry and Tympanometry

An audiometer can be used to detect hearing loss (Procedure 31-5). Audiometers produce pure tones of various decibel (dB) levels and frequencies heard through earphones or an instrument that resembles an otoscope. The decibel is a unit for measuring the intensity of sound. The audiometer

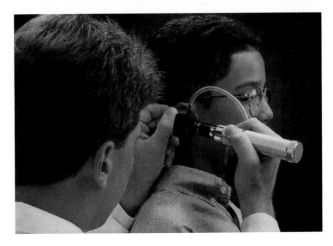

FIGURE 31-8. Examination of the ear with an otoscope. (Reprinted with permission from Willis MC. Medical Terminology: A Programmed Learning Approach to the Language of Health Care. Baltimore: Lippincott Williams & Wilkins, 2002.)

records the results of the test on a special graph. Speech audiometry uses voice tones rather than pure tones to assess hearing. Impedance audiometry evaluates tympanic membrane and ossicle mobility. A probe is inserted into the auditory meatus and emits tones of various intensity levels that bounce back to the probe receiver. If the tympanic membrane and ossicles are normal, the movement is transmitted and rebound is picked up by the receiver to produce a curve on the graph. If the tympanic membrane and ossicles are less mobile than normal, much of the sound transmitted bounces back and is reflected to the instrument to produce a distinct curve on the graph.

Tympanometry works like the audiometer but uses air pressure rather than tones to produce the graph. FIGURE 31-9 illustrates the steps for performing this hearing test.

Tuning Fork Tests

Two tests that may be performed using the tuning fork are the Rinne test and the Weber test. The Rinne test entails lightly tapping the tuning fork, placing the end of it on the mastoid bone, then moving it to the external auditory meatus to determine conductive hearing loss. In normal hearing the sound is louder through the external auditory meatus than the bone. The Weber test entails gently tapping the tuning fork and placing it on the midline of the forehead to differentiate between conductive and sensorineural hearing loss. In conductive loss the sound is louder in the affected ear; in sensorineural loss, the sound is louder in the unaffected ear. Although the physician most likely is the one who performs the tuning fork tests, you should ensure that the tuning fork is available and assist as needed.

THERAPEUTIC PROCEDURES FOR THE EAR

Irrigations and Instillations

Ear irrigations (Procedure 31-6) are performed to relieve pain, to remove debris or foreign objects, or to apply medication solutions. Ear instillations (Procedure 31-7) include a local anesthetic for the pain of otitis externa or otitis media or a topical antibiotic for otitis externa. These medications include the words "for otic use" on the label. For medication irrigations and instillations, observe the principles of medication administration, including checking the medication label for the expiration date.

Checkpoint Question

5. What is an audiometer used for, and how does it work?

COMMON DISORDERS OF THE NOSE AND THROAT

Allergic Rhinitis

Allergic rhinitis is inflammation of the mucous membranes of the nasal passages usually resulting from exposure to an allergen. Symptomatic treatment with antihistamine medication is usually offered to relieve the symptoms. It is also known as hay fever or seasonal allergic rhinitis when it appears in response to seasonal plant pollens. If the symptoms are present year round, it is perennial allergic rhinitis and is usually a reaction to household irritants,

A   B

FIGURE 31–9. Microtymp 2 tympanometric instrument is lightweight and portable and provides a hard copy printout of many middle ear disorders. (A) Press the button, then insert the probe tip into the ear. Watch the LCD screen as it completes the tympanogram in about 1 second. (B) Return the handle to the printer–charger and a printout appears in 5 seconds. (Courtesy of Welch-Allyn.)

Spanish Terminology

el ojo	The eye
los oidos	The ears
la nariz	The nose
la garganta	The throat

such as dust mites and pet dander. The signs are obvious, with paroxysmal sneezing, intense rhinorrhea (nasal drainage), congestion, and watery reddened eyes.

Diagnosis usually entails history and differential diagnosis. Mucous secretions may reveal an increase in immunoglobulin E in response to the allergens. An allergist may isolate the offending protein by skin testing. Allergy treatment entails exposure to the allergen in minute doses to desensitize the immune reaction.

Epistaxis

Commonly known as nosebleed, epistaxis generally occurs from trauma to the nasal membranes, but it may be secondary to another disorder, such as hypertension, malignancy, polyps, or the fragile capillaries associated with pregnancy. Diagnosis necessitates a history and inspection of the nasal mucosa with a nasal speculum (FIG. 31-10). The initial therapy for simple epistaxis is having the patient sit upright with the head slightly forward to avoid postnasal drainage that may lead to nausea. Compress the nares against the septum for 5 to 10 minutes with either ice or a cold, wet compress. Advise the patient to remain still and not to blow the nose until the physician concludes that all danger is past.

Bleeding that continues more than 10 minutes after treatment begins is considered severe. For severe epistaxis, the physician may insert nasal packing or a balloon catheter that may remain in place several hours to several days. For secondary bleeding, treatment of the underlying cause may be indicated. Cautery to an exposed blood vessel helps if that is the only cause.

Nasal Polyps

Nasal polyps are small pendulous tissues that obstruct breathing. Polyps usually occur in the mucous membranes of the nasal passages as a response to long-term allergies. Symptoms include a feeling of fullness or congestion and occasionally a nasal discharge. Diagnosis requires direct examination with a nasal speculum or radiography of the nasal structures. Treatment may be corticosteroids applied either topically or by injection directly into the polyps. The underlying allergy must be treated to prevent recurrence of polyps. If conservative treatment is not effective, conventional or laser surgery is required.

Sinusitis

Sinusitis, or inflammation of one or more of the sinus cavities, can be either acute or chronic. Acute sinusitis is

FIGURE 31–10. Physical examination of the nose with nasal speculum. (Reprinted with permission from Nettina SM. The Lippincott Manual of Nursing Practice. Philadelphia: Lippincott Williams & Wilkins, 2001.)

— Middle turbinate
— Inferior turbinate

PATIENT EDUCATION

Nasal Disorders

Patients need to be alert for any changes in their breathing pattern. The early symptoms of any nasal disorder must be treated as soon as possible to prevent complications. Instruct children not to put small pieces of food or toys in the nose.

Instruct patients about the rebound phenomena of nasal sprays and drops. If used without the advice of a physician, these medications may become addictive. After frequent use, the nasal mucosa responds to withdrawal of the medication with congestion. Nasal preparations should never be used more than 4 times a day for 3 days unless specified by the physician.

usually the result of an upper respiratory infection and is fairly easily resolved. Chronic sinusitis is more persistent and more difficult to control. Either form is particularly common when microorganisms are forced into the moist sinus cavities during hard nose blowing.

Symptoms of sinusitis include the obvious signs of an upper respiratory infection, with the addition of a purulent nasal discharge and facial pain over the sinus areas. Diagnosis requires direct visualization using a nasal speculum, radiography of the sinuses, needle puncture of the sinuses to withdraw a specimen for culture, and ultrasound.

Serious complications in the brain and middle ear may occur if sinusitis is not treated promptly with antihistamines or ephedrine nose drops to shrink mucosal tissue and relieve pressure. Steroidal nasal sprays may also be prescribed. Procedure 31-8 describes the steps for instilling nasal medication. If the cause of the sinusitis is a bacterial infection, antibiotics are prescribed by the physician and effectively relieve symptoms within 7 to 10 days. Chronic sinusitis may require treatment for 4 to 6 weeks. Total blockage of the sinus cavity may result if the disorder is not treated; this may require surgery to puncture the wall between the nose and the involved sinus cavity to allow drainage.

Checkpoint Question

6. What factors may contribute to epistaxis?

Pharyngitis and Tonsillitis

Inflammation of the epithelial tissues of the throat and of the tonsils produces similar symptoms of sore throat and difficulty swallowing. Examination of the throat reveals red, swollen tissues and possibly pustules on the tonsils or in the throat. You may be asked to obtain a throat specimen from these patients for transportation to an outside laboratory for a culture, or you may be required to perform a rapid strep test on the specimen in the office (Procedure 31-9). Treatment of a sore throat may include gargles, an analgesic, and an antibiotic, especially if the throat culture reveals a bacterial infection. Tonsillitis may be treated with an antibiotic, or if the problem is chronic, the tonsils may be surgically removed— a tonsillectomy. This procedure usually includes removal of both pharyngeal tonsils (adenoids) and palatine tonsils.

Laryngitis

Inflammation of the larynx can result from an infection, irritation, or overuse of the voice. The result is hoarseness, cough, and difficulty speaking. Diagnosis is made after a thorough history and visual inspection of the pharynx for redness and signs of infection. Laryngitis may be treated with an antibiotic if it is thought to be caused by a bacterial infection, but more often it is left to resolve on its own. The patient is told to rest the voice and speak as little as possible. A cool-mist humidifier may be helpful in soothing the throat.

LEGAL TIP

A patient calls the office at 4:45 P.M. complaining of a sore throat. Scheduled appointments are running 1 to 2 hours behind. Because it is the middle of flu season, you think it is safe to tell the patient that he has a virus and can be seen in the morning. During the night, the patient's throat closes because of the infection and obstructs his airway. The patient dies, and the autopsy report shows a tonsillar abscess. Could the patient's family sue you? Yes! As a medical assistant, you cannot presume to diagnose medical conditions. You made a medical decision and diagnosed the patient when you decided that the symptoms indicated a virus. Only the physician can make a diagnosis. Always follow office policy regarding telephone advice, and document all phone conversations after bringing them to the physician's attention.

DIAGNOSTIC STUDIES OF THE NOSE AND THROAT

Visual Inspection

Examination of the nose and throat entails visually inspecting the nose using a nasal speculum or viewing the throat using a penlight and tongue depressor. The physician may order radiography and culture to identify infectious microorganisms. The physician may also palpate the lymph nodes in the neck and other neck structures related to the upper airway. You may be responsible for preparing the patient and assisting during the examination.

THERAPEUTIC PROCEDURES FOR THE NOSE AND THROAT

Throat Culture

A throat culture in cases of suspected pharyngitis or tonsillitis can help determine what microorganism is causing the problem. The patient's throat is gently swabbed with a sterile culture swab to obtain the specimen. A sterile swab is necessary to avoid culturing microorganisms not in the throat. After the specimen is obtained, it is either processed in the office with a commercially prepared test kit such as those that check for streptococcal bacteria or sent to a laboratory for analysis. If the specimen is sent to the laboratory, it must be placed in a culture medium, labeled, and sent in a biohazard bag with the appropriate laboratory request. Procedure 31-9 outlines the steps for obtaining the throat culture.

Checkpoint Question

7. Why is it necessary to use a sterile swab to obtain the throat culture specimen?

Measuring Distance Visual Acuity

Purpose: To assess and document the distance visual acuity of a patient in both eyes, with or without corrective lenses.

Equipment: Snellen eye chart, paper cup or eye paddle

Standard: This procedure should take 5 minutes.

Steps	Reason
1. Wash your hands.	Handwashing aids infection control.
2. Prepare the examination area. Make sure the area is well lighted, a distance marker is placed exactly 20 feet from the chart, and the chart is at eye level.	All distance visual acuity testing is done at 20 feet for consistency of results.
3. Greet and identify the patient. Explain the procedure.	Patients who understand the procedure are likely to be compliant and produce an accurate test result.
4. Position the patient at the 20 foot marker.	The patient may stand or sit as long as the chart is at eye level and the patient is 20 feet from it.
5. Observe whether the patient is wearing glasses. If not, ask the patient about contact lenses and mark the results of the test accordingly.	The visual acuity examination is usually performed with patients who need them wearing corrective lenses. If so, the record must indicate that the lenses were worn for the test.
6. Have the patient cover the left eye with the paper cup or the eye paddle. Instruct the patient to keep both eyes open during the test.	The test starts with the left eye covered for consistency. The hand should not be used to cover the eye, since pressure against the eye or peeking through the fingers affects the results. Closing one eye will cause squinting of the other, which changes the vision and skews the findings.
7. Stand beside the chart and point to each row as the patient reads aloud the indicated lines, starting with the 20/200 line. This number is on the right side of the chart next to each line.	It is generally best to start about the second or third row to judge the patient's response. If these lines are read easily, move down to smaller figures. If the patient has difficulty reading the larger lines, notify the physician.
8. Record the smallest line that the patient can read with either 1 or no errors, according to office policy. If the patient reads line 5 with 1 error with the right eye, it will be recorded as OD (ocularis dexter) 20/40–1. If no errors are read at the 20/40 line, it is recorded as OD 20/40. Your physician may prefer that only lines read without any error be counted as correct.	
9. Repeat the procedure with the right eye covered and record as in step 8, using OS (ocularis sinistra). If the patient squints or leans forward while testing either eye, record this observation on the patient record.	
10. Wash your hands and document the procedure.	Procedures are considered not to have been done if they are not recorded.

Charting Example

01/16/2005 4:30 P.M. Visual acuity OD 20/40–1 OS 20/20 with correction Dr. Smart aware. _____
C. Mayers, CMA

Procedure 31-2

Measuring Color Perception

Purpose: To assess and document color perception.

Equipment: Ishihara color plates, gloves

Standard: This procedure should take 5 minutes.

Steps	Reason
1. Wash your hands, put on gloves, and get the Ishihara color plate book.	Handwashing aids infection control. Gloves in this case are to protect not the patient or health care worker but the color plates. Oils from the hands can alter the colors and interfere with testing.
2. Identify the patient and explain the procedure. Ensure that the patient is seated comfortably in a quiet, well-lighted room. Indirect sunlight is best. (Sunlight should not shine directly on the plates; the colors fade with exposure to bright lights.) Patients who wear glasses or contact lenses should keep them on.	The Ishihara tests color perception, not visual acuity. Corrective lenses do not interfere with accurate test results.
3. After opening the book, hold the first plate in the book about 30 inches from the patient and ask if he or she can see the number in the dots on the plate.	The first plate should be obvious to all patients and serves as an example.
4. Record the results of the test by noting the number or figure the patient reports on each plate, using the plate number followed by the response. If the patient cannot distinguish the pattern, record as the plate number followed by the letter X. The patient should not take more than 3 seconds to read the plates and should not squint or guess. These indicate that the patient was unsure and are recorded as X.	
5. Record the results for plates 1 to 10. Plate 11 requires the patient to trace the winding bluish-green line between the two x's. Patients with a color deficit will not be able to trace the line.	If 10 or more of the first 11 plates are read correctly without difficulty, the patient does not have a color deficit. Plates 12, 13, and 14 are usually used to detect the degree of deficiency in patients with red–green color deficiencies.
6. Store the book in a closed, protected area to safeguard the integrity of the colors. Remove your gloves and wash your hands.	Procedures are considered not to have been done if they are not recorded.

Charting Example

12/22/2005 10:30 A.M. Ishihara color deficit testing performed:

Plate 1	12	Plate 7	X (normal 45)
Plate 2	8	Plate 8	X (normal 2)
Plate 3	5 (normal 2)	Plate 9	2 (normal X)
Plate 4	X	Plate 10	X (normal 16)
Plate 5	21 (normal 74)	Plate 11	X (traceable)
Plate 6	X (normal 7)		

_____ B. Cotton, CMA

Instilling Eye Medications

Purpose: Instill and document ophthalmic medications as ordered by the physician.

Equipment: Physician's order and patient record, ophthalmic medication, sterile gauze, tissues, gloves

Standard: This procedure should take 5 minutes.

Steps	Reason
1. Wash your hands.	Handwashing aids infection control.
2. Obtain the patient's medical record, including the physician's order, correct medication, sterile gauze, and tissues.	The medication must specify ophthalmic use. Check the label three times before administering the ophthalmic solution or ointment. Medications formulated for other uses may be harmful if used in the eyes.
3. Greet and identify the patient. Explain the procedure. Ask the patient about any allergies not recorded in the chart.	Identifying the patient prevents errors in treatment.
4. Position the patient comfortably.	The patient may lie or sit with the head tilted slightly back and the affected eye slightly lower to avoid the medication running into the unaffected eye.
5. Put on gloves and pull down the lower eyelid with sterile gauze while asking the patient to look up.	Since there is potential for contact with secretions from the eye, you must wear gloves. Pulling down the lower lid exposes the conjunctival sac to receive the medication. If the patient is looking up and away from the medication, the blink reflex may not be triggered.

Step 5. Pull the lower eyelid down and ask the patient to look up.

6. Instill the medication:	
A. *Ointment:* Discard the first bead of ointment from the container onto a tissue without touching the end of the medication tube to the tissue. Place a thin line of ointment across the inside of the lower eyelid, moving from the inner canthus outward. Release the ointment by twisting the tube slightly. Do not touch the tube to the eye.	The first bead of ointment is considered contaminated. Placing the ointment in the sac avoids touching the eye with the tip of the ointment tube. Twisting the tube releases the ointment.
B. *Drops:* Hold the dropper close to the conjunctival sac (about half an inch away) but do not touch the patient. Release the proper number of drops into the sac. Discard any medication left in the dropper.	Discarding the remaining medication prevents contaminating the remainder of a multiple dose container.

(continues)

Instilling Eye Medications

Steps	Reason
7. Release the lower lid and have the patient gently close the eye and roll it to disperse the medication.	
8. Wipe off any excess medication with the tissue. Instruct the patient to apply light pressure to the puncta lacrimalis for several minutes.	Pressing the puncta prevents the medication from running into the nasolacrimal sac and duct.
9. Properly care for or dispose of equipment and supplies. Clean the work area and wash your hands.	
10. Record the procedure.	Procedures are considered not to have been done if they are not recorded.

Charting Example

10/14/2005 8:45 A.M. Garamycin ophthalmological ointment applied to OS. _____
B. Marker, CMA

Irrigating the Eye

Purpose:	Irrigate the eye as ordered by the physician and document the procedure.
Equipment:	Physician's order and patient's record, small sterile basin, irrigating solution and medication if ordered, protective barrier or towels, emesis basin, sterile bulb syringe, tissues, gloves
Standard:	This procedure should take 10 minutes.

Steps	Reason
1. Wash your hands and put on gloves.	Handwashing aids infection control. You must wear gloves when you may be exposed to body fluids.
2. Assemble the equipment, supplies, and medication if ordered. Check the label three times as recommended for medication administration and make sure the label indicates ophthalmic use. *Note:* If both eyes are to be treated, use separate equipment (solution and bulb syringe) to avoid cross-contamination.	Solutions for the eye must be sterile and must be formulated for ophthalmic use.
3. Greet and identify the patient. Explain the procedure.	Identifying the patient prevents errors in treatment. Patients who understand the procedure are generally cooperative and compliant.
4. Position the patient comfortably, either with the head tilted and the affected eye lower or lying with the affected eye down.	With the affected eye down, there is little chance of contamination running into the unaffected eye.
5. Drape the patient with the protective barrier or towel to avoid wetting the clothing.	

(continues)

Procedure 31-4 *(continued)*

Irrigating the Eye

Steps	Reason
6. Place the emesis basin against the upper cheek near the eye with the towel under the basin. With clean gauze, wipe the eye from the inner canthus outward to remove debris from the lashes.	Debris from the lashes may be washed into the eye.
7. Separate the lids with the thumb and forefinger of your nondominant hand. To steady your hand, you may lightly support your dominant hand, holding the syringe with solution on the bridge of the patient's nose parallel to the eye.	
8. Gently irrigate from the inner to the outer canthus, holding the syringe 1 inch above the eye. Use gentle pressure and do not touch the eye. The physician will order the time or amount of solution to be used.	The solution must flow from the inner to the outer canthus to avoid washing pathogens into the punctum. With the syringe 1 inch above the eye there is little chance of touching the eye and causing discomfort.

Step 8. Hold the syringe 1 inch above the eye.

9. Use tissues to wipe any excess solution from the patient's face.	This prevents the spread of microorganisms.
10. Properly dispose of equipment or sanitize as recommended and remove your gloves. Wash your hands.	Procedures are considered not to have been done if they are not recorded.
11. Record the procedure in the patient's record, including the amount, type, and strength of the solution; which eye was irrigated; and any observations.	

Charting Example

04/16/2005 11:30 A.M. OD irrigated with 500 mL sterile NS, return clear. _____
J. Penta, CMA

Procedure 31-5

Audiometry Testing

Purpose: To accurately assess and document a hearing test using audiometry.

Equipment: Audiometer, otoscope

Standard: This procedure should take 10 minutes.

Steps	Reason
1. Wash your hands.	Handwashing aids infection control.
2. Greet and identify the patient. Explain the procedure. Take the patient to a quiet area or room for testing.	Patients who understand the procedure are likely to be compliant, producing accurate results. A quiet room allows for accurate results without distraction. Determine the signal (raising the hand, saying yes) to indicate that the tones are heard.
3. Using an otoscope or audioscope with a light source, visually inspect the ear canal and tympanic membrane before the examination.	Looking into the ear canal verifies that there are no obstructions, such as cerumen, to interfere with the test. If you see an obstruction, notify the physician and follow any orders for irrigating the ears to remove the obstruction before the test.
4. Choose the correct size tip for the end of the audiometer. Attach a speculum to fit the patient's external auditory meatus, making sure the ear canal is occluded with the speculum in place.	The design of the tip or speculum obviates bulky ear phones. The tip should block any environmental noise during the test.
5. With the speculum in the ear canal, retract the pinna: up and back for adults; down and back for children.	Pulling the pinna up and back for adults and down and back for children straightens the ear canal.
6. Turn the instrument on and select the screening level. There is a pretest tone for practice if necessary. Press the start button and observe the tone indicators and the patient's responses.	The signal (raising the hand, saying yes) was determined before you began the test. The audiometer will proceed down each tone with a light indicator.
7. Screen the other ear.	
8. If the patient fails to respond at any frequency, rescreening is required.	If the patient does not hear a specific tone, a second opportunity should be given.
9. If the patient fails rescreening, notify the physician.	A patient who fails to hear one or more tones may be referred to an audiologist.
10. Record the results in the medical record.	Procedures are considered not to have been done if they are not recorded.

Procedure 31-6

Irrigating the Ear

Purpose: Irrigate the ear as ordered and document the procedure.

Equipment: Physician's order and patient's record, emesis or ear basin, waterproof barrier or towels, otoscope, irrigation solution, bowl for solution, gauze

Standard: This procedure should take 10 minutes.

Steps	Reason
1. Wash your hands.	Handwashing aids infection control.
2. Assemble the equipment and supplies.	Ear irrigation is not a sterile procedure.
3. Greet and identify the patient. Explain the procedure.	Identifying the patient prevents errors in treatment. Ear irrigations are not usually painful, but the flow of the solution may be uncomfortable. The patient may be more cooperative if this is understood.
4. Position the patient comfortably erect.	
5. View the affected ear with an otoscope to locate the foreign matter or cerumen. A. *Adults:* Gently pull up and back to straighten the auditory canal.	The area of treatment must be visualized before irrigation begins. If debris from the external auricle is not removed, it may be washed into the canal.

Step 5. Pull the pinna down and back for children. (Courtesy of Welch-Allyn.)

B. *Children:* Gently pull slightly down and back to straighten the auditory canal.

(continues)

Procedure 31-6   *(continued)*

Irrigating the Ear

Steps	Reason

Step 5. The shape of the ear canal changes with growth. To allow good inspection, position the ear as illustrated.

6. Drape the patient with a waterproof barrier or towel.

Wet clothing would be uncomfortable for the patient.

A

B

Step 6. (A) Place the audiometer tip in the patient's ear. (B) The patient should give a signal when each tone is heard. (Courtesy of Welch-Allyn.)

(continues)

Irrigating the Ear

Steps	Reason
7. Tilt the patient's head toward the affected side.	Tilting the head will facilitate the flow of solution

Step 8. Place the basin under the ear.

Steps	Reason
8. Place the drainage basin under the affected ear.	
9. Fill the irrigating syringe or turn on the irrigating device.	
10. Gently position the auricle as described, using your nondominant hand.	The canal must be straight for visualization and treatment.
11. With your dominant hand, place the tip of the syringe in the auditory meatus and direct the flow of the solution gently up toward the roof of the canal.	Directing the flow against the upper surface prevents pressure against the tympanic membrane and facilitates the outflow of solution.
12. Continue irrigating for the prescribed period or until the desired result (cerumen removal) is obtained.	If the patient complains of pain or discomfort, stop the irrigation and notify the physician.
13. Dry the patient's external ear with gauze. Have the patient sit awhile with the affected ear down to drain the solution.	Solution in the ear is uncomfortable.
14. Inspect the ear with the otoscope to determine the results.	It may be necessary to repeat the procedure and is always necessary to inspect the area to record the results.
15. Properly care for or dispose of equipment and supplies. Clean the work area. Wash your hands.	This prevents the spread of microorganisms.
16. Record the procedure in the patient's chart.	Procedures are considered not to have been done if they are not recorded.

Note: If the tympanic membrane appears to be perforated, do not irrigate without checking with the physician; solution may be forced into the middle ear through the perforation. Remove any obvious debris at the entrance of the canal before beginning the irrigation.

Charting Example
03/17/2005 3:30 P.M. AD irrigated with 500 mL sterile water; return clear with 2 large pieces of yellow-brown cerumen noted. _____ S. Stark, CMA

Charting Example
02/14/2005 9:00 A.M. Audiometry testing performed AU—results in chart. _____
S. Smythe, RMA

Instilling Ear Medication

Purpose: Instill otic medication as ordered and document the instillation.

Equipment: Physician's order and patient's record, otic medication with dropper, cotton balls

Standard: This procedure should take 5 minutes.

Steps	Reason
1. Wash your hands and assemble the equipment.	Handwashing aids infection control.
2. Check the medication label three times as specified for medication administration. The label should specify otic preparation.	Medication for otic instillation is formulated for that purpose.
3. Greet and identify the patient. Explain the procedure.	Identifying the patient prevents errors in treatment. Patients who understand the procedure are generally compliant.
4. Have the patient seated with the affected ear tilted upward.	The medication must be allowed to flow through the canal to the tympanic membrane.
5. Draw up the ordered amount of medication.	

6. Straighten the canal.
 	
  A. *Adults:* Pull the auricle slightly up and back.
 	
  B. *Children:* Pull the auricle slightly down and back.	

7. Insert the tip of the dropper without touching the patient's skin and let the medication flow along the side of the canal.	Touching the patient will contaminate the dropper. The medication should flow gently to avoid discomfort.

Step 7. Insert the tip of the dropper without touching the ear.

8. Have the patient sit or lie with the affected ear up for about 5 minutes after the instillation.	The medication should rest against the tympanic membrane for as long as possible.
9. If the medication is to be retained in the ear canal, insert a moist cotton ball into the external auditory meatus without force.	A slightly moist cotton ball will keep the medication in the canal and not wick it out. Forcing the cotton ball into the ear canal could be painful to the patient.

(continues)

Instilling Ear Medication

Steps	Reason
10. Properly care for or dispose of equipment and supplies. Clean the work area. Wash your hands.	This prevents the spread of microorganisms.
11. Record the procedure in the patient record.	Procedures are considered not to have been done if they are not recorded.

Charting Example

06/15/2005 12:30 P.M. Neosporin otic solution, 2 gtt instilled into AS as ordered. _____ D. Barth, CMA

Procedure 31-8

Instilling Nasal Medication

Purpose: Instill nasal medication as ordered and document the instillation.

Equipment: Physician's order and patient's record, nasal medication, drops or spray, tissues, gloves

Standard: This procedure should take 5 minutes.

Steps	Reason
1. Wash your hands and put on gloves.	Handwashing aids infection control.
2. Assemble the equipment and supplies. Check the medication label three times.	Medications for use in the nasal passages must be formulated for these surfaces.
3. Greet and identify the patient. Explain the procedure and ask the patient about any allergies not documented.	Identifying the patient prevents errors in treatment. Nasal instillations are uncomfortable but should not be painful; patients will be more cooperative if they understand the procedure.
4. Position the patient comfortably recumbent. Extend the patient's head beyond the edge of the examination table or place a pillow under the shoulders. Support the patient's neck to avoid strain as the head tilts back.	The patient must be properly positioned if the medication is to reach the upper nasal passages.
5. Administer the medication.	
A. Hold the dropper upright just above each nostril and dispense one drop at a time without touching the nares. Keep the patient recumbent for 5 minutes.	Touching the dropper to the nostril would contaminate the dropper. For effective treatment, the patient must allow the medication to reach the upper nasal passages.
B. Place the tip of the bottle at the naris opening without touching the patient's skin or nasal tissues and spray as the patient takes a deep breath.	The medication must reach the upper passages; if the patient breathes out while the medication is being sprayed, the medication is exhaled and does not reach the nasal passages.

(continues)

Procedure 31-8   *(continued)*

Instilling Nasal Medication

Steps	Reason
6. Wipe any excess medication from the patient's skin with tissues.	Excess medication around the nares is uncomfortable.
7. Properly care for or dispose of equipment and supplies. Clean the work area. Remove your gloves and wash your hands.	This prevents the spread of microorganisms.
8. Record the procedure in the patient's chart.	Procedures are considered not to have been done if they are not recorded.

Charting Example

06/15/2005 12:00 P.M. Oxymetazoline hydrochloride 0.05% nasal spray, 2 sprays to each nostril as ordered per Dr. Greene. _____ D. Pratt, CMA

Procedure 31-9

Collecting a Specimen for Throat Culture

Purpose: Obtain a throat specimen for analysis in the medical office or for transport to the laboratory.

Equipment: Physician's order and patient's record, tongue blade, sterile specimen container and swab, gloves, commercial throat culture kit (if to be done in the office), completed laboratory request form and biohazard bag for transport (if to be sent to the laboratory for analysis)

Standard: This procedure should take 5 minutes.

Steps	Reason
1. Wash your hands.	Handwashing aids infection control.
2. Assemble the equipment and supplies. Put on gloves.	Follow standard precautions to prevent the transmission of infectious microorganisms.
3. Greet and identify the patient. Explain the procedure.	Identifying the patient prevents errors in treatment.
4. Have the patient sit with a light source directed at the throat.	Good visibility is vital to collection from the area of concern.
5. Carefully remove the sterile swab from the container.	
6. Have the patient say "Ah" as you press down on the midpoint of the tongue with the tongue depressor.	Saying "Ah" raises the uvula out of the way and decreases the gag reflex. If the tongue depressor is placed too far forward, it will not be effective; if it is placed too far back, the patient will gag unnecessarily.

(continues)

Procedure 31-9 (continued)

Collecting a Specimen for Throat Culture

Steps	Reason
7. Swab the areas of concern on the mucous membranes, especially the tonsillar area, the crypts, and the posterior pharynx. Turn the swab to expose all of its surfaces to the membranes. Avoid touching areas other than those suspected of infection.	Pathogens must be collected from sites of concern with a twisting motion for maximum collection. Touching other areas such as the tongue or teeth will alter the substances on the swab.
8. Maintain the tongue depressor position while withdrawing the swab from the patient's mouth.	Keeping the tongue down prevents contaminating the swab unnecessarily.
9. Follow the instructions on the specimen container for transferring the swab or processing the specimen in the office using a commercial kit.	Improper handling of the specimen would alter the results.
10. Properly dispose of the equipment and supplies in a biohazard waste container. Remove your gloves and wash your hands.	This prevents the spread of microorganisms.
11. Route the specimen or store it appropriately until routing can be completed.	
12. Document the procedure.	Procedures are considered not to have been done if they are not documented.

Charting Example

11/20/2005 10:30 A.M. Throat specimen obtained as ordered, rapid strep test negative, specimen to Acme labs for C&S.
_____ M. Mohr, CMA

CHAPTER SUMMARY

Disorders of the eyes, ears, nose, and throat may affect any patient at any age. Although not all patients who have disorders of these structures need a referral to an ophthalmologist or otolaryngologist, you will routinely encounter patients who need to have these conditions properly diagnosed and treated. Severe complications, such as an infection of the brain or hearing loss, can result in patients not receiving adequate attention or not following the physician's instructions for treatment. You will play a vital role by assisting with ear, nose, and throat examinations and educating patients regarding their treatment.

Critical Thinking Challenges

1. The mother of a 10-month old boy explains to you that the baby has had a runny nose and has been fussy for the past 2 days. You notice that he is pulling at his right ear. What equipment do you anticipate that the physician will need for examining the child?

2. A 16-year-old girl complains of a sore throat. Her vital signs are T 102.8 (O), P 112, R 24, and BP 112/84. The physician examines her and tells you to obtain a throat specimen for a rapid strep test to determine whether the pharyngitis is due to an infection with streptococcal bacteria. The patient is reluctant to let you obtain a throat culture, saying it will make her gag and vomit. How do you handle this situation?

3. The school nurse at the local high school phones your office asking for information about a student who has been out of school the past 3 days with conjunctivitis. Specifically, she wants to know whether this student has been diagnosed with this condition or is simply truant. How do you handle this phone call?

Answers to Checkpoint Questions

1. A sty is an infection of the glands of the eyelids; conjunctivitis is an infection of the conjunctiva, the mucous membrane that covers the sclera and cornea.

2. Four common refractive errors are hyperopia (far-sightedness), myopia (nearsightedness), astigmatism (unfocused refraction of light rays on the retina), and presbyopia (age-related vision changes).

3. The E chart is used for patients who cannot read or who do not speak English.

4. Conductive hearing loss stops the flow of sound before the cochlea. Perceptual hearing loss stops the flow of nerve impulses from the cochlea to the brain.

5. An audiometer is used to detect hearing loss. The patient wears earphones and listens for pure tones of various decibel levels and various frequencies. The results of the test are recorded by the audiometer on a graph.

6. Hypertension, malignancy, polyps, and the fragile capillaries associated with pregnancy contribute to epistaxis.

7. A sterile swab is used to obtain the throat culture to prevent obtaining a culture of microorganisms not in the throat.

 WWW.GO   Websites

American Academy of Otolaryngology, Head and Neck Surgery www.entnet.org

Vision Connection www.visionconnection.org

Journal of Pediatric Ophthalmology and Strabismus www.journalofpediatricophthalmology.com

American Foundation for the Blind www.afb.org

Foundation Fighting Blindness www.blindness.org

Prevent Blindness American www.preventblindness.org

American Optometric Association www.aoa.org

Self-help for the hard-of-hearing www.shhh.org

32

Pulmonary Medicine

CHAPTER OUTLINE

COMMON RESPIRATORY
  DISORDERS
  Upper Respiratory Disorders
  Lower Respiratory Disorders
  Common Cancers of the
    Respiratory System

COMMON DIAGNOSTIC AND
  THERAPEUTIC PROCEDURES
  Physical Examination of the
    Respiratory System
  Sputum Culture and Cytology
  Chest Radiography

Bronchoscopy
Pulmonary Function Tests
Arterial Blood Gases

ROLE DELINEATION

ADMINISTRATIVE: ADMINISTRATIVE
  PROCEDURES
- Perform basic administrative medical assisting
  functions

CLINICAL: FUNDAMENTAL PRINCIPLES
- Apply principles of aseptic technique and infection
  control
- Screen and follow up patients' test results

CLINICAL: DIAGNOSTIC ORDERS
- Perform diagnostic tests

CLINICAL: PATIENT CARE
- Adhere to established screening procedures
- Obtain history and vital signs
- Prepare patients for examinations, procedures, and
  treatments
- Assist with examinations, procedures, and treatments
- Recognize and respond to emergencies
- Coordinate care information with other health care
  providers

GENERAL: PROFESSIONALISM
- Display a professional manner and image
- Demonstrate initiative and responsibility
- Work as a member of the health care team
- Prioritize and perform multiple tasks
- Treat all patients with compassion and empathy

CHAPTER COMPETENCIES

LEARNING OBJECTIVES

Upon successfully completing this chapter, you will be able to:
1. Spell and define the key terms.
2. Identify the primary defense mechanisms of the respiratory system.
3. List and describe disorders of the respiratory system.
4. Explain various diagnostic procedures of the respiratory system.
5. Describe the physician's examination of the respiratory system.
6. Discuss the role of the medical assistant with regard to various diagnostic and therapeutic procedures.

PERFORMANCE OBJECTIVES

Upon successfully completing this chapter, you will be able to:
1. Collect a sputum specimen for culture or cytological examination (Procedure 32-1)
2. Instruct a patient in the use of the peak flowmeter (Procedure 32-2)
3. Administer a nebulized breathing treatment (Procedure 32-3)
4. Perform a pulmonary function test (Procedure 32-4)

KEY TERMS

atelectasis	dyspnea	laryngectomy	tidal volume
chronic obstructive pulmonary disease (COPD)	forced expiratory volume (FEV)	palliative	tracheostomy
	hemoptysis	status asthmaticus	
		thoracentesis	

THE RESPIRATORY SYSTEM provides the body with the oxygen that all cells need to perform their functions (FIG. 32-1). It also eliminates carbon dioxide, a waste product, and water from the body. The respiratory system works closely with the cardiovascular system to deliver oxygen to every cell in the body. When a cell is too long deprived of oxygen, the cell dies, and when many cells die, so does the tissue.

The upper airways, tracheobronchial tree, and alveoli come into contact with air from the atmosphere or environment, which can contain dust, pathogenic microorganisms, and other irritants. In healthy individuals, defense mechanisms in the respiratory system help to protect the body from disease and illness caused by these environmental contaminants. TABLE 32-1 summarizes the major defense mechanisms of the respiratory system. Disease can occur, however, when these defenses are overwhelmed by cigarette smoke (Box 32-1), air pollution, infectious organisms, or other irritants.

COMMON RESPIRATORY DISORDERS

Upper Respiratory Disorders

The most common problems of the upper respiratory tract are caused by infectious microorganisms and by allergic reactions that produce inflammation. Acute rhinitis, sinusitis, pharyngitis, tonsillitis, and laryngitis are described in Chapter 31; these are also considered upper respiratory disorders.

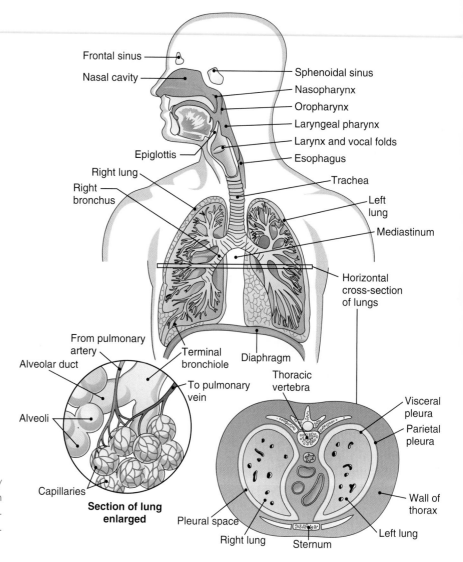

FIGURE 32–1. The respiratory system. (Reprinted with permission from Cohen BJ, Wood DL. Memmler's The Human Body in Health and Disease. Philadelphia: Lippincott Williams & Wilkins, 2000.)

Table 32-1 DEFENSES OF THE RESPIRATORY SYSTEM

Defense	Function
Nasal hairs	Filter large dust particles from the air
Mucous membranes	Trap dust and other particles, add moisture
Turbinates in nose	Whirl air around to increase warming, humidifying, filtering
Epiglottis	Closes over trachea to prevent aspiration during swallowing
Airway reflexes	Trigger cough to clear irritants in pharynx, larynx, trachea
Airway smooth muscles	Constrict when irritation occurs to prevent entry of foreign substances
Macrophage in alveoli	Phagocytize ("eat") bacteria, other foreign cells, debris
Tonsils	Filter air moving through passageways to protect against bacterial invasion; aid in formation of white blood cells

Box 32-1

EFFECTS OF SMOKING ON THE AIRWAYS

Cigarette smoking has many harmful effects on the body. Smoke from a cigarette irritates the airways and causes the membrane to produce more mucus. This increased production of mucus, along with the increase in dust and debris that collects in the mucus, slows down the body's normal clearing processes. The smoke anesthetizes the cilia lining the respiratory tract so they stop waving the debris away. Over time, large amounts of thick, sticky mucus are retained in the lungs, blackening the lung tissue and sealing the alveolar sacs. This thick, tarry mucus causes the patient to cough frequently, especially in the mornings, and to be prone to bronchitis, both acute and chronic, as a result of the destruction of the protective mechanisms of the airway from the heat and tar inhaled in the smoke.

Lower Respiratory Disorders

Diseases of the lower respiratory tract may be acute (sudden in onset with relatively short duration) or chronic (progressing over time or recurring frequently). Acute diseases of the lower respiratory tract include bronchitis and pneumonia. Chronic diseases include asthma, chronic bronchitis, and emphysema. The last two diseases are usually grouped as chronic obstructive pulmonary disease, because most patients have elements of both emphysema and chronic bronchitis.

Bronchitis

Bronchitis is an inflammation of the mucous membranes of the bronchi caused by infection or irritation that induces increased production of mucus in the trachea, bronchi, and bronchioles. The most prominent symptom of bronchitis is a productive cough. If a bacterial or viral infection is present, the sputum may change color from the normal white or clear to yellow, green, gray, or tan. If an infection is suspected, you may be asked to obtain a sputum specimen for culture and sensitivity to determine the causative microorganism and appropriate antibiotic therapy (Procedure 32-1). In many cases, the physician bases a diagnosis of bronchitis on the history and symptoms of the patient without ordering a sputum culture. Treatment generally includes an antibiotic for bacterial infection, smoking cessation, rest, and increased fluid intake. A cough suppressant may be prescribed, especially for use at night, but that is controversial because of the body's need to clear secretions from the airways. Retained secretions can become infected and lead to pneumonia.

Pneumonia

Pneumonia is a bacterial or viral infection in the alveoli, or tiny air sacs that are the site of gas exchange in the lungs. The buildup of fluid and congestion in the alveoli prevents effective gas exchange. Diagnostic testing usually includes analysis of a sputum specimen and chest radiography. Bacterial pneumonias tend to be sudden and severe in onset, causing a fever, cough, chills, and **dyspnea**. Infections caused by bacteria also tend to be local to one lobe or area of the lung. Treatment of bacterial pneumonia primarily is an appropriate antibiotic, bed rest, and medication to relieve symptoms. Pneumonia caused by bacteria often requires hospitalization for administration of intravenous antibiotics and oxygen, especially in the elderly or debilitated patients.

Viral pneumonia is usually more gradual in onset but can be just as serious. Antibiotics are ineffective in treating viral pneumonia; however, the physician may order an antibiotic to prevent a secondary bacterial infection. Viral pneumonia tends to spread throughout the lung fields and often is marked by a fever and productive cough. Treatment may include bed rest or hospitalization.

Checkpoint Question

1. What are the characteristics of bacterial and viral pneumonia?

Asthma

Asthma is a reversible inflammatory process involving primarily the small airways such as the bronchi and bronchioles. Asthma manifests as constriction of the smooth muscle lining the airways, spasms of the bronchi and bronchioles (bronchospasm), swelling of the mucous membranes of the airways, and increased mucus production with productive coughing. All three of these manifestations narrow the airways, making it difficult for the patient to move air into and out of the lungs.

The patient having an asthma attack may have dyspnea, coughing, wheezing, and in severe cases, cyanosis. Patients with asthma usually have exacerbations, or periods of frequent attacks, and remissions, when they are relatively symptom free. Attacks may be triggered by exposure to allergens, such as mold or dust; inhaled irritants, such as cigarette smoke; upper respiratory infections; psychological stress; cold air; or exercise. In some instances the immediate cause of the asthma attack is unknown. While asthma is considered a chronic disorder that occurs in children or adults, many children with asthma outgrow it by adulthood.

PATIENT EDUCATION

Using More Than One Inhaler for Asthma

Asthmatics may use more than one inhaler. One medication is usually a bronchodilator to open the bronchioles and control bronchospasms. Another type of inhaler is a corticosteroid. Steroids help to control inflammation in the bronchioles and generally are prescribed only during a respiratory illness. Teach the patient to use the bronchodilator first, wait 5 minutes, and then use the steroid. Using the steroid inhaler after the bronchodilator allows for more steroid medication to enter the lung tissue, making it more effective.

Some patients are prescribed two inhaled bronchodilators. One type is used daily to prevent asthma attacks, and the other is used as a rescue inhaler. The rescue inhaler should be used only when the asthma cannot be controlled with the daily regimen. Before teaching a patient about the correct pattern for using the inhalers, clarify the information with the physician. Each asthmatic responds differently and requires an individualized approach to care.

Many medications are available to prevent or control the symptoms of asthma, but it is important that they be used properly. On days that the patient has no symptoms of asthma, he or she should use a device called a peak flowmeter (Fig. 32-2) to determine the amount of air moving into and out of the lungs (Procedure 32-2). Instruct the patient to use the peak flowmeter correctly and record the results on a chart or diary provided by the medical office. This record, known as the patient's personal best, assists the physician in establishing and maintaining a medication protocol.

Patients with symptoms of asthma, including wheezing and difficulty breathing, may be prescribed a nebulized breathing treatment with a bronchodilator, a medication to dilate the bronchi, such as albuterol. After the bronchodilator is in the nebulizer administration setup, the machine is turned on and causes the liquid medication to break apart into a fine spray that is inhaled by the patient through a mouthpiece or mask. Procedure 32-3 explains setting up and administering a breathing treatment with a bronchodilator and a nebulizer. Since bronchodilator medications cause an increase in the heart rate, you should monitor the patient's pulse before, during, and after the treatment. If the patient becomes light-headed, discontinue the treatment, have the patient lie down, obtain the vital signs, and notify the physician.

An asthma attack that does not respond to medication is an emergency known as **status asthmaticus**. Because such attacks can be fatal, the patient needs immediate emergency medical services and hospitalization.

Checkpoint Question

2. What factors may trigger an asthma attack?

Chronic Obstructive Pulmonary Disease

Chronic bronchitis and emphysema are most commonly caused by cigarette smoking. As a result, patients who have smoked over a long period often exhibit signs and symp-

FIGURE 32-2.   The peak flowmeter.

> ### LEGAL TIP
>
> Patients with chronic and irreversible diseases, such as COPD, must never be led to believe that the doctor can cure the disease. Avoid making statements such as "everything will be okay" or "the doctor can help you," and otherwise be careful not to indicate that the patient will return to normal function. Legally, the doctor is responsible for your actions, including promises, even if they are innocent and were said only to make the patient feel better. These statements may be taken as a guarantee, and if the results aren't achieved, the patient may file a lawsuit on the grounds that a contract was broken and the promised results were not delivered.

toms of both of these disorders. Chronic bronchitis is a chronic inflammation and swelling of the airways with excessive mucus production, obstruction of the bronchi, and trapping of air behind mucus plugs. The trapping of this air overinflates the alveoli. Chronic bronchitis is not usually an infectious process but instead is produced by chronic irritation of the airways by cigarette smoke or other pollutants. However, because of the increase in sputum and the difficulty these patients have in clearing their sputum, they are prone to develop respiratory infections.

Emphysema is a disease process in which the walls of the damaged alveoli stretch and break down after repeated exposure to irritants such as cigarette smoke and air pollution. The pulmonary capillaries also break down, and the tiny airways leading to each alveolus weaken and collapse. The end result is a sharp reduction in surface area for gas exchange, and once again, air is trapped in the enlarged air sacs that were once clusters of tiny alveoli.

The combination of these diseases, together called **chronic obstructive pulmonary disease** (COPD), produces characteristic symptoms. COPD is a likely cause of shortness of breath, chronic cough, sputum production, and wheezing in the patient with a history of smoking. The onset of these symptoms is usually slow and gradual over years, and the patient may go a long time without realizing that he or she has signs and symptoms of a disease. Many people with COPD have some of the signs and symptoms of asthma, and many of these patients take asthma medications.

Once a patient is diagnosed with COPD, the disease process is not usually reversible. Many patients have a hard time accepting that fact and insist that their physician provide a cure or restore the lungs to normal function. Although the disease is not curable, the progression of COPD can be slowed

PATIENT EDUCATION

Living With COPD

To improve the quality of life, encourage a patient diagnosed with COPD to follow these suggestions:

1. Quit smoking if you haven't already done so! Even though the lungs have been permanently damaged, further deterioration will be reduced if you stop smoking now.
2. Get a flu vaccination each fall and make sure you have had the pneumonia vaccine.
3. Avoid crowds, especially in the winter, when the viruses that cause colds and influenza are prevalent.
4. If pollution is high, stay indoors with the air conditioning on if possible.
5. Use your abdominal muscles instead of your shoulder and neck muscles to avoid strain and fatigue in these muscles.
6. Drink lots of fluids unless the physician has limited your fluid intake. Water is the best fluid. Good fluid intake is the best way to keep the mucus in your airways thin so that it is easy to cough up.
7. Follow a healthy, balanced diet.
8. Avoid doing difficult physical tasks (e.g., vacuuming or mowing the lawn) all in one day. If you must do these chores, do them in short periods spaced throughout the day with frequent rest periods.
9. Organize your home to minimize standing, reaching, and lifting.

and the quality of life improved significantly through education about the disease, a prescribed exercise regimen, proper use of medications, good nutrition, and home oxygen therapy.

Checkpoint Question

3. What two disease processes are present in a patient with COPD?

Tuberculosis

Tuberculosis is an infectious disease spread by respiratory droplets from a person infected with *Mycobacterium tuberculosis*. The patient with active tuberculosis has signs and symptoms such as a productive cough, night sweats, and malaise. Although no tuberculosis vaccine is available, a screening test can be administered to detect a previous infection. However, a patient with a positive screening test for tuberculosis does not necessarily have active disease and there-

fore may not be contagious. The procedure for administering and reading the results of the screening tests (Mantoux and tine tests) for tuberculosis is described in Chapter 26. Patients with symptoms of tuberculosis should be treated as contagious and encouraged to wear a protective mask over the nose and mouth to prevent spreading the disease through infected droplets released into the air during speaking and coughing. In addition, you are required to report any diagnosis of tuberculosis to the local public health department. The treatment for tuberculosis includes a regimen of antibiotic therapy that lasts for months. You should provide emotional support for these patients, since the treatment lasts up to a year, and encourage compliance with the prescribed regimen at each office visit.

Common Cancers of the Respiratory System

Laryngeal Cancer

Cancer of the larynx is seen most commonly in heavy smokers and alcoholics. The presenting symptoms are usually hoarseness that lasts longer than 3 weeks, a feeling of a lump in the throat, or pain and burning in the throat when drinking citrus juice or hot liquids. A patient with laryngeal cancer may be treated with radiation, surgery, or both. Surgery usually is a **laryngectomy**, or removal of the larynx, and formation of a permanent **tracheostomy** stoma (FIG. 32-3). Patients who have had a laryngectomy are unable to speak normally but can be trained to use esophageal speech or a prosthetic speech device.

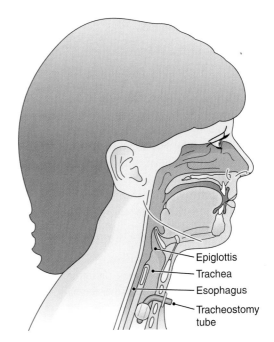

FIGURE 32-3. A tracheostomy tube in place. (Reprinted with permission from Cohen BJ. Medical Terminology: An Illustrated Guide. Philadelphia: Lippincott Williams & Wilkins, 2003.)

WHAT IF

A patient requires home oxygen therapy?

Many patients with severe COPD or end-stage lung cancer are discharged from the hospital with oxygen to use at home. Most surgical supply companies and pharmacies can arrange to have oxygen therapy equipment delivered to the home. The oxygen is usually supplied by a machine called a concentrator that runs on electricity. The concentrator separates oxygen out of room air and concentrates it for delivery to the patient. Attached to the cylinder is a flowmeter, or regulator, that indicates the amount of oxygen being delivered. The patient should be instructed to leave the oxygen at the setting prescribed by the physician. Too much oxygen can be toxic for some patients, such as those with emphysema. A cannula (plastic tube with pronged openings that fit into the nares) is attached to the flowmeter and delivers oxygen to the patient's airways. The company supplying the oxygen should instruct the patient regarding safe home oxygen administration. Since oxygen is highly flammable, you should reinforce safety precautions during oxygen use, including avoiding open flames and sparks. In addition, the supplier should be available 24 hours a day for emergency oxygen maintenance.

Lung Cancer

Lung cancer is one of the most common causes of death in both men and women. Cigarette smoking is believed to be the most common cause; 80% of lung cancer patients are smokers. Prognosis is generally poor for patients with lung cancer, with only 8% of men and 12% of women surviving for 5 years. One of the reasons is that symptoms tend to present rather late in the disease, when it has already had a chance to metastasize, or spread to other organs. Also, many of the symptoms are nonspecific and are seen in most heavy smokers. These symptoms include chronic cough, wheezing, dyspnea, **hemoptysis**, and chest pain.

Diagnosis of lung cancer is made by chest radiography, sputum cytology, bronchoscopy, biopsy, or **thoracentesis**. Treatment is generally **palliative**, giving relief but not a cure, and usually includes surgery, radiation, and chemotherapy. These treatments may improve the patient's prognosis and prolong survival.

Checkpoint Question

4. What factor appears to contribute to both laryngeal cancer and lung cancer?

COMMON DIAGNOSTIC AND THERAPEUTIC PROCEDURES

Physical Examination of the Respiratory System

The traditional examination of the chest consists of four parts: inspection, palpation, percussion, and auscultation. Each is briefly described in the next sections. For the physician to perform this examination efficiently, the patient should be sitting up, and all clothing should be removed from the waist up. The patient should be given a gown and draped appropriately (see Chapter 22).

Inspection

Inspection consists of a visual examination of the chest and the patient's respiratory pattern (TABLE 32-2). During inspection, the physician looks for abnormal shape of the thorax, use of accessory muscles to breathe, surgical scars, cyanosis, and any other visible signs of previous or current respiratory disease.

Palpation

In palpation, the physician uses his or her hands to feel the patient's throat for lumps, areas of tenderness, and location of the trachea, which may be displaced by a tumor. The patient may be asked to say "99" while the physician feels the chest wall in different places to assess the vibrations produced. Solid masses (such as tumors) or fluids (as in pneumonia) increase vibrations, whereas increased air (as seen in emphysema) reduce the vibrations.

Percussion

Percussion is placing a finger or fingers on the chest and striking it with the fingers of the other hand. The physician listens for the sound to determine whether it is normal (res-

Table 32-2	ABNORMAL RESPIRATORY PATTERNS
Pattern	**Description**
Apnea	No respirations
Bradypnea	Slow respirations
Cheyne-Stokes	Rhythmic cycles of dyspnea or hyperpnea subsiding gradually into brief apnea
Dyspnea	Difficult or labored respirations
Hypopnea	Shallow respirations
Hyperpnea	Deep respirations
Kussmaul	Fast and deep respirations
Orthopnea	Inability to breathe except while sitting or standing
Tachypnea	Fast respirations

Table 32-3	ABNORMAL BREATH SOUNDS
Breath Sound	**Description**
Bubbling	Gurgling sounds as air passes through moist secretions in airways.
Crackles (rales)	Crackling sound, usually inspiratory, as air passes through moist secretions in airways. Fine to medium crackles indicate secretions in small airways and alveoli. Medium to coarse crackles indicate secretions in larger airways.
Friction rub	Dry, rubbing or grating sound.
Rhonchi	Low-pitched, continuous sound as air moves past thick mucus or narrowed air passages.
Stertor	Snoring sound on inspiration or expiration; indicates a partial airway obstruction.
Stridor	Shrill, harsh inspiratory sound; indicates laryngeal obstruction
Wheeze	High-pitched musical sound, either inspiratory or expiratory; indicates partial airway obstruction

onant), like that produced by a drum. Dull or flat sounds are heard in patients with consolidation of pulmonary tissue, such as **atelectasis**, pneumonia, or a tumor. A hyperresonant sound is hollow and is heard in patients with emphysema.

Auscultation

Auscultation is listening to the patient's lungs and airway passages with a stethoscope. The physician systematically listens to each side of the chest in each area to compare the sounds bilaterally. The patient should breathe deeply, with an open mouth and the head turned away from the physician's face. The patient is encouraged not to breathe too rapidly to avoid hyperventilation, which can cause dizziness. During auscultation, the physician listens for abnormal or adventitious sounds, such as crackles and wheezes, which may also indicate a disease process (TABLE 32-3).

Checkpoint Question

5. What are the four parts of the chest examination?

Sputum Culture and Cytology

Sputum cultures are obtained to aid with diagnosis and treatment decisions in patients with suspected pneumonia, tuberculosis, or other infectious diseases of the lower airway. A microbiology laboratory will culture and incubate the specimen to identify any pathogenic microorganisms. Sputum specimens obtained for cytology are analyzed in the laboratory for abnormal cells that may indicate precancerous or cancerous conditions of the lung or airway. In all cases, it is important to obtain a specimen that the patient has coughed up and expectorated from the lower airways, with minimal contamination by oral and pharyngeal secretions. The patient is asked to cough deeply and collect the specimen in a sterile container (Procedure 32-1). After instructing the patient on coughing and collecting the specimen, you process the specimen and prepare the laboratory request for transportation to the laboratory for analysis.

Sputum collection for suspected cancer or for tuberculosis may be required over three consecutive mornings. The specimens should be brought into the office as soon as possible to avoid deterioration of the specimen. Most diagnostic specimens are obtained early in the morning, when the greatest volume of secretion has accumulated. If this is not possible, a specimen may also be collected after a nebulized breathing treatment with a bronchodilator (Procedure 32-3). The patient may be weak from illness and thick mucus difficult to bring up, and coughing may exhaust the patient. A cool-mist humidifier may be ordered for use at home to help loosen thick secretions. It is vitally important that the patient understand that the specimen must be collected from the lung fields and not from the mouth. The difference between saliva and sputum should be explained to the patient at his or her level of understanding.

Spanish Terminology

Tose con flema?	Do you cough up any phlegm?
De que color es la flema?	What color is it?
clara	Clear
blanca	White
amarilla	Yellow
verde	Green
oscura	Dark

Chest Radiography

Chest radiography can help in the diagnosis of a large variety of pulmonary problems, including pneumonia, lung cancer, emphysema, tuberculosis, and pulmonary edema. Often the physician orders two views: a posteroanterior (PA) view and a lateral view. This gives the physician a three-dimensional view. If the procedure is performed at the hospital or other outpatient facility, you may have to schedule it and request the results after the radiographs are interpreted by the radiologist.

Bronchoscopy

Bronchoscopy is an endoscopic procedure in which a lighted scope is inserted into the trachea and bronchi for direct visualization. This procedure is considered invasive and requires the patient's written consent. It is usually performed in an outpatient surgical setting, and you may have to schedule it. Bronchoscopy can be used for many diagnostic purposes, such as obtaining sputum specimens, obtaining tissue for biopsy, and visually assessing airway changes caused by chronic pulmonary diseases such as COPD or asthma. It can also be used therapeutically, for example to clear out mucus plugs or to remove a foreign body.

Pulmonary Function Tests

Pulmonary function tests are performed with a spirometer that measures the amount of air a patient can move in and out of the lungs (FIG. 32-4). The patient breathes into a mouthpiece and performs several breathing maneuvers that you explain during the test. By measuring the patient's airflow and comparing the results with predicted values for the patient's height, weight, gender, age, and race, the physician

FIGURE 32–4. A pulmonary function testing machine. (Courtesy of Spirometrics.)

TRIAGE

While working in a medical office, the following three situations are occurring:

A. An 8-year-old child with asthma arrives at the office wheezing. The doctor has ordered a nebulized treatment with a bronchodilator.

B. A 67-year-old man arrives at the office for a scheduled pulmonary function test. The patient's appointment was scheduled for 10 A.M. It is now 10:45 A.M. and the patient is very upset that he has had to wait this long.

C. The doctor has asked you to schedule a 34-year-old patient for a bronchoscopy to be done later this week.

How do you sort these patients? Whom do you see first? Second? Third?

Patient A should be seen first. Anyone who has trouble breathing or a respiratory problem must be treated as a priority. It is important to monitor this patient closely for any changes in condition before, during, and after treatment. Place patient B in an examination room and tell him that you will start his test within 10 minutes or advise him that he can reschedule the test for later this week. Inform patient C that you will schedule her procedure and notify her by phone of the exact date and time. Patients often become anxious about impending tests and can easily become upset with delays. Offer reassurance to the patient as needed.

gains valuable information concerning whether the patient has mild, moderate, or severe obstructive or restrictive disease. The patient's **tidal volume** and **forced expiratory volume** are two measurements that can be obtained during the pulmonary function test. Procedure 32-4 describes the steps for performing the pulmonary function test.

Arterial Blood Gases

Arterial blood gas (ABG) determinations measure the pH and pressures of oxygen and carbon dioxide in arterial blood. The results can indicate whether the patient's lungs are adequately exchanging gases. ABGs can also give information about metabolic acid-base problems, such as diabetic ketoacidosis. Drawing blood from an artery takes special training and is not routinely done in the medical office. However, you may be required to schedule a patient for an arterial puncture at a laboratory or hospital and record the results, which are usually phoned to the office.

Pulse Oximetry

Many medical offices have a pulse oximeter, which quickly and painlessly determines the percentage of oxygen saturation on a patient's capillary blood cells (FIG. 32-5). The pulse oximeter is small, fitting into the palm of the hand, and includes a digital display that notes the patient's pulse rate and oxygen saturation when a sensor cable is attached to the nail bed of the patient's index finger. Pulse oximeter readings should be obtained as a baseline for patients with chronic respiratory conditions and for patients with respiratory signs and symptoms, such as complaints of dyspnea or wheezing. The results should be recorded as a percentage; readings above 95% are considered normal. Although patients with chronic conditions such as emphysema may have readings of 90% or higher, readings below 90% should be reported to the physician immediately.

F I G U R E   3 2 – 5 .   Pulse oximetry is used to measure oxygen saturation of arterial blood. (Reprinted with permission from Cohen BJ. Medical Terminology: An Illustrated Guide. Philadelphia: Lippincott Williams & Wilkins, 2003.)

Checkpoint Question

6. What are the ways the physician can obtain information to help diagnose respiratory disorders?

Procedure 32-1

Collecting a Sputum Specimen

Purpose:	Instruct the patient on the correct procedure for obtaining a sputum specimen and then process the specimen.
Equipment:	Labeled sterile specimen container, gloves, laboratory request, biohazard bag for transporting the specimen.
Standard:	This procedure should take 5 minutes.

Steps	**Reason**
1. Wash your hands and put on clean examination gloves.	Handwashing aids infection control.
2. Assemble the equipment, greet and identify the patient, and explain the procedure. Write the patient's name on a label and affix to the outside of the container.	Identifying the patient avoids errors. Explanations will help gain compliance and ease anxiety.
3. Ask the patient to cough deeply, using the abdominal muscles as well as the accessory muscles to bring secretions from the lungs and not just the upper airways.	The specimen should contain pathogens from the lower respiratory tract rather than from the upper throat.

(continues)

Procedure 32-1 *(continued)*

Collecting a Sputum Specimen

Steps	Reason
4. Ask the patient to expectorate directly into the specimen container without touching the inside and without getting sputum on the outsides of the container. About 5–10 mL is sufficient for most sputum studies.	Touching the inside of the container will contaminate the container. Sputum on the outside of the container may be hazardous.
5. Handle the specimen container according to standard precautions. Cap the container immediately and put it into the biohazard bag for transport to the laboratory. Fill out a laboratory requisition slip to accompany the specimen.	The specimen may be hazardous, and capping the container immediately eliminates the danger of spreading microorganisms. A laboratory requisition will tell the laboratory personnel the type of specimen and specific tests ordered.
6. Properly care for or dispose of equipment and supplies, clean the work area, remove your gloves, and wash your hands.	Standard precautions must be followed throughout the procedure.
7. Send the specimen to the laboratory immediately to avoid compromising the test results.	If you delay, the pathogens may either proliferate, causing overgrowth, or die, causing a false-negative result.
8. Document the procedure.	Procedures are considered not to have been done if they are not documented.

Charting Example

07/03/2004 10:30 A.M. Moderate amount of thick, yellow sputum obtained and sent to ABC laboratory for a C & S as ordered per Dr. Smith. _____ J. Shapiro, CMA

Procedure 32-2

Instructing a Patient on Using the Peak Flowmeter

Purpose: Instruct the patient on the correct procedure for using and recording measurements using the peak flowmeter.

Equipment: Peak flowmeter, recording documentation form

Standard: This procedure should take 5 minutes.

Steps	Reason
1. Wash your hands.	Handwashing aids infection control.
2. Assemble the peak flow meter, disposable mouthpiece, and patient documentation form.	The flowmeter is used to instruct patients in performing a peak flow reading. A disposable mouthpiece should be used. In some offices, the patient is instructed using a peak flowmeter that is given to him or her to take home and use. In this case, no disposable mouthpiece is necessary.

Step 2. A peak flow documentation form.

Steps	Reason
3. Greet and identify the patient and explain the procedure.	Identifying the patient prevents errors.

(continues)

Procedure 32-2   *(continued)*

Instructing a Patient on Using the Peak Flowmeter

Steps	Reason
4. Holding the peak flowmeter upright, explain how to read and reset the gauge after each reading.	In the upright position, the meter is calibrated with numbers and contains a sliding gauge that should move freely up and down the meter next to the numbers.

Step 4. The peak flowmeter and sliding gauge.

Steps	Reason
5. Instruct the patient to put the peak flowmeter mouthpiece in the mouth, forming a tight seal with the lips. After taking a deep breath, the patient should blow hard into the mouthpiece without blocking the back of the flowmeter.	The patient should close the lips around the mouthpiece without biting down. Blocking the back of the flowmeter will interfere with the movement of the gauge.
6. Note the number on the flowmeter corresponding to the level at which the sliding gauge stopped after the patient blew hard into the mouthpiece. Reset the gauge to zero.	A normal range provided with the flowmeter is based on the patient's age, height, and weight. Ideally, the patient's readings should be within this range.
7. Instruct the patient to perform this procedure three times consecutively, in the morning and at night, and to record the highest reading on the form.	The highest reading is the patient's best reading. Recording the readings on the form allows the patient to follow his or her progress based on medication therapy or exposure to allergens.
8. Explain to the patient the procedure for cleaning the mouthpiece by washing with soapy water and rinsing without immersing the flowmeter in water.	Cleaning the mouthpiece is sanitary and prevents the spread of microorganisms.
9. Document the procedure.	Procedures are considered not to have been done if they are not recorded.

Charting Example

12/11/2004 3:30 P.M. Pt. instructed on using a flowmeter—return demonstration without difficulty, verbalized understanding. Given patient documentation form, instructed to record readings in morning and evening. Today's reading 400 LPM. No dyspnea or c/o wheezing, SOB. _____ E. Michael, RMA

Procedure 32-3

Performing a Nebulized Breathing Treatment

Purpose:	Set up and administer a nebulized breathing treatment in the office.
Equipment:	Physician's order, patient's medical record, inhalation medication, saline for inhalation, nebulizer disposable setup, nebulizer.
Standard:	This procedure should take 15 minutes.

Steps	Reason
1. Wash your hands.	Handwashing aids infection control.
2. Assemble the equipment and medication, checking the medication label three times, as when administering any medications.	Checking the medication label three times prevents errors.

Step 2. A nebulizer machine and disposable setup with mouthpiece.

Steps	Reason
3. Greet and identify the patient and explain the procedure.	Properly identifying the patient will avoid errors. Explaining the procedure promotes understanding and compliance.
4. Remove the nebulizer treatment cup from the setup and add the exact amount of medication ordered by the physician.	The physician bases the amount of bronchodilator on the age and weight of the patient.
5. Add 2–3 mL of saline for inhalation therapy to the cup that contains the medication.	The bronchodilator must be mixed with saline before being administered to the patient.

(continues)

Procedure 32-3   *(continued)*

Performing a Nebulized Breathing Treatment

Steps	Reason
6. Place the top on the cup securely, attach the T piece to the top of the cup, and position the mouthpiece firmly on one end of the T piece.	The top of the mouthpiece usually screws onto the bottom of the cup, providing a reservoir for the medication and saline.

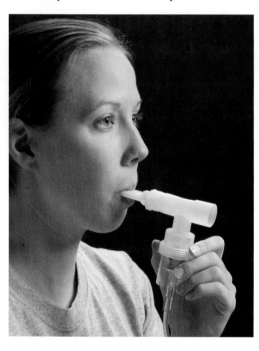

Step 6. The T piece and medication cup.

Steps	Reason
7. Attach one end of the tubing securely to the connector on the cup and the other end to the connector on the nebulizer machine.	
8. Ask the patient to put the mouthpiece in the mouth and make a seal with the lips without biting the mouthpiece. Instruct the patient to breathe normally during the treatment, occasionally taking a deep breath.	The patient may have difficulty breathing or be wheezing but should be encouraged to breathe as normally as possible. Breathing too rapidly may cause hyperventilation. Occasionally taking a deep breath will allow medication to be administered to deeper lung tissues.
9. Turn the machine on. The medication in the reservoir cup will become a fine mist to be inhaled by the patient.	A fine mist will come from the opposite end of the T piece when the patient exhales.
10. Before, during, and after the breathing treatment, take and record the patient's pulse.	Most bronchodilators cause a slight increase in the heart rate. Notify the physician if the increase is significant or if the patient has symptoms such as dizziness.

(continues)

Procedure 32-3 *(continued)*

Performing a Nebulized Breathing Treatment

Steps	Reason
11. When the treatment is over and the medication cup is empty, turn the machine off and have the patient remove the mouthpiece.	The treatment typically takes about 15 minutes.
12. Disconnect the disposable treatment setup and dispose of all parts in a biohazard container. Properly put away the machine.	The setup equipment, including the mouthpiece, may be contaminated with hazardous microorganisms and should be handled and disposed of properly.
13. Wash your hands and document the procedure, including the patient's pulse before, during, and after the treatment.	Procedures are considered not to have been done if they are not recorded. Again, the bronchodilator used for nebulized treatments may cause the heart rate to increase, and the pulse should be noted and recorded during and after the treatment.

Charting Example

11/26/2004 9:15 A.M. Pt. given nebulized breathing treatment with albuterol 2 mg and 3 mL NS for inhalation—pulse before treatment 88, during treatment 100, and after treatment 110. Pt. states she is "breathing easier" after treatment, skin warm and dry, color pink. Dr. Smith notified. _____ J. Barker, CMA

Perform a Pulmonary Function Test

Purpose:	Perform a pulmonary function test and record the procedure.
Equipment:	Physician's order, patient's medical record, spirometer and appropriate cables, calibration syringe and log book, disposable mouthpiece, printer, nose clip.
Standard:	This procedure should take 15 to 30 minutes.

Steps	Reason
1. Wash your hands.	Handwashing aids infection control.
2. Assemble the equipment, greet and identify the patient, and explain the procedure.	Identifying the patient prevents errors, and explaining the procedure promotes compliance.
3. Turn the pulmonary function test machine on, and if the spirometer has not been calibrated according to office policy, calibrate it using the calibration syringe according to the manufacturer's instructions. Record the calibration in the appropriate log book.	The spirometer must be calibrated daily to ensure accurate results.
4. With the machine on and calibrated, attach the appropriate cable, tubing, and mouthpiece according to the type of machine being used.	One cable is plugged into an electrical outlet, and another cable or tube is connected to the spirometer and the patient's mouthpiece.
5. Using the keyboard on the machine, enter the patient's name or identification number, age, weight, height, sex, race, and smoking history.	The spirometer automatically takes these parameters into consideration when providing the results.
6. Ask the patient to remove any restrictive clothing, such as a necktie, and show the patient how to apply the nose clip.	Restrictive clothing can stop the chest from fully expanding, causing an inaccurate result. The nose clip stops air from being expelled from the nose during the test.
7. Ask the patient to stand, breathe in deeply, and blow into the mouthpiece as hard as possible. The patient should continue to blow into the mouthpiece until the machine indicates that it is appropriate to stop blowing. A chair should be available in case the patient becomes dizzy or lightheaded.	Some machines signal to stop blowing with a buzz or beep; however, you may have to instruct the patient if the machine gives only a visual signal. Some patients become lightheaded during this procedure and should be observed closely for signs of difficulty or imbalance.
8. During the procedure, coach the patient as necessary to obtain an adequate reading.	Many patients feel that they have exhaled all air from the lungs when the machine is instructing them to continue. All air must be exhaled to obtain accurate results. The machine will indicate whether the reading or maneuver is adequate.
9. Continue the procedure until three adequate readings, or maneuvers, are performed.	Three maneuvers are usually required to obtain the patient's best result. The patient may rest between readings if necessary.
10. After printing the results, properly care for the equipment and dispose of the mouthpiece into the biohazard container. Wash your hands.	The mouthpiece may be contaminated and must be handled and discarded properly.
11. Document the procedure and place the printed results in the patient's medical record.	The three maneuvers will be recorded on one printout. Procedures are not considered to have been done if not properly recorded.

Charting Example

06/12/2004 3:00 P.M. PFT performed for employment physical as ordered by Dr. John. 3 maneuvers obtained without difficulty. Dr. John notified of results in chart _____ P. Hill, CMA

CHAPTER SUMMARY

The respiratory system provides the body with oxygen, the essential ingredient required for cell metabolism. Without oxygen, cells quickly cease to function and die. The respiratory system also removes carbon dioxide, a chemical that causes acidosis. Because it is open to the atmosphere, the respiratory system is susceptible to infection and irritant injury. You can play an important role in helping the patient to maintain healthy lungs and in assisting the physician to diagnose and treat respiratory disease.

Critical Thinking Challenges

1. Why do you think it is better to inhale through the nose than through the mouth?
2. Mr. Gardner, aged 55, has been diagnosed with COPD and has many questions about his condition. Identify the characteristics of COPD. How do you explain this disease to Mr. Gardner? Develop educational materials on COPD that can be given to all patients with this disorder.

Answers to Checkpoint Questions

1. The onset of bacterial pneumonia is usually sudden and severe; symptoms include fever, cough, chills, and dyspnea. This type of pneumonia is typically local. In contrast, the onset of viral pneumonia is usually gradual; symptoms include fever and a hacking cough. Unlike bacterial pneumonia, viral pneumonia tends to be spread throughout the lung fields.
2. Factors that may trigger an asthma attack are environmental allergens, irritants, infection, stress, cold air, and exercise.
3. The two disease processes in a patient with COPD are chronic bronchitis and emphysema.
4. Cigarette smoking may contribute to both laryngeal cancer and lung cancer.
5. The four parts of the chest examination are inspection, percussion, palpation, and auscultation.
6. The methods of diagnosing respiratory disorders are physical examination, peak flowmeter readings, sputum cultures, chest radiography, bronchoscopy, pulmonary function testing, assessment of arterial blood gases, and pulse oximeter readings.

 Websites

Center for Disease Control and Prevention
   http://www.cdc.gov
American Lung Association http://www.lungusa.org
American Association of Respiratory Care
   http://www.acr.org
American Thoracic Society http://www.thoracic.org
American Cancer Society http://www.cancer.org

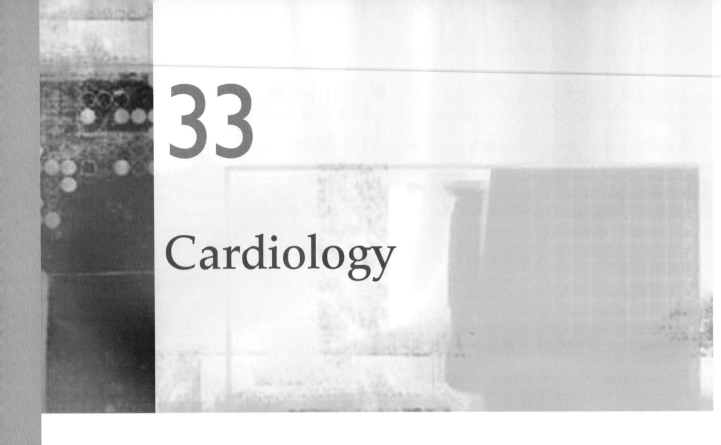

33

Cardiology

CHAPTER OUTLINE

ROLE DELINEATION

ADMINISTRATIVE: ADMINISTRATIVE PROCEDURES
- Perform basic administrative medical assisting functions

CLINICAL: FUNDAMENTAL PRINCIPLES
- Apply principles of aseptic technique and infection control
- Comply with quality assurance practices
- Screen and follow up patient test results

CLINICAL: DIAGNOSTIC ORDERS
- Perform diagnostic tests

CLINICAL: PATIENT CARE
- Adhere to established patient screening procedures
- Obtain patient history and vital signs
- Prepare patient for examinations, procedures, and treatments
- Assist with examinations, procedures, and treatments
- Recognize and respond to emergencies
- Coordinate patient care information with other health care providers

GENERAL: PROFESSIONALISM
- Display a professional manner and image
- Demonstrate initiative and responsibility

- Work as a member of the health care team
- Prioritize and perform multiple tasks
- Treat all patients with compassion and empathy

GENERAL: COMMUNICATION SKILLS
- Recognize and respect cultural diversity
- Adapt communications to individual's ability to understand
- Recognize and respond effectively to verbal, nonverbal, and written communications
- Serve as a liaison

GENERAL: LEGAL CONCEPTS
- Perform within legal and ethical boundaries
- Prepare and maintain medical records
- Document accurately
- Comply with established risk management and safety procedures

GENERAL: INSTRUCTION
- Instruct individuals according to their needs
- Teach methods of health promotion and disease prevention
- Locate community resources and disseminate information

CHAPTER COMPETENCIES

LEARNING OBJECTIVES
Upon successfully completing this chapter, you will be able to:
1. Spell and define the key terms.
2. List and describe common cardiovascular disorders.
3. Identify and explain common cardiovascular procedures and tests.
4. Describe the role and responsibilities of the medical assistant during cardiovascular examinations and procedures.
5. Discuss the information recorded on a basic 12-lead electrocardiogram.
6. Explain the purpose of a Holter monitor.

PERFORMANCE OBJECTIVES
Upon successfully completing this chapter, you will be able to:
1. Perform a basic 12-lead electrocardiogram (Procedure 33-1)
2. Apply a Holter monitor for a 24-hour test (Procedure 33-2)

KEY TERMS

aneurysm	cerebrovascular accident (CVA)	lead	pericarditis
angina pectoris		myocardial infarction (MI)	tachycardia
artifact	congestive heart failure	myocarditis	transient ischemic attack (TIA)
atherosclerosis	electrocardiography	palpitations	
bradycardia	coronary artery bypass graft	percutaneous transluminal coronary angioplasty (PTCA)	
cardiomegaly	endocarditis		
cardiomyopathy			

CARDIOVASCULAR DISEASE is a major cause of illness and death. The cardiologist is a physician who specializes in disorders of the heart, and many patients with chronic cardiac conditions are referred to the cardiology office for treatment and follow-up. However, many of these patients are seen in internal medicine or family practice medical offices also. Because medical assistants see patients who have cardiovascular disorders regardless of the medical specialty, you must understand the cardiovascular system, associated disorders, and common tests and procedures that are ordered for diagnosis and treatment.

COMMON CARDIOVASCULAR DISORDERS

The cardiovascular system consists of the heart (FIG. 33-1) and blood vessels, including the arteries, capillaries, and veins. The rhythmic contractions of the heart pump

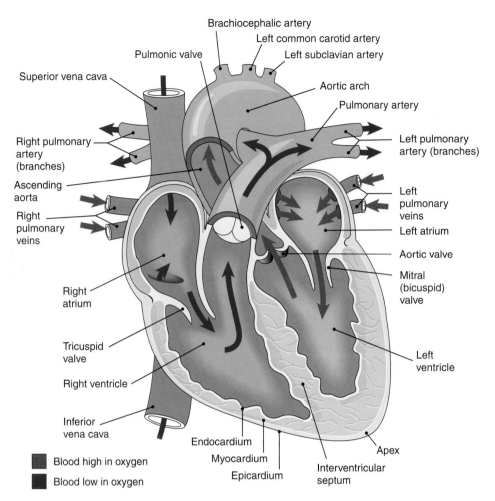

FIGURE 33–1.   The heart and great vessels. (Reprinted with permission from Cohen BJ, Wood DL. Memmler's The Human Body in Health and Disease. Philadelphia: Lippincott Williams & Wilkins, 2000.)

oxygen-rich blood from the lungs throughout the body to oxygenate and nourish the tissues and remove wastes for elimination. While the heart and blood vessels are a closed system for the flow of blood (Fig. 33-2), disorders anywhere in this system may adversely affect other body systems that depend on the cardiovascular system for delivery of oxygen and nutrients. Depending on the body system affected by the lack of oxygen and nutrients being delivered, these can be symptoms of various heart disorders:

- Chest pain
- Dyspnea
- Fatigue
- Diaphoresis
- Nausea and vomiting
- Irregular heartbeat
- Changes in peripheral circulation
- Edema
- Skin ulcers that do not heal
- Pain that increases with walking and decreases with rest
- Changes in skin color

While some of these symptoms can indicate disorders not related to the heart or blood vessels, you should obtain an accurate history and chief complaint and communicate any finding to the physician through complete documentation.

DISORDERS OF THE HEART

Carditis

Cardiac inflammation, or carditis, may affect any of the layers of the heart muscle, and although other factors may be involved, it is usually the result of a systemic infection. **Pericarditis**, an inflammation of the sac that covers the outside of the heart, may be acute or chronic. It is caused by a pathogen, neoplasm, or autoimmune disorder, such as lupus erythematosus or rheumatoid arthritis. Other causes of pericarditis include certain chemicals, radiation, and uremia in patients with kidney failure. Signs and symptoms include a sharp pain in the same locations as with a **myocardial infarction**, except that pain increases on inspiration and on lying down but decreases on sitting up and leaning forward. Dyspnea, tachycardia, neck venous

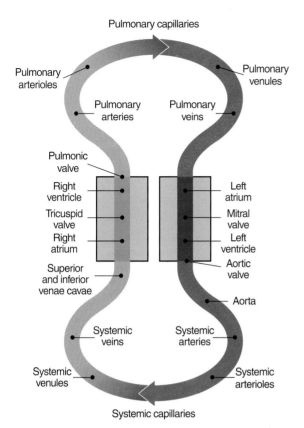

Pulmonary capillaries

Pulmonary arterioles

Pulmonary arteries

Pulmonary venules

Pulmonary veins

Pulmonic valve

Right ventricle

Tricuspid valve

Right atrium

Left atrium

Mitral valve

Left ventricle

Aortic valve

Superior and inferior venae cavae

Aorta

Systemic veins

Systemic arteries

Systemic venules

Systemic arterioles

Systemic capillaries

FIGURE 33–2. Blood vessels form a closed system for the flow of blood. Blood high in oxygen (oxygenated) is shown in red; blood low in oxygen (deoxygenated) is shown in blue. Changes in oxygen content occur as blood flows through capillaries. (Reprinted with permission from Cohen BJ, Wood DL. Memmler's The Human Body in Health and Disease. Philadelphia: Lippincott Williams & Wilkins, 2000.)

distention, pallor, and hypertension are warning signs that serous fluid is compressing the heart and interfering with cardiac function. Treatment is relieving the symptoms and if possible correcting the underlying cause, including administering an antibiotic for bacterial infection.

Myocarditis may be diffused through the heart muscle or may be local to a focal point. Causes include radiation, chemicals, and bacterial, viral, or parasitic infection. Signs and symptoms of early acute episodes are usually nonspecific: fatigue, fever, and mild chest pain. Chronic cases may lead to heart failure with **cardiomegaly** (an enlarged heart muscle), arrhythmias, and valvulitis. Treatment is supportive care and medication as ordered by the physician to kill the responsible pathogen.

Chronic or acute **endocarditis** is infection or inflammation of the inner lining of the heart, the endocardium. The lining of the heart and its valves may gather clusters of platelets, fibrin, and white blood cells to trap the pathogens. These clusters, called vegetations, may break away to become emboli that travel to the spleen, kidneys, lungs, or nervous system. These formations may also scar the valves and

erode the chordae tendinea, small tendons that attach the heart valves to the ventricles. The destruction of these structures may result in reflux, or backflow, of the valves or blood. Diagnosis of endocarditis requires a blood culture to identify the causative agent. Treatment is directed at eliminating the infecting organism.

 Checkpoint Question

1. How does the pain in pericarditis differ from pain of myocardial infarction?

Congestive Heart Failure

Congestive heart failure (CHF) is a condition in which the heart cannot pump effectively. Failure of the right ventricle causes congestion of the peripheral extremities, while failure of the left ventricle leads to pulmonary congestion. Many patients have failure of both sides of the heart; their signs and symptoms include edema of the lower extremities and dyspnea. As blood flow to organs such as the brain and kidneys decreases, patients may also have complaints related to the organs involved. Progressive heart failure results in damage to vital organs and death.

The causes of CHF include coronary artery disease, myocardial disease, valvular heart disease, and hypertension. While there is no cure for it, treatment is aimed at relieving symptoms and preventing permanent damage to vital organs. Medications given to CHF patients include drugs to increase cardiac function and decrease edema.

Myocardial Infarction

Death of any part of the heart muscle, called myocardial infarction (MI), occurs when one or more of the coronary arteries becomes totally occluded, usually by atherosclerotic plaques or by an embolism. An MI may occur suddenly without prior symptoms or in patients with diagnosed atherosclerotic coronary artery disease. Symptoms of myocardial infarction may be similar to those felt during **angina pectoris** in patients with ischemic heart disease, but this disorder is distinguished by pain that lasts longer than 20 to 30 minutes and is unrelieved by rest. Box 33-1 describes criteria that the physician will use to distinguish the chest pain of angina pectoris from the chest pain of MI. Other symptoms include nausea, diaphoresis, weakness, vomiting, and abdominal cramps. The patient may complain of feeling a vise-like grip around the chest cavity. The skin may become cool, clammy, and pale, and the patient may feel anxiety or impending doom. Some patients have nonspecific symptoms such as indigestion and therefore do not seek medical attention. In 20% of patients, the MI may be silent, diagnosed only by routine **electrocardiography** (ECG). It is imperative not to ignore or dismiss complaints by patients with symptoms of MI or to accept the patient's own diagnosis that

Box 33-1

IS IT ANGINA OR MYOCARDIAL INFARCTION?

The pain felt with angina and MI is brought about by myocardial anoxia, or increased need for oxygen to the heart muscle because of exertion, stress, or extremes of heat or cold. Typically, angina is relieved by rest or nitroglycerin, a vasodilator. However, pain from a MI is not relieved by these measures. This is a brief comparison of these two disorders:

	Angina	**Myocardial Infarction**
Description	Moderate pressure deep in the chest; squeezing, suffocating feeling.	Severe deep pressure not relieved by reducing stressors; crushing pressure.
Onset	Pain gradual or sudden; subsides quickly, usually in less than 30 minutes; can be relieved by nitroglycerin, rest, reducing stressors.	Pain sudden; remains after stressors reduced or relieved; not relieved by nitroglycerin, which may be given every 5 min for total of three doses in 10 min
Location	Mid anterior chest, usually diffuse, radiates to back, neck, arms, jaw, epigastric area	Mid anterior chest with same radiating patterns
Signs and symptoms	Dyspnea, nausea, signs of indigestion, profuse sweating	Nausea, vomiting, fear, diaphoresis, pounding heart, palpitations

Any patient who calls the medical office complaining of chest pain must be examined immediately. The office should have an established protocol for handling these calls. The physician must be consulted to decide whether the patient should be directed to the nearest emergency department or come directly to the office.

"it's only indigestion." Although the death of myocardial tissue that occurs during an MI cannot be reversed, early medical intervention may reduce the amount of tissue that dies and increase the patient's chances of survival. Procedures such as **percutaneous transluminal coronary angioplasty** (PTCA) and **coronary artery bypass graft** (CABG) are performed to increase blood flow to the cardiac muscle (Box 33-2).

Cardiac Arrhythmia

When the electrical conduction system of the heart is not functioning normally, cardiac arrhythmias may develop and can be detected on the electrocardiography. Cardiac arrhythmia or dysrhythmia is an abnormal heart rhythm that may occur as a primary disorder or as a response to a systemic problem. Arrhythmia may also be a reaction to a drug toxicity or an electrolyte imbalance. Normally, the sinoatrial (SA) node is the pacemaker of the heart (FIG. 33-3), initiating an electrical impulse in the adult at rest 60 to 100 times a minute. This is sinus rhythm. Arrhythmia may occur if the SA node initiates electrical impulses too fast or too slowly. If the SA node is damaged or the conduction pathway is blocked, the heart will beat too slowly to meet the body's demands. This type of arrhythmia, called **bradycardia**, is characterized by a heart rate less than 60 beats per minute. If the SA node initiates an electrical impulse faster than 100 times per minute, the arrhythmia is called **tachycardia**.

More serious arrhythmias occur when the ventricles beat too fast, a condition known as ventricular tachycardia (VT). This condition occurs when some of the electrical signals originate in the ventricles rather than in the SA node. Once the ventricles begin to beat at a very rapid rate, less blood is pumped out of the heart with each contraction, since the heart's chambers do not have time to fill with blood before the next contraction begins. As less blood is pumped into circulation, less oxygen is carried to the tissues. This lack of adequate blood and oxygen may cause dizziness, unconsciousness, or cardiac arrest.

Another arrhythmia is ventricular fibrillation. Ventricular fibrillation is a medical emergency that occurs when the heart is quivering rather than contracting in an organized fashion. In this condition, very little blood is pumped out of the heart, and the patient will fall unconscious and die very quickly unless a shock with a cardiac defibrillator is administered immediately to restore normal cardiac electrical activity. Automatic external defibrillators (AED) are now available in many medical offices and public places, such as airports and shopping malls. All professional medical assistants should receive certification in cardiopulmonary resuscitation (CPR) and use of the AED, which is relatively easy to operate (Box 33-3). Patients who require frequent defibrillation may benefit from the insertion of an implantable cardiac defibrillator that will automatically deliver an electrical shock to restore normal cardiac conduction. These devices should not be confused with cardiac pacemakers, which help to regulate the normal rhythm of the heart (Box 33-4).

Box 33-2

CORRECTIVE CARDIAC SURGERY

The least traumatic form of cardiac surgery is the *percutaneous transluminal coronary angioplasty (PTCA)*. A double-lumen catheter with a balloon surrounding the upper portion is inserted into a vessel in the groin or axilla. This catheter is threaded into the coronary vessels, with the surgeon watching a fluoroscopic screen while performing the procedure. When the occlusion is found, the balloon is inflated to press the atherosclerotic plaque against the arterial walls and relieve the occlusion. A laser may be used to remove the plaque. A spring or mesh (called a stent) may be inserted and left in place within the vessel to maintain patency. This procedure is less invasive than bypass surgery, but occasionally the artery rebuilds plaque at the site, or the stent may fill with plaque and the artery occlude again.

Coronary artery bypass graft (CABG) is performed by grafting a piece of vessel from another part of the body to the area beyond the occlusion and to the ascending aorta, providing a patent passage for the blood. The surgery requires a still field of surgery, so the heart must be stopped and the patient supported by a cardiopulmonary bypass machine for the length of the operation. The saphenous vein may be used for multiple bypasses; the internal mammary artery is used if the surgery is not extensive. Hospitalization may be as long as 5 to 7 days, and 20% of patients develop a repeat thrombus within 1 year.

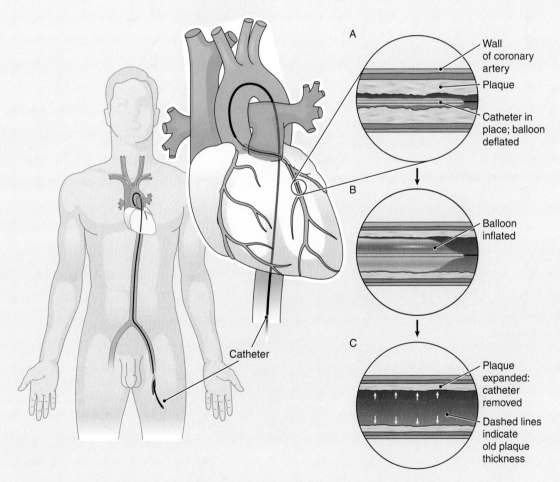

Coronary angioplasty (PTCA). (A) A guide catheter is threaded into the coronary artery. (B) A balloon catheter is inserted through the occlusion. (C) The balloon is inflated and deflated until plaque is flattened and the vessel is opened. (Reprinted with permission from Cohen BJ. Medical Terminology: An Illustrated Guide. Philadelphia: Lippincott Williams & Wilkins, 2003.)

PATIENT EDUCATION

Nitroglycerin

A medication commonly prescribed to increase blood flow to the cardiac muscle is nitroglycerin, a vasodilator. Vasodilators open the lumen of vessels, increasing blood supply to the heart muscle. Patient education should include the following instructions:

- Keep the medication in the dark bottle supplied by the pharmacy, because nitroglycerin can be deactivated if exposed to light.
- Be alert for any side effects, such as light-headedness, syncope, and hypotension. Caution patients not to drive or operate other machinery until these symptoms have passed.
- Be aware that nitroglycerin may be prescribed and dispensed as either tablets or a spray to be used as needed, or it may be ordered as a transdermal patch worn constantly to maintain vasodilation. The usual administration guidelines are for three doses at 5-minute intervals. If pain persists, the patient should be advised to call for emergency medical services.
- Patients with arthritis or visual impairment should use nitroglycerin spray. These patients may find the spray easier to use than tablets, since the tablets are very small.
- Check the expiration date of the medication frequently, and always have an adequate supply available at home and when traveling.
- Encourage patients prescribed nitroglycerin to obtain and wear a Medic-Alert bracelet or necklace. In the event of an emergency, first responders can assist with administering this medication if necessary.
- Ensure that the medication is kept out of the reach of children.

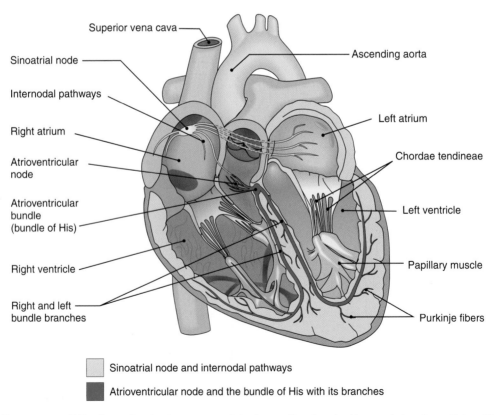

FIGURE 33–3. Conduction system of the heart. (Reprinted with permission from Cohen BJ, Wood DL. Memmler's The Human Body in Health and Disease. Philadelphia: Lippincott Williams & Wilkins, 2000.)

THE AUTOMATIC EXTERNAL DEFIBRILLATOR

The automatic external defibrillator (AED) is becoming more widely supplied in public places and medical offices because of the minimal training required and potential to save the life of a patient with sudden cardiac arrest without waiting for emergency medical services or transportation to a hospital. The device is a small defibrillator in a zippered bag that is usually orange or red with the acronym *AED* written clearly on the front. Inside the bag are also disposable chest pads connected to a cord that is inserted into the connection on the AED. A small washcloth for drying the skin before placing the chest pads if necessary, disposable razor to shave excess chest hair, and examination gloves in the event of possible exposure to blood or other body fluids during the procedure may be added to the AED bag, since these items may be necessary to ensure adequate contact between the patient's skin and the chest pads. In the event that an unconscious patient or victim is found with no pulse (refer to cardiopulmonary resuscitation criteria), the rescuer should apply the chest pads as trained, and using the pictures provided on the pads as a guide, connect the cable to the machine and turn the machine on. The machine has verbal commands to guide the user through the steps necessary to provide an electrical shock if necessary. Do not touch or move the patient while the machine is analyzing the patient's cardiac rhythm or when the machine determines that an electrical shock is necessary.

Checkpoint Question

2. Which two cardiac arrhythmias are emergencies requiring immediate intervention by the medical assistant?

Congenital and Valvular Heart Disease

Valvular disease is an acquired or congenital abnormality of any of the four cardiac valves. Valvular heart disease is characterized by stenosis and obstructed blood flow or by valvular degeneration and backflow of the blood against the course of the circulatory pathway. The valves in the left side of the heart are most often affected. The most common congenital valve diseases include atrial septal defect (ASD), ventricular septal defect (VSD), patent ductus arteriosus (PDA), coarctation of the aorta, aortic or pulmonic stenosis, bicuspid aortic valve, mitral valve prolapse, and tetralogy of Fallot (TABLE 33-1).

Rheumatic heart disease, an acquired valvular disease, presents clinically as a generalized inflammatory disease occurring 10 to 21 days after an upper respiratory infection caused by group A beta-hemolytic streptococci. It is characterized by inflammatory lesions of the connective tissues, particularly in the heart, joints, and subcutaneous tissues. The heart valves are damaged by an abnormal response of the immune system caused by the turbulence of the infected blood. This damage results in a systolic murmur. Although it usually attacks children aged 5 to 15, rheumatic heart disease has declined significantly since the 1940s in North America and Western Europe as a result of improved health care and the availability of antibiotics.

Mitral valve stenosis, a condition that occurs when the leaflet cusps of the mitral valve fuse and thicken, may result from rheumatic heart disease. When the valve cusps thicken and fuse, the result is an abnormally narrow valve, hence mitral regurgitation, or backflow, of blood from the left ventricle into the left atrium. Patients with mitral stenosis often have dyspnea, or shortness of breath, and their ability to exert themselves physically may be limited. Pulmonary edema

ARTIFICIAL PACEMAKERS

When a patient's heart conduction system cannot maintain normal sinus rhythm without assistance, an electrical source can be implanted to assist or replace the sinoatrial node. The permanent or temporary artificial pacemaker is surgically implanted either between the chest wall and the rib cage or within the chest cavity. The pacemaker may be programmed to fire, or initiate an electrical charge, continuously at a predetermined rate or on demand, only when the patient's normal heart rate falls below a preset number.

Pacemaker programming initially occurs when the pacemaker is inserted in an outpatient or inpatient surgical facility. If additional programming or assessment is necessary, the pacemaker may be evaluated by telephone monitoring: the patient uses the telephone receiver to transmit the rate and function of the pacemaker to a physician at the receiving site. If battery function is failing and replacement is not possible or advisable, batteries can be recharged transdermally. A charging unit is placed over the implantation site and plugged into an ordinary electrical outlet. The power cell is recharged through the skin with no discomfort to the patient. Pacemakers are battery operated and usually are manufactured to retain their charge for up to 20 years. Recharging or changing the battery in an implanted pacemaker usually requires an outpatient surgical procedure under a local anesthetic.

Table 33-1	DISEASES OF THE CARDIAC VALVES AND CONGENTIAL CARDIAC DEFECTS	
Disorder	**Description**	**Treatment**
ASD	Abnormal opening between atria, allowing unoxygenated blood in right atrium to mix with oxygenated blood in left atrium; congenital.	Surgery to close.
VSD	Abnormal opening between ventricles, allowing unoxygenated blood in right ventricle to mix with oxygenated blood in left ventricle; congenital.	Surgery to close.
PDA	Abnormal opening between pulmonary artery and aorta; congenital.	Surgery to close.
Coarctation of the aorta	Narrowing of aorta resulting in high blood pressure in upper extremities and low blood pressure in lower extremities; congenital.	Surgery to increase diameter of aorta.
Bicuspid aortic valve	Aortic valve having 2 cusps instead of 3, resulting in incomplete closure between aorta and left ventricle during systole and diastole; congenital.	Surgical replacement of aortic valve.
Aortic or pulmonic stenosis	Narrowing of aortic or pulmonary artery valve leaflets, causing overwork of cardiac muscle and hypertrophy of ventricles; as stenosis increases, valve becomes less flexible	Dilation of stenosed area or surgical replacement of valve.
MVP	Drooping of one or both cusps of mitral (bicuspid) valve into left ventricle during systole, resulting in incomplete closure of valve, backflow of blood from left ventricle into left atrium.	Usually benign; treatment is alleviating any symptoms (palpitations, chest pain). Prophylactic antibiotic may be ordered before dental procedures.
Tetralogy of Fallot	Four defects: pulmonary stenosis, dextroposition of aorta, ventricular septal defect, hypertrophy of right ventricle. Congenital.	Surgery to correct.

ASD, atrial septal defect; VSD, ventricular septal defect; PDA, patent ductus arteriosus; MVP, mitral valve prolapse.

may also develop and cause symptoms such as dyspnea and a productive cough.

Treatment of valvular disease depends on the type and severity of the abnormality. Severe cases may require medication, low-sodium diet, and prophylactic antibiotic before surgery or dental work. If medication is not successful, surgical replacement of the involved valves may be necessary.

Checkpoint Question

3. What microorganism may be responsible for rheumatic heart disease and cardiac valvular damage?

DISORDERS OF THE BLOOD VESSELS

Atherosclerosis

Diseases of blood vessels—arteries or veins—often begin with collection of fatty plaques made of calcium and cholesterol inside the walls of the vessels. These plaques narrow the lumen, or opening, of the blood vessels and impede blood flow. This condition known as **atherosclerosis** is problematic in arteries, as oxygen and nutrients are prevented from reaching various tissues of the body. In addition to the occlusion that occurs with atherosclerosis, the plaques are rougher than the walls of a normal artery and may remain stationary as a thrombus or break away from

Spanish Terminology

Tiene la presión alta?	Do you have high blood pressure?
Tiene dolor en el pecho?	Do you have chest pain?
Ha sentido dolor en el brazo izquierdo?	Have you ever had pain in the left arm?
Tiene mareos?	Do you have dizzy spells?

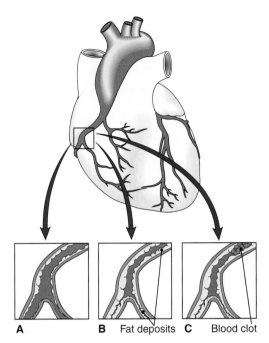

FIGURE 33–4. Coronary atherosclerosis. (A) Fat deposits narrow an artery, leading to ischemia. (B) Blockage of the coronary artery. (C) Formation of a blood clot (thrombus), leading to MI. (Reprinted with permission from Cohen BJ, Wood DL. Memmler's The Human Body in Health and Disease. Philadelphia: Lippincott Williams & Wilkins, 2000.)

the wall of the artery as an embolus (FIG. 33-4). Signs and symptoms of atherosclerosis usually result from ischemia to a body part and may include pain or numbness, loss of normal blood flow, or loss of a palpable pulse to the affected body area.

If the coronary arteries are involved, the condition is coronary artery disease (CAD), the most common type of heart disease and the leading cause of death in men and women in the United States. Patients with CAD may have these symptoms:

- Angina pectoris (pain radiating to the arm, jaw, shoulder, back, or neck, usually felt on exertion and relieved by rest)
- Pressure or fullness in the chest, felt most severely during exertion and relieved by rest
- Syncope (fainting)
- Edema of the extremities, especially the legs
- Unexplained cough, generally without respiratory symptoms
- Excessive fatigue
- Dyspnea

Predisposing conditions for atherosclerosis and coronary artery disease (CAD) include a diet high in saturated fats and a family history of hypercholesterolemia. Other risk factors include cigarette smoking, diabetes mellitus, and hypertension. Consuming a diet low in cholesterol and saturated fats, participating in a moderate exercise pro-

gram, maintaining normal body weight and blood pressure, and not smoking may minimize the chances for developing atherosclerosis and CAD or reduce the progression if a diagnosis has been made. If necessary, the physician may order lipid-lowering medication for patients whose blood cholesterol and triglyceride levels are not affected by dietary or other behavioral changes.

Diagnosis of atherosclerosis is often made by angiography to locate the occlusion and evaluate the degree of obstruction (FIG. 33-5). In this procedure, a catheter is inserted into the blood vessel, and radiographic images are taken as a contrast medium is injected into the vessel. The radiographs are evaluated for the presence and amount of plaque buildup or the presence of a thrombus. Doppler ultrasonography, a test that uses sound waves to produce an image of the blood vessel, may also be ordered to detect atherosclerosis. Doppler ultrasonography, or echocardiography, can be used to determine the ability of the heart to fill and pump blood. This noninvasive test uses sound waves to produce a picture of the heart on a video monitor to detect areas of poor blood flow or damaged muscle.

A relatively new noninvasive test for CAD is electron beam computed tomography (CT), also known as cardiac calcium scoring. In this procedure, CT of the coronary arteries using an electron beam identifies the amount of fat and calcium buildup within the coronary arteries. An elevated score indicates an increased risk for developing CAD, especially if other risk factors are present.

The treatment for atherosclerosis often includes lifestyle changes as described earlier to reverse or prevent further atherosclerotic formations. If the condition is severe, lipid-lowering medication may be prescribed. Surgery to remove the plaque or improve blood flow through an artery may also be indicated for some patients. Your responsibilities will include coordinating diagnostic procedures based on the physician's orders and insurance requirements and teaching patients about behaviors that

FIGURE 33–5. Atherosclerotic coronary occlusion. (Reprinted with permission from Rubin E, Farber JL. Pathology. Philadelphia: Lippincott Williams & Wilkins, 1999.)

can prevent atherosclerosis and CAD. Patients diagnosed with atherosclerosis and CAD require emotional support to encourage compliance with medication and lifestyle changes, such as diet and exercise.

 Checkpoint Question

4. What are four predisposing factors for heart disease?

Hypertension

Patients with a resting systolic blood pressure above 140 mm Hg and a diastolic pressure above 90 mm Hg are said to be hypertensive. Hypertension cannot be diagnosed on the basis of one blood pressure measurement, since other factors, such as emotional upset or anxiety may cause a temporary increase in blood pressure. Since many factors may affect the blood pressure, the physician often requires several blood pressure readings before making the diagnosis of hypertension. However, once the diagnosis is made, you may play a major role in assisting with the control of this condition by regularly monitoring the patient's blood pressure and medication prescriptions; teaching the patient about dietary and lifestyle changes, such as smoking cessation and weight loss; and recording complete and accurate information regarding the medical history each time the patient visits the office.

One type of hypertension, essential hypertension, is a major cause of stroke and renal failure and is a major consequence of atherosclerosis anywhere in the circulatory system. The long-term effects of essential hypertension may include weakening of the arteries throughout the body and enlargement of the left ventricle of the heart. Left ventricular hypertrophy, or enlargement, occurs gradually as the heart works harder to overcome the higher pressure in the arteries. Essential hypertension is often called a silent killer, since the disease is gradual and frequently produces no symptoms in the patient, striking anyone regardless of age, race, sex, or ethnic origin.

Malignant hypertension is severe and sudden in onset and is most common in African-American men under age 40 years regardless of other risk factors. Patients with malignant hypertension have signs and symptoms including diastolic blood pressure higher than 120 mm Hg and blurred vision, headache, and possibly confusion. The physician should be notified immediately if these symptoms are present.

While the cause of essential hypertension may be unknown, its correlation with an elevated serum cholesterol level has been shown. After diagnosis, some patients can control the high blood pressure with a low-sodium, low-fat diet, an exercise program, weight reduction if needed, and antihypertensive and lipid-reducing medications. Diuretic medication may be prescribed to reduce the amount of sodium in the body, which in turn reduces the total fluid volume. The decrease in fluid volume reduces strain on the heart and blood vessels. Patients should also be informed of methods to reduce the cholesterol and triglycerides in their diet.

Patients who have been prescribed antihypertensive medications should be instructed to take that medication as prescribed. Many patients feel that because their blood pressure has reached a manageable level, they do not need to continue the prescribed medication. Explain that the medication is the cause of the lowered blood pressure and that discontinuing the treatment without consulting the physician may jeopardize their recovery.

 Checkpoint Question

5. Which two disorders may result from untreated hypertension?

Varicose Veins

Varicosities, the most common circulatory disease of the lower extremities, occur when the superficial veins of the legs swell and distend (FIG. 33-6). Eventually the valves in the veins fail to close properly, allowing blood to pool and stretch the walls of the veins. People who sit or stand for long periods without moving or contracting their leg muscles are

FIGURE 33–6. Varicose veins of the lower extremities. (Reprinted with permission from Bickley LS, Szilagyi PG. Bates' Guide to Physical Examination and History Taking. Philadelphia: Lippincott Williams & Wilkins, 2003.)

predisposed to varicose veins. A hereditary weakness in the vein walls is also a predisposing factor. Varicosities may also be secondary to deep-vein thrombosis. Signs and symptoms of varicose veins are swelling, aching, and a feeling of heaviness in the legs. Varicosities may also be asymptomatic. Many patients consider varicose veins unattractive and seek treatment even without symptoms.

Treatment of varicose veins is usually conservative, with instructions to avoid standing or sitting for long periods to reduce symptoms and prevent the development of further varicosities. Other helpful measures that may be ordered by the physician include wearing elastic support stockings or wrapping the legs with elastic bandages and elevating the legs for specified periods. Surgery to remove the veins is usually the last approach. A newer treatment technique is injection of a sclerosing agent into small varicose vein segments, but this is not suggested for large areas.

Venous Thrombosis and Pulmonary Embolism

Thrombi, or blood clots, in the peripheral or pulmonary veins commonly affect patients with underlying cardiovascular disease. Risk factors for developing thrombi may be either primary (inherited) or secondary (acquired). Primary causes include hemolytic anemia and sickle cell disease, and secondary factors include long-term immobility, chronic pulmonary disease, thrombophlebitis, varicosities, and defibrillation after cardiac arrest. Oral contraceptives, especially in women who smoke, have also been implicated in young women with none of the usual predisposing factors. A thrombus in the peripheral venous circulatory system may dislodge and become an embolus. This embolus is dangerous to the patient, since the blood clot can lodge in the pulmonary circulation (causing a pulmonary embolism), the cardiac circulation (causing MI), or the cerebral circulation (causing a **cerebrovascular accident**).

Peripheral vascular occlusion may also lead to stasis ulcers, which are caused by breakdown of the skin and underlying tissue due to inadequate circulation to the area. These ulcers develop as deep red discolorations, itching, edema, and large areas of scaling skin leading to fissures and ulcers. Increasing circulation to the lower extremities with use of support stockings, weight reduction, and elevating the limbs may prevent formation of these ulcers.

A blood clot lodged in the pulmonary circulation is a pulmonary embolism. Signs and symptoms of a pulmonary embolism include dyspnea, syncope, and severe pleuritic chest pain with respiration. Diagnosis may include chest radiography, an electrocardiogram, a lung scan, or a pulmonary arteriogram. Doppler studies are used to diagnose deep-vein thrombosis. Depending on the severity, treatment may include bed rest with elevation of the affected extremity, anticoagulant medication such as coumadin, or surgery.

PATIENT EDUCATION

Anticoagulant Therapy

Patients with certain types of cardiac problems are prescribed anticoagulant medications, commonly called blood thinners, used to decrease the risk of a thrombus or embolus developing. Coumadin is a common oral anticoagulant. Lovenox, another anticoagulant, is given as an injection. Teach patients who are prescribed anticoagulants as follows:

- Monitor the mouth, urine, and stool for any signs of bleeding.
- Use a soft-bristle toothbrush.
- Call the office if they notice any signs of bleeding.
- It is important to avoid injuries and falls while taking anticoagulant medications.
- Needle sticks from injections or venipuncture require prolonged application of pressure afterward to control bleeding and bruising.
- It is important to comply with orders for blood work. Anticoagulant medications necessitate frequent tests for blood counts and bleeding times.
- Limit their intake of foods high in vitamin K (asparagus, cabbage, fish, broccoli, cheese, pork, spinach, cauliflower, and rice). These patients should be given a printed flyer on dietary restrictions.
- Avoid taking over-the-counter medications containing aspirin or ibuprofen without consulting the physician. These drugs may cause an increase in bleeding times, interfering with the actions of the anticoagulant.
- Take the medication at the same time every day. If a dose is missed, take it as soon as it is remembered that day, but do not take a double dose.

Checkpoint Question

6. What disease occurs when the superficial veins in the legs become swollen and distended?

Cerebrovascular Accident

Cerebrovascular accident (CVA), sometimes called stroke, results suddenly when damage to the blood vessels in the brain occurs. The damage blocks the circulation, resulting in ischemia, or lack of oxygen, to that part of the brain. Brain tissue dies without adequate oxygen. A common cause of CVA is blockage of the cerebral artery by thrombus or embolus. Hemorrhage, atherosclerotic heart disease, and hypertension are additional causes of CVAs. Unfortunately, CVAs are the most common nervous system disorder in the elderly and one of the leading causes of death in the United States.

Patients who have CVAs usually have varying degrees of weakness or paralysis of one side of the body, with possible involvement of language and comprehension. Symptoms vary according to which artery and which part of the brain is affected. CVAs are fatal when vital centers of the brain are damaged. Once the brain tissue is damaged by a CVA, treatment is aimed at reducing further death of cerebrovascular tissue and assisting the patient to regain any affected function. Patients who have CVAs need many months of rehabilitation, including physical therapy, occupational therapy, and speech therapy. You must remember that although these patients may not be able to communicate effectively with you, they are capable of understanding and should be treated with respect, dignity, and compassion.

Ischemia to small areas of the brain over short periods is known as **transient ischemic attack** (TIA). TIA, or mini-stroke, should be considered a warning sign for a possible impending cerebrovascular accident. TIAs may be caused by atherosclerotic plaques narrowing the arteries supplying blood to the brain, a small embolus that reduces the flow of blood to an area, or spasms of the blood vessels. The symptoms vary according to the arteries affected but usually include the following:

- Mild numbness or tingling in the face or a limb
- Difficulty swallowing
- Coughing and choking
- Slurred speech
- Unilateral visual disturbance
- Dizziness

As many as 50% to 80% of patients who exhibit symptoms of TIAs progress to a stroke. The signs of a major stroke may begin as a TIA and progress to loss of consciousness, hyperpnea (deep, gasping breaths), anisocoria (unequal pupils), and hemiplegia (unilateral paralysis). Any patient who has the signs and symptoms of a TIA or a CVA should be sent to the emergency room following all physician instructions and office policies.

Aneurysm

Weakened blood vessel walls are predisposed to abnormal dilation. Dilation in the form of an **aneurysm** may occur in any vessel, but arteries are most often affected. Because of the high pressure so close to the heart, the aorta is the most common site. The normally elastic vessel wall develops a ballooning effect in one or many forms, all of them dangerous:

- A *dissecting aneurysm* tears the inner walls of the artery and allows blood to leak into the lining of the vessel; the wall will eventually die and tear open.

- A *sacculated aneurysm* balloons from the arterial wall into a sac, which may burst.
- A *berry aneurysm* is usually a congenital defect in a cerebral artery.

Causes of aneurysms include trauma, hypertension, atherosclerosis, certain fungal infections, syphilis, and congenital defects. Symptoms include pain or pressure at the site. Death may occur quickly if the tear is not repaired. Diagnosis is based on a thorough history and examination, an arteriogram or aortogram, computed tomography, or magnetic resonance imaging. Surgical resection is the only option.

Anemia

Deficiencies in hemoglobin or in the numbers of red blood cells result in anemia. Anemia is not considered a disease but is a symptom of an underlying disorder. Anemia can result from any of these:

- Blood loss due to hemorrhage or slow internal bleeding
- A diet low in iron or a malabsorption condition (nutritional anemia)
- Suppressed (by chemotherapeutic medication) or diseased bone marrow, resulting in decreased blood cell formation (aplastic anemia)
- Vitamin B_{12} deficiency due to a lack of intrinsic factor (pernicious anemia)
- Genetic abnormality (sickle cell anemia, thalassemia)
- Destruction of functioning red blood cells by various means, such as liver or spleen dysfunction or toxins (hemolytic anemia)

Symptoms of anemia may include cardiovascular alterations such as tachycardia and pallor, anorexia and weight loss, dyspnea on exertion, and fatigue. Treatment of anemia must address the cause; it can include increasing dietary iron, blood transfusions, and injection of vitamin B_{12} (cyanocobalamin) on a regular basis. Aplastic anemia may require a bone marrow transplant. Unfortunately, genetic abnormalities, such as sickle cell anemia and thalassemia, cannot be corrected at this time.

COMMON DIAGNOSTIC AND THERAPEUTIC PROCEDURES

Testing for cardiovascular disorders may be either invasive or noninvasive. Invasive techniques require entering the body by the use of a tube, needle, or other device. Noninvasive techniques do not require entering the body or puncturing the skin. Depending on the patient's symptoms, testing may be basic and can be done easily during the general physical examination by auscultating the heart and chest cavity. Additional tests the physician may order that you perform in the medical office can include chest radiography or 12-lead ECG. Sometimes initial findings indicate the need for a more sophisticated procedure, such as cardiac catheterization,

Table 33-2 COMMON CARDIOVASCULAR TESTS

Diagnostic Test	Description	Indications
Chest radiography	Noninvasive diagnostic tool using high-energy electromagnetic waves.	Detect and follow cardiovascular, other diseases, response to therapy.
12-Lead ECG	Graph of electrical activity of heart from various angles.	Obtain a baseline or assess acute situation.
Holter monitor	Continuous monitor of heart rhythm via portable device worn for extended period during ADL.	Symptoms of rhythm disturbances not shown on ECG or during physical examination.
Cardiac stress test	ECG of heart rhythm during exercise on graded treadmill or stationary bicycle.	Help diagnose patients with known or suspected heart problems.
Echocardiogram	Ultrasound of heart; sound waves generated by transducer.	Diagnose suspected or known valvular disease, severity of heart failure, cardiomyopathy.
Cardiac catheterization	Insertion of a catheter into the heart.	Diagnose or determine severity of heart disease, atherosclerosis.
Coronary arteriography	Injection of contrast medium into coronary arteries (after cardiac catheterization), allowing visualization via monitor to assess obstruction of arteries.	Assess heart disease and damage after MI.

ADL, activities of daily living; ECG, electrocardiogram.

which is performed at an outpatient surgical center or hospital. TABLE 33-2 describes the most commonly performed cardiovascular tests.

Physical Examination of the Cardiovascular System

The cardiovascular examination is the most basic noninvasive procedure used to assess the heart and blood vessels. When preparing a patient for a cardiovascular examination, you will obtain vital information, including accurate determination of weight, blood pressure, heart and respiratory rates, body temperature, and cardiovascular history (Box 33-5). It is also important to obtain a complete list of the patient's medications and current dosages, including any herbal and vitamin supplements and over-the-counter medications. A brief social and family history should include lifestyle and familial risk factors for cardiovascular disorders. The patient should be questioned regarding a history of smoking tobacco, alcohol intake, family history of heart disease, hypercholesterolemia, diet, and exercise.

The physician or cardiologist usually begins the examination with a review of the patient's history and reason for the office visit. The physician also reviews the patient's vital signs and medications, noting any allergies to medications and other substances. The physician inspects the patient to evaluate the general appearance, noting the circulation and any swelling of the extremities, color of the skin, and jugular vein distention. Palpation is used to evaluate the efficiency of the circulatory pathways and peripheral pulses. Using auscultation with a stethoscope, the physician can evaluate the sounds made as blood flows through the heart and the valves open and close. Abnormal heart sounds, bruits and murmurs, may be detected (Box 33-6).

Box 33-5

OBTAINING A CARDIOVASCULAR PATIENT'S HISTORY: KEY QUESTIONS

By asking the following questions, you can elicit important information from a patient with cardiovascular problems.
- Why are you seeing the cardiologist or physician today?
- What symptoms have you been having?
- How long have you had the pain, discomfort, distress, or unusual sensations? (Patients may not think of chest discomfort as a cardiac symptom.)
- Where is the pain or discomfort? Does it stay in one place or radiate in any direction?
- Is the pain associated with any other symptoms, such as shortness of breath, nausea, weakness, sweating, dizziness?
- If you have been short of breath, does it restrict any of your activities or require you to sleep on additional pillows at night?
- Are you a smoker?
- Do you drink alcoholic beverages?

As you proceed with the interview, keep in mind that patients with cardiovascular problems are usually understandably anxious and concerned. They may bring with them family members who are also concerned or anxious. It is your responsibility to help ease apprehension and to offer reassurance and support when appropriate.

Box 33-6

ABNORMAL HEART SOUNDS

Abnormal heart sounds, called *murmurs*, are sounds the blood makes as it courses through the heart valves. The sounds vary with the severity and location of the abnormality. For instance, they may blow, rasp, rub, bubble, whistle, whoosh, and/or click. A murmur is not a disease, but it may indicate organic heart disease. *Functional murmurs* may only occur during elevations in body temperature or during times of physical stress and are not usually a cause for concern. *Organic murmurs* indicate structural abnormalities of varying degrees and are always present. A cardiologist evaluates the murmur by noting its location in the heart, when it occurs in the cardiac cycle, how long it lasts, and its characteristic sound.

In addition to obtaining important information and data before the physician examines the patient, you must also provide instructions and materials for proper gown wearing and draping. After the examination, the physician may order an ECG, which you will perform and give to the physician for diagnosis.

Checkpoint Question

7. What is a murmur?

Electrocardiogram

One of the most valuable diagnostic tools for evaluating the electrical pathway through the heart is the electrocardiogram, known by the acronym ECG or EKG. The ECG is the graphic record of the electrical current as it progresses

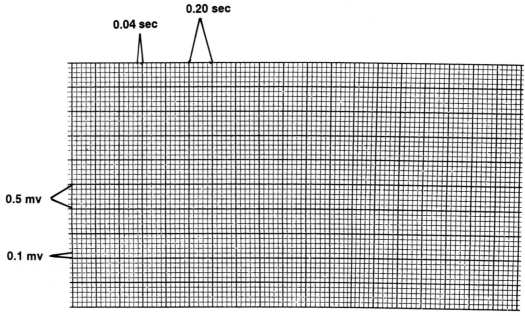

FIGURE 33-7. ECG graph paper. (A) Each small square is 1 mm × 1 mm. Each fifth line is marked darker to make a cube of 5 mm × 5 mm (actual size). (B) Horizontally, the graph paper represents time in seconds. Each small square represents 0.04 seconds and each large square, 0.2 seconds. Five large squares = 1 second (5 × 0.2).

WHAT IF

The physician asks you to perform an ECG on a child?

While pediatric cardiac problems may not be encountered daily in the medical office, obesity, elevated cholesterol and triglyceride blood levels, and type II diabetes are conditions that are seen increasingly frequently in pediatric and family practice offices, and these conditions may require intervention, including electrocardiography. While the placement of the electrodes is similar to that for an adult, smaller electrodes for use on the smaller patient allow for easier placement. A standard ECG can be done on children over 8 or 9 years of age; however, for younger children, the sensitivity, or gain, on the machine should be changed according to the physician's orders or office policy and procedure manual. If the sensitivity or gain is changed, this must be noted on the ECG before it goes into the medical record.

through the heart. It can be performed as part of a routine physical examination or as needed for a patient with chest pain, discomfort, or other signs and symptoms of possible cardiac problems. During the ECG, you are responsible for explaining the procedure to the patient and applying combinations of electrodes, called **leads**, on the patient's limbs and precordial area (anterior chest). ECGs are used to assist in diagnosing ischemia, delays in impulse conduction, hypertrophy of the cardiac chambers, and arrhythmias. They are not used to detect anatomical disorders, such as heart murmurs.

The ECG tracing is printed on graph paper that is either blue or black with a heat-labile white coating. Graph lines are printed over the white coating, appearing as small blocks with thicker lines outlining every five small blocks. On standard ECG paper, each small block is 1 mm². The large blocks are 5 mm² (FIG. 33-7A). Some ECG machines contain a stylus that heats and melts the white coating, exposing the dark background beneath to record the movement of the stylus as the electrical impulses are detected. Newer ECG machines dispense ink from a cartridge into the stylus to mark the ECG tracing paper. The ECG paper may be affected by pressure as well as heat and should be handled carefully to prevent extraneous markings. Each small horizontal block represents time (0.04 seconds), and the vertical small blocks represent voltage (0.1 millivolts). After the heart's electrical markings are traced on the paper, the heart rate and time required for the electrical impulses to spread through the heart can be determined (Fig. 33-7B).

ECG Leads

Over the years, a standard system of electrode placement has evolved and nomenclature has been developed for the recordings from different electrode combinations. Each lead records the electrical impulse through the heart from a different angle. Viewing the conduction of the electrical impulses in these various angles gives the physician a fairly complete view of the entire heart. The standard ECG has 12 leads that produce a three-dimensional record of the impulse wave. Four wires are labeled and color-coded for the limb that the wire should be connected to. The four limb electrodes should be positioned away from bony areas and on muscular areas, such as the calves, outer thighs, and above the elbow. Adjustments may be necessary for patients with amputations, surgery to the extremity, or trauma to the arms or legs (Procedure 33-1).

The right leg (RL) electrode, the grounding lead, helps reduce alternating current (AC) interference and keeps the average voltage of the patient the same as that of the recording instrument. The other three limb leads attached to electrodes on the patient's left leg and arms make up the combinations necessary for the first six views of the heart in the 12-lead ECG. The first three combinations, standard bipolar leads also known as Einthoven leads, allow frontal visualization of the heart's electrical activity from side to side (Box 33-7). Each lead provides specific measurements:

- Lead I measures the difference in electrical potential between the right arm (RA) and the left arm (LA).
- Lead II measures the difference in electrical potential between the right arm (RA) and the left leg (LL).
- Lead III measures the difference in electrical potential between the left arm (LA) and the left leg (LL).

Box 33-8

POSITIONING OF UNIPOLAR PRECORDIAL (CHEST) LEADS

- $LV_1 = (RA + LA + LL)$ to V_1: Fourth intercostal space at right margin of sternum
- $LV_2 = (RA + LA + LL)$ to V_2: Fourth intercostal space at left margin of sternum
- $LV_3 = (RA + LA + LL)$ to V_3: Midway between V_2 and V_4
- $LV_4 = (RA + LA + LL)$ to V_4: Fifth intercostal space at junction of midclavicular line
- $LV_5 = (RA + LA + LL)$ to V_5: Horizontal level of V_4 at left anterior axillary line
- $V_6 = (RA + LA + LL)$ to V_6: Horizontal level of V_4 and V_5 at midaxillary line

Box 33-7

ABBREVIATIONS USED IN PERFORMING ECGS

RA	right arm
LA	left arm
LL	left leg
RL	right leg
V_1–V_6	chest leads
aVR	augmented voltage right arm
aVL	augmented voltage left arm
aVF	augmented voltage left foot or leg

The same limb electrodes provide measurement of the signal between one electrode and the average of the remaining two. These second three combinations, the augmented unipolar limb leads, allow visualization from a frontal view top to bottom:

- Lead aVR (LL + LA) to RA measures the potential at the right arm.
- Lead aVL (LL + RA) to LA measures the potential at the left arm.
- Lead aVF (RA + LA) to LL measures the potential at the left foot.

For a closer look at the electrical conduction through the heart, electrodes are placed directly on the anterior chest wall, but the limb electrodes must remain attached to the patient. The positioning of the chest electrodes must be precise for accuracy. These leads, the unipolar precordial (chest) leads, show the comparison of the chest electrode potential to the average of the three limb electrodes (Box 33-8). All electrodes must connect to the wires of the ECG machine. Each lead is clearly marked on the ECG paper as it is printed,

Box 33-9

PATIENT'S DIARY FOR HOLTER MONITORING

A patient with a Holter monitor must keep a diary of daily activities. When the patient has symptoms, he or she depresses an incident (or event) button on the machine, then records in the diary the activity that caused the incident, including the symptoms. At intervals, the patient also records daily activities such as working quietly at a desk, driving a car, eating a meal, watching television, sleeping. All activities must be noted, including elimination, sexual intercourse, anger, laughter, and so on. Some monitors are equipped with small tape recorders so the patient can keep an audio diary instead of a written one.

Table 33-3   CODING ECG LEADS

Lead	Code	Lead	Code
I	.	V_1	-.
II	..	V_2	-..
III	...	V_3	-...
aVR	-	V_4	-....
aVL	--	V_5	-.....
aVF	---	V_6	-......

or specific codes may be printed on the paper to denote each lead (TABLE 33-3). The recording of the ECG on paper varies from one machine to another, but the principles and techniques are universal (Procedure 33-1).

Checkpoint Question

8. Which three waves represent a cardiac cycle on an ECG?

ECG Interpretation

The physician's interpretation of the standard 12-lead ECG includes an examination of various wave forms associated with the cardiac cycle (FIG. 33-8). Commonly measured components of an ECG tracing are discussed in the following sections.

PR Interval. The time from the beginning of the P wave to the beginning of the QRS complex is called the *PR interval.* This time interval represents depolarization of the atria and the spread of the depolarization wave up to and including the atrioventricular node.

PR Segment. The PR segment represents the period between the P wave and QRS complex.

ST Segment. The distance between the QRS complex and the T wave from the point where the QRS complex ends (J-point) to the onset of the ascending limb of the T wave is called the *ST segment.* On the ECG, this segment is a sensitive indicator of myocardial ischemia or injury.

Ventricular Activation Time. The time from the beginning of the QRS complex to the peak of the R wave, the *ventricular activation time*, represents the time necessary for the depolarization wave to travel from the inner surface of the heart (endocardium) to the outer surface of the heart (epicardium).

During the ECG, the paper speed on the machine should be set at 25 mm per second, which allows the electrical impulses (seen as waves) on the ECG to be measured using the blocks on the ECG paper as a reference (each small horizontal block is 0.04 seconds). Movement of the electricity through the atria is noted and measured on the ECG tracing

FIGURE 33–8. The cardiac cycle waves, segments, and intervals. (Reprinted with permission from Cohen BJ. Medical Terminology: An Illustrated Guide. Philadelphia: Lippincott Williams & Wilkins, 2003.)

as the PR interval (the normal PR interval is 0.12 to 0.20 seconds). Electrical movement through the ventricles is measured and noted on the ECG as the QRS complex, which is normally less than 0.12 seconds. The following elements are taken into consideration:

- Rate: how fast the heart is beating
- Rhythm: regularity of cardiac cycles and intervals
- Axis: position of the heart and direction of depolarization, or electrical movement, through the heart
- Hypertrophy: size of the heart
- Ischemia: decrease in blood supply to an area of the heart
- Infarction: death of heart muscle resulting in loss of function

Under usual diagnostic conditions, the 12-lead ECG provides sufficient data. As the medical assistant, you are responsible for obtaining a good-quality ECG without avoidable **artifacts**. An artifact is an abnormal signal that does not reflect electrical activity of the heart during the cardiac cycle. **Artifact can be due to movement by the patient, mechanical problems with the ECG machine, or improper technique.** TABLE 33-4 describes three types of artifacts and how to prevent them.

Sometimes the physician requests a rhythm strip along with the ECG. A rhythm strip is a long strip of a certain lead or a combination of leads. It may be used to define certain cardiac arrhythmias. While most ECG machines have a button that automatically records the 12 views in the 12-lead ECG, a rhythm strip must be obtained using the manual mode on the ECG machine.

Holter Monitor

In many instances, an ECG that records the electrical activity of the heart for a brief moment in the medical office does not reveal cardiac problems. For diagnosis of intermittent cardiac arrhythmias and dysfunctions, a monitor that records for at least 24 hours is used. **The Holter monitor is small and portable and can be worn comfortably for long periods without interfering with daily activities** (FIG. 33-9). It may be set to record continuously or only when the patient presses a record button when feeling symptoms. This record button is also known as an incident or event button. When applying the Holter monitor, you must instruct the patient to keep a diary of daily activities (Box 33-9). The physician will interpret the ECG tracing recorded by the Holter monitor and compare these findings with activities recorded in the diary to get an accurate view of what activities, if any, precipitate cardiac arrhythmias. Procedure 33-2 describes the steps for applying a Holter monitor.

FIGURE 33–9. A Holter monitor. (Courtesy of Welch Allyn.)

Table 33-4	TYPES OF ARTIFACTS	
Artifact	**Possible Cause**	**How to Prevent Problems**
Wandering baseline	Electrodes too tight or too loose Electrolyte gel dried out Skin has oil, lotion, or excessive hair	Apply electrodes properly Apply new electrodes Prepare skin before applying electrodes
Muscle or somatic artifact	Patient cannot remain still because of tremors or fear	Reassure patient, explain procedure, stress need to keep still; patients with tremo or disease may be unable to stay motionless.
Alternating current artifact	Improperly grounded ECG machine	Check cables to ensure properly grounded machine before beginning test.
	Electrical interference in room	Move patient or unplug appliances in immediate area
	Dangling lead wires	Arrange wires along contours of patient's body

WANDERING BASELINE

Wandering baseline.

SOMATIC MUSCLE TREMOR

Somatic muscle tremor.

AC INTERFERENCE

AC interference.

Chest Radiography

Chest radiography provides valuable basic information about the anatomical location and gross structures of the heart, great vessels, and lungs. It also aids in the evaluation of such disorders as CHF and pericardial effusions. Many patients with CHF have an enlarged heart, especially the ventricles, and pericardial effusions appear as white markings around the heart on the film. Many patients with chronic cardiac conditions also have pulmonary problems, and the chest film can be used to assess the lungs. Any abnormal swelling or growth of the heart or great vessels (aorta, inferior vena cava, superior vena cava, pulmonary arteries) can also be assessed.

Cardiac Stress Test

To measure the response of the cardiac muscle to increased demands of oxygen, the physician may request a cardiac stress test. The heart is usually tested with the patient walking on a treadmill (FIG. 33-10) with periodic increases in the rate or angle of the walk or run, but it may also be done on a stationary bicycle. The patient is attached to an ECG monitor for constant tracing during the test, and the blood pressure is monitored before, during, and after the test. The test is performed according to the physician's orders, and the ECG is interpreted by the physician, but you may be responsible for attaching the electrodes, monitoring and recording the blood pressure, and assisting the physician in watching the patient for signs of light-headedness. Emergency resuscitation equipment should be available in case of cardiac or respiratory difficulties. This test may indicate the need for further cardiac testing. The cardiac stress test may be done as part of a routine physical examination in adults without symptoms or as a diagnostic tool for patients who have intermittent periods of angina pectoris or **palpitations**.

TRIAGE

While working in a medical office, the following three situations are occurring:

A. A 29-year-old woman has been seen by the physician, who orders application of a Holter monitor. She also needs instruction on the importance of completing the diary.

B. A 62-year-old woman needs an ECG. She is complaining of heaviness in her chest.

C. A 17-year-old patient and his mother have just arrived in the office with written orders from an orthopedic surgeon that he needs a "stat preop" ECG. The patient is scheduled for knee surgery in the morning.

How do you sort these patients? Whom do you see first? Second? Third?

Do the ECG for patient B first. Her chest heaviness may be due to a cardiac problem, and the physician should assess this ECG immediately. See patient A next, since she has been waiting. After applying the Holter monitor and explaining the diary, do the ECG for patient C. Every surgeon has standard orders for various tests he or she wants completed before doing surgery. ECGs are commonly ordered and read by a cardiologist or internist before a surgical procedure. Although the written order is written as stat, the test can be done as soon as possible and convenient.

Checkpoint Question

9. What is the purpose of a cardiac stress test?

Echocardiography

An echocardiogram, or echo, uses sound waves generated by a small device called a transducer. These waves travel through the cardiac chambers, walls, and valves and are transmitted back to a screen, where they can be viewed and interpreted. Echocardiograms help the physician to diagnose suspected or known valvular disease in adults and children. Echoes also aid in diagnosing the severity of heart failure and **cardiomyopathy**. In addition, this test can be used to detect injuries to the heart in patients with trauma. Only the most specialized cardiac medical offices have the equipment and personnel (ultrasonographers) to obtain echocardiographs. In most instances, your role is to schedule the outpatient procedure and give the patient any instructions required by the facility. Usually no patient preparations are required for the echocardiography.

Cardiac Catheterization and Coronary Arteriography

Cardiac catheterization is a common invasive procedure used to help diagnose or treat conditions affecting the coronary arterial circulation. It may be performed on patients with shortness of breath, angina, dizziness, palpitations, fluttering in the chest, rapid heartbeat, and other cardiovascular symptoms to determine the severity or cause of the problem. It is often indicated after a cardiac stress test or echocardiogram reveals an abnormality. This procedure is not done in the medical office, but the medical assistant may be responsible for scheduling diagnostic cardiac catheterizations at a local outpatient facility or hospital and giving the patient any instructions required by the outpatient facility. If the procedure is for treatment, it must be done at an inpatient facility that has immediate access to open heart surgical equipment and personnel in the event of an emergency.

During the catheterization, the physician, usually a cardiologist, inserts a flexible tube into a blood vessel in either the arm or the groin and gently guides it toward the heart. When the catheter is in place, coronary arteriography is performed by injecting contrast medium, revealing the heart's chambers, valves, great vessels, and coronary arteries on a monitor. If atherosclerotic plaques are found, an angioplasty may be performed or scheduled for later (Box 33-2).

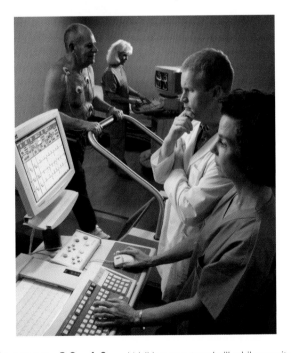

FIGURE 33-10. Walking on a treadmill while monitoring the heart's activity with an ECG machine is one way to determine the heart's ability to adapt to increased work during exercise. (Courtesy of Borgess Medical Center, Kalamazoo, MI.)

Procedure 33-1

Performing a 12-Lead Electrocardiogram

Purpose: Prepare a patient and obtain a 12-lead ECG that is free from artifacts.

Equipment: Physician's order, patient record, ECG machine with cable and lead wires, ECG paper, disposable
                       electrodes that contain coupling gel, gown and drape, skin preparation materials including a razor
                       and antiseptic wipes.

Standard: This procedure should take 20 minutes.

Steps	Reason
1. Wash your hands.	Handwashing aids infection control.
2. Assemble the equipment.	

Step 2. The ECG machine.

Steps	Reason
3. Greet and identify the patient. Explain the procedure.	This avoids errors in treatment and helps gain compliance.
4. Turn the machine on and enter appropriate data, including the patient's name and/or identification number, age, sex, height, weight, blood pressure, and medications.	This information will assist the physician in determining a proper diagnosis.
5. Instruct the patient to disrobe above the waist and provide a gown for privacy. Female patients should also be instructed to remove any nylons or tights.	Clothing may interfere with proper placement of the leads. Patients wearing pants do not have to remove them if they can be pulled up to expose the lower legs.
6. Position the patient comfortably supine with pillows as needed for comfort. Drape the patient for warmth and privacy.	If the patient is uncomfortable, too cool, or improperly draped, movement is likely, which will result in artifact on the ECG tracing.
7. Prepare the skin as needed by wiping away skin oil and lotions with the antiseptic wipes or shaving any hair that will interfere with good contact between the skin and the electrodes.	Skin preparation ensures properly attached leads and helps avoid improper readings and lost time repeating the test.

(continues)

Procedure 33-1 *(continued)*

Performing a 12-Lead Electrocardiogram

Steps	Reason
8. Apply the electrodes snugly against the fleshy, muscular parts of the upper arms and lower legs according to the manufacturer's directions. Apply the chest electrodes, V_1–V_6.	Electrodes that are not snug against the skin or are on bony prominences may cause improper reading and artifact. In case of an amputation or otherwise inaccessible limb, place the electrode on the uppermost part of the existing extremity OR on the anterior shoulder (upper extremity) and groin (lower extremity).

Step 8A. Applying limb electrodes.

Step 8B. Applying chest electrodes.

(continues)

Procedure 33-1 *(continued)*

Performing a 12-Lead Electrocardiogram

Steps	**Reason**
9. Connect the lead wires securely according to the color-coded notations on the connectors (RA, LA, RL, LL, V_1–V_6). Untangle the wires before applying them to prevent electrical artifacts. Each lead must lie unencumbered along the contours of the patient's body to decrease the likelihood of artifacts. Double-check the placement.	Improperly placed leads will result in time lost to an inaccurate reading and retesting.

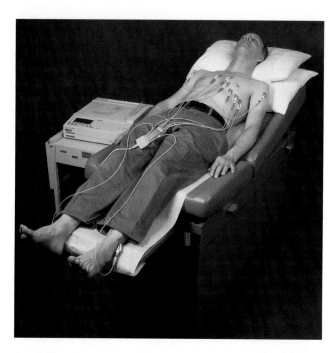

Step 9. The wires should lie along the contours of the patient's body.

10. Determine the sensitivity, or gain, and paper speed settings on the ECG machine before running the test. Set sensitivity or gain on 1 and paper speed on 25 mm/second.	Sensitivity setting of 1 and a paper speed of 25 mm/second are necessary to obtain an accurate ECG. These settings should not be changed without a direct order from the physician and the changes noted on the final ECG tracing.
11. Depress the automatic button on the ECG machine to obtain the 12-lead tracing. The machine will automatically move from one lead to the next without your intervention.	If the physician wants only a rhythm strip tracing, use the manual mode of operation and select the lead manually.

(continues)

Procedure 33-1 (continued)

Performing a 12-Lead Electrocardiogram

Steps	Reason
12. When the tracing is complete and printed, check the ECG for artifacts and a standardization mark.	With sensitivity set on 1, the standardization mark should be 2 small squares wide and 10 small squares high. The standardization mark documents accuracy of operation and provides a reference point.

Normal Standard
Standardization mark
is 10 mm high

One-Half Standard
Standardization mark
is 5 mm high

Double Standard
Standardization mark
is 20 mm high

Step 12. Standardization marks.

Steps	Reason
13. If the tracing is adequate, turn off the machine and remove and discard the electrodes. Assist the patient to a sitting position and help with dressing if needed.	Some patients become dizzy while lying supine.
14. If a single-channel machine was used (each lead produced on a roll of paper, one lead at a time), carefully roll the ECG strip without using clips to secure the roll. This ECG must be mounted on 8 × 11 inch paper or a form before going into the medical record according to the office policy and procedure.	Folding the ECG tracing or applying clips may make marks on the surface, obscuring the reading. Special forms may be purchased specifically for mounting a single-channel ECG strip and placing it in the medical record.
15. Record the procedure in the patient's medical record.	Procedures are considered not to have been done if they are not recorded.
16. Either place the ECG tracing and the patient's medical record on the physician's desk or give it directly to the physician, as instructed.	

Charting Example
12/02/2005 9:45 A.M. Preop 12-lead ECG obtained and placed in chart, given to Dr. Bruno for evaluation. Pt. discharged, no follow-up required at this time. _____A. Perez, CMA

Applying a Holter Monitor

Purpose:	Prepare and instruct a patient on wearing a Holter monitor for continuous cardiac monitoring
Equipment:	Physician's order, patient record, Holter monitor with appropriate lead wires, fresh batteries, carrying case with strap, disposable electrodes with coupling gel, adhesive tape, gown and drape, skin preparation materials including a razor and antiseptic wipes, diary
Standard:	This procedure should take 10 minutes.

Steps	Reason
1. Wash your hands.	Handwashing aids infection control.
2. Assemble the equipment.	
3. Greet and identify the patient. Explain the procedure, reminding the patient that it is important to carry out all normal activities for the duration of the test.	Identifying the patient and explaining the procedure avoids errors in treatment and helps gain compliance. A normal routine is essential to allow the physician to identify areas of concern.
4. Explain the purpose of the incident diary, emphasizing the need to carry it at all times during the test. Ask the patient to remove all clothing from the waist up and put on the gown, and drape appropriately for privacy.	The chest must be exposed for proper placement of the electrodes.
5. With the patient seated, prepare the skin for electrode attachment. Provide privacy. Shave the skin if necessary and cleanse with antiseptic wipes.	Shaving and cleansing the skin will improve adherence of the adhesive on the electrodes.
6. Expose the adhesive backing of the electrodes and follow the manufacturer's instructions to attach each firmly. Apply the electrodes at the specified sites: A. Right manubrium border B. Left manubrium border C. Right sternal border at the fifth rib D. Fifth rib at the anterior axillary line E. Right lower rib cage over the cartilage as a ground lead.	

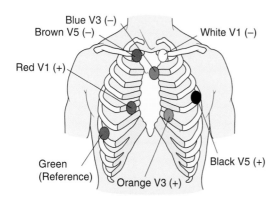

Step 6. Sites for Holter electrodes

Step 6. Place the Holter electrodes as directed by the manufacturer.

(continues)

Procedure 33-2 (continued)

Applying a Holter Monitor

Steps	Reason
7. Check the security of the attachments.	
8. Position electrode connectors down toward the patient's feet. Attach the lead wires and secure with adhesive tape.	Application of adhesive tape over the connections will help ensure that the leads do not work loose during the day.

Step 8. Securely tape each electrode. Tape the lead wires to the patient's body.

9. Connect the cable and run a baseline ECG by hooking the Holter to the ECG machine with the cable hookup.	Check for accurate function of the Holter.
10. Assist the patient to dress carefully with the cable extending through the garment opening. Clothing that buttons down the front is convenient.	This prevents pulling and strain on the leads.
11. Plug the cable into the recorder and mark the diary. If needed, explain the purpose of the diary to the patient again. Give instructions for a return appointment to evaluate the recording and the diary.	
12. Record the procedure in the patient's medical record.	Procedures are considered not to have been done if they are not recorded.

Charting Example

11/28/2004 1:00 P.M. Holter monitor ordered and applied; baseline ECG done. Oral and written instructions given regarding care and use of monitor. Instructions for completion of diary also given. Pt. verbalized understanding of use of monitor and completion of diary. To RTO tomorrow P.M. for removal of the monitor. _____ R. Steele, CMA

CHAPTER SUMMARY

The circulatory system is a closed transport system kept in motion by the force of the beating heart. Nutrients are delivered to cells, cellular wastes are picked up, hormones are directed to target cells, and disease-fighting mechanisms are transported to areas of concern. Since disorders of the cardiac system can affect many systems, including the pulmonary system and the central nervous system, the patient with undiagnosed cardiac disease may complain of lethargy, shortness or breath, or swelling of the extremities. Your responsibility includes obtaining a complete cardiac history from all patients, assisting with the physical examination, and performing or assisting with diagnostic testing. In addition, you may be responsible for scheduling any cardiac procedures that are not performed in your medical office or obtaining necessary referrals from third-party payers when the physician concludes that the patient should be evaluated by a cardiologist. But your most important roles as a medical professional are educating patients at every opportunity to prevent cardiac disease and offering support once a cardiac diagnosis has been made by the physician. It is also important that you maintain CPR certification, since cardiac emergencies can occur in any setting, including the medical office.

Critical Thinking Challenges

1. Draw a diagram of the heart and a cardiac cycle as seen on the ECG. How would you explain an ECG to a patient? How would you assist the patient in relaxing for this procedure?
2. Compare and contrast the signs and symptoms of a CVA and a TIA. Make a list of questions that you would ask a patient or caregiver to determine whether he or she is having a stroke. What kind of help does a patient need at home after a stroke?
3. Explain anemia and identify its symptoms. Why does anemia cause these symptoms? What dietary instruc-

tions should be given to a patient with iron deficiency anemia?
4. Prepare a patient education brochure that describes hypertension and its causes, symptoms, and possible treatments. In this brochure explain why hypertension is often referred to as the silent killer.

Answers to Checkpoint Questions

1. With pericarditis, pain increases with inspiration and movement; pain during MI will not change with patient positioning.
2. Two arrhythmias that require immediate intervention are ventricular tachycardia and ventricular fibrillation.
3. Rheumatic heart disease and cardiac valvular disease may be caused by an upper respiratory infection caused by group A beta-hemolytic streptococci.
4. Four predisposing factors for heart disease are history of elevated cholesterol, smoking, diabetes mellitus, and hypertension.
5. Stroke and renal failure may result from untreated hypertension.
6. Varicose veins occur when the superficial veins in the legs become swollen and distended.
7. A murmur is an abnormal heart sound.
8. P, QRS, and T waves represent a cardiac cycle on an ECG.
9. A cardiac stress test measures the response of the myocardium to increased demands for oxygen.

 Websites

American Heart Association http://www.american
  heart.org
American Red Cross http://www.redcross.org
National Safety Council http://www.nsc.org
American College of Cardiology http://www.acc.org
American Society of Hypertension, Inc. http://www.
  ash-us.org
American Medical Association http://www.ama-assn.org

34

Gastroenterology

CHAPTER OUTLINE

COMMON GASTROINTESTINAL DISORDERS
Mouth Disorders
Esophageal Disorders
Stomach Disorders
Intestinal Disorders
Liver Disorders

Gallbladder Disorders
Pancreatic Disorders

COMMON DIAGNOSTIC AND THERAPEUTIC PROCEDURES
History and Physical Examination of the Gastrointestinal System

Blood Tests
Radiologic Studies
Nuclear Imaging
Ultrasonography
Endoscopic Studies
Fecal Tests

ROLE DELINEATION

ADMINISTRATIVE: ADMINISTRATIVE PROCEDURES
- Perform basic administrative medical assisting functions
- Schedule inpatient and outpatient admissions and procedures

CLINICAL: FUNDAMENTAL PRINCIPLES
- Apply principles of aseptic technique and infection control
- Comply with quality assurance practices

CLINICAL: DIAGNOSTIC ORDERS
- Collect and process specimens
- Perform diagnostic tests

CLINICAL: PATIENT CARE
- Adhere to established patient screening procedures
- Obtain patient history and vital signs
- Prepare patient for examinations, procedures, and treatments
- Assist with examinations, procedures, and treatments
- Coordinate patient care information with other health care providers

GENERAL: PROFESSIONALISM
- Display a professional manner and image
- Demonstrate initiative and responsibility
- Work as a member of the health care team
- Treat all patients with compassion and empathy

GENERAL: COMMUNICATION SKILLS
- Recognize and respect cultural diversity
- Adapt communications to individual's ability to understand
- Recognize and respond effectively to verbal, nonverbal, and written communications
- Serve as a liaison

GENERAL: LEGAL CONCEPTS
- Perform within legal and ethical boundaries
- Document accurately
- Comply with established risk management and safety procedures

GENERAL: INSTRUCTION
- Instruct individuals according to their needs
- Locate community resources and disseminate information

CHAPTER COMPETENCIES

LEARNING OBJECTIVES
Upon successfully completing this chapter, you will be able to:
1. Spell and define the key terms.
2. Describe common disorders of the alimentary canal and accessory organs.
3. Explain the purpose of various diagnostic procedures associated with the GI system.
4. Discuss the role of the medical assistant in diagnosing and treating disorders of the GI system.

PERFORMANCE OBJECTIVES
Upon successfully completing this chapter, you will be able to:
1. Assist with colon procedures (Procedure 34-1).
2. Instruct a patient on collecting a stool specimen (Procedure 34-2).
3. Test a stool specimen for occult blood (Procedure 34-3).

KEY TERMS

anorexia	hepatomegaly	malocclusion	peristalsis
ascites	hepatotoxin	melena	sclerotherapy
dysphagia	insufflator	metabolism	stomatitis
guaiac	leukoplakia	obturator	turgor
hematemesis			

The gastrointestinal (GI) system, or tract, is responsible for the ingestion, digestion, transportation, and elimination of the food we eat (FIG. 34-1). Nutrients are broken down by the action of digestive enzymes into units that can be absorbed through the walls of the GI system into the circulatory and lymphatic systems. This process starts when something is put into the mouth, chewed, and mixed with the enzymes in saliva. Through **peristalsis**, food is pushed along the GI tract, further breaking it down into segments and mixing it with enzymes to hasten the breakdown into nutrients. **Metabolism** is the breakdown of food into usable units through these physical and chemical changes. Any unused food material is eliminated as waste from the GI system as feces.

Disorders of the GI system may affect the alimentary canal, also called the GI tract, or accessory organs such as the liver, gallbladder, and pancreas. This chapter describes common disorders of the GI system and the accessory organs, diagnostic procedures, and your role as a medical assistant. While the physician who specializes in disorders of the GI system is the gastroenterologist, medical assistants working in other offices, including family practice and internal medicine offices, often encounter patients with disorders of this body system.

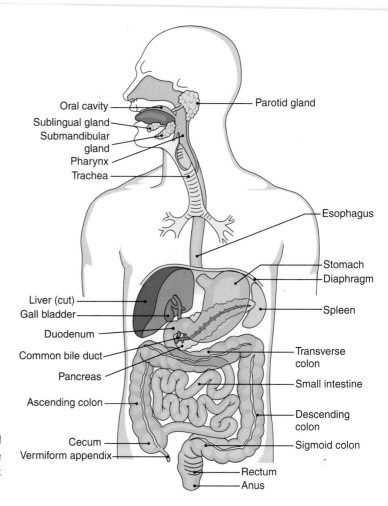

FIGURE 34–1. The digestive system. (Reprinted with permission from Cohen BJ, Wood DL. Memmler's The Human Body in Health and Disease. Philadelphia: Lippincott Williams & Wilkins, 2000.)

COMMON GASTROINTESTINAL DISORDERS

Mouth Disorders

While disorders of the teeth, gums, and oral cavity are typically diagnosed and treated by the dentist, patients requiring a referral to a dentist or oral surgeon may be seen first in the medical office. Physicians and other health care professionals should be aware of these disorders and their importance to nutrition, digestion, and the overall health status of the patient. Your role includes taking an accurate medical history, including inquiring about the condition of the oral cavity and teeth, making referrals as ordered by the physician, and educating patients about the care of the gums and teeth to prevent health problems and loss of teeth.

Caries

Dental caries (tooth decay) is the most widespread disease of the oral cavity. Bacteria allowed to remain on the teeth erode the enamel and allow infection to reach the inner portions of the tooth. Factors that may contribute to the development of dental caries include a poor diet, inade-

quate dental hygiene, and **malocclusion**, abnormal contact between the upper teeth and the lower teeth. Prevention of dental caries includes consuming a balanced diet low in sugars, good oral hygiene as prescribed by the dentist, and frequent professional dental care. Treatment may include drilling the dental caries and replacing the space with a filling or extraction of the affected teeth. Because dental caries can cause discomfort with chewing or biting, they may affect nutrition and ultimately digestion and the overall health of the patient.

Stomatitis

Stomatitis, an inflammation of the oral mucosa, may be caused by a virus, bacteria, or fungus. The two most common forms are herpetic stomatitis, caused by the herpes simplex virus, and candidiasis, caused by the fungus *Candida albicans*.

Herpes simplex is usually self-limiting after the initial exposure to the virus. The virus is usually transmitted hand to mouth, mouth to mouth, or by vector (e.g., shared drinking glasses or eating utensils). The infection presents as a painful sore on the mucosa of the mouth (commonly called a canker sore) or on the lips (commonly called a fever blister or cold sore). After the initial infection, the virus lies dormant for long periods, with exacerbations during illness, stress, over-exposure to the sun, or other trigger. Although there is no cure for herpes simplex, palliative measures such as ointments or creams may be purchased over the counter to relieve the discomfort.

Candida albicans, formerly called *Monilia albicans*, is an opportunistic yeast or fungus. This organism is always present in the mouth but is kept in check by other normal oral bacteria. When the normal bacterial balance in the mouth is altered, *C. albicans* microorganisms multiply, causing an infection that appears as a white substance covering the oral cavity and tongue. Factors that can upset the balance of these microorganisms in the mouth include the use of broad-spectrum antibiotics that kill many bacteria throughout the body, including the mouth, allowing the opportunistic organisms to grow without control. In babies, the disease is called thrush and commonly is due to a favorable environment for the growth of *C. albicans*, as milk changes the pH of the mouth. In adults or infants, treatment with an antifungal agent usually cures the disorder and restores the balance of microbes in the mouth.

Gingivitis

Gingivitis is an inflammation of the gingiva, or gums. It may lead to periodontitis, or inflammation and possible destruction of the supporting structures of the teeth, including the gingiva, periodontal ligament, and mandibular or maxillary bone. In Americans, more teeth are lost to gum disease than to tooth decay. Good oral hygiene and frequent dental care help prevent premature loss of teeth. Once diagnosed, gingivitis is usually treated with an antibiotic.

Oral Cancers

Cancers of the oral cavity are common, especially among individuals who use tobacco products. The constant irritation of the tobacco causes white spots or patches, called **leukoplakia**, to form on the oral mucosa, particularly the lips and tongue. These lesions have clearly defined borders and frequently become malignant. Treatment includes surgery or chemical agents such as radiation or chemotherapy. Although cancer of the lips usually responds well to radiation or surgery, cancers of the margins of the tongue metastasize quickly and are commonly difficult to treat effectively.

Checkpoint Question

1. What are the two most common causes of stomatitis?

Esophageal Disorders

Hiatal Hernia

Hiatal hernia is a common condition that frequently affects people over age 40 years. Weight gain, either recent or prolonged, can be a contributing factor. A hiatal hernia is caused by a defect in the diaphragm that allows a portion of the stomach to slide up into the chest cavity. Normally, the cardiac sphincter, a muscle that separates the end of the esophagus from the beginning of the stomach, prevents gastroesophageal reflux, or backflow of gastric acids, from the stomach into the esophagus. The presence of a hiatal hernia enables the stomach acid to backflow into the esophagus, causing considerable discomfort including indigestion and epigastric pain in the upper abdomen (FIG. 34-2).

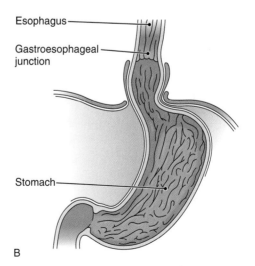

FIGURE 34–2. (A) Normal. (B) Hiatal hernia. The stomach protrudes through the diaphragm into the thoracic cavity, raising the level of the junction between the esophagus and the stomach. (Reprinted with permission from Cohen BJ, Wood DL. Memmler's The Human Body in Health and Disease. Philadelphia: Lippincott Williams & Wilkins, 2000.)

Diagnosis is made by taking a careful medical history, chest radiographs, barium swallow, or endoscopy. Medical treatment is usually preferred to surgical intervention, since surgically corrected hiatal hernias frequently recur. Medical interventions include diet modifications such as small, frequent meals with no food for at least 2 hours before bedtime. In addition, the physician may order antacids, weight loss, elevating the head of the bed, and drug therapy to increase the tone of the cardiac sphincter.

Constant exposure to gastric acid from gastroesophageal reflux can lead to esophagitis, a condition that resembles abraded tissue along the lining of the esophagus. Constant irritation of the lining of the esophagus, also known as Barrett's esophagus, may lead to malignancy. Patients with Barrett's esophagus have a 30% to 40% chance of developing adenocarcinoma. If the source of irritation is gastroesophageal reflux, it will be diagnosed and treated much the same as a hiatal hernia (Box 34-1).

Esophageal Varices

Varicose veins (varices) of the esophagus result from pressure within the esophageal veins. This condition is commonly seen in patients diagnosed with cirrhosis of the liver. Since drainage from the portal vein is impaired by the liver damage, the veins of the esophagus become distended, resulting in varices. The most common and dangerous problem that results from esophageal varices is hemorrhaging if the distended veins rupture. Before a rupture occurs, the treatment of choice is **sclerotherapy**, which uses a chemical agent to cause fibrosing (hardening) of the area around the varices, preventing hemorrhaging. In the event of esophageal hemorrhage, the patient should be transported immediately to the emergency room, where pressure

WHAT IF

Your patient complains of heartburn?

Patients with a complaint of any type of chest pain, including heartburn, should be assessed immediately, since the symptoms of gastroesophageal reflux disease (GERD) may be similar to the chest pain of a patient having cardiac problems. In addition to the chest pain, signs and symptoms of myocardial involvement can include:
- Shortness of breath
- Nausea or vomiting
- Pain that spreads from the chest to the jaw, back or arms

Chest pain that is not cardiac may be diagnosed by the physician as GERD, a chronic disorder characterized by discomfort in the chest (heartburn) due to the backflow of gastric contents into the esophagus. This disorder is caused by a weak lower esophageal sphincter that normally closes after food is swallowed, keeping the material in the stomach. The symptoms of GERD:
- Frequent heartburn or indigestion relieved by antacids
- Hoarseness or laryngitis
- Sore throat
- A feeling of a lump in the throat
- Chronic cough

tubes can be applied directly to the varices to control the bleeding.

Esophageal Cancers

Cancer of the esophagus is most common among older men and is usually fatal. Predisposing factors for this type of cancer include chronic gastroesophageal reflux, smoking, and drinking alcohol. The malignancy narrows the lumen of the esophagus and causes **dysphagia** (difficulty swallowing). As the mass enlarges, swallowing solid food may become extremely painful. Vomiting and weight loss occur as the symptoms progress. A barium swallow with fluoroscopy outlines the lesion, and esophagoscopy with biopsy confirms the diagnosis. If the disease is local, surgical resection, chemotherapy, and radiation are the therapies of choice. No treatment has proven satisfactory, however, and the survival rates are very low.

Checkpoint Question

2. What is a hiatal hernia, and how can it affect the esophagus?

Box 34-1

PREVENTING GASTRIC REFLUX

- Avoid spicy foods and chocolate, especially in the evening.
- Limit caffeine.
- Maintain optimum weight.
- Avoid overeating.
- Wait 1 hour after eating before exercising.
- Do not eat just before going to bed.
- Do not lie down just after eating.
- Stop smoking.
- Place blocks, bricks, or a stack of books under the legs of the bed to elevate the head, chest, and abdomen approximately 12 inches.
- See the physician if symptoms persist.

Stomach Disorders

Gastritis

Gastritis, an inflammation of the lining of the stomach, can be acute or chronic. The most common causes include irritants such as alcohol and certain drugs, including aspirin and nonsteroidal anti-inflammatory medications (NSAIDs). The bacterium *Helicobacter pylori*, also often implicated, is presumed to enter the body through food contaminated with infected fecal material (fecal–oral route) or from eating or drinking from a utensil also used by someone who is infected with the bacteria (oral–oral route). It resides in the mucous lining of the stomach and secretes enzymes that attack the mucous membrane.

Gastritis can cause significant oozing of blood and may result in a positive test for occult (hidden) blood in the stool. In elderly patients, sufficient blood loss can result in anemia. Signs and symptoms of gastritis include evidence of GI bleeding, epigastric discomfort, nausea, and vomiting. Diagnosis is usually made by obtaining a careful and complete history and direct visualization of the gastric mucosa through an endoscopic procedure known as a gastroscopy. Treatment usually involves eliminating the irritant, restoring the proper gastric acidity, and administering antibiotics as prescribed by the physician.

Peptic Ulcers

Ulcers in the GI tract are erosions or sores left by sloughed tissues. These erosions can expose small blood vessels and produce bleeding and pain. Peptic ulcers occur from the exposure of the lining of the stomach and first part of the small intestine (duodenum) to hydrochloric acid (HCl), a caustic chemical produced and secreted by the lining of the stomach that may cause erosion if too much is excreted. As the mucosa erodes, the patient has abdominal pain that intensifies during peristalsis, especially after eating. As the erosions and mucosa become more irritated, the ulcers bleed. The bleeding may range from a slight oozing to life-threatening hemorrhage. Heavy bleeding will lead to **melena**, black tarry stools, or **hematemesis**, vomiting blood. Ulcers in the upper GI tract may perforate into the abdominal cavity with life-threatening consequences such as hypovolemic shock and peritonitis. Chronic ulcerative conditions may also progress to malignancies.

The causes of peptic or gastric ulcers may include the use of chemicals that irritate the gastric mucosa, including aspirin, NSAIDs, and alcohol. Many gastric ulcers are also caused by an infection with *H. pylori*, which can be treated effectively with an antibiotic. Overproduction of gastric HCl also irritates the gastric mucosa and may produce erosions. Gastric acid production is under nerve and hormonal control and increases during times of emotional stress. Diagnosis of an ulcer is similar to the diagnosis of gastritis, including a thorough history and possibly endoscopic examination. The prescribed treatment for ulcers is avoiding the irritants causing the erosion, limiting the production of hydrogen by the gastric cells to neutralize the acid in the stomach, and an antibiotic as prescribed. Surgery to cut or disconnect the vagus nerve (vagotomy), which also reduces the secretion of HCl, may be performed if methods to decrease production of gastric acid are ineffective in treating the ulcer.

Gastric Cancer

Gastric cancer has no known cause, although smoking, excessive alcohol intake, ingesting foods high in preservatives, and genetic predisposition may contribute. Gastric cancer spreads rapidly to adjacent organs (the liver and pancreas) and throughout the peritoneal cavity. Signs and symptoms include chronic indigestion, weight loss, anorexia, anemia, and fatigue. The patient may have hematemesis with bright blood or coffee ground vomitus with dark blood. There may also be dark, bloody stools.

Diagnosis of gastric cancer requires an upper GI series with fluoroscopy, fiberoptic gastroscopy, and biopsy of the lesion or tumor. The extent of the disease can be determined by computed tomography (CT) and biopsy of the suspected metastatic sites, including adjacent organs. Surgery to remove the lesion may range from a subtotal gastric resection (removal of part of the stomach) to a total gastrectomy (removal of the entire stomach). If the cancer has metastasized, other organs may be removed and radiation and chemotherapy may be necessary.

Intestinal Disorders

Gastroenteritis

Gastroenteritis is general inflammation of the stomach, small intestine, and/or colon. This condition is caused by ingesting food or water that contains bacteria, viruses, parasites, or irritating agents such as spices. Food allergies and reactions to certain medications, such as antibiotics, may also inflame these organs. Symptoms include abdominal pain and cramping, nausea, vomiting, diarrhea, and fever.

The symptoms of gastroenteritis are self-limiting in most adults, usually lasting a few hours to a couple of days. However, because of the dehydration that can accompany the diarrhea and vomiting, gastroenteritis may be life-threatening in the elderly, young children, and persons with diabetes mellitus. Treatment is palliative; it includes reducing the work of the GI tract by limiting food intake, treating the nausea, vomiting and diarrhea, and maintaining the fluid balance by hydrating the body as needed. In severe cases, intravenous fluids must be administered to prevent dehydration and death, especially in the young and the elderly. If the cause of the inflammation is a bacterial or parasitic infection, an antibiotic or antiparasitic medication may be prescribed

> ## PATIENT EDUCATION
>
> ### Gastric Bypass Surgery to Treat Obesity
>
> Bariatrics is the study of morbid obesity. A popular surgical procedure to treat obesity is gastric bypass. Here are a few facts about this procedure:
>
> - According to the American Society of Bariatric Surgery (www.asbs.org), candidates for the surgery must be severely obese and have failed to lose weight with other methods.
> - Candidates for gastric bypass surgery must have either a body mass index greater than 40 (approximately 80–100 pounds over the ideal weight for height) or significant medical problems associated with being overweight.
> - The abdomen is incised and the stomach reduced to about the size of a thumb. The large remainder of the stomach is bypassed and the new, smaller stomach is attached directly to the small intestine.
> - The surgery comes with risks and requires lifestyle changes. Anemia and nutritional deficiencies are long-term risks that must be monitored and prevented or corrected.
> - Since weight reduction after this procedure is often quick and dramatic, patients should be encouraged to begin an exercise program following the surgery as indicated by the surgeon.

once the causative microorganism has been identified through a stool culture and analysis.

Duodenal Ulcers

Ulcerative lesions in the duodenum are often caused by exposure to highly corrosive gastric acid that is secreted by the stomach or other irritants that pass through the pylorus to the small intestine. Unlike the stomach, the duodenum has a normally alkaline pH, and the mucosa is not as well protected as the gastric mucosa. When food material passes through the pylorus and brings excessive acid or other irritants with it, an ulcer may form in the duodenum. As with the peptic ulcer, an overproduction of gastric acid may arise from ingestion of highly spicy foods or from overproduction of stress hormones, which also increases production of gastric acid. Treatment for duodenal ulcers is limiting or avoiding the irritating factors and reducing gastric acidity. If these measures are not successful, surgery may be an option. As with peptic ulcers, ulcers in the duodenum left untreated

may perforate the lining of the small intestine or may progress to cancerous lesions.

Malabsorption Syndromes

Malabsorption syndromes prevent the normal absorption of certain nutrients through the walls of the small intestines. Commonly fat is not absorbed. The sign that a patient has a problem with malabsorption of fats includes stools that are frothy and pale. Because fat is necessary for the metabolism of vitamins A, D, E, and K, patients with this disorder require supplemental vitamin therapy.

Celiac sprue is a malabsorption syndrome marked by intolerance to gluten, a protein found in wheat and wheat byproducts. Celiac sprue can develop at any stage of life and often causes diarrhea high in fat. The cause of celiac sprue is not known, but it runs in families, suggesting a genetic factor.

Malabsorption syndromes are treated by addressing the suspected causes and avoiding or replacing the malabsorbed substances.

Checkpoint Question

3. How are peptic and duodenal ulcers different?

Crohn Disease

Crohn disease is an inflammation of deep lining of the bowel ranging from very mild to severe and debilitating. The cause of Crohn disease is unclear, but it is thought to be an autoimmune disorder with a possible genetic link. Crohn disease can affect the small bowel and the colon but is more common in the area of the ileocecal valve. The bowel walls become inflamed and the lymph nodes enlarge, leading to edema of the bowel wall. When the lining of the bowel is swollen, the fluid from the intestinal contents cannot be absorbed, causing diarrhea and cramping, which may lead to more irritation and bleeding. Patients may also have periods of constipation, **anorexia**, and fever.

Although Crohn disease is a chronic disorder, each episode of inflammation causes scarring. The scarring may lead to narrowing of the colon, obstructing the bowel. Bowel obstruction can be life-threatening and is a medical emergency. Diagnosis of Crohn disease necessitates a thorough history and analysis of the blood, which shows an increase in white blood cells and the erythrocyte sedimentation rate. A barium enema, or lower GI, radiographic examination, if ordered by the physician, shows strictures alternating with normal bowel. Sigmoidoscopy and colonoscopy show patchy areas of inflammation within the bowel.

The treatment of Crohn disease is symptomatic; it includes restoration of fluids and electrolytes, administering corticosteroids to reduce inflammation, rest, and a low-fiber diet. Surgery is performed in cases of perforation or hemorrhage. If the situation is severe, a colectomy with an ileostomy may be performed (FIG. 34-3).

Ulcerative Colitis

Like Crohn disease, ulcerative colitis is an inflammatory bowel disease affecting the lining of the colon. It occurs most often in young women but may occur at any age and may affect men also. The cause is not known but is thought to be an abnormal GI immune reaction to foods or microorganisms. Ulcerative colitis is a chronic condition, and the symptoms can be mild or severe with periods of remission.

The tissue that lines the colon becomes congested and edematous, eventually sloughing off and leading to ulcers and bloody diarrhea. Sometimes pus and mucus are present in the stool. Malabsorption of fluids causes weakness, anorexia, nausea, and vomiting. Scarring can occur as the ulcers heal. The colon may produce pseudopolyps, which can be precancerous. Diagnosis may be determined by endoscopic examination or by a barium enema, and biopsy confirms the diagnosis. Colonoscopy is used to evaluate strictures caused by scarring and to assess the risk of cancer.

Treatment of ulcerative colitis requires controlling the inflammation and preventing the loss of fluids and nutrients during periods of exacerbation. If the disease is severe, a corticosteroid is prescribed to relieve the inflammation. Surgery is a last resort and usually involves a proctocolectomy with an ileostomy.

PATIENT EDUCATION

Maintaining Good Bowel Habits

By following these guidelines, patients can prevent common problems of elimination:

- Eat a variety of foods, especially fresh fruits, vegetables, and whole grains. Limit the intake of highly processed foods.
- Drink eight glasses of water a day to keep the stools moist and easy to pass and to hydrate the tissues.
- Get some form of exercise daily. Even a walk around the block will aid muscle tone and help prevent sluggish metabolism.
- Make time for bowel movements when the stimulus is felt. Avoiding or delaying defecation results in loss of moisture from the stool and may make the bowel insensitive to the stimulus.
- Do not use laxatives or enemas. Frequent use may result in a lazy bowel that responds only to these chemical and physical stimuli.

The frequency of bowel elimination is an individual characteristic. If stools are passed only several times a week but are soft, formed, and passed with little effort, there should be no concern about constipation. However, constipation may be a problem if stools are passed daily but are hard, dry, and difficult to pass.

FIGURE 34-3. An ileostomy. The shaded portion indicates the section of the bowel that has been removed or is inactive. (Modified with permission from Cohen BJ. Medical Terminology: An Illustrated Guide. Philadelphia: Lippincott Williams & Wilkins, 2003.)

Irritable Bowel Syndrome

Patients with irritable bowel syndrome frequently complain of bouts of constipation alternating with diarrhea. Although the patient may have signs and symptoms resembling those of Crohn disease or ulcerative colitis, it usually does not result in weight loss, and the prognosis is good. However, this disorder can be debilitating, because there is no warning for the bouts of diarrhea caused by the spastic colon. Women are more likely than men to have this chronic disorder, whose symptoms may range from mild to severe even though endoscopic examination shows no signs of disease. The origin of irritable bowel syndrome is thought to be psychogenic, a reaction to stress and emotions and the actions of the autonomic nervous system, which partly controls the colon. The consumption of specific food irritants may also precipitate an attack; however, the particular food item that triggers symptoms varies from person to person. Diagnosis requires a careful history, both physical and emotional. Other diseases are ruled out by testing. Treatment is stress management and identifying the offending food irritants.

Checkpoint Question

4. Which inflammatory bowel disease can lead to life-threatening bowel obstruction? How?

Diverticulosis

Diverticulosis is a chronic condition of thinning of the bowel wall, causing small out-pouches in the lining of the intestinal wall (FIG. 34-4). This disorder usually occurs in the sigmoid colon but may occur anywhere in the GI tract. The cause has been attributed to a diet deficient in roughage. While many people have diverticulosis without symptoms, the condition becomes more serious when the bowel wall becomes so thin that veins and arteries are exposed. Bleeding can occur when the wall is nicked by a piece of stool and may be severe enough to require surgery to stop the hemorrhage. A diet high in fiber and use of stool softeners may be ordered by the physician to prevent the signs and symptoms in this disorder.

Diverticulosis may progress to diverticulitis, or inflammation of these areas of weakness in the bowel wall. The inflammation is usually caused by fecal material becoming lodged in the thin pockets. The symptoms are fever and abdominal pain. As the bowel becomes swollen and distended, the diseased areas may rupture, exposing the peritoneum to fecal material and resulting in peritonitis. The pouches are visualized on films produced from a barium enema or directly through endoscopic studies.

During the acute phase, treatment includes a bland diet and stool softeners until the inflammation has subsided.

FIGURE 34–4. Diverticulosis of the sigmoid colon. (Reprinted with permission from Neil Hardy, Westpoint, CT.)

Polyps

Colon polyps are masses of benign mucous membrane lining the large intestine that are usually slow growing but may become cancerous. Polyps are usually discovered by a barium enema or during a colonoscopy. If the polyps are discovered at an early stage and removed, cancer of the colon may be prevented. Cancer of the colon may invade the muscle of the bowel and metastasize through the lymph system to other organs.

Hernias

The anterior abdominal wall is covered with various muscles that assist with movement and support and protect the internal structures of the abdomen. When these muscles weaken, the underlying organs or intestines may protrude through the weakened muscle wall, resulting in a hernia. Factors that may increase the risk for developing a hernia include a genetic predisposition to muscular weakness, lifting heavy objects, obesity, and pregnancy. The signs and symptoms of abdominal hernia include a protrusion or bulge over the area of the hernia. Specific types of abdominal hernias are named according to the area of the abdomen: the inguinal hernia occurs in right or left inguinal (groin) areas; the ventral hernia occurs in the front of the abdomen; and the umbilical hernia occurs over the umbilicus. The treatment for abdominal hernias includes surgically repairing the weakened muscle (herniorrhaphy) using grafting material as necessary. To prevent abdominal hernias, encourage the use of abdominal support and good body mechanics when lifting and weight reduction as prescribed by the physician.

The hiatal hernia, or diaphragmatic hernia, occurs when the stomach protrudes up through the diaphragm through a weakened or enlarged cardiac sphincter at the bottom of the esophagus. The symptoms of a hiatal hernia include abdominal pain and indigestion, especially after eating. Surgery to correct a hiatal hernia is not always effective, and the treatment is generally palliative, including eating small, frequent meals and avoiding eating before going to bed.

Appendicitis

The vermiform appendix, a small pouch of tissue protruding from the cecum or first part of the large intestine, is approximately 4 inches long. Although the function of this tissue is not clear, there is no direct involvement with the process of digestion. Appendicitis occurs when the vermiform appendix becomes infected and fills with bacteria, pus, and blood. Adolescents and young adult men are most commonly affected by this condition, but women and young children can also develop appendicitis. The symptoms include severe abdominal pain with tenderness over the right lower quadrant, vomiting, a fever, and an elevated white blood count. A thorough history should be obtained from any patient with these symptoms, and once the physician determines the diagnosis of appendicitis, it is necessary to make arrangements for immediate surgical removal of the infected appendix. If a diagnosis is not made quickly or the appendectomy is delayed, perforation of the appendix and peritonitis can result and make recovery more difficult for the patient.

Hemorrhoids

Hemorrhoids are external or internal dilated veins (varicosities) in the rectum. Internal hemorrhoids may enlarge and may bleed during defecation. A patient with external hemorrhoids may complain of rectal pain and itching and bleeding with bowel movements. Poor abdominal and pelvic floor muscle tone, poor dietary habits including a diet low in fiber, and chronic constipation may cause hemorrhoids. The diagnosis of external hemorrhoids is made by visual inspection, while internal hemorrhoids are diagnosed by anoscopy or proctoscopy. Treatment involves regulating the diet to control constipation, providing local pain relief, using a stool softener, and surgical ligation (hemorrhoidectomy) using standard surgical techniques, laser, or cryosurgery (freezing).

Colorectal Cancers

Cancer of the colon and rectum is often fatal, but the patient's chances for survival are better with early diagnosis and treatment. Although the cause of colorectal cancer is unknown, it has been linked to diets high in animal fats and low in fiber. It is commonly seen in patients with a history of ulcerative colitis or colorectal polyps and affects the first and last parts of the colon more often than other areas (FIG. 34-5). Early signs of colorectal cancer are vague abdominal

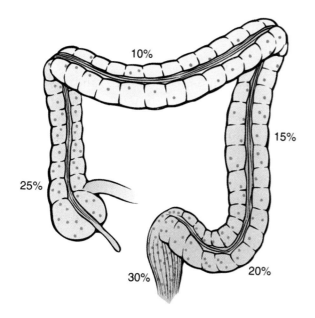

FIGURE 34–5. Percentage distribution of cancer sites in the colon and rectum.

pains with occasional bloody stools. Later signs depend on the section and amount of the colon involved and the degree of metastasis to other organs and tissues.

Many rectal cancers are discovered by a digital examination or an anoscopy, but sigmoidoscopy or colonoscopy is used to determine the extent of involvement. A barium enema with contrast air aids in the diagnosis. Laboratory tests include **guaiac** tests, such as the Hemoccult, which test for occult (hidden) blood in the stool. Surgical removal of the affected area, usually followed by chemotherapy and radiation, is the treatment of choice.

Functional Disorders

Functional disorders of the GI tract include the common disorders constipation, diarrhea, and intestinal gas. Normally, peristalsis causes the products of digestion to move at a constant rate, not too slowly and not too quickly. **Constipation occurs when the lower colon retains fecal material too long so that too much moisture is absorbed, making the stool hard and dry.** Most constipation is caused by poor bowel habits (avoiding defecation and overusing laxatives), low-fiber diet, and inadequate fluid intake. The quality of the stool is more important than the quantity. To avoid constipation, patients should be encouraged to increase oral fluid intake, eat foods high in fiber, such as raw vegetables and fruit, and maintain regular bowel habits. The physician may also prescribe a stool softener and an over-the-counter fiber product as needed.

When the fluid contents of the bowel are rushed through, as in diarrhea, the water and minerals are not reabsorbed into the system and the stool is loose and watery. Bacterial or viral infection or a GI irritant causes the smooth muscles and mucous membranes to work to flush out the bowel as quickly as possible. The treatment for diarrhea includes medication to slow peristalsis, a bland diet, and increasing oral fluids to replace fluids and electrolytes lost in the stool.

Intestinal gas, produced by bacterial decomposition of proteins in the digestive tract, can lead to abdominal discomfort. Gas in the intestinal tract causes a feeling of fullness. The gas may be expelled from the stomach through the mouth (eructation, or belching) or from the intestines through the rectum (flatulence). The production of intestinal gas is due to intolerance of milk products, swallowing air through excessive talking or gum chewing, consuming gas-producing spicy or fatty foods, or slow emptying of the stomach and bowels. The problem can usually be relieved by avoiding the offending foods or behaviors. Various over-the-counter preparations and prescription medications can be used if the problem persists.

Checkpoint Question

5. What causes hemorrhoids?

Liver Disorders

Liver disorders are assessed by observing the cardinal signs of liver dysfunction: jaundice, **ascites** (fluid accumulation in the peritoneal cavity), and **hepatomegaly** (enlargement of the liver). It is vital to obtain a complete medical history from patients with a suspected liver disorder. Particular concern focuses on jaundice, anemia, splenectomy, alcohol use, travel to Third World countries, blood transfusions, use of **hepatotoxins** (drugs that are damaging to the liver), and abuse of controlled substances. Diagnostic tests for liver disorders include the following:

- Liver function tests, including prothrombin time and levels of bilirubin, alkaline phosphatase, albumin, and cholesterol
- Radiography and barium study
- Radioisotope liver scan
- Percutaneous peritoneoscopy and biopsy
- Surgical laparotomy and liver biopsy

Hepatitis

Hepatitis is an inflammation or infection of the liver that may lead to liver destruction and necrosis of hepatic cells. The five types of viral hepatitis are summarized in TABLE 34-1 and listed here:

- *Hepatitis A (HAV)*, the most common type of viral hepatitis, is also known as infectious hepatitis. HAV spreads in food and water contaminated with fecal material or seafood high in coliform bacteria. It is highly contagious, but the prognosis for recovery after an infection with hepatitis A is good.
- *Hepatitis B (HBV)*, also known as serum hepatitis, can be transmitted by contaminated blood and other body fluids. HBV may be so severe that death results, but the use of standard precautions will prevent spread. Fortunately, there is a vaccine to protect against HBV, and it is recommended for all health care workers (see Chapter 1).
- *Hepatitis C (HCV)*, also known as non-A, non-B hepatitis, can be transmitted via blood transfusion or percutaneous contamination. After the initial infection,

HCV frequently progresses to chronic hepatitis that may be asymptomatic but is communicable. As with HBV, the use of standard precautions prevents spread.
- *Hepatitis D (HDV)* occurs only in patients who have had HBV; it cannot survive without HBV.
- *Hepatitis E (HEV)* spreads in food or water contaminated with fecal material and ingested by the unsuspecting individual.

While the viruses responsible for the individual types of viral hepatitis are physically different, the symptoms of all types are similar. They may include fatigue, joint pain, flu-like symptoms with fever, jaundice, dark urine, and light stools. Complications of hepatitis include long-term impaired liver function, chronic hepatitis, liver cancer, and death.

Diagnosis of the various types of viral hepatitis is made by obtaining a complete medical history, blood analysis for hepatitis antibodies, and liver function studies. There is no cure once infection occurs, but the patient is encouraged to rest and take in a supportive diet. Interferon-A is given to some patients to assist the immune system in responding to viral hepatitis. Standard precautions must be observed to protect caregivers and health care workers from contracting hepatitis.

Another cause of hepatitis, toxic hepatitis, is exposure to chemical toxicants or hepatotoxic substances, including certain medications and alcohol. If the offending toxicant is eliminated early enough, the prognosis for recovery is good. The symptoms of toxic hepatitis resemble viral hepatitis, and the diagnosis is similar. A liver biopsy may identify the underlying pathology.

Checkpoint Question

6. How does the cause of viral hepatitis differ from that of toxic hepatitis?

Cirrhosis or Fibrosis

Cirrhosis is a chronic disease characterized by destruction of liver cells and the formation of scar tissue or fibers throughout the liver, altering its function and efficiency.

Table 34-1	TYPES OF VIRAL HEPATITIS	
Virus	**Transmission**	**Precautions**
HAV	Fecal–oral route	Handwashing
HBV	Sera and body fluids	Standard precautions, HBV vaccine
HCV	Blood transfusions Percutaneous contamination	Standard precautions
HDV	Coinfection with HBV	Standard precautions, HBV vaccine
HEV	Fecal–oral route	Handwashing, standard precautions

The causes of cirrhosis include a history of exposure to hepatotoxins, alcoholism, prolonged biliary obstruction, and a history of hepatitis. In the early stages, symptoms include vague GI discomfort. In the late stages, respiratory efficiency decreases because of ascites that forces the abdominal contents against the diaphragm. Bleeding tendencies result from the loss of clotting factors formed in the liver. Dermal pruritus (itching), jaundice, and hepatomegaly are usually present. Diagnosis is made by liver biopsy, liver scan, and blood work. Treatment includes avoiding the hepatotoxins or abstinence from alcohol to prevent further death of hepatic cells, a good diet, vitamin supplements, and supportive care. In cases of liver failure that accompanies increased destruction of liver tissue, the physician may recommend a liver transplant.

Liver Cancer

The liver is rarely a primary site for cancer but is frequently a target site of metastasis. This type of cancer is more common in men than in women and is rapidly fatal. There is no known cause, but primary liver cancers are thought to be due to exposure to carcinogenic chemicals, including hepatotoxins. Patients who have cirrhosis or hepatitis B are more likely than the general population to develop liver cancer.

In the early stages of the disease, patients usually complain of weight loss, weakness, and right upper quadrant pain. Jaundice may be present and will definitely develop as the disease progresses. Diagnosis is confirmed by biopsy, liver function tests, and CT or magnetic resonance imaging (MRI). If the lesion is small and local, resection is possible. Chemotherapy may be used in some instances. If there is no metastasis, a liver transplant may be possible.

Gallbladder Disorders

Cholelithiasis and Cholecystitis

Cholelithiasis is the formation of gallstones made of cholesterol and bilirubin (FIG. 34-6). When the peristaltic action of the gallbladder is sluggish and bile pools in the sac, fluid is absorbed, leaving the solids to concentrate and solidify into stones. Cholecystitis is an acute or chronic inflammation of the gallbladder, usually resulting from an impacted stone in the duct. Cholecystitis or cholelithiasis usually causes pain as peristalsis presses bile against the blockage, especially after a fatty meal.

Signs and symptoms of any gallbladder disorder include acute right upper abdominal quadrant pain that may radiate to the shoulders, back or chest; indigestion; nausea; and intolerance of fatty foods. Later in the illness, jaundice may appear as the ducts to the liver become blocked. Tests to determine the cause of the symptoms include cholecystography after the ingestion of a radiopaque dye, percutaneous transhepatic cholangiography, endoscopic retrograde cholangiopancreatography (ECRP), and duodenal endoscopy.

FIGURE 34–6. Cholelithiasis. The gallbladder has been opened to reveal numerous yellow cholesterol gallstones. (Reprinted with permission from Rubin E, Farber JL. Pathology. Philadelphia: Lippincott Williams & Wilkins, 1999.)

Noninvasive procedures include ultrasound and CT. Flat plate radiographs are not especially accurate for evaluating gallbladder disorders. The treatment may be supportive or palliative, including pain medication and avoiding fatty foods; however, surgical removal of the stones (cholecystectomy) may be necessary, usually through endoscopic laparotomy. Lithotripsy, crushing the gallstones using sound waves, may also be used to break the stones into small pieces that can pass easily through the bile ducts and into the digestive system for elimination.

Gallbladder Cancer

Cancer of the gallbladder is rare and difficult to diagnose. Since the symptoms are similar to those of cholecystitis, this cancer is usually discovered during routine gallbladder tests performed to diagnose general gallbladder disease. The signs and symptoms include right upper quadrant pain, nausea and vomiting, weight loss, and anorexia. However, cholecystitis pain is usually sporadic, while pain due to malignancy is usually chronic and severe. The gallbladder may be palpable and jaundice may be present. It is most common in older women and is rapidly fatal. The cause is not known, but theory suggests that cholelithiasis is a predisposing factor. Diagnosis includes liver function tests, CT, MRI, and cholecystography. Surgical cholecystectomy is the primary treatment, but survival rates are low.

Checkpoint Question

7. How are cholelithiasis and cholecystitis different?

Pancreatic Disorders

Pancreatitis

Pancreatitis is an inflammation of the pancreas that may be related to alcoholism, trauma, gastric ulcer, or biliary tract disease. Signs and symptoms include vomiting and steady epigastric pain radiating to the spine. Signs of progressive disease include abdominal rigidity and decreased bowel activity. Complications include diabetes mellitus, hemorrhage, shock, coma, and death as the digestive enzymes cause the organ to digest itself. Diagnostic blood tests show an increase in serum amylase and glucose levels. Ultrasound and CT are useful for diagnosis. Treatment includes pain relief and medication to reduce pancreatic secretions while the organ recovers. Prognosis depends on the extent and severity of damage to the pancreas.

Pancreatic Cancer

One of the deadliest malignancies is pancreatic cancer, which kills most patients within a year of diagnosis. There is no definitive cause, but it occurs most often in middle-aged African American men who smoke, who have a diet high in fats and proteins, or who are exposed to industrial chemicals for long periods.

Patients complain of weight loss, back and abdominal pain, and diarrhea. Commonly they are jaundiced. Diagnosis is made by laparoscopic biopsy, CT, MRI, endoscopic retrograde cholangiopancreatography (ERCP), and pancreatic enzyme studies. Surgical removal of the pancreas (pancreatotomy), chemotherapy, and radiation therapy are used to treat pancreatic cancer, but the survival rate is very low.

COMMON DIAGNOSTIC AND THERAPEUTIC PROCEDURES

History and Physical Examination of the Gastrointestinal System

Before beginning any patient's care, an adequate history must be obtained. The patient presenting with GI concerns will be assessed for signs (e.g., vomiting) and symptoms (e.g., nausea). From that base, the physician will determine the direction of the diagnostic testing to rule out or to confirm possible diagnosis. The history must include occupation, family history, recent travel to Third World countries, and current medications. Patients should also be required to complete a checklist of concerns, which may include heartburn, GI bleeding, weight gain or loss, history of alcohol use, and laxative and enema use.

The physician will assess skin **turgor** (elasticity), jaundice, edema, bruising, breath odor, size and shape of the abdomen, and presence and quality of bowel sounds. The physician will also palpate abdominal contents.

Blood Tests

Blood work ordered by the physician may include white and red blood cell counts. The red blood cells, hemoglobin, and hematocrit are used to assess possible anemia as the result of GI bleeding. White blood cell counts can help to detect infection, while the erythrocyte sedimentation rate is used to assess inflammatory processes, including inflammation of the GI system.

Blood may also be drawn and sent to the laboratory to determine liver function. Specifically, alkaline phosphatase, serum bilirubin, prothrombin time, and SGPT (serum glutamic pyruvic transaminase) levels are determined in a test collectively known as a liver panel. Pancreatic enzyme studies include evaluation of blood for levels of enzymes normally released by the pancreas, including trypsin, chymotrypsin, steapsin, and amylopsin. Results that fall outside of the normal ranges for these substances indicate pathology and necessitate further testing as determined by the physician.

Radiology Studies

Flat plate radiographs of the abdomen may be ordered for diagnosing GI problems, but without contrast medium, these radiographs are not so useful as contrast radiographs. Radiology studies of the stomach and intestines consist of instilling barium, a radiopaque liquid, into the GI tract orally or rectally to outline the organs and identify abnormalities. The radiographs include standard pictures taken at various intervals after the barium is administered by

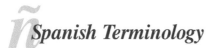

Spanish Terminology

Padece de indigestión?	Do you have indigestion?
Padece de estreñimiento?	Are you constipated?
Tiene diarrea?	Do you have diarrhea?
Ha notado sangre o mucosidad en las hecces fecales?	Have you noticed any blood or mucus in the stools?

mouth or by enema. If a fluoroscope (special type of radiographic equipment) is used, movement of the chalky liquid barium is viewed while it fills the esophagus or colon, giving additional diagnostic information.

The barium swallow (also called an upper GI or UGI) series can reveal abnormal constrictions, masses, and obstruction in the esophagus, stomach, and duodenum. This examination requires that the patient have nothing by mouth (NPO) after midnight the night before the test. A small-bowel series is an extension of the UGI that visualizes the barium flowing through the small intestine to diagnose abnormalities of the first part of the small intestine.

A barium enema, or lower GI study, provides an outline of the colon. It can reveal a blockage, cancerous growths, polyps, and diverticula. Since the lower GI study requires that the colon be empty of stool, the patient must be given specific instructions to follow before the examination. Box 34-2 outlines the standard preparation for a barium enema, which should be orally explained to the patient and given in written form.

Cholecystography is radiography of the gallbladder after the patient takes oral tablets containing a contrast material 12 hours prior to the procedure. The contrast medium is excreted from the liver into the gallbladder, and any abnormalities are viewed on the radiogram. After the initial films are taken, the patient is given a fatty meal that stimulates the contraction of the gallbladder to release bile and contrast medium into the bile ducts. Additional films may be taken to view any obstruction of these ducts by stones. The bile ducts may also be examined using percutaneous transhepatic cholangiography, a test that entails injection of contrast material through a needle inserted through the skin into the hep-

TRIAGE

While you are working in a medical office, the following three situations occur:

A. A 6-year-old boy comes into the office with lower right abdominal pain. The physician wants blood drawn immediately to determine a white blood cell count and rule out appendicitis. The mother of the patient appears concerned.

B. A 58-year-old woman arrives complaining of indigestion. She is having some epigastric discomfort. The physician has ordered an ECG.

C. An 84-year-old woman has brought a stool specimen for a fecal occult blood screening. The doctor is ready to see the patient.

How do you sort these patients? Whom do you see first? Second? Third?

Do patient B's ECG first. A feeling of indigestion or epigastric discomfort can be a sign of cardiac disease. Next draw patient A's blood, since an elevation in the white blood cell count indicates the need for additional tests and/or surgery for appendicitis. Finally, check the stool specimen brought in by the patient for fecal occult blood.

Note: This sequence is the accepted triage standard; however, the physician may opt for the blood work to be done first if he or she considers that patient B's discomfort is probably due to gastric difficulties and has ordered the ECG as a prophylactic measure. This decision is based on the physical examinations of both patients. You and the physician must work as a team to achieve the best outcomes.

Box 34-2

PATIENT PREPARATION FOR BOWEL STUDIES

Many bowel studies, such as barium enema and flexible sigmoidoscopy, require that the bowel be completely clear of fecal matter. With minor variations as directed by the physician, the bowel preparation usually includes the following:

- Liquid diet without dairy products for the full day before the procedure or a clear liquid evening meal
- A laxative or enema the evening preceding the procedure
- Nothing by mouth after midnight except water
- Rectal suppository, Fleet's enema, or cleansing enema the morning of the procedure

If inflammatory processes or ulcerations are suspected inside the bowel, only gentle cleansing will be used to avoid undue discomfort or possible perforation of lesions.

---

atic duct. Once the dye is injected, radiography is performed for diagnosis by the physician.

The role of the medical assistant in radiographic procedures includes determining third-party payer (insurance) requirements for referrals or preauthorization, scheduling the procedure in an outpatient facility, and explaining to the patient the preparations for the examination as necessary. When the test is complete, the radiologist will submit a written report to the referring physician. Follow office policy and procedure for routing the report to the physician for review and advising the patient of the examination results.

Nuclear Imaging

Radionuclides, or radioactive elements, are often used in the diagnosis of disorders of the liver. After the elements are injected into the body, images are taken using a nuclear scanning device, and abnormalities can be detected and evaluated by the radiologist. The injected radionuclide remains radioactive for a short specific period, and there is usually very little if any patient preparation required for this test. The role of the medical assistant includes coordinating any third-party payer requirements such as preauthorization, scheduling the test at a nuclear imaging center or hospital, and following up with the patient when the results are returned to the medical office as indicated in the policy and procedure manual. Test results indicating abnormalities necessitate additional evaluation and testing as determined by the physician.

Ultrasonography

The use of high-frequency sound waves to diagnose disorders of internal structures is used in many specialties, including gastroenterology. Abnormalities in the structure of various digestive accessory organs, such as the liver and gallbladder, can be easily viewed using ultrasonography and require very little if any preparation by the patient. As with other diagnostic tests ordered by the physician, your role includes verifying third-party payer guidelines and obtaining preauthorization if needed. Although ultrasound does not use radiation or radiography, ultrasounds are scheduled in the imaging department of many outpatient or inpatient facilities. Your role includes scheduling the test, advising the patient of the date and time, and following up after the test to obtain results if necessary, ensuring that the physician is aware of the results, and notifying the patient with any findings or additional instructions as ordered by the physician.

Endoscopic Studies

Fiberoptic technology has enabled physicians to pass soft, flexible tubes down the esophagus into the stomach and small intestine or up into the colon for direct visualization of these organs. Supplemental laboratory specimens, including tissue biopsy samples; samples of secretions for gastric analysis, including pH; culture sample to check for bacteria; bile for crystals that may lead to the formation of stones; and cells for cytology, including cancerous or otherwise abnormal cells, can be obtained. Endoscopic examinations are also used to diagnose biliary disorders.

ERCP is used to visualize the esophagus, stomach, proximal duodenum, and pancreas with a flexible endoscope. When the endoscope is in place, dye is injected directly into the ducts of the gallbladder and pancreas, and radiographs are taken to determine patency and function of these structures and the biliary ducts. This procedure is usually performed in a outpatient surgical center under anesthesia. Your role includes scheduling the procedure, advising the patient on any instructions prior to the test, and follow-up when the written report is sent by the gastroenterologist or radiologist.

Anoscopy, which may be performed in the medical office, is insertion of a metal or plastic anoscope into the rectal canal for visual inspection of the anus and rectum and to swab for cultures. The sigmoidoscopy examination provides a visual examination of the sigmoid colon using either a rigid sigmoidoscope or the more widely accepted flexible fiberoptic sigmoidoscope. The rigid sigmoidoscope is about 25 cm (10 inches) long. This instrument is supplied as reusable metal or disposable plastic and is calibrated in centimeters. An **obturator** in the lumen allows the instrument to be inserted with minimal discomfort and can be removed after insertion allowing for better visualization and obtaining specimens. The lens at the end magnifies the view for closer observation of the intestinal mucosa and can be moved aside to allow the physician to swab, suction, or sample the mucosa for biopsy. The handle contains the light source. The scope may be equipped with a hand bulb **insufflator**, a device for blowing air into the colon to expand the walls for easier visualization.

The flexible fiberoptic sigmoidoscope is more popular because it offers better visualization and is less uncomfortable for the patient. The scope is very thin, can bend and maneuver curves, and can be inserted much farther than the rigid scope (FIG. 34-7). The instrument is 35 cm (about 14 inches) or 65 cm (about 26 inches). It usually includes an insufflator and suction in addition to the light source. Though smaller in diameter than the rigid scope, it can also be used to obtain samples and cultures.

FIGURE 34–7. Sigmoidoscopy. The flexible scope is advanced past the proximal sigmoid colon and into the descending colon. (Reprinted with permission from Cohen BJ. Medical Terminology: An Illustrated Guide. Philadelphia: Lippincott Williams & Wilkins, 2003.)

Some physicians prefer that the bowel be as free of feces as possible and may order a light, low-residue meal the evening before the endoscopic examination. An evening laxative may also be ordered to be followed by a cleansing enema on the morning of the procedure. A light breakfast may be allowed, but only if ordered by the physician. Other physicians prefer to view the mucosa as it normally appears, without preparation. Most medical offices note the preferred preparation in the policy and procedure manual. Your role includes informing the patient of the preferred preparation for the procedure, assisting the physician during the procedure, and offering reassurance and support to the patient. Procedure 34-1 describes the steps for assisting with colon procedures in the medical office.

Checkpoint Question

8. What does anoscopy involve, and how does it differ from sigmoidoscopy?

Fecal Tests

As part of the routine examination for some adult patients, many physicians order a stool specimen to test for occult blood. Stool specimens to test for ova (eggs) and parasites are ordered if an infestation is suspected (Box 34-3). Standard precautions must be followed when collecting stool specimens for any purpose.

As a medical assistant, you may be responsible for instructing the patient in the procedure, or you may assist in collection of a stool specimen. Appointments for stool specimens should be scheduled early in the morning. Most people move their bowels shortly after awakening, and delaying the appointment may cause the patient discomfort or may result in loss of the specimen. Some specimens are collected and transported in containers that contain preservatives, and it is your responsibility to ensure that the patient understands and complies with the specific procedure. All specimens collected by the patient at home should be transported to the medical office or laboratory as quickly as possible. Procedure 34-2 describes the steps for instructing a patient to collect a stool specimen.

Screening for Occult Blood

Testing stool for occult, or hidden, blood using a test pack or kit is convenient and readily acceptable to most patients, since the stool for this test is usually collected by the patient at home. This test is used for screening to identify disorders that cause bleeding in the GI tract and is either negative (no blood detected) or positive (blood detected). When a test for occult blood in the stool is positive, the physician orders further diagnostic testing, since there are numerous reasons for blood in the stool, including hemorrhoids, polyps, diverticula, ulcers, and colorectal cancer. Most physicians routinely screen patients over age 50 for occult blood, since the risks for developing cancer of the colon increase in this population.

Several pharmaceutical companies manufacture test packs or kits to detect fecal occult blood. These tests use the guaiac reagent to indicate the presence of blood. Developers are added to the combination of stool and guaiac to turn the test sample an indicated color, usually blue (FIG. 34-8). Each test pack or slide includes an indicator for quality control and must be checked to ensure that the test pack is interpreted accurately. Read the package insert for the specific brand of occult blood kit to become familiar with the procedure, including the quality control indicator. Procedure 34-3 describes the steps in processing occult blood slides.

When explaining how to obtain a stool specimen for the occult blood test, encourage patients to avoid certain foods or medications that may interfere with the testing. For 2 days prior to collecting the stool sample and during the test, the patient should avoid the following foods and medications, which can cause false positive test results:

- Red meat and fruits high in vitamin C
- Certain vegetables that contain peroxidase, including cauliflower, broccoli, lettuce, spinach, and corn
- Aspirin and NSAIDs

Box 34-3

SPECIAL STOOL SPECIMENS

Follow these tips when collecting stool specimens to test for pinworms or parasites or to obtain a swab for culture. Remember to follow standard precautions.

- *Pinworms:* Schedule the appointment early in the morning, preferably before a bowel movement or bath. Pinworms tend to leave the rectum and lay eggs around the anus during the night. Press clear adhesive tape against the anal area. Remove it quickly and place it sticky side down on a glass slide for the physician to inspect.
- *Parasites:* Caution the patient not to use a laxative or enema before the test to avoid destroying the evidence of parasites. If the stool contains blood or mucus, include as much as possible in the specimen container, because these substances are most likely to contain the suspected organism.
- *Stool culture:* A sterile cotton-tipped swab is passed into the rectal canal beyond the sphincter and rotated carefully. Place it in the appropriate culture container or process as directed for smear preparation.

Negative Smears*

Negative and Positive Smears*

Positive Smears*

F I G U R E 3 4 – 8 . Test results for fecal occult blood with the Hemoccult routine screening test. Two samples from the specimen are included on each slide. No detectable blue on or at the edge of any of the smears indicates the test is negative for occult blood. Any trace of blue on or at the edge of one or more of the smears indicates the test is positive for occult blood. (Courtesy of SmithKline Diagnostics, Inc.)

Each test pack, or slide, includes two windows or test areas where stool smears are applied using a wooden or plastic spatula. Many physicians order the patient to collect samples and smear slides from three separate bowel movements. The slide or slides should be brought to the office or mailed in an envelope given to the patient with the test kit. In this situation, instruct the patient to follow the prescribed diet until all of the samples are collected. All slides can be mailed or brought into the office at the same time, since the specimen does not have to be recent.

Procedure 34-1

Assisting With Colon Procedures

Purpose: Prepare the patient and assist with endoscopic colon procedures.

Equipment: Appropriate instrument (flexible or rigid sigmoidoscope, anoscope, or proctoscope), water-soluble lubricant, gown and drape, cotton swabs, suction (if not part of the scope), biopsy forceps, specimen container with preservative, completed laboratory requisition form, personal wipes or tissues, equipment for assessing vital signs, examination gloves.

Standard: This procedure should take 30 minutes.

Steps	Reason
1. Wash your hands.	Handwashing aids infection control.
2. Assemble the equipment and supplies. Write the name of the patient on the label of the specimen container and complete the laboratory requisition.	The name of the patient must be clearly marked on the container and the laboratory requisition form must be complete for accurate identification.
3. Check the light source if a flexible sigmoidoscope is being used. Turn off the power after checking for working order to avoid a buildup of heat in the instrument.	If heat is permitted to build up in the scope, the patient may be burned. If the rigid sigmoidoscope, anoscope, or proctoscope is being used, check the examination light for working order.
4. Greet and identify the patient and explain the procedure. Inform the patient that a sensation of pressure or need to defecate may be felt during the procedure and that the pressure is from the instrument and will ease. The patient may also feel gas pressure when air is insufflated during sigmoidoscopy. *Note:* The patient may have been ordered to take a mild sedative before the procedure.	Identifying the patient prevents errors in treatment. Explaining the procedure helps ease anxiety and ensure compliance.
5. Instruct the patient to empty the urinary bladder.	Pressure from the instrument may injure a full bladder. Urine in the bladder may increase discomfort.
6. Assess the vital signs and record in the medical record.	Colon examination procedures may cause cardiac arrhythmias and a change in blood pressure in some patients. Baseline vital signs will allow you to detect variations from the patient's normal vital signs.
7. Have the patient undress completely from the waist down and put on a gown. Drape appropriately.	
8. Assist the patient onto the examination table. If the instrument is an anoscope or a fiberoptic device, Sims' position or a side-lying position is most comfortable. If a rigid instrument is used, the patient will assume a knee-chest position or be placed on a proctology table that supports the patient in a knee-chest position. *Note:* Do not ask the patient to assume the knee-chest position until the physician is ready to begin. The position is difficult to maintain. Drape the patient.	These positions facilitate the procedure by moving the abdominal organs up into the abdominal cavity rather than the pelvis.

(continues)

Procedure 34-1 *(continued)*

Assisting With Colon Procedures

Steps	Reason
9. Assist the physician as needed with lubricant, instruments, power, swabs, suction, and specimen containers.	
10. During the procedure, monitor the patient's response and offer reassurance. Instruct the patient to breathe slowly through pursed lips to aid in relaxation if necessary.	
11. When the physician is finished, assist the patient into a comfortable position and allow a rest period. Offer personal cleaning wipes or tissues. Take the vital signs before allowing the patient to stand and assist the patient from the table and with dressing as needed. Give the patient any instructions regarding care after the procedure and follow-up as ordered by the physician.	A drop in blood pressure on standing is common after lying in any of these positions for an extended period. If patients complain of dizziness or lightheadedness after sitting up, have them lie down. If any biopsy samples were taken, the patient may have slight rectal bleeding.
12. Clean the room and route the specimen to the laboratory with the requisition. Disinfect or dispose of the supplies and equipment as appropriate and wash your hands.	Follow standard precautions throughout the procedure.
13. Document the procedure.	Procedures are considered not to have been done if they are not recorded.

Charting Example
05/31/2005 12:45 P.M. T 98.6 (O) P 100 R 20 BP 144/86 (L) Sigmoidoscopy performed by Dr. Jacobs and specimen obtained—pt. tolerated well. Specimen to Acme Lab, VS after procedure P 112 R 24 BP 146/86 (L). Pt. denied dizziness after procedure. Discharged per Dr. Jacobs with verbal and written instructions on postprocedural care; pt. verbalized understanding. _____ S. Clay, CMA

Procedure 34-2

Collecting a Stool Specimen

Purpose: Explain the process for collecting a stool specimen to a patient.

Equipment: Stool specimen container (ova and parasite testing), occult blood test kit (occult blood testing), wooden spatulas or tongue blades.

Standard: This procedure should take 10 minutes.

Steps	Reason
1. Wash your hands.	Handwashing aids infection control.
2. Assemble the equipment and supplies. Place the name of the patient on the label on the outside of the container or test slide kit.	Whether the patient is instructed to bring the specimen to the office or transport it to a laboratory, the name of the patient must be clearly marked on the container for accurate identification.
3. Greet and identify the patient and explain the procedure. When obtaining a stool specimen for ova and parasites, the patient should collect a small amount of the first and last portion of the stool after the bowel movement with the wooden spatula or tongue blade and place it in the specimen container without contaminating the outside of the container.	Identifying the patient prevents errors in treatment. The first and last portions of the stool usually contain concentrations of the substances most often required for testing. Having the patient defecate into a disposable plastic container or onto plastic wrap placed over the toilet bowl will assist in collecting the specimen.
4. When obtaining a stool specimen for the occult blood test kit, the patient should place only a small smear on the slide windows after opening the front flap of the test kit.	The stool sample can be obtained from the toilet paper used to wipe after defecating, using the wooden spatula.
5. Explain any dietary, medication, or other restrictions necessary for the collection.	Usually dietary and medication restrictions affect collection of stool for occult blood testing. The policy and procedure manual should list restrictions for other tests.
6. After obtaining the stool sample, store the specimen as directed. Some samples require refrigeration; others are kept at room temperature, and some must be placed in an incubator at a laboratory as soon as possible after collecting.	Check the policy and procedure manual for recommendations for storage and routing of all specimens. Patients instructed to take the specimen to an outside laboratory must be given a complete laboratory requisition form.
7. Document that instructions were given including the routing procedure.	Procedures, including patient instructions, are considered not to have been done if they are not recorded.

Charting Example
06/13/2005 1:00 P.M. Pt. given supplies (specimen pack and wooden spatulas) and instructions on obtaining stools for occult blood; instructions on returning slides also given. Pt. verbalized understanding. _____
P. Jones, CMA

Procedure 34-3

Test a Stool Specimen for Occult Blood

Purpose:	Test stool for occult blood in a sample obtained by the patient and brought or mailed into the office using a test kit.
Equipment:	Gloves, patient's labeled specimen pack, developer or reagent drops.
Standard:	This procedure should take 5 minutes.

Steps	Reason
1. Wash your hands and put on clean examination gloves.	Handwashing aids infection control. Follow standard precautions when handling stool specimens.
2. Assemble the supplies, including the patient's prepared test pack and developer. Check the expiration date on the developing solution.	Proper identification prevents errors. Solution that has expired may yield inaccurate results.
3. Open the test window on the back of the pack and apply 1 drop of the developer or testing reagent to each window according to manufacturer's directions. Read the color change within the specified time, usually 60 seconds.	This ensures accurate results.
4. Apply 1 drop of developer as directed on the control monitor section or window of the pack. Note whether the quality control results are positive or negative as appropriate.	
5. Properly dispose of the test pack and gloves. Wash your hands.	Follow standard precautions throughout the procedure.
6. Record the procedure.	Procedures are considered not to have been done if they are not recorded.

Charting Example

03/28/2005 3:00 P.M. Occult blood slides ×3 returned to office via mail; findings positive. Dr. Franklin notified.
_____ J. Smith, RMA

CHAPTER SUMMARY

All cells of the body require nutrients from food. The organs of the GI system are responsible for ingestion and digestion. Metabolism is breakdown of food into energy units use of the energy by cells. Any disruption of this process is pathological not only to the gastric system but to other body systems and cells. While the medical assistant working in the office of the gastroenterologist encounters many patients with disorders of the GI system, patients with gastric disorders are commonly seen in other offices, including family practice, internal medicine, and pediatrics. A thorough history is essential for an accurate diagnosis. Assisting with various diagnostic procedures, such as colon examinations and stool testing, can also help the physician detect abnormalities in GI function. Of course, patient education regarding diet and prevention of various gastric disorders is also a critical aspect of the professional medical assistant's role and should be considered an ongoing process.

Critical Thinking Challenges

1. Review the preparation of the patient for an upper GI series and a barium enema. Create two handouts that include the following:

   - A description of each procedure
   - A list of reasons for the procedure
   - Preparations required to ensure reliable test results

2. Many endoscopic examinations require the patient to be in an uncomfortable and embarrassing position. How can you help alleviate the stress and anxiety?

3. Mrs. Barnes, a 43-year-old patient, was scheduled for a cholecystography at 11:00 A.M. today and was given all instructions and the oral contrast medium to take the morning of the examination. She calls the office at 10:30 A.M. and tells you that she forgot to take the dye tablets and wants to know whether she should take them now and go in for her test at the appointed time. What do you tell Mrs. Barnes?

Answers to Checkpoint Questions

1. The two most common causes of stomatitis are infections with the herpes simplex virus and the fungus *Candida albicans*.
2. A hiatal hernia is caused by a defect in the diaphragm that lets part of the stomach slide up into the chest cavity. The stomach's cardiac sphincter and the diaphragmatic muscle tone normally prevent gastric acid reflux into the esophagus. Hiatal hernia permits the stomach acid to invade the esophagus, causing irritation.
3. While the ulcerative lesions are similar in appearance and may be caused by the same factors, peptic ulcers are found on the lining of the stomach, and duodenal ulcers are in the first part of the small intestine (the duodenum).
4. Crohn disease can lead to bowel obstruction. With each episode of inflammation, scarring may lead to narrowing of the colon, hence an obstruction.
5. Hemorrhoids may be caused by poor abdominal and pelvic floor muscle tone, poor dietary habits including a diet low in fiber, and chronic constipation.
6. Viral hepatitis is caused by a virus; toxic hepatitis is a toxic reaction to chemical toxicants, certain medications, or alcohol.
7. Cholelithiasis is formation of stones in the gallbladder; cholecystitis is inflammation of the gallbladder, usually due to an impacted stone in the duct.
8. Anoscopy is insertion of an instrument into the rectal canal for visualization of the anus and rectum and to obtain swabs for culture. Sigmoidoscopy is visualization of the sigmoid colon using a rigid or flexible sigmoidoscope.

 Websites

American Society of Bariatric Surgery www.asbs.org

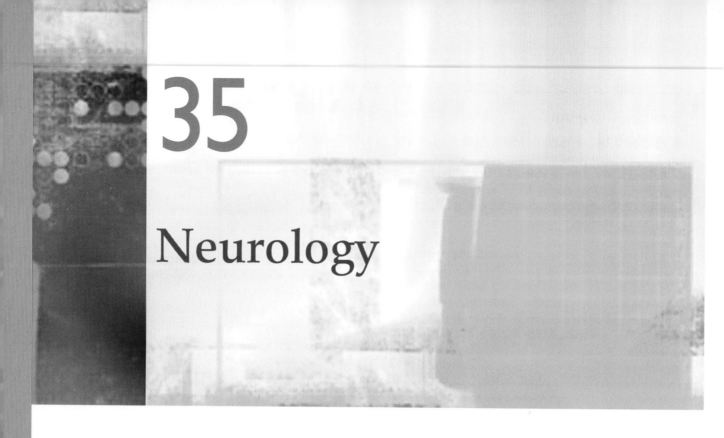

35

Neurology

CHAPTER OUTLINE

COMMON NERVOUS SYSTEM
  DISORDERS
  Infectious Disorders
  Degenerative Disorders
  Seizure Disorders

Developmental Disorders
Trauma
Brain Tumors
Headaches

COMMON DIAGNOSTIC TESTS
  FOR DISORDERS OF THE
  NERVOUS SYSTEM
  Physical Examination
  Radiological Tests
  Electrical Tests
  Lumbar Puncture

ROLE DELINEATION

CLINICAL: FUNDAMENTAL PRINCIPLES
- Apply principles of aseptic technique and infection control
- Screen and follow up patient test results

CLINICAL: PATIENT CARE
- Adhere to established patient screening procedures
- Obtain patient history and vital signs
- Prepare and maintain examination and treatment areas
- Prepare patient for examinations, procedures, and treatments
- Assist with examinations, procedures, and treatments

GENERAL: PROFESSIONALISM
- Work as a member of the health care team
- Prioritize and perform multiple tasks
- Treat all patients with compassion and empathy

GENERAL: COMMUNICATION SKILLS
- Recognize and respond effectively to verbal, nonverbal, and written communications
- Use medical terminology appropriately

GENERAL: LEGAL CONCEPTS
- Perform within legal and ethical boundaries
- Document accurately

GENERAL: INSTRUCTION
- Instruct individuals according to their needs
- Teach methods of health promotion and disease prevention

CHAPTER COMPETENCIES

LEARNING OBJECTIVES

Upon successfully completing this chapter, you will be able to:

1. Spell and define the key terms.
2. Identify common diseases of the nervous system.
3. Describe the physical and emotional effects of degenerative nervous system disorders.
4. Explain the medical assistant's role in caring for a patient having a seizure.
5. List potential complications of a spinal cord injury.
6. Name and describe the common procedures for diagnosing nervous system disorders.

PERFORMANCE OBJECTIVES

Upon successfully completing this chapter, you will be able to:

1. Assist with a lumbar puncture (Procedure 35-1)

KEY TERMS

cephalagia	dysphasia	migraine	seizure
concussion	electroencephalogram	myelogram	spina bifida occulta
contusion	(EEG)	myelomeningocele	
convulsion	herpes zoster	Queckenstedt test	
dysphagia	meningocele	Romberg test	

The nervous system is the chief communication and command center for all parts of the body. The nervous system has two divisions: the central nervous system (CNS) and the peripheral nervous system (PNS). The CNS includes the brain and spinal cord (FIG. 35-1), and the PNS contains the nerves that transmit impulses. Nerves are found throughout the body and in the brain. The autonomic nervous system (ANS), a division of the PNS, functions without voluntary action. Together these divisions of the nervous system allow skeletal movement, maintain vital homeostatic functions such as breathing and heart rate, and promote thought processes including memory and logic. The complexity of the nervous system and its connections with the muscular system make it subject to many disorders that can be difficult to diagnose and treat effectively.

Neurology deals with study of the nervous system and its disorders, and the physician who specializes in this area is a neurologist. The medical assistant who works in a neurology office has many interesting and challenging patients. Also, the medical assistant who works in other medical specialties may also have patients with diseases or disorders of the nervous system. This chapter focuses on some of the common disorders of the nervous system and the role of the medical assistant who works with these patients.

COMMON NERVOUS SYSTEM DISORDERS

Disorders of the nervous system range from minor inconveniences to lethal diseases. The following sections discuss the disorders in groups: infectious, degenerative, convulsive (**seizures**), developmental, traumatic, neoplastic (tumors), and headache.

Infectious Disorders

Meningitis

Meningitis is characterized by inflammation of the meninges covering the spinal cord and the brain. The inflammation can result from either bacterial or viral infection. Viral meningitis is usually not life-threatening and is often short-lived, but bacterial meningitis is often severe and may be fatal. The infection is usually precipitated by an upper respiratory, sinus, or ear infection. Children are the age group most likely to develop meningitis. Meningitis can also result from head trauma when an open wound allows organisms to enter the cranium and nervous system.

Patients with meningitis have a variety of signs and symptoms, including nausea, vomiting, fever, headache, and a stiff neck. Patients may also complain of photophobia, or intolerance to light. A rash with small, reddish purple dots may appear on the body, and as patients become sicker, they may slip into a coma and have seizures.

To diagnose meningitis, the physician usually orders a complete blood count. If the white blood cell count is high, a lumbar puncture is performed and cerebrospinal fluid (CSF) is sent to the laboratory for analysis to determine the infectious organism. The treatment of meningitis depends on the organism causing the infection. The treatment for viral meningitis includes fluids and bed rest, and bacterial meningitis is treated with antibiotics and generally requires hospitalization. The local health department must be notified of the diagnosis, and some states require that an infectious disease form be filed. Check your office policy and procedure manual to determine who is responsible for obtaining, completing, and submitting these reports, keeping in mind that in

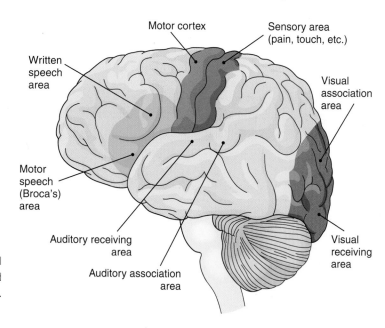

FIGURE 35–1. Functional areas of the cerebral cortex. (Reprinted with permission from Cohen BJ, Wood DL. Memmler's The Human Body in Health and Disease. Philadelphia: Lippincott Williams & Wilkins, 2000.)

many offices it is the medical assistant's responsibility. Depending on the type of meningitis, individuals (family, friends, coworkers, classmates) who have had contact with the patient may require prophylactic treatment.

Checkpoint Question

1. How does the treatment of viral meningitis differ from that of bacterial meningitis?

Encephalitis

Encephalitis is inflammation of the brain. Frequently it results from a viral infection that follows varicella (chickenpox), measles, or mumps. A strain of the virus is transmitted by mosquitoes. This type is primarily seen on the East and Gulf coasts. Symptoms of all forms include drowsiness, headache, and fever. Seizures and coma may occur in later stages. Diagnosis is made via lumbar puncture and analysis of CSF.

Treatment of encephalitis requires hospitalization for intravenous fluid therapy and supportive care. The prognosis is usually good if the diagnosis is made early and treatment begins quickly. As with meningitis, the local health department should be notified to identify those who may have been exposed to the disease.

Herpes Zoster

Herpes zoster, or shingles, is caused by the virus that causes chickenpox and occurs only in those who have had a varicella infection (see Chapter 29). Herpes zoster usually occurs in adults, often in times of physical or emotional stress. The virus, which lies dormant after the initial infection, becomes reactivated and spreads down the length of a nerve, causing redness, swelling, and pain. After about 48 hours, a band of papules develops on the skin following the nerve pathway. These lesions commonly appear on the face, back, and chest and progress to vesicles, pustules, and then dry crusts similar to chickenpox lesions. The lesions may last for 2 to 5 weeks, and the patient may have pain after the lesions disappear.

The treatment of a herpes zoster breakout includes an analgesic or nerve block for pain. Calamine lotion may be applied to the skin to reduce itching. Antiviral medication, such as acyclovir, may be prescribed to alleviate the severity of the disease.

Poliomyelitis

Commonly called polio, this highly contagious and resistant virus affects the brain and spinal cord. The virus can live outside the body for several months, making it almost impossible to eliminate once it has appeared in a community. It is transmitted by direct contact, usually through the mouth. In the United States, its incidence has been greatly reduced by aggressive immunization programs. However, because not all children have received the proper schedule of immunizations and because some adults have not been immunized at all, concern about the disease still exists.

In the acute phase, the patient may complain of a stiff neck, fever, headaches, and a sore throat. Nausea, vomiting, and diarrhea may also occur. As the disease progresses, paralysis may develop. Muscle atrophy leads to eventual deformities. If the respiratory muscles are affected, the patient cannot breathe without artificial assistance.

A new dimension of the disease, postpoliomyelitis muscular atrophy (PPMA) syndrome, has been documented in some individuals who had polio as children. Many of these patients have signs and symptoms similar to those that signaled the onset of the original disease. They usually complain of muscle weakness and a lack of coordination. Typically, patients with PPMA are treated on an outpatient basis with supportive care. No cure is available.

During the acute stage of polio, treatment is palliative and supportive. After this acute stage has resolved, treatment of the patient is rehabilitation of the weakened extremities with a strong emphasis on physical and occupational therapy. To increase mobility, patients are fitted with mechanical supports such as braces and splints. Some patients must wear those devices indefinitely. Emotional support is important for these patients, particularly those with PPMA. Many need counseling to reconcile themselves to body image changes caused by the deformities and to allay fear of dependency.

Activities aimed at preventing polio are essential. You may be responsible for patient education regarding immunizations and keeping them current. The previously used oral polio vaccine contained a weakened form of the polio virus, but today's newer injectable form does not contain a live or weakened form of the virus. In the oral form, the virus could be shed in the stool of the immunized child, and caretakers who were not immunized could contract the disease. This is not possible with the newer form of the vaccine.

Tetanus

Tetanus, commonly called lockjaw, is an infection of nervous tissue caused by the tetanus bacillus, *Clostridium tetani*, which lives in the intestinal tract of animals and is excreted in their feces. The microorganism is also found in almost all soil. An infection occurs after the microbe enters the body through an open wound in the skin, often a puncture wound. Wounds caused by farm equipment involving manure are especially susceptible to a tetanus infection. All deep, dirty wounds should be treated as high risk for tetanus.

Tetanus has a slow incubation period. It may inhabit the body for up to 14 weeks before signs and symptoms appear. Initial symptoms include spasms of the voluntary muscles, restlessness, and stiff neck. As the disease progresses, seizures and **dysphagia** (difficulty swallowing) develop. The facial and oral muscles contract, leaving the mouth sealed with the teeth clenched tightly. Untreated, the respiratory muscles become paralyzed, and the disease is typically fatal.

Prevention is the best defense against tetanus. Wounds should be properly cleaned immediately. Dead tissue around the wound must be removed, and an antibiotic should be given if the wound appears infected. To obtain immunity early in life, immunizations are administered to infants and children on a schedule determined by the American Academy of Pediatrics and the Centers for Disease Control and Prevention. After the initial immunization schedule is complete, the vaccine must be given every 10 years for life. Patients who develop an infection with the tetanus microbe require immediate hospitalization and aggressive antibiotic

therapy. The prognosis is guarded when tetanus has fully developed.

Checkpoint Question

2. What are the initial signs of a tetanus infection?

Rabies

Rabies is caused by a virus that is commonly transmitted by animal saliva through a bite wound from an infected animal and spreads to the organs of the central nervous system. Animals that commonly transmit rabies are skunks, squirrels, raccoons, bats, dogs, cats, coyotes, and foxes. Children are at highest risk for rabies because they are most likely to be bitten by such animals.

The incubation period for rabies ranges from 10 days to many months, depending on the location of the bite. Initial symptoms include fever, general malaise, and body aches. As the disease progresses, mental derangement, paralysis, and photophobia develop. The patient's saliva becomes extremely profuse and sticky, and the throat muscles begin to spasm, making swallowing difficult or impossible, which causes profuse drooling. Muscle spasms of the throat occur at the sight of water or when attempting to drink water, resulting in hydrophobia. The progressive involvement of the tissues of the brain is often fatal.

Immediate treatment of a wound caused by an animal must be the first priority. After the wound is cleansed, the patient should receive an antibiotic and prophylactic vaccine therapy consisting of the human diploid cell vaccine and a rabies immune globulin vaccine. All animal bites must be reported to the city or county animal control center, and you may be responsible for completing and submitting the report. If possible, the animal should be quarantined and evaluated for behavioral changes. If the animal is domestic, a complete veterinary history must be obtained. A copy of the animal's rabies tag and certificate, if available, should be placed in the patient's chart.

Reye's Syndrome

Reye's syndrome, a devastating nervous system illness, typically occurs in children after a viral illness, commonly varicella (chickenpox). Studies have found that the use of aspirin in the presence of a viral illness increases the risk of developing Reye's syndrome. No other antipyretic agents have been implicated in this disorder. Reye's syndrome is not contagious.

While this disorder can affect all organs of the body, it most often affects the liver and the brain. Initial symptoms include vomiting and lethargy, and as the brain swelling continues, confusion, seizures, and coma may develop quickly. The signs and symptoms of Reye's syndrome should be treated as a medical emergency, since early diagnosis and treatment increase the chances of recovering. The prognosis depends on the amount and severity of cerebral edema. Diagnosis is made by obtaining blood samples to determine liver function, including ammonia, aspartate aminotransferase, and alanine aminotransferase levels. Patients with Reye's syndrome require rapid hospitalization, aggressive antibiotic therapy to prevent secondary bacterial infection, and supportive care.

Degenerative Disorders

Multiple Sclerosis

The cause of multiple sclerosis (MS) is unknown, but possible origins include a viral infection, autoimmunity, immunological response, and genetic predisposition. In MS, the myelin sheaths covering many neurons in the body degenerate and are replaced with plaque, which impairs nerve impulse conduction. Multiple sclerosis most commonly occurs in women aged 20 to 40 (Box 35-1). MS is characterized by remissions and exacerbations, but there is no cure. The rate and severity of progression vary greatly among patients.

Typically, patients complain of progressive loss of muscle control. They may also complain of loss of balance, shaking tremors, and poor muscle coordination. Tingling and numbness can also be first signs of the disease. **Dysphasia** may be another sign. As the disease progresses, bladder dysfunction and complaints of visual disturbances are common. Patients may also develop nystagmus (involuntary rapid movement of the eyeball in all directions).

Treatment of MS is palliative. Physical therapy is critical to limit the extent of muscle deterioration and to maintain existing muscle strength. As the disease progresses, the patient is often fitted for prosthetic appliances such as crutches to assist with mobility. Drug therapy includes muscle relaxants and steroids. Because this disease affects persons in the prime of life, patients with MS and their family require psychological support from all of their regular health care providers. Many support groups and counselors specialize in providing therapy for persons with debilitating diseases, including MS, and this information should be shared with patients and families as appropriate.

Amyotrophic Lateral Sclerosis

Commonly known as Lou Gehrig's disease, amyotrophic lateral sclerosis (ALS) causes a progressive loss of motor neurons. It is a terminal disease with no known cause, but a strong familial connection has been observed. ALS occurs most often in middle-aged men. It begins with loss of muscle mobility in the forearms, hands, and legs, then progresses to the facial muscles, causing dysphasia and dysphagia that worsen over time. Death usually occurs 3 to 5 years after the onset of symptoms.

Treatment of ALS consists of keeping the patient comfortable and educating the family. As the disease progresses, it becomes increasingly difficult for the patient to maintain an un-

Box 35-1

MULTIPLE SCLEROSIS: A CASE STUDY

Barbara Smith, aged 28, was happily married with two children, aged 6 months and 4 years. She had no past medical pathology and always considered herself healthy. However, for a month now she had complaints of general weakness and lack of muscle control in her arms and hands. She found it hard to do routine household chores. At first she attributed her tiredness to her young children, but as the symptoms grew worse, she decided to seek medical attention.

Anticipating that her physician would prescribe vitamins and rest, she was shocked when Dr. Fernandez suggested a possible diagnosis of multiple sclerosis. After numerous tests including MRI, CSF analysis, and consultation with a neurologist, the diagnosis was confirmed as multiple sclerosis. Filled with concern, Ms. Smith and her husband questioned Dr. Fernandez about the disease and her prognosis, and he explained that they should expect the disease to have periods of remission and exacerbation. The goal was to increase the time of remission and lessen the severity of attacks during episodes of exacerbation. He explained that during the attacks, the immune system responds by destroying the myelin sheath the surrounds nerve fibers, leaving them exposed, permanently damaged, and unable to function normally. Dr. Fernandez also described the symptoms that Ms. Smith would eventually develop and explained that there is no definitive cure, only palliative treatments such as physical therapy, a muscle relaxant, application of prosthetic appliances, and the administration of steroids and newer medications to suppress the activity of the immune system. He also supplied the Smiths with telephone numbers of local support groups.

Over the next 10 years, Ms. Smith had many remissions and exacerbations. She is now confined to a wheelchair and has great difficulty performing the activities of daily living. She is assisted by a home health aide.

obstructed airway. The family must be taught to prevent and manage choking. Often the physician, with the medical assistant present for emotional support, discusses advance directives, or end-of-life requests with the family and the patient.

Seizure Disorders

Seizures, commonly called convulsions, are involuntary contractions of voluntary muscles caused by a rapid succession of electrical impulses through the brain. Seizures have many causes, including chemical imbalance, trauma, pregnancy-induced hypertension, tumor, and withdrawal from drugs or alcohol. However, many seizures are idiopathic (have no known cause).

Epilepsy is the most common form of seizure disorder. Epilepsy may appear in early childhood or at any life stage. Diagnosis is made through **electroencephalographic** (**EEG**) studies, blood tests, and radiological tests. Epileptic seizures are characterized as either petit mal or grand mal. Petit mal seizures, also called absence seizures or partial seizures, are briefer than grand mal seizures and usually occur only in childhood. The child may appear to fall asleep or drift away momentarily. Some muscle twitching may occur. Then the child awakes and continues the interrupted activity. Petit mal seizures may go undetected for many years.

Grand mal seizures, also called tonic-clonic seizures, are more involved than petit mal seizures. Generally, the patient will go through three phases:

1. The first phase is an aura, or warning that a seizure is impending. The aura may include tingling in the extremities, visual signs (such as flashing lights), or perception of a particular taste or odor. Not all patients have auras, but those who do usually perceive the same aural phenomena each time.
2. The second phase is complete loss of consciousness with extensive muscle twitching or contractions, which may be violent. The patient falls and usually loses control of bladder and bowel functions.
3. The third phase is the postictal phase. The patient slowly regains consciousness but remains drowsy for an extended time.

The primary treatment during the actual seizure is preventing injury to the patient. (See Chapter 28)

Epilepsy is treated with various pharmacological agents that must be taken by the patient regularly to prevent seizure activity. Instruct patients to take their medication every day as prescribed by the physician, never missing a dose. Many epileptic patients who become stabilized and seizure free on medication decide they no longer need the medication. Remind these patients that stopping the medication may lead to the recurrence of seizures.

A patient who has seizures is usually permitted to have a driver's license, but each state has specific regulations requiring that patients be seizure free for a particular length of time. The patient may ask the physician to complete paperwork from the state issuing the driver's license, and you may be asked to assist with completion of these forms.

Febrile Seizures

Febrile (fever) seizures occur in a small number of children, most commonly aged 6 months to 3 years, with an elevated body temperature. Children with febrile seizures must have a complete physical and neurological examination to rule out the possibility of organic origin of the seizures. Children generally outgrow febrile seizures by age 6 or 7 and have no further seizure activity.

WHAT IF

The mother of a 2-year-old who recently had a febrile seizure tells you that she is scared that the child will have another seizure and that it will cause brain damage? Because febrile seizures can be very scary for parents of small children, you can help them cope with these measures:

- Reassure the parents that febrile seizures are common in young children and that they generally are not chronic.
- Allow the parents to be involved in the care of the child. If a seizure occurs in the medical office, urge the parents to hold and comfort the child after the seizure has subsided and the physician has evaluated the child.
- Provide easy-to-understand explanations for all procedures.
- Encourage parents to talk about their fears.
- Remain calm and demonstrate confidence in handling the situation.

Treatment is gently returning the child's body temperature to a more manageable level. Cool compresses are preferable to ice baths or alcohol sponge baths, which may cause hypothermia. Because of the danger of Reye syndrome, these children should not be given salicylates, or products containing aspirin, to reduce the temperature.

Focal, or Jacksonian, Seizures

Focal seizures begin as a small local seizure that spreads to adjacent areas. For instance, the small seizure may begin in the fingers and spread to the hand and arm. The cause of focal seizures must be researched to prevent the progression to general seizures.

Checkpoint Question

3. How do petit mal seizures differ from grand mal seizures?

Developmental Disorders

Neural Tube Defects

Many abnormalities may occur during the embryonic and fetal stages of development. As the embryo develops, the tissue over the neural tube (a tubelike section of the developing embryo) closes and evolves into the components of the CNS. If a developmental failure occurs on the proximal (upper) portion, anencephaly, or the absence of a brain, may result. An abnormality in development in the distal, or caudal, end of the neural tube results in spina bifida. Spina bifida occulta is the most benign form. In this condition, the posterior laminae of the vertebrae fail to close, typically at L-5 or S-1. There are usually no external signs of deformity, although there may be a skin dimple or dark tufts of hair over this area on the lower back. A meningocele occurs when the meninges protrude through the spina bifida. In spina bifida with myelomeningocele, the most severe form, the spinal cord and meninges protrude externally (FIG. 35-2). The main treatment is surgical intervention; prognosis is based on the extent of spinal cord involvement.

Hydrocephalus

Hydrocephalus occurs when the arachnoid and ventricular spaces of the brain contain excessive CSF. Although it occurs most commonly in infants and children as the result of a defect in CSF production or absorption, hydrocephalus sometimes occurs in adults as a result of tumor or trauma. Treatment is surgical insertion of a shunt, which reroutes the excessive CSF from the brain to the right atrium of the heart or the peritoneal cavity. The prognosis is usually good if hydrocephalus is treated aggressively in the early stages, before CNS damage.

Cerebral Palsy

Cerebral palsy describes a group of neuromuscular disorders that result from CNS damage during the prenatal, neonatal, or postnatal period. Although cerebral palsy is not progressive, the damage may become more obvious as developmental delays are discovered. Impairment may range from slight motor dysfunction to catastrophic physical and

LEGAL TIP

Risk Management

Risk management includes those activities performed in the medical office that may help reduce or eliminate litigation or lawsuits. A professional medical assistant can practice risk management by:
- Documenting concisely and accurately immediately following any patient encounter, either in person or on the telephone.
- Being familiar with the office policy and procedure manual and following the guidelines as written.
- Communicating clearly with patients and other health care providers while observing the laws regarding confidentiality.
- Maintaining compliance with state and federal laws with regard to filing insurance claims and billing procedures.
- Practicing within your scope of education and training.

mental disabilities. Prognosis varies with the site of the damage and its severity. Treatment is supportive and rehabilitative. No cure exists.

Trauma

Traumatic injuries are the most common causes of neurological disorders and the leading killer of individuals aged 1 to 24 years. The trauma often is a preventable injury to the head that causes edema in the brain tissue or blows to the posterior neck and back, injuring the spinal cord. You can help prevent these types of injuries and the life-long impairments that accompany permanent damage to the CNS by encouraging parents to require their children to

A , B

C , D

F I G U R E   3 5 – 2 .   Spinal defects. (A) Normal spinal cord. (B) Spina bifida occulta. (C) Meningocele. (D) Meningomyelocele. (Reprinted with permission from Pillitteri A. Maternal and Child Health Nursing: Care of the Childbearing and Childrearing family. 4th ed. Philadelphia: Lippincott Williams & Wilkins, 2003.)

wear a helmet when bicycle riding, skating, skateboarding, and riding in a motor vehicle. Head trauma sustained in a motor vehicle accident often results from the passengers being tossed around the interior of the car or worse yet, ejected from the vehicle. Inexperienced teenage drivers should also be asked about the use of seat belts not just for themselves but their passengers.

Traumatic Brain Injuries

Children are at particularly high risk for head trauma. A child's head is large in proportion to the rest of the body. Therefore, as children fall (as they frequently do), they often fall head first. Children are also prone to traumatic injuries because their reflex systems are immature. Traumatic injuries to the brain include **concussion**, **contusion**, and intracranial hemorrhage. A concussion is a nonlethal brain injury that results from blunt trauma. The patient may momentarily lose consciousness but promptly return to an awake and alert state. The treatment for concussion is rest and observation for signs of a more serious injury, contusion. A contusion is a focal alteration of cerebral circulation. Hemorrhages and extravasation, or pooling, of blood and fluid can result. Loss of consciousness results, and brain damage may occur. The patient may become confused and lethargic and have nausea and vomiting as the intracranial bleeding increases, causing pressure on the brain. Intracra-

Table 35–1	SPINAL CORD INJURIES
Level of Injury	**Resulting Disabilities**
C-1, C-2	Unable to breathe independently; no neck muscle control
C-3, C-4	May manipulate electric wheelchair with mouthpiece; some neck control possible
C-5	Uses wheelchair with hand controls; eats with hand splints; good elbow flexion
C-6	Transfers to wheelchair and bed with little or no assistance; good shoulder control
C-7	Transfers independently to wheelchair and bed; eats with no special devices.
T-1–T-4	Moves from wheelchair to floor with little or no assistance; normal upper extremity function.
T-5–L-2	Limited walking with bilateral leg braces and crutches.
L-3–L-4	Walks with short leg braces with or without crutches.
L-5–S-3	Walks independently with no equipment if foot strength is good.

C, cervical; L, lumbar; S, sacral; T, thoracic.

nial hemorrhage is bleeding of a vessel inside the skull due to trauma, congenital abnormality, or aneurysm.

Traumatic brain injuries are diagnosed with radiographic studies. Treatment for contusions and hemorrhages can be surgery, drug therapy, and supportive care. The prognosis for all brain injuries depends on the extent of damage and the location of the injury.

Spinal Cord Injuries

Spinal cord injuries are most common among individuals 15 to 35 years of age. Most spinal cord injuries are due to trauma from a motor vehicle accident, diving accident, or fall. A complete spinal cord injury is one in which the cord is transected and no neurological abilities remain below the point of injury. An incomplete spinal cord injury is one in which the cord is injured or partially severed, causing minor to severe disability below the point of injury (TABLE 35-1). The higher in the spinal cord the injury, the more serious the complications and paralysis for the patient (TABLE 35-2).

In caring for patients who may have a spinal cord injury, the initial consideration is to prevent further damage. Accident victims with suspected spinal cord injuries must be kept immobile until proper emergency medical service personnel are present. Treatment in the emergency department is focused on stabilization, and patients usually require an extended hospitalization and rehabilitation, depending on the extent of the damage to the spinal cord.

In the physician's office, recovering trauma patients may receive follow-up treatment and evaluation. These patients

PATIENT EDUCATION

Spinal Cord and Traumatic Brain Injuries

Spinal cord and traumatic brain injuries are common in young people. Both types of injuries can produce serious and even fatal results. As a medical assistant, you must take an active role in educating your community, patients, and friends about prevention of these injuries:

- Use seat belts in automobiles for all passengers.
- Secure infants and young children in approved car seats.
- Avoid alcohol when participating in sporting activities and driving.
- Obey traffic signs and speed limits.
- Avoid illicit drug use and any medication that impairs awareness.
- Wear a helmet while bicycling and riding a motorcycle.
- Never dive head first into water that is shallow or unclear.

Table 35-2	TYPES OF PARALYSIS	
Type	**Causes**	**Result**
Hemiplegia	Cerebrovascular accident; trauma to one side of brain; tumors	Paralysis on one side of body, opposite the side of involvement
Paraplegia	Spinal cord trauma; spinal tumors	Paralysis of any part of the body below the point of involvement
Quadriplegia	Spinal cord trauma; spinal tumors	Paralysis of all limbs (usually cervical or high thoracic vertebra involvement)

are monitored for changes in their reflexes and evaluated for physical therapy and occupational therapy. The goal of long-term care is to prevent complications, which can include skin ulcerations (pressure ulcers), hypostatic pneumonia, bladder infection, muscle contractures, and psychological depression. Most of the physical complications are treated with physical therapy and good care either in the home or in the long-term rehabilitation facility. The mental and emotional complications require intensive therapy by counselors who specialize in treating patients with debilitating disorders.

Checkpoint Question

4. How does a complete spinal cord injury differ from an incomplete one?

Brain Tumors

A brain tumor may be either malignant or benign and may be a secondary or metastatic site. If the brain tumor is the primary site, it is named for the site of origin (e.g., glioma, meningioma, medulloblastoma). Both malignant and benign tumors can produce serious complications for the patient because of the limited space inside the cranium. Generally the patient has vague complaints of headaches, blurred vision, personality changes, or memory loss. In more advanced cases, seizures, blindness, and dysphagia may be evident. The type of tumor and its location affect the presenting symptoms, their severity and onset, and the prognosis.

Diagnosis is made primarily with radiological studies. The treatment can include surgery, radiation therapy, chemotherapy, or a combination of radiation and chemotherapy.

Headaches

It is estimated that 70% of the population has **cephalagia**, or headaches. Headaches have a variety of origins, including stress, trauma, bone pathology, infection (e.g., sinus), or vascular disturbance. In many instances, the cause is never known.

Migraine headaches are one of the most common types. Migraine can be triggered by stress, high altitude, smoking, certain smells, or ingested chemicals (caffeine, alcohol, certain food additives), but in many situations the cause is unknown. Many patients who have migraines have an aura, or sensory perception such as flashing lights or wavy lines, before onset. Once the migraine headache begins, the symptoms usually include a unilateral temporal headache, photophobia, diplopia (double vision), and nausea. Generally these headaches are treated with an analgesic, and the patient may be instructed to rest in a dark, quiet room. The physician may also prescribe medication to arrest the headache and symptoms when the migraine begins. These medications, sometimes called abortive headache medications, include the triptans (sumatriptan succinate [Imitrex] and naratriptan hydrochloride [Amerge]) or ergotamines (ergotamine titrate with caffeine [Cafergot] or dihydroergotamine mesylate[Migranal]).

TRIAGE

While you are working in a medical office, the following three situations occur at the same time:

A. Patient A is a 35-year-old woman who came to the office with a severe migraine. She is sitting in the darkened examination room with an emesis basin because she has been nauseated and vomiting this morning. The physician has ordered an injection of sumatriptan succinate (Imitrex).

B. Patient B is a 46-year-old patient who came to the office for an injection of anesthetic into the spinal column to relieve chronic pain caused by an injury that occurred on the job 2 years ago.

C. Patient C is phoning about a bill received after an office visit last month. The patient is angry and demanding to speak to the physician immediately.

How do you sort these patients? Whom do you see first? Second? Third?

Patient C should quickly be referred to the office manager or billing supervisor in a calm and professional manner. In most offices the clinical medical assistant does not have enough information about the patient's account to determine the nature of the problem. Next patient A should be given the injection and allowed to remain in the examination room until the medication has taken effect or she feels able to leave. While she is resting in the quiet, darkened room after the injection, you can prepare patient B and the treatment room.

Other common types of headaches:

- *Tension headaches* are associated with contraction of the muscles of the neck and scalp due to stress. The treatment is a muscle relaxant, analgesic, and reversing the precipitating factors. Biofeedback techniques may also be useful to assist with coping with stress that cannot be avoided.
- *Cluster headaches* are similar to migraine headaches but typically occur at night. They are usually short lasting but may recur as often as 4 or 5 times a night for several weeks and then not again for weeks or months. Treatment is a muscle relaxant, analgesic, and stress relief techniques.

COMMON DIAGNOSTIC TESTS FOR DISORDERS OF THE NERVOUS SYSTEM

The physician may perform a variety of tests to evaluate a patient's neurological status. These tests may be invasive or noninvasive and may include radiological and electrical tests along with physical examination.

Physical Examination

The physical examination, a key component of diagnosis of nervous system disorders, includes the following evaluations:

- Mental status and orientation
- Cranial nerve assessment
- Sensory and motor functions
- Reflex assessment

The patient's mental status is evaluated by routine questioning to establish mental alertness and orientation. For example, the examiner may ask the patient to count to 10 and to state the president's name and the year.

Cranial nerves are assessed according to the methods described in TABLE 35-3. Visual acuity may be tested on a chart such as the Snellen eye chart, and the results can indicate a refractive error or a more serious neurological disorder. Sensory function is tested with the pin versus soft brush method for spinal nerves and cranial nerves. The instrument commonly used is the Buck neurological hammer (FIG. 35-3). With the patient's eyes closed, the physician uses the pin and brush to determine the patient's ability to distinguish between sensations. The physician evaluates sensory reception

Table 35–3 CRANIAL NERVES

Nerve (Number)	Type	Functions	Examination Methods
Olfactory (I)	Sensory	Smell	Test each nostril for smell reception, interpretation
Optic (II)	Sensory	Vision	Test vision for acuity, visual fields
Oculomotor (III)	Motor	Pupil constriction, raise eyelids	Test papillary reaction to light, ability to open and close eyes
Trochlear (IV)	Motor	Downward, inward eye movement	Test for downward, inward eye movement
Trigeminal (V)	Motor	Jaw movements, chewing, mastication	Ask patient to open and clench jaws while palpating the jaw muscles
	Sensory	Sensation on face, neck	Test face and neck for pain sensations, light touch, temperature
Abducens (VI)	Motor	Lateral movement of eyes	Test ocular movement in all directions
Facial (VII)	Motor	Muscles of face	Ask patient to raise eyebrows, smile, show teeth, puff out cheeks
	Sensory	Sense of taste on anterior two-thirds of tongue	Test for taste sensation with various agents
Acoustic (VIII)	Sensory	Hearing	Test hearing ability
Glossopharyngeal (IX)	Motor	Pharyngeal movement, swallowing	Ask patient to say "ah," yawn to observe upward movement of soft palate; elicit gag response, note ability to swallow
	Sensory	Taste on lower third of tongue	Test for taste with various agents
Vagus (X)	Motor	Swallowing, speaking	Ask patient to swallow, speak; note hoarseness
Accessory (XI)	Motor	Movement of shoulder muscles	Ask patient to shrug against resistance
Hypoglossal (XII)	Motor	Movement, strength of tongue	Ask patient to protrude tongue, push tongue against cheek

F I G U R E   3 5 – 3 .   The Buck neurological hammer. The pin and brush fit inside the frame of the hammer and are used to assess sensation. (Courtesy of MDF Instruments, Inc.)

and determines whether there is a reception difference on either side of the body.

Motor functioning is tested by watching the patient walk. Many disorders can be detected by observing a patient's gait. Part of this assessment includes the **Romberg test**. The patient is asked to stand with feet together and with the eyes closed. A positive Romberg sign is noted if the patient sways or is unsteady.

The last part of the examination is reflex testing (TABLE 35-4). FIGURE 35-4 depicts the correct method for tendon reflex testing. Reflexes are scored on this scale:

- 0   No response
- 1+   Diminished response
- 2+   Normal
- 3+   Brisker than normal
- 4+   Hyperactive with clonus, which is the repetitive jerking of a muscle and indicates a neurological disorder

Patients with weak or slow responses to stimuli applied during reflex testing may require additional testing to determine the source of the problem. Since the muscles require electrical impulses from the nervous system to contract, the physician must determine whether the problem is with the muscles or if there is a disorder of the nervous system.

Radiological Tests

The most common noninvasive radiological tests include computed tomography (CT) and magnetic resonance imaging (MRI). These tests may be done with a contrast medium or dye. The contrast medium helps differentiate between the soft tissue areas of the nervous system and the tumors, lesions, or hemorrhages that may blend in with their supporting tissues.

A myelogram is an invasive radiological test in which dye is injected into the CSF. The spinal cord is filmed, and any abnormalities, such as tumors or damage from injury, can be detected. The blood vessels of the brain can be visualized on radiographic film by injecting dye through a femoral artery catheter threaded up to the carotid artery in a test called cerebral angiogram.

Radiography of the skull may be used to rule out many possible disorders and is diagnostic for fractures.

Electrical Tests

The EEG is a noninvasive test that records electrical impulses in the brain. A variety of electrodes are placed on the patient's scalp, and tracings of brain wave activity are recorded. Typically, the patient is given a mild sedative to induce a quiet state. This test is used to assess hyperactive electrical responses in the brain as seen in patients with seizure disorders. In the inpatient acute care setting, EEG is used to determine brain activity in patients who are on life support but who may be brain dead and have no chance for recovery.

Checkpoint Question

5. What are the differences between a myelogram and an EEG?

Lumbar Puncture

A lumbar puncture is used to diagnose infectious inflammatory or bleeding disorders affecting the brain and spinal cord or as a means of injecting pain control medication into the spinal column near the nerves producing the pain. A needle is inserted into the subarachnoid space at L4-5, below the level of the spinal cord (FIG. 35-5).

Table 35–4	REFLEX TESTING		
Reflex	**Method of Testing**	**Expected Response**	**Location**
Brachioradialis	Tap styloid process of radius	Flexion of elbow	C-5, C-6
Biceps	Tap biceps tendon	Flexion of elbow	C-5, C-6
Triceps	Tap triceps	Extension of elbow	C-7
Patellar	Tap patellar tendon	Extension of leg	L-2, L-4
Achilles	Tap Achilles tendon	Plantarflexion of foot	S-1
Corneal	Light touch on corneoscleral corner	Closure of eyelid	CN V, VII

C, cervical; L, lumbar; S, sacral; CN, cranial nerve.

A   B   C   D

FIGURE 35-4. Techniques for eliciting major tendon reflexes. (A) Biceps reflex. (B) Triceps reflex. (C) Patellar reflex. (D) Ankle or Achilles reflex.

Third lumbar vertebra
Dura mater
Subarachnoid space
Cauda equina

FIGURE 35-5. Technique for lumbar puncture. The L-3 to L-5 spaces are just below the line connecting the anterior and superior iliac spines (Taylor C, Lillis CA, LeMone P. Fundamentals of Nursing, 2nd ed. Philadelphia: Lippincott, 1993:543.)

ñ Spanish Terminology

Es buena su memoria?	Is your memory good?
Le duele la cabezo?	Have you any pain in the head?
Tiene usted vértigo?	Do you feel dizzy?
Voltese a su lado izquierdo (derecho).	Turn on your left (or right) side.

If CSF is removed and sent to the laboratory, it may be tested for glucose, protein, bacteria, cell counts, and red blood cells, which indicate intracranial bleeding. It may also be performed to evaluate intracranial pressure. An obstruction to CSF flow can be determined with the **Queckenstedt test**. For this test, you will be directed to press against the patient's jugular veins in the neck (right, left, or both) while the physician monitors the pressure of CSF. If CSF pressure increases when the jugular vein is compressed, the finding is normal. If no increase in pressure occurs, the flow of CSF is blocked.

If a lumbar puncture is performed in the medical office, your responsibility includes assisting the patient into a side-lying curled position or a supported forward-bending sitting position and maintaining sterility of the items used during the puncture (see Chapter 24). The physical position is uncomfortable and difficult to maintain, and you should help the patient to relax as much as possible by encouraging slow, deep breathing during the procedure. The steps for assisting the physician with a lumbar puncture are described in Procedure 35-1.

If CSF has been removed, the physician may require that the patient lie flat for 6 to 12 hours to prevent a spinal headache. In addition, the patient may require intravenous fluid and pain medication. For these reasons, the lumbar puncture is more commonly performed in outpatient clinics than in the medical office.

Procedure 35-1

Assisting With a Lumbar Puncture

Purpose: To prepare and assist the physician during lumbar puncture.

Equipment: Sterile gloves, examination gloves, 3- to 5-inch lumbar needle with stylet (physician will specify gauge and length), sterile gauze sponges, specimen container, local anesthetic and syringe, needle, adhesive bandages, fenestrated drape, sterile drape, antiseptic, skin preparation supplies (razor), biohazard sharps container, biohazard waste container.

Standard: This procedure should take 20 minutes.

Steps	Reason
1. Wash your hands.	Handwashing aids infection control.
2. Assemble the equipment, identify the patient, and explain the procedure.	Identifying the patient helps prevent errors in treatment. Explaining the procedure helps ease anxiety.
3. Check that the consent form is signed and in the chart. Warn the patient not to move during the procedure. Tell the patient that the area will be numb but pressure may still be felt after the local anesthetic is administered.	Because this is an invasive procedure, informed consent should be obtained and the form kept in the chart. Although there is little chance of damage to the spinal cord, movement may injure the patient and will probably contaminate the field.
4. Have the patient void. Direct the patient to disrobe and put on a gown with the opening in the back.	Emptying the bladder will decrease discomfort during the procedure. The back must be exposed for the procedure.
5. Prepare the skin unless this is to be done with sterile preparation. If the physician prefers to prepare the skin using sterile forceps after gloving, you may have to add sterile solution to the field (see Chapter 6). Assist as needed with administration of the anesthetic.	Before beginning, assess the lumbar region. If the site is hairy, it may be necessary to shave the skin before the procedure. Strict medical and surgical asepsis must be observed to reduce the risk of introducing microorganisms into the nervous system.
6. When the physician is ready, prepare the sterile field and assist with the initial preparations. Assist the patient into the appropriate position.	These positions widen the space between the vertebrae to allow entrance of the needle. Your presence will help ensure that the patient does not move.

(continues)

Procedure 35-1 *(continued)*

Assisting With a Lumbar Puncture

Steps	Reason
A. For the side-lying position, stand in front of the patient and help by holding the patient's knees and top shoulder. Ask the patient to move so the back is close to the edge of the table. B. For the forward-leaning, supported position, stand in front of the patient and rest your hands on the shoulders as a reminder to remain still. Ask the patient to breathe slowly and deeply.	
7. Throughout the procedure, observe the patient closely for signs such as dyspnea or cyanosis. Monitor the pulse at intervals and record the vital signs after the procedure. Note the patient's mental alertness and any leakage at the site, nausea, or vomiting. Assess lower limb mobility.	
8. When the physician has the needle securely in place, help the patient to straighten slightly to ease tension and to allow a normal CSF flow.	
9. If specimens are to be taken, put on gloves to receive the potentially hazardous body fluid. Label the tubes in sequence as you receive them. Label them also with the patient's identification and place them in biohazard bags.	Standard precautions must be followed.
10. If the Queckenstedt test is to be performed, you may be required to press against the patient's jugular veins in the neck (right, left, or both) while the physician monitors the pressure of CSF.	Normally, the pressure of CSF will rise and drop rapidly as the veins in the neck are compressed. If an obstruction is present, the rise and return to normal may be slow or there may be no response to the external application of pressure.
11. At the completion of the procedure, cover the site with an adhesive bandage and assist the patient to a flat position. The physician will determine when the patient is ready to leave the examining room and the office.	Some patients have headache after the procedure and must be monitored carefully during the recovery period.
12. Route the specimens as required. Clean the examination room and care for or dispose of the equipment as needed. Wash your hands.	Standard precautions must be followed throughout the procedure.
13. Chart all observations and record the procedure.	Procedures are considered not to have been done if they are not recorded.

Charting Example

02/12/04 8:30 A.M. Patient positioned and draped for lumbar puncture. VS 120/80 (R), 86, 18. LP performed by Dr. Alexander. _____

9:00 A.M. LP complete. Pt. tolerated procedure well. CSF specimen to lab Post LP VS 114/74 (R) 76, 16. _____

9:30 A.M. Pt. denies discomfort. No n/v No leakage at LP site. Bandage clean and dry. Pt and wife given discharge instructions. Verbalized understanding. Pt d/c per Dr. Alexander. _____ B. Ryan, CMA

CHAPTER SUMMARY

The nervous system is complex and works with both conscious and unconscious functions. It allows us to perform the activities of daily living, records our memories, helps us think rationally, moves us through our external environment, and coordinates our internal environment. Nervous system disorders can be grouped into several types: infectious, degenerative, convulsive, developmental, traumatic, neoplastic, and headache. Common diagnostic tests include radiological studies (e.g., CT, MRI), EEG, physical examination, prenatal screening, lumbar puncture, and skull radiography. Although many positive strides are being made in the diagnosis and care of neurological disorders, medical assistants must be aware that neurological disorders can be physically and psychologically devastating for patients and their families.

Critical Thinking Challenges

1. Research and prepare a patient education fact sheet about migraine headaches: the possible triggers, the causes, and the treatments, including abortive headache medications.
2. A 3-year-old girl comes to the office with varicella zoster (chickenpox). She has a fever, and the physician orders acetaminophen. The child's mother asks, "Why can't she have aspirin instead?" How do you respond?
3. Your patient, a 21-year-old man, was in a motor vehicle accident last year, and a spinal cord injury left him paraplegic. Explain how this injury has most likely affected his life, not just physically but emotionally and psychologically. How do you handle any anger or apathy directed at you or the physician?

Answers to Checkpoint Questions

1. Viral meningitis is treated with fluids and bed rest, and bacterial meningitis requires antibiotic medication and hospitalization.
2. The initial symptoms of a tetanus infection include spasms of the voluntary muscles, restlessness, and a stiff neck.
3. Petit mal seizures are briefer than grand mal seizures. Grand mal seizures are more extensive than petit mal seizures and have three phases: an aura, or warning, of an impending seizure; complete loss of consciousness; and the postictal phase, during which the patient slowly regains consciousness.
4. A complete spinal cord injury is total transection of the spinal cord, with no neurological abilities remaining below the point of injury. An incomplete spinal cord injury is one in which the cord is not completely severed, with minor to severe neurological disabilities below the point of injury.
5. An EEG is a noninvasive electrical test of brain waves. A myelogram is an invasive radiological test in which dye is injected into the CSF to help detect abnormalities.

Websites

Centers for Disease Control and Prevention
www.cdc.gov/ncidod/dvrd/rabies/
National Reye Syndrome Foundation www.reyessyndrome.org
National Institutes of Health www.nlm.nih.gov/medlineplus/seizures.html
North Pacific Epilepsy Research www.seizures.net
Association for Spina Bifida and Hydrocephalus www.asbah.org
Spina Bifida Association of America www.sbaa.org
National Institutes of Health www.nlm.nih.gov/medlineplus/cerebralpalsy.html

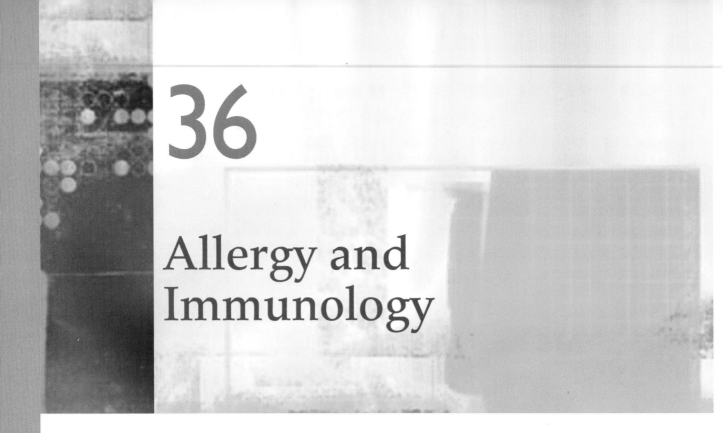

36

Allergy and Immunology

CHAPTER OUTLINE

ROLE DELINEATION

ADMINISTRATIVE: ADMINISTRATIVE PROCEDURES
- Perform basic administrative medical assisting functions
- Understand and adhere to managed care policies and procedures

CLINICAL: FUNDAMENTAL PRINCIPLES
- Apply principles of aseptic technique and infection control
- Comply with quality assurance practices
- Screen and follow up patient test results

CLINICAL: DIAGNOSTIC ORDERS
- Collect and process specimens
- Perform diagnostic tests

CLINICAL: PATIENT CARE
- Adhere to established patient screening procedures
- Obtain patient history and vital signs
- Prepare patient for examinations, procedures, and treatments
- Assist with examinations, procedures, and treatments
- Coordinate patient care information with other health care providers

GENERAL: PROFESSIONALISM
- Display a professional manner and image
- Demonstrate initiative and responsibility
- Work as a member of the health care team
- Prioritize and perform multiple tasks
- Adapt to change
- Treat all patients with compassion and empathy

GENERAL: COMMUNICATION SKILLS
- Recognize and respect cultural diversity
- Adapt communications to individual's ability to understand
- Recognize and respond effectively to verbal, nonverbal, and written communications
- Use medical terminology appropriately
- Serve as a liaison

GENERAL: LEGAL CONCEPTS
- Perform within legal and ethical boundaries
- Document accurately
- Implement and maintain federal and state health care legislation and regulations
- Comply with established risk management and safety procedures

GENERAL: INSTRUCTION
- Instruct individuals according to their needs
- Teach methods of health promotion and disease prevention
- Locate community resources and disseminate information

GENERAL: OPERATIONAL FUNCTIONS
- Perform routine maintenance of administrative and clinical equipment

CHAPTER COMPETENCIES

LEARNING OBJECTIVES
Upon successfully completing this chapter, you will be able to:
1. Spell and define the key terms.
2. Describe disorders of the lymphatic and immune systems.
3. Identify laboratory tests and clinical procedures related to the lymphatic and immune systems.
4. Describe what is meant by immunity.
5. Explain what a vaccine is and identify some of the common vaccines in use today.
6. Discuss HIV, ARC, and AIDS.

KEY TERMS

acquired immunodeficiency syndrome (AIDS)	antihistamine	immunity	toxoid
allergen	attenuated	interferon	vaccine
allergy	complement	Kaposi sarcoma	Western blot
antibodies	ELISA	opportunistic infection	
antigen	histamine	retrovirus	
	immune globulins	titer	

THE LYMPHATIC AND IMMUNE SYSTEMS

OUR ENVIRONMENT contains a large variety of infectious agents, such as viruses, bacteria, fungi, and parasites. Any of these agents can cause pathological damage and if allowed to multiply unchecked, may kill their host. In a normal individual with an intact immune system, most infections do not last long and rarely result in permanent damage.

Some medical assistants choose to work in medical practices that specialize in allergy and immunology, and patients with disorders of the immune system are seen in all types of medical practices. In the allergy and immunology specialty office, you may see patients with a variety of disorders related to acute or chronic disorders of the immune system, including allergic reactions or symptoms. This chapter focuses on some common disorders of the lymphatic and immune systems.

The Lymphatic System

The lymphatic system and certain special blood cells make up the immune system. Together, these systems protect us from the pathogens in our environment (FIG. 36-1). Specifically, the lymphatic system includes lymph fluid, lymph vessels, and lymph nodes, which filter and destroy pathogens removed from the tissues. The tonsils, spleen, and thymus are

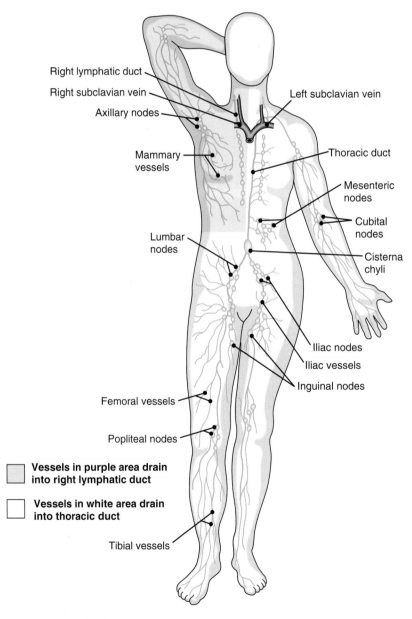

F I G U R E   3 6 – I .   The lymphatic system. (Reprinted with permission from Cohen BJ. Medical Terminology: An Illustrated Guide. Philadelphia: Lippincott Williams & Wilkins, 2003.)

Table 36-1	IMPORTANT LYMPH NODES, LOCATIONS, AND IMMUNE RESPONSES	
Nodes	**Location**	**Immune Response**
Cervical	Neck	Enlarged during upper respiratory, facial, scalp infections
Axillary	Axillae (armpits)	May be enlarged after infection of upper extremities, breasts; cancer cells from breasts often metastasize to axillary nodes
Tracheobronchial	Near trachea, large bronchial tubes	May become solid masses of blackened tissue in severely polluted areas
Mesenteric	Between layers of peritoneum that form mesentery	Filter lymph from abdominal and pelvic organs
Inguinal	Groin	Receive drainage from lower extremities, external genitalia; when enlarged, called buboes, as in bubonic plague

organs of the lymphatic and immune systems. They function as filters, removing microorganisms, as do the lymph nodes found throughout the body. TABLE 36-1 describes the location and immune response of various lymph nodes.

The Immune System

The body is protected from microorganisms by two types of defenses. These defenses can work against any invading pathogen (nonspecific defenses), or they may work against only a particular pathogen (specific defenses). Nonspecific defenses include the body's first line of protection, commonly called the barrier defenses. These mechanical and chemical barriers include the following:

- Intact skin
- Respiratory barriers (nostril hairs, cilia, and mucus)
- Digestive enzymes
- Acidity of the genitourinary tract
- Tears, which are slightly bactericidal
- Protective reflexes (coughing, sneezing, vomiting, and diarrhea)

Other nonspecific defenses include phagocytosis, fever, inflammation, and the production of interferon. **Interferon** is produced by cells that are infected with viruses, and although interferon cannot prevent the entry of viruses into cells, it

does block reproduction of infected cells. Three types of human interferon, alpha, beta, and gamma, were first produced in amounts sufficient for clinical research in the 1970s. Studies have shown that alpha-interferon may be useful in the treatment of AIDS.

Specific defenses include **immunity**, the body's ability to fight off a microorganism once infection has occurred. Two types of lymphocytes—B cells and T cells—produced by the immune system play a major role in immunity. B cells are produced in the bone marrow and mature in the spleen and lymph nodes; T cells are produced in the thymus gland and circulate between blood and lymph.

Antigens and Antibodies

Antigens are chemical markers that identify cells. Human cells have their own antigens that identify all of the cells in an individual as self. When antigens are foreign, or other than self, the body recognizes them as dangerous and attempts to destroy them. Infections with bacteria, viruses, fungi, protozoa, malignant cells, and organ transplants produce antigens that activate immune responses.

In response to foreign antigens, the body produces certain proteins called **antibodies**. These proteins, also called **immune globulins** or gamma-globulins, are produced by plasma cells. Antibodies do not destroy foreign antigens but attach and label them for destruction by other types of white blood cells called phagocytes. When a B cell is confronted with a specific type of antigen, it transforms into a plasma cell or memory cell. Memory cells can quickly produce antibodies if the same antigen appears again. These antibodies, or immune globulins, described in TABLE 36-2, produce humoral immunity. In addition, antibodies can activate several proteins in the blood, called **complement**, that prompt the inflammatory process. These proteins promote vasodilation, attract white blood cells to the area of infection, destroy antigens, and prevent the spread of bacteria. TABLE 36-3 describes several laboratory tests for antibodies that are useful in confirming a diagnosis.

T cells are antigen specific, meaning that each one responds usually to only one antigen. A type of immunity, cell-mediated immunity, depends on T lymphocytes, which can multiply rapidly in response to an antigen. This antigen usually has been brought to the T cell by a macrophage, or cell responsible for engulfing and digesting the microorganism. Unfortunately, T cells also react to beneficial foreign tissues, such as skin grafts and transplanted organs. Another type of T cell secretes a chemical called interleukin that stimulates B cells and other T lymphocytes to destroy the invading antigen.

Checkpoint Question

1. What are antigens? What does the body form in response to foreign antigens?

Table 36-2   IMMUNOGLOBULINS

Immunoglobulin	Properties, Functions
IgA	Found in exocrine excretions, such as milk, tears, mucous secretions; probably a protective mechanism for mucosa
IgD	Plasma preparation from persons with a high concentration of Rh antibodies; given to Rh-negative mothers soon after delivery of an Rh-positive infant to prevent hemolytic disease of the newborn in subsequent pregnancies
IgE	Found in mast cells of respiratory, gastrointestinal tracts; important in allergic responses; elevated during allergic response
IgG	Main immunoglobulin in human serum; produces antibodies for various pathogens; elevated during infection; activates complement to complete immune response; frequently given to provide immediate temporary immunity against various pathogens
IgM	Formed in early stages of almost all immune reactions; controls ABO blood group antibodies; helps to stimulate production of complement

Types of Immunity

Genetic, or natural, immunity is programmed in the DNA and does not involve antibodies. Some individuals are born with a natural, inherent immunity to certain diseases, and in some cases the immunity is specific to a particular species. For example, scarlet fever, measles, diphtheria, and influenza do not affect animals that come into contact with humans with these illnesses. In the same way, many animal infections, such as distemper, do not affect humans who come into contact with diseased animals.

Another type of immunity, acquired immunity, involves antibodies and may be either natural or artificial. This immunity may be acquired either passively or actively.

*   *Passive acquired natural immunity* comes from another source, such as across the placenta from the mother to the fetus or through breast milk to a nursing infant.
*   *Passive acquired artificial immunity* is produced by injection of gamma-globulins, or antibodies, after a presumed exposure to an infectious pathogen. Gamma-globulins are not vaccines and do not stimulate immune mechanisms but provide immediate temporary antibody protection. TABLE 36-4 lists some gamma-globulins.
*   *Active acquired natural immunity* develops in a person who contracts a specific disease, causing the body to produce antibodies and memory cells.
*   *Active acquired artificial immunity* is produced by administration of a **vaccine**, which stimulates the production of antibodies and memory cells to prevent specific diseases by killing the pathogen if it enters the body. Vaccines contain antigens to which the immune system responds, much as it would to an exposure to a disease.

Vaccines can be made with organisms killed by heat or with live organisms. If live organisms are used, they must be treated in the laboratory to weaken them; they are **attenuated**. Another type of vaccine is made from a form of the toxin produced by a disease microorganism. The toxin is altered with heat or chemicals to reduce its harmfulness, but it can still function as an antigen to induce immunity. Such an altered toxin is called a **toxoid**.

Booster shots are follow-up administrations of vaccines to maintain a high level, or **titer**, of antibodies in the blood. In some cases, active immunity acquired by artificial means does not last a lifetime, making it necessary to boost the body's production of antibodies against a specific disease. An example of a vaccine that requires more than one dose to assure immunity is the vaccine for mumps, measles, and rubella which is given as one injection to infants and repeated during childhood.

Table 36-3   ANTIBODY-SPECIFIC LABORATORY TESTS

Test	Purpose
Complement fixation test	Measures severity of infection; helps indicate extent and effectiveness of antigen–antibody reactions.
Antibody titer	Measures amount of specific antibody in the blood; if in several weeks antibody level is up, infection is current
Fluorescent antibody test	Antibodies from blood sample stained or marked by fluorescent material, permitting rapid diagnosis of various kinds of infections.

Spanish Terminology

Tiene alergias?	Do you have any allergies?
Tiene difficultad al respirar?	Are you having any difficulty in breathing?
Tiene una infección.	You have an infection.
Necesita una vacuna.	You need a vaccine.

Checkpoint Question

2. What are three types of vaccines?

COMMON LYMPHATIC DISORDERS

Lymphadenitis

Any disease of the lymphatic system is lymphadenopathy; lymphadenitis is an inflammatory condition that commonly results from a bacterial or viral infection. Symptoms include enlarged, tender lymph nodes. This enlargement is caused by drainage of microorganisms or toxins from the infection into the lymph nodes. The site of origin of the infection can often be determined by the location of the affected node. For example, enlarged inguinal lymph nodes typically result from infections of the external genitalia, while enlarged cervical lymph nodes may result from an upper respiratory infection. Treatment of lymphadenitis is directed at eliminating the primary infection.

Mononucleosis

Mononucleosis, caused by Epstein-Barr virus (EBV), affects the entire lymphatic system. Symptoms include fatigue, asthenia (weakness), sore throat, and enlarged tender lymph nodes. Mononucleosis is usually transmitted by direct oral contact and primarily affects young adults. In addition to the medical history and physical examination, the diagnosis of mononucleosis is usually made by obtaining a blood specimen and sending the specimen to the serology department of the laboratory (see Chapter 46). The physician may order a Monospot antibody test, an EBV antibody test, or a complete blood count. The presence of more than 10% atypical T lymphocytes (a specific type of lymphocyte) in the blood and a total white blood cell count of 15,000 to 20,000 cells per cubic millimeter are further signs of the disease. Recovery usually takes 4 to 8 weeks. As with any virus, treatment is symptomatic and palliative.

Checkpoint Question

3. In lymphadenitis, why do the lymph nodes become enlarged and tender?

Hodgkin Disease

Hodgkin disease commonly affects young men and is characterized by lymphadenopathy, splenomegaly, fever, weakness, anorexia, and weight loss. Although it can originate in any lymphoid tissue, it usually begins in the lymph nodes of the supraclavicular, high cervical, or mediastinal areas. The diagnosis is often made by identifying a malignant cell, the Reed-Sternberg cell, in the lymph nodes. If the disease is local, the treatment of choice is radiotherapy using high-dose radiation. If the disease is more widespread, chemotherapy is given alone or in combination with radiation therapy. There is a high probability of cure with available treatments.

COMMON IMMUNE DISORDERS

Allergies

An **allergy** is an individual's hypersensitivity reaction to a particular antigen called an **allergen**. Allergens include plant pollens, foods, chemicals, antibiotics, other medications, and mold spores. While not everyone responds to these substances adversely, those with allergies may have reactions ranging from mild, such as seasonal rhinitis or hay fever, to severe, including anaphylaxis, a total collapse of the respiratory and circulatory systems. These allergens may be inhaled, ingested, injected, or absorbed into the skin. Because of the complexity of the antibody response, the first contact builds up the memory cells, which produce a reaction on the next contact with the allergen.

Table 36-4	GAMMA GLOBULINS
Globulin	**Function**
Tetanus immune globulin	Prevents tetanus infection after exposure in patients not immunized
Immune serum globulin	May prevent infectious hepatitis after exposure
Immune globulin Rh$_0$ (concentrated human antibody)	Prevents formation of antibodies against Rh factor in Rh-negative mother after birth of Rh-positive baby
Rabies antiserum (human or horse)	Treat victims of rabid animal bites

TRIAGE

While you are working in a medical office, the following three situations occur:

A. Patient A is a new patient being seen today for symptoms of seasonal allergies, including watery eyes and nasal congestion for the past week. The physician has examined him and asked you to obtain some antihistamine drug samples to give to him before he is discharged.

B. Patient B received an allergy injection approximately 10 minutes ago and is requesting to leave to avoid being caught in traffic and late to work. The receptionist has offered to discharge him for you.

C. Patient C has been ordered to have some blood drawn for mononucleosis screening.

How do you sort these patients? Whom do you see first? Second? Third?

Although patients A and B appear more important in terms of requiring immediate clinical contact, you should take time to explain the importance of waiting at the medical office to patient B, since serious allergic reactions after injections with allergens can occur up to 30 minutes after administration. The receptionist, while attempting to be helpful, should not be permitted to discharge this patient prematurely. Next, the antihistamine medication should be obtained as ordered by the physician, and patient A should receive a thorough explanation of the dosage, administration, and side effects before being discharged. Patient C should be taken care of last, since a blood draw takes patience and a distraction-free environment.

In sensitive individuals, the antigen–antibody reaction may cause the release of an excessive amount of **histamine**, a substance normally found in the body in response to injured cells. The release of histamine in response to exposure to an allergen causes an inflammatory reaction, including increased capillary permeability, hence edema. It may also cause contraction of involuntary muscles, particularly those in the bronchial tree, and the resultant bronchospasm may become life-threatening. **Antihistamine** medications sometimes reduce the symptoms of mild to moderate allergic reactions, but individuals with breathing difficulties should receive immediate care by emergency services personnel.

Autoimmunity

Normally the body can recognize proteins that belong to itself and produces antibodies only when foreign proteins invade. In autoimmune diseases, however, the body fails to recognize its own proteins and produces antibodies that destroy its own cells and tissues. Examples of autoimmune diseases include rheumatoid arthritis, chronic thyroiditis, lupus erythematosus, and pernicious anemia. Diabetes mellitus, colitis, and multiple sclerosis are also thought to be caused by autoimmune processes. There is no cure for autoimmune diseases.

Immunodeficiency Diseases

Failure of any of the components of the immune system results in an immune deficiency. This may be genetic and may be apparent soon after birth, or it may be acquired as the result of a disease process or chemotherapy of various carcinomas. The deficiency may affect any part of the immune system, and severity varies.

Acquired immunodeficiency syndrome, AIDS, is an infectious disease that overwhelms the body's immune system. Human immunodeficiency virus (HIV) is the pathogen that causes AIDS by destroying T-helper cells and suppressing the body's cell-mediated immune response. HIV is a **retrovirus**, which means that it enters the cell, infiltrates the cell's RNA, and transfers its own DNA to the cell's DNA by means of an enzyme called transcriptase. The change in DNA prevents the affected cell from functioning normally. It can function only to nourish and incubate more HIV. Patients infected with HIV are predisposed to life-threatening infections and malignancies.

The incubation period of an initial infection with HIV ranges from a few months to several years. An infected person may unknowingly spread HIV to others before any symptoms appear. HIV is not spread by casual contact; it is most often transmitted through an exchange of blood or body fluids that may result from sexual contact, sharing a contaminated needle, transfusion of contaminated blood, or accidental injury from a sharp instrument used in an invasive procedure. It may also travel across the placenta from an infected

WHAT IF

A mother voices concern over her teenage daughter's diagnosis of mononucleosis?

The mother may be concerned because mononucleosis is sometimes called the kissing disease. However, the virus is spread through contact with contaminated saliva, which can occur through other activities besides kissing, such as sharing drinking cups.

mother to her infant. A person with HIV may go through the following stages as the infection progresses to AIDS:

1. Acute infectious stage, with generally mild flulike symptoms.
2. Latent period, without symptoms.
3. Complaints of weight loss, lymphadenopathy, fever, diarrhea, anorexia, fatigue, and skin rash.
4. Onset of immunodeficiency disorders, such as Kaposi's sarcoma and *Pneumocystis carinii* pneumonia (possibly the initial stages of full-blown AIDS).

The infectious diseases associated with AIDS are called **opportunistic infections** because HIV lowers the body's resistance and provides an opportunity for infection by bacteria and parasites, and abnormal cell development that is usually contained by normal defenses. Some opportunistic infections associated with AIDS are candidiasis (a yeastlike fungus often seen in the mouth, respiratory tract, and skin), herpes simplex (a viral infection causing small, painful blisters on the skin of the lips, nose, or genitalia), and *Pneumocystis carinii* pneumonia (a one-celled microorganism causing lung infection with fever, cough, chest pain, and sputum production).

Although it is a direct result of HIV infection, AIDS combines several disease processes. Alone, none is considered to be specific to AIDS, but each of these signs and symptoms is a reason for concern in the HIV-positive individual. Box 36-1 describes some of the signs and symptoms frequently associated with AIDS. Patients who are HIV positive are treated prophylactically according to laboratory data, including the T-cell count. As a medical assistant, you must be knowledgeable about AIDS, especially its transmission, both for your own protection and for the protection of your patients. A good understanding of this disease and the meth-

---

Box 36-1

SIGNS AND SYMPTOMS FREQUENTLY ASSOCIATED WITH HIV AND AIDS

Malignancies

Kaposi sarcoma is a cancer arising from the lining cells of capillaries. It produces bluish red nodules on the skin, particularly on the lower limbs. Cancer of the lymph nodes, called lymphoma, is also associated with HIV infection.

Periods of Severe Fatigue

Even though everyone has periods of some fatigue, these periods are not normally prolonged or unexplained. Extreme fatigue that lasts more than several weeks should be considered a warning sign of a health problem.

Sudden, Unexplained Weight Loss

As a rule, an unexplained weight loss of 10 pounds or more in less than 60 days should be cause for concern.

Night Sweats

Drenching night sweats and chills with fever often occur with AIDS, tuberculosis, and other serious illnesses.

Diarrhea

Diarrhea that persists for more than a week is common among AIDS patients.

Bruising or Bleeding

The blood of an HIV-positive person has an unusually long clotting time. HIV-positive patients have a tendency to bleed or bruise easily; even minor injuries can result in severe bruising. The mucous membranes may bleed with no evidence or history of trauma or injury.

Coughing, Shortness of Breath, Other Respiratory Symptoms

Pneumocystis carinii pneumonia is a type of pneumonia associated closely with AIDS. It begins as a cough, either dry or productive, and persists for weeks, leading to severe shortness of breath. The persistent cough may be accompanied by chills, fever, tightness in the chest, increased pulse, and increased respirations. *P. carinii* pneumonia is considered to be the most frequent life-threatening opportunistic infection in persons with AIDS.

Persistent Generalized Lymphadenopathy

When a person has AIDS, the lymph system is unable to control the infections associated with the disease. The lymph glands and nodes become enlarged in an effort to control the disease. Lymphadenopathy is manifested as enlarged, hard, painful nodes in various parts of the body.

Oral Thrush

Candida albicans thrives in the suppressed immune system. Although AIDS patients frequently have thrush, esophageal thrush is the most significant indicator of HIV infection. A condition called hairy leukoplakia—lesions on each side of the tongue with grayish white patchy discolorations—often is observed in HIV-positive patients.

(continues)

Box 36-1 *(continued)*

Neurological Problems

Patients who have AIDS are subject to a variety of nervous system disorders, including headaches, stiff neck, general pain, and weakness or numbness of the extremities. They may also have depression, delusions, hallucinations, paranoia, and dementia.

Malignancies associated with HIV.

PATIENT EDUCATION

AIDS Prevention

When providing instructions about AIDS prevention, explain to your patient that it is safest, of course, to abstain from sex. However, if that is not an option, instruct your patient to have sex only with a partner who is known not to be infected, who has sex with no one but the patient, and who does not use needles or syringes. Also tell the patient to use a latex condom and a spermicide. Generally, instruct patients to do the following:

- Avoid contact with another person's blood, body fluids, semen, and vaginal secretions.

- Avoid sharing needles, syringes, and any objects that come in contact with blood or body fluids.

- Avoid using alcohol and drugs. Use of these substances can hinder clear thinking and lead to unwise decision making.

ods for preventing its transmission helps prevent misinformation, rumor, apathy, and fear. Furthermore, obtaining an accurate medical history from patients at risk for HIV or AIDS is important. TABLE 36-5 offers some suggestions for interview questions.

Checkpoint Question

4. How is HIV spread?

COMMON DIAGNOSTIC AND THERAPEUTIC PROCEDURES

Allergy Testing

As a medical assistant, you may be responsible for allergy testing. You should obtain a careful history of allergic episodes, set up the allergens as ordered by the physician, assist with or perform the allergy testing, and follow up with patient education. Because of the potential for anaphylaxis after purposeful exposure to allergens during the testing,

Table 36-5   OBTAINING AN ACCURATE HISTORY FROM A PATIENT AT RISK FOR HIV OR AIDS

A patient who is at risk for HIV or AIDS may be reluctant to provide you with an accurate social history. Here are some helpful hints for obtaining an accurate history.

Instead of asking...	Ask...	Rationale
Do you have sex with prostitutes?	Have you ever paid for sexual activities?	Some patients do not admit using a prostitute but acknowledge paying for sexual favors.
Do you do IV drugs?	Do you do skin popping? Steroid injections?	Some patients do not perceive skin popping steroid injections as IV drug use.
Do you practice safe sex?	What method of safe sex do you use? Do you use a condom? Do you reuse condoms?	Some patients perceive using birth control as practicing safe sex; birth control per se offers no protection against HIV.
Are you a homosexual?	What is your sexual preference? Do you have sex with members of your sex?	Some patients may not perceive themselves as homosexuals or do not want to be labeled.

Box 36-2

ALLERGY TESTING SAFETY PRECAUTIONS

Although allergy testing is usually performed in a controlled setting, there is always a possibility of anaphylaxis. A well-equipped emergency cart or tray must be as close to the testing site as possible. A basic setup should include the following:

- Injectable epinephrine with syringes and needles
- Various sizes of airways
- Oxygen, masks, and Bag-mask device
- A tourniquet

Some sites may require tracheotomy equipment, a defibrillator, electrocardiography machine, and intravenous equipment.

FIGURE 36-3. A wheal produced by a positive allergy test. (Reprinted with permission from Goodheart HP. Goodheart's Photoguide of Common Skin Disorders, 2nd ed. Philadelphia: Lippincott Williams & Wilkins, 2003.)

emergency equipment and medications should be close at hand during and after the test procedure (Box 36-2).

Allergy skin test methods include scratch tests, intradermal injections, and patch tests. The scratch or puncture tests are usually done on the outer surface of the upper arm or back to detect allergies to substances in the environment, such as pollen or mold, and to certain animals, such as cats and dogs. The skin surface is labeled or numbered in rows 1.5 to 2 inches apart (FIG. 36-2). A short scratch is made with

a needle or lancet and a drop of each allergen is placed on each scratch. The patient may have 50 or more tests at a time, following a certain pattern so that the site of each allergen is identified. The test sites are examined after 15 to 20 minutes. A positive test for allergy is indicated by development of a wheal at the site (FIG. 36-3). Patients should not leave the office for at least 30 minutes after allergy testing so they can be observed for delayed allergic reactions.

Intradermal tests are done by injecting 0.01 to 0.02 mL of specific allergen extract on the anterior forearm; 10 to 15 tests may be done on each arm. These are thought to be more accurate than the scratch or puncture method.

Patch tests determine the cause of contact dermatitis. A small amount of suspected allergen is placed on the anterior forearm, covered with cellophane, and taped down. The patient may have 20 to 30 tests at a time. Results are read after 24 hours.

The results of each of these tests depend on the reactions and are usually graded according to comparison with guides supplied by the manufacturers of the allergens. Laboratory blood tests, which are more expensive and invasive, test for specific antibodies in the blood, usually ingestants for suspected food allergies. You may be responsible for collection and transportation of blood specimens.

Laboratory Testing for HIV

ELISA, or enzyme-linked immunosorbent assay, is used to screen blood for antibodies to the AIDS virus. A positive result indicates probable exposure to the virus and the possibility that the virus is in the blood. Since false-positive results can occur with ELISA, the **Western blot** test is used to confirm positive findings and is considered to be diagnostic. Your responsibility in this testing is usually confined to collecting the specimen by phlebotomy and routing it to the proper laboratory.

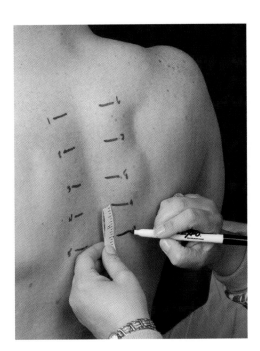

FIGURE 36-2. In preparation for allergy testing, the skin surface is numbered in rows 1.5 to 2 inches apart.

LEGAL TIP

HIV Testing

Testing for HIV has many legal implications. The laws vary from state to state, but they generally include:

- Patients must sign an informed consent form before being tested.
- Pre- and posttest counseling, usually by a state approved HIV counselor, regardless of the test results.
- Most laws have specific standards that mandate by whom, when, and how HIV test results can be given.
- To ensure confidentiality, most laboratories will use a numeric or other coding system rather than the patient's name on the lab requisition form.
- Laboratories that perform HIV testing must be approved by the state for this testing.

CHAPTER SUMMARY

An intact immune system is our best protection against constant exposure to microorganisms that may be dangerous to our health. Disorders of the immune system include those that are acquired through diseases, such as HIV infection, or as a result of suppression of the immune system by certain medications such as chemotherapy agents. Patients with disorders of the immune system may be particularly susceptible to communicable diseases, and you should take extra precautions to prevent the spread of microorganisms through adequate medical aseptic techniques, such as handwashing.

Allergy, a common disorder of the immune system, produces signs and symptoms ranging from mild to severe. Since some medications can cause life-threatening allergic reactions in the susceptible, you should always observe your patients closely following administration of a medication and immediately report any adverse reaction to the physician.

Critical Thinking Challenges

1. Your patient has been diagnosed with breast cancer. Why is it important for the physician to order a biopsy of lymph nodes in the axillary area?
2. Research and report on the reasons for not obtaining blood pressure or a blood specimen from an arm that has had lymph nodes removed from the axilla.
3. The mother of your patient questions the need for booster shots for her young son. How do you impress on her the importance of immunizations? Explain in terms that a lay person would understand.

Answers to Checkpoint Questions

1. Antigens are chemical markers that identify cells. Foreign antigens must be destroyed. The body forms antibodies that attach to these antigens, marking them for destruction.
2. Three types of vaccines are live attenuated, killed, and altered toxin (toxoid).
3. Lymphadenitis usually results from an infection. The enlarged lymph nodes are caused by increased drainage of microorganisms or toxins from the infection into the lymph nodes.
4. HIV is transmitted through an exchange of blood or body fluids that may result from sexual contact, sharing a contaminated needle, transfusion, or accidental injury from a sharp instrument used in an invasive procedure. It also can be transmitted across the placenta from infected mother to infant.

 Websites

American Academy of Allergy Asthma and Immunology
    http://www.aaaai.org/
Food Allergy & Anaphylaxis Network http://www.food allergy.org/
National Institute of Allergy and Infectious Diseases
    http://www.niaid.nih.gov/
Asthma and Allergy Foundation of America
    http://www.aafa.org/
Epstein-Barr Virus and Infectious Mononucleosis
    http://www.cdc.gov/ncidod/diseases/ebv.htm
CDC Divisions of HIV/AIDS Prevention
    http://www.cdc.gov/hiv/dhap.htm

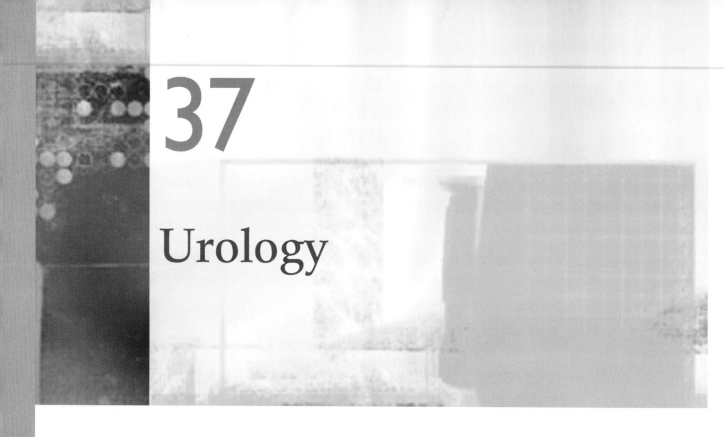

37

Urology

CHAPTER OUTLINE

COMMON URINARY DISORDERS
Renal Failure
Calculi
Tumors
Hydronephrosis
Urinary System Infections

COMMON DISORDERS OF THE MALE REPRODUCTIVE SYSTEM
Benign Prostatic Hyperplasia
Prostate Cancer
Testicular Cancer
Hydrocele
Cryptorchidism
Inguinal Hernia
Infections
Impotence

COMMON DIAGNOSTIC AND THERAPEUTIC PROCEDURES
Urinalysis
Blood Tests
Cystoscopy, or Cystourethroscopy
Intravenous Pyelogram and Retrograde Pyelogram
Ultrasound
Rectal and Scrotal Examinations
Vasectomy

ROLE DELINEATION

ADMINISTRATIVE: ADMINISTRATIVE PROCEDURES
• Perform basic administrative procedures
• Understand and adhere to managed care policies and procedures

CLINICAL: FUNDAMENTAL PRINCIPLES
• Apply principles of aseptic technique and infection control
•• Comply with quality assurance practices
• Screen and follow up patient test results

CLINICAL: DIAGNOSTIC ORDERS
• Collect and process specimens
• Perform diagnostic tests

CLINICAL: PATIENT CARE
• Adhere to established patient screening procedures
• Obtain patient history and vital signs
• Prepare and maintain examination and treatment areas
• Assist with examinations, procedures, and treatments
• Coordinate patient care information with other health care providers

GENERAL: PROFESSIONALISM

- Display a professional manner and image
- Demonstrate initiative and responsibility
- Work as a member of the health care team
- Prioritize and perform multiple tasks
- Adapt to change
- Treat all patients with compassion and empathy

GENERAL: COMMUNICATION SKILLS

- Recognize and respect cultural diversity
- Adapt communications to individual's ability to understand
- Recognize and respond effectively to verbal, nonverbal, and written communications
- Use medical terminology appropriately
- Serve as a liaison

GENERAL: LEGAL CONCEPTS

- Perform within legal and ethical boundaries
- Prepare and maintain medical records
- Document accurately
- Comply with established risk management and safety procedures

GENERAL: INSTRUCTION

- Instruct individuals according to their needs
- Explain office policies and procedures
- Teach methods of health promotion and disease prevention

GENERAL: OPERATIONAL FUNCTIONS

- Perform inventory of supplies and equipment
- Perform routine maintenance of administrative and clinical equipment

CHAPTER COMPETENCIES

LEARNING OBJECTIVES

Upon successfully completing this chapter, you will be able to:

1. Spell and define the key terms.
2. Identify and explain the primary organs of the urinary system.
3. List and describe the disorders of the urinary system and the male reproductive system.
4. Describe and explain the purpose of various diagnostic procedures associated with the urinary system.
5. Discuss the role of the medical assistant in diagnosing and treating disorders of the urinary system and the male reproductive system.

PERFORMANCE OBJECTIVES

Upon successfully completing this chapter, you will be able to:

1. Perform a female urinary catheterization (Procedure 37-1)
2. Perform a male urinary catheterization (Procedure 37-2)
3. Instruct a male patient on the self testicular examination (Procedure 37-3)

KEY TERMS

anuria	enuresis	nephrostomy	pyuria
blood urea nitrogen	hematuria	nocturia	retrograde pyelogram
catheterization	impotence	oliguria	specific gravity
cystoscopy	incontinence	prostate-specific antigen	ureterostomy
dialysis	intravenous pyelogram (IVP)	proteinuria	urinalysis
dysuria	lithotripsy	psychogenic	urinary frequency

The process of metabolism creates waste products that must be eliminated from the body. Several body systems contribute to preventing a buildup of the end products of metabolism, including the gastrointestinal system, the respiratory system, and the integumentary system. The urinary system also removes waste from the blood while regulating fluid volume, important electrolytes, blood pressure, and pH (acid-base) balance (FIG. 37-1). Disorders of the filters of the urinary system, the kidneys, are diagnosed through various urine and blood tests and radiographs. Patients with kidney problems are typically referred to a nephrologist, a physician who specializes in the physiology of the kidneys. Disorders of the anatomy, or physical characteristics, of the urinary system are referred to another type of specialist, a urologist. Since the male reproductive system is so in inextricably linked to the urinary system, disorders of the male reproductive system are also often referred to the urologist. This chapter does not review the anatomy and

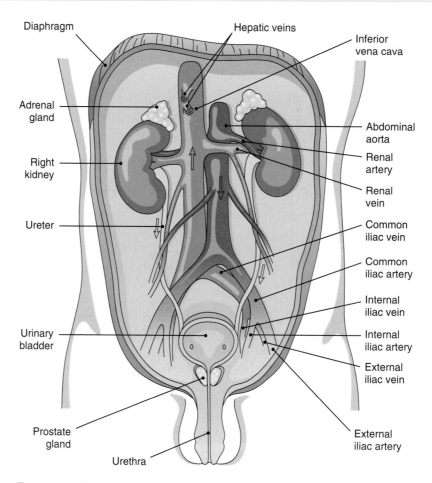

FIGURE 37–1. Urinary system with blood vessels. (Reprinted with permission from Cohen BJ, Wood DL. Memmler's The Human Body in Health and Disease. Philadelphia: Lippincott Williams & Wilkins, 2000.)

physiology of the urinary system but focuses on common disorders, diagnostic procedures, and treatments associated with the urinary and male reproductive systems.

COMMON URINARY DISORDERS

Renal Failure

Renal failure is an acute or chronic disorder of kidney function manifested by the inability of the kidney to excrete wastes, concentrate urine, and aid in homeostatic electrolyte conservation. In acute renal failure, the patient has **oliguria** and a corresponding rise in nitrogen-containing wastes in the blood. The causes of acute renal failure include a serious loss of fluid due to severe burn or hemorrhage, trauma, toxic injury to the kidney, and an obstruction beyond the level of the collecting tubules.

Chronic renal failure is a gradual loss of nephrons with corresponding inability of the kidney to perform its functions. It may result from another disease process, such as systemic lupus erythematosus, diabetic neuropathy, radiation, or renal tuberculosis. The patient has general weakness, edema of the lungs and tissues, and neurological symptoms such as

confusion progressing to seizures and coma as the wastes, or toxins, not filtered by the kidneys build up in the blood.

Treatment for both acute and chronic renal failure may involve renal **dialysis** to remove nitrogenous waste products and excess fluid from the body. Dialysis dependence may be short term in an acute illness or long term in end-stage renal disease. Without functional nephrons, wastes must be filtered through membranes other than those in the renal tissues. Two methods are used: hemodialysis and peritoneal dialysis.

With hemodialysis, toxins are removed from the blood by routing the patient's blood through a dialysis machine containing synthetic filters and a dialysate, a substance used to balance the electrolyte concentration in the blood. The machine can be regulated to remove or retain certain substances as needed for the individual patient. This type of dialysis requires that the patient's circulatory system be accessed as often as 3 times a week for 3 to 4 hours at a time. Therefore, most patients receive a surgical fistula, or graft, between an artery and a vein to make entry with a needle during the procedure easier for the patient. The fistula is often placed in one of the arms, and this arm should not be used for taking blood pressures or for blood draws.

Patients receiving peritoneal dialysis often perform the procedure at home. An appropriately balanced dialysate is administered through a catheter into the abdominal cavity, allowed to remain in the abdominal cavity for a specified time, and then drained into a collecting bag. As the dialysate flows from the peritoneal cavity, it brings with it filtered wastes and excess fluid removed from the patient's blood through the blood vessels in the abdominal cavity. Patients who have had extensive abdominal surgery with disruption of the peritoneal membranes are not good candidates for this type of dialysis. Peritoneal dialysis allows the patient the freedom to move about and continue a more normal lifestyle at home than with hemodialysis, which requires that the patient go to an outpatient facility several times a week. However, an abdominal catheter may result in an altered body image and psychological depression. The surgical opening on the abdomen can also become infected, leading to peritonitis, a serious infection in the abdominal cavity.

Neither type of dialysis is a cure for the underlying renal dysfunction, but both can prolong life almost indefinitely. Chronic renal failure frequently involves other systems as well as the urinary system and requires treatment for that involvement.

Calculi

Calculi are stone formations that may be found anywhere in the urinary system and may range from granular particles to staghorn structures that fill the renal pelvis. Stones seem most likely to form if the urine is alkaline; the symptoms vary with the size and location of the stone. Hematuria may be present if rough edges of calculi abrade the mucous membrane lining the urinary system. The patient has flank pain if a stone lodges in one of the ureters.

Treatment may not be needed if the stones are small enough to be flushed out with increased fluid intake. Large stones may require surgery or **lithotripsy**, a procedure in which ultrasound is used to crush the stones. In either case, the chemical makeup of the stones is evaluated for the forming components, and the patient's diet may be adjusted to prevent recurrence (Box 37-1).

Checkpoint Question

1. What are calculi, and when are they more likely to form?

Tumors

The urinary system may be a primary or secondary site for tumors. Tumors are more common in the urinary bladder but may also occur in the kidney. Symptoms vary but usually include hematuria and an unexplained abdominal mass. Treatment is based on the extent and type of tumor and may include surgery, chemotherapy, radiation, or a combination.

Box 37-1

DIAGNOSING AND TREATING CALCULI: A CASE STUDY

Clark Watkins, a 45-year-old white man, has severe right flank pain radiating to the suprapubic and inguinal regions of the abdomen. He has a fever of 100.3°F, nausea, and some vomiting. Urinalysis shows gross and microscopic hematuria and calcium crystal casts; it is clear of pyuria and white blood cells.

Dr. Brown performs in-office ultrasonography, and the results suggest renal calculi. He orders IVP, which reveals sand-to-gravel calculi.

Your role is to provide patient education. Demonstrate to Mr. Watkins the procedure for filtering his urine and provide him with the strainer so he can bring in the solid material for analysis. Mr. Watkins's diet will be altered in accordance with the composition of the stones. He may be referred to a dietitian or given a diet list after counseling with Dr. Brown. Encourage Mr. Watkins to increase his fluid intake to flush the stones and to walk frequently to assist peristalsis in the ureters and passing the stones. Urge him to drink fruit juices, especially cranberry juice, in addition to water, and discourage caffeine drinks. He may need an antiemetic if nausea and vomiting interfere with fluid intake. Caution him to watch for signs of infection and obstruction, including cloudy urine, which may contain pus, and fever.

Hydronephrosis

Hydronephrosis is distention of the renal pelvis and calyces resulting from an obstruction in the kidney or ureter that causes a backup of urine. The symptoms include flank pain, hematuria, pyuria, fever, and chills. To restore the flow of urine, the stricture must be corrected, if possible, through **cystoscopy**. If it is not possible to restore the flow of urine to the urinary bladder, it may be necessary to perform a **nephrostomy** (opening the kidney and placement of a catheter in the kidney pelvis) or **ureterostomy** (surgical creation of an opening to the outside of the body from the ureter).

Urinary System Infections

Glomerulonephritis is inflammation of the glomerulus, or filtering unit, of the kidney. Symptoms range from very mild edema of the extremities, **proteinuria**, **hematuria**, and oliguria to complete renal failure. It is occasionally seen in children 1 to 4 weeks after a streptococcal infection as the large streptococcal antibodies are trapped in the small capillaries of the glomerulus, causing irritation and inflammation. Glomerulonephritis in adults may be chronic, with scarring

PATIENT EDUCATION

Urinary Tract Health

As the medical assistant, you will teach patients about everyday habits related to good general health. Encourage patients with urinary system symptoms to follow these suggestions to avoid urinary tract infections in the future:

For All Patients

- Drink lots of fluids, which help remove waste products from the fluid compartments. We are all generally advised to drink 8 glasses of water a day so that tissues are well hydrated, feces are soft, and infections in the lower urinary system are relatively unlikely.
- Empty your bladder when you feel the need. Urine held beyond comfort causes bladder stress and irritation. Allowing urine to stagnate in the bladder increases the risk of infection.
- Cranberry juice and vitamin C help acidify the urine and make the urinary system less attractive to bacteria.

Especially for Women

- Avoid using perfumed products in the perineal area. The female urinary meatus is very short and prone to irritation. Urethral infections quickly become bladder infections with irritation.
- Avoid tight-fitting lower garments, especially nylon underwear. Loose-fitting cotton underwear absorbs moisture and allows for airflow, making both bladder and vaginal infections less likely.
- Wipe carefully from front to back after using the toilet. Wash with soap and water and rinse well if infections are a recurrent problem.
- If you are prone to urinary tract infections, void immediately after sexual intercourse to flush the area of bacteria that might have intruded into the urethra. Avoid tub baths, particularly bubble baths; showers are less likely to contribute to infections.

and hardening of the glomeruli from repeated episodes of acute glomerulonephritis, and may lead to renal failure. Symptoms of the chronic form include proteinuria, casts in the urine (see Chapter 43), and hematuria. Treatment is usually symptomatic, and if an infection is involved, an antibiotic is prescribed.

Pyelonephritis is inflammation of the renal pelvis and the body of the kidney. It usually results from an ascending infection from the ureters and may be acute or chronic.

Symptoms include those of any infection, such as chills and fever, nausea, and vomiting, but also include flank pain and **pyuria** (pus in the urine).

Medication to acidify the urine and make the system less hospitable to bacteria may be the treatment of choice for pyelonephritis. In addition, an antibiotic may be prescribed.

Cystitis is an inflammation of the urinary bladder. This condition is far more common in women than in men because a woman's urethra is shorter. Symptoms begin with **urinary frequency**, **dysuria**, and urgency and progress to chills, fever, nausea, vomiting, and flank pain. The causative microorganism is identified with a urine culture, and the treatment usually is an antibiotic once the causative microorganism has been identified.

Urethritis is inflammation of the urethra that may occur before the signs and symptoms of cystitis appear, or it may indicate a sexually transmitted disease, such as gonorrhea or nongonococcal urethritis. The treatment for cystitis is also effective for urethritis. Other signs and symptoms of the urinary system and the possible causes are listed in TABLE 37-1.

Checkpoint Question

2. Why are women more likely than men to have cystitis?

COMMON DISORDERS OF THE MALE REPRODUCTIVE SYSTEM

Male patients with disorders of the reproductive system often have signs and symptoms pertaining to the urinary sys-

WHAT IF

A mother brings her 5-year-old daughter to the office with complaints of burning on urination? What questions do you ask? How do you educate the mother and child?

First, ask if the child urinates when she feels the urge or if she holds her urine. Some young girls are inclined to hold their urine long past the time to void, setting up a perfect situation for bacterial growth. Caution the child to go to the bathroom when the need arises, making sure to use terms she can understand. Next, ask the mother if she uses bubble bath in the child's bath water. Young girls have a very short urethra and are prone to urethritis if they bathe in water with certain types of bubble bath. Finally, explain that the child must learn to wipe from front to back to avoid urinary tract infections.

Table 37–1	Symptoms of Urinary Tract Disorders and Possible Causes
Symptoms	**Possible Causes**
Anuria	Renal failure, acute nephritis, lead or mercury poisoning, complete obstruction of urinary tract
Burning during voiding	Urethritis
Burning during and after voiding	Cystitis
Dysuria	Infection
Enuresis	Normal to age 3 years
Frequency	Infection, diabetes
Hematuria	Diseases of glomeruli, trauma, neoplasm, calculi
Incontinence	Infection, uterine prolapse, nerve damage, neoplasm, senility
Nocturia	Infection, prostatic hypertrophy, abdominal pressure (pregnancy), diabetes
Oliguria	Acute nephritis, dehydration, fever, urinary obstruction, neoplasm
Polyuria	Diabetes mellitus, diabetes insipidus, diuretic use, high fluid intake
Proteinuria	Disease of glomeruli or protein metabolism, infection, nephrotic syndrome
Pyuria	Infection
Renal colic	Calculi
Urgency	Infection, disease of the prostate

tem. If you work in a family practice or internal medicine office, you may care for male patients with reproductive system disorders, or these patients may be referred to urology for specific treatment or surgery. Common disorders include benign prostatic hyperplasia, carcinoma of the prostate gland, and testicular cancer.

Benign Prostatic Hyperplasia

As most men reach their middle years, the prostate begins to enlarge, or hypertrophy. Benign prostatic hyperplasia is a noncancerous enlargement of the prostate gland that occurs commonly in men over age 40. Diagnosis is with a digital rectal examination, which should be performed as part of the routine physical examination in men after age 40. Using a gloved hand and water-soluble lubricant, the physician will insert the index finger into the rectum and palpate the prostate for size, shape, and consistency.

As the prostate gland enlarges, it presses on the urethra and urinary bladder, causing urinary symptoms such as frequency and **nocturia**. While this condition is not usually a serious problem, it can be treated medically or surgically by partially or completely removing the prostate gland. The surgical procedure, prostatectomy, can be performed transurethrally or through a surgical opening into the suprapubic area of the lower abdomen. If the prostate is removed transurethrally, the procedure is a transurethral resection of the prostate. Box 37-2 describes the surgical techniques used to treat prostatic hypertrophy in more detail.

Box 37-2

SURGICAL INTERVENTION FOR PROSTATIC HYPERTROPHY

Transurethral Resection of the Prostate

A cystoscope with an electrocautery wire cutting loop, a resectoscope, is inserted through the urethra and rotated through the prostate to remove pieces of the gland. The pieces are washed out with irrigating fluid introduced through the scope. There is no abdominal incision, making this a relatively safe procedure for the high-risk patient. The whole organ is not usually removed for this surgery; therefore, the obstruction frequently returns. This is not a choice for malignancies.

Suprapubic Prostatectomy

Performed through the abdominal wall and bladder, suprapubic prostatectomy allows the surgeon to peel out the whole organ through a wide surgical field and to check the bladder for involvement. This approach is the choice for large prostate glands or for malignancies. As in all surgeries, there are postoperative risks, particularly for the elderly. These include pain, hemorrhage, urinary leakage, and prolonged convalescence.

(continued)

Box 37-2 (continued)

Perineal Resection

An incision between the scrotum and the anus is a short, direct route to the prostate without interfering with the bladder and is preferred for some large malignancies. It appears to be relatively nontraumatic for the very old or infirm. Surgeons find that the field offers less room to maneuver than with the suprapubic approach. It is not a good choice for young men, because impotence and urinary and fecal incontinence are frequent postoperative complications. The proximity of the anal area also increases the risk of infection.

Retropubic Resection

A low abdominal incision above the pubis but below the bladder avoids trauma to the bladder and thereby allows a shorter convalescence than with the suprapubic approach. It also provides better removal options than the transurethral approach. It is a good choice if pathology is limited to the prostate, with no bladder involvement.

Prostate Cancer

Prostate cancer, like most cancers, is best treated when detected early. In the early stages of the disease, many men are asymptomatic. As a result, male patients over age 40 should be encouraged to have yearly physical examinations that include a digital rectal examination, which often allows the physician to palpate an enlarged gland. If the prostate gland is enlarged, a biopsy of the prostate may be advised to determine the cause of the enlargement.

Another diagnostic test often ordered as part of the routine physical examination is the **prostate-specific antigen**, or PSA, blood test. PSA is normally found in the blood of all men, but its level increases with any inflammation of the prostate, including cancer. While the cause of prostate cancer is not known, it is most common in men over age 50, with 75% of diagnoses in men over age 75. Treatment depends on the extent of the malignancy and the patient's age and general health status. Prostate cancer is often treated by a combination of surgery, chemotherapy, and radiation.

Checkpoint Question

3. Does the patient with benign prostatic hyperplasia have an elevated PSA level? Why or why not?

Testicular Cancer

Although testicular cancer accounts for only about 1% of all malignancies, the metastatic and mortality rates are high. This type of cancer is most often seen in men aged 15 to 34. The cause of testicular cancer is unknown, but predisposing factors may include cryptorchidism, infection, genetic factors, and endocrine abnormalities. The symptoms are gradual and painless and may initially only involve a vague feeling of scrotal heaviness.

Once a diagnosis of testicular cancer has been made, treatment may be orchiectomy, or surgical removal of the testicle. Chemotherapy and radiation may also be used.

Hydrocele

Hydrocele, a collection of fluid in the scrotum and around the testes, may result from trauma or infection or may simply be due to aging. Diagnosis is based on symptoms and inspection. If the condition is extremely uncomfortable, aspiration of the excessive fluid may be required, and if the condition persists, surgical intervention may be the treatment of choice. In most cases, no treatment is necessary and the fluid is reabsorbed by the body. Hydrocele is common in male infants but generally subsides without treatment.

Cryptorchidism

Normally, the testes descend from the abdominal cavity into the scrotal sac in the male fetus by the eighth month of gestation. In a small percentage of male infants, one or both of the testes fail to descend by the time of delivery (FIG. 37-2). Cryptorchidism refers to either one or both undescended testes. Surgical correction, known as orchiopexy, is usually performed before age 4 years, preferably at 1 or 2 years. If an undescended testis is not surgically corrected, it results in sterility of the undescended organ and may increase the risk of testicular malignancy later in life.

FIGURE 37-2.   Possible locations of undescended testicles.

urine is needed, such as for pregnancy testing. The urinalysis includes a physical and chemical evaluation, **specific gravity**, and a microscopic examination (see Chapter 43). If an infection is suspected, the physician may also order a urine culture.

The patient may produce the urine specimen by performing a clean-catch midstream procedure after receiving instructions from you on the proper procedure for collecting the specimen. In some cases, the physician may order a urine specimen obtained by **catheterization**, introduction of a sterile flexible tube into the urinary bladder (FIG. 37-3).

FIGURE 37–3.   Types of catheters. *From the top:* No. 24 indwelling catheter, No. 16 indwelling catheter, No. 16 straight catheter, coudé catheter, self-contained catheterization specimen collection unit.

FIGURE 37–4.   Sterile water is inserted into the indicated lumen to inflate the balloon of the indwelling catheter. When the balloon is inflated, the catheter will remain within the bladder.

In the medical office a straight catheter is used for catheterization and removed once the urine specimen is obtained. Some patients have an indwelling catheter inserted at another facility, such as a hospital. Indwelling catheters are similar to straight catheters, but these types are kept in place by a balloon on the end of the catheter inflated after placement in the bladder (FIG. 37-4). Indwelling catheters are not usually inserted in the medical office.

Catheters are sized 8 to 10 fr for children and 14 to 20 fr for adults. Procedures 37-1 and 37-2 describe the procedure for performing a catheterization in females and males, respectively, in the medical office, and Box 37-3 explains some principles of urinary catheterization.

Blood Tests

Serum levels of uric acid, **blood urea nitrogen** (**BUN**), or creatinine may be indicated for diagnosis of some disease processes of the urinary system. It will likely be your responsibility to draw the patient's blood and process it on site or direct it to the proper testing facility (see **Chapter 44**).

Cystoscopy, or Cystourethroscopy

Cystoscopy is direct visualization of the bladder and urethra with a lighted instrument called a cystoscope (FIG. 37-5). Cystoscopy allows the physician to diagnose many disorders of the lower urinary tract, such as tumors and inflammation. You may be responsible for providing preoperative instructions to the patient as directed by the physician. This procedure is usually done under local anesthesia and may be performed in the urologist's office, but some physicians prefer to have the patient receive a general anesthetic and outpatient hospitalization.

Box 37-3

PRINCIPLES OF CATHETERIZATION

Catheterization is usually a last resort for obtaining a urine specimen. Even under the most aseptic conditions, there is a risk of introducing infection into the urinary system. However, some patients require catheterization when there is no other alternative. For example, catheterization is required in these circumstances:

- It is impossible to obtain a clean-catch midstream specimen for urinalysis.
- The residual urine, or urine left in the bladder after urination, must be measured.
- Medication must be instilled into the bladder to treat an infection.
- The patient has urinary retention or cannot urinate.

Urinary catheter types and sizes vary. They are made of plastic or rubber. If the patient has prostatic hypertrophy, the physician may order a coude catheter, which is slightly curved and a bit stiffer than the other types, so that it is easier to advance it beyond the obstructing enlarged prostate gland.

Checkpoint Question

5. What is the most common test for disorders of the urinary system in the medical office?

Intravenous Pyelogram and Retrograde Pyelogram

An intravenous pyelogram (IVP) is radiographic examination of the kidneys and urinary tract using a radiopaque dye injected into the circulatory system. This dye is filtered by the kidneys to serve as a contrast medium and enhance visualization of the renal structures. Although this procedure is not done in the medical office, you will schedule the examination at the appropriate facility and give the patient instructions to be followed before the procedure. Specifically, the patient is required to cleanse the bowels with a laxative the night before the test and to have an enema the morning of the procedure, since feces may prevent adequate visualization of the kidneys. In addition, the patient is asked not to eat or drink anything for at least 8 hours before the dye is injected, to increase the blood concentration and visibility of the dye.

Question the patient carefully about possible iodine allergy, including allergic reactions to seafood, particularly shellfish. Encourage the patient to increase fluid intake after the test to flush out the dye and counteract any dehydration caused by the preliminary cleansing.

A retrograde pyelogram is similar to the IVP except that the dye is not injected intravenously but is introduced through a catheter in the ureters through a cystoscope. This test is commonly used when IVP is contraindicated because of poor kidney function. Like IVP, this test is not performed in the medical office, but you may be responsible for making arrangements with the appropriate facility and giving the patient any necessary instructions.

Checkpoint Question

6. How does a retrograde pyelogram differ from an intravenous pyelogram?

Ultrasound

Ultrasound is noninvasive use of sound waves to show stones and obstructions in the urinary system and tissues. No special preparation is required other than an explanation of the procedure to the patient. If ordered by the physician, you may be responsible for scheduling this procedure with the appropriate facility.

Rectal and Scrotal Examinations

For the male patient seen in the physician's or urologist's office, you will assist with examination of the reproductive organs by instructing the patient to disrobe from the waist down and providing him with appropriate draping. The physician will inspect and palpate the scrotum for lumps and inguinal hernia. Using a gloved hand and water-soluble lubricant, the physician will perform a digital rectal examination, inserting the index finger into the rectum and palpating the prostate for size, shape, and consistency.

At home, male patients should perform the testicular self-examination, since this is the best method for early detection of

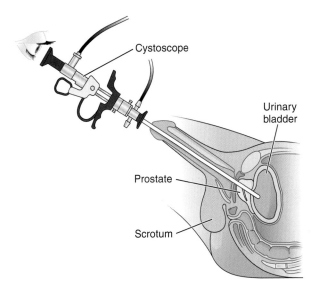

FIGURE 37-5. The interior of the urinary bladder as seen through a cystoscope. (Modified with permission from Cohen BJ. Medical Terminology: An Illustrated Guide. Philadelphia: Lippincott Williams & Wilkins, 2003.)

Spanish Terminology

Orina sin querer?	Do you pass water involuntarily?
Es necesario una muestra de su orina.	Need a urine specimen.
Sera incomodo.	It will be uncomfortable.

testicular cancer. The American Cancer Society recommends that all men perform this examination frequently, possibly weekly, and you are responsible for teaching the patient about this disease and the self-examination. You should explain that the best time for the self-examination is following a warm shower or bath, when the scrotal sac is relaxed (Procedure 37-3). If lumps or thickened areas are palpated during the examination, instruct the patient to notify the physician immediately.

Vasectomy

A popular form of reproductive control is the vasectomy, or surgical removal of all or a segment of the vas deferens to prevent the passage of sperm from the testes. This procedure is frequently performed in the medical office, and you will assist by instructing the patient on preoperative orders as indicated by the physician. Some physicians order light preoperative sedation and may require that the patient have nothing by mouth after midnight on the day of the procedure. On the day of the procedure, you should assist the physician by providing the appropriate surgical tray or instruments and assist the disrobed patient into the lithotomy position with appropriate draping materials to provide privacy. The physician will make two small incisions near the scrotal sac, pull each vas deferens (from the right and left testes) through the incision, clamp each vas deferens proximally and distally, and surgically cut and remove a segment of each. The remaining vas deferens ducts are placed back in the scrotal sac after the clamps are removed and the site is sutured.

Ejaculation and sexual function are not affected by this procedure. The volume of sperm in the ejaculate is so small that its absence is not noticeable. The sperm produced by the testes after this procedure are absorbed in the testes. Since sterility may not be immediate, the patient should be advised to use another form of birth control, such as a condom, until sperm counts confirm that the ejaculate is free of sperm. You should advise the patient to return to the office for periodic sperm counts until no sperm are found in the ejaculate.

Procedure 37-1

Female Urinary Catheterization

Purpose:	Using sterile aseptic technique, perform a straight catheterization on a female torso model.
Equipment:	Straight catheterization tray with 14- or 16-fr catheter, sterile tray, sterile gloves, antiseptic, specimen cup with lid, lubricant, sterile drape, examination light, anatomically correct female torso model, biohazard container
Standard:	This procedure should take 15 minutes.

Steps	Reason
1. Wash your hands.	Handwashing aids infection control.
2. Identify the patient, explain the procedure, and have the patient disrobe completely from the waist down; provide a gown and adequate draping.	Identifying the patient helps prevent errors in treatment. The privacy of the patient should be maintained at all times.
3. Place the patient in the dorsal recumbent or lithotomy position, draping carefully to prevent unnecessary exposure. Carefully open the tray and place it between the patient's legs. Shine the examination light on the perineum.	The dorsal recumbent or lithotomy position allows the best view of the perineum and urinary meatus. Placing the tray between the legs of the patient allows easy access to the catheter and supplies. Adequate lighting is essential.

(continues)

Procedure 37-1 *(continued)*

Female Urinary Catheterization

Steps	Reason
4. Remove the sterile glove package and put on the sterile gloves without contaminating them.	
5. Carefully remove the sterile drape and place it under the buttocks of the patient without contaminating your gloves.	If the sterile drape is item on top of the tray, it may be carefully lifted out of the tray by the edge with the clean hands and carefully placed under the buttocks. This drape is a barrier to protect the examination table from spills.
6. Open the antiseptic swabs and place them upright inside the catheter tray. Open the lubricant and squeeze a generous amount onto the tip of the catheter while it lies in the catheter tray.	The antiseptic swabs should be opened before beginning the actual catheterization. Placing the package upright prevents the antiseptic from spilling. Lubricant applied to the catheter allows for easier insertion.
7. Remove the sterile urine specimen cup and lid and place them to the side of the tray without contaminating your gloves.	Urinary catheterization is a sterile procedure.
8. Using your nondominant hand, carefully expose the urinary meatus by spreading the labia. This hand is now contaminated and must not be moved out of position until the catheter is in the bladder.	
9. Using your sterile dominant hand, pick up the catheter and carefully insert the lubricated tip into the urinary meatus approximately 3 inches. The other end of the catheter should be left in the tray, which will collect the urine that drains from the bladder.	The adult female urethra is approximately 2 to 3 inches long. Once urine begins flowing into the catheter tray, the catheter is in far enough.
10. Once the urine begins to flow into the catheter tray, hold the catheter in position with your nondominant hand by releasing the labia and moving your fingers down onto the catheter. Use your dominant hand to direct the flow of urine into the specimen cup if a specimen is needed.	
11. When the urine flow has slowed or stopped OR 1000 mL has been obtained, carefully remove the catheter by pulling it straight out.	No more than 1000 mL of urine should be removed from the bladder, since doing so may cause painful spasms of the bladder. Most patients do not have 1000 mL.
12. Wipe the perineum carefully with the drape that was under the buttocks. Dispose of the urine appropriately and discard the catheter, tray, and supplies in a biohazard container.	Once the catheter is removed, it is not necessary to keep your dominant hand sterile.
13. If a urine specimen was obtained, properly label the specimen container and complete the laboratory requisition. Process the specimen according to the guidelines of the laboratory.	

(continues)

Procedure 37-1 (continued)

Female Urinary Catheterization

Steps	Reason
14. Remove your gloves and wash your hands.	Standard precautions must be followed throughout the procedure.
15. Instruct the patient to dress and give any follow-up information regarding test results as necessary.	
16. Document the procedure in the patient's medical record.	Procedures are considered not to have been done if they are not recorded.

Charting Example

02/14/2005 9:15 A.M. Catheterization with a 14-fr straight cath, 300 mL dark amber urine obtained, specimen to Acme lab for C & S. _____ S. Strobb, CMA

Procedure 37-2

Male Urinary Catheterization

Purpose: Using sterile aseptic technique, perform a straight catheterization on a male torso model.

Equipment: Straight catheterization tray with 14- or 16-fr catheter, sterile tray, sterile gloves, antiseptic, specimen cup with lid, lubricant, sterile drape, examination light, anatomically correct male torso model, biohazard container.

Standard: This procedure should take 15 minutes.

Steps	Reason
1. Wash your hands.	Handwashing aids infection control.
2. Identify the patient, explain the procedure, and have the patient disrobe completely from the waist down while providing a gown and adequate draping.	Identifying the patient helps prevent errors in treatment. The privacy of the patient should be maintained at all times.
3. Place the patient supine, draping carefully to prevent unnecessary exposure. Carefully open the tray and place it to the side of the patient on the examination table or on top of the patient's thighs.	The male urinary meatus is on the glans penis. Placing the tray on top of the patient's legs allows easy access to the catheter and supplies.
4. Remove the sterile glove package and put on the sterile gloves without contaminating them.	
5. Carefully remove the sterile drape and place it under the glans penis.	If the sterile drape is the top item in the tray, it may be carefully lifted out of the tray by the edge with clean hands and placed under the penis. This drape is a barrier to protect the examination table and patient from any spills.

(continues)

Procedure 37-2 *(continued)*

Male Urinary Catheterization

Steps	Reason
6. Open the antiseptic swabs and place them upright inside the catheter tray. Open the lubricant and squeeze a generous amount onto the tip of the catheter as it lies in the bottom of the catheter tray.	The antiseptic swabs should be opened before beginning the catheterization. Placing the package upright helps prevent the antiseptic from spilling. Lubricant on the catheter allows for easier insertion.
7. Remove the sterile urine specimen cup and lid and place them to the side of the tray without contaminating your gloves.	Urinary catheterization is a sterile procedure.
8. Using your nondominant hand, carefully pick up the penis, exposing the urinary meatus. This hand is now contaminated and must not be moved out of position until the catheter is inserted into the urinary bladder.	
9. Using your sterile dominant hand, pick up the catheter and carefully insert the lubricated tip into the urinary meatus approximately 4 to 6 inches. The other end of the catheter should be left in the tray, which will collect the urine that drains from the bladder.	The adult male urethra is approximately 4 to 6 inches long. Once urine begins flowing into the catheter tray, the catheter is in far enough.
10. Once the urine begins to flow, hold the catheter in position with your nondominant hand. Use your dominant hand to direct the flow of urine into the specimen cup if a specimen is needed.	
11. When the urine flow has slowed or stopped OR 1000 mL has been obtained, carefully remove the catheter by pulling it straight out.	No more than 1000 mL of urine should be removed from the bladder, since doing so may cause painful spasms of the bladder.
12. Wipe the glans penis carefully with the drape and dispose of the urine, catheter, tray, and supplies appropriately in a biohazard container.	Once the urinary catheter has been removed, it is not necessary to keep the dominant hand sterile.
13. If a urine specimen was obtained, properly label the container and complete the laboratory requisition. Process the specimen according to the guidelines of the laboratory.	
14. Remove your gloves and wash your hands.	Standard precautions must be followed throughout the procedure.
15. Instruct the patient to dress and give any follow-up information regarding test results as necessary.	
16. Document the procedure in the patient's medical record.	Procedures are considered not to have been done if they are not recorded.

Charting Example

6/17/2005 3:00 P.M. Catheterization with 14-fr straight cath, 600 mL light amber urine obtained, specimen to Acme lab. _____ J. Jones, CMA

Procedure 37-3

Instructing a Male Patient on the Testicular Self-Examination

Purpose: Teach a male patient to perform the testicular self-examination.

Equipment: A patient instruction sheet if available, testicular examination model or pictures.

Standard: This procedure should take 10 minutes.

Steps	Reason
1. Wash your hands.	Handwashing aids infection control.
2. Identify the patient and explain the procedure.	Identifying the patient prevents errors in treatment.
3. Using the testicular model or pictures, explain the procedure, telling the patient to examine each testicle by gently rolling the testicle between the fingers and the thumb with both hands while checking for lumps or thickenings.	Both hands should be used to check each testicle to ensure complete palpation of all areas. Lumps and thickened areas are not normal and should be reported to the physician.

Step 3. Gently roll the testes in a horizontal plane between the thumb and fingers.

Step 3. Follow the same procedure and palpate upward along the testis.

(continues)

Procedure 37-3 *(continued)*

Instructing a Male Patient on the Testicular Self-Examination

Steps	Reason
4. Explain that the epididymis is a structure on top of each testicle and should be palpated to avoid incorrectly identifying it as an abnormal growth or lump.	If the epididymis is not correctly identified, the patient may palpate it during the examination and erroneously believe it is an abnormal growth.

Step 4. Locate the epididymis, a cordlike structure on the top and back of the testicle that stores and transports sperm.

Steps	Reason
5. Instruct the patient to report any abnormal lumps or thickenings to the physician.	
6. Allow the patient to ask questions about the self-examination.	The patient should always be encouraged to ask questions to ensure understanding.
7. Document the procedure in the patient's medical record.	Procedures are considered not to have been done if they are not recorded.

Charting Example

12/13/2005 10:15 A.M. Pt. given verbal and written instructions on the testicular self-examination; verbalized understanding. _____ C. Brook, CMA

CHAPTER SUMMARY

The urinary system performs many vital functions to maintain the internal environment of the body. Female and male patients often come to the medical office for signs and symptoms of the urinary system, especially infection of the urinary bladder and urethra. The urinary system is also evaluated during a complete physical examination even if no symptoms are present, since substances such as glucose, blood, or protein are not normally found in urine and can indicate diseases of other body systems. Because of the structure and function of the male reproductive system, many disorders of the male reproductive system involve the urinary system. If you work in a urology office, you will often encounter many of the disorders described in this chapter. But the medical assistant who works with adults or children in other settings may also have patients with problems of the urinary system, and for this reason you should be familiar with the common diseases, treatment methods, and diagnostic procedures.

Critical Thinking Challenges

1. Differentiate between peritoneal dialysis and hemodialysis. Why are some patients poor risks for peritoneal dialysis? What can you ask the patient to determine whether or not the peritoneal catheter is functioning or infected?
2. Research the newest pharmacological agents used to treat impotence and explain the method of action, usual dosages, and side effects.
3. A male patient in your office has just been diagnosed with a low sperm count, and the physician has recommended that he switch from briefs to boxer shorts. How do you think this will affect his sperm count, and why?

4. Create a patient education brochure explaining the procedure for performing the testicular self-examination.

Answers to Checkpoint Questions

1. Calculi are stoney formations that are most likely to form when the urine is alkaline.
2. In women, the urethra is short, allowing more bacteria to reach the bladder. Also, the urethra is within the labia, which can harbor other microorganisms.
3. The patient with benign prostatic hyperplasia probably has an elevated PSA, since this substance is elevated when the prostate gland is inflamed for any reason.
4. Microorganisms that may cause infections in the male reproductive system include staphylococci, streptococci, *Escherichia coli*, Chlamydia, and *Neisseria gonorrhoeae*.
5. The urinalysis is the test most commonly performed in the medical office to diagnose disorders of the urinary system.
6. With a retrograde pyelogram, dye is introduced through a catheter inserted into the urinary bladder and ureters, not injected intravenously, as with the IVP.

 Websites

Brady Urological Institute, Johns Hopkins Medical Institutions http://urology.jhu.edu/
Urology Channel http://www.urologychannel.com/
National Kidney and Urologic Diseases Information Clearinghouse
    http://kidney.niddk.nih.gov/kudiseases/pubs/impotence
Urology Notes http://www.urologyinstitute.com/html/kidney
Prostate Cancer Research Institute http://www.prostatecancer.org/

38

Obstetrics and Gynecology

CHAPTER OUTLINE

ROLE DELINEATION

ADMINISTRATIVE: ADMINISTRATIVE
PROCEDURES
- Perform basic administrative medical assisting
  functions
- Understand and adhere to managed care policies and
  procedures

CLINICAL: FUNDAMENTAL PRINCIPLES
- Apply principles of aseptic technique and infection
  control

- Comply with quality assurance practices
- Screen and follow up patient test results

CLINICAL: DIAGNOSTIC ORDERS
- Collect and process specimens
- Perform diagnostic tests

CLINICAL: PATIENT CARE
- Adhere to established patient screening procedures
- Obtain patient history and vital signs

- Prepare and maintain examination and treatment areas
- Prepare patient for examinations, procedures, and treatments
- Assist with examinations, procedures, and treatments
- Coordinate patient care information with other health care providers

GENERAL: PROFESSIONALISM

- Display a professional manner and image
- Demonstrate initiative and responsibility
- Work as a member of the health care team
- Prioritize and perform multiple tasks
- Adapt to change
- Treat all patients with compassion and empathy

GENERAL: COMMUNICATION SKILLS

- Recognize and respect cultural diversity
- Adapt communications to individual's ability to understand

- Recognize and respond effectively to verbal, nonverbal, and written communications
- Use medical terminology appropriately
- Serve as a liaison

GENERAL: LEGAL CONCEPTS

- Perform within legal and ethical boundaries
- Prepare and maintain medical records
- Document accurately
- Comply with established risk management and safety procedures

GENERAL: INSTRUCTION

- Instruct individuals according to their needs
- Explain office policies and procedures
- Teach methods of health promotion and disease prevention

CHAPTER COMPETENCIES

LEARNING OBJECTIVES

Upon successfully completing this chapter, you will be able to:

1. Spell and define the key terms.
2. List and describe common gynecological and obstetric disorders.
3. Identify your role in the care of gynecological or obstetric patients.
4. Describe the components of prenatal and postpartum patient care.
5. Explain the diagnostic and therapeutic procedures associated with the female reproductive system.
6. Identify the various methods of contraception.
7. Describe menopause.

PERFORMANCE OBJECTIVES

Upon successfully completing this chapter, you will be able to:

1. Instruct the Patient on the breast self-examination (Procedure 38-1).
2. Assist with the pelvic examination and Pap smear (Procedure 38-2).
3. Assist with colposcopy and cervical biopsy (Procedure 38-3).

KEY TERMS

abortion	dysmenorrhea	laparoscopy	pessary
amenorrhea	dyspareunia	lightening	polymenorrhea
amniocentesis	Goodell's sign	lochia	primigravida
Braxton-Hicks contractions	gravid	menorrhagia	primipara
Chadwick's sign	gravida	menarche	proteinuria
colpocleisis	gravidity	menses	puerperium
colporrhaphy	hirsutism	metrorrhagia	rectocele
colposcopy	human chorionic	multipara	salpingo-oophorectomy
culdocentesis	gonadotropin (HCG)	nulligravida	
curettage	hysterosalpingogram	nullipara	
cystocele	labor	parity	

The female reproductive system is responsible for the development and maintenance of primary and secondary sexual characteristics and for sexual reproduction. Gynecology and obstetrics are the two medical specialties concerned with female sexual and reproductive functions. Gynecology is a specialty of medicine that deals with development and disorders of the female reproductive system, including the internal and external organs. Obstetrics is the branch of medicine that cares for female patients through pregnancy, childbirth, and the postpartum period. The organs of the female internal reproductive system are shown in FIGURE 38-1.

Puberty is the onset of production of cyclical hormones that cause secondary sexual characteristics, including **menses**, or menstruation. The age at which a girl begins menses is **menarche**. The menstrual cycle, which is about 28 days, comprises a series of complex events in the internal organs controlled by hormones secreted by the anterior pituitary gland and the ovaries (FIG. 38-2). Always remind and encourage patients, especially adolescents, to record and track the menstrual cycle, since the regularity of the cycle is often critical to the physician's assessment of the patient's gynecological health. In addition, the first day of the last menstrual period (LMP) is necessary for calculating an approximate due date in the pregnant patient. This chapter discusses some of the common disorders of the female reproductive system and caring for the obstetric patient in the medical office before and after delivery.

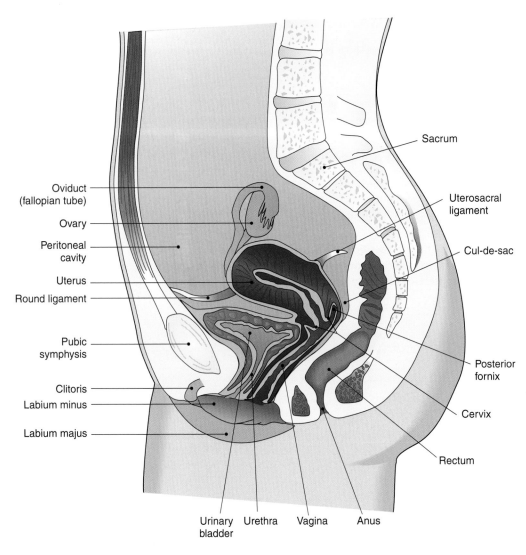

FIGURE 38–1.   Female reproductive system. (Reprinted with permission from Cohen BJ, Wood DL. Memmler's The Human Body in Health and Disease. Philadelphia: Lippincott Williams & Wilkins, 2000.)

FIGURE 38–2. The menstrual cycle. (Reprinted with permission from Cohen BJ, Wood DL. Memmler's The Human Body in Health and Disease. Philadelphia: Lippincott Williams & Wilkins, 2000.)

GYNECOLOGICAL DISORDERS

Dysfunctional Uterine Bleeding

Dysfunctional uterine bleeding is abnormal or irregular uterine bleeding, including heavy, irregular, or light bleeding caused by an endocrine imbalance. Abnormal uterine bleeding includes the following:

- **Menorrhagia**, excessive bleeding during menses
- **Metrorrhagia**, irregular bleeding at times other than menses
- **Polymenorrhea**, abnormally frequent menses
- Postmenopausal bleeding, bleeding after menopause that is not associated with tumor, inflammation, or pregnancy

Diagnosis of dysfunctional uterine bleeding consists of ruling out other causes, such as hormonal imbalance, tumor, or another condition of the endometrial lining of the uterus. Treatment includes hormone therapy and oral contraceptives, or **curettage** (scraping) of the uterine cavity, depending on the cause. Hysterectomy, surgical removal of the uterus, may be the treatment of choice for patients who do

not respond to conservative therapy, who are at increased risk for adenocarcinoma, and who do not desire pregnancy.

Checkpoint Question

1. What is the difference between menorrhagia and metrorrhagia?

Premenstrual Syndrome

Characterized by a wide variety of physical, psychological, and behavioral signs and symptoms, premenstrual syndrome (PMS) occurs on a regular, cyclic basis (Box 38-1). For diagnostic purposes, the patient must have a complex of signs and symptoms associated with PMS that occur during the 7 to 10 days before menses. These signs and symptoms must be severe enough to interfere with interpersonal relationships and routine activities. PMS usually diminishes a few hours after the onset of menses, and the cause is idiopathic (unknown). Diagnosis is based on the physician's assessment of the history and physical examination. Patients should chart their symptoms for several months on a calendar that includes the menstrual cycle.

Box 38-1

SYMPTOMS OF PREMENSTRUAL SYNDROME

The hormonal flux associated with the menstrual cycle affects body systems other than the reproductive system. The cascade of events results in this series of symptoms:

- Hypoglycemia, a drop in blood sugar that results in headaches, nausea, and fatigue, and may explain the food cravings many women have. Increasing carbohydrate intake ensures a steady blood glucose level, which may ease the symptoms.
- Fluid retention in all parts of the body, with edema, weight gain, mastalgia, sinusitis, backache, and headache. Reducing salt intake alleviates some of the edema.
- Sodium and potassium imbalance causing fatigue, irritability, and depression during cyclical fluctuation of these chemotransmitters. Encourage patients to be sure they get enough dietary forms of these minerals.
- Decreased immunity may lead to rhinitis and other upper respiratory infections, acne, and herpes outbreaks.

You can have a dramatic influence on the patient's ability to cope with PMS by providing emotional support, teaching the patient about it, and encouraging regular exercise, which may help minimize it. In addition, certain dietary restrictions, such as eliminating caffeine, salt, and animal fats, can decrease the severity of PMS. Patients also should be encouraged to get adequate rest and avoid unnecessary stress.

Endometriosis

Endometriosis is a condition of unknown cause in which endometrial tissue grows outside the uterine cavity. Endometrial tissue may be found in the fallopian tubes, the ovaries, the uterosacral ligaments, and in rare cases, in other parts of the abdominal cavity. The patient, who is often of reproductive age, complains of infertility, **dysmenorrhea**, pelvic pain, and **dyspareunia**. The patient's symptoms and physical findings may indicate endometriosis, but the diagnosis and the severity must be confirmed by direct visualization, usually by way of a **laparoscopy** (FIG. 38-3).

Treatment of endometriosis may relieve the pelvic pain, but some treatments reduce fertility. The type of therapy depends on the age of the patient, the severity of the symptoms, and the patient's desire for future pregnancy. Hormone and drug therapy to suppress the growth of the tissue and laparo-

scopic excision of the tissue using laser or cautery may be used to treat endometriosis. For patients with severe symptoms, the treatment of choice may be a hysterectomy with possible bilateral **salpingo-oophorectomy**, or surgical removal of the fallopian tubes and ovaries.

Checkpoint Question

2. What are some symptoms of endometriosis?

Uterine Prolapse and Displacement

Prolapse of the uterus is an abnormal condition in which the uterus droops or protrudes down into the vagina. Often, the condition is accompanied by **cystocele**, **rectocele**, or both. Cystocele is herniation of the urinary bladder into the vagina, and rectocele is herniation of the rectum into the vagina. The degree of prolapse is usually described as mild, moderate, or severe, or grade I, II, or III. A commonly used method classifies the prolapse in degrees:

- First-degree prolapse occurs when the uterus has descended to the level of the vaginal orifice.
- Second-degree prolapse occurs when the uterine cervix protrudes through the vaginal orifice.

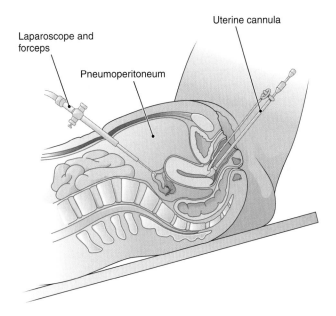

FIGURE 38–3. Laparoscopy. The laparoscope is inserted through a small incision in the abdomen. A forceps is inserted through the scope to grasp the fallopian tube. To improve the view, a uterine cannula is inserted into the vagina to push the uterus upward. Insufflation of gas creates an air pocket, and the pelvis is raised, which forces the intestines higher into the abdomen. (Reprinted with permission from Cohen BJ. Medical Terminology: An Illustrated Guide. Philadelphia: Lippincott Williams & Wilkins, 2003.)

- Third-degree prolapse occurs when the entire cervix and uterus protrude beyond the vaginal orifice.

Diagnosis of uterine prolapse is made during a pelvic examination, at which time the degree of prolapse can be determined. While many women do not have symptoms, others complain of pelvic pressure, dyspareunia, urinary problems, or constipation. Surgical treatment may include vaginal hysterectomy, **colporrhaphy** (suture of the vagina), or **colpocleisis** (surgery to occlude the vagina). Medical management for patients who are elderly or a poor risk for surgery includes hormone therapy to strengthen the muscular floor of the pelvis and the use of a **pessary**. A pessary is a device that is inserted into the vagina and fits around the cervix to support the uterus. You should instruct the patient on the proper procedure for caring for the device by removing it according to the physician's orders and washing it with soap and warm water before reinserting it into the vagina.

The uterus is normally tilted slightly forward over the bladder with the cervix at a right angle to the direction of the vagina. The uterus is movable, and stress on the supporting ligaments occasionally tilts it from its natural position. This is called uterine displacement (FIG. 38-4). The symptoms of uterine displacement may include pressure in the rectal area or against the bladder and are not usually severe, just troublesome to the patient. Treatment follows the same protocol as required for uterine prolapse. In some instances, the uterus may simply be stitched back into its original position in a hysteropexy.

Leiomyomas

Leiomyomas are benign tumors of the uterus, including fibroid tumors, myomas, and fibromyomas. These tumors may be in any of the uterine tissue layers— endometrium, myometrium, or perimetrium—and they vary greatly in size. Most patients are asymptomatic, but large tumors tend to distort the uterus and are relatively likely to be symptomatic. Symptoms may include abnormal bleeding, pelvic pressure and discomfort, constipation, urinary frequency, and infertility.

A presumptive diagnosis is based on the patient's symptoms and physician's assessment, which initially includes bimanual examination and sounding of the uterus. Sounding of the uterus requires the physician to do a pelvic examination and insert a uterine sound (a long slender instrument) into the uterine cavity. Obstruction or resistance may be due to the tumor pressing into the uterine cavity. Treatment of leiomyoma depends on the size of the tumor or tumors. Small asymptomatic tumors are monitored to detect excessive growth. Depending on the patient's age and desire for pregnancy, myomectomy or hysterectomy may be indicated.

Checkpoint Question

3. How are uterine prolapse and uterine displacement different?

Ovarian Cysts

Numerous types of ovarian cysts, including functional cysts and polycystic ovaries, are benign. Functional ovarian cysts, which are fairly common, include the follicular cyst. This is a fluid-filled sac that causes few if any problems. The patient is most often asymptomatic unless the cyst is large or ruptures. Functional cysts are usually detected during surgery, and treatment is simply puncture or excision.

A　　　　　　　　　**B**　　　　　　　　　**C**

FIGURE 38–4. Retrodisplacements of the uterus. (A) The normal position of the uterus as detected on palpation. (B) In retroversion the uterus turns posteriorly as a whole. (C) In retroflexion the fundus bends posteriorly above the cervical end.

In contrast, polycystic ovary syndrome (Stein-Leventhal syndrome) is a more troublesome and complex disorder. It affects both ovaries and is most often found in adolescent girls and young women, who have numerous symptoms of an endocrine imbalance. The signs include anovulation, irregular menses or **amenorrhea** (no menses), and **hirsutism**, an abnormal or excessive growth of hair. Diagnosis is based on pelvic examination, ultrasonography, laparoscopy, or exploratory laparotomy. Treatment is difficult and depends on the signs and symptoms and the patient's desire for future pregnancy. Management of this disorder includes hormone therapy or oral contraceptives.

Gynecological Cancers

The malignant tumors affecting the female reproductive system and their characteristics, diagnosis, and treatment are outlined in TABLE 38-1. For patient education, you should know the American Cancer Society's recommendations regarding the frequency of pelvic and breast examinations and Pap smears. You should obtain current brochures and literature on various types of cancers from the American Cancer Society and have them readily available to patients.

Cervical and breast cancers have an excellent prognosis when detected and treated early, but left untreated or diagnosed in later stages, these cancers are deadly. Instruct and encourage all female patients to perform a breast self-examination every month (Procedure 38-1). Patients should also be encouraged to have a complete physical that includes a breast examination by the physician and a pelvic examination and Papanicolaou (Pap) test, a screening test for early detection of cancer of the cervix, as indicated by the American College of Obstetricians and Gynecologists (ACOG). Specifically, since August 2003, ACOG recommends that the first Pap test and pelvic be performed about 3 years after the first sexual intercourse or by age 21, whichever comes first, and annually until age 30 years. Women over age 30 who have had three negative Pap tests can be screened every 2 to 3 years or annually if desired.

Initially, the abnormal growth of cancerous cells in the cervix is asymptomatic, which further necessitates early detection during the physical examination and Pap smear. The Pap test is a grading of any abnormal tissue scraped from the cervix using a classification system such as the one described in TABLE 38-2. Some laboratories use another system, the Bethesda system, to provide a more descriptive narrative of the abnormal cells. Atypical (abnormal) cells seen may also be described as ASCUS (*a*typical *s*quamous *c*ells of *u*ndetermined *s*ignificance). Regardless of the method used by the laboratory to classify the Pap test results, not all abnormal results indicate cancer. However, since this is a deadly disease, it must be ruled out using further diagnostic studies such as **colposcopy**, a magnified examination of the cervical tissue with a special instrument called a colposcope. Other reasons for an abnormal Pap result include inflammation of the cervix and some sexually transmitted diseases such as human papilloma virus (HPV) infection.

Table 38-1   CANCERS OF THE FEMALE REPRODUCTIVE SYSTEM

Cancer	Warning Signs	Risk Factors	Early Detection	Treatment
Breast	Breast changes: lumps, pain, thickening, swelling, retraction, dimpling	Over age 40, history of breast cancer, early menarche, nulliparity, first birth at late age	Monthly self-examination, mammogram by age 40, q 2 years 40–49, q year after 50	Lumpectomy, mastectomy, radiation, chemotherapy
Cervical	Often asymptomatic; irregular bleeding, abnormal vaginal discharge	Intercourse at early age, multiple sex partners, cigarette smoking, history of STDs such as HPV	Annual Pap smear	Cryotherapy, electrocoagulation, local excision, surgery, radiation, chemotherapy
Endometrial	Irregular bleeding outside of menses, unusual vaginal discharge, excessive bleeding during menses, postmenopausal bleeding	Obesity, early menarche, multiple sex partners, late menopause, history of infertility, family history	Endometrial biopsy at menopause for high-risk women	Progesterone therapy, surgery, radiation, chemotherapy
Ovarian	Often asymptomatic; abdominal enlargement, vague digestive disorders, discomfort, gas distention	Risk increases with age (especially after 60), nulliparity, history of breast cancer	Periodic complete pelvic examination	Surgery, radiation, chemotherapy

Table 38–2	CLASSIFICATIONS OF PAPANICOLAOU TESTS

Class	Characteristics
I	Normal test, no atypical cells
II	Atypical cells but no evidence of malignancy
III	Atypical cells possible but not conclusive for malignancy
IV	Cells strongly suggest malignancy
V	Strong evidence of malignancy

Infertility

Female infertility is more difficult to diagnose than male infertility. Most testing begins by eliminating the male as the infertile party, then focuses on the female partner. Testing is usually not started until after 1 year of unprotected intercourse without conception.

The causes of infertility may include uterine or cervical abnormalities, tubal occlusion or scarring, a hormonal imbalance, or psychological factors. Diagnosis requires a complete history and physical examination. An endometrial biopsy may diagnose anovulation; progesterone blood levels may indicate hormonal deficiencies; or hysterosalpingography may indicate tubal occlusion or uterine abnormalities. Treatment necessitates identifying and correcting the problem. Procedures such as in vitro fertilization may also be recommended, again depending upon the nature of the problem.

Checkpoint Question

4. What two factors greatly affect the prognosis of all cancers?

Sexually Transmitted Diseases

Many of the diseases transmitted through sexual contact have serious consequences. The most deadly of these is acquired immunodeficiency syndrome (AIDS), although other sexually transmitted diseases (STDs) also continue to be a problem. Since STDs are easily transmitted, all STDs must be reported to the local health department by the medical office. This may be your responsibility, or the physician may be required to report the disease according to local policy or the policy of the medical office. In some areas, you may have to file a form or written report; others have a phone reporting system. You need to be familiar with your office policy and procedure manual regarding this requirement and the local laws on reporting. The patient should be encouraged to notify sexual partners so that they may also receive treatment for the appropriate STD.

AIDS

AIDS is an infectious disease that overwhelms the body's immune system. The pathogen that causes AIDS is the human immunodeficiency virus (HIV), which destroys T-helper cells, lowering the body's ability to fight infection. Transmission of HIV most often occurs through an exchange of blood or body fluids, including a sexual act with an HIV-positive partner. A person who is HIV positive may go through the following stages as the infection progresses to AIDS:

1. Acute infectious state with generally mild flulike symptoms.
2. Latent period without symptoms but still infectious.
3. Weight loss, lymphadenopathy, fever, diarrhea, anorexia, fatigue, and skin rashes.
4. Onset of immunodeficiency disorders, such as Kaposi's sarcoma and *Pneumocystis carinii* pneumonia.

Although new treatments prolong the HIV-positive individual's life, there is no cure. Research to find more effective treatments and a possible cure is ongoing.

Chlamydia

Chlamydia infections cause urethritis in men, cervicitis in women, and lymphogranuloma venereum in both, all caused by the organism *Chlamydia trachomatis*. Chlamydia is the

PATIENT EDUCATION

AIDS Prevention

When providing instructions about AIDS prevention, explain to your patient that it is safest, of course, to abstain from sex. Encourage your patients to have sex only with a partner who is known not to be infected, who has sex with no one but the patient, and who does not use needles or syringes. Also, tell the patient to use a latex condom and a spermicide if it is not known whether the sexual partner is infected. Generally, instruct patients thus:

- Avoid contact with another person's blood, body fluids, semen, and vaginal secretions.
- Avoid sharing needles, syringes, and any objects that come into contact with blood or body fluids.
- Avoid using alcohol and drugs. Use of these substances can hinder clear thinking and lead to unwise decision making.

ñ Spanish Terminology

¿Cuando fue el primer día de su ultimo periodo menstrual?	When was the first day of your last menstrual period?
¿Usa usted un dispositivo anticonceptivo?	Do you use a contraceptive device?
¿Cuando se le hizo la ultima mamografía?	When was your last mammogram?
¿Ha tenido usted la menopausia?	Have you gone through menopause?

most common STD in the United States. Female patients may be asymptomatic or may have vague flulike symptoms that are difficult to diagnose without specific reason to suspect infection. In severe cases, there may be extensive lymph gland involvement known as lymphogranuloma venereum. Chlamydia is one of the leading causes of pelvic inflammatory disease, causing tubal scarring and eventual infertility in women. Infants born to mothers with chlamydial infections may have conjunctivitis and pneumonia. The fetus may spontaneously abort, deliver prematurely, or be stillborn.

Diagnosis is made by a swab culture of the site sent to the laboratory for identification of the microorganism. The disease is treated with an antibiotic such as doxycycline, tetracycline, or sulfamethoxazole until the patient tests negative for the presence of the pathogen.

Condylomata Acuminata

Condylomata acuminata is a viral infection of the genital area causing the growth of soft, papillary warts that appear in a wide variety of places, including the vulva, vagina, cervix, and perineum. The cause is HPV. The genital warts usually appear about 3 months after exposure. Biopsy of the condyloma is appropriate to rule out the slight possibility of a malignancy. Although HPV is difficult to eradicate, cryotherapy (freezing the involved area) or laser ablation (burning with laser) has moderate success. Genital warts have been implicated as a risk for cervical cancer.

Gonorrhea

Gonorrhea is the second most common STD. It is caused by a gram-negative diplococcus, *Neisseria gonorrhoeae*. The symptoms appear in the genitalia 2 to 8 days after exposure. In some female patients, the Bartholin and Skene glands fill with pus, and the infection may spread to the cervix. However, female patients may be asymptomatic and unaware of the disease. The disease may lead to salpingitis with scarring and adhesions or pelvic inflammatory disease. Infants born to mothers infected with gonorrhea may develop purulent conjunctivitis with corneal ulcerations that result in blindness. All infants are now treated prophylactically in the newborn nursery.

Diagnosis is based on the symptoms and through a culture of the drainage if present. Once diagnosed, gonorrhea may be treated with penicillin, although penicillin-resistant strains are now appearing.

Syphilis

After AIDS, syphilis is the most serious STD. It is caused by a spirochete, *Treponema pallidum*. The first sign is a chancre or ulcerated lesion at the primary site of infection on the genitalia. This chancre appears several days to several weeks after infection, heals very quickly, and may not be noticed. Although the chancre heals quickly, the spirochete spreads quickly through the bloodstream and becomes systemic, with far-reaching consequences. The second phase is identified by a rash that may appear anywhere on the body. The patient continues to be infectious at this stage, but treatment with penicillin will stop the progression of the disease to the next, or tertiary, phase. If left untreated, the rash will disappear and the syphilis may lie dormant for years. At some point, however, the patient will experience cardiovascular damage, central nervous system involvement, and death.

Infants born with syphilis caused by transplacental infection are commonly mentally retarded, deaf, blind, or deformed. Many babies spontaneously abort or are delivered stillborn.

Herpes Genitalis

Herpes genitalis is caused by the herpes simplex virus 2 (HSV2), is characterized by painful vesicular lesions in the vaginal, vulvar, or anorectal area, and has no cure. This genital infection usually appears within 3 to 7 days after exposure. The infected patient may present with painful vesicles in the genital region that rupture and leave equally painful ulcers that eventually heal in about 10 days. In addition, the patient may have swollen and tender lymph nodes and flulike symptoms. After the lesion heals, the patient may be in remission for years, or the symptoms may recur with each stressful situation. Patients with herpes genitalis should be advised to avoid sexual contact during episodes of vesiculation because the exudate is highly contagious. Although there is no cure, the condition is somewhat controlled with an antiviral agent such as acyclovir.

Infants born vaginally to mothers with active lesions may develop the disease within a few weeks of birth. The virus spreads rapidly to the organs of the infant, and up to 90% of infected infants die.

Box 38-2

INFECTIOUS AGENTS IN VULVOVAGINITIS

- *Trichomonas vaginalis*: Known as trich, this protozoan causes an STD. The signs are a thin, frothy, greenish or gray vaginal discharge with an odor. Signs and symptoms include dysuria with urinary frequency and intense pruritus. Treatment is oral metronidazole for both partners.
- *Candida albicans*: Also known as monilia, this fungus grows best in the presence of glucose. The signs include a thick, curdlike discharge with white patches on the vaginal walls, usually with no odor. Intense itching is usual. The pathogen is found in the intestines and is most likely to affect the patient during the secretory phase of the menstrual cycle. It is very common during pregnancy and in patients receiving antibiotic therapy. Treatment requires nystatin vaginal suppositories, which may be purchased without a prescription.
- *Gardnerella vaginitis*: This gram-negative bacillus causes a gray discharge with a foul odor. It is treated with metronidazole.

Vulvovaginitis, Salpingitis, and Pelvic Inflammatory Disease

Although vulvovaginitis, salpingitis, and pelvic inflammatory disease can be caused by infections other than sexually transmitted diseases, these disorders are commonly caused by infections transmitted sexually. Vulvovaginitis is inflammation of the vulva and vagina and is one of the common complaints of female patients. Symptoms often include pruritus, burning of the vulva or the vagina (or both), and increased vaginal discharge. On examination, the vulva and vagina are reddened. The type of discharge often indicates the cause of the disorder (Box 38-2). The causative agent is confirmed by a microscopic examination of a vaginal smear or by culture of the vaginal discharge. Effective treatment depends on the cause.

Salpingitis is a bacterial infection of the fallopian tubes that is most often transmitted by sexual intercourse. Young sexually active women, women with multiple sexual partners, and women with intrauterine devices are at increased risk for salpingitis. Numerous microorganisms may cause salpingitis, but the most common microbes include *N. gonorrhoeae*, *C, trachomatis*, genital mycoplasma, and normal flora bacteria. Salpingitis is sometimes called pelvic inflammatory disease when the surrounding structures, including the pelvic peritoneum, uterus, ovaries, and surrounding tissues are inflamed. Signs and symptoms include varying degrees of abdominal pain and tenderness with or without fever

and leukocytosis, an abnormal increase in the white blood cell count.

Cultures for gonorrhea and tests for Chlamydia are essential for antibiotic therapy. **Culdocentesis** may be necessary to obtain purulent drainage and determine the exact cause of the infection. Laparoscopy may be performed to determine the extent of the infection. Treatment for mild infections includes antibiotic and analgesic therapy, bed rest, and removal of the source of infection. In patients with pyosalpinx (pus in the fallopian tubes), tubal obstruction, abscess, and serious inflammation and edema, treatment may be a hysterectomy with bilateral salpingectomy-oophorectomy or an incision and drainage.

Checkpoint Question

5. Which sexually transmitted disease is associated with a female reproductive cancer?

COMMON DIAGNOSTIC AND THERAPEUTIC PROCEDURES

The Gynecological Examination

As part of the gynecological examination, the physician examines the patient's breasts, performs a pelvic examination, and obtains a Pap smear. Because of the risk of contracting infection from body fluids, especially blood, you and the physician must observe standard precautions, wearing protective barriers such as gloves as appropriate during the examination. When scheduling the appointment, instruct the patient not to douche, use vaginal medication, or have sexual intercourse for 24 hours before the examination. If a Pap smear will be performed, the appointment should be scheduled about 1 week after the end of menses. When the patient arrives for the scheduled appointment, spend time with the patient to establish rapport, especially with new patients and patients with special needs, such as the young, elderly, and disabled. A procedure that is rushed or seems hurried to the patient may diminish the professional image of the office and the patient's attitude toward the physician and staff.

The physician usually begins the examination by examining the breast and surrounding tissue, including the axillae and chest tissue up to the clavicle. This tissue is inspected for dimpling or size disparity and palpated for lumps or thickenings. Next, the physician examines the external and internal female genitalia to identify or diagnose any abnormal conditions (Procedure 38-2). Although the dorsal lithotomy position provides the best visibility for the physician, this position may be difficult for elderly or some disabled persons. Elevating the head of the table to 30° may be easier for the patient while allowing the physician to do a thorough examination. The elevation of the table does not seem to have any disadvantages, and often the patient finds this position more comfortable, but consult with the physician if the lithotomy position is not possible. If elevating the head of the examination table is not appropriate, an alternative position, such as Sim's, may be necessary.

When preparing for the pelvic examination, ensure first that the vaginal speculum is warm and is the correct size for the patient. Warm the speculum by running it under warm water or by storing it on an electric heating pad set on a low setting. Some examination tables are equipped with a special warming drawer for the vaginal specula that heats them automatically as long as the examination table is plugged into an electrical outlet. Selecting an appropriate vaginal speculum is important to maintain the patient's comfort and to facilitate the examination. Although the patient's age and size are the primary factors, the largest speculum that is comfortable for the patient provides the best visibility. Two sizes may be set out to give the physician a choice. Vaginal specula come in pediatric, small, medium, and large sizes, and a variety of sizes should be available in each examination room.

Checkpoint Question

6. What procedures does the physician perform as part of a complete gynecological examination?

WHAT IF

The first Pap smear or gynecological examination for young women may cause great anxiety. What if an 18-year old is to have her first Pap smear today? How should you handle the situation?

Bring the patient into the room and encourage her to talk about her feelings. Do not have her change into an examining gown until she has had an opportunity to speak with the physician or practitioner about the procedure. Some young patients want their mother present; others do not. If the patient's mother is present, ask her to meet her daughter's wishes about remaining in the room. You are more likely to be given an accurate sexual history if the mother is not present. The physician may require the presence of another health care worker, like the medical assistant, during the examination; however, some physicians feel comfortable performing the examination without assistance. If you remain in the room, you will have an opportunity to provide reassurance and information. Male physicians should have a female health care worker in the room during the examination as a legal precaution.

Colposcopy

Colposcopy is visual examination of the vaginal and cervical surfaces using a stereoscopic microscope called a colposcope. It is often performed to evaluate patients with atypical Pap smear results to locate the origin of abnormal cells, to select areas for cervical, endocervical, or endometrial biopsy, to assess cervical lesions, or for follow-up in patients with a history of cervical dysplasia or cervical cancer.

If a biopsy is to be done, be sure that written consent has been obtained. When possible, label specimen containers and complete laboratory request forms before the procedure. Have the completed forms and labeled containers ready in the examination room for use after the specimen is obtained. Although there is usually very little or no bleeding from the biopsy, chemical cautery using silver nitrate or Monsel solution should be available to control bleeding as necessary. The patient preparation for colposcopy with cervical biopsy is similar to that required for the pelvic examination (Procedure 38-3).

Hysterosalpingography

Hysterosalpingography is a diagnostic procedure in which the uterus and uterine tubes are radiographed after injection of a contrast medium. The radiograph is called a **hysterosalpingogram**. This test is often performed to determine the configuration of the uterus and the patency of the fallopian tubes for patients with infertility. Although this test is not usually performed in the physician's office, you may be responsible for scheduling the procedure and explaining to the patient any preparations, where to go, and when.

Dilation and Curettage

Dilation and curettage (D & C) may be performed to remove uterine tissue for diagnostic testing, to remove endometrial tissue, to prevent or treat menorrhagia, or to remove retained products of conception after a spontaneous **abortion** or miscarriage. During the procedure, the cervical canal is widened with a uterine sound and the lining of the uterus is scraped with a curet. This procedure usually requires anesthesia and may be performed as an inpatient or outpatient procedure. The patient must sign a preoperative consent form and you may be asked to give any preoperative instructions as directed by the physician. Preoperative instructions may include advising the patient of the need for a perineal pad, not a tampon, to be worn postoperatively and information regarding the signs of infection, hemorrhage, or other follow-up care according to the specifications of the physician.

OBSTETRIC CARE

Unlike other physicians, obstetricians are frequently called to the hospital to deliver infants during regular office hours. In the absence of the physician, you must use good judgment when pregnant patients come into the office for a scheduled appointment or call with questions and concerns. For instance, you may have to determine whether a situation can wait for the physician's return, another physician should be consulted, the patient should go to the hospital, or with the physician's permission you should advise the patient how to manage the problem. Protocols listed in the policy and procedure manual for actions to be taken in specific situations help ensure that in the physician's absence, safe procedures are followed for your patients and help protect you and your physician from errors in treatment.

Diagnosis of Pregnancy

Many patients suspect that they are **gravid**, or pregnant, because they have signs. However, early signs of pregnancy may indicate other disorders and therefore are considered presumptive until a conclusive diagnostic procedure is done. Presumptive signs include amenorrhea, nausea, vomiting, breast enlargement and tenderness, fatigue, and urinary

Table 38-3	SIGNS AND SYMPTOMS OF PREGNANCY	
Presumptive Signs	**Probable Signs**	**Conclusive Signs**
Cessation of menses	HCG in urine, blood	Fetal heart tones
Nausea and vomiting	Braxton-Hicks contractions	Fetal movement detected by examiner
Breast tenderness	Enlargement of abdomen	Visualization of the fetus
Breast enlargement	Uterine changes	
Patient feels quickening or fetal movement	Goodell's sign	
Fatigue	Chadwick's sign	
Urinary frequency		

frequency. Probable signs include **human chorionic gonadotropin** (**HCG**) in the maternal urine or blood, changes in the uterus and cervix, **Braxton-Hicks** contractions, and enlargement of the uterus (TABLE 38-3). Braxton-Hicks contractions are irregular uterine contractions that occur fairly frequently but do not affect the cervix like the contractions of active labor. These contractions are normal, and although the patient may or may not be aware, the physician can feel the contractions during a bimanual examination or while palpating the abdomen. The diagnosis of pregnancy is confirmed by the physician or the image of a fetus on ultrasonography.

Cervical changes that occur during pregnancy include softening of the cervix, known as **Goodell's sign**; increased vascularity of the cervix and vagina causing a bluish-violet color (**Chadwick's sign**); and formation of a mucous plug. The mucous plug forms in the cervical os (opening) and protects the developing fetus and the amniotic sac from the external environment. With the onset of labor, the mucous plug is expelled with a small amount of blood and is often referred to as the bloody show.

TRIAGE

While you are working in a gynecology medical office, the following three situations arise:

A. Patient A's pharmacist calls about her birth control prescription refill.

B. Patient B, a new patient, is possibly pregnant, and you have an empty examination room.

C. The physician, a woman, would like you to set up for a Pap smear and pelvic examination for patient C.

How do you sort these situations? What do you do first? Second? Third?

First, have another medical assistant take the call from the pharmacist or have the receptionist take a message. This is clearly not an emergency, and if you have to call back, you can do so at a more convenient time. Next you should prepare the setup for the Pap smear and pelvic examination for patient C. Assembling the items to be used during this examination should not require much time, and once the setup is ready, the physician can perform the examination without your assistance. Finally, call patient B to the examination room and take a thorough medical history and vital signs. Since patient B is new, she may require reassurance and answers to her questions and concerns about her possible pregnancy or the office in general.

Checkpoint Question

7. Why are presumptive signs and symptoms of pregnancy not considered to be conclusive?

First Prenatal Visit

A pregnant patient's initial prenatal visit is extensive and critical to the ongoing assessment of the pregnancy. You and the physician obtain a thorough and detailed history of the patient, including information about previous pregnancies and deliveries and general health status (Box 38-3). To elicit complete and accurate information, the health history interview should be conducted in a private room where there will be no interruptions.

Box 38-3

PARITY VERSUS GRAVIDITY

The prenatal history must include information regarding the patient's previous pregnancies to help predict the outcome of this one. The term **parity** refers to the number of live births, and **gravidity** refers to any pregnancy, regardless of its length and outcome. The pregnant, or gravid, woman is a **gravida**, usually with an indicator of the number. A woman who has never been pregnant is a **nulligravida**, while the woman who is pregnant for the first time is a **primigravida**. The number of live births is also given a prefix indicator, such as **nullipara** (has never borne a living child), **primipara** (first living child), and **multipara** (many live births).

These numbers are listed for the physician's review as gr (or simply g), p, pret (preterm or premature), and ab (abortion, spontaneous or induced). For example, a woman who is pregnant for the third time, has lost no pregnancies, and carried her previous pregnancies to term is listed as gr iii, pret 0, ab 0, p ii. (Arabic numbers are also acceptable.)

A woman who is pregnant for the fifth time and who has delivered one set of twins and two single infants, has had no premature infants, and has lost one pregnancy spontaneously would be listed as gr v, pret 0, ab i, p iv.

The first prenatal visit includes confirmation of pregnancy, complete history and physical, determination of the estimated date of delivery, assessment of gestational age, identification of risk factors, and patient education. The estimated date of delivery is a prediction of the due date, assuming the pregnancy progresses normally (Box 38-4). Normal gestation is 37 to 40 weeks. Infants born before the 37th week are considered to be premature. Those born after the 41st week are postmature.

The complete physical examination and laboratory tests include a pelvic examination with Pap smear, pregnancy test, clinical pelvimetry, and laboratory blood tests. You should reinforce the physician's instructions to the patient and encourage patients to call the office if they have further questions or concerns.

Patients should be instructed to notify the physician if any of the following occur:

- Vaginal bleeding or spotting
- Persistent vomiting
- Fever or chills
- Dysuria
- Abdominal or uterine cramping

Box 38-4

DETERMINING THE ESTIMATED DATE OF CONFINEMENT OR EXPECTED DATE OF DELIVERY

The EDC is also called the expected date of delivery (EDD). Because of the negative connotations of the word *confinement* and because women are no longer confined during pregnancy or the postpartum period, terminology for the due date is changing to reflect current maternity trends. Many methods are used for determining this projected date. Nagele's rule requires an arithmetic calculation using the following formula:
=The first day of the last menstrual period (LMP) – 3 months + 7 days + 1 year
Example: LMP = May 3, 2003

LMP =	5	3	2003
	−3	+7	+1
Due date =	2	10	2004

A simpler method is adding 9 months and 7 days to the first day of the LMP. Try that method with the example.

The third common method is to use a gestational wheel. Using the inner wheel, line up the first day of the LMP on the outer wheel with the appropriate arrow and read around the wheel to the indicated milestones in the pregnancy. Many wheels indicate the date of conception and times recommended for blood work and other testing, and all show the date that delivery is expected.

Gestational wheel.

- Leaking amniotic fluid
- Alteration in fetal movement
- Dizziness or blurred vision
- Other problems

In addition, advise the pregnant patient to avoid taking any medications or drugs, even over-the-counter preparations, without consulting the physician. Many factors, including medications, nicotine, and alcohol, can put the developing fetus at risk. Depending on maternal exposure to the substance and the stage of fetal development, development may be so altered as to cause deformities or damage to other internal organs and may threaten the life of the fetus.

The first prenatal examination is done to establish a detailed baseline of the patient's physical condition. This is a complete physical examination with a pelvic examination, screening for *N. gonorrhoeae*, chlamydial infection, cervical cancer, syphilis, and tuberculosis. The first prenatal visit also includes the following:

- Blood work. The Venereal Disease Research Laboratory, rapid plasma reagin, or other test for syphilis; complete blood count with hematocrit, hemoglobin, and white blood cell count with differential; blood type with Rh factor; antibody screen; and other tests as necessary.
- Tuberculosis screening. Tine test or purified protein derivative injection.
- Urinalysis. Glucose, albumin, and acetone testing.

Subsequent Prenatal Visits

If the pregnancy is progressing as expected and without complications (FIG. 38-5), the patient is scheduled for office visits at 12, 16, 20, 24, and 28 weeks of gestation. The patient is usually seen every 2 weeks during the last 2 months and once a week after the 36th week of gestation. This schedule may be altered according to the patient's condition. TABLE 38-4 outlines the specific examination and procedures to be performed during subsequent prenatal visits. The height of the fundus (FIG. 38-6) is also palpated at each visit to assess fetal growth.

Checkpoint Question

8. The pregnant patient should be advised to contact the physician when what problems occur?

Onset of Labor

Labor is the physiological process leading to expelling the fetus from the uterus. About 4 weeks before the onset of labor, **lightening** indicates that the fetus has descended further into the pelvis, and the patient may appear to be carrying the baby lower in the abdomen. The actual onset of labor is characterized by regular uterine contractions that become more intense and more frequent with time. True

LEGAL TIP

Fetal Protection

Many medications that might be considered beneficial to the pregnant female may be dangerous to the developing fetus. It is important, therefore, for the professional medical assistant to carefully question female patients who might be pregnant or who are known to be pregnant about any medications including drugs purchased over-the-counter. This information should be passed along to the physician. The Food and Drug Administration (FDA) has developed a method to classify drugs that are dangerous to the fetus. These categories are listed on package inserts that accompany prescription drugs and in various drug reference books such as the Physician's Desk Reference. The categories and a description of dangerous effects on the fetus are listed as follows:

- Category A - Research indicates that there is probably no risk at any point in the pregnancy
- Category B - Animal research indicates no fetal risk but human studies are not complete
- Category C - Research on animals shows this drug to be a danger. Human studies are inconclusive or no studies are available.
- Category D - There is clear precedence for risk but the drug may be used if there is no substitution
- Category X - There is clear evidence of risk and the drug should not be used by pregnant women

labor is distinguished from false labor by its effect (dilation and effacement) on the cervix and the increased frequency and intensity of contractions. Another indication of true labor is bloody show, the expulsion of the mucous plug from the cervical os. The patient may call to say her water broke, which indicates rupture of the amniotic sac, another indication of impending labor and delivery.

Whatever signs or symptoms of labor occur, you should know how to advise the patient. The physician makes the decision to send the patient to the hospital, to come to the medical office, or to stay home and wait. You relay the information from the patient to the physician. The office's policy and procedure manual should include specific instructions regarding how the physician wants pregnant patients managed if the physician is not immediately available.

The onset of labor should be discussed with the patient so she knows what to expect and how to manage the situation. Always have the patient's medical record available when talking with the patient or the physician. It is critical to the decision-making process to know the patient's estimated

FETAL DEVELOPMENT*

1st Lunar Month (4 weeks)

The embryo is 4 to 5 mm in length.
Trophoblasts embed in decidua.
Chorionic villi form.
Foundations for nervous system,
    genitourinary system, skin,
    bones, and lungs are formed.
Buds of arms and legs begin to form.
Rudiments of eyes, ears, and nose appear.

2nd Lunar Month (8 weeks)

The fetus is 27 to 31 mm in length
    and weighs 2 to 4 g
Fetus is markedly bent.
Head is disproportionately large as
    a result of brain development.
Sex differentation begins.
Centers of bone begin to ossify.

3rd Lunar Month (3 months)

The fetus average length is 6 to 9
    cm, and weight is 45 g.
Fingers and toes are distinct.
Placenta is complete.
Fetal circulation is complete.

4th Lunar Month (4 months)

The fetus is 12 cm in length and
    weighs 110 g.
Sex is differentaited.
Rudimentary kidneys secrete urine.
Heartbeat is present.
Nasal septum and palate close.

5th Lunar Month (5 months)

The fetus is 19 cm in length and
    weighs approximately 300 g.
Lanugo covers entire body.
Fetal movements are felt by mother.
Heart sounds are perceptible by
    auscultation.

6th Lunar Month (6 months)

The fetus is about 23 cm in length
    and weighs 630 g.
Skin appears wrinkled.
Vernix caseosa appears.
Eyebrows and fingernails develop.

7th Lunar Month (7 months)

The fetus is about 27 cm in length
    and weighs about 1100 g.
Skin is red.
Pupillary membrane disappears
    from eyes.
The fetus has an excellent chance
    of survival.

8th Lunar Month (8 months)

The fetus is 28 to 30 cm in length
    and weighs 1.8 kg.
Fetus is viable.
Eyelids open.
Fingerprints are set.
Vigorous fetal movement occurs.

9th Lunar Month (9 months)

The fetus' average length is 32 cm;
    weight is about 2500 g.
Face and body have a loose
    wrinkled appearance because
    of subcutaneous fat deposit.
Lanugo disappears.
Amniotic fluid decreases.

10th Lunar Month

The average fetus is 36 cm in length
    and weighs 3000 to 3600 g.
Skin is smooth.
Eyes are uniformly slate colored.
Bones of skull are ossified and
    nearly together at sutures.

* All length given are crown to rump.

FIGURE 38–5. Fetal development.

Table 38-4	SCHEDULE OF PRENATAL VISITS
Month	**Frequency**
1–6	Monthly
7–8	Every 2 weeks
9	Weekly
Included in visit	**When done**
Weight	Each visit
Blood pressure	Each visit
Fundal height	Each visit
Fetal heart rate	Each visit
Check of edema	Each visit
Pelvic examination	Middle of ninth month, weekly as indicated
Inquiry about symptoms, signs, problems	Each visit
Prenatal education	Each visit
Nutrition and appetite	Each visit
Urinalysis for glucose, albumin	Each visit
Hematocrit, hemoglobin	32–34 weeks (more often for anemia)
Urine culture	Per signs, symptoms
Rh titers	Initially
AFP	15–20 weeks
Blood glucose	24–28 weeks
Ultrasonography	For fetal age, best 8–16 weeks

From Reeder, SJ, Martin LL, Koniak D. Maternity Nursing, 17th ed. Philadelphia: Lippincott Williams & Wilkins, 1992:403.

date of delivery and physical condition. Many patients today are choosing options for delivery other than a standard hospital delivery with the physician present. Options include midwife assistance, a birthing center, water birth, and home delivery. The patient must be informed about the advantages and risks of all of these and together with the physician make a decision that takes into account the well-being of the mother and the newborn.

Postpartum Care

The postpartum period, the **puerperium**, runs from childbirth until involution, when the reproductive structures return to normal. It may take as long as 6 weeks. Once the patient is discharged from the hospital, her care will be managed at the medical office. Hospital reports received in the medical office for the patient's record usually contain certain acronyms and abbreviations related to labor and delivery and the postpartum period. Box 38-5 explains these special terms.

The time for the first postpartum visit depends on the type of delivery and the patient's condition when discharged from the hospital. The needs of postpartum patients today may be greater than in the past because the length of stay in the hospital is typically shorter, with some patients discharged within 24 hours after delivery. Usually the patient is scheduled for the postnatal visit within 4 to 6 weeks of delivery if there were no complications.

At the postpartum visit, the physician performs a complete gynecological and breast examination. Allow plenty of time for counseling the patient regarding her new role as a parent. Many patients have questions and concerns regarding breast-feeding, birth control, menstruation, and parenting. Before the examination, obtain the patient's weight and vital signs and samples for urinalysis and possibly hematocrit and hemoglobin. During the examination, the physician assesses any uterine discharge. **Lochia**, a discharge from the uterus after delivery, progresses through the following stages:

- Lochia rubra. Blood-tinged discharge within 6 days of delivery
- Lochia serosa. Thin, brownish discharge lasting about 3 to 4 days after the lochia rubra
- Lochia alba. White postpartum discharge that has no evidence of blood and may last up to week 6

The amount of lochia should diminish considerably during the puerperium. The patient should be instructed to notify the physician if there is any abnormality of the lochial progression.

FIGURE 38–6. Height of the fundus at corresponding gestational dates varies greatly from patient to patient. Those shown are most common. A convenient rule of thumb is that at 5 months' gestation, the fundus is usually at or slightly above the umbilicus. (Reprinted with permission from Weber J. Health Assessment in Nursing. Philadelphia: Lippincott Williams & Wilkins, 2003.)

Box 38-5

ACRONYMS AND ABBREVIATIONS USED IN LABOR AND DELIVERY AND THE POSTPARTUM PERIOD

Following is a brief list of terms frequently used in the medical record.

AROM	Artificial rupture of membranes
AVD	Assisted vaginal delivery
CPD	Cephalopelvic disproportion
L & D	Labor and delivery
NSVD	Normal spontaneous vaginal delivery
PROM	Premature rupture of membranes
SROM	Spontaneous rupture of membranes
VBAC	Vaginal birth after cesarean

Terms for presentations

LOA	Left occiput anterior
LOP	Left occiput posterior
ROA	Right occiput anterior
ROP	Right occiput posterior

Fetal descriptors

AGA	Appropriate for gestational age
LBW	Low birth weight
LGA	Large for gestational age
SGA	Small for gestational age

Checkpoint Question

9. What is lochia? Name and describe the three types.

OBSTETRIC DISORDERS

Ectopic Pregnancy

Gestation in which a fertilized ovum implants somewhere other than in the uterine cavity is an ectopic pregnancy. Usually an ectopic pregnancy occurs in the fallopian tube, and when it does, it may be called a tubal pregnancy. Other sites of implantation include the abdomen, the ovaries, and the cervical os. The patient may have signs of early pregnancy, including breast enlargement or tenderness, nausea, and absent or delayed menses. Pelvic pain, syncope, abdominal symptoms, painful sexual intercourse, and irregular menstrual bleeding begin fairly early in the pregnancy. If an ectopic pregnancy is not diagnosed early, there is the potential for rupture of the fallopian tube, which causes hemorrhage into the abdominal cavity and the possibility of shock and death. Diagnostic procedures include urine or serum human chorionic gonadotropin pregnancy test, ultrasound to determine the location of the pregnancy, laparoscopy to visualize the enlarged tube, and perhaps culdocentesis to confirm abdominal bleeding. Treatment is surgical excision of the ectopic pregnancy through either a laparoscopy or laparotomy.

Hyperemesis Gravidarum

Nausea and vomiting, commonly called morning sickness, are expected during early pregnancy and usually can be treated with small frequent meals, adequate hydration, and reassurance. However, if the vomiting becomes unrelenting and leads to dehydration, electrolyte imbalance, and weight loss, the diagnosis is hyperemesis gravidarum. Occasionally the patient must be hospitalized. At early prenatal visits you may have to discern between morning sickness and the more serious hyperemesis gravidarum by obtaining a complete description of the nausea and vomiting. Of course, the physician makes the diagnosis and orders appropriate treatment, including antiemetics or intravenous fluids if necessary.

Abortion

One of the common disorders of pregnancy is first-trimester spontaneous abortion, also called an early pregnancy loss or miscarriage. With early diagnosis of pregnancy, it is now known that the spontaneous abortion occurs more often than previously thought. An induced abortion is intentional, while a spontaneous abortion occurs because of fetal or maternal conditions without any outside interference in the pregnancy.

A spontaneous abortion is defined as the loss of pregnancy before the fetus is viable. You need to be familiar with the early signs and symptoms of an impending spontaneous abortion to advise a patient who calls until the physician can be contacted. The first symptom is usually vaginal bleeding, followed by uterine cramps and low back pain. Without telling the patient that she may be in danger of spontaneously aborting her pregnancy (this is diagnosing), you may instruct the patient to come to the medical office, go to the emergency room, or remain at home on bed rest until the physician returns the call, depending on the office policy and procedure.

Preeclampsia and Eclampsia

Hypertension that is directly related to the pregnancy is termed pregnancy-induced hypertension (PIH). The two types of PIH are preeclampsia and eclampsia. Preeclampsia is characterized by **proteinuria**, edema of the lower extremities, and hypertension after the 20th week of gestation. As the condition progresses, the patient may complain of blurred vision, headaches, edema, and vomiting. Medical management includes restricted activities, increased bed rest, sexual abstinence, antihypertensive therapy, and well-balanced meals with an increase in protein and a decrease in sodium. Close monitoring of the patient is important, and it requires scheduling the patient for more frequent office visits. The risk of developing eclampsia increases as the pregnancy advances.

Eclampsia is almost always preceded by preeclampsia but has a sudden onset. In eclampsia, the clinical signs of preeclampsia are still present but become more extreme. Eclampsia is always characterized by seizures that may be followed by coma, hypertensive crisis, and shock. The progression of preeclampsia to eclampsia constitutes a medical emergency. Management of eclampsia includes stabilizing the patient and may require induced delivery of the baby, regardless of gestational age.

Placenta Previa and Abruptio Placentae

Placenta previa is a condition in which the placenta is implanted either partially or completely over the internal cervical os, making delivery of the fetus before the placenta difficult. During the second or third trimester of pregnancy, the patient may have painless vaginal bleeding, which may be minimal, such as spotting, or profuse. Placenta previa is easily diagnosed by prenatal ultrasound. Medical management includes bed rest and drug therapy if the patient is preterm. If the patient is near term and if the bleeding is severe and poses a danger to the mother or fetus, then delivery of the baby is essential, usually by cesarean (Box 38-6).

The premature separation or detachment of the placenta from the uterus is abruptio placentae. Depending on the severity of the separation, symptoms include pain, uterine tenderness, bleeding, signs of impending shock, and fetal distress or death. If abruptio placentae is confirmed, the baby is usually delivered by cesarean section.

Checkpoint Question

10. What is placenta previa, and how is it managed in a preterm patient?

COMMON OBSTETRIC TESTS AND PROCEDURES

Pregnancy Test

Many over-the-counter pregnancy tests check for HCG in the urine. Chapter 43 has more information about urine pregnancy tests.

Alpha Fetoprotein

Levels of alpha fetoprotein (AFP) are obtained from maternal serum to screen the fetus for defects in the neural tube, a part of the fetus that develops into the brain and spinal cord. The test is performed at 16 to 18 weeks of gestation and is used for screening purposes. Elevated AFP levels may indicate nervous system deformities, including spina bifida, but falsely elevated tests can be caused by more than one fetus or incorrect gestational dates. Positive results indicate the need for further studies including **amniocentesis** and fetal ultrasound.

Amniocentesis is insertion of a needle through the abdomen and into the gravid uterus to remove fluid from the amniotic sac. This fluid is analyzed for a variety of nervous system disorders. It can also be used to diagnose genetic problems, estimate gestational age, or assess lung maturity of the fetus. It may be performed in the office, and if so, you are responsible for preparing the patient, assisting the physician, preparing the specimen for transportation to the laboratory, and giving the patient any postprocedural instructions from the physician. Although some obstetric offices have a sonographer on staff, fetal ultrasounds may have to be scheduled in an outpatient facility.

Fetal Ultrasonography

An ultrasound of the fetus is use of high-frequency sound waves to create an image of internal structures. Fetal ultrasound is performed to assess the size, gestational age, position, and number of fetuses as well as fetal structures and development. Some abnormal maternal and fetal conditions, such as ectopic pregnancy, placenta previa, neural tube defects, and cardiac defects may be diagnosed by ultrasound. The gender of the fetus may also be determined, although this is not typically a justification for performing an ultrasound.

Box 38-6

CESAREAN SECTION

Sometimes a normal vaginal delivery is not possible or advisable, such as in these situations:
- Cephalopelvic disproportion: the baby's head is too large for the birth canal.
- Placenta previa.
- Poor presentation other than an occipital presentation, such as transverse (the baby lying across the cervix) or breech (a buttocks first presentation).
- Failure to progress: inefficient labor or the cervix will not dilate.
- Infant or maternal distress.

In these situations, the infant is delivered by cesarean section. An incision is made through the abdominal wall into the uterus and the infant is removed. It was once believed that women who had delivered by cesarean section should not be allowed to deliver vaginally because it was feared that the uterine scar might rupture. Current surgical techniques have lessened that fear, and many women now deliver vaginally after a cesarean delivery.

Table 38-5   MAIN METHODS OF CONTRACEPTION

Method	Description	Advantages	Disadvantages
Surgical			
Vasectomy, tubal ligation	Tubes carrying gametes cut	Nearly 100% effective, no chemical or mechanical devices	Not easily reversible, rare surgical complications
Hormonal			
Pill	Oral estrogen or progesterone to prevent ovulation	Highly effective, requires no last-minute preparation	Alters physiology, serious side effects possible
Injection	Inject synthetic progesterone q 3 mo to prevent ovulation	Highly effective, lasts 3–4 months	Alters physiology; possible side effects menstrual irregularity, amenorrhea; expensive
Implant	Synthetic progesterone under skin to prevent ovulation; may not be available except to women already using	Highly effective; lasts 5 years	Alters physiology; possible side effects menstrual irregularity, amenorrhea; expensive
Patch	Patch with progesterone, estrogen worn on skin 3 weeks in 4 to prevent ovulation	Use is simple; does not require pill or injection	Should be replaced same day of week; pregnancy can occur if patch off more than 24 hours or left on more than 1 week
Ring	Small, flexible ring in vagina releases synthetic progesterone, estrogen to prevent pregnancy for 1 mo	Does not require pill, injection; does not interfere with sexual intercourse	Side effects may include bleeding between periods, breast tenderness, other symptoms associated with hormone therapy
IUD	T-shaped plastic device with copper or progesterone	Spontaneous sexual intercourse	Heavy or long menstrual periods; cramping during, after insertion; periodic check for placement by feeling for string
Barrier			
Male condom	Sheath fits over erect penis, contains ejaculate	Easily available, does not affect physiology, protects from STDs	Must be applied before intercourse, may slip or tear
Female condom	Sheath that fits into vagina, held in place with rings	Easily available, protects from STDs	More expensive than male condom, must be inserted before intercourse
Diaphragm, spermicide	Rubber cap fits over cervix; prevents entrance of sperm	Does not affect physiology; some protection against STDs	Must be inserted before intercourse, requires fitting by physician
Other			
Spermicide	Chemical to kill sperm; best used with a barrier method	Easily available, does not affect physiology, some protection from STDs	Local irritation, must be used just before intercourse
Fertility awareness	Abstinence while fertile per menstrual history, basal temperature, quality of cervical mucus	Does not affect physiology; accepted by certain religions	High failure rate, requires careful record keeping
Emergency contraception	Morning-after pill reduces risk of pregnancy up to 120 hours after unprotected sex	May prevent pregnancy after unprotected sexual intercourse	Nausea, vomiting; no protection from STDs; may not prevent ectopic pregnancy; the closer to ovulation, the greater chance of pregnancy

Contraction Stress Test and Nonstress Test

A contraction stress test (CST) is performed in the third trimester to determine how the fetus will tolerate uterine contractions. Uterine contractions may be induced by the woman stimulating her nipples, known as the nipple-stimulating CST, or the contractions can be induced by the administration of oxytocin, called an oxytocin-stimulated CST. In both tests, the fetal heart tones and movement are monitored in relation to the uterine contractions. Although the contractions are meant to be temporary, the CST is usually performed in the hospital in the event continued contractions and delivery occur.

The nonstress test (NST) is a noninvasive obstetric procedure used to evaluate the fetal heart tones and movement in relation to spontaneous uterine contractions. The NST may be safely performed in the medical office, whereas the CST is usually performed in the hospital setting.

CONTRACEPTION

Numerous methods of contraception (birth control) are available (TABLE 38-5). The decision to practice contraception and the selection of an appropriate method involves many factors, including the patient's religious, cultural, and personal beliefs. In addition, the health history, financial situation, and motivation of the patient may be important considerations for the patient, the spouse or partner, and the physician. To reinforce the physician's advice and instructions, you should understand the various methods, including the indications, risk factors, cost, and effectiveness. Both you and the physician should be prepared to educate and advise the patient regarding the choice of contraception.

Menopause

Menopause, also called the climacteric period, is the stage of life during which ovulation ceases because of decreasing ovarian function. This period, characterized by the cessation of the menstrual cycle, usually occurs around

PATIENT EDUCATION

Kegel Exercises

The patient's age, gravidity, and past childbearing take their toll on the muscles of the perineum. Kegel exercises can increase the tone of this area. Stronger perineal support helps eliminate stress incontinence and supports the vaginal walls to avoid uterine prolapse.

Explain to the patient that she can do Kegel exercises at any time, such as when standing in the grocery line, waiting at a stop light, or sitting in class. Instruct her to tighten the vaginal opening and buttocks as if she were stopping the flow of urine. This position should be held for about 3 seconds. The patient should work up to doing the exercises in as many as 15 to 20 repetitions four or five times a day.

45 to 50 years of age. Changes in the menstrual cycle in early menopause include oligomenorrhea, amenorrhea, dysfunctional uterine bleeding, and hot flashes, flushing, or perspiration.

The decrease in circulating estrogen has been implicated as a risk factor for atherosclerosis, coronary heart disease, and osteoporosis. Supplemental estrogen, known as HRT or hormonal replacement therapy, protects against the cardiovascular and skeletal disorders and decreases the menopausal symptoms, such as hot flashes, depression, and drying of the vaginal mucosa. In addition to an active exercise program, dietary calcium, and a healthy and moderate lifestyle, HRT helps menopausal women retain optimum health and vitality. For those with only minor menopausal symptoms, weight-bearing exercises, a healthy diet, and vitamin and mineral supplements have eased the transition through the menopausal stage. Women in this stage of life should continue to have regular pelvic examinations, Pap smears, breast examinations, and mammograms.

Instructing the Patient on the Breast Self-Examination

Purpose: Properly instruct the female patient on the procedure for performing a breast self examination.

Equipment: Patient education instruction sheet if available; breast examination model if available

Standard: This procedure should take 5 minutes.

Steps	Reason
1. Wash your hands.	Handwashing aids infection control.
2. Explain the purpose and frequency of examining the breasts.	The purpose is to check for lumps, dimples, and thickened areas that can indicate malignancy and allow for early diagnosis and treatment. The patient should be encouraged to examine her breasts at the same time each month, about a week after the menstrual cycle.
3. Describe the three positions necessary for the patient to examine the breasts: in front of a mirror, in the shower, and lying down.	Inspecting and palpating the breasts in a variety of positions allows for a thorough examination of all breast tissue.
4. Explain that she should disrobe and inspect the breasts in front of a mirror with her hands on her hips and with her arms raised above her head. Advise the patient to look for any changes in contour, swelling, dimpling of the skin, or changes in the nipple.	Regular inspection shows what is normal and gives the patient confidence for the examination.

Step 4 A. Inspect both breasts in front of a mirror with the hands on the hips.

Step 4B. Inspect both breasts with the arms raised over the head.

(continued)

Procedure 38-1 *(continued)*

Instructing the Patient on the Breast Self-Examination

Steps	Reason
5. In the shower, the patient should feel each breast with her hands over wet skin, using the flat part of the first three fingers. Instruct her to use her right hand to lightly press over all areas of her left breast and her left hand to examine her right breast, checking for any lumps, hard knots, or thickenings.	Palpating the breasts in the shower allows the hands to glide more easily over wet skin.

Step 5. Examine the breasts in the shower.

6. After showering, the patient should lie down and examine her right breast after placing a pillow or folded towel under her right shoulder and placing her right hand behind her head. With her left hand, she should use the flat part of the fingers to palpate the breast tissue, using small circular motions beginning at the outermost top of her right breast and working clockwise around the breast.	Placing a pillow or folded towel under the right shoulder distributes the breast tissue more evenly on the chest.

Step 6 A. While lying down, palpate each breast carefully.

(continued)

Instructing the Patient on the Breast Self-Examination

Steps	**Reason**

Step 6 B. Palpate the breast using the flat part of fingers in a circular motion.

Steps	Reason
7. Encourage the patient to palpate the breast carefully by moving her fingers in toward the nipple, while palpating every part of the breast, including the nipple.	Breast tissue extends from the clavicle to the end of the rib cage and from the sternum to underneath the axilla.
8. Repeat the procedure for the left breast, placing a pillow or folded towel under the left shoulder and the left hand behind the head.	
9. Gently squeeze each nipple between the thumb and index finger. Report any discharge to the physician.	

Step 9. Squeeze each nipple gently.

(continued)

Instructing the Patient on the Breast Self-Examination

Steps	Reason
10. Explain to the patient that she should promptly report any abnormalities to the physician.	
11. Document the patient education	Procedures are considered not to have been done if they are not recorded.

Charting Example

4/12/2005 2:15 P.M. Pt. given written and verbal instructions on performing the monthly breast self-examination. She verbalized understanding. Advised to contact the office for any problems or abnormalities _____ E. Smith, RMA

(Figures in step 4A, 4B, 5, 6A, and 9 are reprinted with permission from Pillitteri A: Maternal and Child Nursing. Philadelphia: Lippincott, Williams & Wilkins, 2003. The figure in step 6 B is reprinted with permission from Weber J and Kelley J: Health Assessment in Nursing. Philadelphia: Lippincott Williams & Wilkins, 2003.)

Assisting with the Pelvic Examination and Pap Smear

Purpose:	Prepare the examination room and the female patient for a pelvic examination and Pap smear and assist the physician as needed.
Equipment:	Gown and drape; appropriate size vaginal speculum; cotton-tipped applicators; water-soluble lubricant; examination gloves; examination light; tissues; materials for Pap smear: cervical spatula and/or brush, glass slides, fixative solution, laboratory request form, identification labels OR materials required by laboratory; Biohazard container.
Standard:	This procedure should take 15 minutes.

Steps	Reason
1. Wash your hands.	Handwashing aids infection control.
2. Assemble the equipment and supplies.	The vaginal speculum can be warmed under warm running water, on a heating pad set on warm, or in a warming drawer found on some examination tables. Lubricant must not be used on the vaginal speculum before insertion, since this will cause inaccurate Pap smear results.
3. Label each slide with the date and type of specimen on the frosted end with a pencil.	Each slide should be labeled *C* for cervical, *V* for vaginal, or *E* for endocervical, depending on where the physician obtains the cells for examination.
4. Greet and identify the patient. Explain the procedure.	Identifying the patient prevents errors. Explaining the procedure may reduce anxiety.

(continued)

755

Procedure 38-2

Assisting with the Pelvic Examination and Pap Smear

Steps	Reason
5. Ask the patient to empty her bladder and if necessary, collect a urine specimen.	An empty bladder will make the examination more comfortable.
6. Provide the patient with a gown and drape and ask her to disrobe from the waist down.	If the patient is also having a breast examination, she should be instructed to disrobe completely and put the gown on with the opening in the front. This allows easier access for the breast examination.
7. Position the patient in the dorsal lithotomy position with her buttocks at the bottom edge of the table.	Because this position is embarrassing and may stress the legs and back, assist the patient into this position only when the physician is ready to do the examination.
8. Adjust the drape to cover the patient's abdomen and knees, exposing the genitalia, and adjust the light over the genitalia for maximum visibility.	Good visibility is essential for a thorough examination.
9. Assist the physician with the examination as needed by handing instruments and supplies as needed.	Anticipating the physician's needs during the procedure promotes a more thorough and efficient examination
10. After applying examination gloves, hold the microscope slides while the physician obtains and makes the smears.	

Step 10. Hold the slide by the frosted end to receive the smears.

| 11. Spray or cover each slide with fixative solution by holding the slide 4 to 6 inches from the can and spraying lightly once across the slide or dropping the fixative onto the slide. | Spraying the fixative solution too close to the slide will distort the cells or blow them off the slide. The fixative is necessary to preserve the cervical scrapings for cytology analysis. |

(continued)

Procedure 38-2 (continued)

Assisting with the Pelvic Examination and Pap Smear

Steps	Reason
12. When the physician removes the vaginal speculum, have a basin or other container ready to receive it.	

Step 12. Receive the used instruments in a basin or other container to transfer to the soaking solution for sanitizing.

| 13. Apply lubricant across the physician's two fingers without touching the end of the lubricant container to the physician's gloves. | Water-soluble lubricant helps make the manual examination more comfortable. |

Step 13. Apply about 1 to 2 inches of water-soluble lubricant to the physician's gloved fingers.

(continued)

Procedure 38-2 (continued)

Assisting with the Pelvic Examination and Pap Smear

Steps	Reason
14. Encourage the patient to relax during the bimanual examination as needed.	The patient may be more relaxed during the examination if you are supportive.

Step 14. Technique for bimanual examination of the pelvic organs in women. (Reprinted with permission from Smeltzer SC and Bare BG: Textbook of Medical-Surgical Nursing. Philadelphia: Lippincott Williams & Wilkins, 2000.)

Steps	Reason
15. After the examination, help the patient slide up to the top of the examination table and remove both feet at the same time from the stirrups.	Injury can be prevented if the patient moves up the table before removing feet from the stirrups. Removing both feet at the same time puts less strain on the patient.
16. Offer the patient tissues to remove excess lubricant and help her sit if necessary, watching for signs of vertigo.	Excess lubricant can be uncomfortable. Some patients, especially the elderly, may be dizzy on sitting up.
17. Ask the patient to get dressed and assist as needed. Provide for privacy as the patient dresses.	
18. Reinforce any physician instructions regarding follow-up appointments and advise the patient on the procedure for obtaining the laboratory findings from the Pap smear.	For quality management, let the patient know when to schedule follow-up appointments and when and how laboratory findings will be obtained.
19. Properly care for or dispose of equipment and clean the examination room. Wash your hands.	Procedures are considered not to have been done if they are not recorded.
20. Document your responsibilities during the procedure, such as routing the specimen, patient education, and so on.	

Charting example:
2/27/2005 3:00 P.M. Pt. Pap and pelvic today per Dr. Todd. Cervical and vaginal slides sent to Acme lab for cytology. Pt. given written and oral instructions on obtaining results. _____ B. Lewis, CMA

Procedure 38-3

Assisting with the Colposcopy and Cervical Biopsy

Purpose: Prepare the examination room and the female patient for a colposcopy with cervical biopsy

Equipment: Gown and drape, vaginal speculum, colposcope, specimen container with preservative (10% formalin), sterile gloves in appropriate size, sterile cotton-tipped applicators, sterile normal saline solution, sterile 3% acetic acid sterile povidone-iodine (Betadine), silver nitrate sticks or ferric subsulfate (Monsel solution), sterile biopsy forceps or punch biopsy instrument, sterile uterine curet, sterile uterine dressing forceps, sterile 4 × 4 gauze, sterile towel, sterile endocervical curet, sterile uterine tenaculum, sanitary napkin, examination gloves, examination light, tissues, biohazard container.

Standard: This procedure should take 20 to 30 minutes.

Steps	Reason
1. Wash your hands.	Handwashing aids infection control.
2. Verify that the patient has signed the consent form.	Colposcopy with biopsy is an invasive procedure that requires written consent.
3. Assemble the equipment and supplies.	
4. Check the light on the colposcope.	Properly functioning equipment is crucial to the quality of the examination.
5. Set up the sterile field without contaminating it.	A biopsy is an invasive procedure requiring asepsis.
6. Pour sterile normal saline and acetic acid into their sterile containers. Cover the field with a sterile drape.	Items that can be placed on the sterile field include the sterile cotton-tipped applicators and sterile containers for the solutions. Covering the sterile field maintains sterility as you prepare the patient.
7. Greet and identify the patient. Explain the procedure.	Identifying the patient prevents errors. Explaining the procedure may ease anxiety.
8. When the physician is ready to proceed, assist the patient into the dorsal lithotomy position. If you are to assist the physician from the sterile field, put on sterile gloves after positioning the patient.	Correct positioning is essential for a clear view of the cervix.
9. Hand the physician the applicator immersed in normal saline, followed by the applicator immersed in acetic acid.	Acetic acid swabbed on the area improves visualization and aids in identifying suspicious tissue.
10. Hand the physician the applicator with the antiseptic solution (Betadine).	The area to be sampled for biopsy must be swabbed with an antiseptic solution to reduce microorganisms and pathogens in the area.
11. If you did not apply sterile gloves to assist the physician, apply clean examination gloves and receive the biopsy specimen into the container of 10% formalin preservative.	Because the specimen may be hazardous, standard precautions must be observed.
12. Provide the physician with Monsel solution or silver nitrate sticks to stop any bleeding if necessary.	If bleeding occurs, a coagulant, such as Monsel solution or silver nitrate, may have to be applied.

(continued)

Procedure 38-3 *(continued)*

Assisting with the Colposcopy and Cervical Biopsy

Steps	Reason
13. When the physician is finished with the procedure, appropriately assist the patient from the stirrups and to a sitting position. Explain to the patient that a small amount of bleeding may occur. Have a sanitary napkin available.	Bleeding with a cervical biopsy is usually minimal, and a small sanitary pad should be sufficient.
14. Label the specimen container with the patient's name and date and prepare the laboratory request.	The specimen must be properly identified, and the laboratory request must be complete.
15. Ask the patient to get dressed and assist as needed. Provide for privacy as the patient dresses.	
16. Reinforce any physician instructions regarding follow-up appointments, and tell the patient how to obtain the biopsy findings.	For quality management, let the patient know when to schedule follow-up appointments and when and how laboratory findings will be provided.
17. Properly care for or dispose of equipment and clean the examination room. Wash your hands.	
18. Document your responsibilities during the procedure, such as routing the specimen, patient education, and so on.	Procedures are considered not to have been done if they are not recorded.

Charting Example

10/15/2005 10:45 A.M. Colposcopy performed per Dr. Lyttle; cervical biopsy obtained and sent to Acme lab for cytology. Minimal bleeding post procedure; pt. given sanitary pad, oral and written instructions on post-procedure care. Verbalized understanding. _____ J. Pratt, CMA

CHAPTER SUMMARY

Assisting in obstetrics and gynecology is a challenging and fascinating area of medicine. The female reproductive system is highly complex, involving dramatic changes in growth and development and the ability to produce a healthy newborn. This chapter describes the examination of the female reproductive system and your role in assisting the patient and the physician in this specialized examination. In addition, it discusses a variety of disorders related to the female reproductive system and normal patterns such as menarche and menopause. Finally, it addresses caring for the pregnant patient and disorders or conditions sometimes seen in pregnancy.

Regardless of the reason for the gynecological examination, the medical office visit may be an emotional and intimidating experience. As a professional medical assistant, you are in a unique position to provide the patient with reassurance and emotional support that may prove to be comforting to the patient and rewarding to you.

Critical Thinking Challenges

1. A multiparous patient who is married and has a history of cigarette smoking desires a highly effective method of contraception. What are her bests choices for contraception? Explain which choice is best and why.
2. Your patient has both genital herpes and condylomata acuminata. She wants to know whether these disorders are contagious and how they can be cured. How do you respond to these questions?
3. Research the effects of maternal exposure to various substances and prepare a poster describing your findings that could be used to educate pregnant women and those considering pregnancy.
4. In addition to the contraceptives listed in this chapter, what options are available today? List the contraceptives available today, including the advantages and risks associated with each.
5. What gynecological procedures can be performed by the physician during a laparoscopy? How is the recovery different from recovery from a laparotomy?

Answers to Checkpoint Questions

1. Menorrhagia is excessive bleeding during menses, and metrorrhagia is irregular bleeding at times other than menses.
2. The symptoms of endometriosis include infertility, dysmenorrhea, pelvic pain, and dyspareunia. The cause is unknown.
3. Uterine prolapse is an abnormal condition in which the uterus droops or protrudes down into the vagina. Displacement of the uterus involves an abnormal tilting of the uterus in the pelvic cavity.
4. The prognosis of all cancers is much better with early diagnosis and treatment.
5. Genital warts have been implicated as a risk factor for cervical cancer.
6. The complete gynecological examination includes a breast examination and a pelvic examination with a Pap smear.
7. The presumptive signs and symptoms of pregnancy are not conclusive because they may indicate other conditions in the female reproductive system.
8. The pregnant patient should notify the physician if she has vaginal bleeding or spotting, persistent vomiting, fever or chills, dysuria, or abdominal or uterine cramping, leaking amniotic fluid, altered fetal movement, dizziness, or blurred vision.
9. Lochia, a discharge from the uterus after delivery, progresses through several types: lochia rubra (blood tinged), lochia serosa (thin, brownish), lochia alba (white).
10. Placenta previa is a condition in which the placenta is implanted either partly or completely over the cervical os. In a preterm patient, the condition is managed with bed rest and drug therapy.

 Websites

American College of Obstetricians and Gynecologists
http://www.acog.org

National Center for HIV, STD, and TB Prevention
http://www.cdc.gov/nchstp/dstd/disease_info.htm

American Social Health Association
http://www.ashastd.org/stdfaqs

American Infertility Association http://www.americaninfertility.org

American Cancer Society http://www.cancer.org

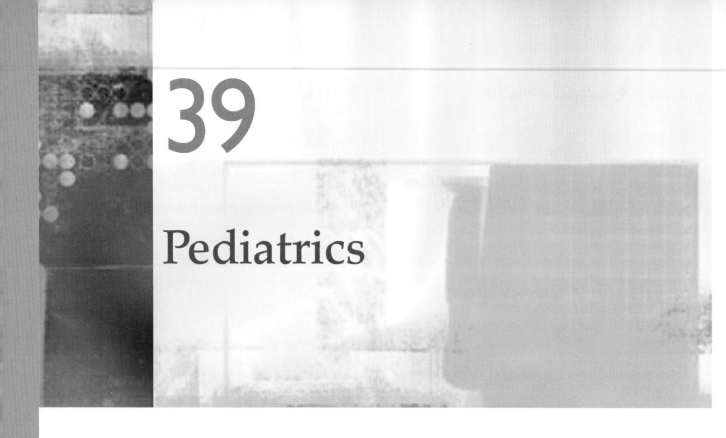

39

Pediatrics

CHAPTER OUTLINE

ROLE DELINEATION

ADMINISTRATIVE: ADMINISTRATIVE
PROCEDURES

CLINICAL: FUNDAMENTAL PRINCIPLES
• Apply principles of aseptic technique and infection control
• Comply with quality assurance practices
• Screen and follow up patient test results

CLINICAL: DIAGNOSTIC ORDERS
• Collect and process specimens
• Perform diagnostic tests

CLINICAL: PATIENT CARE
• Adhere to established patient screening procedures
• Obtain patient history and vital signs
• Prepare and maintain examination and treatment areas
• Prepare patient for examinations, procedures, and treatments
• Assist with examinations, procedures, and treatments
• Maintain medication and immunization records
• Recognize and respond to emergencies
• Coordinate patient care information with other health care providers

GENERAL: PROFESSIONALISM
- Display a professional manner and image
- Demonstrate initiative and responsibility
- Work as a member of the health care team
- Prioritize and perform multiple tasks
- Treat all patients with compassion and empathy

GENERAL: COMMUNICATION SKILLS
- Recognize and respect cultural diversity
- Adapt communications to individual's ability to understand
- Recognize and respond effectively to verbal, nonverbal, and written communications
- Use medical terminology appropriately
- Serve as a liaison

GENERAL: LEGAL CONCEPTS
- Perform within legal and ethical boundaries
- Prepare and maintain medical records
- Document accurately
- Comply with established risk management and safety procedures

GENERAL: INSTRUCTION
- Instruct individuals according to their needs
- Teach methods of health promotion and disease prevention

GENERAL: OPERATIONAL FUNCTIONS
- Perform routine maintenance of administrative and clinical equipment

CHAPTER COMPETENCIES

LEARNING OBJECTIVES
Upon successfully completing this chapter, you will be able to:
1. Spell and define the key terms.
2. List safety precautions for the pediatric office.
3. Explain the difference between a well-child and a sick-child visit.
4. List types and schedule of immunizations.
5. Describe the types of feelings a child might have during an office visit.
6. List and explain how to record the anthropometric measurements obtained in a pediatric visit.
7. Identify two injection sites to use on an infant and two used on a child.
8. Describe the role of the parent during the office visit.
9. List the names, symptoms, and treatment for common pediatric illnesses.

PERFORMANCE OBJECTIVES
Upon successfully completing this chapter, you will be able to:
1. Measure infant weight and length (Procedure 39-1)
2. Measure head and chest circumference (Procedure 39-2)
3. Apply a pediatric urine collection device (Procedure 39-3).

KEY TERMS

aspiration	immunization	pediatrics	sick-child visit
autonomous	neonatologist	psychosocial	varicella zoster
congenital anomaly	pediatrician	restrain	well-child visit

THE PEDIATRIC PRACTICE

Medical assistants who work in an office where infants and children are seen must understand that the needs of children and adolescents are often different from those of adult patients. Pediatrics is the medical specialty devoted to the care of infants, children, and adolescents. This care includes diagnosis and treatment of childhood diseases, prevention of accidents and trauma, and monitoring the physical and **psychosocial**, or mental and emotional, development of the child. These patients are not simply small adults; however, they may contract some of the illnesses that are seen in adult patients. Pediatric patients are also susceptible to a unique array of illnesses and problems not present in adults. Some young patients have **congenital anomalies** that are life-threatening or debilitating. Because children have immature nervous systems, faster metabolism, and accelerated growth patterns, they are subject to complications that may not occur in adult patients.

A **pediatrician** is a physician who is specially trained to care for both the well child and diseases of infants, children, and adolescents. While most traditional pediatricians treat all children up through the teen years, pediatric specialists include **neonatologists**, physicians who treat only newborns, and physicians who specialize in the treatment of adolescents. In addition, the medical assistant working in the family practice will see patients of all ages, including children.

Safety

A pediatric office decorated and furnished in a manner appropriate to children's physical and psychosocial needs creates an unthreatening and possibly even inviting environment. Child-size furniture helps these patients feel comfortable and welcome. Popular toys evoke happy associations. Safe toys allow for hands-on activity while the child is waiting to see the physician. Popular storybooks and magazines give parents an opportunity to read quietly to a child who may not feel well enough to play. Some offices are designed with separate waiting areas for sick children and well ones to prevent transmission of communicable diseases between patients.

Safety is a prime concern for choosing toys and equipment for a pediatric office. Waiting room toys should be examined frequently and replaced when damaged or soiled. All toys should be washable and should be cleaned according to office policy to reduce the risk of disease transmission. Try to see the office from a child's viewpoint. If necessary, get down to a child's level to discover dangers such as sharp table corners and exposed electrical outlets, which an adult might overlook.

The examination room should also be designed for children's safety. Keep all medical equipment out of a child's reach, and never leave a young child alone in the examining room. Follow these tips to ensure your patient's safety:

- Place infant scales on a sturdy table, and never leave an infant alone on a scale.
- Store any disinfectants away from patient care areas.
- Store and dispose of all sharps in proper containers.
- Practice stringent handwashing and standard precautions with every patient. Many childhood diseases are highly contagious and can be transmitted by poor medical asepsis.

Checkpoint Question

1. What are three safety precautions that should be used in a pediatric office?

Types of Pediatric Office Visits

The Well-Child Office Visit

Well-child visits are regularly scheduled office visits whose goal is to maintain the child's optimum health. These visits, scheduled to correspond with the immunization schedule, include a complete examination and an evaluation of the child's neurological and psychosocial development. The neurological examination consists of the physician checking for the presence or absence of various reflexes. TABLE 39-1 describes various infant reflexes and the normal responses typically assessed at the well-child infant visit. In addition to the reflexes, the physician observes for development appro-

TRIAGE

While working in a family practice office, you have to complete these three tasks:

A. Patient A is a 2-month-old who has just been placed in examination room 1. You are to take the vital signs and measurements, including length, weight, and head circumference.

B. Patient B is a 14-month-old who was seen today and diagnosed with otitis media. The physician has asked you to give the parent a prescription for an antibiotic and schedule a referral with an ear, nose, and throat physician for possible myringectomy and tubes.

C. A mother is on the phone, concerned because patient C, her newborn, is vomiting.

How do you sort these tasks? What do you do first? Second? Third?

First, speak to the mother of patient C. This infant will dehydrate very quickly, and the situation must be assessed promptly and efficiently. Give advice about increasing fluids or giving pediatric electrolyte solutions *only* after assessing the situation, consulting with the physician, and receiving instructions from the physician to pass along to the mother. Next deal with patient B by giving the parent the prescription and clarifying any other orders from the physician. The information regarding the referral can be given to the parent to make the arrangements, or you may make the appointment later in the day, when time permits. Of course, the required paperwork for the referral must be faxed to the referral physician, and this may be delegated to an administrative assistant according to the office policy and procedure manual.

See patient A after Patient B is discharged. When obtaining a history for a well-child checkup, you want to give the parent your undivided attention and take extra time to establish rapport with the parent and the infant.

priate for the age of the infant or child. The child is observed or the caregiver is questioned about areas such as social development, fine motor development, gross motor development, language, and nutrition using a guide such as the Denver II (FIG. 39-1). Any other concerns on the part of the caregiver are also addressed at these visits.

The well-child visit also provides an opportunity to administer **immunizations** to protect children from diseases that in the past caused early death or long-term health

Table 39-1 INFANT REFLEXES AND RESPONSES

Reflex	Response
Sucking or rooting	Stroking the cheek causes the infant to turn toward the stroke with its mouth open to suck. This reflex subsides by 3–6 months.
Moro or startle	A loud noise or sudden change in position causes the infant to look startled; the back arches, the arms and legs fly out and then quickly come back close to the body, and the infant cries. The Moro reflex results in the thumbs and forefingers forming a **C** while the other fingers spread open (in the startled reflex, the fingers remain clenched). Both reflexes disappear by 6 months.
Grasp	Stroking the infant's palm causes the fingers to grasp; stroking the plantar surface causes the toes to flex to grasp. The palmar grasp disappears by 3 months. The plantar grasp disappears by 9–12 months.
Tonic neck or fencing	With the infant supine, the physician turns the head to either side. The arm and leg on the side the infant is facing will flex, and the limbs on the opposite side will extend. This reflex disappears by 3–4 months.
Placing or stepping	The physician holds the infant upright at the edge of the examining table with the heel just below the edge. When the tops of the feet touch the table edge, the infant will place each foot up on the table and make walking movements. This reflex disappears by 6 weeks.
Babinski	When the plantar surface of the foot is stroked, the toes flare outward. This reflex disappears by 12 months.

The absence of a response or a hyperresponse may indicate a neurological deficit.

problems. Immunizations produce immunity by slowly introducing an altered form of the disease-producing bacteria or virus into the body, which stimulates the body to produce antibodies to protect against the specific disease. Immunizations are available for these diseases:

- Hepatitis B (HBV). 0.5 mL intramuscularly (IM) given at birth, 1 month, and 6 months.
- Diphtheria, tetanus, acellular pertussis (DTaP). 0.5 mL given IM at 2 months, 4 months, 6 months, 15 to 18 months, and 4 to 6 years. Children over age 7 years and adults should receive Td (tetanus, diphtheria).
- Poliomyelitis (IPV). 0.5 mL given subcutaneously (SC) at 2 months, 4 months, 6 to 12 months, and 4 to 6 years.
- Mumps, measles, and rubella (MMR). 0.5 mL given SC at 12 to 15 months and 4 to 6 years, depending on state law.
- Haemophilus influenzae type B (HiB). 0.5 mL given IM in 3 or 4 doses, depending on the manufacturer. Three doses are given at 2 months, 4 months, and 12 to 15 months. Four doses are given at 2 months, 4 months, 6 months, and 12 to 15 months.
- **Varicella zoster** (VZV), also known as chicken pox. 0.5 mL SC given twice: at 12 months, one dose. At age 13 years or according to state law, 2 doses at least 28 days apart.
- Hepatitis A. 0.5 mL IM given to children and 1.0 mL IM given to adults (refer to vaccine package insert to determine ages and doses).
- Pneumococcus. 0.5 mL IM in 4 doses at 2 months, 4 months, 6 months, and 12 to 15 months. Children over age 12 months receiving the vaccine for the first time

should receive 2 doses at least 2 months apart. Children aged 24 months to 9 years receive only one dose.
- Influenza. May be given nasally as live attenuated influenza vaccine (LAIV) or IM as trivalent inactivated influenza vaccine (TIV). The dose is based on the age of the child (refer to package inserts for each type of vaccine). While this vaccine was not recommended for all children in the past, beginning in the fall of 2004 the American Academy of Pediatrics recommends that all children aged 6 to 23 months receive this vaccination yearly.
- Meningococcus. 0.5 mL given SC to older adolescents who will be moving into college dormitories or residence halls. It is not recommended for children under age 2 and is not a required pediatric immunization.

Vaccine manufacturers have established protocols that must be followed to ensure full immunity to the specific diseases. If you are responsible for administering vaccines, you must read all package inserts and become familiar with the correct administration and possible adverse effects before administering the medication. In addition, you must give the parent or caregiver of the child the written vaccine information statement (VIS) about each vaccine you are administering. In some cases, it may be necessary to obtain written consent before administering the vaccine. The VIS for individual vaccines describes the disease and provides information specific to the immunization, such as recommended ages and adverse reactions (FIG. 39-2).

Immunization schedules are developed by the American Academy of Pediatrics (AAP) and the Centers for Disease Control and Prevention, and they change periodically as new

(text continued on page 771)

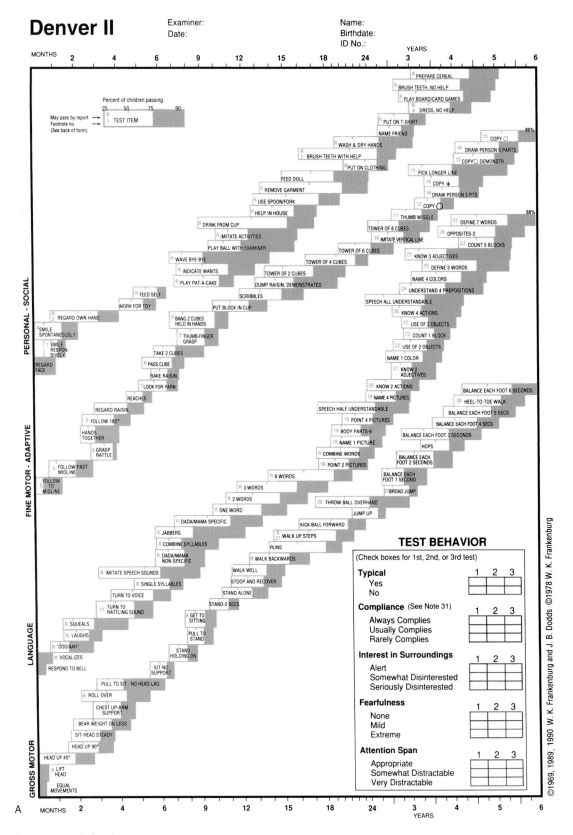

FIGURE 39–1. (**A**) The Denver Developmental Screening Test II.

DIRECTIONS FOR ADMINISTRATION

1. Try to get child to smile by smiling, talking or waving. Do not touch him/her.
2. Child must stare at hand several seconds.
3. Parent may help guide toothbrush and put toothpaste on brush.
4. Child does not have to be able to tie shoes or button/zip in the back.
5. Move yarn slowly in an arc from one side to the other, about 8″ above child's face.
6. Pass if child grasps rattle when it is touched to the backs or tips of fingers.
7. Pass if child tries to see where yarn went. Yarn should be dropped quickly from sight from tester's hand without arm movement.
8. Child must transfer cube from hand to hand without help of body, mouth, or table.
9. Pass if child picks up raisin with any part of thumb and finger.
10. Line can vary only 30 degrees or less from tester's line. V
11. Make a fist with thumb pointing upward and wiggle only the thumb. Pass if child imitates and does not move any fingers other than the thumb.

12. Pass any enclosed form. Fail continuous round motions.
13. Which line is longer? (Not bigger.) Turn paper upside down and repeat. (pass 3 of 3 or 5 of 6)
14. Pass any lines crossing near midpoint.
15. Have child copy first. If failed, demonstrate.

When giving items 12, 14, and 15, do not name the forms. Do not demonstrate 12 and 14.

16. When scoring, each pair (2 arms, 2 legs, etc.) counts as one part.
17. Place one cube in cup and shake gently near child's ear, but out of sight. Repeat for other ear.
18. Point to picture and have child name it. (No credit is given for sounds only.)
    If less than 4 pictures are named correctly, have child point to picture as each is named by tester.

19. Using doll, tell child: Show me the nose, eyes, ears, mouth, hands, feet, tummy, hair. Pass 6 of 8.
20. Using pictures, ask child: Which one flies?... says meow?... talks?... barks?... gallops? Pass 2 of 5, 4 of 5.
21. Ask child: What do you do when you are cold?... tired?... hungry? Pass 2 of 3, 3 of 3.
22. Ask child: What do you do with a cup? What is a chair used for? What is a pencil used for?
    Action words must be included in answers.
23. Pass if child correctly places <u>and</u> says how many blocks are on paper. (1, 5)
24. Tell child: Put block **on** table; **under** table; **in front of** me, **behind** me. Pass 4 of 4.
    (Do not help child by pointing, moving head or eyes.)
25. Ask child: What is a ball?... lake?... desk?... house?... banana?... curtain?... fence?... ceiling? Pass if defined in terms of use, shape, what it is made of, or general category (such as banana is fruit, not just yellow). Pass 5 of 8, 7 of 8.
26. Ask child: If a horse is big, a mouse is __? If fire is hot, ice is __? If the sun shines during the day, the moon shines during the __? Pass 2 of 3.
27. Child may use wall or rail only, not person. May not crawl.
28. Child must throw ball overhand 3 feet to within arm's reach of tester.
29. Child must perform standing broad jump over width of test sheet (8½ inches).
30. Tell child to walk forward, ⟲⟳⟲⟳➔ heel within 1 inch of toe. Tester may demonstrate.
    Child must walk 4 consecutive steps.
31. In the second year, half of normal children are noncompliant.

B **OBSERVATIONS:**

FIGURE 39–1. *(continued)* (**B**) Instructions for the test. Test kits, test forms, and reference manuals, which must be used to ensure accuracy, may be ordered from Denver Developmental Materials Incorporated, P.O. Box 6919, Denver CO 80206-0919. (Reprinted with permission from William K. Frankenburg, M.D.)

DIPHTHERIA TETANUS & PERTUSSIS VACCINES

W H A T   Y O U   N E E D   T O   K N O W

1 Why get vaccinated?

Diphtheria, tetanus, and pertussis are serious diseases caused by bacteria. Diphtheria and pertussis are spread from person to person. Tetanus enters the body through cuts or wounds.

DIPHTHERIA causes a thick covering in the back of the throat.
• It can lead to breathing problems, paralysis, heart failure, and even death.

TETANUS (Lockjaw) causes painful tightening of the muscles, usually all over the body.
• It can lead to "locking" of the jaw so the victim cannot open his mouth or swallow. Tetanus leads to death in about 1 out of 10 cases.

PERTUSSIS (Whooping Cough) causes coughing spells so bad that it is hard for infants to eat, drink, or breathe. These spells can last for weeks.
• It can lead to pneumonia, seizures (jerking and staring spells), brain damage, and death.

Diphtheria, tetanus, and pertussis vaccine (DTaP) can help prevent these diseases. Most children who are vaccinated with DTaP will be protected throughout childhood. Many more children would get these diseases if we stopped vaccinating.

DTaP is a safer version of an older vaccine called DTP. DTP is no longer used in the United States.

2 Who should get DTaP vaccine and when?

Children should get 5 doses of DTaP vaccine, one dose at each of the following ages:

✓ 2 months   ✓ 4 months   ✓ 6 months
   ✓15-18 months   ✓ 4-6 years

DTaP may be given at the same time as other vaccines.

3 Some children should not get DTaP vaccine or should wait

• Children with minor illnesses, such as a cold, may be vaccinated. But children who are moderately or severely ill should usually wait until they recover before getting DTaP vaccine.

• Any child who had a life-threatening allergic reaction after a dose of DTaP should not get another dose.

• Any child who suffered a brain or nervous system disease within 7 days after a dose of DTaP should not get another dose.

• Talk with your doctor if your child:
   - had a seizure or collapsed after a dose of DTaP,
   - cried non-stop for 3 hours or more after a dose of DTaP,
   - had a fever over 105°F after a dose of DTaP.

Ask your health care provider for more information. Some of these children should not get another dose of pertussis vaccine, but may get a vaccine without pertussis, called **DT**.

4 Older children and adults

DTaP should not be given to anyone 7 years of age or older because pertussis vaccine is only licensed for children under 7.

But older children, adolescents, and adults still need protection from tetanus and diphtheria. A booster shot called **Td** is recommended at 11-12 years of age, and then every 10 years. There is a separate Vaccine Information Statement for Td vaccine.

Diphtheria/Tetanus/Pertussis   7/30/2001

FIGURE 39—2. Vaccine Information Statement (VIS) for DtaP. (Courtesy of the Centers for Disease Control and Prevention.)

5 | What are the risks from DTaP vaccine?

Getting diphtheria, tetanus, or pertussis disease is much riskier than getting DTaP vaccine.

However, a vaccine, like any medicine, is capable of causing serious problems, such as severe allergic reactions. The risk of DTaP vaccine causing serious harm, or death, is extremely small.

Mild Problems (Common)
- Fever (up to about 1 child in 4)
- Redness or swelling where the shot was given (up to about 1 child in 4)
- Soreness or tenderness where the shot was given (up to about 1 child in 4)

These problems occur more often after the 4th and 5th doses of the DTaP series than after earlier doses. Sometimes the 4th or 5th dose of DTaP vaccine is followed by swelling of the entire arm or leg in which the shot was given, lasting 1-7 days (up to about 1 child in 30).

Other mild problems include:
- Fussiness (up to about 1 child in 3)
- Tiredness or poor appetite (up to about 1 child in 10)
- Vomiting (up to about 1 child in 50)

These problems generally occur 1-3 days after the shot.

Moderate Problems (Uncommon)
- Seizure (jerking or staring) (about 1 child out of 14,000)
- Non-stop crying, for 3 hours or more (up to about 1 child out of 1,000)
- High fever, over 105°F (about 1 child out of 16,000)

Severe Problems (Very Rare)
- Serious allergic reaction (less than 1 out of a million doses)
- Several other severe problems have been reported after DTaP vaccine. These include:
  - Long-term seizures, coma, or lowered consciousness
  - Permanent brain damage.
  These are so rare it is hard to tell if they are caused by the vaccine.

Controlling fever is especially important for children who have had seizures, for any reason. It is also important if another family member has had seizures. You can reduce fever and pain by giving your child an *aspirin-free* pain reliever when the shot is given, and for the next 24 hours, following the package instructions.

6 | What if there is a moderate or severe reaction?

What should I look for?

Any unusual conditions, such as a serious allergic reaction, high fever or unusual behavior. Serious allergic reactions are extremely rare with any vaccine. If one were to occur, it would most likely be within a few minutes to a few hours after the shot. Signs can include difficulty breathing, hoarseness or wheezing, hives, paleness, weakness, a fast heart beat or dizziness. If a high fever or seizure were to occur, it would usually be within a week after the shot.

What should I do?

- Call a doctor, or get the person to a doctor right away.
- Tell your doctor what happened, the date and time it happened, and when the vaccination was given.
- Ask your doctor, nurse, or health department to file a Vaccine Adverse Event Reporting System (VAERS) form. Or call VAERS yourself at **1-800-822-7967** or visit their website at **http://www.vaers.org.**

7 | The National Vaccine Injury Compensation Program

In the rare event that you or your child has a serious reaction to a vaccine, a federal program has been created to help pay for the care of those who have been harmed.

For details about the National Vaccine Injury Compensation Program, call **1-800-338-2382** or visit the program's website at **http://www.hrsa.gov/osp/vicp**

8 | How can I learn more?

- Ask your health care provider. They can give you the vaccine package insert or suggest other sources of information.

- Call your local or state health department's immunization program.

- Contact the Centers for Disease Control and Prevention (CDC):
  - Call **1-800-232-2522** (English)
  - Call **1-800-232-0233** (Español)
  - Visit the National Immunization Program's website at **http://www.cdc.gov/nip**

U.S. DEPARTMENT OF HEALTH & HUMAN SERVICES
Centers for Disease Control and Prevention
National Immunization Program

Vaccine Information Statement
DTaP (7/30/01)   42 U.S.C. § 300aa-26

F I G U R E 3 9 – 2 . *(continued).*

Recommended Childhood and Adolescent Immunization Schedule — United States, January – June 2004

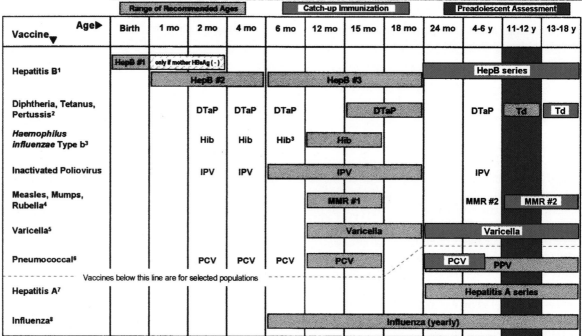

Vaccine ▼	Age ▶	Birth	1 mo	2 mo	4 mo	6 mo	12 mo	15 mo	18 mo	24 mo	4-6 y	11-12 y	13-18 y
						Catch-up Immunization					*Preadolescent Assessment*		
Hepatitis B[1]		HepB #1	only if mother HBsAg (-)								HepB series		
				HepB #2			HepB #3						
Diphtheria, Tetanus, Pertussis[2]				DTaP	DTaP	DTaP		DTaP			DTaP	Td	Td
Haemophilus influenzae Type b[3]				Hib	Hib	Hib[3]	Hib						
Inactivated Poliovirus				IPV	IPV		IPV				IPV		
Measles, Mumps, Rubella[4]							MMR #1				MMR #2	MMR #2	
Varicella[5]							Varicella				Varicella		
Pneumococcal[6]				PCV	PCV	PCV	PCV			PCV	PPV		
Hepatitis A[7]											Hepatitis A series		
Influenza[8]							Influenza (yearly)						

Vaccines below this line are for selected populations

This schedule indicates the recommended ages for routine administration of currently licensed childhood vaccines, as of December 1, 2003, for children through age 18 years. Any dose not given at the recommended age should be given at any subsequent visit when indicated and feasible. ▮ Indicates age groups that warrant special effort to administer those vaccines not previously given. Additional vaccines may be licensed and recommended during the year. Licensed combination vaccines may be used whenever any components of the combination are indicated and the vaccine's other components are not contraindicated. Providers should consult the manufacturers' package inserts for detailed recommendations. Clinically significant adverse events that follow immunization should be reported to the Vaccine Adverse Event Reporting System (VAERS). Guidance about how to obtain and complete a VAERS form can be found on the Internet: http://www.vaers.org/ or by calling 1-800-822-7967.

1. Hepatitis B (HepB) vaccine. All infants should receive the first dose of hepatitis B vaccine soon after birth and before hospital discharge; the first dose may also be given by age 2 months if the infant's mother is hepatitis B surface antigen (HBsAg) negative. Only monovalent HepB can be used for the birth dose. Monovalent or combination vaccine containing HepB may be used to complete the series. Four doses of vaccine may be administered when a birth dose is given. The second dose should be given at least 4 weeks after the first dose, except for combination vaccines which cannot be administered before age 6 weeks. The third dose should be given at least 16 weeks after the first dose and at least 8 weeks after the second dose. The last dose in the vaccination series (third or fourth dose) should not be administered before age 24 weeks.

Infants born to HBsAg-positive mothers should receive HepB and 0.5 mL of Hepatitis B Immune Globulin (HBIG) within 12 hours of birth at separate sites. The second dose is recommended at age 1 to 2 months. The last dose in the immunization series should not be administered before age 24 weeks. These infants should be tested for HBsAg and antibody to HBsAg (anti-HBs) at age 9 to 15 months.

Infants born to mothers whose HBsAg status is unknown should receive the first dose of the HepB series within 12 hours of birth. Maternal blood should be drawn as soon as possible to determine the mother's HBsAg status; if the HBsAg test is positive, the infant should receive HBIG as soon as possible (no later than age 1 week). The second dose is recommended at age 1 to 2 months. The last dose in the immunization series should not be administered before age 24 weeks.

2. Diphtheria and tetanus toxoids and acellular pertussis (DTaP) vaccine. The fourth dose of DTaP may be administered as early as age 12 months, provided 6 months have elapsed since the third dose and the child is unlikely to return at age 15 to 18 months. The final dose in the series should be given at age ≥4 years. **Tetanus and diphtheria toxoids (Td)** is recommended at age 11 to 12 years if at least 5 years have elapsed since the last dose of tetanus and diphtheria toxoid-containing vaccine. Subsequent routine Td boosters are recommended every 10 years.

3. Haemophilus influenzae type b (Hib) conjugate vaccine. Three Hib conjugate vaccines are licensed for infant use. If PRP-OMP (PedvaxHIB or ComVax [Merck]) is administered at ages 2 and 4 months, a dose at age 6 months is not required. DTaP/Hib combination products should not be used for primary immunization in infants at ages 2, 4 or 6 months but can be used as boosters following any Hib vaccine. The final dose in the series should be given at age ≥12 months.

4. Measles, mumps, and rubella vaccine (MMR). The second dose of MMR is recommended routinely at age 4 to 6 years but may be administered during any visit, provided at least 4 weeks have elapsed since the first dose and both doses are administered beginning at or after age 12 months. Those who have not previously received the second dose should complete the schedule by the 11- to 12-year-old visit.

5. Varicella vaccine. Varicella vaccine is recommended at any visit at or after age 12 months for susceptible children (i.e., those who lack a reliable history of chickenpox). Susceptible persons age ≥13 years should receive 2 doses, given at least 4 weeks apart.

6. Pneumococcal vaccine. The heptavalent **pneumococcal conjugate vaccine (PCV)** is recommended for all children age 2 to 23 months. It is also recommended for certain children age 24 to 59 months. The final dose in the series should be given at age ≥12 months. **Pneumococcal polysaccharide vaccine (PPV)** is recommended in addition to PCV for certain high-risk groups. See MMWR 2000;49(RR-9):1-38.

7. Hepatitis A vaccine. Hepatitis A vaccine is recommended for children and adolescents in selected states and regions and for certain high-risk groups; consult your local public health authority. Children and adolescents in these states, regions, and high-risk groups who have not been immunized against hepatitis A can begin the hepatitis A immunization series during any visit. The 2 doses in the series should be administered at least 6 months apart. See MMWR 1999;48(RR-12):1-37.

8. Influenza vaccine. Influenza vaccine is recommended annually for children age ≥6 months with certain risk factors (including but not limited to children with asthma, cardiac disease, sickle cell disease, human immunodeficiency virus infection, and diabetes; and household members of persons in high-risk groups [see MMWR 2003;52(RR-8):1-36]) and can be administered to all others wishing to obtain immunity. In addition, healthy children age 6 to 23 months are encouraged to receive influenza vaccine if feasible, because children in this age group are at substantially increased risk of influenza-related hospitalizations. For healthy persons age 5 to 49 years, the intranasally administered live-attenuated influenza vaccine (LAIV) is an acceptable alternative to the intramuscular trivalent inactivated influenza vaccine (TIV). See MMWR 2003;52(RR-13):1-8. Children receiving TIV should be administered a dosage appropriate for their age (0.25 mL if age 6 to 35 months or 0.5 mL if age ≥3 years). Children age ≤8 years who are receiving influenza vaccine for the first time should receive 2 doses (separated by at least 4 weeks for TIV and at least 6 weeks for LAIV).

For additional information about vaccines, including precautions and contraindications for immunization and vaccine shortages, please visit the National Immunization Program Web site at www.cdc.gov/nip/ or call the National Immunization Information Hotline at 800-232-2522 (English) or 800-232-0233 (Spanish).

Approved by the Advisory Committee on Immunization Practices (www.cdc.gov/nip/acip), the American Academy of Pediatrics (www.aap.org), and the American Academy of Family Physicians (www.aafp.org).

FIGURE 39–3. An Immunization Schedule. (Courtesy of the American Academy of Pediatrics.)

Table 39-2 **COMMON CHILDHOOD ILLNESSES**

Illness	Signs and Symptoms	Cause	Treatment
Common cold	Congestion, cough, malaise, sore throat, fever	Virus	Increase PO fluids, rest, cold mist humidifier, antihistamine, decongestant
Gastroenteritis	Vomiting, diarrhea, fever	Virus or bacterium	Increase PO fluids, medication to relieve symptoms
Otitis media	Earache (may accompany or follow a cold), reduced hearing, fever, tugging at the affected ear in infants	Virus or bacterium	Increased PO fluids, antihistamine, decongestant, antibiotic for bacterial infection

vaccines become available (FIG. 39-3). These schedules should be posted prominently in the office and replaced as necessary with the latest information. For various reasons, some children are not on the suggested immunization schedule, but all children must be current with their immunizations before they are permitted to attend public school.

The Sick-Child Office Visit

A **sick-child visit** occurs whenever an infant or child requires medical treatment for signs or symptoms of illness or injury. The goal of these visits is diagnosis and treatment of the child's immediate illness or injury. After examining the child, the physician may pursue diagnostic tests and treatments including radiography, laboratory tests, medication, or simply the reassurance that the illness will run a predictable and manageable course. TABLE 39-2 lists three common childhood illnesses and their causes, signs and symptoms, and treatments.

Checkpoint Question

2. What is the difference between well-child and sick-child visits?

LEGAL TIP

Before treating a minor patient, generally a person un der age 18 years, parental permission must be obtained. The exceptions to this rule:
- Pregnancy or prenatal care
- Sexually transmitted disease
- Rape
- Life-threatening injury

Emancipated minors (children under age 18 years who support themselves financially), minors enlisted in the armed services, and married minors may obtain treatment without parental consent. You are responsible for knowing your state's laws regarding the treatment of minors.

CHILD DEVELOPMENT

Psychological Aspects of Care

Understanding a child's psychological needs and development helps you provide safe and effective care. During an office visit, the patient may have the same feelings as adults: fear and powerlessness. However, depending on the child's age and ability to understand, the behaviors associated with these feelings are different from those of the adult patient. Specifically, children may have these feelings:

- Fear that something painful and frightening will be done
- Anxiety about repetition of a previous bad experience
- Guilt and feelings of being punished for being bad or misbehaving
- Powerlessness and loss of physical autonomy
- Curiosity about new surroundings and experiences

Some children verbalize these feelings, while others can express them only by crying and resisting the approach of the medical staff. As a professional medical assistant, you can reassure patients and family members by demonstrating your understanding of the child's feelings and displaying a kind and gentle manner. Include the child in the explanation of procedures on an age-appropriate level. Children who are encouraged to "help" during the examination or procedure (such as holding the adhesive bandage before receiving an injection) may also feel part of the examination and may be more cooperative.

Parents are a source of support and comfort to a child. Their presence minimizes stress in unfamiliar surroundings. Encourage parents to remain with young children and to assist in care when appropriate. For instance, ask the parent to stand beside the child as you weigh him or her. Many children are more compliant if much of the preliminary workup is performed while the parent **restrains**, or holds, the child (FIG. 39-4).

As a child develops and becomes more **autonomous**, or independent, a parent's immediate presence may be less meaningful as long as the child knows that the parent is close by. Many adolescent patients prefer to be alone with the physician to demonstrate their independence and to discuss matters that they may not be comfortable talking about with the parent present. Depending on the maturity of the adolescent, ask the patient, not the parent, if the parent should be present during the examination.

Checkpoint Question

3. What kinds of feelings might a pediatric patient experience during an office visit?

Physiological Aspects of Care

To anticipate age-appropriate behavior and to provide proper psychological support and physical care, you must have a broad knowledge of child growth and development patterns. Never expect a child to react or respond beyond his or her developmental age. For example, a 2-year-old is naturally reluctant to be examined and may resist your advances. Many 4- or 5-year-olds are curious and willing to cooperate if you turn the examination into a game. Children older than 4 years should understand the need to comply, but this age group may still have to be restrained during some procedures, such as injections. A normal child's growth and development of mind, body, and personality follow an orderly progression. TABLE 39-3 describes the stages of growth and development and lists special considerations for the medical assistant.

The nervous system is complete but immature at birth. During regular visits to the pediatrician, the infant is tested

FIGURE 39-4. Much of the examination can be performed while the mother holds the baby.

for infantile automatisms—reflexes found in the newborn that disappear later in childhood. Examples include the Moro (or startle) reflex and the rooting reflex. The absence of infantile automatisms or continuation of these reflexes beyond infancy suggests central nervous system dysfunction and requires further testing. One of the most popular tools for evaluating specific gross and fine motor coordination is the Denver Developmental Screening Test (DDST) II (Fig. 39-1). The DDST II evaluates children from the most basic reflexes to complex interpersonal reactions. If you perform the assessment, you should be trained in proper testing to evoke the most diagnostic response. The indicators are registered in a vertical line drawn at the child's age. Children should register within the normal range for their age. The DDST does not measure intelligence levels.

THE PEDIATRIC PHYSICAL EXAMINATION

Typically, you prepare the patient for examination, and you may also assist with the examination by restraining the child. Often you are responsible for documenting much of the history and the chief complaint and for collecting specimens for diagnostic testing. When approaching the patient, you should have a calm and cheerful manner and use a firm but gentle touch to increase the patient's feeling of security. Involve the parents as much as possible during the examination and keep them in the infant or child's view to reduce anxiety for both the patient and the parent.

During the examination, the physician will systematically review the body systems of the patient. The general appearance of the infant or child is assessed, the heart and lungs auscultated, the eyes, ears, nose, and throat inspected, and developmental issues appropriate for the age of the child discussed with the parent or caregiver. The child who is preschool age or older will have vision and hearing tested. Your role includes obtaining relevant data from the parent, obtaining anthropometric measurements, and performing hearing and vision screening tests as appropriate. Of course,

WHAT IF

A child's mother complains that her baby vomits everything he eats?

If the vomiting is projectile, the child may have pyloric stenosis, a disorder usually seen in infants several days to several months old. Diagnosis is usually made by parental history, physical examination, and radiography. The physician often can palpate an olive-shaped lump in the right upper quadrant of the abdomen while the child is supine. Surgery (pyloroplasty) is the treatment. Although pyloric stenosis is not an emergency, surgery is usually scheduled promptly to prevent dehydration. Inform the parents about the disorder and reassure them as needed.

Vomiting may also be caused by gastroenteritis, or an infection of the stomach and intestines caused by a bacterium or virus. These infants may also have diarrhea. Regardless of the cause, infants may dehydrate very quickly and should be seen by the physician without delay.

Table 39-3 PEDIATRIC GROWTH AND DEVELOPMENTAL STAGES

Age	Growth	Stage	Development	MA Considerations
Infancy (0–1 yr)	Triples birth weight; increases physical control of body; sits and stands; may walk by 1st birthday	Trust	Newborn can see, hear, smell, feel pain, communicate. Protective mechanisms include blink reflex, pulling in for warmth, pulling away from pain or restraint. Development cephalic to caudal: head control; then full body control (e.g., rolling over, crawling, walking); then motor development (e.g., picking up small objects). Fastest period of growth, development, from total dependence to walking and talking.	Involve parent; keep parent in child's view; Approach child slowly; use soft, soothing voice; speak reassurance; advise parents to call about fever over 100.5°F rectally, diarrhea, vomiting, failure to nurse or take a bottle. Encourage appropriate use of car seat as required by law in most states.
Toddler (1–3 yr)	Growth rate slows; Body proportions change; Language skills begin	Autonomy	Growth levels off but exploration and social development continue. Negativism precedes autonomy. The child will begin to seek relationships and is acutely aware of strangers.	Use all skills above; explain procedures so child can understand; expect resistance; use firm, direct approach; ignore negative behavior; restrain to maintain child's safety; allow child to hold security object. Warn parents of increased potential for accidents. Continue to encourage use of car seat and proper restraint in motor vehicle.
Preschool (3–6 yr)	Language and self-control develop; motor skills increase	Initiative	Socialization continues, with fairly clearly marked stages of social development in next 10 years. Many early-stage problems resolve; except for usual communicable diseases, generally a time of good health. Diseases such as leukemia, Hodgkin disease, various sarcomata may present, but these years usually spent establishing relationships with peers, exercising autonomy, completing growth process.	Use all skills above; Encourage child to speak feelings; explain why procedure being done; have child help as much as possible (e.g., hold equipment). Advise parents to be alert for risks of accidents and trauma with riding toys such as tricycles and bicycles. Encourage the use of helmet. *Children over 40 lb or 4 yr can use booster seat until age 8 or 4 ft 9 in tall. Check your state laws.*
School age (6–12 yr)	Social skills develop; Peer group becomes important; Self-concept develops	Industry		Involve child in decision making; involve child in care, e.g., collecting specimens, choosing which procedure first; encourage and support questions. Children may indicate what hurts and how they feel, so include child when asking questions. *Encourage use of booster seat to age 8 and seat belt thereafter according to state law.*
Adolescent (12–18 yr)	Emotional changes; identity, place in world being defined	Identity		Discuss procedures so adolescent can understand; adolescents may resist authority figures; be sure patient education includes smoking, alcohol, perhaps birth control and STDs. At physician's discretion, this information may be discussed without parent. As children in this age group begin to drive, encourage use of seat belts for self and passengers.

STD, sexually transmitted disease; MA, medical assistant.

you will be responsible for recording this information in the patient's medical record.

The Pediatric History

A child's medical history differs greatly from an adult patient's history. During the early years, it is important to know the history of the mother's pregnancy, labor, and delivery. The length of the pregnancy, any maternal illnesses or complications, neonatal complications, and risk factors must be recorded as predictors of the infant's health and development. Most newborn charts contain a copy of the delivery record or birth summary outlining the delivery with the Apgar score and progress notes from the newborn nursery (Box 39-1). As the child grows, the history expands to include childhood illnesses, developmental milestones, immunizations, and nutritional status.

Obtaining and Recording Measurements and Vital Signs

Before the physical examination is conducted, you should obtain some or all of the following measurements: height or length, head and chest circumference, weight, temperature, and the pulse and respiratory rate. The blood pressure may or may not be required, depending on the child's age and the preference of the examiner. The measurements and schedule for obtaining them should be detailed in the office policy and procedure manual.

In a well-child visit, you typically measure the child's height or length, head and chest circumference, and weight. These measurements show the child's growth and development patterns and are good indicators of health status. Weight is the most frequently obtained measurement in pediatrics, often needed by the physician to assess nutritional status and determine medication dosages. Head and chest measurements may alert the physician to cardiac or intracranial abnormalities. Procedures 39-1 and 39-2 describe the steps for obtaining the weight, length, and head and chest circumference.

After obtaining these measurements, you may be required to graph the weight, height or length, and head circumference on a growth chart in the patient's medical record (FIG. 39-5). These charts are designed to show the child's growth patterns using data obtained at each well-child visit. Once the measurements are plotted, the child's percentile can be determined. The percentile is used to compare the patient's growth with those of children of the same age. The head circumference is not included on growth charts for children older than 36 months, and chest circumference is usually not graphed.

Checkpoint Question

4. Why is it important to track a child's anthropometric measurements?

Box 39-1

THE APGAR SCORE

Named for pediatrician Virginia Apgar, the Apgar score is a method for describing the general health of newborns at 1 minute and 5 minutes after delivery. Signs assessed:
- Heart rate
- Respiratory effort
- Muscle tone
- Response to a suction catheter in the nostril
- Color

A perfect score for each sign is 2; a total absence of any sign is 0. A perfect score of 10 indicates the following:
- Heart rate is greater than 100 beats per minute.
- Respirations are eupneic or the baby is crying.
- Muscle tone is good and the baby is active.
- Baby coughs or sneezes in response to suction catheter.
- Skin is completely pink, with no acrocyanosis.

Most babies have 1-minute scores of 7 to 9, because many have a bit of acrocyanosis until respiration is fully established. Babies with 1-minute scores below 4 usually require medical assistance, particularly respiratory intervention with oxygen.

The Apgar score is not considered an indicator of future intelligence or health problems. Rather, it is used by the obstetrician, pediatrician, and delivery room personnel to assess newborns who may require closer observation or intervention.

Pediatric Vital Signs

Temperature. A child's temperature may be measured by the axillary, oral, rectal, or tympanic method (FIG. 39-6). If the child is compliant, the axillary route is satisfactory, but the tympanic method has gained popularity because it is rapid, reliable, and most readily accepted at all ages. Oral measurement may be used with an older child but should not be used if the child is congested, coughing, vomiting, or uncooperative. The rectal route should not be used for newborns and small infants or if the child has diarrhea.

Pulse and Respiration. The pulse rate reflects the heart rate and usually is easily measured. Pulse rate can be affected by activity, body temperature, emotion, and illness. The pulse of children under 2 years of age should be assessed apically. To do this, place the stethoscope on the chest between the sternum and left nipple. Count the rate for 1 full minute. For children older than 2 years, take the radial pulse. Expect the child's heart rate to be considerably higher than an

**Birth to 36 months: Girls
Head circumference-for-age and
Weight-for-length percentiles**

NAME _____

RECORD # _____

Published May 30, 2000 (modified 10/16/00).
SOURCE: Developed by the National Center for Health Statistics in collaboration with
the National Center for Chronic Disease Prevention and Health Promotion (2000).
http://www.cdc.gov/growthcharts

A

FIGURE 39-5. Growth charts. (**A**) For girls birth to 36 months for length, weight, and head circumference.

2 to 20 years: Boys
Stature-for-age and Weight-for-age percentiles

F I G U R E   3 9 – 5 .   *(continued)* (**B**) For boys 2 to 20 years for height and weight. (Courtesy of the Centers for Disease Control and Prevention.)

FIGURE 39–6. The axillary temperature is readily acceptable to most children and is considered accurate if the child is compliant.

Table 39-5	NORMAL RESPIRATORY RATES FOR CHILDREN
Age	**Rate/Minute**
Newborn	30–35
1–2 yr	25–30
4–6 yr	23–25
8 yr and older	16–20

adult's. A newborn may have a pulse rate of 100 to 180 beats per minute, and with fever a rate of 200 beats per minute or more is not unusual. As the child matures, the rate will slow. By age 2, a child's rate may range from 70 to 100 beats per minute. By puberty, the rate is comparable to that of an adult. TABLE 39-4 details normal pulse rates for children.

Measure respiratory rate by observing the rise and fall of the child's chest. It is not necessary to disguise the fact that you are counting respirations as with adults. Because infants breathe using the abdominal muscles more than the chest, observe abdominal movements and count for 1 full minute. For children over age 2 years, use the same method as adults: count the respiratory rate for 30 seconds and multiply by two. Expect a newborn's respiratory rate to be as high as 35 per minute (TABLE 39-5). Like the pulse rate, the respiratory rate will slow as the child matures. At age 2 years it will be about 25, and by puberty it will be comparable to an adult's.

Blood Pressure. Blood pressure measurements are not required for most pediatric patients but may be appropriate at times. Blood pressure is the most difficult measurement to obtain in an infant or child because it is so difficult to prevent movement. Infants and children have smaller ex-

tremities than adults and require a smaller cuff. Because of their soft, nonresistant vessels and smaller bodies, children have lower blood pressure than adults. You may have problems determining the diastolic pressure in some children using a standard sphygmomanometer. In children less than 1 year of age, expect a blood pressure of about 90/50. The blood pressure will gradually rise as the child matures. By age 10, a child's blood pressure will be in the low normal range of 110/60 (TABLE 39-6). Blood pressure checks become routine when children are about school age.

 Checkpoint Question

5. How does a child's pulse and respiratory rate differ from an adult's?

Using Restraints

During the examination and certain procedures, you may need to help restrain the child. Restraining is sometimes necessary to protect the child from injury and to help the physician complete the examination in a timely manner. Many children understandably resist the examination or procedure because they are frightened and do not want to be touched. Calm and gentle restraint is in the best interest of everyone involved (FIG. 39-7).

ADMINISTERING MEDICATIONS

Administering medications to children challenges you and the parents who are responsible for home administration. Medication dosages for children are calculated by weight or

Table 39-4	NORMAL PULSE RATES FOR CHILDREN
Age	**Rate/Minute**
Newborn	100–180
3 mo–2 yr	80–150
2–10 yr	65–130
10 yr and older	60–100

Table 39-6	NORMAL BLOOD PRESSURE FOR CHILDREN	
Age	**Systolic**	**Diastolic**
Newborn	<90	<70
1–5 yr	<110	<70
10 yr and older	<120	<84

In millimeters of mercury.

FIGURE 39-7. Mummy restraint. Place the child diagonally on a small receiving blanket. (**A**) Wrap the right corner across the torso, covering the right arm and shoulder. Pull it snugly under the child's left arm and tuck it under the child's body. (**B**) Pull the left corner across the child's left arm and shoulder and tuck it snugly under the torso at the back so that the child's weight secures the end. (**C**) Wrap the end of the blanket up around the child.

by body surface area. However, because children vary in weight, age, and fat-to-muscle ratio, they metabolize and absorb medication at varying rates. As a result, the physician prescribes medication according to how much the child weighs, and you must give only the amount prescribed. To prevent errors, always check drug dosage calculations for an infant or child with another staff member. The formulas for calculating pediatric dosages are described in Chapter 8. Before administering any medication, you should know the safe amount, correct administration procedure, intended actions, and side effects. In most pediatric practices, the physician uses only 50 or so medications that are suitable for children, making it relatively easy for you to learn all that is necessary about each medication. As for any medication, the seven "rights" of drug administration remain the same: the *right patient, right drug, right dose, right route, right time, right method*, and *right documentation.*

Oral Medications

Use caution when administering oral medications to a child to prevent **aspiration**. Hold infants in a semireclining position, not lying down. Place the medication in the mouth beside the tongue. Depending on the child's age, use a medication spoon, syringe, dropper, or medicine cup. Many children will suck medication from a syringe easily and safely. Administer small amounts of medication, allowing the child time to swallow. Always explain to children who are old enough to understand why medications are important, then proceed in a swift and safe manner to give the medication.

Injections

Medications are given to infants and children by injection when there is no choice. Children commonly fear injections more than any other medical procedure. You should approach the child in a calm and firm manner, but never lie to the child or say that the injection will not hurt. Although it is important for the child to know that an injection is about to be given, you can prevent some anxiety by not letting the child see the syringe. Offer the child an age-appropriate explanation, then quickly give the medication. After administering any medication, praise and comfort the child.

Most children's injections are given in the vastus lateralis, at least until age 2 years (FIG. 39-8). The dorsogluteal site is not used for children under age 2 years because the muscles have not developed well. Chapter 8 lists the steps in administering an intramuscular injection.

 Checkpoint Question

6. How is medication dosage calculated for children?

COLLECTING A URINE SPECIMEN

Because infants and small children cannot void into a specimen container on command, if a urine specimen is needed, you must use a collection device. Procedure 39-3 describes the procedure for applying it. Once applied, the device should be left in place until the infant urinates. The infant may wear a diaper over the collection device until the specimen is obtained.

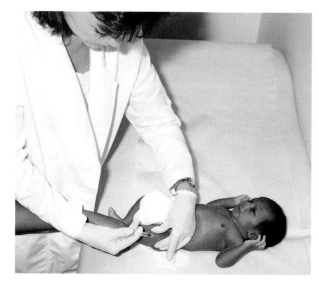

FIGURE 39-8. The vastus lateralis is the site of choice for infant injections.

UNDERSTANDING CHILD ABUSE

A child's social and physical well-being may be compromised by physical or emotional abuse or neglect or by sexual abuse. Abuse is thought to be the second most common cause of death in children under age 5 years. Although many children are permanently disabled or seriously injured as a result of physical abuse, many more carry emotional scars that will never heal.

The Federal Child Abuse Prevention and Treatment Act mandates that threats to a child's physical and mental welfare be reported by anyone having contact with children in a professional or employment setting (e.g., teachers, physicians, nurses, medical assistants, day care workers). Health care workers, teachers, social workers, and others who work with children are protected against liability if they report their suspicions in good faith. Medical assistants should be aware of the signs of abuse—either obvious indications or subtle warnings—that must be pursued for the child's safety.

These are the obvious indications of child abuse:

- Reports of physical or sexual abuse by the child
- Previous reports of abuse in the family with current indicators
- Conflicting stories about the "accident" or injury from the parents and the child
- Injuries inconsistent with the history
- Injuries blamed on siblings or someone other than the parent
- Repeated emergency room visits for injuries
- Fractures, burns, or skeletal injuries of a suspicious nature

These indications of child abuse are hidden or not apparent:

- Dislocations

WHAT IF

You notice bruises and burn marks on the chest and back of the 3-year-old girl you are assessing?

If you suspect a child is being abused, approach the child and the parent in a calm and supportive manner. Discuss any suspicions about the cause of a child's injuries privately with the physician right away. State laws vary regarding the procedure for reporting abuse; local regulations should be outlined in the policies and procedures manual. As a medical assistant, you have an ethical and moral responsibility to report suspected cases of abuse or neglect.

- Nervous system trauma, particularly shaken baby syndrome
- Internal injuries, particularly to the abdominal area

These are behavioral indications of child abuse:

- Too-willing compliance, overeagerness to please
- Passive avoidance, such as refusing to make eye contact, shrinking from contact
- Extremely aggressive, demanding, rage-filled behavior
- Role reversal, parenting the parent
- Developmental delay (the child may be using energy needed for maturation to defend against abuse)

These are the warning signs of child abuse:

- Malnutrition
- Poor growth pattern
- Poor hygiene
- Gross dental disorders
- Unattended medical needs

PEDIATRIC ILLNESSES AND DISORDERS

Because children do not have a well-developed immune system, they are particularly susceptible to viruses and bacterial infections. As a result, sick-child visits occur frequently during early childhood. Some infants and small children have febrile seizures during illness because of the child's immature nervous system. This does not mean that the child will be prone to seizures as he or she matures. Parents should be instructed how to obtain a child's temperature and be encouraged to call the office for any evidence of a fever. All parents should be advised never to give aspirin to young children with viral fever, since aspirin has been associated with Reye syndrome. This syndrome causes encephalopathy and fatty infiltration of the internal organs and may cause either mental retardation or death. Check with the physician about the type of medication to use before suggesting any antipyretic, including over-the-counter medications.

Impetigo

A common skin disorder in children is impetigo, a contagious bacterial infection that may be caused by either Staphylococcus or Streptococcus. The lesions commonly occur on the face, neck, and other exposed areas of the body. Patches of exudative vesicles produce honey-colored crusts. These vesicles leave red areas when the crusts are removed.

The treatment for impetigo is washing the area two to three times a day and applying a topical antibiotic. An oral antibiotic may be prescribed for severe cases. Discourage scratching and advise parents to keep separate and wash frequently any towels, washcloths, and bed linens to prevent the spread of the disease.

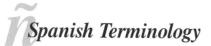

Spanish Terminology

Ha tenido la criatura alguna enfermedad o lesiónes?	Has the child had any illnesses or injuries?
Necesitamos una muestra de su orina.	We need a urine specimen.
Que vacunas se han dado a la criatura?	Which immunizations has the child received?
Tose el niño por la noche?	Does the child cough at night?
Con que frecuencia evacua la criatura?	How often does the child have a bowel movement?

Meningitis

Inflammation of the meninges covering the spinal cord and the brain, meningitis can result from either a bacterial or a viral infection. Viral meningitis is usually not life-threatening and is short lived, but bacterial meningitis is often severe and may be fatal. The infectious process is usually precipitated by an upper respiratory, sinus, or ear infection, and since these infections commonly occur in children under age 5 years, they are the most likely age group to develop meningitis. Meningitis can also result from head trauma in which an open area allows the microorganisms to enter the nervous system. Older adolescents living in college dormitories or residence halls are also at high risk for meningitis and should be immunized before leaving for college.

The signs and symptoms of meningitis include nausea, vomiting, fever, headaches, and a stiff neck. A rash with small, reddish purple dots may appear on the body. As the patient becomes sicker, he or she may become comatose and develop seizures. To diagnose meningitis, the physician usually orders a complete blood count, and if the white blood cell count is elevated, a lumbar puncture is performed to withdraw cerebrospinal fluid for analysis. The treatment of meningitis is based on the microorganism. Viral meningitis is treated with oral fluids and bed rest, and bacterial meningitis is treated with an antibiotic and generally hospitalization.

Checkpoint Question

7. How does treatment of viral meningitis differ from that of bacterial meningitis?

Encephalitis

Encephalitis is inflammation of the brain that frequently results from a viral infection following chickenpox, measles, or mumps. A strain of the virus is transmitted by mosquitoes. This type is primarily seen on the East and Gulf coasts. Symptoms of all forms include drowsiness, headache, and fever in the early stages; however, seizures and coma may occur in the later stages. Diagnosis is by a lumbar puncture and analysis of the cerebrospinal fluid. Treatment requires hospitalization for intravenous therapy

and supportive care, but the prognosis is usually good if the diagnosis is made early and treatment begins quickly.

Tetanus

Tetanus, commonly called lockjaw, is an infection of nervous tissue caused by the tetanus bacillus, *Clostridium tetani*, which lives in the intestinal tract of animals and is excreted in their feces. The organisms are found in almost all soil. The bacilli enter the body through a puncture wound or open area in the skin. Wounds caused by farm equipment in which manure is present are especially susceptible to tetanus. All deep, dirty wounds should be treated as high risk for tetanus.

Checkpoint Question

8. What is the best way to prevent polio?

Cerebral Palsy

Cerebral palsy is a term for a group of neuromuscular disorders that result from central nervous system damage sustained during the prenatal, neonatal, or postnatal period of development. Although cerebral palsy is not progressive, the damage may become more obvious as developmental delays are discovered. Impairment may range from slight motor dysfunction to catastrophic physical and mental disabilities. Prognosis varies with the site of the damage and its severity. Treatment is supportive and rehabilitative. There is no cure.

Croup

Laryngotracheobronchitis, also known as croup, is a disease primarily seen in children 3 months to 3 years of age. It is caused by a viral infection of the larynx resulting in swelling and narrowing of the airway. This results in difficulty breathing characterized by a high-pitched crowing wheeze (stridor) on inspiration and a sharp barking cough. Treatment may include hospitalization, cool mist vaporizer, and medication to decrease the swelling.

PATIENT EDUCATION

Middle Ear Infections

Explain to the child's parents that children have short, straight eustachian tubes. Upper respiratory infections, particularly with coughing, may force microorganisms into the middle ear spaces. As the infection grows, the eustachian tubes swell and eventually close. Exudate from the mucous membrane continues to be produced, causing fluid to build with resulting pressure and pain.

Bacterial otitis media (middle ear infection) has been associated with and may be caused by putting the child to bed with a bottle of milk, juice, or formula. The drink and bacteria set up a medium for growth within the eustachian tube.

Epiglottitis

Swelling of the epiglottis may resemble croup, but it is usually more serious and may be life-threatening if it progresses to complete obstruction of the airway. It occurs most frequently in children aged 2 to 6 years, although it can be seen in all age groups. It is caused by a bacterial infection, usually *Haemophilus influenzae*. A child diagnosed with epiglottitis in the medical office must be transported immediately to the hospital, since the first priority is maintaining and possibly establishing an airway. As with any medical emergency in the office, you must be prepared to assist the physician as needed while contacting the emergency medical services for transport. In addition, the parents of the sick child will need support and guidance during this emotional time.

Cystic Fibrosis

Cystic fibrosis is an inherited disease that affects the exocrine glands of the body, changing their secretions and making the mucus extremely thick and sticky. Although it affects several areas of the body, the most serious complications of cystic fibrosis are usually respiratory. Children with this disease are prone to repeated respiratory infections because of the difficulty in clearing the mucus from their airways. Treatment of cystic fibrosis includes medication to reduce the thickness of secretions and frequent breathing treatments to maintain open airways. Many new treatments are being developed, and much exciting research into prevention and cure is under way.

Checkpoint Question

9. Why is epiglottitis considered a medical emergency?

Asthma

As discussed in Chapter 32, asthma is a reversible inflammatory process of the bronchi and bronchioles. When a patient with asthma has dyspnea, it is due to bronchospasm and constriction of the smooth muscle lining the airways. Patients have an increase in mucus production with a productive cough. It becomes difficult for the patient to move air into and out of the lungs. In children, attacks may be triggered by exposure to an allergen in the environment such as mold or dust, an inhaled irritant such as cigarette smoke, or upper respiratory infection. Many children who develop asthma outgrow it by adulthood.

The treatment for asthma includes the administration of bronchodilators through an inhaler, which may not be appropriate for a small child or infant, or through a machine (nebulizer) (see Chapter 32 for more information about nebulized breathing treatments). An infant or small child will not be able to hold the mouthpiece tightly between the lips during the treatment; however, masks are available. As with adult patients taking bronchodilators, the pulse rate should be monitored before, during, and after the treatment.

PATIENT EDUCATION

Coping With Febrile Seizures

Febrile (fever) seizures can be very scary for parents of small children. Here's how you can help parents cope:

- Reassure the parents that febrile seizures are common in young children and that they generally do not become chronic.
- Provide easy-to-understand explanations for all procedures.
- Encourage parents to speak about their fears.
- If the seizure occurs in the medical office, urge the parents to hold and comfort the child once the child is stabilized.

You too will probably be anxious if a seizure occurs in the office, but you must remain calm and demonstrate confidence in handling the situation.

Otitis Media

Otitis media, an inflammation or infection of the middle ear, is frequently caused by an upper respiratory infection (URI) in infants and children. This disorder is particularly common in infants and children because of the relatively horizontal position of the eustachian tube between the nasopharynx and middle ear (see Chapter 31). Symptoms include severe pain, fever of varying degrees, and mild to moderate hearing loss. Infants may be fussy and tug at their ears. Any elevation in a child's temperature should be a warning to check for otitis media.

Diagnosis is usually made by inspecting the tympanic membrane with an otoscope, which reveals a reddened, bulging tympanic membrane. If the suspected pathogen is bacterial, an antibiotic may be prescribed. With the exception of aspirin, analgesics are often recommended for the relief of the pain. If nasal congestion is present, a decongestant may reduce some of the swelling. In severe chronic cases, surgery may be performed to relieve pressure, and tubes may be inserted through the tympanic membrane to equalize the pressure.

Tonsillitis

Pharyngitis, or a sore throat, may be caused by inflammation of the tissues of the throat and/or the tonsils (see Chapter 31). Inspection of the throat may reveal the tissue to be red and swollen, possibly with pustules on the tonsils or in the throat. When a diagnosis of tonsillitis is made, you may be asked to take a sample for a throat culture to rule out streptococcus bacteria as the causative pathogen. If the throat culture is positive for streptococcus, an antibiotic will be ordered. If the throat culture is negative but the infection appears bacterial, an antibiotic may still be prescribed. Chronic tonsillitis may be treated by surgical removal of the tonsils—a tonsillectomy—by a surgeon who specializes in disorders of the ears, nose, and throat.

Checkpoint Question

10. Why is otitis media more common in children than adults?

Obesity

According to the American Academy of Pediatrics (AAP), obesity in children has become an epidemic. The importance of assessing the weight and length of infants and children and plotting this information on the appropriate growth chart is essential in assisting the physician in early recognition; however, prevention of obesity is even more important in preventing long-term complications, such as heart disease and diabetes. You must ask parents or caregivers during each visit to the office about the eating patterns, nutrition status, and activity levels of the child and offer education and support when necessary or as indicated by the physician. Since children develop eating habits early in life and take these habits into adulthood, you should teach parents about eating in moderation and increasing physical activity as a means to reduce the weight of an overweight child or prevent abnormal gains in weight. If the physician prescribes a specific diet or reduces caloric intake, you should offer support and guidance to the caregiver as needed.

Attention Deficit Hyperactivity Disorder

Attention deficit hyperactivity disorder (ADHD) is a condition of the brain affecting boys more frequently than girls and causing difficulty in controlling behavior. The problematic behavior in children with ADHD includes these signs of inattention in the school-age child:

- Daydreaming or difficulty paying attention
- Easy distraction
- Inability to complete tasks
- Forgetfulness
- Reluctance to perform tasks that require mental effort
- Low grades in school

The hyperactivity is often seen thus:

- Excessive talking
- Inability to sit quietly for any length of time
- Breaking rules regarding running or jumping

In addition to inattention and hyperactivity, children with ADHD are often impulsive and behave irrationally to others, even after being repeatedly warned about a specific behavior, dangerous or not. These children have difficulty taking turns and may be disruptive, shouting out answers before being called on in the classroom.

The diagnosis for a child with ADHD is often based on a thorough history of the child's behaviors, including reports from teachers or other professionals who work with the child. The AAP publishes guidelines for diagnosing ADHD in children aged 6 to 12 years. There is no one test for diagnosing this disorder; instead, the diagnosis is based on certain behaviors in several settings (i.e., school and home). Once the physician has made the diagnosis, an individual treatment plan is devised; it may include behavior therapy, psychological counseling for the child and the family, education about ADHD, coordination of the treatment plan with the family and involved teachers, and stimulant medications.

Procedure 39-1

Obtaining an Infant's Length and Weight

Purpose: Accurately determine the length and weight of an infant.

Equipment: Examining table with clean paper, tape measure, infant scale, protective paper for the scale, appropriate growth chart.

Standard: This procedure should take 10 minutes.

Steps	Reason
1. Wash your hands.	Handwashing aids infection control.
2. Explain the procedure to the parent and ask him or her to remove the infant's clothing except for the diaper.	
3. Place the child on a firm examination table covered with clean table paper. If using a measuring board, cover the board with clean paper.	Measurements may not be correct if the surface is not firm. Clean paper prevents cross-infection.
4. Fully extend the child's body by holding the head in the midline. Grasp the knees and press flat onto the table gently but firmly. Make a mark on the table paper with your pen at the top of the head and at the heel of the feet.	Most infants assume a flexed position, requiring you to extend the legs for accurate measurement. If you need assistance, ask the parent or a coworker to hold the child in position. A foot board against the soles will give the most accurate measurement.
5. Measure between the marks in either inches or centimeters, according to the preference of the physician	
6. Record the child's length on the growth chart and in the patient's chart.	Procedures are considered not to have been done if they are not recorded. To plot the measurement on the growth chart, find the child's measurement in inches or centimeters and move in that line across to the age column. Make a mark where the two values intersect.
7. Either carry the infant or have the parent carry the infant to the scales.	
8. Place protective paper on the scale and balance the scale.	Protective paper prevents transmission of microorganisms. The balance beam must be centered before each use.
9. Remove the diaper just before laying the infant on the scale.	For the most accurate weight, infants should be weighed without any clothing. However, cool air against the infant's skin may cause voiding. Some offices permit the infant to be weighed in the diaper as long as it is dry and clean.

(continued)

Procedure 39-1   *(continued)*

Obtaining an Infant's Length and Weight

Steps	Reason
10. Place the child gently on the scale. Keep one of your hands over or near the child on the scale at all times.	

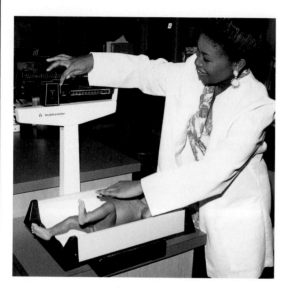

Step 10A. Infants are weighed lying down.

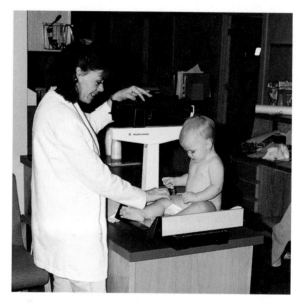

Step 10B. Infants who can sit may be weighed while sitting if this is less frightening for them.

Steps	Reason
11. Quickly but carefully move the counterweights to balance the apparatus exactly.	This will ensure accurate measurement.
12. Pick up the infant and instruct the parent to replace diaper if removed for the weight.	
13. Record the weight on the growth chart and in the patient's chart.	Procedures are considered not to have been done if they are not recorded. To plot the measurement on the growth chart, find the child's measurement in pounds or kilograms, then move in that line across to the age column. Make a mark where the two values intersect.
14. Wash your hands.	

Charting Example

02/08/2005 10:00 A.M. Length 79.5 cm, Wt. 26 lb. 10 month-old _____ J. DeBard, CMA

Procedure 39-2

Obtaining the Head and Chest Circumference

Purpose: Accurately determine the head and chest circumference of an infant.

Equipment: Paper or cloth measuring tape, growth chart

Standard: This procedure should take 5 minutes.

Steps	Reason
1. Wash your hands.	Handwashing aids infection control.
2. Place the infant supine on the examination table or ask the parent to hold the child.	

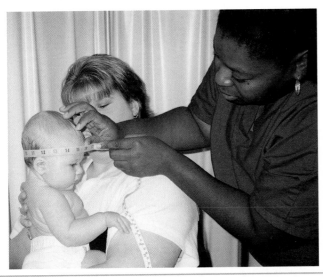

Step 2. Ask the parent to hold the child.

3. Measure around the head above the eyebrow and posteriorly at the largest part of the occiput.	For an accurate reading, measure the largest circumference.

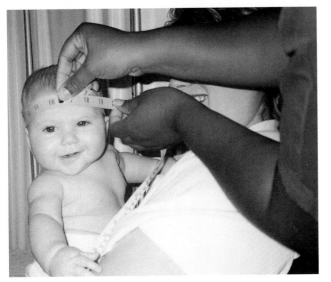

Step 3. Measure around the head above the eyebrow and posteriorly at the largest part of the occiput.

(continued)

Procedure 39-2   *(continued)*

Obtaining the Head and Chest Circumference

Steps	Reason
4. Record the child's head circumference on the growth chart and in the patient's chart.	Procedures are considered not to have been done if they are not recorded. To plot the measurement on the growth chart, find the child's measurement in inches or centimeters, then move in that line across to the age column. Make a mark where the two values intersect.
5. With the clothing removed from the chest, measure around the chest at the nipple line, keeping the measuring tape at the same level anterior and posterior.	The tape should be at the same level to ensure the most accurate reading.

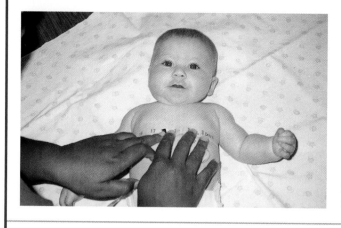

Step 5. Measure around the chest at the nipple line, keeping the measuring tape at the same level anteriorly and posteriorly.

Steps	Reason
6. Record the child's chest circumference on the growth chart and in the patient chart.	Procedures are considered not to have been done if they are not recorded. To plot the measurement on the growth chart, find the child's measurement in inches or centimeters, then move in that line across to the age column. Make a mark where the two values intersect.
7. Wash your hands.	

Note: If the head and chest growth are within normal limits, this measurement is not usually required after 12 months.

Charting Example
10/15/2005 9:45 A.M. Wt. 14 lb. Length 24 in. Head 15 in, Chest 17 in. _____ B. Brady, CMA

Procedure 39-3

Applying a Urinary Collection Device

Purpose: Correctly apply a urinary collection device to a child.

Equipment: Gloves, personal antiseptic wipes, pediatric urine collection bag, completed laboratory request slip, biohazard transport container.

Standard: This procedure should take 5 minutes.

Steps	Reason
1. Wash your hands and assemble the equipment and supplies.	Handwashing aids infection control.
2. Explain the procedure to the parents.	
3. Place the child supine. Ask for help from the parents as needed.	The child may be more cooperative if a parent helps.
4. After putting on gloves, clean the genitalia with the antiseptic wipes:	
A. For girls: Cleanse front to back with separate wipes for each downward stroke on the outer labia. The last clean wipe should be used between the inner labia.	Cleansing front to back will remove debris from the area and avoid introducing bacteria into the urethra.
B. For boys: Retract the foreskin if the baby has not been circumcised. Cleanse the meatus in an ever-widening circle. Discard the wipe and repeat the procedure. Return the foreskin to its proper position.	Cleansing outward will avoid introducing bacteria into the urethra. Returning the foreskin to the correct position will prevent constriction of the penis.
5. Holding the collection device, remove the upper portion of the paper backing and press it around the mons pubis. Remove the second section and press it against the perineum. Loosely attach the diaper.	The collection device must be securely attached to ensure collection of the next voiding. Reattaching the diaper will avoid soiling if the child has a stool.
6. Give the baby fluids unless contraindicated and check the diaper frequently.	
7. When the child has voided, remove the device, clean the skin of residual adhesive, and diaper.	Adhesive left on the skin may be irritating.
8. Prepare the specimen for transport to the laboratory or process it according to the office policy and procedure manual.	
9. Remove your gloves and wash your hands.	Standard precautions must be followed when handling body fluids.
10. Record the procedure.	Procedures are considered not to have been done if they are not recorded.

Charting Example

08/16/2005 11:45 A.M. Urine collection device applied; approximately 50 mL clear amber urine obtained after 20 minutes. Specimen sent to Acme Laboratory for urinalysis. _____ S. Schein, CMA

CHAPTER SUMMARY

Working with children offers many rewards; however, the special developmental needs and unique physiology of children makes these patients challenging and must always be taken into consideration. This chapter focuses on the skills necessary to assist the pediatrician or physician in a family practice office, whether the child is being seen for a well-child visit or for a sick-child visit. However, even though the developmental stages of children follow a normal progression, some children progress faster or more slowly than the "norm," and parents should be discouraged from comparing children of the same age.

Many childhood diseases can be prevented through an effective immunization program, and you should always be ready to answer questions regarding diseases and transmission and the vaccine to prevent those diseases. This chapter also focuses on immunizations and the role of the medical assistant in administering these vaccines. Common childhood diseases not preventable with vaccines are described. You must take every precaution when working with children to prevent the spread of these diseases whenever possible.

Critical Thinking Challenges

1. During years of practice, Dr. Hernandez has found that many new parents are unfamiliar with basic child care needs. He decides to publish a short booklet for his new parents describing various aspects of child care. The booklet should be informative and professional and show genuine concern for children. Using your creativity and your knowledge of child care, develop a sample booklet for Dr. Hernandez's patients after choosing two of these topics:

   * General safety tips
   * Types of office visits
   * Immunizations (what they are, why they are important, at what ages they are given, side effects and adverse effects)
   * What a parent can expect during an office visit
   * Brief explanation of child development
   * Tips for administering oral medications to children

2. Using the following data and an appropriate growth chart, mark the appropriate percentile for the following:

   * A 4-month-old girl whose head circumference is 43 cm

   * A 3-year-old girl who is 91 cm tall
   * A 7-month-old girl who weighs 16.5 pounds

Answers to Checkpoint Questions

1. These are safety precautions for a pediatric practice:

   * Keep all medical equipment out of a child's reach.
   * Never leave a child alone in the examining room.
   * Place infant scales on a sturdy table and never leave a child alone on a scale.
   * Store disinfectants away from patient care areas.
   * Dispose of all sharps in proper containers.
   * Practice stringent handwashing and standard precautions with every patient.

2. Well-child visits are scheduled at regular intervals and are designed to maintain the child's optimum health. Sick-child visits are scheduled as needed with the goal of diagnosing and treating a child's immediate illness or injury.

3. A child may feel fear, anxiety, guilt, powerlessness, or curiosity during an office visit.

4. A child's anthropometric measurements show the growth and are good indicators of the health status.

5. A child's pulse and respiratory rates are higher than an adult's.

6. Medication dosage in children is calculated by weight or by body surface area.

7. For viral meningitis, fluids and bed rest are encouraged. For bacterial meningitis, an antibiotic is prescribed and hospitalization may be required.

8. The best way to prevent polio is through immunization.

9. Epiglottitis is a medical emergency because the small airways of the infant or child can become occluded or blocked as the epiglottis swells, causing respiratory arrest.

10. Otitis media is common in infants and children because of the horizontal position of the eustachian tube. Microorganisms travel easily from the mouth, throat, and nasal passages to the middle ear.

 Websites

American Academy of Pediatrics www.aap.org
Advisory Committee on Immunization Practices
   www.cdc.gov/nip/publications/acip-list.htm
National Center for Health Statistics
   www.cdc.gov/growthcharts/
Vaccine Information Statements www.cdc.gov/nip/
   publications.vis

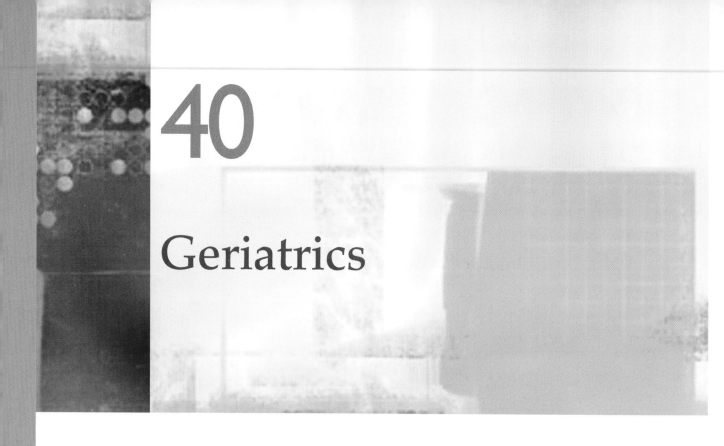

40

Geriatrics

CHAPTER OUTLINE

ROLE DELINEATION

**ADMINISTRATIVE: ADMINISTRATIVE
PROCEDURES**
- Perform basic administrative medical assisting
  functions
- Schedule, coordinate, and monitor appointments

CLINICAL: FUNDAMENTAL PRINCIPLES
- Apply principles of aseptic technique and infection
  control
- Screen and follow up patient test results

CLINICAL: PATIENT CARE
- Adhere to established patient screening procedures
- Prepare patient for examinations, procedures, and
  treatments
- Assist with examinations, procedures, and treatments
- Recognize and respond to emergencies
- Coordinate patient care information with other
  health care providers

GENERAL: PROFESSIONALISM

- Display a professional manner and image
- Demonstrate initiative and responsibility
- Work as a member of the health care team
- Treat all patients with compassion and empathy

GENERAL: COMMUNICATION SKILLS

- Adapt communications to individual's ability to understand
- Serve as a liaison

GENERAL: LEGAL CONCEPTS

- Perform within legal and ethical boundaries
- Document accurately
- Comply with established risk management and safety procedures

GENERAL: INSTRUCTION

- Instruct individuals according to their needs
- Teach methods of health promotion and disease prevention
- Locate community resources and disseminate information

CHAPTER COMPETENCIES

LEARNING OBJECTIVES

Upon successfully completing this chapter, you will be able to:

1. Spell and define the key terms.
2. Explain how aging affects thought processes.
3. Describe methods to increase compliance with health maintenance programs among the elderly.
4. Discuss communication problems that may occur with the elderly and list steps to maintain open communication.
5. Recognize and describe the coping mechanisms used by the elderly to deal with multiple losses.
6. Name the risk factors and signs of elder abuse.
7. Explain the types of long-term care facilities available.
8. Describe the effects of aging on the way the body processes medication.
9. Discuss the responsibility of medical assistants with regard to teaching elderly patients.
10. List and describe physical changes and diseases common to the aging process.

KEY TERMS

activities of daily living (ADL)	compliance	Kegel exercises	presbyopia
biotransform	degenerative joint disease (DJD)	keratosis (senile)	senility
bradykinesia	dementia	kyphosis (dowager's hump)	syncope
cataracts	dysphagia	lentigines	transient ischemic attack (TIA)
cerebrovascular accident (CVA)	gerontologist	osteoporosis	vertigo
	glaucoma	potentiation	
		presbycusis	

CONCEPTS OF AGING

As the elderly population has increased, established concepts about aging have also changed. The greeting card image of a cozy, gray-haired grandmother in her rocking chair is being replaced by a trim, active woman rushing out the door with a briefcase or tennis racket under her arm. **Gerontologists**, specialists in aging, describe many of the elderly today as healthy enough to maintain homes well into their 80s and 90s. The branch of medicine that deals with the elderly population is geriatrics, and while some physicians today are treating only geriatric patients, any physician in family practice or internal medicine will take care of the elderly. Other specialties, such as ophthalmology, also treat many geriatric patients daily. Box 40-1 outlines some myths and stereotypes about the elderly. How many are far from typical of this age group today?

Stereotyping the elderly is a subtle and usually unconscious way to disassociate ourselves from the prospect of growing old. Although other cultures respect their elderly for their wealth of wisdom and experience, the American media perpetuate myths and stereotypical reactions by implying that graying hair and wrinkles in the skin are repulsive and should be avoided at all costs. Those costs include billions of dollars spent on delaying the physical signs of aging. Consider how the following situations take on new meaning when applied to different age groups.

Box 40-1

MYTHS AND STEREOTYPES ABOUT THE ELDERLY

Myths
- Old people are weak and sick.
- Old people can no longer learn.
- Old people have no more contributions to make.
- Old people are boring.
- Old people are a drag on the economy.
- Old people are always lonely.
- Old people cannot live alone.
- Old people cannot be trusted to make rational decisions.
- Old people have lost all interest in life.

Stereotypes
- Old people have sensory losses.
- Old people have erratic sleep patterns and nap a lot.
- Old people do everything slower.
- Old people have lost stature and slump a lot.
- Old people cannot remember what happened this morning but can recall everything that happened 40 years ago.

- You are running late again. Dashing out of the door, you remember that you left the keys to the car on the kitchen table—again.
- You stride purposefully from the bedroom into the kitchen with a specific goal in mind, only to reach the kitchen without any idea why you were in such a hurry to get there.

We have all done these things and will no doubt do them again. However, if these things are done by an elderly person, they are considered to be a sign of approaching **senility** or **dementia**. While some memory loss and difficulty with thought processes are inevitable as a result of aging, memory loss in the elderly is often the result of various disease processes and medications. The next section describes some techniques that you can use to enhance compliance with patients who have difficulty with thought processes, whether the cause is natural aging or a specific disease or medication regimen.

REINFORCING MEDICAL COMPLIANCE IN THE ELDERLY

Working with elderly patients who may have problems with memory loss or thought processes is extremely important to ensure that they take their medications as prescribed and follow the physician's instructions precisely. A patient who has good rapport with the office staff is likely to be truthful about the need for memory aids, and compliance may be increased. A patient who has difficulties with memory may benefit from these approaches:

- Write out instructions in easy-to-understand terms.
- Use large print.
- Have the patient repeat instructions to you for reinforcement.
- Ask the patient to show you how he or she will perform a procedure before leaving the office.
- Give the patient a copy of a large appointment calendar and list the times and days for treatments and medications, to be crossed off as completed.

Many chronic illnesses that affect the elderly require medication or treatment for the remainder of the patient's life. In these situations, the patient may not notice much improvement, making compliance over a long period problematic. You should reinforce the fact that although the patient may not return to his or her former health status, the prescribed treatment will maintain health at a manageable level. A patient's diabetes or heart disease will not be cured, but treatment will help the patient maintain a reasonable standard of health and independence.

It is important that each time a patient visits the medical office, you ask for a complete account of all medications being taken, including prescribed and over-the-counter medications, herbal supplements, and vitamins. To maintain a complete and accurate list of these medications, you may have patients bring all medications to the office at each visit and ask the patient to state how often each is taken. If you ask, "Mrs. Jones, are you still taking your heart medicine?" she may answer yes whether or not she is actually taking the medication as prescribed. In addition to difficulty with thought processes and occasional forgetfulness, some patients simply grow tired of the constraints that illness and medications impose on their lives, and some must make the financial choice between medication and food on the table. Assisting the patient to find ways to fit health requirements into a fairly normal lifestyle or coordinating with community resources to relieve financial constraints will help to ensure that treatment plans are followed and that the patient achieves the best level of health possible.

Checkpoint Question

1. What are some reasons a patient may not comply with a prescribed treatment plan?

REINFORCING MENTAL HEALTH IN THE ELDERLY

With the recognized correlation between physical and mental health, we must be acutely aware of the patient's mental status in patients who have acute or chronic physical problems. Some elderly patients are adapting to new roles of dependency after a lifetime of social interaction, career objectives, and family development. Some have been relieved of social responsibility whether they welcome it or not, and if they are ill, they must take on a dependent role. Adjusting to pain or disability is often easier than adjusting to loss of social interaction or dependency.

Paradoxically, if you open yourself to patients, including the elderly, and you are accessible and caring, you are likely to be the object of anger simply because you are seen as a safe outlet for venting frustrations. A suffering patient is less likely to release pent-up rage at someone who may respond with hostility or corresponding anger; consequently, the patient may hold in and the problem is compounded. Making yourself available to field these emotions can be as therapeutic as any treatment administered to this patient. To do this effectively:

1. Maintain open communication, freely discussing hopes and fears realistically, listening attentively, and offering advice without diagnosing or offering false hope.
2. By listening and being supportive to the patient and family members, help the patient to cope with and express feelings of guilt for being ill, anger at self and others nearby, and the loss of health and independence.
3. Work toward maintaining the patient's positive self-image by reinforcing the positive qualities of the patient's physical health or personal situation as appropriate.

4. Assist family members to maintain a positive support system by listening to concerns and possibly serving as a liaison for outside social services or resources if available.
5. Without being discouraging or offering false hope, prepare the patient for the possibility that a return to the previous state of health may not be feasible.
6. Direct the patient and family to specific support groups, such as the American Heart Association, the American Cancer Society, or another group specific to the patient's problem to assist them with acquiring information about the patient's condition.

Checkpoint Question

2. How can you help promote good mental health in your elderly patients?

PATIENT EDUCATION

Herbal Supplements

The herb gingko, also known as ginkgo biloba, maidenhair tree, kew tree, fossil tree, ginkyo, and yinhsing, is advertised in the United States as a natural way to improve memory and concentration. It is for this reason that the elderly have been targeted for the purchase of this product. After all, it can be purchased over the counter at many pharmacies and health food stores, and so many patients do not consider it a medication. However, it is extremely important that you obtain a thorough history from your patients each time they visit the office and specifically ask about any over-the-counter medications, including herbs and vitamin supplements. This drug may improve memory in some patients, but it causes an increase in clotting time in anyone who takes it and should not be used by patients with bleeding or clotting disorders. Any patient being scheduled for a surgical procedure must also be asked about the use of herbs. Patients who are taking the following medications should avoid taking gingko:

- Warfarin (coumadin)
- Aspirin
- Nonsteroidal anti-inflammatory drugs (NSAIDs), such as ibuprofen, naproxen, and indomethacin

The physician should be informed if any patient taking this herbal supplement, since reactions with other medications in addition to those listed could have serious consequences.

COPING WITH AGING

Although most elderly people are generally healthy and satisfied with their lives, those who live in long-term care facilities or whose health and economic situation are unstable have every right to feel overwhelming stress and grief. Stress will compromise the immune system, raise the blood pressure and blood sugar level, and strain the heart and lungs—all at a time when the patient needs all available resources to fight a debilitating disease process. You can help patients to cope with stress by listening to their fears and concerns, respecting their right to have these feelings, and helping them to reduce the stressors in their lives. Keep in mind that the coping mechanisms (e.g., denial, projection, repression) used to protect ourselves from stress may become more pronounced with age.

The ability of patients to cope with their losses is in direct relation to the importance of the losses and their own personal habits for coping with loss in the past. Be aware of a patient's loss of specific senses, abilities, or important things in life, such as sight, hearing, movement, perception, health, employment, home, and spouse. Also, be alert to the loss of nonspecific things—life purpose, goals, a sense of achievement, self-worth, recognition, security. Some elderly patients react to these losses by disengaging emotionally and relinquishing all decision making to family members. This may compound their grieving and lead to a sense of hopelessness and resignation. To prevent this reaction, involve elderly patients, like all patients, as much as possible by allowing them to have a voice in decisions that will affect their care. The elderly who are encouraged to make decisions and take responsibility for themselves are happier, more sociable, and live longer than those who are not.

LEGAL TIP

Advance Directives

An advance directive is a legal document outlining the wishes of an adult should he/she become mentally incompetent or otherwise unable to communicate decisions about end-of-life care. Although physicians as medical professionals are dedicated to sustaining life, a patient's autonomy must be respected at all times, including decisions to avoid or terminate life-sustaining procedures or equipment. As unpleasant as the prospect of death may be, documenting and communicating the wishes of the patient to the physician will assist with avoiding any confusion about the wishes of the patient should a life-threatening situation arise. Also, if the patient has an advanced directive on file somewhere other than the medical office, this should be noted in the patient's medical record.

Alcoholism

Some elderly, like adults coping with other losses, turn to alcohol as a way to escape dealing with the various losses associated with aging. Because alcohol slows brain activity and impairs mental processes, coordination, and judgment, a patient who comes to the office under the influence of alcohol may be mistaken for having dementia (mental deterioration), a transient ischemic attack (TIA), or central nervous system impairment. Also, many medications taken by the elderly affect the central nervous system and react badly with alcohol, compounding the problem. For example, alcohol increases the effect of opioids, barbiturates, and depressants of all types, and caretakers may not recognize this reason for the **potentiation**.

Identifying an elderly patient who is using or abusing alcohol may require the entire office to work as a team with the patient's family or caregiver to seek causes of various symptoms, such as impaired judgment or coordination. As often as necessary you should reinforce with elderly patients and their caregivers the effects of alcohol on mental processes and undesirable interactions with medication. In addition, the patient and responsible caregivers may require a referral to a mental health professional or other community resource to deal effectively with alcohol abuse. You may be required to make this referral as ordered by the physician.

Suicide

When ill health, multiple losses, and deep depression become too much for the patient to bear, suicide may seem preferable to life. Unlike suicide among younger people, suicide among the elderly is likely to be well planned and successful. Most elderly suicides are white men over age 65, especially those who have recently lost a spouse to death or divorce. These suicides are not usually a cry for help but a genuine effort to end life. Watch for these signs of intent:

- Deepening confusion and scattered attention
- Increasing anger, hostility, or isolation
- Increase in alcoholism or requests for opioids or sedatives
- Marked loss of interest in matters of health
- Secretive behavior
- Sharp mood swings from deep depression to euphoria
- Giving away favored objects

Always take seriously a patient who expresses an intent to commit suicide, and communicate this to the physician. You should work with the health care team to restore mental health as aggressively as to restore physical health.

Checkpoint Question

3. What are some signs of suicidal intent?

Ñ Spanish Terminology

Asi se toma este medicamento.	This is how you take this medication.
¿Tiene usted dolor junto con la rigidez?	Do you have pain with the stiffness?
La auxiliar sanitaria le ayudara con su cuidado personal.	The home health aide will help with your personal care.
Ha notado usted algún cambio en su habilidad de recordar cosas?	Have you noticed a change in your memory?

LONG-TERM CARE

Although many elderly are able to live in their own homes, some enter long-term care facilities if they cannot return to health and independence. These are three main types of long-term care:

- *Group homes* or *assisted living facilities* for the elderly who are able to tend to their own **activities of daily living** (ADL) (e.g., bathing, dressing, eating), but who need companionship and light supervision for safety.
- *Long-term care facilities* for those who need help with most areas of personal care and moderate medical supervision. Many of these patients are ambulatory but have a chronic disease that makes living at home alone impossible.
- *Skilled nursing facilities* for those who are gravely or terminally ill and need constant supervision. If the illness is acute and short term, the patient may return to an intermediate stage of care after recovery and possibly to full independence.

Expect some elderly patients to react to a move to long-term care with sorrow and a deep sense of loss. The patient may show the signs and symptoms of grief: poor appetite, headaches, insomnia, deep depression, and vague aches and pains. Report all signs and symptoms to the physician. Many physicians continue to care for patients residing in long-term care facilities. You may be responsible for blocking time in the daily schedule for the physician to visit these patients, and you may receive phone calls at the medical office from facilities regarding changes in patient's care and physical condition.

Checkpoint Question

4. How are long-term facilities and skilled nursing facilities different?

ELDER ABUSE

Although elder abuse is not as widely publicized as child abuse, it is thought to be almost as prevalent. The following are common risk factors for elder abuse:

- Multiple chronic illnesses that stress the family's physical, emotional, and financial resources

- Senile dementia that precludes reasoning or interaction
- Bladder or bowel incontinence
- Age-related sleep disturbances that interfere with the caretaker's rest
- Dependence on the caretaker for ADL

Elder abuse and neglect may take several forms, but family members (adult children and spouses) are the typical perpetrators.

- Passive neglect may result from the caretaker's ignorance regarding the patient's physiological and psychological needs.

WHAT IF

A patient's relative asks you about options for home care for an elderly parent?

Explain that many options allow patients to remain in their home. One option is the use of home health aides. Some insurance plans pay for this service. Home health aides do light housecleaning and cooking and promote patient safety. A second option is a community resource center. Some communities have senior citizen programs that provide transportation for shopping, doctor appointments, and entertainment. These programs get the older patient out of the house, preventing boredom and enhancing self-esteem. A third option is day care for the elderly. These programs keep the patient safe, entertained, and cared for during the day. The advantages of day care are that it relieves the caregiver of the need to place a parent in a long-term care facility, keeps the patient safe during the day, and allows the relative the freedom to continue employment or attend to personal needs. Community programs for senior citizens are good sources of information for caregivers or for relatives searching for respite or permanent care.

- Active neglect may take many forms, including over-medicating to render the patient passive and easier to care for or depriving the victim of adequate nutrition to decrease physical resources.
- Psychological abuse may include threatening imprisonment in the home, perhaps locking in a room, or physical abuse, withholding food or medication, or physical isolation.
- Financial abuse may involve only small amounts of money or entire substantial estates. The patient's financial resources may be embezzled, squandered, or frankly stolen, leaving the victim destitute.
- Physical abuse may be as simple as pinches and slaps or may be life-threatening, may be sexual, and may be so well concealed that even perceptive health care providers do not suspect it.

If you suspect abuse or neglect, you are responsible ethically and legally for bringing it to the attention of the physician, who should assess the situation and if it is confirmed, notify the proper authorities. Most states require that health care professionals report all suspected cases of elder abuse to the department of social services, just as is required for suspected child abuse. The entire medical staff may be held responsible if the abuse is not reported immediately. These signs may indicate elder abuse:

- Wounds of suspicious origin in various stages of healing
- Signs of restraints having been used, such as wrist or ankle abrasions or bruising
- Neglected large, deep pressure ulcers
- Poor hygiene or poor nutrition with little or no effort at correction
- Dehydration not caused by a disease process
- Untreated injury or medical condition
- Excessive and unwarranted agitation or apathetic resignation

Some elderly patients fear reprisal or abandonment by their caregivers, just as children do, and are reluctant to complain of any improprieties. Separate the caregiver from the patient for the examination if possible, and treat the patient with the utmost compassion and care. Document all findings with full descriptions. It may be necessary to photograph the suspected injuries.

Checkpoint Question

5. What are the types of elder abuse?

MEDICATIONS AND THE ELDERLY

The need to teach some elderly patients about self-medication is a challenge that will become increasingly common as the general population ages. At the same time that elderly patients need more medications for various disorders, the body is coping with the stress of illness, disease, or injury along with slowing of many bodily functions. The gastrointestinal system is no longer moving medications along as efficiently because peristalsis has slowed. The circulatory system is not absorbing the dissolved medication from the intestines or the injection site and delivering it to the target tissue as quickly. The liver does not **biotransform** (convert) the medication as quickly, so that it remains in the body longer than might be desirable and possibly adds to cumulative effect. Finally, the kidneys are receiving less blood, so that less medication is filtered and removed from the body. All of these decreases in body systems can result in possible toxic effects of medications in the elderly.

Your responsibility is to elicit information from the patient about all medications they are taking: prescribed and over-the-counter medications, including herbal or vitamin supplements. Follow these guidelines to help ensure that your elderly patient adheres to the prescribed medication regimen:

1. Explain all side effects, precautions, interactions, and expected actions in a manner the patient can understand.
2. Explain the proper dosage and how to measure it. For patients with failing eyesight, mark plastic measuring cups with indelible ink at the correct level so they can easily see it.
3. Write out a schedule and suggest methods to help the patient remember. Suggestions may include a daily dose pack available at pharmacies, an egg carton with hours for taking the medications marked on the cups, and a calendar marked with the medications and hours, to be checked off after taking the medication.
4. Tell the patient to take the most important medication first. If it is not possible to take the other medications at this time, it may be acceptable to skip a dose of less important medication.
5. Encourage the patient not to rush when taking medications. The patient should be sitting or standing, not reclining. One pill should be taken at a time with lots of water. If the medication is difficult to swallow, have the patient try putting the pill on the back of the tongue and drinking water with a straw.
6. A patient who has difficulty reading or has failing eyesight can ask the pharmacist for large print on the label. This makes medication errors less likely. Child-proof containers are not necessary if there are no children in the home, and the patient may find them difficult to open.
7. Explain that the medication must be taken until it is gone (if this is the case). No medication should be taken by other family members or saved for another illness.
8. Encourage patients to take an active role in therapy. Teach them to apply ointments or transdermal patches or to give themselves injections. A patient who feels in charge is more likely to complete a course of

medication or to remain on the medication for the long term than one who feels passive.

Checkpoint Question

6. How can you help your elderly patients follow the medication regimen prescribed by the physician?

SYSTEMIC CHANGES IN THE ELDERLY

Although longevity is considered largely hereditary, environmental factors play a significant part in how long and how well we will live. An obese, physically inactive smoker is much less likely to be in good health than a nonsmoker whose diet is well balanced and who exercises. In addition, certain occupational hazards, such as black lung disease from coal mining, may shorten a life that should have lasted for decades longer.

The aging changes are thought to be programmed into our cells along with our genetic material. Hypotheses suggest that when cells reach a specific reproduction level, they either do not replace themselves or replicate more slowly or ineffectively. These changes manifest themselves at varying rates for all persons, but follow a recognized order as outlined in TABLE 40-1.

DISEASES OF THE ELDERLY

The degenerative conditions noted in Table 40-1 are typically part of the aging process. Many of these changes cause problems that must be managed by the health care team; others are mere inconveniences for the patient. Diseases related to ag-

WHAT IF

You are organizing your charts at the beginning of the day, and you notice that one of your patients, an 88-year-old man, has HOH (hard of hearing) stamped on the front of his chart. How can you best communicate with him?

When speaking to an elderly patient who is hearing impaired, it is important not to shout. Instead, get closer to the patient, face the patient directly, and speak slowly and distinctly. Try to give written instructions whenever possible, and encourage the patient to ask questions for clarification. Avoid speaking to the hard-of-hearing patient with your back to the light, since this may cast shadows and preclude lipreading.

ing are described in the preceding chapters on specialties. The following sections describe two conditions commonly associated with aging that may appear in the middle years as well.

Parkinson's Disease

Parkinson's disease is a slow, progressive neurological disorder affecting specific cells of the brain that produce the neurotransmitter dopamine. The initial symptoms frequently include muscle rigidity, involuntary tremors, and difficulty walking. Parkinson's disease affects men more than women and is estimated to affect in some form approximately 1 in 100 persons over age 60. This disease may progress for 10 years or more before resulting in complete debilitation or death.

Normally, dopamine and acetylcholine, another neurotransmitter, are in balance and produce smooth, controlled muscle movement. With lower levels of dopamine, acetylcholine is not counterbalanced. This leads to involuntary movements of muscles and inability to control these movements. While the causes of Parkinson's disease are unknown, researchers are working to determine whether there is a genetic component. Some evidence suggests that certain toxins may cause the disease. These toxins may be environmental or related to certain medications. These are the signs and symptoms of Parkinson's disease:

- Muscle rigidity
- **Bradykinesia** (abnormally slow voluntary movements)
- Difficulty walking, with a shuffling, mincing gait
- Forward-bending posture with no normal arm swing
- Laryngeal rigidity with a monotone voice
- Pharyngeal rigidity with dysphagia and drooling
- Facial muscle rigidity with a masklike, expressionless face and infrequent blinking reflex, causing frequent eye infections
- Small tremors in the fingers in a characteristic pill-rolling action. These start unilaterally and stop with purposeful action in the affected hand. Tremors are greatest during times of stress and anxiety and are diminished at sleep or rest. Muscles resist passive stretching and become rigid with passive manipulation (FIG. 40-1).

The diagnosis of Parkinson's disease is usually made by excluding other causes. Testing may show decreased levels of dopamine in the urine. A symptomatic history is the primary method of diagnosing after all other possibilities have been ruled out. Parkinson's disease has no cure. Treatment is symptomatic, supportive, and palliative. Medications include the following:

- Levodopa (L-dopa). Dopamine replacement crosses the blood-brain barrier to restore balance with acetylcholine. Individualized doses are gradually increased as symptoms progress. Levodopa is fairly effective for

(text continued on page 801)

T a b l e   4 0 - 1   EFFECTS OF AGING ON BODY SYSTEMS

	Systemic Changes	Manifestations	How You Can Help
Integumentary system	Loss of subcutaneous fat	Wrinkling, sagging, decreased ability to maintain hydration, reduced protection against temperature change	Encourage drinking plenty of fluids, dressing appropriately for weather
	Loss of pigment	Less protection against sun damage, paler skin, graying hair	Encourage use of sunscreen with appropriate UV protection
	Loss of elasticity	Increased skin dryness, risk of trauma	Suggest good lubricating lotion, bathing less often. Caution patient to guard against injuries.
	Receding capillaries	Sallow skin, thickened nails	Suggest ways to guard against injuries.
	Slower reproduction of hair, skin cells	Balding; thin, fine hair; slower healing	
	Diminished oil, sweat production	Dry, fragile skin; intolerance to heat	Encourage use of good lubricating lotion, bathing less often. Suggest ways to avoid overheating.
	Erratic pigment, cell production	Senile **lentigines, keratoses**	Teach patient to conduct skin checks, to notify physician of concerns.
Musculoskeletal System	Loss of muscle strength, size	Loss of strength, flexibility, endurance	Suggest frequent exercise appropriate to age and ability.
	Loss of bone density, typical loss of height with osteoporosis.	Vertebral compression with diminished height, **kyphosis; osteoporosis** with frequent fractures	Explain weight-bearing exercise. Encourage home safety check to avoid falls. Physician may recommend calcium supplement, dietary consultation, estrogen replacement.
	Degenerative joint cartilage	Less clear margins with spurs of bone that restrict movement, **degenerative joint disease,** arthritis	Physician may limit phosphorus intake.
Nervous system	Slow nerve conduction	Slow reaction time, slow learning, slow perception of pain with resulting increase in injuries	Allow extra time as needed and teach about hazards of delayed reaction times. Aim teaching at comprehension level. Encourage home safety checks.
	Reduced cerebral circulation	Loss of balance, **vertigo,** frequent falls	Have patient install bath rails, remove throw rugs, conduct home safety check. Encourage use of walking aid.
	Referred circulatory problems	Increase in cardiovascular diseases (atherosclerosis, arteriosclerosis) reflected as CVA, cerebral hypoxia, TIA	Teach patient and family about danger signs for CVA, TIA.
Cardiovascular system	Atherosclerosis, arteriosclerosis, narrowing of blood vessels	Loss of peripheral circulation, fatty plaques with risk of MI, CVA, cold extremities, slow healing time, hypertension.	Encourage exercise; balanced, low-fat, low-salt diet; dressing appropriately for weather; home safety check.
	Slow response to demands for increased output	Complaints of fatigue on exertion	Help patient pace exercise and exertion.
	Diminished function	Pulmonary involvement with edema, dyspnea	Explain about low-salt diets and orthopneic positions.
Respiratory system	Stiffening costal cartilage	Decreased expansion, contraction; barrel chest; decreased lung capacity	Explain about smoking hazards, emphysema. Encourage moderate exercise.
	Decreased gas exchange	Fatigue, breathlessness on exertion; impaired healing due to insufficient oxygen, **syncope**	Encourage exercise as appropriate and use of walking aid. Caution about upper respiratory infection, encourage home safety check.
	General loss of muscle mass	Difficulty coughing deeply, may lead to pneumonia	Encourage drinking adequate fluids to liquefy respiratory secretions.

System	Change	Effect/Symptom	Intervention
Gastrointestinal system	Drying of secretions, including saliva	Dry mouth, **dysphagia**	Teach oral hygiene, adequate fluid intake
	Decreased enzyme activity	Incomplete digestion, poor conversion of nutrients with malnourishment	Encourage small, frequent well-balanced meals.
	Slower peristalsis	Constipation, flatulence, indigestion	Suggest increase in fluid, fiber intake. Warn about laxative dependency.
	Loss of teeth	Poor chewing, choking on large pieces, loss of appetite, poor nutrition	Refer to a dentist; teach good oral hygiene. Suggest dietary counseling.
Urinary system	Decreased bladder capacity.	Urinary frequency	Encourage patient to respond to initial urge to void
	Decreased bladder muscle tone	Urinary retention with urinary tract infection or incontinence	Suggest exercises for strengthening pelvic floor. Urge patient to empty bladder completely when voiding.
	Fewer functioning nephrons	Less blood flowing through kidneys to be cleaned of wastes, creating possibly lethal levels of medications or normal body wastes.	Suggest increase in fluid intake to maintain hydration.
Endocrine system	Decreased enzyme activity	Menopause, glucose intolerance with NIDDM, slower metabolism	Physician will supplement as needed.
Immune system	Diminished production of T cells, B cells	Loss of resistance to illness	Encourage age-appropriate immunization.
	Diminished ability of body to distinguish self from foreign substances	Increase in autoimmune diseases	Explain symptoms of autoimmunity.
	Diminished other defenses (e.g., GI enzymes)	Overload on compromised immune system, frequent serious illnesses	Encourage age-appropriate immunizations, guarding against communicable diseases.
Eyes	Less time spent in deep sleep	Less restful sleep, more frequent naps	Encourage rest periods as needed.
	Diminished lens accommodation	**Presbyopia**	Obtain referral to ophthalmologist. Recommend adequate lighting, large-print books, brochures, pamphlets
	Lens cloud	**Cataracts** (lens opacity) that dim vision as less light reaches the retina	Obtain referral to ophthalmologist. Recommend adequate lighting.
	Loss of ciliary function	**Glaucoma** (increased intraocular pressure), intolerance to light or glare, poor night vision	Obtain referral to ophthalmologist. Recommend adequate lighting, avoidance of night driving.
Ears	Loss of auditory hair cells (organ of Corti)	Hearing loss in upper frequencies, problems distinguishing sibilants	Obtain referral to otologist. Speak clearly, facing patient, in area with few distractions.
	Ossicle becomes fixed	**Presbycusis**	Obtain referral to otologist. Speak clearly, facing patient, in area with few distractions.
Other senses	Diminished sense of smell	Loss of appetite, poor nutrition	Suggest dietary consultation.
	Diminished sense of taste	Loss of appetite, poor nutrition, perhaps increased use of salt, other seasonings	Suggest dietary consultation. Encourage use of seasonings other than salt
Female reproductive system	Decreased egg production	Menopause	Physician may prescribe supplemental estrogen.
	Decreased estrogen Production	Hot flashes; thinner, drier vaginal walls with itching, painful intercourse; osteoporosis	Physician may prescribe supplemental estrogen.
	Poor perineal muscle tone	Rectocele, cystocele, stress incontinence	Suggest **Kegel exercises** to strengthen pelvic floor.

(continues

Table 40-1 *(continued)*

	Systemic Changes	Manifestations	How You Can Help
Male reproductive system	Smaller penis, testicles	Loss of libido	Physician may refer patient for counseling.
	Atherosclerosis, arteriosclerosis	Impotence	Physician may refer patient for counseling. Explain good nutrition to avoid atherosclerosis
	Benign prostatic hypertrophy (BPH)	Urgency, frequency, nocturia, retention	Encourage patient to have yearly checks for BPH.

A 10 years postmenopause

B 15 years postmenopause Height loss 1.5"

C 25 years postmenopause Height loss 3.5"

Typical loss of height associated with osteoporosis and aging. (Courtesy of Wilson Research Foundation.)

CVA, cerebrovascular accident; TIA, transient ischemic attack; MI, myocardial infarction; GI, gastrointestinal; NIDDM, non–insulin dependent diabetes mellitus; BPH, benign prostatic hypertrophy.

Lentigines, liver spots; keratoses, skin thickening; kyphosis, dowager hump; vertigo, whirling sensation, dizziness; presbyopia, loss of near vision; cataracts, lens opacity; glaucoma, increased intraocular pressure; sibilants, ch, s, sh, z sounds; presbycusis, hearing loss.

a time but gradually loses its effectiveness. Unfortunately, levodopa has serious side effects, including nausea, vomiting, tachycardia, and arrhythmias. It has severe adverse reactions with alcohol.

- Anticholinergics. These drugs decrease the levels of acetylcholine so that depleted levels of dopamine are not so out of balance. This method works best in mild, early stages.
- Antihistamines with anticholinergic action. In the early, mild stages, this method of lowering acetylcholine levels to balance with low levels of dopamine alleviates symptoms.

Since 1997, a procedure known as deep brain stimulation has been used to treat tremor and rigidity. In this procedure, electrodes are surgically placed in certain areas of the brain and connected by wires to an impulse generator that is implanted under the skin of the chest. This transmitter sends electrical impulses to the electrodes in the brain, blocking the impulses that cause the tremors. Although this procedure is effective for controlling involuntary movements and tremors, it is generally not used if medication can control the patient's symptoms. Like all other methods, this treatment is palliative and not curative.

Parkinson's patients retain their mental and cognitive functions unless an organic brain disturbance is also present. They are aware of the outward signs of the disease and may be embarrassed and emotionally depressed. They require great psychological support from the medical staff, family, and support groups. You can help in these ways:

- Encourage the patient to participate in all ADL.
- Promote independence.
- Be aware that because rigidity extends to the gastrointestinal tract, the patient may have dysphagia and constipation. Suggest that the patient increase fluid intake, eat a balanced diet, and increase fiber intake.
- Tell the patient that a decreased cough reflex can lead to choking. Suggest that the patient take small bites and chew each mouthful of food carefully before attempting to swallow.
- Encourage the patient to use eating aids such as a no-spill cup, plate with high sides, and special utensils. High toilet seats and handrails in the bath also help increase the patient's independence and safety.
- Listen to the patient. Intelligence is still intact and needs to be stimulated.
- Educate the patient about safety factors. The forward-bending posture and altered gait frequently lead to falls. Encourage these patients to hold on to handrails and pick up feet carefully to avoid falling. Also, the home should be free from rugs and loose cords that may cause accidental tripping.
- Enlist the help of support groups. Include the caregiver and urge respite care when exhaustion and stress become overwhelming.

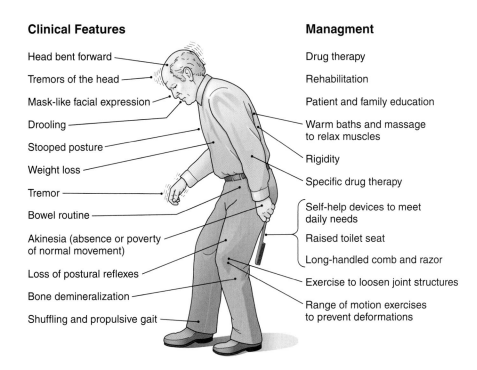

Clinical Features

- Head bent forward
- Tremors of the head
- Mask-like facial expression
- Drooling
- Stooped posture
- Weight loss
- Tremor
- Bowel routine
- Akinesia (absence or poverty of normal movement)
- Loss of postural reflexes
- Bone demineralization
- Shuffling and propulsive gait

Managment

- Drug therapy
- Rehabilitation
- Patient and family education
- Warm baths and massage to relax muscles
- Rigidity
- Specific drug therapy
- Self-help devices to meet daily needs
- Raised toilet seat
- Long-handled comb and razor
- Exercise to loosen joint structures
- Range of motion exercises to prevent deformations

FIGURE 40–1. The Parkinson's patient.

Checkpoint Question

7. How can you assist a patient with Parkinson's disease?

Alzheimer's Disease

Roughly half of the cases of dementia in the elderly are due to Alzheimer's disease. The symptoms of Alzheimer's disease may be similar to those caused by TIA, cerebral tumor, and dementia other than Alzheimer's. The cause of Alzheimer's is not known.

The symptoms of Alzheimer's disease may begin as early as age 40, with a gradual loss of memory and slight personality changes. The changes may occur over as long as 15 years and are frequently so gradual that diagnosis is difficult and may be made only by ruling out all other possibilities. Autopsy reveals organic brain changes, including a loss of neurons and neurotransmitters. Plaques or deposits may be present as a residue of the neural cell deterioration.

Alzheimer's disease has seven recognized stages. The progression from one stage to the next may be gradual. Some stages may last for years, but a patient may pass through other stages so quickly that the progression goes unnoticed. Expect varying levels of response from patients in these different levels (TABLE 40-2). When caring for Alzheimer's patients, you must remember that anger and hostility are symptoms of the disease, not to be taken personally. Be sure to do the following:

- Respond with the utmost patience and compassion
- Speak calmly and without condescension
- Never argue with the patient, even if the patient blames you unfairly for something the patient forgot.
- Do not expect the patient to remember you from previous visits. Reintroduce yourself.
- Explain even common procedures as if the patient has never had them explained.

- Approach quietly and professionally in an unthreatening manner and remind the patient who you are and what you must do.
- Speak in short, simple, direct sentences, and explain only one action at a time.
- Keep a list of support contacts for family members to call.

Home care agencies usually offer respite care, which can be vitally important for caregivers, who need to maintain their own mental and physical health. An exhausted, distraught family member may not be thinking clearly. The most therapeutic action may be for you to assist the family with proper contacts to help make caring for a family member with this devastating disease less traumatic.

MAINTAINING OPTIMUM HEALTH

No one realistically expects to have the same strength and agility at age 70 as at age 20. With attention to exercise and good nutrition, however, it is possible to maintain a good level of fitness that adds to quality of life.

Exercise

Exercise plays a vital role in maintaining overall physical and mental health (TABLE 40-3). Older patients should begin an exercise program only after a thorough physical examination and should follow the physician's recommendation. Provide the following guidelines for elderly patients who are starting an exercise program with the physician's approval:

1. Before exercise, always warm up cold muscles for at least 10 minutes. Slow and rhythmic movements, such as walking, raise the heart rate and increase metabolism. Then do slow, easy stretching to lengthen sluggish muscles.

Table 40-2   LEVELS OF ALZHEIMER DISEASE

Level	Description
I, II	Presenile dementia may end here, with no further progression. Brain changes insignificant; only remarkable symptom may be forgetfulness. ADL done with reasonable ease.
III	Patient losing ability to remember facts, faces, and names but still aware enough to recognize problem, become increasingly frustrated and angry. Most ADL still performed reasonably well.
IV	Late confusional or mild Alzheimer. Patient beginning to misplace things, has increasing difficulty remembering, neglects ADL. Most aware of a problem but deny any concern.
V	Early dementia or moderate Alzheimer. Patient must have custodial care, has severe memory lapses, disorientation, anger, great frustration.
VI	Middle dementia or moderately severe Alzheimer with severe memory loss, no self-care at any level, disoriented most of the time with immense anger, hostility, combativeness. Fear of water.
VII	Late dementia. patient requires full-time care, rarely seen in the office. Unless home care is an option, physician will probably visit long-term care facility. Patient rarely speaks, almost never intelligibly; incontinent; may require tube feeding.

TRIAGE BOX

While you are working in a medical office, the following three patients are waiting:

A. Patient A is a 76-year-old woman who is active but underweight, with a history of osteoporosis. She is here for a physical examination, and the doctor has just instructed you to obtain some blood work for laboratory analysis.

B. Patient B is an 87-year-old man brought in by his daughter, who takes care of him in her home since his stroke 3 years ago. His wife is deceased and his daughter is concerned because his memory seems to be failing him.

C. Patient C is a 90-year-old man residing in an assisted living facility with his wife, who is 88. They were brought to the office today because the husband is due for a blood pressure check and possible medication adjustment. They are alert and sharp mentally, although both move more slowly than usual and the wife requires a walker.

How would you sort these patients? Whom do you see first? Second? Third?

When working with elderly patients, it is important to remember not to rush them or appear inattentive. Since patient B is having new symptoms and may require a longer time with the physician, you should check him in first and get vital signs and any appropriate medical information from both the patient and his daughter. The husband and wife should be seen next, since all that is required is a brief chief complaint and obtaining vital signs. When both the husband and wife are comfortable and safely seated, you may leave them alone until the doctor is available to see them. Patient A should be seen last, since obtaining blood from the elderly requires special attention to detail and patience. Once the blood sample is obtained, she may be discharged after checking the medical record to assure that no physician orders have been missed.

Table 40-3 BENEFITS OF EXERCISE

System	Benefits
Cardiovascular	Increases endurance Lowers cholesterol to avoid atherosclerosis Maintains vascular elasticity to delay arteriosclerosis
Musculoskeletal	Increases bone mass to reduce osteoporosis Decreases fat–muscle ratio and increases metabolism Retains strength and flexibility to ensure mobility, improve posture
Nervous	Improves mental health by reducing stress, fatigue, tension, boredom Maintains or restores balance to reduce risk of falls
Endocrine	May decrease need for insulin or oral hypoglycemic medication in diabetes

4. Breathe deeply and evenly. If you cannot carry on a conversation, slow down. Never hold your breath while you exercise.

5. Rest when you get tired. Do not try to exercise to the point of exhaustion.

6. Keep a record of your progress. It is motivational to watch your performance improve.

7. Exercise with a friend, with a group, or to music that you enjoy (FIG. 40-2).

8. Make exercise a part of your daily routine, but do not make it a chore. Do something vigorous every day and take pride in it.

FIGURE 40-2. Participating in group exercise helps to maintain overall physical and mental health.

2. Begin by exercising for brief periods. Exercise only 5 to 10 minutes a day the first week, then progress to 10 to 15 minutes a day the next week. Gradually work up to about 30 to 45 minutes of pleasantly challenging strength and cardiovascular endurance activity after about a month. This routine reduces the chance of injury and is likely to be an attainable goal.

3. Stop if you feel pain, shortness of breath, or dizziness. Never try to work through pain.

Diet

Many elderly patients have difficulty maintaining good nutrition. Reduced activity means a corresponding decrease in hunger. Decaying teeth or poorly fitting dentures cause pain, making it hard to chew. Saliva production decreases, making it harder to swallow. The senses of smell and taste diminish, interfering with the cephalic phase of digestion. Many elderly patients eat alone or are not able to enjoy the socializing that adds immeasurably to the pleasure of eating.

A balanced diet is vital to good health at any age. Although activity levels, hence calorie requirements, are lower among the elderly, vitamin and mineral requirements do not decrease with age. Efforts must be made to increase the nutritional level of the elderly. Smaller, more frequent meals may be easier to digest than infrequent large meals. Water should be encouraged to maintain hydration and to aid digestion and elimination.

Talk to patients or their families about valuable services such as Meals on Wheels, which delivers nutritious meals to the home daily or 5 days a week. This program ensures that at least one well-balanced meal a day is available. Most services prepare meals to meet special dietary needs, such as low sodium or low fat. The program volunteer is alert to the needs of the patient and will report to a coordinator if the patient does not answer the door or seems ill or confused. This resource helps reassure the family that the patient's nutritional and social needs are being met.

Safety

Alert the patient and caregivers to hazards in the home of an elderly patient and offer the following suggestions:

- Remove any scatter rugs, especially on highly polished floors.
- Never allow electrical cords to cross passageways.
- Remove or reduce clutter as much as possible.
- Strengthen handrails on stairs and install them in tubs and near the commode.
- Install a telephone by the bedside and near a favorite chair. Consider a telephone in the bathroom also.
- Install and carefully maintain smoke alarms and carbon monoxide detectors throughout the house.
- Establish a system in which someone calls and checks on the patient every day. Many communities have programs in which volunteers call the sick or elderly daily to check on their needs and offer a few minutes of conversation. If the patient fails to answer, someone goes to the home to check on the patient. This service ensures that the patient is never without contact for long. Lifeline, an emergency service, is another option that increases the feeling of safety for patients who live alone.

CHAPTER SUMMARY

In the early 1900s the leading causes of death were infant mortality and infectious diseases. Today, the major causes of death are cardiovascular disease, trauma, and homicide. The median age of the population has steadily increased, with the average life span growing by about 25 years since early 1900s. With the advances being made in health care, the life span has increased with each generation since World War II. These increases will likely continue, producing a major force in shaping the health care industry in this country for many years to come.

Medical assistants who work in most medical offices today come into frequent contact with elderly patients. While this age group should not be stereotyped into passive, dependent roles, you should be alert to the normal physiological changes of aging and adjust your communication techniques accordingly. This chapter covers some of these expected physiological changes and diseases that do not affect all elderly patients. Working with geriatric patients with diseases such as Parkinson's or Alzheimer's necessitates that you understand the disease process and develop excellent interpersonal skills.

Critical Thinking Challenges

1. Mrs. Moss, aged 78, lives with her son and daughter-in-law and their two school-age children. She has dysphagia and a poor appetite. Identify ways in which Mrs. Moss can improve or maintain her nutritional status while participating in the family meals.
2. Mr. Brown is 90, and his wife is 86. They live alone, and Mrs. Brown is the primary caregiver. During the physical examination, Mr. Brown is found to have several large decubital ulcers. Summarize the various types of elder abuse or neglect. What is likely the problem in this case? Explain how you would handle this situation.
3. The pharmacist calls you at the office and says he has an elderly patient waiting to have a prescription for a high blood pressure medication filled. This prescription was filled just 2 weeks ago, but the patient says he is "all out of my medicine." What do you advise the pharmacist to do?

Answers to Checkpoint Questions

1. Elderly patients may not comply with treatment plans because of memory loss from normal aging or because they are growing tired of the constraints im-

posed on their life by illness. Some patients may have financial difficulties that force them to choose between medication and food on the table.

2. You can help your elderly patients maintain good mental health by encouraging open communication, helping them deal with their feelings, promoting a positive self-image, helping family members to be supportive, and suggesting support groups as needed.

3. The signs of suicidal intent include deepening confusion, increasing anger, increased alcohol or drug use, lack of interest in health, secretive behavior, sharp mood swings, and giving away personal possessions.

4. Long-term care facilities are for individuals who need help with personal care and some medical supervision. Skilled nursing facilities are for gravely or terminally ill individuals who need constant supervision.

5. Elder abuse may be passive or active neglect or it can be psychological, financial, or physical.

6. To help your elderly patient follow the prescribed medication regimen: provide a full explanation of the medication in a way that the patient understands; explain the proper dosage and techniques for measuring; develop a written schedule for taking the medication; instruct the patient to take the most important medica-

tion first; tell the patient not to rush when taking the medication; have the patient ask the pharmacist for large print on the label; explain the appropriate use of the medication; and encourage patients to take an active role in their therapy.

7. To assist a patient with Parkinson's disease, encourage activity and independence, promote good nutrition and hydration, caution the patient about the potential for choking, educate the patient about safety, use therapeutic communication skills, and enlist the help of support groups for the patient and their caregivers.

 Websites

The Center for Social Gerontology http://www.tcsg.org
American Association of Retired Persons
   http://www.aarp.org
National Center on Elder Abuse http://elderabuse
   center.org
National Institute on Aging http://www.nia.nih.org
Centers for Medicare and Medicaid Services
   http://www.cms.hhs.gov

The Clinical Laboratory

Performing Laboratory Procedures

41

Introduction to the Clinical Laboratory

CHAPTER OUTLINE

ROLE DELINEATION

GENERAL: PROFESSIONALISM
- Display a professional manner and image.
- Demonstrate initiative and responsibility.

GENERAL: COMMUNICATION SKILLS
- Use medical terminology appropriately

GENERAL: LEGAL CONCEPTS
- Perform within legal and ethical boundaries
- Document accurately
- Implement and maintain federal and state health care legislation and regulations
- Comply with established risk management and safety procedures
- Recognize professional credentialing criteria

GENERAL: OPERATIONAL FUNCTIONS
- Perform inventory of supplies and equipment
- Perform routine maintenance of administrative and clinical equipment

CLINICAL: FUNDAMENTAL PRINCIPLES
- Comply with quality assurance practices

CLINICAL: DIAGNOSTIC ORDERS
- Collect and process specimens

CHAPTER COMPETENCIES

LEARNING OBJECTIVES
Upon successfully completing this chapter, you will be able to:

1. Spell and define the key terms.
2. List reasons for laboratory testing.
3. Outline the medical assistant's responsibility in the clinical laboratory.
4. Name the kinds of laboratories where medical assistants work and the functions of each.
5. List the types of personnel in laboratories and describe their jobs.
6. Name the types of departments found in most large laboratories and give their purposes.
7. Explain how to use a package insert to determine the procedure for a laboratory test.
8. List the equipment found in most small laboratories and give the purpose of each.
9. List and describe the parts of a microscope.
10. Explain the significance of the Clinical Laboratory Improvement Amendments and how to follow their regulations to ensure quality control.
11. Define OSHA and state its purpose.
12. List the laboratory safety guidelines.

PERFORMANCE OBJECTIVE
Upon successfully completing this chapter, you will be able to:
1. Care for the microscope (Procedure 41-1).

KEY TERMS

aerosol	Clinical Laboratory	National Committee for	quality control (QC)
anticoagulant	Improvement	Clinical Laboratory	reagents
calibration	Amendments (CLIA)	Standards (NCCLS)	reportable range
capillary action	material safety data sheet	normal values	specimens
centrifugal force	(MSDS)	quality assurance (QA)	

THE MEDICAL LABORATORY provides the physician with some of medicine's most powerful diagnostic tools. Laboratory staff analyze blood, urine, and other body samples to facilitate identification of diseases and disorders. Results of laboratory testing are compared with normal or reference values (acceptable ranges for a healthy population) to determine the relative health of body systems or organs. Blood levels of various medications are determined to adjust dosages to therapeutic levels. Bacteria, viruses, parasites, and other microorganisms are identified to begin the treatment process. (See Appendix F for a list of commonly performed laboratory tests and their **normal values**.)

Laboratory testing is most commonly used for the following:

- Detecting and diagnosing disease
- Following the progress of a disease and its response to treatment
- Meeting legal requirements (e.g., drug testing, a marriage license)
- Monitoring a patient's medication and treatment
- Determining the levels of essential substances in the body
- Identifying the cause of an infection
- Determining a baseline value
- Preventing disease

As a medical assistant, you have an important role in laboratory analysis—even when testing is performed at sites other than the medical office. In general, you may be responsible for the following:

- Informing patients of the proper procedure or preparation for obtaining laboratory **specimens** (samples, such as blood or urine, used to evaluate a patient's condition)
- Obtaining a quality specimen
- Arranging for appropriate transport if the specimen is to be analyzed at another site
- Performing common laboratory tests in the physician's office or clinic
- Documenting and maintaining a **quality assurance** (**QA**) program designed to ensure thorough patient care and a **quality control** (**QC**) protocol designed to monitor and evaluate testing procedures, supplies, and equipment to ensure accuracy in laboratory performance
- Maintaining laboratory instruments and equipment to manufacturers' standards

Medical assistants also may control purchase of laboratory supplies and selection of **reagents**, substances used to produce a reaction in tests. In addition, you may be in charge of biohazard safety and waste disposal for the workplace. This chapter outlines the basic information you will need to ensure the quality of the laboratory testing in your facility.

TYPES OF LABORATORIES

Three types of laboratories significant to the medical assistant are reference, hospital, and physician office laboratories (POLs). Hospital and reference laboratories may perform hundreds of specialized tests and may process thousands of specimens per day. In contrast, POLs perform only a few types of tests on a limited number of patients.

Reference Laboratory

A reference or referral laboratory is a large facility, similar to a factory, in which thousands of tests of various types are performed each day. A reference laboratory's direct patient contact is limited to its own satellite specimen procurement stations. It also receives specimens from physicians' offices, hospitals, and clinics across the region it serves. The specimens are delivered by special courier, U.S. mail, or other ground or air transportation delivery service. Specimens sent to reference laboratories must be packaged

PATIENT EDUCATION

Specimen Collection

Before collecting a specimen, instruct the patient on the proper preparation for testing. For instance, does the test require that the patient fast or follow a specific dietary regimen? Does the test require stopping any medications or modifying dose patterns? Is the timing of collection imperative, or will a random sample be sufficient? Failure to inform the patient properly before testing may result in erroneous (invalid) test results, which can cause a delay in treatment or incorrect diagnosis.

At the time of specimen collection, tell the patient:

- The name of the test (e.g., blood cell count)
- The type of specimen required (e.g., blood, stool, urine)

Be sure to tell the patient approximately how long it will take for the results to be available and how and by whom the patient will be contacted regarding the results.

Patient education requirements for drawing an HIV test vary from state to state, although most require pretest and posttest counseling. Most states do not allow HIV test results to be given over the telephone.

FIGURE 41-1. Transport containers are constructed to maintain the integrity of the specimen and to protect those who are responsible for the care and handling of possibly hazardous bodily fluids and substances.

to withstand rough handling, pressure changes, and temperature extremes during shipment. Packaging includes placement in a special leak-proof secondary transport container (FIG. 41-1) that meets federal regulations for transportation of biohazardous materials.

Tests are performed in bulk test runs, and results and reports are managed by information systems. Reference laboratories usually are not responsible for reporting test results to patients. Test results generally are returned to the referring physician, who relays the results to the patient.

Employees of reference laboratories have specific job descriptions. Specimen processors accept (receive) the specimens and log patient data and specimen information into the computer, which assigns each specimen an accession (testing) number. Processors also centrifuge, separate, and prepare aliquots (a portion of a specimen used for testing) if indicated and send them to the correct departments for testing.

Testing is performed by medical technologists, medical laboratory technicians, or laboratory assistants, depending on the complexity of the procedure. Most testing is performed in large batches on automated instruments. Test personnel are responsible for QC procedures, such as checking instruments, performing daily maintenance, and running control specimens. Test duties include loading specimens and reagents into the instruments to perform test runs and managing test results by accepting or rejecting, recording, and reporting results of QC and patient specimens.

Customer (or client) services personnel answer questions from sites submitting specimens, track specimens, report results, add or delete tests requested by physicians, and troubleshoot problems primarily by phone. Medical assistants may work in specimen processing or client services. They may also be employed in testing, provided they meet the Clinical Laboratory Improvements Amendments of 1988 (CLIA 1988) federal requirements, which include documented testing experience and supervision by a CLIA-qualified person.

Hospital Laboratory

The hospital laboratory serves inpatients (patients who stay overnight or longer) and outpatients (patients who come for services and leave the same day).

The hospital laboratory staff includes phlebotomists to collect and sometimes process blood specimens, laboratory assistants to collect and process specimens and perform limited testing, and medical laboratory technicians and medical technologists to perform most of the testing. Laboratories also have receptionists or secretaries, who process outpatients and manage the large volume of requisitions, test results, and other information and paperwork generated daily. Medical assistants work as laboratory secretaries, receptionists, phlebotomists, or laboratory assistants.

Hospital test menus are restricted to the most commonly requested tests and tests for which results are needed immediately. Less commonly ordered tests are sent to reference laboratories. Whether the test is performed on site or sent to a reference laboratory, results generally are available within 24 to 48 hours. Results for some of the less common or more sophisticated tests may take a week or longer.

Laboratory Request Forms

Hospital and reference laboratories provide request forms appropriate to their individual operations (FIG. 41-2). All forms should be convenient to use, with clear instructions for complete patient and physician identification to avoid errors. Most request forms cover a variety of tests, so that a single form can be used for tests in hematology, chemistry, immunology, and so on. Some forms serve as both request and report form, listing expected values by test. Many requisitions now contain bar codes that allow fast, accurate processing and reduce specimen identification errors. Most hospitals use computer-generated forms that also contain specimen labels. Box 41-1 lists the information required on all laboratory request forms.

Physician Office Laboratory

The most common type of laboratory is the POL, which may vary greatly in size and quality. POLs generally perform a limited number of waived (or low complexity) to moderate-complexity tests (discussed later in the chapter).

FIGURE 41-2. Laboratory request forms.

Box 41-1

LABORATORY REQUEST FORMS: COMMONLY REQUIRED INFORMATION

- Patient's database. This includes name, address, social security number, and the medical office identification number to avoid errors with identical names. Other identifying information may be included.
- Patient's birth date and gender. Many test results vary with age and sex.
- Date and time of collection. Often test results are affected by the passage of time or the time of day the specimen was collected.
- Physician's name and address or identification number. Results may have to be reported immediately; this information also avoids errors in reporting.
- Checklist of the test or tests to be performed. These may be grouped under one heading as a profile, such as a thyroid profile or a liver profile, which includes more than one test to determine the state of health of one organ, or a general health profile, such as a complete blood count.

Other required information may include the source of the specimen, such as culture swabs for microbiology tests; medications the patient is taking that may alter certain test results (e.g., anticoagulants affecting prothrombin time); directions for reporting (e.g., an immediate need should be marked STAT); and total volume of a 24-hour urine specimen.

Samples for less common or high-complexity tests may be obtained here but are sent to hospital or reference laboratories for testing.

The most common tests in this type of laboratory are urinalysis, blood cell counts, hemoglobin and hematocrit, and blood glucose or cholesterol levels. In POLs, pregnancy tests and quick screening tests for diseases such as mononucleosis and strep throat are also available. Like hospital and reference laboratories, POLs use forms that list normal ranges for various tests (Fig. 41-3).

A POL may have medical assistants who in addition to other tasks perform laboratory duties: collecting samples, performing tests, managing QC, maintaining instruments, keeping accurate records, and reporting results. Medical assistants may perform all of these tasks, only if a physician monitors QC and abnormal results. The chapters in this unit will introduce you to the skills and knowledge necessary to operate a POL.

Checkpoint Question

1. What is a reference laboratory, and how does it differ from a POL? Name and describe the kinds of positions that a medical assistant may hold in a reference laboratory.

LABORATORY DEPARTMENTS

Most large laboratories are divided into departments. This makes it easier to divide the workload and to group similar kinds of tests. Small laboratories, such as POLs, may have only one department. Even so, understanding the basic divisions of laboratory testing may make it easier to understand the nature of the tests and the information they provide.

Below is a list of common laboratory departments, possible subdivisions, and the kinds of testing performed in each.

Hematology

The hematology department performs tests on blood and blood-forming tissues. The various types of cells in the blood and the amount or number of each type of cell are determined. Common tests include complete blood count, white blood cell count, red blood cell count, platelet count, hemoglobin, hematocrit, differential, erythrocyte sedimentation rate, and reticulocyte count.

Coagulation

Often a part of the hematology department, coagulation testing entails evaluating how well the body reacts when blood vessels are injured. The most common tests are prothrombin time, partial prothrombin time, fibrinogen, and bleeding time. These tests also are used to monitor levels of **anticoagulant** drugs, such as heparin and coumadin, during medication therapy. An anticoagulant is anything that prevents or delays blood clotting.

Clinical Chemistry

The clinical chemistry department measures chemical substances in blood or serum. These substances may include hormones, enzymes, electrolytes, gases, medicines and drugs, sugars, proteins, fats, and waste products. The most common tests in small laboratories are glucose, cholesterol, blood urea nitrogen, and electrolytes.

Toxicology

Toxicology is often a separate department in the chemistry laboratory. Toxicology testing entails measuring blood levels of both therapeutic drugs and drugs of abuse.

A

LABORATORY DATA SHEET

(Patient Identification)

	LAB TEST	ADULT NORMAL RANGE	DATES AND RESULTS
BLOOD	WBC x 10³	4.8-10.8	
	RBC x 10⁶	M 4.4-6.0 / F 4.2-5.4	
	Hgb gm	M 13.0-17.0 / F 12.0-16.0	
	Hct %	M 41-51 / F 37-47	
	MCV m3	80-96	
	MCH mmg	27-31	
	MCHC %	32-36	
	Polys %	25-62	
	Band %	0-22	
	Lymph %	20-53	
	Mono %	2-12	
	Eos %	0-2	
	Sed Rate (West)	M 0-10 mm/hr. / F 0-20 mm/hr.	
URINE	Color	amber	
	Sp. G	1.001-1.035	
	pH	4.6-8.0	
	Protein	0	
	Sugar	0	
	Ketones	0	
	Bilirubin	0	
	Blood	0	
	WBC	0-5/HPF	
	RBC	0-3/HPF	
	Bacteria	0	
CULTURES	Vag. Saline	0 trich.	
	KOH	0 monilia	
	Uncult	0	
	Throat	0 Gp. A Strep	
	G.C.	0	

B

LABORATORY DATA SHEET

(Patient Identification)

LAB TEST	ADULT NORMAL RANGE	DATES AND RESULTS
Gluc. (Random)		
Gluc. (Fasting)	65-110 mg/dl	
Gluc. 2 hr. pc.	Less than 120	
BUN	10-25 mg/dl	
Creatinine	0.7-1.4 mg/dl	
Na	135-145 meq/L	
K	3.5-5.0 meq/L	
Cl	95-105 meq/L	
CO_2	24-32 meq/L	
Uric A.	2.5-8.0 mg/dl	
T. Protein	6.0-8.0 g/dl	
Albumin	3.5-5.0 g/dl	
Globulin	2.5-3.2 g/dl	
A/G	0.9-1.9	
Calcium	8.5-11.0 mg/dl	
Phos.	2.5-4.5 mg/dl	
Chol.	150-300 mg/dl	
Trig.	30-200 mg/dl	
Alk. Phos.	30-115 U/L	
SGOT	7-40 U/L	
SGPT	7-40 U/L	
LDH	100-225 U/L	
T. Bili.	0.2-1.5 mg/dl	
D. Bili.	0.2-0.5 mg/dl	
Ind. Bili.	0.2-1.0 mg/dl	
T_4 RIA	3.8-11.4 meg %	
T_3 Uptake	25-35 %	
T_7 Index	0.9-3.9 units	
TSH	2-10 microunits/ml	

FIGURE 41-3. Laboratory data sheet. Normal values are provided for the various tests.

Urinalysis

The urinalysis department often is housed within the chemistry, hematology, or microbiology department. The most common urinalysis is the complete urinalysis (UA), an evaluation of the physical, chemical, and microscopic properties of urine. UA can be performed manually or by automated instruments. Urine pregnancy tests also may be performed in this department.

Immunohematology

Commonly called the blood bank, this department is found only in hospitals and blood donor centers. The immunohematology department performs blood typing and compatibility testing of patient's blood with blood products for transfusion purposes. Blood products prepared, stored, and dispensed include whole blood, packed red cells, platelets, fresh-frozen plasma, cryoprecipitate (substances that settle out of blood after freezing), and Rh immune globulin, such as RhoGAM. Other services may include autologous donation (donation of blood by prospective patients for their own use), tissue typing for transplant purposes, and paternity testing.

Immunology

Testing in the immunology department is based on the reactions of antibodies formed against certain diseases in the presence of proteins called antigens. Recent advances

LEGAL TIP

Test Results

While working in a laboratory, you will have access to the results of many confidential blood and urine tests, such as tests for HIV, drugs, pregnancy, and sexually transmitted diseases. You have an ethical responsibility not to communicate any results to unauthorized persons. Only patients and their physicians are entitled to the results. The only exception is the provision in state laws requiring the reporting of certain test results for public safety; however, reporting this information is not the responsibility of the medical assistant.

in serology testing have produced quick and accurate tests for diagnosing many diseases, including syphilis, human immunodeficiency virus (HIV), mononucleosis, and streptococcus A and B.

Microbiology

The microbiology department identifies the various microorganisms that cause disease. Through sensitivity testing, this department identifies which antibiotics will successfully treat infections grown from patients' specimens. Microbiology may include one or more of the following:

- Bacteriology, the study of bacteria
- Virology, the study of viruses
- Mycology, the study of fungi and yeasts
- Parasitology, the study of parasitic protozoa and worms

Anatomical and Surgical Pathology

The anatomical and surgical pathology department studies tissue and body fluid specimens from aspirations, autopsies, biopsies, organ removal, and other procedures to identify or evaluate the effects of cancer and other diseases. The following are common subdivisions of pathology, which may be individual departments in larger institutions.

Histology

Histology is the study of the microscopic structure of tissue. In histology, samples of tissue are prepared, stained, and evaluated under a microscope to determine whether disease is present. Types of histology specimens include tissue obtained through biopsy and surgical frozen sections that must be evaluated immediately to determine whether further surgery is needed.

Cytology and Cytogenetics

Cytology is the study of the microscopic structure of cells. In cytology, the individual cells in body fluids and other specimens are evaluated microscopically for the presence of disease, such as cancer. The most common cytology test is the Papanicolaou (Pap) test, in which vaginal secretions containing cells brushed or scraped from the cervix are evaluated.

Cytogenetics is a type of cytology in which the genetic structure of the cells obtained from tissue, blood, or body fluids, such as amniotic fluid, are examined or tested for chromosome deficiencies related to genetic disease.

Checkpoint Question

2. What departments may be found in a large laboratory? Summarize the testing done in each one.

LABORATORY PERSONNEL

Within the various departments of reference and hospital laboratories, specially trained professionals oversee laboratory operations or perform testing required by physicians. Each professional position requires a particular level of education and training and has specific responsibilities (Box 41-2).

PHYSICIAN OFFICE LABORATORY TESTING

Many tests can be performed in an office laboratory that meets the standards set forth by Congress in the 1988 **Clinical Laboratory Improvement Amendments** (**CLIA**) and in modifications of the original amendment (discussed later in the chapter). Most tests performed in the POL fall into one of two general categories: tests performed on a semiautomated machine and tests conducted with a self-contained kit. Tests in these categories vary among manufacturers.

The best source of information for safe and accurate testing is the package insert shipped inside the test kit or the instrument reagents and QC instructions specific for various office test instruments. Box 41-3 outlines the type of information contained in test package inserts. For many kit tests, the package insert is the only information provided to guide the performance of the test and to evaluate the results. The package insert information should be combined with routine laboratory practice in a written procedure for each test performed in the laboratory. The Commission on Office Laboratory Accreditation (discussed later in this chapter) provides step-by-step instructions for writing a clinical procedure that meets CLIA standards.

Understanding key information needed for test performance and QC makes package inserts a simple and integral part of office laboratory testing. Ask your laboratory procedures instructor for examples of package inserts from pregnancy test kits or serology test kits for practice in obtaining this information.

LABORATORY EQUIPMENT

Laboratory equipment and supplies for performing physician office tests come in hundreds of types and sizes. It is not necessary to become familiar with every possible type of laboratory equipment. However, a few basic pieces are common to most small laboratories. These include the following:

- Automated cell counter
- Microscope
- Chemistry analyzer
- Centrifuge
- Incubator
- Refrigerator or freezer
- Glassware

Box 41-3

UNDERSTANDING KIT PACKAGE INSERTS

Test package inserts provide the following basic pieces of information:

- Procedure. Explains the test method in numbered steps, usually with illustrations.
- Test principles. Outlines the test.
- Specimen required. Tells whether the test is done on blood, urine, or other body fluids and what collection method is acceptable.
- Reagents needed (or included). Lists the reagents in the kit and any other reagents or materials necessary to perform the test.
- Quality control. States recommendations for testing procedures to ensure that test results are accurate.
- Expected values. Lists normal values for comparison to results obtained.
- Interferences. Explains any factors that may alter test results or compromise test accuracy.

Cell Counter

A cell counter is an automated analyzer used to test blood specimens. The simplest cell counter counts only red and white blood cells and performs hemoglobin and hematocrit testing. Specimens are inserted individually, and results may be printed or read from a screen (see Chapter 45).

Cell counters also include more complex analyzers that accept hundreds of specimens and perform 12 to 15 tests and calculations on each specimen. Medical assistants test specimens using a cell counter if they have received documented training in its use from a CLIA-qualified person.

Checkpoint Question

3. Why are package inserts crucial for safe and accurate testing?

Microscope

The microscope is used to identify and count cells and microorganisms in blood and various other body specimens. Learning how to use a microscope properly requires time and repeated practice. The compound microscope is the type most commonly used in the medical office. The compound microscope is a two-lens system in which ocular and objective lenses together provide the total magnification. A light source illuminates the objects as they are magnified. FIGURE 41-4 shows a microscope and its various parts.

FIGURE 41-4. Basic components of the standard light microscope. (Courtesy of Nikon, Melville, NY.)

The *frame*, which consists of the arm and base, is the basic structural component of the microscope. The ocular at the top of the instrument is for the user's eye. It is marked with its magnification, usually ×10. Binocular microscopes (two eyepieces) minimize eyestrain and have adjustments to allow for variations in spacing between the user's eyes.

To bring the object to be viewed into focus, the *coarse adjustment knob* is used with the lower-powered objective to focus on the object; the *fine adjustment knob* is used with the higher-powered objective or the oil immersion lens for the greatest definition. Always focus in two steps. First look at the slide and objective from the side (not through the ocular or oculars), bringing the slide very close to the lens. Then look through the ocular or oculars as you move the slide farther from the lens to bring it into focus. This procedure will prevent damage to the lens from contact with the slide.

The *nosepiece* houses three or four objective lenses and rotates to bring the objective into working position. Pressure to the objectives should never be used to rotate lenses. Only the grip should be used to make this adjustment. The magnification power is marked on each objective. The shorter, or low-power, objective, magnifies ×10. The higher power magnifies ×40 for closer observation. With the use of oil, the third objective, called the oil immersion lens, magnifies ×100. Some microscopes have a fourth objective with a ×4 lens to scan larger specimens. To determine the total magnification of a specimen, multiply the magnification of the working objective by the magnification of the ocular lens (×10):

Low power: $10 \times 10 = 100$
High power: $40 \times 10 = 400$
Oil immersion: $100 \times 10 = 1000$

The *stage* is the flat surface that holds the slide for viewing. An opening in the solid surface allows illumination of the slide from below. Many stages have clips to hold the slide in place and to allow manual movement of the slide as needed. Some stages mechanically adjust the position vertically or horizontally by moving adjustment knobs, also called X and Y axis knobs.

The *condenser* concentrates the light rays to focus on the slide. The condenser is adjustable. In the lower position, the light focus is reduced; in the higher position, it is increased.

The *diaphragm*, in the condenser, consists of interlocking plates that adjust into a variable-sized opening, or iris, to regulate the amount of light from the source in conjunction with the condenser. The more highly magnified the slide must be, the greater the need for light.

The *light source* is housed in the base.

Microscopes are delicate, expensive instruments. To ensure that the microscope used in your clinical laboratory is kept in good working order, you must handle it properly and maintain it according to the manufacturer's standards (Procedure 41-1). Be sure to place it in a low-traffic area and away from any source of vibration, such as a centrifuge. It should always be covered when not in use.

Checkpoint Question

4. How do the three objective lenses of the microscope differ?

Chemistry Analyzers

Like cell counters, traditional chemistry analyzers vary from simple instruments that perform one or a few tests and require manual operation to complex analyzers that perform 30 or more tests per sample and are operated by computer.

Advances in laboratory instrumentation have led to the development of portable and even hand-held devices for point-of-care testing. These devices are especially suited to POL testing because they are simple to operate, require only small amounts of sample for testing, and provide results in minutes. The machine computes the result and displays it on a screen and/or provides a printout of results.

For high-volume testing and to perform a large variety of tests, a number of bench-top chemistry analyzers are suitable for POL testing. Several use dry reagent technology, in which all reagents are impregnated into a special strip or card. The strip or card is inserted into the machine and a drop of whole blood or serum is applied to the strip with an automated pipette. Other analyzers use wet reagent systems with special reagent packs required for each type of test. These machines can usually be interfaced with an office computer to allow for storage and retrieval of results. Whatever the analyzer, the operator must follow the specific manufacturer's instructions for proper care and use.

Centrifuges

A centrifuge uses centrifugal force, or spinning to exert force outward, to separate liquids into their component parts. A whole blood specimen, when centrifuged, is separated into a bottom layer of heavy red blood cells, a thin middle layer of platelets and white blood cells called the buffy coat (FIG. 41-5), and a top liquid layer that is the lightest of the components. The top layer is serum if the specimen was allowed to clot before centrifuging or plasma if the specimen was anticoagulated and not allowed to clot.

Tubes must always be balanced in the centrifuge. If an uneven number of tubes are to be spun, a tube with water must counterbalance the odd tube. Try to place tubes with approximately the same level of liquid in opposing spaces. All tubes must be securely capped. Never start centrifugation until the lid is locked (many will not start until the lid is securely locked). NEVER open the centrifuge until all motion has stopped, and NEVER stop the spin with your hand. Follow the manufacturer's recommendations for cleaning, oiling, and maintaining the equipment. As with all equipment, read the instructions before operation.

A special type of centrifuge called a microhematocrit centrifuge is used to perform a hematocrit test. A special capillary tube filled with blood is spun in the centrifuge. Clay is inserted to seal one end of the tube, and this end is positioned to the outside of the centrifuge to contain the specimen within the capillary tube. The percentage of packed red blood cells compared to the total volume of specimen is determined, and the result is the hematocrit. This is further discussed in the chapter on hematology.

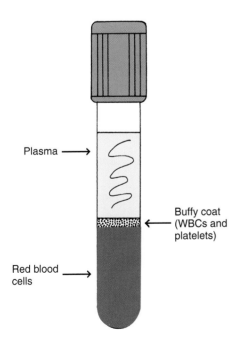

Plasma

Buffy coat (WBCs and platelets)

Red blood cells

FIGURE 41-5. Centrifuged blood specimen. (Reprinted with permission from McCall R. Phlebotomy Essentials. Baltimore: Lippincott Williams & Wilkins, 2003.)

Incubator

Microbiology specimens require a suitable environment to thrive and reproduce. Culture media inoculated with specimens are stored in an incubator for approximately 24 hours to allow microbes to reproduce to a large enough quantity to be identified. The incubator is set at about body temperature (99°F or 37°C), and a daily log is maintained to record the incubator temperature.

Refrigerators and Freezers

Laboratory refrigerators and freezers are similar to those used in the home, but their uses are very different. They are used to store reagents, kits, and specimens. The temperature is critical and must be measured and recorded daily. Food should never be stored in these refrigerators because of the possibility of biohazard contamination. These also vary in size and can be purchased according to office needs and space.

Glassware

For general purposes, the term glassware also includes the disposable plastic supplies used in many medical offices. As with all other medical supplies, sizes and shapes vary with the purpose. Many forms are named for their inventor or for their use. The term glassware includes the following items:

- Beaker. Container with wide mouth for mixing, holding, or heating liquids. Beakers come in various sizes and are used for measurements that need not be exactly precise.
- Flask. Container with narrow neck and a rounded base for holding or transporting liquid in a laboratory. Names include Florence, volumetric, and Erlenmeyer. Volumetric flasks, which have **calibration** lines etched on the neck, are used for critical measurements.
- Glass slide and coverslip. Used with the microscope for holding the specimen to be viewed and usually disposable.
- Graduated cylinder. Used for measuring substances or solutions.
- Petri dish or plate. Shallow, covered dish filled with a solid medium to support the growth of microorganisms.
- Pipette (pipet). Narrow glass or plastic tube, sometimes graduated, open at both ends, used to transport or measure small amounts of liquid. Some pull liquid in by **capillary action**, others by mechanical suction (FIG. 41-6). Pipettes marked TC (to contain) are designed to hold a certain volume; those marked TD (to deliver) are designed to dispense a certain volume. Names include Pasteur, serological, volumetric, and Mohr. Box 41-4 describes how to use a pipette.
- Test tube. Cylindrical container open at one end and rounded or pointed on the other, used for holding laboratory specimens.

FIGURE 41-7 displays various kinds of glassware.

FIGURE 41-6. Assorted pipettes. Pipettes on the right have attached or integrated suction. The bulb at the tip is used for suction with standard pipettes.

LABORATORY SAFETY

Technicians must always be safety conscious when using laboratory equipment. All specimens studied in the laboratory should be considered hazardous and must be treated as such. A technician who is aware of the types of hazards in the clinical laboratory is likely to work safely and avoid injury.

There are three basic types of hazards in the laboratory:

- Physical hazards (fire, broken glass, liquid spills)
- Chemical hazards (acids, alkalis, chemical fumes)
- Biological hazards (diseases such as HIV, hepatitis, and tuberculosis)

Physical hazards include fires caused by an electrical malfunction. Staff must be able to find and operate fire extinguishers and identify fire escape routes. Maintaining and using electrical equipment by the manufacturer's instructions will reduce fire hazards. Avoid using extension cords and overloading electrical circuits. Before servicing any electrical equipment, unplug the instrument.

Box 41-4

HOW TO USE A PIPETTE

Hold the pipette upright, not at an angle, with the tip slightly under the surface of the liquid. Use a slight suction on the suction apparatus until the meniscus is slightly above the desired level. Maintain the level by holding your finger over the top of the tube or maintaining constant pressure on the mechanical apparatus. Raise the pipette from the liquid and wipe the tip with a tissue. Allow the bottom of the meniscus curve to reach the desired calibration by releasing a small amount of the liquid into a waste receptacle. With the pipette vertical, place the side of the pipette against the receiving vessel and allow the contents to drain.

Some pipettes, such as the Unopette, have a premeasured amount of reagent supplied. The whole unit is discarded in a biohazard receptacle after use. Reusable glass pipettes and the mechanical components of automated pipettes should be cleaned according to the manufacturer's instructions. Some may be autoclaved after soaking and rinsing, whereas some require special chemical disinfection or sterilization.

Correct and incorrect pipette positions.

(continued)

Box 41-4 (continued)

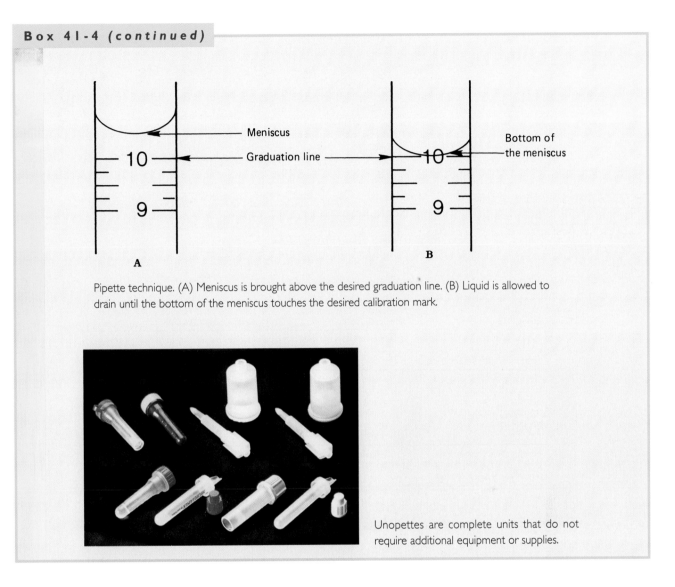

Pipette technique. (A) Meniscus is brought above the desired graduation line. (B) Liquid is allowed to drain until the bottom of the meniscus touches the desired calibration mark.

Unopettes are complete units that do not require additional equipment or supplies.

Chemical hazards can be minimized by labeling all chemicals with the **material safety data sheet (MSDS)** information. MSDS provide the manufacturer's instructions for storage, handling and disposal of the chemical. They describe the risks associated with the product and indicate steps necessary to prevent exposure. An up-to-date volume of MSDS for all chemicals used in the laboratory is the focal part of the facility's chemical hygiene plan. The plan should also include chemical safety protocols specific to that facility.

Hazardous chemicals may have additional labels of precaution. The National Fire Protection Association developed a classification system to identify areas where hazardous chemicals and other materials are stored. This system uses a diamond-shaped symbol, divided into four quadrants, to represent different types of hazards (FIG. 41-8). The BLUE section indicates health hazards; the RED section indicates fire hazards; and the YELLOW section indicates reactive hazards. The WHITE is left blank unless there is a specific hazard such as an oxidizer, water reactive, or radiation hazard. There will be a number from 0 (no hazard) to 4 (serious hazard) in each colored section. Hazardous materials classification posters should be prominently displayed in all laboratory areas.

FIGURE 41-7. Glassware. *Left to right:* beakers, Erlenmyer flasks, graduated cylinders, volumetric flasks. *Front:* test tube.

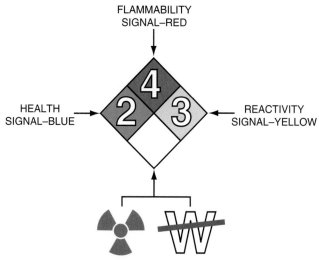

FLAMMABILITY
SIGNAL–RED

HEALTH
SIGNAL–BLUE

REACTIVITY
SIGNAL–YELLOW

RADIOACTIVE OR WATER REACTIVE

Identification of Health Hazard Color Code: **BLUE**		Identification of Flammability Color Code: **RED**		Identification of Reactivity (Stability) Color Code: **YELLOW**	
	Type of possible injury		Susceptibility of materials to burning		Susceptibility to release of energy
SIGNAL		SIGNAL		SIGNAL	
4	Materials that on very short exposure could cause death or major residual injury even though prompt medical treatment was given.	4	Materials that will rapidly or completely vaporize at atmospheric pressure and normal ambient temperature, or that are readily dispersed in air and that will burn readily.	4	Materials that in themselves are readily capable of detonation or of explosive decomposition or reaction at normal temperatures and pressures.
3	Materials that on short exposure could cause serious temporary or residual injury even though prompt medical treatment was given.	3	Liquids and solids that can be ignited under almost all ambient temperature conditions.	3	Materials that in themselves are capable of detonation or explosive reaction but require a strong initiating source or that must be heated under confinement before initiation or that react explosively with water.
2	Materials that on intense or continued exposure could cause temporary incapacitation or possible residual injury unless prompt medical treatment is given.	2	Materials that must be moderately heated or exposed to relatively high ambient temperatures before ignition can occur.	2	Materials that in themselves are normally unstable and readily undergo violent chemical change but do not detonate. Also materials that may react violently with water or that may form potentially explosive mixtures with water.
1	Materials that on exposure would cause irritation but only minor residual injury even if no treatment is given.	1	Materials that must be preheated before ignition can occur.	1	Materials that in themselves are normally stable, but that can become unstable at elevated temperatures and pressures or that may react with water with some release of energy, but not violently.
0	Materials that on exposure under fire conditions would offer no hazard beyond that of ordinary combustible material.	0	Materials that will not burn.	0	Materials that in themselves are normally stable, even under fire exposure conditions, and that are not reactive with water.

FIGURE 41-8. Hazardous materials rating system. (Reprinted with permission from McCall R. Phlebotomy Essentials. Baltimore: Lippincott Williams & Wilkins, 2003.)

Biological hazards refer to specimens capable of transmitting disease. Personal protective equipment (PPE) used per Occupational Safety and Health Administration (OSHA) requirements and strict compliance with handwashing protocols are the best tools for preventing exposure.

Methods for handling each of these hazards must be outlined in detail in your facility's policy and procedure manual. Each member of the staff must be familiar with safety protocols to ensure that risks are kept to a minimum.

Occupational Safety and Health Administration

OSHA is a federal agency in the U.S. Department of Labor that monitors and protects the health and safety of workers. OSHA standards are federal regulations that protect workers by eliminating or minimizing chemical, physical, and biological hazards and preventing accidents. OSHA standards supersede all other regulatory agency requirements. Two OSHA standards of particular importance to medical laboratories are the Occupational Exposure to Blood-borne Pathogens Standard and the Hazardous Communication (HazCom) Standard, or the "right to know law."

Prevention of disease transmission in a medical facility is often called infection control or biohazard risk management. The OSHA Blood-borne Pathogens Standard requires all medical employers to provide training for their employees in techniques that will protect them from occupational exposure to infectious agents, including blood-borne pathogens. Safety manuals must be available or incorporated into the policies and procedures manual to guide employees in correct procedures and emergency protocols.

In addition, OSHA standards require that all workers who are at risk for exposure to potentially hazardous material wear PPE supplied by the employer and readily available for use. PPE includes the following:

- Gloves
- Gown
- Apron
- Face shield
- Goggles
- Glasses with side shields
- Mask
- Lab coat

Workers who are sensitive to allergens such as latex must be supplied with latex-free equipment.

All PPE must be appropriate to the level of exposure. (Review the use of standard precautions in Chapter 1.) A medical assistant performing phlebotomy or assisting with collection of most tissue samples is safe with glove protection. Situations that may result in splashes, splatters, or spreading of an **aerosol** (particles suspended in gas or air), however, require full coverage, including a face shield and footwear, such as shoe covers.

According to OSHA requirements, employers are required to provide free immunization against hepatitis B virus and other blood-borne pathogens if vaccines are available to employees within 10 days of being assigned to duties with possible exposure to blood-borne pathogens. Patient care and laboratory test duties carry the risk of exposure to blood-borne pathogens. Exposure can occur if the skin is pierced or if any body fluid splashes into the eyes, nose, mouth, other opening, or abrasion.

The OSHA HazCom Standard requires all hazardous materials to be labeled by their manufacturers. Hazardous

chemicals must be labeled with a warning, such as "danger"; a statement of the hazard, such as "flammable"; precautions to avoid exposure; and first aid measures for exposure incidents. In addition, manufacturers must supply a MSDS for their products. Employers are responsible for obtaining or developing a protocol for each hazardous agent used on site. This protocol should include an MSDS supplied by the manufacturer for each substance used in the medical office. The extensive information on the MSDS includes items such as storage guidelines, flammability, and exposure precautions. These sheets should be maintained in an office binder near the site of use and should be reviewed routinely by all office staff (Box 41-5).

Checkpoint Question

5. What are three types of hazards found in the laboratory? Give suggestions for preventing exposure to them.

Box 41-5

MATERIAL SAFETY DATA SHEET

An MSDS is required for each of the hazardous materials at a particular site. In the laboratory, these can include disinfectants, cleaning compounds, laboratory chemicals, and some office supplies (e.g., toners, printing compounds). All of these must be labeled as hazardous, with the contents listed on the label. Protocols for each hazardous agent used on site must be listed on the MSDS with the following information:

- Product name and identification. Include all names (trade and generic) by which it may be known.
- Hazardous components. List all hazardous components if the agent contains more than one.
- Health hazard data. Note the risks to those using the agent.
- Fire and explosive data. If this is a volatile agent, note what precautions are necessary to prevent an accident.
- Spill and disposal procedures. Note how to handle spills and disposal to avoid danger.
- Recommendations for personal protection equipment. Note whether gloves, gown, face shield, or other equipment should be worn during use of this agent.
- Handling, storage, and transportation precautions. List any special precautions that must be observed.

Safety Guidelines

These guidelines are some of the most important safety factors required in all laboratories. Follow them carefully to protect yourself, your coworkers, and your patients.

1. Never eat, drink, or smoke in the laboratory area.
2. Never touch your face, mouth, or eyes with your gloves or with items such as a pen or pencil used in the laboratory.
3. Do not apply makeup or lipstick or insert contact lenses in the laboratory.
4. Wear gloves and appropriate protective barriers whenever contact with blood, body fluids, secretions, excretions, broken skin, or mucous membranes is possible. If splatters, splashes, spills, or exposure to aerosols is possible, wear appropriate PPE.
5. Label all specimen containers with biohazard labels.
6. Store all chemicals according to the manufacturer's recommendations. Discard any container with an illegible label. Never store chemicals in unlabeled containers.
7. Wash hands frequently for infection control. Always wash hands before and after gloving and before leaving the work site.
8. Clean reusable glassware and other containers with recommended disinfectant or soap and dry thoroughly before reuse. Wear gloves to prevent cuts.
9. Avoid inhaling the fumes of any chemicals found in the laboratory or wearing contact lenses when working with these types of chemicals. Use of chemicals with hazardous fumes should be limited to facilities equipped with a fume hood.

10. Know the location and operation of all safety equipment, such as fire extinguishers, eyewashes (FIG. 41-9), and safety showers. Keep fire extinguishers close at hand, because many chemicals are flammable.
11. Use safe practices when operating laboratory equipment. Read the manuals and know how to operate the equipment. Avoid contact with damaged electrical equipment.
12. Disinfect all laboratory surfaces concurrently and at the end of the day with a 10% bleach solution or appropriate disinfectant. Never allow clutter to accumulate.
13. Dispose of needles and broken glass in sharps containers. Use biohazard containers for any other contaminated articles.
14. Use mechanical pipetters, but never the mouth, to apply suction to the pipette.
15. Use the proper procedure for removing chemical or biological spills. If the spill is chemical, follow the manufacturer's directions; commercial kits are available for such cleanups (FIG. 41-10). If the spill is biological:

   • Put on gloves.
   • Cover the area with disposable material, such as paper towels to soak up the spill; discard in a biohazard container.
   • Flood the area with disinfecting solution, allowing it to sit for 10 to 15 minutes.
   • Wipe up the solution.
   • Dispose of all waste in a biohazard container.

A   B

F I G U R E   4 1 - 9 .   Eyewash basin. (A) Press the lever at the right of the basin. (B) The stream of water forces the caps from the nozzles. Lower your face and eyes into the stream and continue to wash the area until the eyes are clear.

FIGURE 41-10. Spill cleanup kits. (Reprinted with permission from McCall Phlebotomy Essentials. Baltimore: Lippincott Williams & Wilkins, 2003.)

16. Avoid spills:

- Pour carefully (palm the label).
- Pour at eye level if possible or practical; never pour close to the face.
- Tightly cap all containers immediately after use.

17. Use a splatter guard or splash shield whenever there is any risk of splatter or exposure to aerosols. Spills, splatters, and exposure to aerosols commonly occur in these circumstances:

- Taking the stopper off a blood collection tube
- Transferring blood from a collection syringe to a specimen receptacle
- Conducting centrifugation
- Preparing a smear
- Flaming the inoculation loop

18. When removing a stopper, hold the opening away, use gauze around the cap, and twist gently. Avoid glove contact with the specimen.

19. Immediately report to your supervisor any work-related injury or biohazard exposure.

20. Follow all guidelines for standard precautions and the requirements of the various types of transmission-based precautions as described in Chapter 1.

21. When opening a tube or container, hold the mouth away from you to avoid aerosols, splashes and spills.

Checkpoint Question

6. How would you clean up a biological spill?

Incident Reports

When there is an occurrence in the medical setting for which liability could be considered, an incident report should be completed. An incident report is indicated if a patient, employee, or visitor is injured, if an employee is stuck with a contaminated needle, in case of medication error, or if blood is drawn from the wrong patient. The incident report should be completed by the staff member involved in the incident or closest to the patient or visitor involved in the incident.

Information necessary on an incident report includes the injured person's name, address, telephone number, and date of birth; the date and time; name and address of the facility where the incident occurred; and a brief description of the incident, including any diagnostic procedures or treatments performed. Witnesses to the incident should be listed with names, addresses, and phone numbers for insurance investigation if necessary. In addition to the signature of the person completing the form, a supervisor or doctor should review and sign the form in accordance with the office incident report policy.

CLINICAL LABORATORY IMPROVEMENT AMENDMENTS

With the goals of standardizing laboratory testing and enforcing quality protocols, Congress originally passed the Clinical Laboratory Improvement Amendments (CLIA) in 1988 to establish regulations governing any facility that performs testing for the diagnosis, prevention, or treatment of human disease or for assessment of patients' health

WHAT IF

Your laboratory is not in compliance with OSHA's safety regulations?

In such a situation, your health and that of your colleagues is in jeopardy. OSHA developed the guidelines to protect you from serious injury or death. OSHA can impose significant fines for noncompliance. Continued noncompliance may result in loss of the laboratory's license. In some situations, the physician may not be allowed to file for Medicare compensation. Other situations may incur large fines. To bring the laboratory back into compliance, any citations must be addressed and corrected. OSHA inspectors will revisit the site and reconsider licensure.

status. While final modification of the amendments was made on January 24, 2003, with an effective date of April 24, 2003, the amendments maintain their original name, CLIA '88.

Standards were developed to cover all laboratories from large regional laboratories to the smallest POL. The Centers for Medicare and Medicaid Services (CMS) regulate all laboratory testing (except research) performed on humans in the United States through CLIA. The Division of Laboratory Services of the Survey and Certification Group in the Center for Medicaid and State Operations is responsible for implementing the CLIA program.

CLIA regulations set standards for the following:

- Laboratory operations
- Application and user fees
- Procedures for enforcement of the amendment
- Approval of programs for accreditation

Levels of Testing

CLIA regulations established the three levels of testing discussed next based on the complexity of the testing method.

Waived Tests

Waived tests are low-complexity tests that require minimal judgment or interpretation. They include many tests simple enough for the patient to perform at home (e.g., dipstick urinalysis and glucose monitoring). If these are the only types of tests performed on site, the laboratory can apply for a certificate of waiver (CLIA Waiver Registration), but it still must follow all manufacturers' recommendations for each piece of equipment or product used for testing.

The following are a few of the tests listed in the waived category:

- Urine dipstick or reagent tablets
- Fecal occult blood packets
- Ovulation testing in packets with color comparison charts
- Urine pregnancy testing kits using color comparison charts
- Nonautomated erythrocyte sedimentation rate tests
- Nonautomated copper sulfate testing for hemoglobin
- Centrifuged microhematocrits
- Low-complexity blood glucose determination testing
- Hemoglobin by single analyte instruments with self-contained reagent and specimen interaction and direct measurement and readout

Many additional tests, including rapid strep kits, have waived methodologies available, but the Food and Drug Administration (FDA) has not provided waived status to every manufacturer. The most up-to-date listing of available waived tests can be found on the CMS Web site.

Moderate-Complexity Tests

Most of the testing performed in large, established laboratories has moderate complexity. These are some moderate-complexity tests commonly performed in POLs with moderate-complexity certification:

- Urine and throat cultures
- Automated testing for cholesterol, high-density lipoproteins, and triglycerides
- Gram staining
- Microscopic urinalysis
- Automated hematology procedures with or without a differential requiring no operator intervention during the analytic process and no interpretation of a histogram
- Manual white blood cell count differentials without identification of atypical cells
- Automated coagulation procedures that do not require intervention during analysis
- Automated chemistry procedures that do not require intervention during analysis
- Automated urinalyses that do not require intervention during analysis

A subcategory of moderate-complexity testing called provider-performed microscopy (PPM) requires POLs to have a special registration certificate. PPM can be performed only by a physician or dentist or by a nurse midwife, nurse practitioner, or physician assistant under the direct supervision of a physician. PPM tests include the following:

- All direct wet-mount preparations to be tested for bacteria, fungi, parasites, and human cellular elements
- All potassium hydroxide preparations
- Pinworm examinations
- Fern tests
- Postcoital direct qualitative examinations of vaginal or cervical mucus
- Urine sediment examinations
- Nasal smear examinations for granulocytes
- Fecal leukocyte examinations
- Qualitative semen analysis (limited to the presence or absence of sperm and detection of motility)

High-Complexity Tests

High-complexity tests, which are rarely performed in medical offices, include the following:

- Advanced cell studies (cytogenetics)
- Cytology (e.g., Pap tests)
- Histocompatibility
- Histopathology
- Manual cell counts

If the level of testing to be performed is in question, it must be considered high complexity until its level can be designated by CMS. CMS publishes a list of all tests in the moderate-complexity category. States may establish stricter rules than those set by the governing body, but they may not adopt less strict rules.

Laboratory personnel must also meet the educational levels set forth by CLIA. These guidelines and their updates can be found in the Federal Register.

As a source of CLIA '88 compliance support for POLs, the Commission on Office Laboratory Accreditation (COLA) was established. COLA was subsequently granted deemed status under CLIA. The Joint Commission on Accreditation of Healthcare Organizations (JCAHO) also recognized COLA's laboratory accreditation program and granted it deemed status under JCAHO standards. COLA works to support the health care industry by providing knowledge and resources for maintaining quality laboratory operations.

Laboratory Standards

Laboratories that perform moderate- or high-complexity testing may be inspected in an unannounced visit every year by representatives from CMS or the Centers for Disease Control and Prevention (CDC) under the direction of the Department of Health and Human Services. As discussed later, they must meet all standards set by CLIA.

Patient Test Management

It must be proved that a system is in place to ensure that the specimens are properly maintained and identified and that the results are accurately recorded and reported. Policies must be written for standards of patient care and employee conduct. Each test performed will be evaluated for safety, reliability, and diagnostic indication for its performance.

Policy and procedure manuals will clearly outline patient preparation, specimen handling, how tests are to be performed, alternatives to the usual testing methods for specific situations, and what to do in the event of questionable testing results.

Quality Control

A comprehensive QC program monitors each phase of the laboratory process, including specimen collection, specimen processing, testing, and reporting results. The programs also monitor reagents, instruments, and personnel in addition to actual test performance. Each laboratory must have its own written policies and procedures that include instructions to ensure that all QC standards for monitoring the accuracy and quality of each test are in place for all levels of testing the laboratory conducts. The protocols ensure reliable findings and identification and elimination of errors.

Control Sample Manufacturers provide specimens comparable to human specimens with known reference ranges. Testing control samples at the same time the patient specimen is tested or when a new reagent kit is received ensures that all components are performing as required. Reagent and instrument manufacturers document frequencies for performing QC on their products. The performance of these controls must be recorded in the QC log book.

The **National Committee for Clinical Laboratory Standards** (NCCLS) establishes rules to ensure the safety, standards, and integrity of all testing performed on human specimens. FIG. 41-11 is an example of an NCCLS form on which control sample testing can be recorded. If controls do not fall in the range given in the manufacturer's package insert, testing *cannot* be conducted. The cause must be discovered and corrected before reporting any patient

LEGAL TIP

Chain of Custody

While working in a laboratory, you may be responsible for collecting drug screen specimens or other tests that become legal evidence with a documented chain of custody. Chain of custody (COC) systems are designed to account for each specimen at all times. Specimens in the system are documented with a COC form, a statement signed by each successive person in the chain of custody. COC collections should be completed following the step-by-step instructions on the testing laboratory's COC requisition. The instructions are similar to this:

- Client name's and identification.
- Which urine drug screen test is requested.
- Client's signature with date and time of collection.
- Collector's signature with date and time of collection.
- Whether or not specimen collection was witnessed.
- Specimen temperature (90.5–99.8°F is acceptable).
- Tamper seals affixed and signed as indicated on the requisition. The seal should be attached to one side of container, go across the lid, and attach again to the other side of the container.
- COC requisition in packet of tamper-proof bag.
- Specimen in pouch of tamper-proof bag.
- Tamper-proof bag sealed and transported to testing facility.

These requirements for collection of the specimen must also be fulfilled:

- Client must present picture identification. Client must empty pockets prior to specimen collection.
- Water supply must be turned off to the restroom used for specimen collection and a dye added to the toilet water to prevent client from using toilet water to replace specimen.
- Minimum required specimen volume is usually 35 mL.

Quality Control Log

Test: _____   Control Lot Number: _____

Date	Control Value	Performed By	Accept	Reject	Corrective Action Taken

FIGURE 41-11. Quality control log. (Reprinted with permission from *Physician's Office Laboratory Guidelines and Procedure Manual*, 3rd ed. Wayne, PA: National Committee for Clinical Laboratory Standards, 1995.)

results. Start by checking the reagents and controls for expiration dates, accurate reconstitution, and expiration dates once reconstituted. Next check to see that the testing instrument is clean and functioning properly. If all of this has been done, reconstitute or open a new control sample or reagent and begin the process again.

Management of Reagents Reagents are chemicals used to produce a reaction. All reagents have a manufacturer's lot number and expiration date. These must be recorded in a QC log book with the date received, the date opened, and the initials of the person who opened the package. If the reagent consistently performs inappropriately, the lot number will help the manufacturer identify defects. All supplies and equipment, reagents, and testing components must be labeled with identification, storage requirements, date of preparation or when opened, and expiration date.

Instrument Calibration Laboratory equipment is sensitive and requires strict compliance with operation and maintenance standards. Manufacturers provide maintenance schedules and methods for evaluating performance. Maintenance of equipment and supplies must be documented in the QC log book; this includes maintenance either by an

employee or by a manufacturer's representative. Any corrective action required for equipment or supply malfunction must be documented. FIGURES 41-12 and 41-13 show sample NCCLS forms on which this information can be recorded.

Instruments are designed to produce results within a documented **reportable range**. If the QC results are not within the stated reference range, the instrument's calibration should be checked by the manufacturer's instructions, and patients' and QC specimens should be retested. If the calibration is correct and the results of QC specimens run in the same manner as the patients' specimens are within the stated reference range, the patients' results are correct. The flow chart in FIGURE 41-14 shows how you can evaluate test results for errors.

The laboratory's procedure manual must state the manufacturer's recommendation for the performance of calibration procedures, and supporting documentation must show that controls are performed as directed. Some procedures may require that controls be performed at each testing. Documentation must show the action taken to verify results, what was done when a problem arose, what the solution to the problem was, when the testing equipment was serviced and by whom, and what was done.

FIGURE 41-12. Preventive maintenance record form. (Reprinted with permission from *Physician's Office Laboratory Guidelines and Procedure Manual,* 3rd ed. Wayne, PA: National Committee for Clinical Laboratory Standards, 1995.)

FIGURE 41-13. Instrument history record. (Reprinted with permission from *Physician's Office Laboratory Guidelines and Procedure Manual*, 3rd ed. Wayne, PA: National Committee for Clinical Laboratory Standards, 1995.)

Quality Assurance

The laboratory's policy and procedure manual should cover recommendations for continuing education for the laboratory personnel and evaluation methods for ensuring that workers are competent. The qualifications and responsibilities of all laboratory workers are specified by CLIA, with education and training requirements for all levels of personnel. Employers must ascertain the educational background of employees, provide opportunities for continuing education, and conduct or provide for proficiency testing. This information must be documented and available for inspection by CLIA representatives.

Proficiency Testing

Proficiency testing facilitates external evaluation of the laboratory. To continue testing and maintain Medicare eligibility, all laboratories, even those conducting only waived tests, must participate in three proficiency tests a year and must be available for at least one on-site inspection. Three times a year, the laboratory is shipped specimens prepared by an approved agency. These specimens must be tested by the same procedures used for patients' evaluation and the results mailed to the proficiency testing agency. The proficiency testing agency evaluates the results and provides feedback on performance.

Quality Control Log Book

To record compliance with CLIA measures, a record must be kept of each control sample and standard test. The log must show the date and time of the test, the control or standard results expected, what results were obtained, and the action taken for correction, if any. Documentation must be consistent, and the records must be retained for at least 2 years. Computer software programs are also available for maintaining this data.

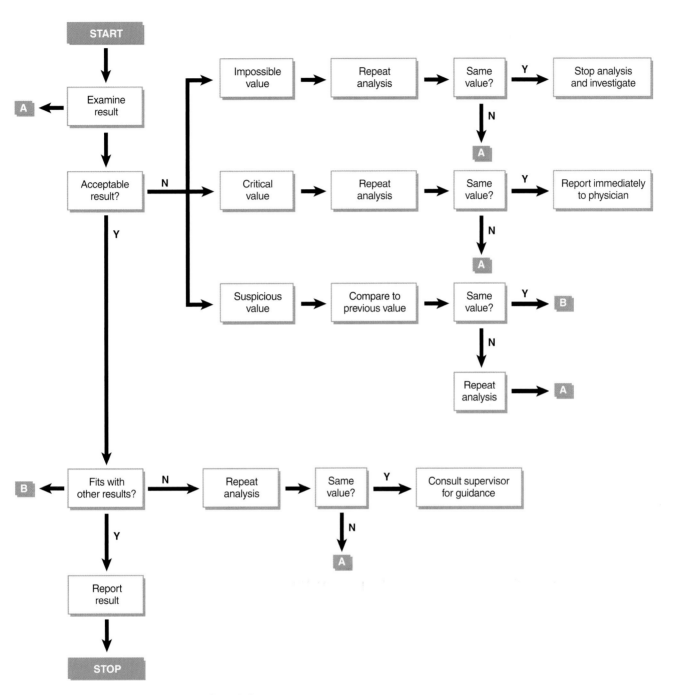

FIGURE 41-14. Flow chart for evaluation of test result for random error: a simple strategy for determining whether an individual test result is reasonable and correlates with other results. Y, yes; N, no. A and B (*far left*) show interconnection between evaluation of repeat testing and where decision-making strategy should resume. For example, if an impossible value is obtained and repeat analysis does not show same value, uppermost horizontal line of chart says that testing procedure should return to symbol A, where the steps are begun again with *examine result*. (Adapted from Cembrowksi GS. Use of patient data for quality control. Clin Lab Med 6:715, 1986).

Procedure 41-1

Caring for a Microscope

Purpose: To protect the integrity and function of laboratory equipment

Equipment: Lens paper, lens cleaner, gauze, mild soap solution, microscope

Steps	Reason
1. Wash your hands.	Handwashing aids infection control.
2. Assemble the equipment.	
3. If you need to move the microscope, carry it in both hands, one holding the base and the other holding the arm.	
4. Clean the ocular areas, following these steps:	
A. Place a drop or two of lens cleaner on a piece of lens paper. Never use tissue or gauze, because either may scratch the ocular areas.	
B. Wipe each eyepiece thoroughly with the lens paper. To prevent transfer of oils from your skin, do not touch the ocular areas with your fingers.	
C. Wipe each objective lens, starting with the lowest power and continuing to the highest power (usually an oil immersion lens). If the lens paper appears to have dirt or oil on it, use a clean section of the lens paper or a new piece of lens paper with cleaner.	Wiping in this manner ensures that you progress from the cleanest area (eyepieces) to the least clean area (oil immersion lens).
D. Using a new piece of dry lens paper, wipe each eyepiece and objective lens so that no cleaner remains.	Removing the cleaner completely prevents distortion by residue.
5. Clean the areas other than the oculars:	This removes oil and dirt from mechanical and structural surfaces.
A. Moisten gauze with mild soap solution and wipe all areas other than the oculars, including the stage, base, and adjustment knobs.	
B. Moisten another gauze with water and rinse the washed areas.	
6. To store the cleaned microscope, ensure that the light source is turned off. Rotate the nosepiece so that the low-power objective is pointed down toward the stage. Cover the microscope with the plastic that came with it or a small trash bag.	This protects the mechanism and surfaces between uses.

Note: To maintain precision focusing, the microscope should be used in a low-traffic area and away from any source of vibration, such as a centrifuge.

Note: Follow the manufacturer's recommendations for changing the light bulb and servicing the microscope.

CHAPTER SUMMARY

As the CLIA list of waived tests continues to grow, medical assistants can provide numerous laboratory findings to aid diagnosis. By maintaining an up-to-date working knowledge of the CLIA standards, medical assistants can validate and document the quality and dependability of the results they report. Maintaining awareness of the types of hazards in the clinical laboratory allows the medical assistant to perform these critical tasks safely.

Critical Thinking Challenges

1. Review the laboratory safety rules and create a poster summarizing these rules for display in the laboratory.
2. List all items that must be documented in the laboratory. Design a form to meet these requirements. Who should complete the form? Where should it be kept? Explain your responses.
3. Working with another student, develop a plan of action to use in case your controls do not come into range and how to go about correcting a problem.

Answers to Checkpoint Questions

1. A reference laboratory is a large facility that serves a particular region, performing thousands of specialized tests daily. In contrast, the POL performs only a few kinds of common tests; some specimens may be sent to a reference laboratory for testing. Medical assistants working in reference laboratories may be employed as specimen processors, sorting specimens and entering data into computers. They may also work as customer service personnel, answering telephones, tracking specimens, and reporting results to the centers from which the specimens were collected.

2. A large laboratory may have the following departments:

   - Hematology, testing for abnormalities of blood and blood-forming tissues
   - Coagulation, measuring clotting time
   - Clinical chemistry, measuring chemicals in blood
   - Toxicology, measuring drug levels in blood
   - Urinalysis, evaluating physical, chemical, and microscopic properties of urine
   - Immunohematology, performing blood typing and compatibility testing for transfusion
   - Immunology, evaluating antibody reactions
   - Microbiology, identifying pathogens
   - Anatomical and surgical pathology, studying tissue and body fluid specimens to identify or evaluate the effects of disease

3. Because tests vary among manufacturers, the package insert is the best source of information on performing the test and evaluating the results.
4. The low-power objective lens magnifies objects ×10 and is used for scanning. The high-power objective lens magnifies objects ×40 and is used for close observation. The oil immersion lens magnifies objects ×100 for close visualization.
5. The three basic types of hazards are physical (e.g., fire, broken glass, and liquid spills), chemical (e.g., acids, alkalis, and chemical fumes), and biological (e.g., diseases such as HIV, hepatitis, and tuberculosis).
6. To clean up a biological spill, first put on gloves. Cover the area with disposable material, such as paper towels; discard these in an appropriate container. Next, flood the area with disinfecting solution and allow it to sit for 10 to 15 minutes. Wipe up the spill. Dispose of all waste in a biohazard container.

 Websites

Commission on Office Laboratory Accreditation
  www.cola.org
Centers for Medicare and Medicaid Services
  www.cms.hhs.gov/clia/waivetbl.pdf

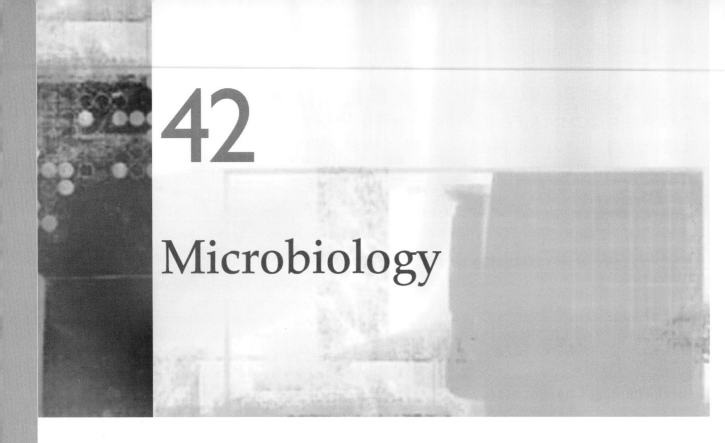

42

Microbiology

CHAPTER OUTLINE

ROLE DELINEATION

CLINICAL: FUNDAMENTAL PRINCIPLES
- Apply principles of aseptic technique and infection control

CLINICAL: DIAGNOSTIC ORDERS
- Collect and process specimens
- Perform diagnostic tests

GENERAL: LEGAL CONCEPTS
- Perform within legal and ethical boundaries
- Document accurately
- Comply with established risk management and safety procedures

CHAPTER COMPETENCIES

LEARNING OBJECTIVES

Upon successfully completing this chapter, you will be able to:

1. Spell and define the key terms.
2. List and describe primary microorganisms.
3. Identify various bacterial illustrations.
4. Describe how bacteria are named.
5. Describe the classifications of fungi, rickettsiae, chlamydiae, protozoa, and metazoa.
6. State the factors necessary for microbial growth.
7. Describe the medical assistant's responsibilities in microbiological testing.
8. List the most common types of microbiological specimens collected in the physician's office laboratory.
9. State the differences between mixed cultures, secondary cultures, and pure cultures.
10. Describe the different types of medium used for microbial testing.
11. List the steps used in caring for media plates.
12. List each step in Gram staining and state the purpose of each step.
13. State the purpose of sensitivity testing and give the meaning of sensitive, resistant, and intermediate results.

PERFORMANCE OBJECTIVES

Upon successfully completing this chapter, you will be able to:

1. Label and identify specimens for transportation and handling (Procedure 42-1).
2. Prepare a wet-mount slide.
3. Prepare a dry specimen smear (Procedure 42-2).
4. Prepare a specimen with Gram stain (Procedure 42-3).
5. Inoculate a tube of broth medium.
6. Inoculate a culture and conduct sensitivity testing (Procedure 42-4).

KEY TERMS

aerobic	cocci	obligate	rickettsia
anaerobic	diplococci	opportunistic	secondary culture
agar	flagella (sing. flagellum)	pathogens	spirochetes
bacteriology	media	parasitology	staphylococci
bacilli (sing. bacillus)	morphology	Petri plate	streptococci
centesis	mycology	primary cultures	virology
Chlamydiae	nosocomial infections		

MICROBIOLOGY LITERALLY means the study of small life, such as bacteria, parasites, and fungi. Most are too small to be seen without a microscope. Microorganisms likely to present health problems are those that thrive at temperatures between 96°F and 101°F in a fairly neutral environment. Of course, many normal flora (bacteria that are not pathogenic) live and thrive on the human body without causing disease. Microorganisms that are capable of producing disease are called **pathogens**. As a medical assistant, to protect yourself, the physician, patients, and all coworkers from **nosocomial infections** (infections acquired in a medical setting), you need to be aware of the organisms present around us and their potential for causing disease.

Bacteria require the following five elements for survival: nutrients, warmth, moisture, darkness, and oxygen (aerobes) or lack of O_2 (anaerobes). The human body provides all five elements. These same five elements are simulated in the microbiology laboratory with the use of culture **media** and an incubator.

Medical microbiology is performed using cultures and smears of patients' specimens referred to the laboratory. The specimens may be taken from wounds or other areas, such as the throat, vagina, urethra, or skin, by using a swab, a stick topped with cotton or other absorbent manmade fiber. Specimens may be drawn from the body by **centesis** (surgical puncture) or by venipuncture. Specimens are also excreted from the body as sputum, stool, or urine.

As a medical assistant, you will frequently collect specimens or assist the physician with the collection. You may collect specimens from wounds or from the throat, but the physician usually collects specimens from the eye, ear, rectum, or reproductive organs. In all instances, you must practice aseptic technique to ensure the integrity of the specimen. In addition, standard precautions are necessary to protect all health care workers and patients.

MICROBIOLOGICAL LIFE FORMS

Bacteria

Bacteriology is the science and study of bacteria. Organisms have both a genus and species name. The genus is always spelled with a capital letter, and the species begins with a lowercase letter (*Staphylococcus aureus*). In print the name is italic or underlined. The name reflects the characteristics of the bacterium or the name or place associated with its discovery.

Several groups of bacteria, including the spore-forming bacteria, are significant in medical microbiology. Bacteria are unicellular (one-celled) simple organisms, each with its own characteristics. Bacteria do not require a host for their life stages as long as they have the five survival requirements. The organisms can be identified by their distinct shapes, or **morphology** (TABLE 42-1); chemical tests; and other means, such as motility tests.

Cocci (spherical bacteria) are responsible for many diseases. Some species of **staphylococci** are found on all surfaces of the skin and many mucous membranes. They are generally not pathogenic unless they reach an area that is usually sterile, where they may cause abscess formation or other form of infection. Species of **streptococci** may cause sore throat, scarlet fever, rheumatic fever, many pneumonias, and various skin infections. **Diplococci** cause bacterial meningitis, gonorrhea, and some of the pneumonias.

Bacilli (bacteria with a rod shape) are usually **aerobic** (requiring oxygen to live) and may be gram positive or gram negative; some form spores. Diseases caused by bacilli include tetanus, botulism, gas gangrene, tuberculosis, pertussis, salmonellosis, certain pneumonias, and otitis media.

Spirochetes are long, spiral, flexible organisms; spiral bacteria are classified as spirilla if they are rigid rather than flexible. Spirochetes are responsible for syphilis and Lyme disease.

Vibrios are very motile comma-shaped bacteria. They cause cholera. FIGURE 42-1 shows the various forms of bacteria.

Bacterial Spore Formation

Some of the microorganisms in our environment produce spores to protect themselves under adverse conditions. The bacterium, usually a bacillus, forms a capsule around it-

self and enters a resting state that allows it to resist most means of asepsis. When conditions are favorable for reproduction, the spore reverts to its active form and resumes its life cycle. These are examples:

- *Clostridium botulinum* (food poisoning)
- *Clostridium tetani* (tetanus)
- *Clostridium perfringens* (gas gangrene)
- *Bacillus anthracosis* (anthrax)

Spores are destroyed by autoclaving with the proper components of heat, steam, pressure, and time (see Chapter 41).

Checkpoint Question

1. What are the four main categories of bacteria?

Rickettsias and Chlamydiae

Specialized forms of bacteria that fit in a category of their own are the **rickettsias** and the **chlamydiae**. Both are smaller than bacteria but larger than viruses. Because they both require a living host for replication and survival, they are referred to as **obligate** intracellular parasites. Rickettsias cause Rocky Mountain spotted fever. The chlamydiae cause trachoma and lymphogranuloma venereum.

Fungi

Mycology is the science and study of fungi. Infectious fungi are small organisms like bacteria with the potential to produce disease in susceptible hosts. Some fungi are microscopic, but many can be seen without the aid of a microscope. Fungi resemble plants, whereas bacteria appear to resemble one-celled animals. Fungi may be in the form of yeasts or molds in the human body. They are **opportunistic**, usually becoming pathogenic when the host's normal flora can no longer counterbalance the colony's growth.

Fungal diseases, called mycoses or mycotic infections, include these:

Molds

- Aspergillus. Often affects the ear but may affect any organ or surface; may be fatal if widespread.
- Blastomycosis. Usually asymptomatic but may cause skin ulcers or bone lesions and may spread to the viscera.
- Coccidioidomycosis. May cause acute flulike respiratory symptoms or may become chronic and infect almost any body part.
- Histoplasmosis. Spreads through contaminated soil; usually asymptomatic but may lead to pneumonia.
- Tinea. Cutaneous mycoses (e.g., tinea pedis [athlete's foot], tinea corporis [ringworm of the body], tinea capitis [ringworm of the scalp], and tinea unguium [nail fungus]).

Table 42-1	CATEGORIZING BACTERIA
Morphology	**Types**
Round (spherical)	Cocci
Grapelike clusters	Staphylococci
Chain formations	Streptococci
Paired	Diplococci
Single	Micrococci
Rod-shaped	Bacilli
Somewhat oval	Coccobacilli
End-to-end in chains	Streptobacilli
Spiral	Spirochetes
Flexible (usually with **flagella**, whiplike extremities that aid movement)	
Rigid	
Curved rods (comma-shaped)	Spirilla
	Vibrios

FIGURE 42-1. Forms of bacteria. (A) Gram-positive staphylococci. (B) Streptococci in short chains. (C) Gram-positive diplococci. (D) Gram-negative bacilli. (E) A long, rod-shaped bacterium. (F) Gram-positive spore-forming bacilli. (G) The spirochete *Treponema pallidum* responsible for syphilis. (H) *Vibrio*.

FIGURE 42-2. The fungus *Candida albicans*.

Yeasts

Candidiasis causes thrush (skin and mouth), vaginitis, and endocarditis. It may be spread by contact (FIG. 42-2).

Viruses

Virology is the study of viruses, the smallest microorganisms. Viruses cause influenza, infectious hepatitis, rabies, polio, and acquired immunodeficiency syndrome (AIDS). They are so small that they can be seen only with an electron microscope, not the usual bright-field microscope found in the medical office. They require a living host for survival and replication and are referred to as obligate intracellular parasites. Because viruses are not susceptible to antibiotics, most are extremely difficult to treat. Antiviral therapies are being developed for many of the viruses, and researchers continue to work on cures for many viral diseases, such as AIDS and herpes.

Protozoa

Single-celled parasitic animals that may be diagnosed in the **parasitology** laboratory are the protozoa. These microorganisms and conditions they cause include the following:

- Entamoeba: diarrhea, dysentery, and liver and lung disorders
- Giardia: giardiasis, diarrhea, and malabsorption of nutrients
- Trichomonas: trichomoniasis, vaginitis, and urinary tract infection
- Plasmodium: malaria
- Toxoplasma: toxoplasmosis and fetal abnormalities

Metazoa

Metazoa include helminths, nematodes, and arthropods. The helminth family includes roundworms, flatworms, and flukes. Most survive almost anywhere in the human body or may migrate through the body until they find a place to settle. Helminths can cause schistosomiasis, liver fluke infestations, and beef or pork tapeworm infestation. The nematodes cause roundworm infestations, gastrointestinal obstruction, bronchial damage, pinworm infestation, and trichinosis. Arthropods include mites, lice, ticks, and fleas along with bees, spiders, wasps, mosquitoes, and scorpions. All may cause injury by their bites or stings, and several are also capable of transmitting disease by their bite or sting.

MICROBIOLOGICAL TESTING: THE MEDICAL ASSISTANT'S ROLE

Your role in microbiological testing may be extensive. Although this role varies from office to office and sometimes from state to state, it will include both administrative and clinical responsibilities.

Administrative duties in microbiological testing:

- Routing specimens
- Handling and filing reports
- Ensuring patients' safety and education
- Billing and insurance filing

Clinical skills:

- Collecting and processing specimens
- Assisting the physician and patient as needed
- Maintaining standard precautions and safety
- Terminal cleaning after testing is complete

SPECIMEN COLLECTION AND HANDLING

Laboratory tests are most often performed on specimens that are easily obtained from the body, such as blood, urine, feces, sputum, and other body secretions and fluids. The specimen gives the physician a view of the condition of the system from

WHAT IF

Your patient asks you how to prevent cutaneous mycoses, such as tinea pedis?

Explain to your patient that tinea pedis is a common fungal infection. Then offer the following suggestions, which can aid prevention:

- Practice good basic hygiene.
- Thoroughly dry between the toes.
- Do not share footwear.
- Use antifungal powder between the toes and in shoes.
- Wear foot protection when using public showers.

which the specimen was obtained. For instance, a urine culture will indicate the infectious process at work within the urinary system; a sputum culture will grow the organism responsible for the patient's respiratory signs and symptoms.

As a medical assistant, you may be responsible for collecting most of the specimens in the medical office. To ensure that the office or reference laboratory receives a sample that will indicate the disease process for which the specimen was collected, you must collect the specimen from the appropriate site using the proper method. You also must handle the specimen so that it will yield accurate findings (Box 42-1).

Types of Specimens

Microbiology entails extensive work with cultures of the referred biological specimen. **Cultures are media that will support the growth of microorganisms. The organisms are encouraged to replicate under controlled conditions for the purpose of diagnosing disease.** These may be **primary cultures**, which come directly from the patient's specimen and are used to investigate any or all of the microorganisms found at the specimen site. Or they may be **secondary cultures**, also called subcultures, suspicious organisms taken from the primary culture and encouraged to grow for more extensive study. Pure cultures contain only one type of organism and may be a primary or secondary culture.

You may have to collect blood to be examined for microorganisms. Care must be taken in any instance of venipuncture, of course, but for the purpose of culture, the specimen must remain uncontaminated or the findings will not be diagnostic or

will produce an inaccurate diagnosis (see Chapter 44). The yellow-stopper tube should be anticoagulated with sodium poly ethanol sulfonate unless the pathogen is suspected to be *Neisseria gonorrhoeae*. In adults, usually 10 to 20 mL is collected; in children, 1 to 5 mL is collected. Sometimes specimens are collected in blood culture bottles. In this case take care to ensure that the liquid in the bottle does not touch the inner part of the needle. This will eliminate the possibility of entry of the liquid into the patient's bloodstream.

Sputum is often tested for diagnosis of respiratory diseases. It should be the first morning specimen, collected by deep coughing, taking care that saliva is not also expectorated into the container. You may be responsible for explaining to the patient the proper procedure for sputum collection (see Chapter 32).

Wound specimens may be collected by you or the physician. It may be necessary to collect wound specimens from several sites in the wound area (see Chapter 29).

Other commonly obtained specimens include throat cultures (see Chapter 32), urine cultures (see Chapter 43), and stool specimens (see Chapter 34).

Box 42-1

GUIDELINES FOR SPECIMEN COLLECTION AND HANDLING

- Follow standard precautions for specimen collection as outlined by the Centers for Disease Control and Prevention.
- Review the requirements for collecting and handling the specimen, including the equipment, the type of specimen to be collected (e.g., exudate, blood, mucus), the amount required for laboratory analysis, and the procedure to be followed for handling and storage.
- Assemble the equipment and supplies. Use only the appropriate specimen container as specified by the medical office or laboratory.
- Ensure that the specimen container is sterile to prevent contamination of the specimen by organisms not present at the collection site.
- Examine each container before use to make sure that it is not damaged, the medium is intact and moist, and it is well within the expiration date.
- Label each tube or specimen container with the patient's name and/or identification number, the date, the name or initials of the person collecting the specimen, the source or site of the specimen, and any other information required by the laboratory. Use an indelible pen or permanent marker. Make sure you print legibly, document accurately, and include all pertinent information.

Checkpoint Question

2. What are the differences between mixed cultures, secondary cultures, and pure cultures?

Types of Culture Media

Media (liquid, solid or semisolid preparations) support the growth of microorganisms for easy identification. The microorganism will proliferate for diagnosis of disease when it has been provided an environment for optimal growth.

Various types of media are prepared with a mixture of substances that nourish pathogens. All of the suspected microorganism's requirements for replication must be present. The medium provides nutrients, moisture, and the proper pH. The temperature and darkness are maintained by an incubator (FIG. 42-3). The presence or absence of oxygen is provided by the type of incubator, oxygen for aerobes and carbon dioxide for anaerobes. As stated earlier, some media are solid, some are semisolid, and some are liquid, or broth.

The medium may contain additives to support the growth of specific organisms and inhibit the growth of others; these are selective media. Nonselective media will grow almost any microorganism.

Media designed for **anaerobic** bacteria (bacteria that live without oxygen) may contain a tablet that generates carbon dioxide and eliminates oxygen in the closed environment of the medium container. Many laboratories use special sealed jars containing a pouch of chemicals that maintain an anaerobic environment. In some instances, the plate may be placed in a jar with a lighted candle. The jar is tightly sealed

FIGURE 42-4. The Bio-Bag anaerobic culture set. It includes a plate of CDC-anaerobic blood agar in an oxygen-impermeable bag. The system contains its own gas-generating kit and cold catalyst. (Courtesy of Becton Dickinson, Franklin Lakes, NJ).

and the candle consumes the available oxygen and gradually burns itself out. FIGURE 42-4 displays one type of anaerobic culture set.

Specimens submitted for laboratory study are most frequently cultured on blood agar, a solid medium prepared by adding 5% sheep's blood to **agar**, a firm, jellolike transparent and colorless substance made from seaweed. The agar congeals the blood and forms a firm surface to support the growth of microorganisms. The firm surface makes it easy to observe the culture growth. The blood adds the nourishment required for replication of the microorganisms.

A **Petri plate** is a glass or plastic dish used to hold a solid culture medium, such as blood agar. The plate is fitted with a cover to maintain the integrity of the specimen. Petri plates are clear and allow visual examination of a culture as it grows. Agar is also placed in sterile glass tubes and allow to harden at an angle. These are agar slants. The flat angled surface is where the medium is to be inoculated.

A liquid or broth medium is usually provided in a small jar or tube. Many special broth media are supplied with swabs to be used for specimen collection and are enclosed in special envelopes for transporting the specimen.

Caring for the Media

Commercially prepared culture media in disposable plastic Petri plates are available for use in medical offices. The plates are supplied in a plastic sleeve and must be stored in the refrigerator with the side containing the medium on top. (FIG. 42-5). The plates should be stored in the plastic wrapper to keep the medium moist. Petri plates stored with the

FIGURE 42-3. Standard laboratory incubator. (Courtesy of So-Low Environmental Equipment, Cincinnati, OH.)

FIGURE 42-5. Solid media are supplied on Petri plates wrapped in a plastic sleeve. Petri plates are always stored medium side up.

medium down may form condensation on the lids that will drip onto the surface, making it too moist for an accurate culture. Check the expiration date and the condition of the medium surface before using the plates. Discard any plates that are past the expiration date or any medium that has dried or cracked. When the shipment arrives, date each sleeve. Rotate the media in the refrigerator so that the oldest is in front and used first, based on the date it expires, not the date it was received. *Note:* The temperature of the refrigerator should be checked and recorded daily. Be sure not to overfill the refrigerator or allow media to be placed against the back wall or sides. This will raise the temperature.

Culture media may also be prepared in the medical office from a commercially available dehydrated form. Be sure to follow manufacturer's guidelines and use strict sterile technique. **Whether prepared in the office or commercially, a culture medium is effective for 72 hours once it has been inoculated with a specimen. Transportation or on-site testing within that time frame is essential.**

Agar must be refrigerated until needed, then warmed to room temperature before use. A cold plate or tube will kill many microorganisms, most of which require a warmer temperature for growth. Most physician offices are equipped with an incubator set at about 99°F (37°C), or just about body temperature. Check and record the incubator temperature daily.

Checkpoint Question

3. Why is it important to store the Petri plates with the medium side uppermost?

Transporting the Specimen

Many pathogens are not particularly fragile, but care must be taken to transport or process the specimen as soon as possi-

ble so the organisms do not die off. The sooner the specimen is processed, the sooner the pathogen can be identified and treatment can begin. Some microorganisms, such as *N. gonorrhoeae*, are very fragile and must be cultured under controlled conditions as quickly as possible.

Specimens to be processed in outside or regional laboratories must be placed in transport medium, such as the Culturette (Marion Scientific) (FIG. 42-6) or Precision Culture CATS (Precision Dynamics). All directions appropriate for the specimen are stated on the package. Most transport systems are designed to be self-contained and include a plastic tube with a sterile swab and transport medium appropriate for the type of specimen (FIG. 42-7). Most are stored at room temperature. Because transported specimens will be handled by a large laboratory, special care must be taken in filling out all identification slips and information. Procedure 42-1 describes the steps for preparing a specimen for transport.

Properly prepared transport media may be mailed or routed by a courier. The outside laboratory may provide a mailing or shipping container, either cardboard or plastic foam, to protect the specimen during transport. A label indicating the presence of a biohazardous biological specimen is attached to the outside of the container. In many instances, specimens are collected and transported on days that ensure their arrival during the business week to avoid having them remain in transit until the start of a new week. Delays in testing may cause some of the microorganisms to die or to overproliferate, possibly compromising the results of the test.

For the most reliable results, laboratory tests should be performed on fresh specimens within 1 hour after collection. When this is not possible, the specimen must be stored properly to preserve the physical and chemical properties necessary for accurate diagnosis. Specimens should never be subjected to extreme temperature changes. TABLE 42-2 lists general guidelines for handling and storing specimens commonly collected in the medical office.

FIGURE 42-6. Transport media.

FIGURE 42-7. (A) Place the swab in a Culturette tube. (B) Crush the ampule of medium at the bottom of the tube.

Table 42-2	HANDLING AND STORING COMMONLY COLLECTED SPECIMENS	
	Handling	**Storage**
Urine	Clean-catch midstream with care to avoid contaminating the inside of the container; must not stand more than 1 hr after collection.	Refrigerate if cannot be tested within 1 hr; add preservative at direction of laboratory; preservatives not usually used for urine culture.
Blood	Handle carefully, as hemolysis may destroy microorganisms; collect in anticoagulant tube at room temperature; specimen must remain free of contaminants; see laboratory manual for proper anticoagulant.	For most specimens, refrigerate at 4°C (39°F) to slow changes in physical and chemical composition.
Stool	Collect in clean container. To test for ova and parasites, keep warm.	Deliver to laboratory immediately. If delayed, mix with preservative provided or recommended by laboratory, or use transport medium.
Microbiology specimens	Do not contaminate swab or inside of specimen container by touching either to surface other than site of collection. Protect anaerobic specimens from exposure to air	Transport specimen as soon as possible. If delayed, refrigerate at 4°C (39°F) to maintain integrity.

Observe standard precautions while handling any of these specimens.

MICROSCOPIC EXAMINATION OF MICROORGANISMS

Smears and Slides

Specimens grown on a culture may be spread onto a glass slide to be inspected under a microscope. Sometimes a special treatment with stain or fixative will be applied to aid in identification. Some pathogens are more easily identified if they are allowed to move freely in a wet mount (Box 42-2). These should always be viewed immediately, or within 30 minutes of collection.

If multiple smears are to be made from one culture, the colonies to be observed should be numbered on the back of the Petri plate or plates. Number the slides with corresponding numbers with a diamond-tipped pen on the frosted edge of the slide for proper identification of the culture sites (Procedure 42-2).

GRAM STAINING: A DIAGNOSTIC TOOL

Identification by Staining

Staining the microorganisms may help the physician narrow the field of possible pathogens and initiate treatment before a culture has been incubated (Box 42-3). Most bacteria are colorless and hard to see or identify without special treatment such as staining.

The Gram stain process was developed by Hans Gram, a Dutch physician who discovered that after staining with crystal violet and safranin, certain bacteria (cocci and bacilli) retain crystal violet dye. These bacteria can be seen with the use of a bright-field microscope. Bacteria that re-

---

Box 42-2

PREPARING A WET MOUNT SLIDE

To prepare a wet mount, follow these steps:
1. Place a drop of the specimen on a glass slide with sterile saline or 10% potassium hydroxide (KOH).
2. Place a coverslip over the specimen to reduce evaporation.
3. To decrease evaporation, coat the rim of the coverslip with petrolatum.
4. Inspect the slide by microscope using the high-power objective lens with diminished light.

Wet mount slide preparation. (A) A drop of fluid containing the organism is placed on a glass slide. (B) The specimen is covered with a coverslip ringed with petroleum jelly.

A

B

GRAM STAINING: A DIAGNOSTIC TOOL

Gram staining provides important diagnostic information. Even before a culture can be incubated, a physician may tentatively diagnose a patient's disease and begin treatment based on the results of Gram staining, the organism's morphology, and the patient's reported symptoms. These are some common diseases and their Gram stain findings:

Gram Positive	Gram Negative
Strep throat	Whooping cough (pertussis)
Scarlet fever	*Escherichia coli* (some forms of cystitis)
Diphtheria	*Haemophilus influenzae*
Meningitis	Certain pneumonias
Tetanus	Gonococcus
Botulism	Salmonella
Certain pneumonias	Shigella
Gardnerella vaginitis	Cholera
Staphylococcal skin lesions	
Toxic shock syndrome	

tain the purple color are said to be gram positive. Those that do not retain the crystal violet will stain red with the safranin stain, also called the counterstain. These are said to be gram negative. Procedure 42-3 details the steps for Gram staining a smear slide. The Gram stain is read with the use of a bright field microscope. The report should include morphology (cocci or bacilli), gram reaction (gram positive if blue, gram negative if red), and the arrangement (chains or clusters). In most offices the Gram stain is read and reported by the physician, but the medical assistant needs to be able to observe the slide to ensure it can be read. If there is a problem, he or she may have to make and stain a new slide.

Microbiological Inoculation

Microbiological inoculation is introduction of a microorganism into culture medium and placement in a hospitable environment. To ensure that the specimen is placed on or in the culture medium in the proper manner to encourage maximal growth, you will inoculate it with the specimen swab or remove a portion of the specimen with a sterile inoculating loop (FIG. 42-8). The culture plates are streaked using a qualitative or quantitative technique. Broth or semisolid medium is considered to be inoculated when the swab or loop is inserted below its surface (FIG. 42-9).

Generally, a swab is used when the specimen is lifted directly from the site to the medium. An inoculating loop is used when lifting a colony from a culture to inoculate a secondary culture. The specific colonies will be lifted from the primary culture plate and streaked onto the second plate to be incubated again for a pure culture and further study. Procedure 42-4 describes the steps for culture inoculation.

Checkpoint Question

4. Why are bacteria stained?

Sensitivity Testing

The suspected pathogen is inoculated in a broth medium from the pure or secondary culture and incubated for 18 to 24

FIGURE 42-8. Bacteriology loops for inoculation and transfer of bacterial cultures. (Courtesy of Becton Dickinson, Franklin Lakes, NJ).

hours. With a sterile swab, suspend some of this growth in a liquid medium to a turbidity of approximately 2+ (enough that printed material is barely visible through the suspension). Dip another sterile swab in the suspension and spread it over the entire surface of the Muller Hinton or blood agar plate. Impregnate the plate with the various antibiotic disks. After the plate has been incubated for the prescribed length of time (usually another 18–24 hours), it will be inspected for a zone of no growth around each disk. Those that exhibit a margin with no bacterial growth indicate that the pathogen is sensitive or susceptible to this medication. If there is no zone around the disk, the organism is said to be resistant to that antibiotic. If there is a small zone, it may be reported as intermediate. The antibiotic of choice will be the one with the largest zone of inhibition (no growth) (FIG. 42-10).

Streptococcal Testing

Streptococcal pharyngitis (strep throat) in children and young adults is one of the most common infections in the medical office. Because of the need for rapid diagnosis to begin appropriate treatment, many kits are available to test quickly for the pathogen group A beta-hemolytic streptococcus or *Streptococcus pyogenes*. The results are read in a few minutes while the patient waits. Treatment can begin at once.

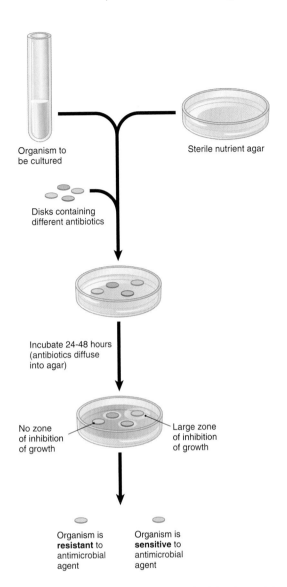

FIGURE 42-10. Disk diffusion method for determining the sensitivity of bacteria to antimicrobial agents.

The theory behind the rapid tests for streptococcus relies on the antigen–antibody reaction, which causes a change on the testing material. The manufacturer provides quick, easy-to-follow instructions. Quality control measures are included with the test kit. See Chapter 46 for further discussion of strep testing.

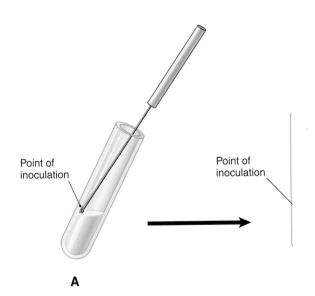

A

FIGURE 42-9. Technique for inoculating a tube of broth medium. (A) Slant and inoculate the side of the tube as shown. (B) Replace the tube upright. This submerges the inoculation site.

Checkpoint Question

5. What is the purpose of sensitivity testing?

Procedure 42-1

Preparing a Specimen for Transport

Purpose: To maintain and ensure the viability of a specimen for testing purposes.

Equipment: Appropriate laboratory requisition, specimen container, mailing container.

Steps	Reason
1. Assemble the equipment.	
2. Complete the laboratory request form.	All information must be written in the appropriate blanks. If information is not applicable or not available, indicate it on the slip. Do not leave any questions unanswered.
3. Wash hands and put on gloves.	Handwashing aids infection control.
4. Check the expiration date and condition of the transport medium.	Out-of-date medium must not be used. If the medium appears to be dried or looks different from normal, do not use it.
5. Peel the envelope away from the transport tube about one-third of the way and remove the tube.	Often the envelope is used to package the specimen. This will be indicated on the package.
6. Label the tube with the date, patient's name, source of the specimen, and initials of the person processing the specimen.	The specimen container must be identified to accompany the laboratory slip.
7. Obtain the specimen as directed by the physician or receive it from the physician.	The specimen may be obtained by various methods and from many sites.
8. Return the swab to the tube and follow the manufacturer's recommendation for immersion in the medium.	Instructions vary and are specific to the manufacturer. All instructions must be followed to ensure accurate test results.
9. Remove and dispose of gloves and wash hands.	
10. Package for transport as directed on the packaging. Some specify returning the tube to the peel-apart envelope.	The laboratory slip and all components of the transport system must be together to avoid misidentification.
11. Route the specimen.	The specimen may be mailed or sent by carrier.

Charting Example

05/04/2004 1:00 P.M. Culture sample taken by swab from left lower leg wound. Yellow-green drainage noted. Sample sent by courier to Wakefield lab for culture. _____ O. Campbell, CMA

Procedure 42-2

Preparing a Dry Smear

Purpose: To aid in the identification of microorganisms in a specimen.

Equipment: Specimen, Bunsen burner, slide forceps, slide, sterile swab or inoculating loop, pencil or diamond-tipped pen.

Steps	Reason
1. Wash your hands.	Handwashing aids infection control.
2. Assemble the equipment.	
3. Label the slide with the patient's name and the date on the frosted edge with a pencil.	Labeling will ensure proper identification. Pencil markings will not rinse off during staining.
4. Put on gloves and face shield. Hold the edges of the slide between the thumb and index finger. Starting at the right side of the slide and using a rolling motion of the swab or a sweeping motion of the inoculating loop, gently and evenly spread the material from the specimen over the slide. The material should thinly fill the center of the slide within half an inch of each end.	Wear the face shield to avoid splatters from the inoculating loop. Spread the material thinly to avoid obscuring the slide with too much material. Rolling ensures that as much of the specimen as possible is deposited on the slide. Sweeping the loop accomplishes the same purpose. Confining the specimen to the area within half an inch of the edges avoids contaminating the gloves.

Step 4. Use a rolling motion to deposit the specimen material on the slide.

Steps	Reason
5. Do not rub the material vigorously over the slide.	Doing so may destroy fragile microorganisms.
6. Dispose of the contaminated swab or inoculating loop in a biohazard container. If you are not using a disposable loop, sterilize it as follows: A. Hold the loop in the colorless part of the flame of the Bunsen burner for 10 seconds. B. Raise the loop slowly (to avoid splattering the bacteria) to the blue part of the flame until the loop and its connecting wire glow red.	The swab and the loop contain body fluid and are considered biohazardous.

(continued)

Procedure 42.2   *(continued)*

Preparing a Dry Smear

Steps   **Reason**

Step 6B. Fire the loop and its connecting wire.

   C. If reusing the loop, cool it so the heat will not kill
      the bacteria that must be allowed to grow. Do not
      wave the loop in the air because doing so may
      expose it to contamination. Do not stab the
      medium with a hot loop to cool; this creates an
      aerosol.

7. Allow the smear to air dry in a flat position for at
   least half an hour. Do not blow on the slide or wave it
   about in the air. Heat should not be applied until the
   specimen has been allowed to dry. Some specimens
   (e.g., Pap smear) require a fixative spray.

The cells will dry slowly at room temperature. If you
blow on the slide, you may contaminate the
specimen with bacteria from your mouth. Fixative
may be sprayed from 4 to 6 inches to protect the
cells from contaminants or to keep them from
becoming dislodged. Heat at this point may destroy
the microorganisms.

8. Hold the dried smear slide with the slide forceps.
   Pass the slide quickly through the flame of a Bunsen
   burner three or four times. The slide has been fixed
   properly when the back of the slide feels slightly
   uncomfortably warm to the back of the gloved hand.
   It should not feel hot.

Passing the slide through the heat kills the
microorganisms and attaches them firmly to the
slide so they do not wash off during staining and
are not dislodged during viewing. Excessive heat
may distort the specimen cells.

(continued)

Procedure 42-2 *(continued)*

Preparing a Dry Smear

Steps	Reason
Step 8. Pass the slide through the flame.	
9. Examine the smear under the microscope or stain it according to office policy. Usually the physician examines the slide for identification.	
10. Dispose of equipment and supplies in appropriate containers. Remove and dispose of gloves and wash your hands.	

Note: Direct smears are slides made straight from the patient. When observing the stained slide, you will see epithelial cells and bacterial cells. Indirect smears are slides made from the culture grown for 18 to 24 hours after incubation and contain only bacterial cells.

Charting Example
07/23/04 10:00 A.M. Specimen taken from nostril and prepared as a direct smear. Gram-positive cocci in chains. Dr. York read the slide. _____ B. White, RMA

Procedure 42-3

Gram Staining a Smear Slide

Purpose: To aid in the identification of pathogens in a specimen

Equipment: Crystal violet stain, staining rack, Gram iodine solution, wash bottle with distilled water, alcohol-acetone solution, counterstain (e.g., Safranin), absorbent (bibulous) paper pad, specimen on a glass slide labeled with a diamond-tipped pen, immersion oil, microscope, Bunsen burner, slide forceps, stopwatch or timer

Steps	Reason
1. Wash your hands.	Handwashing aids infection control.
2. Assemble the equipment.	
3. Make sure the specimen is heat-fixed to the labeled slide and the slide is room temperature (see Procedure 42-2).	Labeling the slide with a diamond-tipped pen or pencil ensures that the identification will not wash off.
4. Put on gloves.	
5. Place the slide on the staining rack with the smear side up.	The staining rack collects the dye as it runs off the slide for disposal.
6. Flood the smear with crystal violet. Time with the stopwatch or timer for 30 to 60 seconds.	

Step 6. Flood the slide with crystal violet to stain the bacteria purple.

(continued)

Procedure 42-3 *(continued)*

Gram Staining a Smear Slide

Steps	Reason

7. Hold the slide with slide forceps.

   A. Tilt the slide to an angle of about 45° to drain the excess dye.

Step 7A. Tilt the slide to drain off excess dye.

   B. Rinse the slide with distilled water for about 5 seconds and drain off excess water.

Washing off the stain stops the coloring.

Step 7B. Rinse with water.

(continued)

Procedure 42-3   *(continued)*

Gram Staining a Smear Slide

Steps	Reason
8. Replace the slide on the slide rack. Flood the slide with Gram iodine solution and time for 30 to 60 seconds.	The iodine acts as a mordant and fixes, or binds, the crystal violet to the gram-positive bacteria. The stain will be permanent in the receptive gram-positive cells after it is fixed with the iodine solution.

Step 8. Flood with Gram iodine solution.

9. Using the forceps, tilt the slide at a 45° angle to drain iodine solution. With the slide tilted, rinse the slide with distilled water from the wash bottle for about 5 to 10 seconds. Slowly and gently wash with the alcohol-acetone solution until no more stain runs off.	The alcohol-acetone removes the crystal violet stain from the gram-negative bacteria. The gram-positive bacteria retain the purple dye. If the process is carried on too long or too vigorously, dye may leach out of the gram-positive bacteria and lead to incorrect findings.

Step 9. Rinse with alcohol-acetone solution until no more purple stain runs off.

(continued)

Procedure 42-3 (continued)

Gram Staining a Smear Slide

Steps	Reason
10. Immediately rinse the slide with distilled water for 5 seconds and return the slide to the rack.	Rinsing stops the decolorizing.

Step 10. Immediately rinse alcohol-acetone solution.

Steps	Reason
11. Flood with Safranin or suitable counterstain. Time-process for 30 to 60 seconds.	The gram-negative bacteria stain pink or red with the counterstain.

Step 11. Flood with Safranin or counterstain.

(continued)

Procedure 42-3   *(continued)*

Gram Staining a Smear Slide

Steps	**Reason**
12. Drain the excess counterstain from the slide by tilting it at a 45° angle.	Moisture or excess solution may obscure the slide and hinder identification.

A. Rinse the slide with distilled water for 5°seconds to remove the counterstain.

Step 12A. Rinse clear of counterstain.

B. Gently blot the smear dry with bibulous paper. Take care not to disturb the smeared specimen. Wipe the back of the slide clear of any solution. It may be placed between the pages of a bibulous paper pad and gently pressed to remove excess moisture.

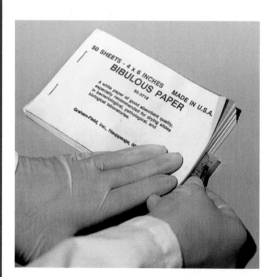

Step 12B. Blot gently with bibulous paper.

(continued)

Procedure 42-3 (continued)

Gram Staining a Smear Slide

Steps	Reason
13. Inspect the slide using oil immersion objective lens for greatest magnification. The physician interprets the slide.	
14. Properly care for or dispose of equipment and supplies. Clean the work area. Remove gloves and wash your hands.	

Note special precautions: Results may be misinterpreted if a reagent is defective or near expiration or if the timing factors in the staining process are not as directed. The bacteria may overstain, or color may leach from the cells if care is not taken to observe the time limits. The results will not be accurate if the specimen was not heated properly (killing the bacteria) or was not incubated long enough or if the general technique was not performed correctly. Prepared smears of known gram-positive and gram-negative organisms are processed with the patient's specimen for quality control. See Procedure 42-2 for charting example.

Procedure 42-4

Inoculating A Culture

Purpose: To introduce a portion of a specimen into the culture medium for growth and replication of microorganisms and produce isolated colonies.

Equipment: Specimen on a swab or loop, china marker or permanent laboratory marker, sterile or disposable loop, Bunsen burner, labeled Petri dish (the patient's name should be on the side of the plate containing the medium, because it is always placed upward to prevent condensation from dripping onto the culture).

Steps	Reason
1. Assemble the equipment.	
2. Put on gloves and the face shield.	Wear the face shield to avoid splatters from the inoculating loop.
3. Label the medium side of the plate with the patient's name, identification number, source of specimen, time collected, time inoculated, your initials, and date.	Because culture incubation may take 24–72 hours, dating ensures that the plate is read at the proper time. Labeling the medium side will prevent misplacing culture in the incorrect lid.
4. Remove the Petri plate from the cover (the Petri plate is always stored with the cover down), and place the cover on the work surface with the opening up. Do not open the cover unnecessarily.	Each time the cover is removed, there is a chance of contamination. Having the cover's opening upward avoids contamination from the work surface.

(continued)

Procedure 42-4   *(continued)*

Inoculating A Culture

Steps	Reason
5. Using a rolling and sliding motion, streak the specimen swab clear across half of the plate, starting at the top and working to the center. Dispose of the swab in a biohazard container. If the inoculating loop is used for lifting a secondary culture, streak in the same manner.	The specimen will spread in gradually thinning colonies of bacteria.

Step 5. Use a rolling, sliding motion to transfer the specimen to the plate.

Step 5. Pattern of specimen deposition for a qualitative culture

6. Dispose of this loop. If your office does not use disposable inoculating loops, sterilize the loop as described in step 6 of Procedure 42-2.

(continued)

Procedure 42-4 *(continued)*

Inoculating A Culture

Steps	**Reason**
7. Turn the plate a quarter-turn from its previous position. Pass the loop a few times in the original inoculum then down into the medium approximately a quarter of the surface of the plate. Do not enter the originally streaked area after the first few sweeps.	The loop draws into the clean surface a bit of the specimen that was streaked in the first part of the procedure.

Step 7. Draw the loop at right angles to the midpoint of the plate.

Step 7. Pattern of specimen deposition for a qualitative culture

8. Dispose of this loop. If you are not using a disposable loop, flame loop and allow it to cool again.	The loop must be flamed again to avoid contamination from the previous pass.
9. Turn the plate another quarter-turn so that now it is 180° to the original smear. Working in the previous manner, draw the loop at right angles through the most recently streaked area. Again, do not enter the originally streaked area after the first few sweeps.	The loop pulls out gradually thinning bits of the specimen to isolate colonies. Large groups of colonies close together are more difficult to identify than isolated colonies.

Step 9. Turn the plate another quarter-turn and streak in the same manner.

Step 9. Pattern of specimen deposition for a qualitative culture

(continued)

Procedure 42-4   *(continued)*

Inoculating A Culture

Steps	Reason

Pale yellow colonies of *Staphylococcus aureus* on a properly streaked plate.

NOTE: For quantitative cultures, streak the plate with the specimen from side to side across the middle of the media. Then, with a sterile loop, streak the entire plate back and forth across the initial inoculate.

Streak the plate with the specimen from side to side across the middle.

This is the initial inoculation for this type of streaking.

Streak the entire plate back and forth across the initial inoculate.

This allows bacteria to grow in a way that colonies can be counted—thus going a quantative result.

(continued)

Procedure 42-4 *(continued)*

Inoculating A Culture

Steps	Reason
10. If the plate is to be used for sensitivity, follow these steps: A. Using sterile forceps or an automatic dispenser, place the specified disks on areas of the plate equidistant from each other. 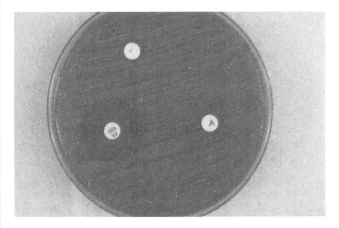 Step 10. A sensitivity culture showing area of resistance and areas of susceptibility. B. Press them gently with the sterilized loop or forceps until good contact is made with the surface of the agar.	
11. Properly care for or dispose of equipment and supplies. Remove gloves and wash your hands.	
12. Incubate for the specified time. Read the results and record as directed by office policy.	

Note: All sensitivity testing should be done on isolates of pure culture.

Charting Example

7/14/04 9:15 A.M. Swab specimen taken of (L) heel wound, transferred to culture medium for incubation. To be read 7/16/04. Pt instructed on wound care and infection control; verbalized understanding of instructions.
_____ G. Gray, RMA

CHAPTER SUMMARY

Microbiology in the physician's office lab is a vital part of the practice. The key thing to remember is that you must begin with a good specimen. This means that the medical assistant must take great care not to contaminate the specimen with anything but only have the microorganisms from that patient. There are many types of testing media, quality control procedures and safety guidelines to follow in the dealing with microbiology. You must be aware of how microorganisms are named, how they may react in various atmospheres and how to maintain the integrity of each specimen before it is tested. Since the Gram's Stain is an initial part to most microbiology tests it is important that you become proficient in making these slide specimens. Some specimens are sent to outside labs for testing. You must follow all collection and handling guidelines in dealing with such specimens.

Critical Thinking Challenges

1. You are asked to give a brief talk to a group of elementary school children on microbiological life forms. Develop an age-appropriate discussion of this topic. How would you make it possible for the children to correlate the presence of microbes with the need to wash their hands?

2. Write a policy that explains how to care for media and how to transport specimens. Be sure to include who can participate in this process.

3. Create a patient education brochure for streptococcal pharyngitis infections. Include information about what it is, how it is transmitted, signs and symptoms, and the testing procedure.

Answers to Checkpoint Questions

1. The four main categories of bacteria are cocci, bacilli, spirochetes, and vibrios.

2. Mixed cultures are used to investigate any or all of the microorganisms found at a site. Secondary cultures remove from the mixed cultures only those organisms that need to be encouraged to grow for more extensive study. Pure cultures contain only one organism and may be either a primary or a secondary culture.

3. If Petri plates are stored with the medium downward, condensation may form on the lids and drip onto the surface, making it too moist for an accurate culture.

4. Staining bacteria helps the physician narrow the field of possible pathogens and begin treatment before a culture has been incubated. Most bacteria are colorless and hard to see or identify without special treatment such as staining.

5. Sensitivity testing is done to determine which antibiotic inhibits bacterial growth.

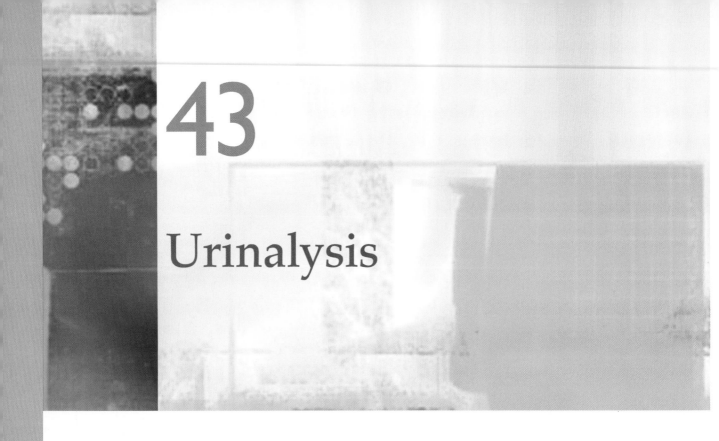

43

Urinalysis

CHAPTER OUTLINE

ROLE DELINEATION

CLINICAL: FUNDAMENTAL PRINCIPLES
- Apply principles of aseptic technique and infection control
- Comply with quality assurance practices

CLINICAL: DIAGNOSTIC ORDERS
- Collect and process specimens
- Perform diagnostic tests

CLINICAL: PATIENT CARE
- Prepare patient for examinations, procedures, and treatments

GENERAL: LEGAL CONCEPTS
- Perform within legal and ethical boundaries
- Document accurately

GENERAL: INSTRUCTION
- Instruct individuals according to their needs

CHAPTER COMPETENCIES

LEARNING OBJECTIVES

Upon successfully completing this chapter, you will be able to:

1. Spell and define the key terms.
2. Describe the methods of urine collection.
3. List and explain the physical and chemical properties of urine.
4. State the conditions that can be detected by abnormal urinalysis findings.
5. List and describe the components that can be found in urine sediment and describe their relationships to chemical findings.

PERFORMANCE OBJECTIVES

Upon successfully completing this chapter, you will be able to:

1. Explain to and/or assist a patient in obtaining a clean-catch midstream urine specimen (Procedure 43-1).
2. Explain the method of obtaining a 24-hour urine collection (Procedure 43-2).
3. Determine color and clarity of urine (Procedure 43-3).
4. Accurately interpret chemical reagent strip reactions (Procedure 43-4).
5. Perform copper reduction test (Procedure 43-5).
6. Perform a nitroprusside reaction (Acetest) for ketones (Procedure 43-6).
7. Perform acid precipitation test (Procedure 43-7).
8. Perform diazo tablet test (Ictotest) for bilirubin (Procedure 43-8).
9. Prepare urine sediment (Procedure 43-9).
10. Prepare urine sediment for microscopic examination.

KEY TERMS

ammonia	electrolytes	hemoglobinuria	precipitation
bilirubinuria	Ehrlich units	lyse	quantitative
creatinine	esterase	nitroprusside	sulfosalicylic acid
culture	galactosuria	particulate matter	threshold
diurnal variation	glycosuria	phosphates	urates

A URINALYSIS IS A PHYSICAL and chemical examination of urine to assess renal function and other possible problems. Because so many urinalyses are done in the office laboratory, proficiency in this skill is essential for the medical assistant. As indicated by clinical symptoms or physical and chemical findings in the urine, a microscopic examination may be added. The microscopic procedure is not designated by CLIA as a waived test. Insight into many systemic diseases or conditions can be gained from urinalysis. Diabetes mellitus, shock, malnutrition, preeclampsia, and blood transfusion reactions are several of the disorders that can be diagnosed or assessed by an examination of the urine. As with all body fluids, urine must be handled using OSHA-mandated personal protective equipment and safety guidelines.

SPECIMEN COLLECTION METHODS

Proper collection of a urine specimen varies with the test to be performed. Unless otherwise specified by the physician, a freshly voided specimen is all that is necessary. This is called a random urine. The patient voids the urine into a clean, dry container. To diagnose a urinary tract infection (UTI), the specimen is collected either as clean-catch midstream or by catheter and submitted to the laboratory in a sterile container with a lid. Detecting the microorganism causing disease may require that a **culture** be performed. A culture is a laboratory test in which microorganisms are grown in a nutrient medium to be identified and tested for antibiotic susceptibility. All cultures require the specimen not be contaminated during the preliminary testing process. Proper patient instruction in the clean-catch procedure avoids contamination with microorganisms from the perineal area, which would produce misleading results in urine culture or microscopic analysis.

Once the urine is collected, many of its elements deteriorate within 1 hour. If testing cannot be performed within this time, the specimen is refrigerated at 4° to 8°C for up to 4 hours. Multiplication of microorganisms in an unrefrigerated specimen changes the pH from acidic to alkaline. Glucose in the urine may be used as a nutrient by the microorganisms, resulting in a false-negative or lowered glucose result.

The timing of collection is sometimes an important consideration. First-morning urine specimens are the most concentrated and are useful for many tests that are more easily read with concentrated components (e.g., pregnancy testing); 2-hour postprandial (after a meal) specimens are used for glucose testing.

Clean-Catch Midstream Urine Specimen

A clean-catch midstream urine is the most commonly ordered random specimen. It is useful when the physician suspects an infection, because any microorganisms present after this collection will be from the urinary tract and not from contamination such as the perineal area. This specimen can be used for a culture if nothing has been allowed to contaminate the urine, such as a pipette or reagent strip. Collection is done after the urinary meatus and surrounding skin have been cleansed. The urine is voided into a sterile container. The clean-catch midstream procedure for males differs from the procedure for females (Procedure 43-1).

Bladder Catheterization

Another method for aseptic urine collection is catheterization. A thin sterile tube (catheter) is inserted into the bladder through the urethra. This procedure usually is performed by a physician or a nurse. Some medical assistants may be trained by their physicians to perform catheterizations. Bladder catheterization is recommended when the patient cannot give a urine specimen in a sterile manner using the clean-catch method. (See Chapter 37.)

Suprapubic Aspiration

Suprapubic aspiration is the least common method of urine collection. A needle is inserted into the bladder through the skin of the abdominal wall above the symphysis pubis, and urine is withdrawn (aspirated). This method is not common and is performed by a physician.

24-Hour Urine Collection

Because substances such as proteins, creatinine, and electrolytes are excreted with diurnal variation during a 24-hour period, a 24-hour collection is a better indicator of values than a random specimen. (Creatinine is a substance formed from creatine metabolism. Electrolytes are elements that dissolve in the blood and carry an electrical charge.) To obtain this kind of specimen, the patient collects all voided urine within a 24-hour period (Procedure 43-2). Providing an information sheet with written instructions for collecting a 24-hour urine specimen helps ensure the patient's compliance.

PATIENT EDUCATION

Instructions for 24-hour Urine Collection

The following instructions can be given to patients to ensure proper collection:

Instructions to Patients

- Instructions must be followed exactly. Your test results are based on the total amount of urine excreted by your body over a 24-hour period. Not following instructions will result in inaccurate results reported to your physician.
- Some tests have dietary and/or drug restrictions. Check with your physician or the laboratory before starting the collection. Drink the amount of fluid you normally would during the 24-hour collection period.
- The physician or laboratory will give you a special container to collect the urine. A preservative may be in the container. Do not throw away the preservative. Preservatives may be caustic or toxic. Do not void directly into the container. Be very careful not to spill the preservative on you or anything else.* Refrigerate the container during collection. The urine must be kept cold.

Day 1

- Empty your bladder into toilet. Record this specific date and time on your 24-hour urine container.
- Collect all specimens during the day, evening, and night for the entire 24-hour period. Add all of the specimens to the container. Gently shake the container after each urine specimen is added. Keep the urine container refrigerated during the collection period and until you take it to the physician or laboratory for testing.

Day 2

- Exactly 24 hours later, completely empty your bladder and add this specimen to the container. This last specimen completes your 24-hour collection. Record the ending date and time on the container. Replace the cap and tighten firmly. Refrigerate the specimen until you can turn it in. Take the specimen to the physician or laboratory as soon as possible.
- If you were on a special diet for this test, you may resume your normal diet after the specimen is collected.

* If you do spill the preservative, immediately wash with large amounts of water. You will have to get a new container from your physician or laboratory to collect the specimen.

Table 43-1	EXPECTED RANGE FOR PHYSICAL PROPERTIES
Property	**Expected Range**
Color	Pale yellow to amber
Clarity	Clear
Odor	Slightly aromatic but not fruity, no ammonia
Specific gravity	1.001–1.035

Checkpoint Question

1. What is the time frame for testing urine that is not refrigerated? Why is this important?

PHYSICAL PROPERTIES OF URINE

The physical properties include the urine's color, appearance (such as clarity or turbidity), specific gravity, and odor. While the odor may not be included in the urinalysis report, these odors can alert the experienced medical assistant to specific conditions. A diabetic patient's urine may smell sweet, and bacteria may give urine a foul odor. Color and clarity are assessed visually and are subjective, meaning the individual performing the testing will determine whether these properties can be considered within the normal range (TABLE 43-1).

Color

Urine color can be affected by many things: diet, drugs, diseases, and the concentration of the urine. The normal color of urine is a pale straw color to dark yellow. The yellow color is due to the pigment urochrome. Pale urine is typically very dilute and is seen after high fluid intake and after di-

uretic therapy. Likewise, deep, dark yellow can signify highly concentrated urine, such as when fluids are withheld or the patient is dehydrated. It also may mean that the patient recently took a multiple vitamin pill.

Clarity

Normal, freshly voided urine is usually clear (transparent). Haziness or turbidity (cloudiness) indicates the presence of particulate matter. Some alkaline urine may appear turbid because of a high concentration of **phosphates**. Some acidic urine may become turbid (cloudy) on standing as a result of **precipitation** of **urates** (nitrogenous compounds resulting from the body's metabolism of protein). Turbidity caused by either of these is considered normal. Red or white blood cells, bacteria, or mucus can also cause turbidity.

Laboratories vary in terminology used to express clarity or turbidity of urine. Common terminology dictates that when a small amount of turbidity is present, so that black lines on white paper can be seen through the specimen, it is hazy. As turbidity increases and these black lines can no longer be seen, it is called cloudy (Procedure 43-3). The three terms most commonly used to describe clarity are clear, hazy, and cloudy. TABLE 43-2 summarizes the common causes of variations in the color and clarity of urine.

Specific Gravity

The specific gravity reflects the concentration of a urine specimen. The weight of the urine is compared to the weight of water. Normal urine is slightly heavier than water. If you were to compare the weight of distilled water to itself, the specific gravity of the water would be 1.000. Urine, which contains cells and elements such as sodium, potassium, and chloride, is heavier than water. Specific gravity for a normal urine specimen is 1.003 to 1.035.

Table 43-2	COMMON CAUSES OF VARIATIONS IN THE COLOR AND CLARITY OF URINE
Color and Clarity	**Possible Causes**
Yellow-brown or green-brown	Bile in urine (as in jaundice)
Dark yellow or orange	Concentrated urine, low fluid intake, dehydration, inability of kidney to dilute urine, fluorescein (intravenous dye), multivitamins, excessive carotene
Bright orange-red	Pyridium (urinary tract analgesic)
Red or reddish-brown	Hemoglobin pigments, pyrvinium pamoate (Povan) for intestinal worms, sulfonamides (sulfa-based antibiotics)
Green or blue	Artificial color in food or drugs
Blackish, grayish, smoky	Hemoglobin or remnants of old red blood cells (indicating bleeding in upper urinary tract), chyle, prostatic fluid, yeasts
Cloudy	Phosphate precipitation (normal after sitting for a long time), urates (compound of uric acid), leukocytes, pus, blood, epithelial cells, fat droplets, strict vegetarian diet

In addition to these causes, foods such as blackberries, rhubarb, beets, and those with red dye are common causes of dark or reddish urine that might resemble hematuria.

Urine with low specific gravity is dilute. As stated previously, this may result from a high fluid intake. Abnormal conditions that produce dilute urine are diabetes insipidus and kidney infection or inflammation.

Urine with high specific gravity is concentrated. A patient who is dehydrated, perhaps from sweating, vomiting, or diarrhea, may produce a concentrated specimen because the body is trying to conserve water. High specific gravity can occur in diabetes mellitus.

Specific gravity can be determined by a variety of methods. The oldest are the urinometer, a floating measuring instrument which requires 10 mL or more of urine, and the refractometer, which requires a drop of urine and is read using a scale that measures the amount of light bent by the particles in the urine. The specific gravity pad on the reagent strip also takes a drop of urine, and the color change is compared to a chart to determine the value. This allows specific gravity to be determined in combination with the other chemical assays on the reagent strip and is the most common and efficient method of measurement.

 Checkpoint Question

2. What are the three physical properties of urine, and which two are assessed visually?

CHEMICAL PROPERTIES OF URINE

Urine contains chemicals produced in the body and ingested from the environment. The reagent strip produces 10 chemical measurements. If more **quantitative** (measurement of a specific amount or quantity) information is needed (e.g., protein), the test is performed in the chemistry laboratory (see Chapter 47). TABLE 43-3 gives the expected value for each chemical property. Detecting and measuring chemical properties can facilitate the diagnosis of many conditions. Included in the discussion of each urine chemistry are the disease processes that might be indicated by abnormal readings.

Table 43-3	EXPECTED RANGE OF CHEMICAL PROPERTIES
Property	**Expected Range**
Glucose	Negative
Bilirubin	Negative
Ketones	Negative
Blood	Negative
pH	5.0–8.0
Protein	Negative to trace
Urobilinogen	0.1–1.0 EU/dL
Nitrite	Negative
Leukocyte esterase	Negative

Box 43-1

URINE CONFIRMATORY TESTING

Reagent strip tests are screening tests. Confirmation with a more sensitive and/or specific method may be requested to follow up some positive results. Your laboratory will have a specific procedure outlining the performance of confirmation tests.

Analyte	**Common Confirmatory Test**
Protein	Sulfosalicylic acid test
Ketones	Acetest
Bilirubin	Ictotest
Glucose	Clinitest

Several manufacturers produce reagent strips that can be dipped into urine. These strips have chemicals embedded in pads that react with the chemicals in the urine. A reagent pad will change color as the chemical reaction takes place. All reagent pad colors are compared with a color chart to interpret the reactions at the specific time indicated for each reaction (Procedure 43-4). Confirmation of positive reagent strip reactions (e.g., bilirubin, protein) are sometimes part of laboratory protocol as defined by the facility where the test is performed. Box 43-1 lists several types of confirmation tests.

pH

The kidneys excrete acids produced during normal metabolic processes. Hydrogen ions and **ammonia** are excreted as well. Ammonia is produced by decomposition of nitrogen. The kidneys regulate the acid-base balance of the body by reabsorbing water, sodium, chloride, potassium, bicarbonate, glucose, calcium, and amino acids. Because the body produces more acids than bases, urine is usually acidic.

Expected values for urine pH can range from 5.0 (acidic) to 8.0 (slightly basic). The typical value for freshly voided urine is slightly acidic at 6.0. While acidic urine is normal, it also occurs with a high-protein diet and uncontrolled diabetes. Alkaline urine (above 7.0) can occur after meals and with a vegetarian diet, certain renal diseases, and urinary tract infection. Usually pH is tested with the reagent strip.

Glucose

Glucose is filtered and reabsorbed in the kidneys. If plasma renal **threshold** levels exceed 180 g/dL, not all of the glucose will be reabsorbed, and detectable amounts of it will be present in the urine. This can vary and requires measuring the actual blood level for a diagnostic assessment. The amount of glucose in urine corresponds to plasma levels;

RENAL THRESHOLD AND GLYCOSURIA

Glucose is resorbed in the proximal convoluted tubule. When blood glucose levels exceed 180 mg/dL, depending on the individual, not all of the glucose can be reabsorbed into the bloodstream.

Rarely does a healthy person's blood glucose level exceed this threshold value. Diabetics, however, may pass some glucose in their urine because of the high level in their blood. A frequently used term, *spilling sugar*, means that not all of the sugar is reabsorbed and some is excreted in the urine.

normal urine does not contain glucose. Glucose-negative urine corresponds to a plasma level of less than 180 mg/dL. In a hyperglycemic state, such as diabetes mellitus, **glycosuria** (glucose in urine) can occur if plasma levels are greater than 180 mg/dL (Box 43-2).

The copper reduction method (Clinitest) has been used for many years to detect reducing sugars in urine (Procedure 43-5). This test is used to detect any reducing sugar (sugar that gives up electrons easily in chemical reactions), such as glucose, galactose, lactose, or fructose. Its use is significant to children aged 2 years or less to screen for **galactosuria**. (Galactosuria, or increased level of galactose in the blood and urine, is a condition in newborns lacking an enzyme that metabolizes galactose.) The results of this test may be inaccurate, because other sugars and ascorbic acid (vitamin C) can react with the reagent. The reagent strips are specific for glucose and are preferred for their accuracy; however, the Clinitest tablets may be used as confirmation for chemical reagent strips. *Note:* The reaction produces heat, so always use a glass tube.

Ketones

Ketones are a group of chemicals produced during fat metabolism. In normal circumstances, energy is derived primarily from carbohydrate metabolism. In conditions of insufficient carbohydrates, as in starvation, low-carbohydrate diet, and inadequately managed diabetes, fats are used and ketones are produced.

In normal urine, ketones are typically too low to be measurable. A positive ketone test indicates that the body is burning more fat than normal. A **nitroprusside** reaction is used to detect ketones (Procedure 43-6). (Nitroprusside is a nitrogen cyanic compound that reacts with ketones.) This is the method used on both reagent strips and tablet tests. Many laboratories choose to confirm results with the nitroprusside tablet (Acetest).

Proteins

Small quantities of proteins are found in normal urine. Proteinuria (increased amounts of protein in the urine) is an important indicator of renal disease. Reagent strips are used to determine the presence of proteins in urine. Other events that can cause protein in urine include strenuous physical exercise, pregnancy, infection, hematuria (blood in urine), pyuria (white cells in urine), and multiple myeloma. Microscopic examination of the urine can help determine whether the proteinuria is caused by bacteria, casts, or cellular elements.

Turbidity or precipitation tests confirm a protein on the reagent strip (Procedure 43-7). The most common confirmation test is observing the amount of cloudiness when equal amounts of urine and **sulfosalicylic acid** are mixed. The urine used must be centrifuged to remove all particulate matter before adding the acid.

If the amount of protein is negligible and produces a negative reagent strip reaction, there should be no cloudiness when the sulfosalicylic acid is added to the urine. When the concentration of urine protein reaches approximately 20 mg/dL, turbidity will result as sulfosalicylic acid combines with the urine. As protein levels increase, so will the degree of turbidity during the reaction with the acid.

Blood

Small numbers of red blood cells are occasionally observed in urine. Intact capillaries in the glomerulus usually do not allow the passage of cells into the Bowman's capsule. Hematuria not due to contamination from menstrual flow indicates bleeding in the urinary tract that may result from renal disorders, certain neoplasms, urinary tract infection, or trauma to the urinary tract. Reagent strips test for blood in the urine, and confirmation is made by microscopic examination.

The reagent strip reacts to hemoglobin, which is the primary constituent of red cells. **Hemoglobinuria** may occur with transfusion reaction, chemical toxicity, or burn. The strip also reacts to myoglobin, a protein found in muscles. Myoglobin may be released into the bloodstream from crushing injury or other trauma and then be excreted in the urine.

Bilirubin

Bilirubin is formed during breakdown of hemoglobin. It is processed in the liver before being excreted into the intestines. Urine contains very low levels of bilirubin, reflecting the usual low serum levels. Bilirubinuria (bilirubin in the urine) can occur with certain liver diseases (e.g., hepatitis), biliary tract obstruction, and hemolytic states, such as transfusion reactions.

The reagent strip is designed to react to bilirubin; however, dark yellow urine can make it difficult to read the reaction, because bilirubin is also a yellow pigment. Many laboratories confirm a positive strip result by a diazo tablet method (Ictotest) (Procedure 43-8).

Important note: Bilirubin is a highly unstable substance and will break down with exposure to light. Specimens must be shielded from light and processed as soon as possible to avoid deterioration of the specimen.

Urobilinogen

When bilirubin is secreted into the intestines in the bile, bacterial action converts it to urobilinogen. Some of this is reabsorbed into the bloodstream and excreted by the kidneys. The remaining urobilinogen leaves the body in the feces.

Small amounts of urobilinogen are normally found in urine, usually 0.1 to 1.0 **Ehrlich units**/dL (mg/dL). (The Ehrlich unit is unique for urobilinogen.) As with bilirubin, increased levels of urobilinogen can be found with conditions that have a high rate of red cell destruction. Also, bowel obstructions cause the feces to remain in the intestines for longer periods, resulting in greater reabsorption of urobilinogen along with the rest of the fluid portion. Urobilinogen levels rise both in urine and in serum when this occurs. Liver impairment can also lead to increased levels of urobilinogen because some of the urobilinogen that is reabsorbed from the intestinal tract is processed by the liver and excreted in the feces. Urobilinogen is tested by reagent strip.

Checkpoint Question

3. What does a positive bilirubin test indicate?

Nitrite

Some types of bacteria that infect the urinary tract have an enzyme that can reduce nitrate to nitrite. This factor is used to assess the presence of bacteria in urine. In the nitrite test, urine is applied to a reagent pad. If bacteria are present, nitrates will be converted to nitrites, and the resulting color development can be observed. A positive nitrite test result indicates bacteriuria, which occurs with urinary tract infections.

Leukocyte Esterase

Leukocytes in the urine indicate a urinary tract infection. Phagocytic white cells, such as neutrophils, are called to the kidney to fight the infection. These leukocytes contain an enzyme called **esterase**. This is detected with the leukocyte esterase reaction on the reagent strip. Normal urine may contain a few white cells but not in sufficient numbers to produce a positive leukocyte esterase test.

Checkpoint Question

4. Which two indicators on a dipstick suggest a urinary tract infection?

URINE SEDIMENT

The microscopic examination of urine can corroborate the findings of the urinalysis and may produce new data with diagnostic value. Cells and other structures are noted and counted during a microscopic examination. Microscopic examination of urine is not a CLIA-waived procedure.

Urine sediment is prepared by centrifuging urine and saving the button of cells and other particulate matter that collects in the bottom of the tube. This button is resuspended, and a drop of this suspension is placed on a slide and viewed with a microscope. Making a sediment concentrates all the structures in the urine so that it is unlikely that any components will be missed (Procedure 43-9).

A slide system used in conjunction with a unique centrifuge tube is available to examine sediments. This provides some standardization of the procedure so that the numbers in the findings have meaning with regard to abnormal results. Glass slides, with or without coverslips, may still be used by some laboratories.

Structures Found in Urine Sediment

The following structures may appear in the urine: red blood cells, white blood cells, bacteria, epithelial cells, crystals, casts, and others (Fig. 43-1). Correlations with chemical properties of the urine are described as appropriate.

Red Blood Cells

The presence of red cells in urine, as stated previously, can occur with a number of conditions, including renal damage. When sediment contains red cells, the reagent strip should be positive for blood. Protein may also be positive if hemolysis is occurring. A positive reagent strip test for blood with no red cells seen microscopically may occur with various kinds of hemolysis, such as with transfusion reactions and sickle cell crisis (see Chapter 45). As stated earlier, myoglobin will cause a positive reaction.

White Blood Cells

Leukocytes in the sediment indicate a urinary tract infection. The leukocyte esterase test on the chemical strip will be positive when white cells are present in significant numbers. The protein test may be positive if some of the white blood cells **lyse** (break apart) or if the infection is damaging the renal tubules, as in glomerulonephritis.

Bacteria

Bacteria are always present on the skin but not usually in the bladder. Urine normally does not contain bacteria if a clean-catch specimen is collected properly. The presence of significant amounts (more than a trace) of bacteria in a urine specimen is considered an indication of a urinary tract infection.

CELLS IN URINE

Epithelial Cells Three types of epithelial cells may appear in urine sediment: renal tubular, transitional and/or squamous. Other types of cells may appear in urine but are difficult to identify due to morphologic changes caused by urine. Tubular cells are approximately ⅓ larger than white blood cells. Transitional epithelial cells may arise from the renal pelvis, ureters, bladder or urethra. They tend to be pear-shaped. Squamous cells are large and flat with a prominent nucleus. They originate in the urethra.

RENAL TUBULAR

TRANSITIONAL

SQUAMOUS

RBCs Red blood cells may originate from any part of the renal system. The presence of large numbers of RBCs in the urine suggests infection, trauma, tumors, renal calculi, etc. However, the presence of 1 or 2 RBC/(HPF) in the urine sediment, or blood in the urine from menstrual contamination, should not be considered abnormal.

RBCs

WBCs White blood cells in the urine (pyuria) may originate from any part of the renal system. The presence of more than 5 WBCs per HPF may suggest infection, cystitis, or pyelonephritis.

RENAL TUBULAR & WBC (SEDI-STAIN*)

WBCs

CASTS IN URINE

Hyaline Casts Hyaline casts are formed from a protein gel in the renal tubule. Hyaline casts may contain cellular inclusions. Hyaline casts will dissolve very rapidly in alkaline urine. Normal urine sediment may contain 1 to 2 hyaline casts per low power field (LPF).

HYALINE

Granular Casts Granular casts are casts with granules present throughout the cast matrix. They are quite refractile. If the granules are small, the cast is defined as a finely granular cast. If granules are large, it is termed a coarsely granular cast. Granular casts can appear in urine in normal or abnormal states.

GRANULAR

RBC Casts RBC casts are pathologic and their presence is usually indicative of severe injury to the glomerulus. Rarely, transtubular bleeding may occur, forming RBC casts. RBC casts are found in acute glomerulonephritis, lupus, bacterial endocarditis and septicemias. "Blood" casts are granular and contain hemoglobin from degenerated RBCs.

RBC CASTS

WBC Casts WBC casts occur when leukocytes are incorporated within the cast matrix. WBC casts will usually indicate an infection, most commonly pyelonephritis. They may also be seen in glomerular diseases. WBC casts may be the only clue to pyelonephritis.

WBC CASTS

CRYSTALS FOUND IN ACID URINE

Uric Acid Crystals Uric acid has birefringent characteristics; therefore, it polarizes light, giving multi-colors. Uric acid crystals are found in acid urine. Uric acid may assume various forms, e.g., rhombic, plates, rosettes, small crystals. The color may be red-brown, yellow or colorless. Although increased in 16% of patients with gout, and in patients with malignant lymphoma or leukemia, their presence does not usually indicate pathology or increased uric acid concentrations.

URIC ACID (BRIGHTFIELD)

FIGURE 43-1. Atlas of urine sediment.

CRYSTALS FOUND IN ACID URINE

URIC ACID (POLARIZED)

Leucine/Tyrosine Crystals   Leucine and tyrosine are amino acids which crystallize and often appear together in the urine of patients with severe liver disease. Tyrosine usually appears as fine needles arranged as sheaves or rosettes and appear yellow. Leucine is usually yellow, oily-appearing spheres with radial and concentric striations.

TYROSINE (BRIGHTFIELD)

LEUCINE (BRIGHTFIELD)

Cystine Crystals   Cystine crystals are thin, hexagonal-shaped (6-sided) structures. They appear in the urine as a result of a genetic defect. Cystine crystals and stones will appear in the urine in cystinuria and homocystinuria. Cystine crystals are frequently confused with uric acid crystals. Cystine crystals do not polarize light.

CYSTINE (BRIGHTFIELD)

CYSTINE (POLARIZED)

CRYSTALS FOUND IN ACID, NEUTRAL AND ALKALINE URINE

Calcium Oxalate   Calcium oxalate crystals most frequently have an "envelope" shape and appear in acid, neutral or slightly alkaline urine. They appear in the urine after the ingestion of certain foods, i.e., cabbage, asparagus.

CALCIUM OXALATE (BRIGHTFIELD)

Hippuric Acid   Hippuric acid crystals are colorless or pale yellow. They occur as needles, six-sided prisms, or star-shaped clusters. They appear in urine after the ingestion of certain vegetables and fruits with benzoic acid content. They have little clinical significance.

HIPPURIC ACID (BRIGHTFIELD)

CRYSTALS FOUND IN ALKALINE URINE

Ammonium Biurate or Ammonium Urates   Ammonium urates are yellow-brown in appearance and occur in urine as spheres or spheres with spicules ("thorny apples"). Both forms are frequently seen together. They appear in urine when there is ammonia formation in the urine present in the bladder. They are considered to have little clinical significance.

AMMONIUM URATES (BRIGHTFIELD)

Triple Phosphate   Triple phosphate crystals are common in urine sediment. They have a "coffin-lid" shape, are colorless and appear in alkaline urine. The ingestion of fruit may cause triple phosphate to appear in urine.

TRIPLE PHOSPHATE (BRIGHTFIELD)

BACTERIA, FUNGI, PARASITES IN URINE

Bacteria   Bacteria in the urine (bacteriuria) can result from contaminants in collection vessels, from periurethral tissues, the urethra, or from fecal or vaginal contamination as well as from true urinary infection.

BACTERIA

Yeast   Yeast cells vary in size, are colorless, ovoid, and are often budding. They are often confused with RBCs. *Candida albicans* is often seen in diabetes, pregnancy, obesity and other debilitating conditions.

YEAST

Trichomonas Vaginalis   Trichomonas vaginalis is a flagellate protozoan which affects both males (urethritis) and females (vaginitis).

TRICHOMONAS VAGINALIS

FIGURE 25-1. *(continued)*

A positive nitrite test result on the reagent strip correlates with some categories of bacteria in the sediment. Since not all bacteria produce nitrites, a negative nitrate reaction does not mean that the specimen is free of bacteria.

Epithelial Cells

Epithelial cells cover the skin and organs and line pathways, such as the digestive and urinary tracts. Their shapes vary according to their location of origin. **Epithelial cells normally slough off and are found in the urine, but increased amounts can indicate an irritation, such as inflammation somewhere in the urinary system.** The three types of epithelial cells in the urine are squamous, transitional, and renal. Squamous epithelial cells cover external skin surfaces and are considered a normal finding in urine, since urine comes in contact with skin during urination. Transitional epithelial cells line the bladder and are seen with infections of the lower urinary tract, such as cystitis. Renal epithelial cells line the nephrons and are seen with infections and inflammations of the upper urinary tract.

There is no chemical test for epithelial cells. However, if renal epithelial cells are seen in urinary sediment, damage to the renal tubules is likely, and the protein test may be positive.

Crystals

Crystals are made up of a chemical substance in the urine in sufficient quantities to form a solid three-dimensional structure that can be seen microscopically. **The three most common crystals found in urine sediment—calcium oxalate, uric acid (both of which occur in urine with a pH below 7.0), and triple phosphate (found in urine above pH 7.0)—are not independently pathological.** Uric acid crystals can, however, be seen with fever, leukemia, or gout. Crystals can contribute to the formation of stones in the urinary tract.

Casts

Cast formation occurs in the tubules of the nephron. **When protein is present in sufficient quantities, it will cement together whatever solutes or cells are in the tubule as well; this is called a cast.** Most casts eventually break free and flow into the urine. **The type of cast can indicate certain pathologies.** For instance, in pyelonephritis, white cells that are present to combat the infection become trapped in the protein network and form white cell casts. Casts are counted using low-power magnification with reduced light and are reported as a number per low-power field.

Checkpoint Question

5. What are three of the most common crystals found in urine?

Other Structures

Other structures can be found in urine sediment. Yeast in the urine can result from vaginal contamination of the specimen or may be the causative agent of a urinary tract infection, especially in a diabetic patient. The parasite *Trichomonas vaginalis* is a contaminant from the genital tract of an infected person. Mucus may be present if there is an inflammation in the urinary tract. Mucus threads are usually reported in quantities, such as few, moderate, or many. Spermatozoa may be found when there has been a recent emission.

URINE PREGNANCY TESTING

Human chorionic gonadotropin (HCG) is a hormone secreted by the developing placenta shortly after conception. Its appearance and rapid rise in concentration in the mother's serum and urine make it an excellent marker for confirming a pregnancy.

Pregnancy test kits have progressed from older agglutination-inhibition assays to immunoassays that can detect levels as low as 25 mIU/mL. These levels are typically seen within 10 to 12 days after fertilization, sometimes before the first missed period. All pregnancy tests measure some part of the HCG molecule. Most test kits simply require the addition of urine to the test and are very easy to use. Newer urine pregnancy test kits use enzyme-linked immunosor-

WHAT IF

A patient asks you what drugs can be detected in the urine? What do you say?

Many employers are requiring routine urine drug testing for their employees. Urine tests are preferred to blood tests because they are less expensive and are noninvasive. The following drugs can be detected in the urine: amphetamines, barbiturates, benzodiazepines, cocaine, marijuana, opioids, PCP, and methadone. If you must obtain urine specimens for drug testing, it is essential that you ensure security of the urine and confidentiality of the results.

bent assay (ELISA). ELISA kits use a solid-phase antibody specific for one site on the HCG molecule. A second labeled antibody is directed to another site on the molecule. When HCG antigen is present, a specific antibody–antigen–antibody–enzyme complex will form. The enzyme complex produces a color change and indicates the presence of HCG.

The first-morning urine specimen is the specimen of choice because the urine is most concentrated at that time. Many laboratories test the specific gravity and do not report a negative pregnancy result if it is below 1.005, because the urine may be too dilute to detect low HCG serum levels.

Urine Drug Testing

Each urine specimen submitted for drug testing must be analyzed using an initial test approved for commercial use by the Food and Drug Administration. Several techniques are available to screen for the five drug classes. Two tests are required to prove a positive drug result. The initial test eliminates negative urine specimens from further testing. A negative specimen either contains no drug or has a concentration less than a specified cutoff level. Gas chromatography/mass spectrometry (GC/MS) technology is used for confirmation testing.

Procedure 43-1

Obtaining a Clean-Catch Midstream Urine Specimen

Purpose: To minimize contamination of a voided urine specimen.

Equipment: Sterile urine container labeled with patient's name, bedpan or urinal (if necessary), gloves if you are to assist patient.

Steps	Reason
1. Wash your hands. If you are to assist the patient, put on gloves.	Handwashing aids infection control.
2. Assemble the equipment.	
3. Identify the patient and explain the procedure. Ask for and answer any questions.	
4. If the patient is to perform the procedure, provide the necessary supplies.	
5. Have the patient perform the procedure.	
A. Instruct the male patient:	
i. If uncircumcised, expose the glans penis by retracting the foreskin, then clean the meatus with an antiseptic wipe. The glans should be cleaned in a circular motion away from the meatus. A new wipe should be used for each cleaning sweep.	The antiseptic solution removes bacteria from the urinary meatus and the surrounding skin. Wiping away from the meatus will remove bacteria from the area; wiping toward the meatus or returning to the area with a used wipe would reintroduce bacteria to the site.
ii. Keeping the foreskin retracted, initially void a few seconds into the toilet or urinal.	Organisms in the lower urethra and at the meatus will be washed away. Collecting the middle of the stream ensures the least contamination with skin bacteria.

(continued)

Procedure 43-1 *(continued)*

Obtaining a Clean-Catch Midstream Urine Specimen

Steps	Reason
iii. Bring the sterile container into the urine stream and collect a sufficient amount (about 30–100 mL). Instruct the patient to avoid touching the inside of the container with the penis.	Touching the inside with the penis may contaminate the specimen.
iv. Finish voiding into the toilet or urinal.	Prostatic fluid may be expressed at the end of the stream and may contaminate the specimen.
B. Instruct the female patient: i. Kneel or squat over a bedpan or toilet bowl. Spread the labia minora widely to expose the meatus. Using an antiseptic wipe, cleanse on either side of the meatus, then the meatus itself. Use a wipe only once in a sweep from the anterior to the posterior surfaces, then discard it.	The antiseptic solution removes bacteria from the urinary meatus. Bringing a wipe back to the surface already cleaned will recontaminate the area. The antiseptic solution is washed away before the specimen is collected at midstream.
ii. Keeping the labia separated, initially void a few seconds into the toilet.	Organisms remaining in the meatus will be washed away.
iii. Bring the sterile container into the urine stream and collect a sufficient amount (about 30–100 mL).	
iv. Finish voiding into the toilet or bedpan.	
6. Cap the filled container and place it in a designated area.	Transport the specimen in a biohazard container for testing.
7. Properly care for or dispose of equipment and supplies. Clean the work area. Remove gloves and wash your hands.	

Charting Example
05/31/2004 1:30 P.M. Pt instructed in midstream collection of urine with antiseptic wipe. U/A: Color, straw; clarity, clear; specific gravity, 1.020; dipstick negative; pH 7.0. _____ S. Miller, CMA

Procedure 43-2

Obtaining a 24-hour Urine Specimen

Purpose: To determine the quantity and proportion of substances in a 24-hour urine sample.

Equipment: Patient's labeled 24-hour urine container (some patients require more than one container),
            preservatives required for the specific test, chemical hazard labels, graduated cylinder that holds at
            least 1 L, serological or volumetric pipettes, clean random urine container, gloves, fresh 10% bleach
            solution, patient log form.

Steps	Reason
1. Wash your hands.	Handwashing aids infection control.
2. Assemble the equipment.	
3. Identify the type of 24-hour urine collection requested and check for any special requirements, such as any acid or preservative that should be added. Label the container appropriately.	Proper identification avoids errors. Special additives protect the integrity of the specimen.

Step 3: 24-hour specimen containers. Each type is used for specific tests.

Steps	Reason
4. Add to the 24-hour urine container the correct amount of acid or preservative using a serological or volumetric pipette.	This prevents altered findings due to incorrect preparation.
5. Use the provided label or make a label with spaces for the patient's name, beginning time and date, and ending time and date so that the patient can fill in the appropriate information.	This ensures that the patient documents the testing times.
6. Instruct the patient to collect a 24-hour urine sample as follows:	

   A. Void into the toilet, and note this time and date
      as beginning.

   B. After the first voiding, collect each voiding and
      add it to the urine container for the next 24 hours.

   C. Precisely 24 hours after beginning collection,
      empty the bladder even if there is no urge to void.

   D. Note on the label the ending time and date.

(continued)

Procedure 43-2   *(continued)*

Obtaining a 24-hour Urine Specimen

Steps	Reason
7. Explain to the patient that depending on the test requested, the 24-hour urine may have to be refrigerated the entire time. Instruct the patient to return the specimen to you as soon as possible after collection is complete.	Proper care of the specimen prevents degradation of the urine components, which may alter findings.
8. Record in the patient's chart that supplies and instructions were given to collect a 24-hour urine specimen and the test that was requested.	This documents patient education and instructions.
9. When you receive the specimen, verify beginning and ending times and dates before the patient leaves. Check for any acids or preservatives to be added before the specimen goes to the testing laboratory.	This protects the integrity of the specimen.
10. Put on gloves.	
11. Pour the urine into a cylinder to record the volume. Pour an aliquot of the urine into a clean container to be sent to the laboratory. (Label the specimen with the patient's identification.) Record the volume of the urine collection and the amount of any acid or preservative added on the sample container and on the laboratory requisition. If permitted, you may dispose of the remainder of the urine.	
12. Record the volume on the patient's log form.	
13. Clean the cylinder with fresh 10% bleach solution, then rinse with water. Let it air dry. If you are using a disposable container, be sure to dispose of it in the proper biohazard container.	
14. Clean the work area and dispose of waste properly. Remove protective equipment and wash your hands.	

Note: Some containers come with the preservative already added. In either case, be sure the patient is instructed not to discard preservative and not to allow it to be handled.

Warning! Use caution when handling acids and other hazardous materials. Be familiar with the material safety data sheets for each chemical in your site.

Note: Depending on the type of office and laboratory, you may not need the aliquot.

Charting Example
3/8/2004 9:30 A.M. Pt instructed to collect urine for 24 hours and verbalized understanding. Pt was given container and written instructions to begin collecting at 8:00 A.M. on 3/9 and to end on 3/10 at 8:00 A.M. Will bring specimen in on 3/10. _____ M. Smith, CMA

3/10/2004 10:10 A.M. Pt returned with 24-hour specimen collection. Total volume is 1850 mL. Labeled 50-mL aliquot to reference laboratory. _____ M. Smith, CMA

Procedure 43-3

Determining Color and Clarity of Urine

Purpose:	To determine by visual inspection the presence of particulate and soluble matter in a urine specimen.
Equipment:	Gloves, impervious gown, face shield, 10% bleach solution, patient's labeled urine specimen, clear tube, usually a centrifuge, white paper scored with black lines.

Steps	Reason
1. Wash your hands.	
2. Assemble the equipment.	
3. Put on gloves, impervious gown, and face shield.	
4. Verify that the names on the specimen container and the report form are the same.	This prevents reporting errors.
5. Pour 10–15 mL of urine into the tube.	This provides an adequate quantity for testing and allows for visual assessment of the urine.
6. In bright light against a white background, examine the color. The most common colors are straw (very pale yellow), yellow, dark yellow, and amber (brown-yellow).	The intensity of the yellow color, which is due to urochrome, depends on urine concentration. (Table 43-2 has information about other urine colors.)
7. Determine clarity. Hold the tube in front of the white paper scored with black lines. If you see the lines clearly (not obscured), record as clear. If you see the lines but they are not well delineated, record as hazy. If you cannot see the lines at all, record as cloudy.	The lines help discern clarity by providing contrast.
8. Properly care for or dispose of equipment and supplies. Clean the work area using a 10% bleach solution. Remove gloves, gown, and face shield. Wash your hands.	

Note: Rapid determination of color and clarity is necessary because some urine turns cloudy if left standing.

Bilirubin, which may be found in urine in certain conditions, breaks down when exposed to light. Protect the specimen from light if urinalysis is ordered but testing is delayed.

If further testing is to be done but is delayed more than an hour, refrigerate the specimen to avoid alteration of chemistry.

Charting Example

05/31/2005 2:45 P.M. Random urine collected. Yellow/clear. _____ H. Henderson, RMA

Procedure 43-4

Chemical Reagent Strip Analysis

Purpose: To determine the level of constituents in a patient's urine to aid in the diagnosis of urinary or metabolic disorders

Equipment: Patient's labeled urine specimen, chemical strip (such as Multistix or Chemstrip), manufacturer's color comparison chart, stopwatch or timer, gloves, impervious gown and face shield, 10% bleach solution

Steps	Reason
1. Wash your hands.	
2. Assemble the equipment.	
3. Put on gloves, impervious gown, and face shield.	
4. Verify that the names on the specimen container and the report form are the same.	
5. Mix the patient's urine by gently swirling the covered container.	
6. Remove the reagent strip from its container and replace the lid to prevent deterioration of strips by humidity.	
7. Immerse the reagent strip in the urine completely, then immediately remove it, sliding the edge of the strip along the lip of the container to remove excess urine.	Immersing the reagent strip resuspends particulate matter in urine. Immediate removal of the strip prevents colors from leaching during prolonged exposure to urine.
8. Start your stopwatch or timer immediately.	Reactions must be read at specific intervals as directed on the package insert and on the color comparison chart.
9. Compare the reagent pads to the color chart, determining results at the intervals stated by the manufacturer. Example: Glucose is read at 30 seconds. To determine results, examine that pad 30 seconds post dipping and compare with color chart for glucose.	

(continued)

Procedure 43-4   *(continued)*

Chemical Reagent Strip Analysis

Steps	Reason

2161

Multistix® 10 SG

Reagent Strips for Urinalysis

For In Vitro Diagnostic Use

READ PRODUCT INSERT BEFORE USE.
IMPORTANT: Do not expose to direct sunlight.
Do not use after 12/99.

COLOR CHART

Bayer

TESTS AND READING TIME

Test / Reading Time							
LEUKOCYTES 2 minutes	NEGATIVE		TRACE	SMALL +	MODERATE ++	LARGE +++	
NITRITE 60 seconds	NEGATIVE		POSITIVE	POSITIVE	(Any degree of uniform pink color is positive)		
UROBILINOGEN 60 seconds	NORMAL 0.2	NORMAL 1	mg/dL 2	4	8	(1 mg = approx. 1EU)	
PROTEIN 60 seconds	NEGATIVE	TRACE	mg/dL 30 +	100 ++	300 +++	2000 or more ++++	
pH 60 seconds	5.0	6.0	6.5	7.0	7.5	8.0	8.5
BLOOD 60 seconds	NEGATIVE	NON-HEMOLYZED TRACE	NON-HEMOLYZED MODERATE	HEMOLYZED TRACE	SMALL +	MODERATE ++	LARGE +++
SPECIFIC GRAVITY 45 seconds	1.000	1.005	1.010	1.015	1.020	1.025	1.030
KETONE 40 seconds	NEGATIVE	mg/dL	TRACE 5	SMALL 15	MODERATE 40	LARGE 80	LARGE 160
BILIRUBIN 30 seconds	NEGATIVE		SMALL +	MODERATE ++	LARGE +++		
GLUCOSE 30 seconds	NEGATIVE	g/dL (%) mg/dL	1/10 (tr.) 100	1/4 250	1/2 500	1 1000	2 or more 2000 or more

©1997 Bayer Corporation, Diagnostics Division, Tarrytown, NY 10591   5   Rev. 12/97   0401123

Step 9: Multistix package insert. (Courtesy of Bayer Corporation, Elkhart, IN.)

Steps	Reason
10. Read all reactions at the times indicated and record the results.	This adheres to strict time-sensitive testing protocol.
11. Discard the reagent strips in the proper receptacle. Discard urine unless more testing is required.	

(continued)

Procedure 43-4 *(continued)*

Chemical Reagent Strip Analysis

Steps	Reason
12. Clean the work area with 10% bleach solution. Remove gown, gloves, and face shield. Wash your hands.	

Warning: Do not remove the desiccant packet in the strip container; it ensures that minimal moisture affects the strips. The desiccant is toxic and should be discarded appropriately after all of the strips have been used.

Notes: The manufacturer's color comparison chart is assigned a lot number that must match the lot number of the strips used for testing. Record this in the quality assurance (QA/QC) log.

False-positive and false-negative results are possible. Review the manufacturer's package insert accompanying the strips to learn about factors that may give false results and how to avoid them.

Aspirin may cause false-positive ketones. Document any medications the patient is taking. If the patient is taking pyridium, do not use a reagent strip for testing, because the medication will interfere with the color.

Outdated materials give inaccurate results. If the expiration date has passed, discard the materials.

Procedure 43-5

Clinitest for Reducing Sugars

Purpose: To determine the presence of reducing sugars when testing by reagent strip is not appropriate

Equipment: Patient's labeled urine specimen, transfer pipettes, distilled water, positive and negative controls, stopwatch or timer, five-drop Clinitest color comparison chart, Clinitest tablets (tightly sealed or new bottle), daily sample log, 16 × 125 mm glass test tubes, patient report form or data form, test tube rack, impervious gown, gloves, face shield, 10% bleach solution

Steps	Reason
1. Wash your hands.	
2. Assemble the equipment.	
3. Put on impervious gown, gloves, and face shield.	
4. Identify the specimen to be tested, and record patient and sample information on the daily log.	
5. Record the patient's identification information, catalog and lot numbers for all test and control materials, and expiration dates on report or data form.	This complies with CLIA QA/QC requirements
6. Label test tubes with patient and control identification, and place them in the test tube rack.	Proper labeling avoids misidentification.
7. Using a transfer pipette, add 10 drops of distilled water to each labeled test tube in the rack. Add drops by holding the dropper vertically to ensure proper delivery.	
8. Add 5 drops of the patient's urine or control sample to the appropriately labeled tube, using a different transfer pipette for each.	This prevents diluting the urine with water or contaminating the water with urine.
9. Open the Clinitest bottle and shake a Clinitest tablet into the lid without touching it. Drop the tablet from the lid into the test tube. Repeat for all patient and control samples being tested. Close the Clinitest bottle.	Touching the tablet may result in a false result. The Clinitest bottle must be tightly capped at all times because moisture causes the tablets to deteriorate, affecting test results.
10. Observe reactions in the test tubes as the mixture boils. After the reaction stops, wait 15 seconds, then gently swirl the test tubes.	This mixes the contents so you can read the results.
11. Compare results for the patient specimen and controls with the 5-drop method color chart immediately after shaking. (If positive or negative controls do not give expected results, the test is invalid and must be repeated.)	This ensures testing accuracy.

(continued)

Procedure 43-5 *(continued)*

Clinitest for Reducing Sugars

Steps	Reason

5-Drop Method Standard Procedure

DIRECTIONS FOR TESTING:

1. Collect urine in clean container. With dropper in upright position, place **5 drops** of urine in test tube. Rinse dropper with water and add 10 drops of water to test tube.

2. Drop one tablet into test tube. Watch while complete boiling reaction takes place. Do not shake test tube during boiling, or for the following 15 seconds after boiling has stopped. **3.** At the end of this 15-second waiting period, shake test tube gently to mix contents. Compare

color of liquid to Color Chart below. Ignore sediment that may form in the bottom of the test tube. Ignore changes after the 15-second waiting period. **4.** Write down the percent (%) result which appears on the color block that most closely matches the color of the liquid.

NEGATIVE	1/4%	1/2%	3/4%	1%	2% or more

Step 11: Clinitest package insert. (Courtesy of Bayer Corporation, Elkhart, IN.)

12. Clean the work area with 10% bleach, and dispose of all waste properly. Remove gown, gloves, and face shield. Wash your hands.

Warning! Always use glass test tubes, never plastic. Do not touch the test tube bottoms; they become very hot during the test reaction.

Notes: Watch carefully during the boiling to see if the tube contents pass through all of the colors on the five-drop color chart, resulting in a final color that reflects a lower score than one seen during the reaction. This pass-through phenomenon should be reported as "exceeds 2%." If your office requires a precise quantitative result on samples that exhibit the pass-through phenomenon, perform the two-drop method according to the Clinitest package insert, using the 2-drop color chart for interpretation.

Clinitest may be used as a confirmatory test when dipstick urine tests for glucose result in a trace value or greater or cannot be interpreted and on children under age 2 who are being tested for problems with glucose metabolism regardless of dipstick result.

Certain medications (ascorbic acid) and reducing substances other than glucose (galactose and lactose) may cause false-positive results. If this occurs, further testing is necessary.

Charting Example

04/21/2004 9:00 A.M. Random urine tested for glucose. Clinitest, results 3/4%. _____
N. Peterson, CMA

Procedure 43-6

Nitroprusside Reaction (Acetest) for Ketones

Purpose: To determine the level of ketones in the urine to aid diagnosis of diseases and disorders of fat metabolism

Equipment: Patient's labeled urine specimen, white filter paper, plastic transfer pipette, Acetest tablet, manufacturer's color comparison chart, gloves, impervious gown, face shield, 10% bleach solution

Steps	Reason
1. Wash your hands.	
2. Assemble the equipment.	
3. Put on gloves, impervious gown, and face shield.	
4. Identify the specimen to be tested and record patient and sample information on the daily log.	
5. Record on report or data form the patient's identification information, catalog and lot numbers for all test and control materials, and expiration dates.	This complies with CLIA QA/QC requirements.
6. Shake an Acetest tablet into the cap and put it on the filter paper. Replace the cap.	Dispensing the tablet in this manner prevents contamination of the tablet or bottle contents. The white background of the filter paper allows for contrast.
7. Swirl urine specimen to mix. Using a transfer pipette, place 1 drop of well-mixed urine on top of the tablet.	When the urine and the tablet meet, the reaction begins.
8. Wait 30 seconds for the complete reaction.	Nitroprusside reaction occurs if ketones are present.
9. Compare the color of the tablet to the color chart, and record the results as negative, trace, small amount, moderate amount, or large amount.	Nitroprusside reaction gives a color change of varying degrees of purple if ketones are present. The color correlates to the amount of ketones in the urine.

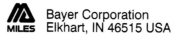   Bayer Corporation
MILES   Elkhart, IN 46515 USA

Colors shown below are for use with ACETEST Reagent Tablets only.

Step 9: Acetest package insert. (Courtesy of Bayer Corporation, Elkhart, IN.)

10. Properly care for or dispose of equipment and supplies. Clean the work area with 10% bleach solution. Remove gloves, gown, and face shield, and wash hands.

Charting Example

11/20/2004 8:00 A.M. Urine specimen collected and tested for ketones; results showed large amount. Dr. Wendt notified. _____ B. Evans, CMS

Acid Precipitation Test for Protein

Purpose:	To determine levels of protein in the urine to aid in diagnosis of diseases and disorders that increase protein metabolism
Equipment:	Patient's labeled urine specimen, test tube rack, clear test tubes, transfer pipettes, positive and negative controls, stopwatch or timer, daily sample log, 3% sulfosalicylic acid (SSA) solution, patient report form or data form, impervious gown, gloves, face shield, 10% bleach solution.

Steps	Reason
1. Wash your hands.	
2. Assemble the equipment.	
3. Put on impervious gown, gloves, and face shield.	
4. Identify the patient's specimen to be tested, and record patient and sample information on the daily log.	Proper identification and recording avoids errors and complies with QA/QC requirements.
5. Record on report or data form the patient's name or identification, catalog and lot numbers for all test and control materials, and expiration dates.	This complies with QA/QC requirements.
6. Label the test tubes with patient and control identification, and place in test tube rack.	Proper labeling avoids misidentification.
7. Centrifuge the patient sample at 1,500 rpm for 5 minutes.	
8. Add 1–3 mL supernatant urine (top portion of spun urine) or control sample to appropriately labeled tube in rack. Repeat for all samples and controls, using a clean transfer pipette for each.	Using a clean pipette avoids contamination of pipettes, samples, and controls.
9. Add an equal amount of 3% SSA to sample quantity in each tube. Use a clean transfer pipette for each addition if your 3% SSA does not have a repeating dispenser.	Adding equal amounts of 3% SSA reduces errors in testing.
10. Mix the contents of the tubes and let stand for a minimum of 2 minutes but no longer than 10 minutes. Use a stopwatch or timer to make sure you perform the next step within the appropriate time frame.	The reactants must be mixed together. Adherence to timing guidelines is necessary for accuracy in testing.
11. Mix the contents of tubes again, then observe the degree of turbidity in each test tube and assign a score as follows: Neg: No turbidity or cloudiness; urine remains clear Trace: Slight turbidity 1+: Turbidity with no precipitation 2+: Heavy turbidity with fine granulation 3+: Heavy turbidity with granulation and flakes 4+: Clumps of precipitated protein The specimen may be matched against a McFarland standard for objective assessment.	

(continued)

Procedure 43-7   *(continued)*

Acid Precipitation Test for Protein

Steps	Reason
12. Clean work area with 10% bleach solution, and dispose of all waste properly. Remove gown, gloves, and face shield. Wash your hands.	

Notes: This is a confirmatory test used for specimens with dipstick urine test results greater than trace value for protein.

If positive and negative controls do not give expected results, the test is invalid and must be repeated.

Charting Example

03/28/2005, 9:00 A.M. Urine specimen collected and tested for protein; results 3+ using acid precipitation test.
_____ R. McDonald, CMA

Procedure 43-8

The Diazo Tablet Test (Ictotest) for Bilirubin

Purpose:	To determine any bilirubin excreted by the kidneys to aid in diagnosis of liver, gallbladder, or hemolytic diseases
Equipment:	Patient's labeled urine specimen, clean paper towel, transfer pipette, diazo (Ictotest) tablets, stopwatch or timer, Ictotest white mats, impervious gown, gloves, face shield, 10% bleach solution

Steps	Reason
1. Wash your hands.	
2. Assemble the equipment.	
3. Put on impervious gown, gloves, and face shield.	
4. Verify that the names on the specimen container and the report form are the same.	
5. Place an Ictotest white mat on a clean, dry paper towel.	The mat provides a testing surface. The paper towel must be dry because moisture may cause a false result.
6. Using a clean transfer pipette, add 10 drops of urine to the center of the mat. (If the urine is red, it may be difficult to read the reaction properly. In this event, pour an aliquot of the urine into a urine tube or test tube, and centrifuge as if preparing urine sediment. Use 10 drops of supernatant in this step.)	
7. Shake a tablet into the bottle cap and put in the center of the mat. Do not touch the tablet with your hands.	Touching the tablet contaminates it and may cause a false-positive result.

(continued)

Procedure 43-8 *(continued)*

The Diazo Tablet Test (Ictotest) for Bilirubin

Steps	Reason
8. Recap the bottle immediately.	The bottle must be recapped to prevent deterioration of the contents.
9. Using a clean transfer pipette, place 1 drop of water on the tablet and wait 5 seconds.	
10. Add another drop of water to the tablet so that the solution formed by the first drop runs onto the mat.	This allows the diazo chemical to react with the urine.
11. Within 60 seconds, observe for either a blue or purple color on the mat around the tablet. Either color indicates a positive result. Pink or red indicates a negative result.	

Step 11: Ictotest package insert. (Courtesy of Bayer Corporation, Elkhart, IN.)

12. Clean the work area with 10% bleach solution, and dispose of waste properly. Remove gown, gloves, and face shield. Wash your hands.	

Notes: Quality control must be performed daily and recorded appropriately. Follow office policies and procedures for compliance with QA/QC requirements.

The specimen should be free of pyridium, chlorpromazine, and other drugs that interfere with color interpretation.

The tablets must be protected from exposure to light, heat, and moisture to prevent deterioration.

Charting Example
3/23/2005 9:30 A.M. Urine specimen collected and tested for bilirubin using diazo test. Results positive.
_____ K. Rogers, RMA

Procedure 43-9

Preparing Urine Sediment

Purpose: To aid in the determination and identification of formed elements and solid particles in a urine specimen

Equipment: Patient's labeled urine specimen, urine centrifuge tubes, transfer pipette, centrifuge (1,500–2,000 rpm), impervious gown, gloves, face shield, 10% bleach solution

Steps	Reason
1. Wash your hands.	
2. Assemble the equipment.	
3. Put on impervious gown, gloves, and face shield.	
4. Verify that the names on the specimen container and the report form are the same.	
5. Swirl specimen to mix. Pour 10 mL of well-mixed urine into a labeled centrifuge tube or standard system tube. Cap the tube with a plastic cap or parafilm.	
6. Centrifuge the sample at 1500 rpm for 5 minutes.	Centrifugation ensures that cellular and particulate matter is pulled to the bottom of the tube.
7. When the centrifuge has stopped, remove the tubes. Make sure no tests are to be performed first on the supernatant. Remove the caps and pour off the supernatant, leaving 0.5–1.0 mL of it. Suspend the sediment again by aspirating up and down with a transfer pipette, or follow manufacturer's directions for a standardized system.	The concentrated urine is now prepared for microscopic examination.
8. Properly care for and dispose of equipment and supplies. Clean the work area with 10% bleach solution. Remove gown, gloves, and shield. Wash your hands.	

Notes: If the urine is to be tested by chemical reagent strip, perform the dip test before spinning the urine.

Preparing a urine specimen of less than 3 mL for sediment is not recommended because that is not enough urine to create a true sediment. However, some patients cannot provide a large amount of urine. In such cases, document the volume on the chart under sediment to ensure proper interpretation of results.

Centrifuge maintenance requires periodic checks to ensure that the speed and timing are correct. Document this information on the maintenance log.

CHAPTER SUMMARY

Urine tests help the physician determine or rule out abnormalities to make a correct diagnosis. The medical assistant ensures a properly collected clean-catch midstream specimen by thoroughly instructing the patient in the collection procedure. Another important factor the medical assistant can influence is the elapsed time from collection to examination in the laboratory. Changes over time after collection include (1) decreased clarity due to crystallization of solutes, (2) rising pH, (3) loss of ketone bodies, (4) loss of bilirubin, (5) dissolution of cells and casts, and (6) overgrowth of contaminating microorganisms. Urinalysis may not reflect the findings of absolutely fresh urine if the sample is more than 1 hour old. Proper performanceof the urinalysis, including confirmation tests as indicated, is an important function of the medical assistant.

Answers to Checkpoint Questions

1. Urine should be tested within 1 hour of collection. (If testing cannot be performed within 1 hour, refrigerate the specimen at 4°–8°C until testing can be performed.) If the urine is not properly refrigerated, the specimen can deteriorate.
2. The three reported physical properties of urine are color, clar ed visually.
3. A positive biliruin test can indicate problems such as liver disease, hepatitis and bile duct destruction.
4. Positive nitrates and leukocytes on a dipstick would suggest a urinary tract infection.
5. Three of the most common crystals found in urine are calcium oxalate, uric acid, and triple phosphate.

Critical Thinking Challenges

1. Most laboratories pour off a portion of a urine specimen to test rather than dipping the chemical reagent strip directly into the urine container. Why?
2. Why is the first morning specimen preferred for urine pregnancy testing?

 Websites

London Health Sciences Centre—Urinalysis Showcase
www.lhsc.on.ca/lab/renal/showcase.htm
Virtual Hospital—Urinalysis www.vh.org/adult/provider/
pathology/CLIA/UrineAnalysis/UrineAnalysis.html

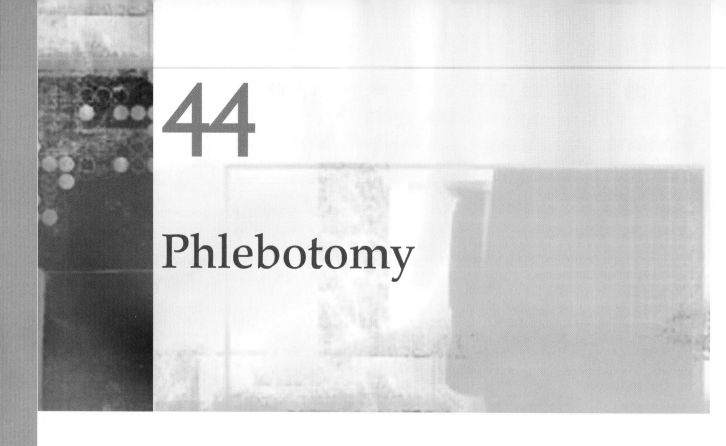

44

Phlebotomy

CHAPTER OUTLINE

ROLE DELINEATION

CLINICAL: FUNDAMENTAL PRINCIPLES
- Apply principles of aseptic technique and infection control
- Comply with quality assurance practices

CLINICAL: DIAGNOSTIC ORDERS
- Collect and process specimens
- Perform diagnostic tests

CLINICAL: PATIENT CARE
- Adhere to established patient screening procedures

GENERAL: PROFESSIONALISM
- Display a professional manner and image
- Prioritize and perform multiple tasks

GENERAL: COMMUNICATION SKILLS
- Adapt communications to individual's ability to understand

CLINICAL: LEGAL CONCEPTS
- Perform within legal and ethical boundaries
- Document accurately

CHAPTER COMPETENCIES

LEARNING OBJECTIVES

Upon successfully completing this chapter, you will be able to:

1. Define and spell the key terms.
2. Identify equipment and supplies used to obtain a routine venous specimen and a routine capillary skin puncture.
3. List the major anticoagulants, their color codes, and the suggested order in which they are filled from a venipuncture.
4. Describe the location and selection of the blood collection sites for capillaries and veins.
5. Explain the importance of correct patient identification and complete specimen and requisition labeling.
6. Describe the steps in preparation of the puncture site for venipuncture and skin puncture.
7. Describe care for a puncture site after blood has been drawn.
8. List precautions to be observed when drawing blood.

PERFORMANCE OBJECTIVES

Upon successfully completing this chapter, you will be able to:

1. Obtain a blood specimen from a patient by venipuncture (Procedure 44-1).
2. Obtain a blood specimen from a patient by skin puncture (Procedure 44-2).
3. Use a butterfly collection system.

KEY TERMS

anticoagulant	gauge	Luer adapter	sharps container
antecubital space	gel separator	multisample needle	syncope
antiseptic	hematoma	order of draw	
bevel	hemoconcentration	palpate	
evacuated tube	hemolysis	prophylaxis	

SUCCESSFULLY OBTAINING blood specimens requires study and practice. Blood is collected by several methods, including arterial puncture, skin puncture, and venipuncture. This chapter describes blood collection equipment and supplies for safe venipuncture and skin puncture. Use of arterial specimens is limited to the evaluation of respiratory function. You must perform blood collection in the safest manner possible. Blood is a biohazardous material, so it should be handled with standard precautions and appropriate barrier precautions.

Needlestick injuries contribute to the overall burden of health care worker injuries. Estimates indicate that 600,000 to 800,000 such injuries occur annually, and about half go unreported. Needlestick injuries may expose workers to blood-borne pathogens, such as human immunodeficiency virus (HIV), hepatitis B virus, and/or hepatitis C virus. A health care worker's risk of infection depends on the pathogen, the severity of the needlestick injury, and the use of vaccination before the exposure and **prophylaxis** (protective treatment for the prevention of disease once exposure has occurred) after it. Become familiar now with the instructions for immediate action from the Centers for Disease Control and Prevention (CDC) in case of a needlestick injury (Box 44-1).

GENERAL BLOOD DRAWING EQUIPMENT

Blood Drawing Station

A blood drawing station is equipped for performing phlebotomy procedures on outpatients or patients in medical offices sent by their physicians for laboratory testing (FIG. 44-1). This station includes a table close at hand for supplies and a chair or bed for the patient. The table should be at a convenient height for working with enough space to hold numerous supplies. Phlebotomy chairs are available from several manufacturers. The chair should be comfortable and have adjustable armrests to allow proper positioning of either arm. A safety device locks the armrest in place in front of the patient to prevent falling from the chair if fainting occurs. A bed or reclining chair should be available for patients with a history of fainting and to perform heel sticks or other procedures on infants and small children.

Gloves

Guidelines from the CDC and the Occupational Safety and Health Administration (OSHA) require that gloves be worn during phlebotomy procedures. **A new pair of gloves must** be used for each patient and removed when the procedure is finished. Nonsterile, disposable latex, nitrile, vinyl, or polyethylene gloves are acceptable.

Standard precautions require handwashing after glove removal. Good glove fit enhances safe manipulation. Gloves that are dusted with powder can be a source of contamination for some tests, especially those collected by capillary puncture. Some users have allergic responses to glove powder. Powder in latex gloves can facilitate suspension of latex particles in the air, posing danger to those with latex allergy.

Antiseptics

Antiseptics inhibit the growth of bacteria. They are safe for use on human skin and are used to clean the skin before skin puncture or venipuncture. The most commonly used antiseptic for routine blood collection is 70% isopropyl alcohol. Other antiseptics used for blood collection are povidone iodine, 0.5% chlorhexidine gluconate, and benzalkonium chloride.

Spill Kit Supplies and Instructions

The supplies available in a biohazard spill kit should include but are not limited to the following:

- A copy of these biohazardous spill cleanup instructions
- Nitrile disposable gloves
- Laboratory coat
- Absorbent material, such as absorbent paper towels, granular absorbent material
- All-purpose disinfectant, such as normal household bleach (diluted 1:10) or an iodophor
- Bucket for diluting disinfectant (can be used to store the kit contents when not in use)
- Dustpan, broom, hand broom (for picking up broken glass and other contaminated sharps)

- Sharps waste containers
- Biohazard waste bags

All reusable items should be autoclavable or compatible with the disinfectant used. Most of the listed items and other biohazard spill control items are sold in biohazardous-spill control kits.

When cleaning blood spills, you should wear disposable gloves of sufficient sturdiness that they will not tear while you clean. If the gloves develop holes, tears or splits, remove them, wash hands immediately, and put on fresh gloves. Disposable gloves must never be washed or reused.

Spills of blood and blood-contaminated fluids should be properly cleaned using either a chemical germicide approved for use as a hospital disinfectant and tuberculocidal at recommended dilution or a solution of 5.25% sodium hypochlorite (household bleach) diluted 1:10 with water.

Cleaning up Blood and Body Fluids

1. Secure spill area.
2. Locate a spill cleanup kit.
3. Wear gloves during cleanup.
4. Pour or place adsorbent material over the spill.
5. Use a scoop or dustpan to pick up material.
6. Wipe blood up with an absorbent towel.
7. Apply a disinfectant to the area.
8. Double-bag all cleanup materials in red biohazard bags for disposal.

Cleaning up Glass, Blood, and Body Fluids

- Wear double gloves or utility gloves if there is broken glass in a blood or fluid spill.
- Pick up the glass with a mechanical device, such as forceps, or scoop it up with a broom and dustpan or cardboard. (DO NOT USE YOUR HANDS TO PICK UP THE GLASS!)
- Place the broken glass in a sharps (needle disposal) container.
- Follow steps listed earlier for cleaning up blood or fluid spills.

FIGURE 44-1.   A well-stocked blood drawing station.

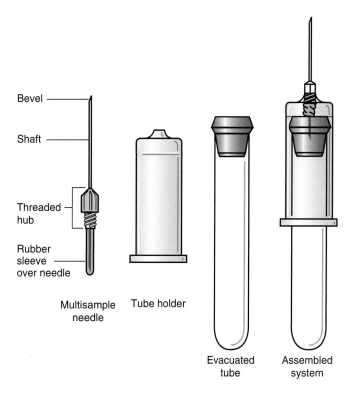

FIGURE 44-2. Traditional components of the evacuated tube system. (Reprinted with permission from McCall R. Phlebotomy Essentials. Baltimore: Lippincott Williams & Wilkins, 2003.)

Gauze Pads

Clean 2 × 2 gauze pads folded in fourths are used to hold pressure over the puncture site. Cotton or rayon balls may be used but are not recommended because of their tendency to stick to the site and cause bleeding when removed.

Bandages

An adhesive bandage (e.g., Band-Aid) is used to cover the site once the bleeding has stopped. If a patient is allergic to adhesive bandages, use paper, cloth, or knitted tape over a folded gauze square. Do not use a bandage on infants under 2 years of age because of the danger of aspiration and suffocation. Latex-free bandages are available in case of latex allergy.

Needle and Sharps Disposal Containers

Regardless of safety features, immediately dispose of used needles, lancets, and other sharp objects in a puncture-resistant, leakproof disposable container called a sharps container. These containers are usually marked as biohazard and are red or bright orange for easy identification. Needles should never be cut, bent, or broken before disposal.

Checkpoint Question

1. What are disinfectants and antiseptics used for?

VENIPUNCTURE EQUIPMENT

Venipuncture procedures require the use of the following special equipment.

Tourniquets

The tourniquet constricts the flow of venous blood in the arm and makes the veins more prominent, so they are easier to find and penetrate with a needle. The tourniquet is a soft, pliable rubber strip, usually 1 inch wide and 15 to 18 inches long. It can easily be released with one hand, does not cut into the patient's arm, and is inexpensive enough that a new tourniquet can be used for each patient.

Needles

OSHA requires needles to have safety features to minimize accidental needlesticks. Manufacturers provide needles with various features to facilitate this requirement. Users can select products that both meet requirements and provide ease of use.

Sterile, disposable, single-use-only needles are used for venipuncture. They are silicon-coated, which enables them to penetrate the skin smoothly. The end of the needle that pierces the vein is cut on a slant or **bevel**. The bevel allows the needle to penetrate the vein easily and prevents coring, removal of a portion of skin or vein. The long, cylindrical portion of the needle is called the shaft, and the end that connects to the blood-drawing apparatus is called the hub.

FIGURE 44-3. BD Eclipse multisample safety needle attached to traditional tube holder. (Courtesy Becton-Dickinson, Franklin Lakes, NJ).

The **gauge** of a needle indicates the size of the lumen (bore size or opening) of the needle. The larger the gauge number, the smaller the diameter of the needle (e.g., 20 gauge is larger than 25 gauge). Selection of the gauge is based on the size and condition of the patient's vein. A 21- to 22-gauge needle is used for most routine blood collection. Never use a 24-gauge needle to collect blood, as the lumen is too small and will rupture blood cells, causing **hemolysis** of the specimen.

BLOOD COLLECTION SYSTEMS

Two blood collection systems are commonly used for venipuncture: the vacuum or **evacuated tube** system and the syringe system.

Evacuated Tube System

The evacuated tube system consists of a tube holder (adapter) and evacuated tube needle. This is a closed system allowing the patient's blood to flow from the vein through the needle and into the collection tube without exposure to the air. This system facilitates collecting multiple tubes with a single venipuncture. Evacuated tube systems are composed of three components: a **multisample needle** (allows collection of multiple tubes of blood during one venipuncture), a plastic needle holder that holds the collection tubes, and various collection tubes (FIG. 44-2).

With beveled points on both ends, multisample needles are threaded in the middle to screw into the needle holder. One end of the needle is longer and is exposed for piercing the patient's skin and entering the vein. The shorter end penetrates the rubber stopper of the collection tube and with its retractable rubber sleeve prevents leakage of blood during tube changes. The sleeve is pushed back when it goes into the stopper; it allows blood to flow into the tube and recovers the end of the needle when the tube is removed. A multisample needle with safety features in shown in FIGURE 44-3.

The holder, sometimes called an adapter, has an indentation about half an inch from the hub (FIG. 44-4). This indentation marks the point where the short, sleeved end of the needle starts to enter the rubber stopper of the tube. A large opening at the other end of the holder accepts the blood collection tube. There are flanges (extensions) on the sides of the rim of the holder to aid in tube placement and removal. Holder safety features include a shield that covers the needle or device that retracts the needle into the holder after it is withdrawn from the vein (FIG. 44-5).

Evacuated tubes contain a vacuum with a rubber stopper sealing the tube. These tubes are made of glass or plastic and range in size from 2 to 15 mL. Tube size is selected according to the patient's age, amount of blood needed, and the size and condition of the patient's vein. The tubes are sterile to prevent contamination of the specimen and the patient.

Because of the vacuum inside the tube, evacuated tubes fill with blood automatically. The vacuum is premeasured by the manufacturer to draw the precise amount of blood into the

FIGURE 44-4. Traditional needle and tube holders. (Reprinted with permission from McCall R. Phlebotomy Essentials. Baltimore: Lippincott Williams & Wilkins, 2003.)

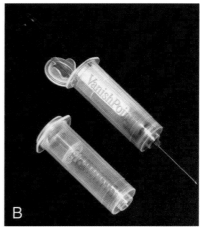

FIGURE 44-5. Safety tube holders. (A) Venipuncture Needle-Pro with needle-sheathing device. (B) Vanish point tube holder with needle-retracting device. (Retractable Technologies, Little Elm, TX.)

tube. The tube fills until the vacuum is exhausted, so that a tube that has lost all or part of its vacuum will not fill completely, if at all.

Tube Additives

Different laboratory tests require different types of blood specimens. Some tests require serum samples; for these the blood is drawn into a tube that allows clotting. Other tests require whole blood or plasma, and these samples are drawn into a tube that contains an **anticoagulant** additive because it prevents clotting.

An additive is any substance (other than the tube coating) that is placed in a tube. Additives have specific functions. Below is a list of the most common additives and their functions:

- Anticoagulants prevent the blood from coagulating or clotting.
- Clot activators enhance coagulation.
- Thixotropic **gel separator**, an inert substance, forms a physical barrier between the cellular portion of a specimen and the serum or plasma portion after the specimen has been centrifuged.

The evacuated tube system uses color-coded stoppers as a means of identifying the additive content of each type of tube (TABLE 44-1). It is necessary to use the correct anticoagulant because improper anticoagulant use can alter test results.

Syringe System

Syringes are made of glass or disposable plastic and vary in volume from 1 to 50 mL. Choose a syringe whose volume will accommodate all of the blood necessary for the tests the physician has requested.

The barrel of the syringe is graduated in milliliters. Pulling on the plunger of the syringe creates a vacuum in the barrel.

The plunger often sticks and is hard to pull. A technique called breathing the syringe makes the plunger easier to move. To do this, before beginning the procedure, pull back the plunger to about halfway up the barrel, then push it back. This makes the plunger move more smoothly and reduces the tendency to jerk when it is first pulled after insertion into the vein.

The vacuum created by pulling on the plunger while a needle is in a patient's vein fills the syringe with blood. Pulling the plunger slowly and resting between pulls allows the vein time to refill with blood.

Using a syringe for blood collection requires transfer of blood to a collection tube. Various brands of devices ensure safety during the transfer of blood from a syringe into an evacuated tube. Force on the syringe plunger is not required because the vacuum in the tube will draw the specimen from the syringe.

Blood specimens collected by syringe must be transferred to evacuated tubes following proper order of draw (discussed later in the chapter).

Winged Infusion Set

The butterfly collection system, or winged infusion set, has a stainless steel beveled needle with attached winged-shaped plastic extensions connected to a 6- to 12-inch length of tubing. The most common butterfly needle sizes are 21 to 23 gauge and half an inch to three-quarters of an inch long. Butterflies come with attachments to be used with syringes and a special multisample **Luer adapter** (a device for connecting a syringe or evacuated holder to the needle) that allows them to be used in an evacuated tube system (FIG. 44-6). The set is an essential tool for collecting blood from difficult or small veins, such as hand veins or fragile veins of children and the elderly. FIGURE 44-7 shows how to use the butterfly system.

Table 44-1   EVACUATED TUBE SYSTEM: COLOR CODING

BD Vacutainer™ Tubes With Hemogard™ Closure	BD Vacutainer™ Tubes With Conventional Stopper	Additive	Inversions at Blood Collection*	Laboratory Use	Your Lab's Draw Volume/Remarks
		• Clot activator and gel for serum separation	5	BD Vacutainer™ SST™ Tube for serum determinations in chemistry. Tube inversions ensure mixing of clot activator with blood. Blood clotting time 30 minutes.	
		• Lithium heparin and gel for plasma separation	8	BD Vacutainer™ PST™ Tube for plasma determination in chemistry. Tube inversions prevent clotting.	
		• None (glass) • Clot activator (plastic tube with Hemogard closure)	0 5	For serum determinations in chemistry and serology. Glass serum tubes are recommended for blood banking. Plastic tubes contain clot activator and are not recommended for blood banking. Tube inversions ensure mixing of clot activator with blood and clotting within 60 minutes.	
		• Thrombin	8	For stat serum determinations in chemistry. Tube inversions ensure complete clotting which usually occurs in less than 5 minutes.	
		• Sodium heparin • Na₂EDTA • None (serum tube)	8 8 0	For trace-element, toxicology and nutritional-chemistry determinations. Special stopper formulation provides low levels of trace elements (see package insert).	
		• Sodium heparin	8	For plasma determinations in chemistry.	
		• Lithium heparin • Potassium oxalate/sodium fluoride	8 8	Tube inversions prevent clotting. For glucose determinations. Oxalate and EDTA anticoagulants will give plasma samples.	
		• Sodium fluoride/ Na₂ EDTA • Sodium fluoride (serum tube) • Sodium heparin (glass) • K₂EDTA (plastic)	8 8 8 8	Sodium fluoride is the antiglycolytic agent. Tube inversions ensure proper mixing of additive and blood. For lead determinations. This tube is certified to contain less than .01 μg/mL/(ppm) lead. Tube invasions prevent clotting.	
		• Sodium polyanethol sulfonate (SPS)	8	SPS for blood culture specimen collections in micro-biology. Tube inversions prevent clotting.	
		• Acid citrate dextrose additives (ACD): **Solution A -** 22.0g/L trisodium citrate. 8.0g/L citric acid, 24.5g/L dextrose **Solution B -** 13.2g/L trisodium citrate,	 8 8	 ACD for use in blood bank studies, HLA phenotyping, DNA and paternity testing.	

(continues)

Table 44-1 (CONTINUED)

BD Vacutainer™ Tubes With Hemogard™ Closure	BD Vacutainer™ Tubes With Conventional Stopper	Additive	Inversions at Blood Collection*	Laboratory Use	Your Lab's Draw Volume/Remarks
		4.8g/L citric acid, 14.7g/L dextrose • Liquid K$_3$EDTA (glass) • Spray-dried K$_2$EDTA (plastic)	 8 8	K$_3$EDTA for whole blood hematology determinations. K$_2$EDTA for whole blood hematology determinations and immunohematology testing (ABO grouping, Rh typing, antibody screening). Tube inversions prevent clotting.	
		• Spray-dried K$_2$EDTA	8	For whole blood hematology determinations and immunohematology testing (ABO grouping, RH typing, antibody screening). Designed with special cross-match label for required patient information by the AABB. Tube inversions prevent clotting.	
		• .05M sodium citrate (≈3.2%) • .129M sodium citrate (3.8%) • Citrate, theophylline, adenosine, dipyridamole (CTAD)	3–4 3–4 3–4	For coagulation determinations. NOTE: Certain tests may require chilled specimens. Follow your institution's recommended procedures for collection and transport. CTAD for selected platelet function assays and routine coagulation determination. Tube inversions prevent clotting.	

Partial-draw Tubes (2 ml and 3 ml, 13 × 15 mm) **Small-volume Pediatric Tubes** (2 ml: 10.25 × 47 mm, 3 ml: 10.25 × 64 mm)

		• None	0	For serum determinations in chemistry and serology. Glass serum tubes are recommended for blood banking. Plastic tubes contain clot activator and are not recommended for blood banking. Tube inversions ensure mixing of clot activator with blood and clotting within 60 minutes	
		• Sodium heparin • Lithium heparin • Liquid K$_3$EDTA (glass) • Spray-dried K$_2$EDTA (plastic)	8 8 8 8	For plasma determinations in chemistry. Tube inversions prevent clotting. K$_3$EDTA for whole blood hematology determinations. K$_2$EDTA for whole blood hematology determinations and immunohematology testing (ABO grouping, Rh typing, antibody screening). Tube inversions prevent clotting.	
		• .105M sodium citrate (=3.2%) • .129M sodium citrate (3.8%)	3–4	For coagulation determinations. Tube inversions prevent clotting. NOTE: Certain tests may require chilled specimens. Follow your institution's recommended procedures for collection and transport of specimen.	

BD Vacutainer Systems
Preanalytical Solutions
1 Becton Drive
Franklin Lakes, NJ 07417 USA
www.bd.com

BD Technical Services: 800.631.0174 *Invert gently, do not shake
BD, BD Logo and all other trademarks are property of Becton, Dickinson and Company. ©2002 BD.
Printed in USA 01/02 VS5229-4

FIGURE 44-6. Winged infusion sets. *Left:* Attached to a syringe. *Right:* Attached to evacuated tube holder by means of a Luer adapter. (Reprinted with permission from McCall R: Phlebotomy Essentials. Baltimore: Lippincott Williams & Wilkins, 2003.)

FIGURE 44-7. Procedure for using butterfly in a hand vein. (A) Hand with tourniquet in place reveals prominent vein. (B) With the skin pulled taut over the knuckles, the needle is inserted into the vein until there is a flash of blood in the tubing. (C) Using the nondominant hand, a wing of the butterfly is held against the patient's hand to steady the needle while the blood collecting tube is pushed onto the blood collecting needle. (D) Once the proper tubes have been drawn, gauze is placed over the vein and the needle is removed. (Reprinted with permission from McCall R: Phlebotomy Essentials. Baltimore: Lippincott Williams & Wilkins, 2003.)

Checkpoint Question

2. What are three chemical substances that may be added to collection tubes? Explain the function of each.

ORDER OF DRAW

A designated order of draw is recommended to avoid contamination of nonadditive tubes by additive tubes, cross-contamination between different types of additive tubes, contamination with tissue thromboplastin, and microbial contamination.

The National Committee for Clinical Laboratory Standards (NCCLS) is an organization of representatives from the health care community, industry, and government who use consensus to develop voluntary guidelines and standards for the laboratory. NCCLS recommends one order of draw for both collection of evacuated tubes and filling evacuated tubes from a syringe (TABLE 44-2).

SKIN PUNCTURE (MICROCOLLECTION) EQUIPMENT

Capillary puncture or skin puncture requires penetration of the capillary bed in the dermis of the skin with a lancet or other sharp device. The small specimen volumes required by point-of-care instruments allow more laboratory tests to be collected by skin puncture. The equipment used to collect the specimen depends on the test being performed.

Table 44-2 NCCLS ORDER OF DRAW, STOPPER COLOR, AND RATIONALE FOR COLLECTION ORDER

Order of Draw	Tube Stopper Color	Rationale for Collection Order
Blood cultures (sterile collections)	Yellow sodium polyanetholesulfonate (SPS) (or sterile media containers)	Minimizes chance of microbial contamination
Plain (nonadditive) tubes	Red	Prevents contamination by additives in other tubes.
Coagulation tubes	Light blue	Second or third position in order of draw prevents tissue thromboplastin contamination. Must be the first additive tube in the order because all other additive tubes affect coagulation tests.
Serum separator gel tubes (SSTs)	Red and gray rubber Gold plastic	Prevents contamination by additives in other tubes. Comes after coagulation tests because silica particles activate clotting and affect coagulation tests. Carryover of silica into subsequent tubes can be overridden by the anticoagulant in them.
Plasma separator gel tubes (PSTs)	Green and gray rubber Light green plastic	Contains heparin, which affects coagulation tests and interferes in collection of serum specimens. Causes the least interference in tests other than coagulation tests.
Heparin tubes	Green	Same as PST.
Ethylenediaminetetraacetic acid (EDTA) tubes	Lavender	Causes more carryover problems than any other additive. Elevates sodium and potassium levels. Chelates and decreases calcium and iron levels. Elevates prothrombin time and partial thromboplastin time results.
Oxalate/fluoride tubes	Gray	Sodium fluoride and potassium oxalate elevate sodium and potassium levels, respectively. Comes after hematology tubes because oxalate damages cell membranes and causes abnormal red blood cell morphology.

FIGURE 44-9.   Microcollection tubes and clay sealant.

Microhematocrit tubes for sampling specimens directly from a lavender-top tube are plain; those used for collecting hematocrit specimens directly from a capillary puncture are coated with ammonium heparin. Plain tubes have a blue band on one end of the capillary tube, and ammonium heparin–coated tubes have a red band. A plastic or clay sealant is used to close one end of the tube (FIG. 44-9).

Lancets

A sterile disposable lancet is used to pierce the skin to obtain drops of blood for testing. Lancets are designed to control depth of puncture and have safety features to reduce accidental sharps injuries. Manufacturers offer lancets in a range of lengths and depths to facilitate varying puncture situations and sample requirements. FIGURE 44-8 shows several types of lancets used for microcollection.

Microcollection Containers

Micro containers consist of small, round-bottomed nonsterile plastic tubes and color-coded stoppers that indicate the presence or absence of an additive. The color coding is identical to that of blood collection tubes used in venipuncture. Micro containers are used for filling, measuring, stoppering, centrifuging, and storing blood, all in one container. Samples for bilirubin are collected in an amber-colored plastic tube that protects the blood from light.

Microhematocrit Tubes

Microhematocrit tubes are narrow-bore glass or plastic disposable capillary tubes used for hematocrit determinations. They fill by capillary action and hold 50 to 75 mL of blood.

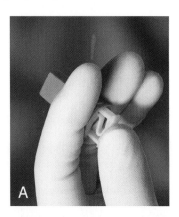

FIGURE 44-8.   Several types of finger and heel puncture lancets. (A) Vacutainer Genie Lancets. (Becton-Dickinson, Franklin Lakes, NJ.) (B) Tenderlett toddler, junior, and adult lancet devices. (Courtesy of ITC, Edison, NJ.) (C) Tenderfoot toddler, newborn, preemie, and micro-preemie heel incision devices. (Courtesy of ITC, Edison, NJ.)

Filter Paper Test Requisitions

Another microcollection device is filter paper that is part of a test requisition. It is used to test newborns for genetic defects, such as hypothyroidism and phenylketonuria. The filter paper is printed with circles that must be filled with blood (FIG. 44-10). The lateral surface of the newborn's heel is punctured and the blood droplet is absorbed into individual circles on a filter paper card. A large drop of blood must be applied from one side of the paper, and the blood must soak through to the other side.

The specimen should air dry in a horizontal position and not be stacked with other collection requisitions.

Warming Devices

Important especially for heel sticks, warmers increase blood flow before the skin is punctured. Heel-warming devices (FIG. 44-11) provide a temperature not exceeding 42°C.

Alternatively, a diaper or towel may be wet with warm tap water and used to wrap the hand or foot before skin puncture. Do not use water so hot that it might burn the patient.

PATIENT PREPARATION

Gaining the patient's trust and confidence and putting the patient at ease will help minimize anxiety and divert attention from any discomfort associated with the procedure. To do this, display a cheerful, confident, and pleasant manner, introduce yourself, explain the procedure in simple terms, and communicate effectively with the patient. Many patients know from experience where it is easiest to find an accessible vein. In conjunction with your knowledge and skill, choosing the best site will make the procedure less traumatic. Talk quietly with the patient and progress through the procedure with confidence.

After identifying the patient and explaining the procedure, verify that the patient has followed any dietary instructions

F I G U R E   44-10.   Newborn screening specimen forms. (A) Initial specimen form. (B) Second specimen form. (Courtesy of Daniel Gray, State of New Mexico Scientific Laboratory, Albuquerque.)

FIGURE 44-11. Infant heel warmer. (Reprinted with permission from McCall R. Phlebotomy Essentials. Baltimore: Lippincott Williams & Wilkins, 2003.)

or restrictions ordered by the physician or required by the test requested. Fasting, the most common dietary restriction, requires the patient to refrain from eating for a certain period, usually from midnight until specimen collection the following morning. It is essential to emphasize that fasting does not require the patient to refrain from drinking water. Hydration is important to make veins palpable and accessible for venipuncture.

If the patient indicates that fasting instructions or dietary restrictions were not followed, notify the physician for a decision whether or not to proceed with the venipuncture. If you are instructed to proceed in obtaining the specimen, write "nonfasting" on both the test requisition and the specimen label.

Always believe patients who say they faint during venipuncture. Have these patients lie down during the procedure. This reduces the chance of **syncope** (fainting), and if the patient does faint, he or she will not fall. If the patient is sitting and feels faint or mentions feeling weak, have him or her lower the head and take deep breaths. Never draw blood from a patient who is likely to faint unless the physician is in the office.

One of the most important steps in specimen collection is identification of the patient. Ask the patient to state his or her name, date of birth, or any other information to verify identity. After you collect the blood specimen, label the sample with the patient's first and last names, an assigned identification number if available, the date and time, and your initials to verify who drew the sample.

Checkpoint Question

3. How should you label the patient's blood sample?

PERFORMING A VENIPUNCTURE

The forearm veins in the **antecubital space** (the inside of the elbow) are commonly used for venipuncture. The three main veins in this area are the cephalic, median cubital, and basilic (FIG. 44-12). The primary vein for venipuncture is the median cubital vein.

Begin the procedure by washing your hands and putting on gloves. Equipment and supplies should be assembled near the phlebotomy chair. The tourniquet should be placed 3 to 4 inches above the planned venipuncture site and secured with a half-bow knot (FIG. 44-13). Apply the tourniquet tightly enough to slow venous blood flow without affecting arterial blood flow. The half-bow makes it easy to remove the tourniquet with one hand. Rapid removal is important in collection procedures and emergencies. Leaving the tourniquet in place longer than 1 minute will change the blood components as a result of **hemoconcentration**. Velcro closure, rubber tubing, or a blood pressure cuff may also be used as a tourniquet.

Ask the patient to make a fist so that the veins in the arm become more prominent. Do not allow the patient to open and close the fist because it will cause hemoconcentration (pooling of blood components) and lead to erroneous test results.

WHAT IF

Your patient feels faint while you are drawing blood?

1. Remove the tourniquet and withdraw the needle as quickly as possible.
2. Talk to the patient to divert attention from the procedure and to help keep him or her alert.
3. Have the patient lower the head and breathe deeply while you physically support the patient to prevent injury in case of collapse.
4. Loosen a tight collar or tie if possible.
5. Apply a cold compress or washcloth to the forehead and back of the neck.
6. Call for the physician if the patient does not respond.

Modified with permission from McCall R. Phlebotomy Essentials. Baltimore: Lippincott Williams & Wilkins, 2003.

Right arm in anatomic position

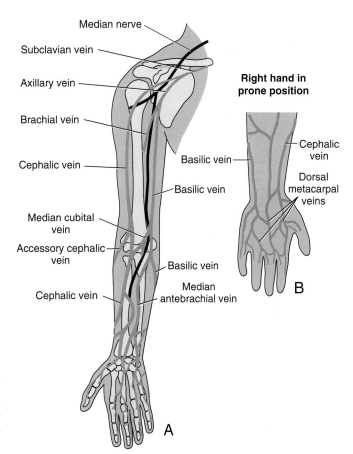

Right hand in prone position

Median nerve

Subclavian vein

Axillary vein

Brachial vein

Cephalic vein

Basilic vein

Basilic vein

Cephalic vein

Dorsal metacarpal veins

Median cubital vein

Accessory cephalic vein

Basilic vein

Cephalic vein

Median antebrachial vein

A

B

FIGURE 44-12. (A) Principal veins of the arm, including major antecubital veins subject to venipuncture. (B) Forearm, wrist, and hand veins subject to venipuncture. (Reprinted with permission from McCall R. Phlebotomy Essentials. Baltimore: Lippincott Williams & Wilkins, 2003.)

Selection of the Venipuncture Site

While some veins are visible, the best choice for venipuncture is found by touch. Use the tip of the index finger to **palpate** (feel) veins to determine their suitability. Palpating helps locate veins and determine their size, depth, and direction. If no suitable antecubital vein can be found, release the tourniquet and repeat the procedure to this point on the other arm.

If no suitable antecubital vein is found in either arm, check hand veins and finally wrist veins. Massaging the arm from wrist to elbow increases blood flow and makes veins more palpable. Warming the site with a warm towel can produce the same effect.

The complete procedure for performing a venipuncture is outlined in Procedure 44-1.

When a blood sample cannot be obtained, you may have to change the position of the needle. FIGURE 44-14 shows proper and improper needle positions. Rotate the needle half a turn; the bevel of the needle may be against the wall of the vein. If the needle has not penetrated the vein, slowly advance it farther into the vein. If the needle has penetrated too far into the

vein, pull it back a little. The tube may not have sufficient vacuum; try another tube before withdrawing the needle.

Never attempt a venipuncture more than twice. If a blood specimen cannot be obtained in two tries, do not try a third time. Have another person attempt the draw or do a microcollection (skin puncture) if possible. Box 44-3 lists some common errors in venipuncture that you need to guard against.

Complications of Venipuncture

The most common complication of venipuncture is **hematoma** formation caused by blood leaking into the tissues during or after venipuncture. Hematomas are painful, cause unsightly bruising, and can cause compression injuries to nerves. Box 44-2 describes situations that may trigger hematoma formation. If a hematoma begins to form during the venipuncture, release the tourniquet immediately, withdraw the needle, and hold pressure on the site for at least 2 minutes. Cold compresses reduce pain and swelling.

FIGURE 44-13.   Tourniquet application. (A) Proper tourniquet placement with tension applied. (B) Both tourniquet sides grasped between thumb and forefinger of the right hand. (C) Left side of tourniquet crossed over the right side with both sides held between the thumb and index finger of the left hand. (D) Left end of tourniquet tucked under right side, forming loop. (E) Properly tied tourniquet. (Reprinted with permission from McCall R. Phlebotomy Essentials. Baltimore: Lippincott Williams & Wilkins, 2003.)

Accidental puncture of an artery is recognized by the blood's bright red color and the pulsing of the specimen into the tube. In this case, it is important to hold pressure over the site for a full 5 minutes after the needle is removed.

Aseptic techniques used to prevent infection of the venipuncture site include the following:

- Not touching the site after cleaning
- Removing the needle cap at the last possible minute prior to venipuncture
- Not opening bandages ahead of time

Permanent nerve damage may result from poor site selection, movement of the patient during needle insertion, inserting the needle too deeply or quickly, or excessive blind probing.

PERFORMING A SKIN PUNCTURE

Adult skin punctures are performed when no veins are accessible, to save veins for procedures such as chemotherapy, and for point-of-care testing. Technology now allows some tests to be performed on very small blood samples, but some results are more accurate on venipuncture specimens than on capillary specimens. Tests that cannot be performed on skin puncture specimens include most erythrocyte sedimentation rate methods, coagulation studies on plasma, cultures, and tests that require large blood volumes.

The skin puncture is the preferred method to obtain blood from infants and children. Venipuncture on infants and children may damage veins and surrounding tissues. Restraining the infant or child may cause injury.

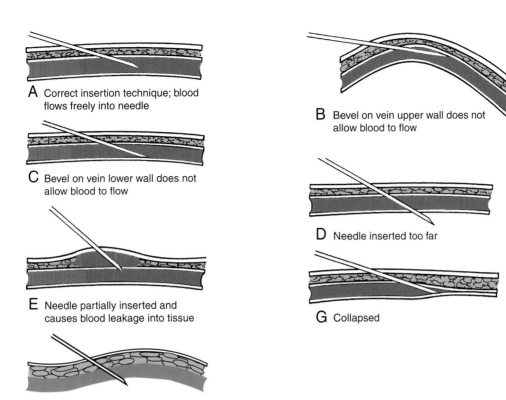

A Correct insertion technique; blood flows freely into needle

B Bevel on vein upper wall does not allow blood to flow

C Bevel on vein lower wall does not allow blood to flow

D Needle inserted too far

E Needle partially inserted and causes blood leakage into tissue

G Collapsed

F When a vein rolls, the needle may slip to the side of the vein without penetrating it

FIGURE 44-14. Proper and improper needle positioning. (A) Needle correctly positioned in a vein; blood flows freely into the needle. (B) Bevel on the upper wall of the vein prevents blood flow. (C) Bevel on the lower wall of the vein prevents blood flow. (D) Needle inserted too deep runs through the vein. (E) Partially inserted needle causes blood to leak into tissue. (F) Needle slipped beside the vein, not into it; occurs when a vein rolls to the side. (G) Collapsed vein prevents blood flow. (Reprinted with permission from McCall R. Phlebotomy Essentials. Baltimore: Lippincott Williams & Wilkins, 2003.)

The complete procedure for performing a skin puncture is outlined in Procedure 44-2.

Complications of Skin Puncture

Obtaining a specimen without clots is a challenge in microcollection. The body's clotting system is activated to stop the bleeding as soon as the skin is punctured. If an anticoagulated specimen is required, it should be drawn first to get an adequate volume before the blood begins to clot. Any other additive specimens are collected next, and clotted specimens are collected last. If the blood has begun to produce microscopic clots while you are filling the last tube, this is not a problem, because clotting is required in this tube. Box 44-4 lists some common sources of errors in microcollection that you need to guard against.

Box 44-2

SITUATIONS THAT MAY TRIGGER HEMATOMA FORMATION

1. The vein is fragile or too small for the needle.
2. The needle penetrates all the way through the vein.
3. The needle is only partly inserted into the vein.
4. Excessive or blind probing is used to find the vein.
5. The needle is removed while the tourniquet is still on.
6. Pressure is not adequately applied after venipuncture.

Reprinted with permission from McCall R. Phlebotomy Essentials. Baltimore: Lippincott Williams & Wilkins, 2003.

Checkpoint Question

4. What is the proper order of draw when using the evacuated tube system? Why is this important?

Box 44-3

SOURCES OF ERROR IN VENIPUNCTURE

Errors in Venipuncture Preparation
- Improper patient identification
- Failure to check patient adherence to dietary restrictions
- Failure to calm patient prior to blood collection
- Use of improper equipment and supplies
- Inappropriate method of blood collection

Errors in Venipuncture Procedure
- Failure to dry the site completely after cleansing with alcohol
- Inserting needle bevel side down
- Use of needle that is too small, causing hemolysis of specimen
- Venipuncture in an unacceptable area
- Prolonged tourniquet application
- Wrong order of tube draw
- Failure to mix blood collected in additive-containing tubes immediately
- Pulling back on syringe plunger too forcefully
- Failure to release tourniquet prior to needle withdrawal

Errors after Venipuncture Completion
- Failure to apply pressure immediately to venipuncture site
- Vigorous shaking of anticoagulated blood specimens
- Forcing blood through a syringe needle into tube
- Mislabeling of tubes
- Failure to label appropriate specimens with infectious disease precaution
- Failure to put date, time, and initials on requisition
- Slow transport of specimens to laboratory

Box 44-4

SOURCES OF ERROR IN SKIN PUNCTURE

- Misidentification of patient
- Puncturing wrong area of infant heel
- Puncturing bone in infant heel
- Puncturing fingers of infants
- Puncturing wrong area of adult finger
- Contaminating specimen with alcohol or Betadine
- Failure to discard first blood drop
- Excessive massaging of puncture site
- Collecting air bubbles in pH or blood gas specimen
- Hemolyzing specimen
- Failure to seal specimens adequately
- Failure to chill specimens requiring refrigeration
- Erroneous specimen labeling
- Failure to document skin puncture collection on the requisition or in the computer
- Failure to warm site
- Delaying specimen transport
- Bruising site as a result of excessive squeezing

Procedure 44-1

Obtaining a Blood Specimen by Venipuncture

Purpose: To obtain blood for diagnostic purposes and/or monitoring of prescribed treatment

Equipment: Needle, syringe, and test tubes or evacuated tubes; tourniquet; sterile gauze pads; bandages; needle and adaptor; sharps container; 70% alcohol pad or other antiseptic; permanent marker or pen; appropriate biohazard barriers (e.g., gloves, impervious gown, face shield)

Steps	Reason
1. Check the requisition slip to determine the tests ordered and specimen requirements.	This ensures proper specimen collection.
2. Wash your hands.	Handwashing aids infection control.
3. Assemble the equipment. Check the expiration date on the tubes.	Assembling the equipment ensures that everything you need is available. Expired tubes may no longer have a vacuum; additives may no longer be functional.
4. Greet and identify the patient. Explain the procedure. Ask for and answer any questions.	Identifying the patient prevents errors. Explaining the procedure helps ease anxiety and ensure compliance.
5. If a fasting specimen is required, ask the patient the last time he or she ate.	For fasting specimens, patient should not have eaten within at least 8 hours.
6. Put on nonsterile latex or vinyl gloves.	Standard precautions must be observed.
7. Break the seal of the needle cover and thread the sleeved needle into the adaptor, using the needle cover as a wrench. Tap the tubes that contain additives to ensure that the additive is dislodged from the stopper and wall of the tube. Insert the tube into the adaptor until the needle slightly enters the stopper. Do not push the top of the tube stopper beyond the indentation mark. If the tube retracts slightly, leave it in the retracted position. If using a syringe, tighten the needle on the hub and breathe the syringe.	This ensures proper needle placement and tube positioning and prevents loss of vacuum in the evacuated tubes or sticking of the plunger in the barrel of the syringe.
8. Instruct the patient to sit with a well-supported arm.	Veins in the antecubital fossa are most easily located when the arm is straight. The tourniquet makes the veins more prominent. Making a fist raises the vessels out of the underlying tissues and muscles.

(continued)

Obtaining a Blood Specimen by Venipuncture

Steps

Reason

A. Apply the tourniquet around the patient's arm 3–4 inches above the elbow.

Step 8A. Apply the tourniquet 3 to 4 inches above the elbow.

B. Apply the tourniquet snugly, but not too tightly.

Step 8B. Pull the tourniquet snugly around the arm.

(continued)

Obtaining a Blood Specimen by Venipuncture

Steps	Reason

C. Secure the tourniquet by using the half-bow knot.

Step 8C. Secure the tourniquet by using the half-bow.

D. Make sure the tails of the tourniquet extend upward to avoid contaminating the venipuncture site.

Step 8D. The tourniquet should extend upward.

(continued)

Procedure 44-1   *(continued)*

Obtaining a Blood Specimen by Venipuncture

Steps	Reason
E. Ask the patient to make a fist and hold it but not to pump the fist.	
9. Select a vein by palpating. Use your gloved index finger to trace the path of the vein and judge its depth.	The index finger is most sensitive for palpating.

Step 9. Trace the path of the vein.

Steps	Reason
10. Release the tourniquet after palpating the vein if it has been left on for more than 1 minute.	The tourniquet should not be left on for more than 1 minute at a time during the procedure.
11. Cleanse the venipuncture site with an alcohol pad, starting in the center of puncture site and working outward in a circular motion. Allow the site to dry or dry the site with sterile gauze. Do not touch the area after cleansing.	The circular motion helps avoid recontamination of the area. Puncturing a wet area stings and can cause hemolysis of the sample.
12. If blood being drawn for culture will be used in diagnosing a septic condition, make sure the specimen is sterile. To do this, apply alcohol to the area for 2 full minutes. Then apply a 2% iodine solution in ever-widening circles. Never move the wipes back over areas that have been cleaned; use a new wipe for each sweep across the area.	Ensuring sterility of the specimen will aid accurate diagnosis.
13. Reapply the tourniquet if it was removed after palpation. Ask patient to make a fist.	Tourniquet time greater than 1 minute may alter findings.

(continued)

Procedure 44-1   (continued)

Obtaining a Blood Specimen by Venipuncture

Steps	Reason
14. Remove the needle cover. Hold the syringe or assembly in your dominant hand, thumb on top of the adaptor and fingers under it. Grasp the patient's arm with the other hand, using your thumb to draw the skin taut over the site. This anchors the vein about 1–2 inches below the puncture site and helps keep it in place during needle insertion.	Anchoring the vein allows for easier needle penetration and less pain.
15. With the bevel up, line up the needle with the vein approximately one-quarter to half an inch below the site where the vein is to be entered. At a 15–30° angle, rapidly and smoothly insert the needle through the skin. Remove your nondominant hand and slowly pull back the plunger of the syringe. Or place two fingers on the flanges of the adapter and with the thumb push the tube onto the needle inside the adapter. When blood begins to flow into the tube or syringe, release the tourniquet and allow the patient to release the fist. Allow the syringe or tube to fill to capacity. When blood flow ceases, remove the tube from the adapter by gripping the tube with your nondominant hand and place your thumb against the flange during removal. Twist and gently pull out the tube. Steady the needle in the vein. Try not to pull up or press down on the needle while it is in the vein. Insert any other necessary tubes into adapter and allow each to fill to capacity.	The sharpest point of the needle is inserted first. Proper tube filling ensures correct ratio of blood to additive. Removal of the tourniquet releases pressure on the vein and helps prevent blood from seeping into adjacent tissues and causing a hematoma.

Step 15. Insert the needle at a 15 to 30° angle.

(continued)

Procedure 44-1 *(continued)*

Obtaining a Blood Specimen by Venipuncture

Steps	Reason
16. Release the tourniquet and remove the tube from the adapter before removing the needle from the arm.	Removing the last tube from the adapter before removing the needle from the vein prevents any excess blood from dripping from the tip of the needle onto the patient. Pressure decreases the amount of blood escaping into the tissues.

A. Place a sterile gauze pad over the puncture site at the time of needle withdrawal. Do not apply any pressure to the site until the needle is completely removed.

Step 16A. Place a sterile gauze pad over the site.

B. After the needle is removed, apply pressure or have the patient apply direct pressure for 3–5 minutes. Do not bend the arm at the elbow.

Bending the arm increases the chance of blood seeping into the subcutaneous tissues.

Step 16B. Apply pressure for 3 to 5 minutes

(continued)

Procedure 44-1 *(continued)*

Obtaining a Blood Specimen by Venipuncture

Steps	Reason
17. Transfer the blood from a syringe into the tubes in the proper order of draw via the transfer device and allow the vacuum to fill the tubes. Do not hold the tube while using the transfer device; place it in a tube rack and carefully insert the device through the stopper. If the vacuum tubes contain an anticoagulant, they must be mixed immediately by gently inverting the tube 8–10 times. Do not shake the tube. Label the tubes with the proper information.	Mixing anticoagulated tubes prevents clotting of blood. Proper labeling of blood specimens avoids mixup of samples.
18. Check the puncture site for bleeding. Apply a dressing, a clean 2 × 2 gauze pad folded in quarters held in place by an adhesive bandage or 3-inch strip of tape.	
19. Thank the patient. Instruct the patient to leave the bandage in place at least 15 minutes and not to carry a heavy object (such as a purse) or lift heavy objects with that arm for 1 hour.	Courtesy helps the patient have a positive attitude about the procedure and the physician's office.
20. Properly care for or dispose of all equipment and supplies. Clean the work area. Remove gloves and wash your hands.	Standard precautions must be followed throughout the procedure to prevent the spread of microorganisms.

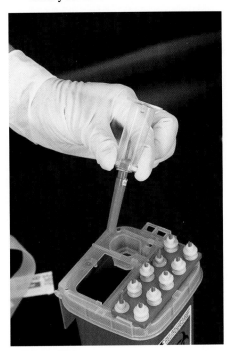

Step 20. Properly care for or dispose of all supplies.

(continued)

Procedure 44-1   (continued)

Obtaining a Blood Specimen by Venipuncture

Steps	Reason
21. Test, transfer, or store the blood specimen according to the medical office policy.	
22. Record the procedure.	Procedures are considered not performed if they are not recorded.

Charting Example

05/31/2005 10:00 A.M. OP venipuncture for platelet count, dx code ###.## per Dr. Jacobs. _____
J. Simpson, RMA

Procedure 44-2

Obtaining a Blood Specimen by Skin Puncture

Purpose:	To obtain blood for diagnostic purposes and/or monitoring of prescribed treatment
Equipment:	Sterile disposable lancet or automated skin puncture device, 70% alcohol or other antiseptic, sterile gauze pads, microcollection tubes or containers, heel-warming device if needed, appropriate biohazard barriers (e.g., gloves, impervious gown, face shield)

Steps	Reason
1. Check the requisition slip to determine the tests ordered and specimen requirements.	This ensures proper specimen collection.
2. Wash your hands.	Handwashing aids infection control.
3. Assemble the equipment.	Having the equipment ready will speed collection so the blood does not clot before the entire specimen has been collected.
4. Greet and identify the patient. Explain the procedure. Ask for and answer any questions.	Identifying the patient prevents errors. Explaining the procedure helps ease anxiety and ensure compliance.
5. Put on gloves.	Standard precautions must be observed.

(continued)

Obtaining a Blood Specimen by Skin Puncture

Steps

6. Select the puncture site (the lateral portion of the tip of the middle or ring finger of the nondominant hand, lateral curved surface of the heel, or the great toe of an infant). The puncture should be made in the fleshy central portion of the second or third finger, slightly to the side of center, and perpendicular to the grooves of the fingerprint. Perform heel puncture only on the plantar surface of the heel, medial to an imaginary line extending from the middle of the great toe to the heel, and lateral to an imaginary line drawn from between the fourth and fifth toes to the heel. Use the appropriate puncture device for the site selected.

Reason

The ring and middle fingers are less calloused than the forefinger. The lateral part of the tip is the least sensitive part of the finger. A puncture made across the fingerprints will produce a large, round drop of blood. In an infant skin puncture, the area and the depth designated reduces the risk of puncturing the bone.

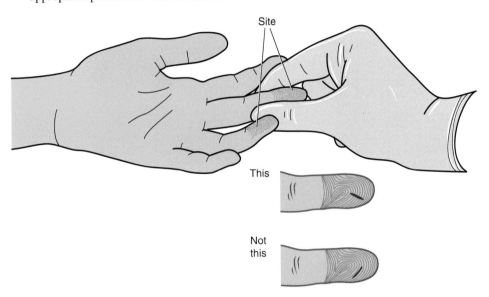

Step 6. Recommended site and direction of finger puncture. (Reprinted with permission from McCall R: Phlebotomy Essentials. Baltimore: Lippincott Williams & Wilkins, 2003)

Step 6. Acceptable areas for heel punctures on newborns.

(continued)

Procedure 44-2   *(continued)*

Obtaining a Blood Specimen by Skin Puncture

Steps	Reason
7. Make sure the site chosen is warm and not cyanotic or edematous. Gently massage the finger from the base to the tip.	Massaging the area increases the blood flow. Good circulation at the chosen site yields a better blood sample for analysis.
8. Grasp the finger firmly between your nondominant index finger and thumb, or grasp the infant's heel firmly with your index finger wrapped around the foot and your thumb wrapped around the ankle. Cleanse the selected area with 70% isopropyl alcohol and wipe dry with a sterile gauze pad or allow to air dry.	The area must be dry to eliminate alcohol residue, which can cause the patient discomfort and interfere with test results. Maintaining your hold at the site prevents the patient from contaminating the cleansed puncture area and allows you to have control of the puncture site.

A   B

Step 8. Grasp the finger firmly. Cleanse the site with alcohol and dry with a sterile gauze pad.

(continued)

Procedure 44-2 *(continued)*

Obtaining a Blood Specimen by Skin Puncture

Steps	Reason
9. Hold the patient's finger or heel firmly and make a swift, firm puncture. Perform the puncture perpendicular to the whorls of the fingerprint or footprint. Dispose of the used puncture device in a sharps container.	The proper puncture will allow the blood to form a rounded drop that can be easily collected.
A. Wipe away the first drop of blood with a sterile dry gauze.	The first discarded drop may be contaminated with tissue fluid or alcohol residue.

Step 9A. Wipe away the first drop of blood.

B. Apply pressure toward the site but do not milk the site.	Milking the site will dilute the specimen with tissue fluid.
10. Collect the specimen in the chosen container or slide. Touch only the tip of the collection device to the drop of blood. Blood flow is encouraged if the puncture site is held downward and gentle pressure is applied near the site. Cap microcollection tubes with the caps provided and mix the additives by gently tilting or inverting the tubes 8–10 times.	Scraping the collection device on the skin activates platelets and may cause hemolysis. Mixing the specimens prevents clotting. Touching the tube to the site may cause contamination.

Step 10. Touch only the tip of the collection tube to the drop of blood.

(continued)

Procedure 44-2   *(continued)*

Obtaining a Blood Specimen by Skin Puncture

Steps	Reason
11. When collection is complete, apply clean gauze to the site with pressure. Hold pressure or have the patient hold pressure until bleeding stops. Label the containers with the proper information. Do not apply a dressing to a skin puncture of an infant under 2 years of age. Never release a patient until the bleeding has stopped.	Proper labeling prevents mixup of specimens. Younger children may develop a skin irritation from the adhesive bandage. Also, a young child may put the bandage in the mouth and choke.

Step 11. Apply pressure with clean gauze.

Steps	Reason
12. Thank the patient. Instruct the patient to leave the bandage in place at least 15 minutes.	Courtesy helps the patient have a positive attitude about the procedure and the physician's office.
13. Properly care for or dispose of equipment and supplies. Clean the work area. Remove gloves and wash your hands.	Standard precautions must be followed throughout the procedure.
14. Test, transfer, or store the specimen according to the medical office policy.	
15. Record the procedure.	Procedures are considered not to have been done if they are not recorded.

Note: Several precautions should be observed to produce the most accurate specimen. The greatest concern with microcollection specimens is hemolysis, the rupture of erythrocytes with the release of hemoglobin. Do not squeeze or milk the heel or finger to increase blood flow. Never scrape the microcollection device on the skin; allow the container to touch only the drop of blood. Also, be careful to avoid additional sources of errors, which are listed in Box 26-4.

Charting Example

07/12/2005 9:00 A.M. OP fingerstick from prothrombin time dx ###.## per Dr. Robins. _____
S. Smith, CMA

CHAPTER SUMMARY

You must always have a professional attitude and be sympathetic to the fears and anxieties of the patient in all areas of patient care. For many patients, venipuncture is particularly frightening. Demonstrate compassion and understanding to allay their fears. Your skill and knowledge, coupled with a caring approach, will help ensure that the patient's experience in phlebotomy is not unpleasant.

The quality of the test result is only as good as the quality of the specimen. Medical assistants are responsible for collecting specimens properly and testing them accurately. The office laboratory can provide a challenge and opportunity to work with the physician in improving and promoting the health of the patient.

Critical Thinking Challenges

1. Your patient complains of serious pain when you insert the needle into the vein. Explain the steps you will take to make the patient more comfortable.

2. How can you help ease patient anxiety about venipuncture? Explain exactly what steps you will take.

3. Your patient asks you how long you have been drawing blood and whether you are "good." How do you respond? Justify your response.

Answers to Checkpoint Questions

1. Disinfectants are used to kill bacteria on equipment and surfaces. Antiseptics are safe for people and are used to clean the skin before skin puncture or venipuncture.

2. Common additives include anticoagulants (prevent the blood from coagulating, or clotting); clot activators (enhance coagulation); and thixotropic gel separator (after centrifugation forms a physical barrier between the cellular portion of a specimen and the serum or plasma portion).

3. You should label the blood sample with the patient's first and last names, an identification number, the date and time, and your initials to verify who drew the sample.

4. When using the evacuated tube system, the proper order of draw is blood culture tubes, plain red, light blue, red/gray and gold, green, lavender, gray. It is important to follow the correct order of draw to avoid contamination between additives.

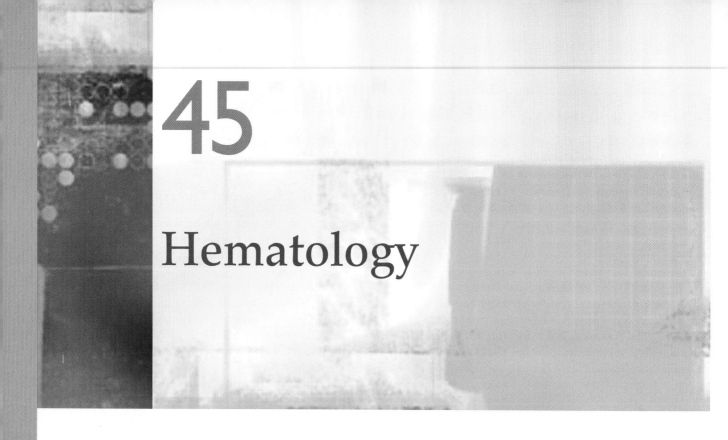

45

Hematology

CHAPTER OUTLINE

FORMATION OF BLOOD CELLS

HEMATOLOGICAL TESTING

COMPLETE BLOOD COUNT
   White Blood Cell Count and
      Differential
   Red Blood Cell Count
   Hemoglobin

Hematocrit
Mean Cell Volume
Mean Cell Hemoglobin and Mean
   Cell Hemoglobin Concentration
Platelet Count

ERYTHROCYTE
  SEDIMENTATION RATE

COAGULATION TESTS
   Prothrombin Time
   Partial Thromboplastin Time
   Bleeding Time

ROLE DELINEATION

CLINICAL: FUNDAMENTAL PRINCIPLES
- Apply principles of aseptic technique and infection control
- Comply with quality assurance practices

CLINICAL: DIAGNOSTIC ORDERS
- Collect and process specimens
- Perform diagnostic tests

CLINICAL: PATIENT CARE
- Adhere to established patient screening procedures

GENERAL: PROFESSIONALISM
- Display a professional manner and image
- Prioritize and perform multiple tasks

GENERAL: COMMUNICATION SKILLS
- Adapt communications to individual's ability to understand

GENERAL: LEGAL CONCEPTS
- Perform within legal and ethical boundaries
- Document accurately

CHAPTER COMPETENCIES

LEARNING OBJECTIVES

Upon successfully completing this chapter, you will be able to:

1. Spell and define the key terms.
2. List the parameters measured in the complete blood count and their normal ranges.
3. State the conditions associated with selected abnormal complete blood count findings.
4. Explain the functions of the three types of blood cells.
5. Describe the purpose of testing for the erythrocyte sedimentation rate.
6. List the leukocytes seen normally in the blood and their functions.
7. Explain the hemostatic mechanism of the body.
8. List and describe the tests that measure the body's ability to form a fibrin clot.
9. Explain how to determine the prothrombin time and partial thromboplastin time.

PERFORMANCE OBJECTIVES

Upon successfully completing this chapter, you will be able to:

1. Use a Unopette system for diluting blood specimens (Procedure 45-1).
2. Perform a manual white blood cell count (Procedure 45-2).
3. Make a peripheral blood smear (Procedure 45-3).
4. Stain a peripheral blood smear (Procedure 45-4).
5. Determine a white blood cell differential (Procedure 45-5).
6. Perform a red blood cell count (Procedure 45-6).
7. Perform a hemoglobin determination (Procedure 45-7).
8. Perform a microhematocrit determination (Procedure 45-8).
9. Determine a Wintrobe erythrocyte sedimentation rate (Procedure 45-9).
10. Determine a bleeding time (Procedure 45-10).

KEY TERMS

anisocytosis	folate	hemolytic anemia	sickle cell anemia
enzyme	granulocytes	hemostasis	thrombocytes
erythrocyte	hematocytometer	leukocytes	thromboplastin
erythropoietin	(hemocytometer)	morphology	
femtoliter	hematopoiesis	poikilocytosis	

THE HEMATOLOGY LABORATORY analyzes the blood cells, their quantities, and their characteristics for diagnosis and management of many conditions. Anemias, leukemias, and infections are some of the more common disorders detected and managed by hematological testing. In addition, hematology includes the study of **hemostasis**, or the ability of the patient to maintain blood in a fluid state within the vessels. Thus, the hematology laboratory is helpful in evaluating individuals who have difficulty forming a clot and those who form clots spontaneously within their blood vessels.

FORMATION OF BLOOD CELLS

Blood is made up of two parts, fluid (plasma) and three general types of cells, **erythrocytes** (red blood cells, or RBCs), **leukocytes** (white blood cells, or WBCs), and **thrombocytes** (platelets) (FIG. 45-1).

Blood cells are formed in the bone marrow. The long bones, skull, pelvis, and sternum manufacture most of these cells. Other blood cell–making sites are the liver and spleen. The yolk sac of the developing fetus also produces blood cells. (The yolk sac is the structure that nourishes the embryo until the seventh week, when the placenta takes over.)

Hematopoiesis (blood cell production) starts with very young, immature cells within the marrow that eventually divide and differentiate (acquire distinct or individual characteristics and mature). These cells become erythrocytes, leukocytes, and thrombocytes according to the body's needs. Each type of cell has a particular function, discussed later in this chapter. Hematopoiesis is influenced by hormones and requires adequate nutrients, such as iron, to produce functional cells. Once these cells have reached maturity, they are released from the bone marrow and travel into the bloodstream.

Checkpoint Question

1. What is hematopoiesis, and how is it influenced?

HEMATOLOGICAL TESTING

While hematological testing is often used to diagnose and manage disease of the blood cells and coagulation proteins, it is also useful in the study of other diseases, such as metabolic, nutritional, immunological, and neoplastic disorders. Common hematological tests include the complete

FIGURE 45-1. (A) A blood smear. (B) RBCs (large, round cells) and platelets (stained purple). (C) Segmented neutrophil. (D) Neutrophil band. (E) Lymphocyte. (F) Monocyte. (G) Eosinophil. (H) Basophil.

blood count (CBC), erythrocyte sedimentation rate (ESR or sed rate), and coagulation tests. CLIA (Clinical Laboratory Improvement Amendments) regulations limit the types of hematology testing medical assistants can perform. The list of tests medical assistants can perform, updated regularly by Centers for Medicare & Medicaid Services (CMS), includes these items:

- Erythrocyte sedimentation rate (not automated)
- Hematocrit (all spun microhematocrit procedures)
- Hemoglobin (selected methods)
- Prothrombin time (selected methods)

COMPLETE BLOOD COUNT

The CBC, or hemogram, is one of the most frequently ordered tests in the laboratory. It consists of a number of parameters, including these:

- WBC count and differential
- RBC count
- Hemoglobin (Hgb) determination
- Hematocrit (Hct) determination

- Mean cell volume (MCV)
- Mean corpuscular hemoglobin (MCH)
- Mean corpuscular hemoglobin concentration (MCHC)
- Platelet count

A dilution of whole blood may be prepared from either a free-flowing finger puncture (see Chapter 44) or from a specimen anticoagulated with ethylenediaminetetraacetic acid (EDTA) (Procedure 45-1). Each kind of blood cell (white, red, and platelets) can be counted using a counting chamber called a **hematocytometer** or a **hemocytometer** (FIG. 45-2). The dilution and diluting fluid used is different for each of the counts. Manual cell counts have been largely replaced by automated cell counters (FIG. 45-3, Box 45-1). Many models are available to suit the diverse needs of large reference laboratories and smaller physician office laboratories.

White Blood Cell Count and Differential

WBCs (leukocytes) provide the main line of defense against foreign invaders such as bacteria and viruses. Some types circulate in the peripheral blood, and others migrate into tis-

FIGURE 45-2. The Neubauer hemacytometer.

sues and cavities to perform their functions. The normal range for a WBC count is 4300 to 10,800/mm³. Test results may depend on the method used for testing, and normal reference intervals vary among regions and populations. A patient's WBC count can be determined by use of the hematocytometer counting chamber (Procedure 45-2) or an automated cell counter.

Diminished numbers of leukocytes (leukopenia) can result from several factors:

- Chemical toxicity
- Nutritional deficiency
- Chronic or overwhelming infection
- Certain malignancies

FIGURE 45-3. Coulter Ac-T diff2 Hematology Analyzer. (Courtesy of Beckman-Coulter, Fullerton, CA.)

Box 45-1

AUTOMATED BLOOD CELL COUNTERS

A number of biotechnology companies have instruments that can count and size blood cells. Beckman Coulter and Bayer are two of these companies. Although each has its own specific method, the main operating principles are similar.

A portion of whole blood (anticoagulated with EDTA) is taken in and diluted. These dilutions are moved into counting chambers, where they are drawn through tiny holes (apertures). As the cells pass through the holes, an electrical current, a light beam, or a laser beam is interrupted. The instrument registers the interruption as a cell. It can tell the size of the cell by the length of time the beam is interrupted or the amount of light scatter.

These instruments have become so sophisticated that a white blood cell differential now can be reported accurately. Hemoglobin is also measured, along with other parameters, such as mean corpuscular hemoglobin, adding to the diagnostic value of the complete blood count.

Patients with pronounced leukopenia may be vulnerable to infections. Leukocytosis (increased numbers of WBCs) can stem from many sources:

- Infection
- Inflammatory condition
- Certain drugs
- Injury to tissue
- Certain malignancies

The WBC differential determines the amounts of various WBC types in the peripheral blood. These types include the following:

- Neutrophils (Fig. 45-1, *C* and *D*)
- Lymphocytes (Fig. 45-1*E*)
- Monocytes (Fig. 45-1*F*)
- Eosinophils (Fig. 45-1*G*)
- Basophils (Fig. 45-1*H*)

Because all of these types of leukocytes are colorless, a drop of blood is smeared on a glass slide and then stained so that they can be seen with a microscope. Once the peripheral blood is stained, 100 WBCs are counted, tallied according to type, and reported as percentages (Procedures 45-3 to 45-5). These cell types fall into three general categories: **granulocytes** (subdivided into neutrophils, eosinophils and basophils, so called because of granules in their cytoplasm that have distinctive staining characteristics) **lymphocytes**, and

monocytes. Each of the three has a distinct purpose in fighting infection.

Checkpoint Question

2. What is leukopenia, and what are four conditions that may cause it?

Neutrophils

Neutrophils—also called polymorphonuclear neutrophils, polys, segmented neutrophils, or segs—are the most abundant leukocytes and are the main granulocyte. Following their release from the bone marrow, they circulate in the blood for about 7 hours. They then move into the tissues, where they perform their function. Neutrophils defend against foreign invaders by phagocytizing them. The invaders are destroyed inside the cells by digestive **enzymes** in the granules. (Enzymes are substances that speed reactions.) These digestive enzymes eventually kill the neutrophil too. The normal percentage of neutrophils is 50% to 70%; their numbers increase in patients with bacterial infections.

When stained, the neutrophil has a light pink cytoplasm. This is due to the many small granules it contains. Its dark purple nucleus is segmented, and the typical number of lobes is 2 to 5. A hypersegmented neutrophil is one that has more than five lobes or segments. This can indicate a vitamin B_{12}, or **folate**, deficiency. (Folate, a salt of folic acid, is an essential nutrient.) A band (or stab) is a younger, less mature version of the neutrophil. The band's appearance is the same as that of the more mature counterpart, but its nucleus is not segmented. The percentage of bands is 0% to 5%. Higher percentages of bands may indicate any of various acute conditions that necessitate immediate attention. In combination with leukocytosis, this is called a left shift.

Checkpoint Question

3. What is the function of neutrophils?

Lymphocytes

Lymphocytes (lymphs) are the second most numerous WBC. The main function of lymphocytes is to recognize that a particular cell or particle is foreign to the body and to make antibodies specific to its destruction. The antibodies coat this foreign mass, resulting in one of two possible outcomes: the phagocytic system is activated to destroy the pathogen, or the complement system (a series of chemicals in the blood) is activated to destroy the cellular invaders by puncturing holes in their membranes. The normal percentage of lymphocytes is 20% to 35%. Higher numbers, especially of atypical ones, can signal a viral infection such as infectious mononucleosis. The life span of the lymphocyte is generally 3 to 4 days, longer than that of the neu-

trophil. However, some have much longer lives, spanning into years or even decades.

The lymphocyte is the smallest of the leukocytes. When stained, it has a small, round dark purple nucleus. The surrounding cytoplasm is scant and sky blue. Atypical lymphs are larger, with more cytoplasm that is either darker or lighter.

Monocytes

Monocytes (or monos) are the third most abundant leukocytes. Like neutrophils, monocytes phagocytize foreign material. They also aid the lymphocyte in providing the humoral response (destruction of foreign particles by antibodies). Monocytes stay in the bloodstream for about 3 days and then move into tissues.

The shape of the monocyte nucleus varies but tends to be indented or horseshoe-shaped. It is much larger than the lymphocyte and closer in size to the neutrophil. When stained, the monocyte's cytoplasm is gray blue and has a ground-glass appearance. The normal percentage of monocytes is 3% to 8%. Monocytosis (increase in monocytes) occurs with inflammatory responses and certain bacterial infections, such as syphilis and tuberculosis. Monocytopenia may occur after administration of certain drugs or an overwhelming infection.

Eosinophils

Eosinophils (or eos) are fourth in abundance. Their function is not completely understood. The normal percentage of eosinophils is 0% to 6%. They are higher in allergic reactions and some infections, especially parasitic. The eosinophil has a bilobed nucleus with large red granules in the cytoplasm.

Basophils

Basophils (or basos) are the least numerous, fewer than 1% of circulating WBCs. The nucleus is either bilobed or trilobed, and on staining, very large dark blue-purple granules are seen in the cytoplasm. Basophils appear to be a factor in allergic asthma, in contact allergies, and in hypothyroidism and chronic myeloid leukemia.

Checkpoint Question

4. Elevated eosinophils and basophils are both seen with what condition?

Red Blood Cell Count

RBCs (erythrocytes) transport gases (mainly oxygen and carbon dioxide) between the lungs and the tissues. Their special structure, a biconcave disk containing hemoglobin, lets them readily exchange gases in the tissues and lung fields. As blood moves through the capillary bed of the lungs, RBCs release carbon dioxide that was picked up at the tissues and then binds oxygen. As the blood leaves the lungs and circulates to the organs, oxygen is released from the RBCs into the tissues. At the same time, carbon dioxide (the byproduct of metabolism) diffuses into the blood and is brought back to the lungs to be exhaled.

RBCs are made in the bone marrow along with all other blood cells. Their production is influenced by the hormone **erythropoietin**, which is released from the kidneys. When tissue hypoxia is detected, this hormone migrates to the marrow to increase RBC production (erythropoiesis), which corrects the anemia by releasing more RBCs into the circulation. Other factors can also influence the quality and quantity of erythropoiesis. For example, vitamin B_{12} and folic acid are required for the cells to mature properly. The globin molecule needs iron to make functional hemoglobin. Initially, erythrocytes have a nucleus, but as they mature, the nucleus is pushed out and the color of their cytoplasm changes from blue to red. The mature RBC is a pale red biconcave disk that can squeeze through very small capillaries. The average RBC lives about 120 days.

Measurements of RBCs and associated parameters provide a useful guide for detecting anemia, which can be caused by decreased erythrocyte production (as in iron deficiency), increased RBC destruction (as in hemolytic anemia), or blood loss. The normal range of RBCs for men is 4.6 to 6.2 million/mm^3 and for women, 4.2 to 5.4 million/mm^3 (Procedure 45-6).

A WBC differential count with peripheral blood includes a report on RBC **morphology** or appearance. This report contains comments on the variation in size (**anisocytosis**) and shape (**poikilocytosis**) of the RBCs. TABLE 45-1

PATIENT EDUCATION

Iron Deficiency Anemia

Patients who have iron deficiency anemia should be taught proper dietary management. They should be instructed to eat foods high in iron, such as liver, oysters, kidney beans, lean meats, turnips, egg yolks, whole wheat bread, carrots, raisins, and dark greens. A vitamin supplement with iron can be added to the diet. Patients should be warned that iron supplements can cause constipation and dark stools.

describes some common erythrocyte abnormalities and their associated conditions.

Hemoglobin

Hemoglobin is the functioning unit of the red blood cell. Each hemoglobin molecule contains four protein chains called globins. Alpha and beta are the most common types of globin chains, with some gamma (fetal) in newborns. Defects in the globin chains result in abnormal hemoglobins such as S (sickle) found in persons having **sickle cell anemia** or carrying the sickle trait. In the folds of each globin is a heme unit that contains one iron molecule; the iron can reversibly bind gases such oxygen and carbon dioxide. The iron also gives RBCs their distinctive red color. There are millions of hemoglobin molecules in each RBC. The normal

Table 45-1   ERYTHROCYTE ABNORMALITIES

Abnormality	Associated Conditions
Hypochromasia—diminished hemoglobin in RBCs; appear paler with more area of central pallor.	Anemias (especially iron deficiency), **thalassemia** (a hemolytic anemia)
Hyperchromasia—increased hemoglobin in RBCs; appear to have less or no area of central pallor.	**Megaloblastic anemia** (characterized by large, dysfunctional RBCs), hereditary **spherocytosis** (condition in which nearly all the RBCs are spherocytes)
Polychromasia—some RBCs have a blue color.	Hemolysis, acute blood loss
Microcytosis—RBCs are smaller than usual.	Iron deficiency anemia, thalassemia
Macrocytosis—RBCs are larger than normal.	B_{12} and folate deficiencies, megaloblastic anemias
Elliptocytes/ovalocytes—RBCs are distinctly oval in shape.	Hereditary **elliptocytosis**, iron deficiency anemia, **myelofibrosis** (disorder in which bone marrow tissue develops in abnormal sites), sickle **cell anemia** (hereditary anemia characterized by the presence of sickle-shaped RBCs)
Target cells—RBCs resemble a target with light and dark rings.	Liver impairment, anemias (especially thalassemia), **hemoglobin C disease** (genetic blood disorder)
Schistocytes—RBCs are fragmented.	Hemolysis, burns, **intravascular coagulation** (clot formation within the vessels)
Spherocytes—RBCs show no area of central pallor.	Hereditary spherocytosis, hemolytic anemias, burns
Burr cells—RBCs have small, regular spicules (sharp points).	Artifact as blood dries, **hyperosmolarity** (a condition of increased numbers of dissolved substances in the plasma)

FIGURE 45-4.   HemoCue Plasma/Low Hemoglobin Analyzer. (Courtesy of HemoCue, Mission Viejo, CA.)

range for hemoglobin is 13 to 18 g/dL (or g/100 mL) in men and 12 to 16 g/dL in women. Anemia is detected with a hemoglobin measurement, which is a direct indicator of the body's ability to oxygenate tissues. The manual method of determining hemoglobin measurement is described in Procedure 45-7. There are also point-of-care methods approved for use by medical assistants. An example is the HemoCue System (FIGURE 45-4).

Hematocrit

The hematocrit is the percentage of RBCs in whole blood. It is expressed as a percentage. For example, a hematocrit of 40% indicates that 40% of the total blood volume consists of RBCs. The remaining 60% is plasma, WBCs, and platelets.

To measure the hematocrit, the blood is centrifuged to pack the RBCs and the percentage is read. Automated instruments do not measure the hematocrit but rather calculate it from the RBC count and MCV. The purpose of measuring the hematocrit is to detect anemia. The normal range is 45% to 52% in men and 37% to 48% in women (Procedure 45-8).

Checkpoint Question

5. A patient has a hematocrit of 20%. What does this percentage signify?

Mean Cell Volume

Because RBCs vary in size, MCV measures the average size of RBCs. For example, a patient with a MCV of 85 **femtoliters** may have RBCs that range in size from 75 fL to 95

fL but that average 85 fL. The MCV can be an indicator of anemias such as those caused by the nutritional deficiencies that affect RBC production. The normal range for MCV is 80 to 95 fL.

Microcytosis (MCV below 80 fL) is most commonly caused by iron deficiency. This finding coupled with RBC count, hemoglobin, and hematocrit will indicate anemia and may lead to a diagnosis of iron deficiency anemia. Likewise, macrocytosis (MCV above 95 fL) may be caused by a deficiency of vitamin B_{12} or folic acid. These abnormalities can also result in anemia. Liver disorders sometimes raise the MCV.

Mean Cell Hemoglobin and Mean Cell Hemoglobin Concentration

MCH and MCHC indicate relative hemoglobin concentration in the blood. Both the MCH and MCHC are calculated. RBCs with inadequate amounts of hemoglobin are termed hypochromic. The MCH is derived from the ratio of hemoglobin to the number of RBCs in the specimen. The normal range for MCH is 27 to 31 picograms. An increase may be seen in macrocytic anemias, and a decrease is consistent with microcytic, hypochromic anemias.

The MCHC is derived from the ratio of hemoglobin to hematocrit. The normal range for MCHC is 32 to 36 g/dL. The MCHC is reduced in true hypochromic anemia and may be increased when spherocytes (RBCs with high hemoglobin content) are present.

Platelet Count

Platelets (thrombocytes), like other blood cells, are made in the bone marrow. However, they are not actually cells but cell fragments that adhere to damaged endothelium. Platelets are essential to hemostasis because they not only aid in sealing wounds and stopping bleeding until a clot can form but also help initiate the clotting factors to form the more stable fibrin clot.

The normal range for platelets is 200,000 to 400,000/mm³. Thrombocytopenia (decreased platelets) can be caused by a variety of conditions and may be associated with increased bleeding. The bleeding is usually from many small capillaries. The risk of bleeding increases as the platelet count decreases. Treatment requires a specific diagnosis of the cause of the thrombocytopenia, which may be anemia, infectious disease, drug, acute leukemia, radiation treatment, or chemotherapy. Thrombocytosis (increased platelets) is most often benign. It can be seen after splenectomy or during inflammatory disease. Marked thrombocytosis (above 1 million/mm³) may be associated with an increased clotting tendency or severe bleeding if the platelet function is impaired.

Platelets are much smaller than RBCs. They stain a light purplish blue, have an irregular shape, and contain visible granules but no nucleus.

ERYTHROCYTE SEDIMENTATION RATE

The ESR measures the rate in millimeters per hour at which RBCs settle out in a tube. Place anticoagulated blood in a calibrated glass column and allow to settle undisturbed for 1 hour. At the end of the hour the distance the RBCs have fallen is measured. Although there are several methods for determining the ESR, such as the Wintrobe and the Westergren methods, the principle remains the same. Procedure 45-9 describes the steps in a Wintrobe ESR. FIGURE 45-5 outlines the steps for the Westergren method.

The normal range for men is 0 to 10 mm/hour, and for women, 0 to 20 mm/hour. Elevations in ESR values are not specific for any disorder but indicate either inflammation or any other condition that causes increased or altered proteins in the blood (e.g., rheumatoid arthritis). The more rapidly the RBCs fall in the column, the greater the degree of inflammation. Physicians use this as a guideline when monitoring the course of inflammation in rheumatoid arthritis. The ESR can also be elevated with infection and pregnancy.

FIGURE 45-5. Westergren Dispette System for ESR determination. *Left:* After mixing four parts EDTA-anticoagulated whole blood with one part 0.85% saline, mixture is poured into a vial. *Center:* Dispette is placed in vial using a twisting motion until blood reaches bottom of safety autozeroing plug. *Right:* Vial and Dispette are placed upright in a special rack for 60 minutes before reading the ESR. (Courtesy of Ulster Scientific, Highland, NY.)

COAGULATION TESTS

Coagulation tests measure the ability of whole blood to form a clot. Coagulation proteins in the blood act in sequential order when stimulated by cell membrane disruptions (cuts, tears, or other injuries) to form a clot. This clot stabilizes the platelet plug, which is the first link in the chain of events that occur on injury. Both the platelet plug and the fibrin clot are needed for continued hemostasis. When vascular damage occurs, the following sequence of events occurs:

1. *Vasoconstriction.* The vein constricts to reduce blood loss.
2. *Platelet plug formation.* The platelets adhere to the wound and form a plug, temporarily slowing or stopping the blood flow.
3. *Fibrin clot formation.* When activated, the clotting factors form an insoluble clot at the wound site. (The two most common tests for determining how well a fibrin clot can form are prothrombin time and partial thromboplastin time, discussed in the next sections.)
4. *Clot lysis and vascular repair.* Another set of proteins slowly dissolves the fibrin clot as the surrounding endothelial tissue of the blood vessel wall replicates to repair the damage.

Prothrombin Time

The prothrombin time (PT) is a test in which calcium and **thromboplastin** (a complex substance that starts the clotting process) are added to the patient's plasma and the clotting time observed. The normal range is 12 to 15 seconds, but each laboratory establishes its own range. Among the factors that may prolong a patient's PT are liver disease, vitamin K deficiency, and coumarin (oral anticoagulant) therapy.

The PT is the primary monitor of coumarin anticoagulant therapy. The PT is reported along with its corresponding International Normalized Ratio (INR) to standardize results. The INR is a mathematical calculation that compares the patient's PT to a reference standard. Several point-of-care instruments allow medical assistants to determine prothrombin time and INR in the office (FIG. 45-6).

Partial Thromboplastin Time

The partial thromboplastin time (PTT) is a two-stage test in which first partially activated thromboplastin is incubated with the patient's plasma and then calcium is added. The clotting time is then determined. The normal range is 32 to 51 seconds, but each laboratory establishes its own range, so there may be a slight variation. PTT may be prolonged in certain factor deficiencies, especially those that cause hemophilia. Heparin (anticoagulant) therapy also prolongs the PTT. Thus, it is used to monitor dosages.

FIGURE 45-6.   The Hemochron Jr. signature analyzer for determination of prothrombin times. (Courtesy of ITC, Edison, NJ.)

Bleeding Time

The bleeding time test determines the time required for blood to stop flowing from a very small wound. An incision is made on the inside of the forearm with an automated cutting device, such as a Simplate, to a depth of 1 mm. Normal bleeding times range from 2 to 6 minutes (Procedure 45-10).

Although it is a nonspecific test, prolonged bleeding times can occur with low platelet numbers or impaired platelet function. Ingestion of aspirin or other anti-inflammatory medication can also inhibit platelet function. Long bleeding time may indicate the use of medication or a disease state such as uremic syndrome. Bleeding times are often determined before surgery when the patient's personal or family history includes increased bruising or bleeding. A laboratory

WHAT IF

Your patient is taking coumarin and does not return for scheduled prothrombin tests? What should you do?

Let the physician know. The physician will determine whether a refill prescription should be called in to the pharmacy. Document all phone conversations with the patient, including the date, time, and message. Also document the patient's responses, quoting him or her whenever possible. The patient should be informed of the dangers of self-dosing coumarin, such as excessive bleeding with overdose or clotting with underdose. Make sure the patient understands the purpose of the medication and why blood tests are so important. Determine why the patient is not coming in for blood work; the reason may be as simple as transportation. Many communities have visiting nurse associations or hospital outreach programs whose staff members will draw blood for patients in the home.

test screens for platelet function on an anticoagulated whole blood sample. This is decreasing the need for bleeding times.

 Checkpoint Question

6. What are the two most common tests used to determine how well a fibrin clot will form?

Procedure 45-1

Preparing a Whole Blood Dilution Using the Unopette System

Purpose: To prepare a dilution of whole blood for manual cell counts

Equipment: Unopette system, gauze

Steps	Reason
1. Wash your hands.	
2. Assemble the equipment.	
3. Using the shield on the capillary pipette, pierce the diaphragm in the neck of the reservoir, pushing the tip of the shield firmly through the diaphragm before removing it with a twisting motion. Fill the pipette with free-flowing whole blood obtained through skin puncture or from a properly obtained, well-mixed EDTA (lavender top) tube specimen. (See Chapter 44 for performing a skin puncture.)	

Step 3A. Puncture diaphragm. (Courtesy of Becton Dickinson Vacutainer Systems, Rutherford, NJ.)

Step 3B. Remove shield from pipette assembly with a twist. (Courtesy of Becton Dickinson Vacutainer Systems, Rutherford, NJ.)

(continued)

Procedure 45-1   *(continued)*

Preparing a Whole Blood Dilution Using the Unopette System

Steps	Reason

Step 3C. Draw sample into pipet from free-flowing skin puncture or tube. (Courtesy of Becton Dickinson Vacutainer Systems, Rutherford, NJ.)

Steps	Reason
4. If filling from a tube, place the tip of the Unopette just below the surface of the blood. Allow capillary action to fill the Unopette system completely.	The tube must be filled completely to obtain the proper concentration of blood to diluent.
5. Wipe off the pipette with gauze, being careful not to draw it across the tip.	Wiping the assembly free of blood removes surface contaminants. The gauze may absorb some of the blood sample if it comes in contact with the pipette tip, causing erroneous results.
6. Squeeze the reservoir gently to expel the air but none of the specimen. Place your finger over the opening of the pipette's overflow chamber.	Air in the reservoir will prevent the blood from entering the chamber; expressing the air creates a vacuum that assists in filling the unit. Covering the opening prevents loss of the specimen.

Step 6. Squeeze reservoir slightly to force out some air. (Courtesy of Becton Dickinson Vacutainer Systems, Rutherford, NJ.)

Steps	Reason
7. Maintain pressure on the reservoir and your finger position on the pipette, and insert the pipette into the reservoir.	Entry into the reservoir must be provided for the blood to combine with the diluent.

(continued)

Procedure 45-1 *(continued)*

Preparing a Whole Blood Dilution Using the Unopette System

Steps	Reason
8. Release the reservoir pressure. Then remove your finger from the pipette.	The vacuum draws the blood into the reservoir to begin the reaction.
9. Gently press and release the reservoir several times, forcing the diluent into but not out of the overflow chamber.	Gentle swishing action rinses blood from the pipette without destroying the fragile cells and ensures accurate dilution. Solution escaping the overflow chamber adversely affects the dilution ratio and becomes a source of contamination.

Step 9. Squeeze reservoir gently two or three times. (Courtesy of Becton Dickinson Vacutainer Systems, Rutherford, NJ.)

Steps	Reason
10. Place your index finger over the opening of the overflow chamber and gently invert or swirl the container several times. Remove your finger and cover the opening with the pipette shield.	The specimen must be well mixed to ensure proper results, but gentle mixing is necessary to maintain the integrity of the cells. Covering the unit prevents leakage and evaporation.

Step 10. Cover opening with index finger and gently invert to mix. (Courtesy of Becton Dickinson Vacutainer Systems, Rutherford, NJ.)

11. Label with the required information.

Procedure 45-2

Performing a Manual White Blood Cell Count

Purpose: To determine the number of leukocytes per cubic millimeter in a blood sample to aid in the diagnosis and treatment of infectious processes or blood dyscrasias

Equipment: Unopette system for WBC count, moist filter paper or moist cotton ball, Neubauer hemacytometer, Petri dish, cover glass, hand tally counter, gauze

Steps	Reason
1. Wash your hands.	Handwashing aids infection control
2. Assemble the equipment.	
3. Prepare a whole blood dilution according to Procedure 45-1.	
4. At the proper interval, mix the contents again by gently swirling the assembly.	
5. Remove the pipette from the Unopette reservoir and replace it as a dropper assembly.	The dropper adaptor allows the diluted specimen to charge the hemacytometer.

Step 5. Convert to dropper assembly. (Courtesy of Becton Dickinson Vacutainer Systems, Rutherford, NJ.)

6. Invert the reservoir and gently squeeze the sides, discarding the first 3 or 4 drops.	The capillary lumen must be cleaned of blood that might not be adequately mixed.
7. Charge the hemacytometer by touching the tip of the assembly to the **V**-shaped loading area of the covered chamber. Control the flow gently, and do not overfill. Do not allow the specimen to flow into the **H**-shaped moats that surround the platform loading area.	Forceful charging may cause bubble formation or may overfill the chamber; either will make counting and identifying the cells very difficult.

(continued)

Procedure 45-2 *(continued)*

Performing a Manual White Blood Cell Count

Steps	Reason

Step 7. Charge the hemacytometer. (Courtesy of Becton Dickinson Vacutainer Systems, Rutherford, NJ.)

Steps	Reason
8. Place the hemacytometer and the moistened filter paper or cotton ball in the Petri dish, and cover the entire assembly for 5 to 10 minutes.	The added moisture keeps the cells moist and allows the cells to settle for counting.
9. Place the prepared hemacytometer on the microscope stage, and turn to the ×100 magnification.	The specimen is ready for the cell count.
10. Use a zigzag counting pattern: starting at the top left, count the top row left to right. At the end of the top row, drop to the second row, and count from right to left.	The traditional counting pattern avoids omitting or overcounting cells.
11. Using the tally counter, count all of the WBCs within the boundaries and those that touch the top and left borders. Do not count those that touch the bottom or right borders.	Using this protocol prevents an inaccurate estimation of cells.

(continued)

Procedure 45-2   (continued)

Performing a Manual White Blood Cell Count

Steps   **Reason**

Step 11A. The ruled area of the Neubauer hemacytometer. There are nine large (1 mm) squares. Each of the large corner squares is subdivided into 16 squares and is marked W to indicate use for counting leukocytes. The large center square is subdivided into 25 smaller squares, each 0.04 mm. The squares marked R were used for counting erythrocytes when they were counted manually. The higher magnification of this center square (bottom) illustrates all 25 0.04-mm squares marked P where platelets are counted. (Courtesy of Becton Dickinson Vacutainer Systems, Rutherford, NJ.)

Step 11B. Rules for microscopic counting of leukocytes on the Neubauer hemacytometer; 1 mm^2 is illustrated. Leukocytes are counted in 9 of these 1-mm squares. Leukocytes that touch the top or left triple boundary lines are counted; those that touch the bottom or right boundaries are not. Solid circle, cells counted; open circle, cells not counted. (Courtesy of Becton Dickinson Vacutainer Systems, Rutherford, NJ.)

(continued)

Procedure 45-2 *(continued)*

Performing a Manual White Blood Cell Count

Steps	Reason
12. Record the number. Return the tally counter to 0, and move to the next square until all nine squares have been counted. If the numbers do not match within 10%, the hemacytometer was improperly charged and the test must be repeated. Count the opposite side of the hemacytometer.	Comparing the results between squares as you go helps ensure accuracy of testing results.
13. Add the total from both sides of the hemacytometer and divide by 2. Add 10% to the averaged total.	The calculation is simpler if you allow for a total of 10 squares rather than 9.
14. Multiply this figure by 100.	The result is the total WBCs per cubic millimeter.
15. Clean the hemacytometer and cover glass with 10% bleach solution, and wipe dry with lens paper.	
16. Clean the work area. Remove your PPE, and wash your hands.	Handwashing aids infection control.

Note: When performing a manual WBC count, always refer to the manufacturer's directions for counting and calculating results.

Charting Example

05/24/2005 3:15 P.M. Venipuncture to left antecubital vein. Hematology results as follows:

WBC 4880/mm^3
WBC diff:
Neutrophils 60%
Lymphocytes 25%
Monocytes 5%
Eosinophils 8%
Basophils 2%
RBC 4.6

Hgb 17
Hct 50%
MCV 88
Platelets 250,000
ESR 16
PT 18
Ptt 45

_____ J. Lowe, RMA

Making a Peripheral Blood Smear

Purpose: To prepare a blood sample for microscopic examination.

Equipment: Clean glass slides with frosted ends, pencil, well-mixed whole blood specimen, transfer pipette

Steps	Reason
1. Wash your hands.	Handwashing aids infection control.
2. Assemble the equipment.	
3. Greet and identify the patient. Explain the procedure. Ask for and answer any questions.	
4. Put on gloves, impervious gown, and face shield.	
5. Obtain an EDTA (lavender-top tube) blood specimen from the patient, following the steps for venipuncture described in Chapter 44.	
6. Label the slide on the frosted area.	The slide must be labeled with the patient's name or identification number; the frosted end will retain the markings.
7. Place a drop of blood 1 cm from the frosted end of the slide.	

Step 7. Drop of blood on slide with spreader slide placed in front. (Reprinted with permission from McCall R: Phlebotomy Essentials Baltimore: Lippincott Williams & Wilkins, 2003.)

8. Place the slide on a flat surface. With the thumb and forefinger of the dominant hand, hold the second (spreader) slide against the surface of the first at a 30° angle. Draw the spreader slide back against the drop of blood until contact is established. (*Note:* The angle of the spreader slide may have to be greater than 30° for large or thin drops of blood and less than 30° for small or thick drops.) Allow the blood	A flat surface allows for smooth movements. A 30° angle allows the blood to be spread in a thin film for viewing.

(continued)

Making a Peripheral Blood Smear

Steps	Purpose

to spread under the edge, then push the spreader slide at a moderate speed toward the other end of the slide, keeping contact between the two slides at all times.

Step 8. Spreader slide with drop of blood spreading to its edges. (Reprinted with permission from McCall R: Phlebotomy Essentials Baltimore: Lippincott Williams & Wilkins, 2003.)

9. Allow the slide to air dry. (The figures show properly and improperly prepared smears.)

Step 9. A properly prepared smear will yield a slide that is easy to read. (Reprinted with permission from McCall R: Phlebotomy Essentials Baltimore: Lippincott Williams & Wilkins, 2003.)

10. Properly care for or dispose of equipment and supplies. Clean the work area. Remove gloves, gown, and face shield, and wash your hands.

Note: Too much blood will make the smear invalid.

Procedure 45-4

Staining a Peripheral Blood Smear

Purpose: To aid in identifying the types of blood cells in a patient sample for diagnosis and treatment of infectious processes and blood dyscrasias.

Equipment: Staining rack, Wright's stain, Giemsa stain, prepared slide, tweezers.

Steps	Reason
1. Wash your hands.	
2. Assemble the equipment.	
3. Put on gloves, impervious gown, and face shield.	
4. Obtain a recently made dried blood smear.	A smear that is more than 2 hours old may have deteriorated.
5. Place the slide on a stain rack blood side up.	This provides a stable surface for staining.
6. Flood the slide with Wright's stain. Allow the stain to remain on the slide for 3 to 5 minutes or for the time specified by the manufacturer.	Wright's stain contains alcohol to fix blood to the slide and to stain the cells according to their characteristics.
7. Using tweezers, tilt the slide so that the stain drains off. Apply equal amounts of Giemsa stain and water. A green sheen will appear on the surface. Allow the stain to remain on the slide for 5 minutes or the time specified by the manufacturer.	This buffers the Wright's stain and enhances staining.
8. Holding the slide with tweezers, gently rinse the slide with water. Wipe off the back of the slide with gauze. Stand the slide upright and allow it to dry.	This rinses and removes the excess stain for viewing under a microscope.
9. Properly care for or dispose of equipment and supplies. Clean the work area. Remove gloves, gown, and face shield, and wash your hands.	

Note: Some manufacturers provide a simple one-step method that consists of dipping the smear in a staining solution, then rinsing. Directions provided by the manufacturer vary with the specific test.

Procedure 45-5

Performing a White Blood Cell Differential

Purpose: To identify and quantify leukocytes present in a blood sample for diagnosis and treatment of infectious processes and blood dyscrasias.

Equipment: Stained peripheral blood smear, microscope, immersion oil, paper, recording tabulator

Steps	Reason
1. Wash your hands.	
2. Assemble the equipment.	
3. Put on gloves.	
4. Place the stained slide on the microscope. Focus on the feathered edge of the smear and scan with the low-power objective to ensure an even distribution of cells and proper staining.	Stage mounting sets up the slide to be read. Scanning the slide is a quality control procedure.
5. Carefully turn the nosepiece to the high-power objective and bring the slide into focus using the fine adjustment.	
6. Place a drop of oil on the slide and rotate the oil immersion lens into place. Focus and begin to identify any leukocytes.	Oil is always used with the oil immersion lens, which has the highest magnification, to provide a path for the light source.
7. Record on a tally sheet or tabulator the types of white cells found.	Tallying the types seen is necessary to record accurate percentages.
8. Move the stage so that the next field is in view. Identify any white cells in this field, and continue to the next field to identify all that are present until 100 white cells have been counted.	Many fields must be viewed before 100 cells have been counted. The systematic movement of the stage so that another field comes into view ensures that this is accomplished correctly.
9. Calculate the number of each type of leukocyte as a percentage.	Since 100 cells are counted, each represents one percentage point.
10. Properly care for or dispose of equipment and supplies. Clean the work area. Remove gloves, and wash your hands.	

Note: A WBC differential is performed by a trained laboratory technologist. Abnormal cells can appear in the peripheral blood; recognizing them is an important diagnostic procedure that requires specific training. (See Procedure 45-2 for charting example.)

Procedure 45-6

Performing a Manual Red Blood Cell Count

Purpose:	To determine the number of erythrocytes per cubic millimeter in a blood sample for diagnosis and treatment of anemias and blood dyscrasias.
Equipment:	Unopette system for red cell count, clean, lint-free hemacytometer, cover glass, gauze, moist filter paper or moist cotton ball, Petri dish, microscope, hand tally counter

Steps	Reason
1. Wash your hands.	
2. Assemble the equipment.	
3. Prepare a whole blood dilution according to Procedure 45-1.	
4. At the proper interval, mix the contents again by gently swirling the assembly.	Stage mounting sets up the slide to be read. Scanning the slide is a quality control procedure.
5. Remove the pipette from the Unopette reservoir and replace it as a dropper assembly.	
6. Invert the reservoir and gently squeeze the sides, discarding the first 3 or 4 drops.	Oil is always used with the oil immersion lens, which has the highest magnification, to provide a path for the light source.
7. Charge the hemacytometer by touching the tip of the assembly to the **V**-shaped loading area of the covered chamber. Control the flow gently, and do not overfill. Do not allow the specimen to flow into the **H**-shaped moats that surround the platform loading area.	Tallying the types seen is necessary to record accurate percentages.
8. Place the hemacytometer and the moistened filter paper or cotton ball in the Petri dish, and cover the entire assembly for 5 to 10 minutes.	Many fields must be viewed before 100 cells have been counted. The systematic movement of the stage so that another field comes into view in order ensures that this is accomplished correctly.
9. Place the prepared hemacytometer on the microscope stage, and turn to the ×100 magnification.	Since 100 cells are counted, each represents one percentage point.
10. Place the hemacytometer on the microscope stage so that the ruled area can be surveyed with the low-power objective. Focus the microscope, then progress to the ×400 magnification to count the RBCs.	The slide is ready for evaluation.
11. Count the RBCs in the four corner squares and the center square following zigzag pattern. Starting at the top far left, count the top row left to right. At the end of the top row, drop to the second row, and count from right to left. Continue this pattern until all of the rows are counted. Count cells touching the upper and left side, but do not count those on the lower and right side.	The traditional counting pattern avoids omitting or overcounting cells.

(continued)

Procedure 45-6 *(continued)*

Performing a Manual White Blood Cell Coun

Steps	Reason
12. Tally the count and record the number. Return the counter to 0 and count the next grid. Count the opposite side of the hemacytometer.	
13. The count within the squares should not vary by more than 20 cells. If the variance is greater, the test must be repeated.	Comparing results as you count helps ensure accuracy of testing.
14. Average the two sides and multiply the result by 10,000.	This calculation gives the total number of RBCs per cubic millimeter.
15. Clean the hemacytometer and cover glass with 10% bleach and wipe dry with lens paper. Dispose of or care for any other equipment and supplies appropriately. Clean the work area. Remove gloves and gown and wash your hands.	

Note: Read and follow the manufacturer's instructions for this procedure. (See Procedure 45-2 for charting example.)

This procedure is rarely performed in the office. It has largely been replaced by a hemoglobin measurement, hematocrit determination, or automated CBC.

Procedure 45-7

Performing a Hemoglobin Determination

Purpose: To determine the oxygen-carrying capacity of the blood in a patient sample for diagnosis and treatment
               of anemia

Equipment: Hemoglobinometer, applicator sticks, whole blood

Standard:

Steps	Reason
1. Wash your hands.	
2. Assemble the necessary equipment.	
3. Put on gloves, gown, and face shield.	
4. Obtain an EDTA (lavender-top tube) blood specimen from the patient, following the steps for capillary puncture described in Chapter 44.	
5. Place a drop of well-mixed whole blood obtained by skin puncture on the glass chamber of the hemoglobinometer. Slide the coverslip into the holding clip over the chamber.	This prepares the sample for the hemoglobin determination.
6. At one of the open edges, push the applicator stick into the chamber. Gently move the stick around until the specimen no longer appears cloudy.	This lyses the red cells, releasing the hemoglobin.
7. Slide the chamber into the hemoglobinometer. Remove the face shield.	The chamber must be in the receiving slot for the color comparison reading.
8. With your left hand, hold the meter and press the light button. View the field through the eyepiece. With your right hand, move the dial until the right and left sides match in color intensity. Note the hemoglobin level indicated on the dial.	The chamber must be illuminated to compare the colors. Matching fields indicate that the amount of hemoglobin in the sample matches the internal standard.
9. Clean the chamber and work area with 10% bleach solution. Dispose of equipment and supplies appropriately. Remove gloves and gown and wash your hands.	

Note: For quality assurance, calibration chambers are included in the hemoglobinometer kit and are used to verify proper function of the meter. This procedure may vary with the instrument. Some manufacturers offer a digital readout that is less subjective and is therefore considered more accurate and easier to use.

Charting Example

12/02/2005 10:30 A.M. Pt c/o no energy. Periods have been heavy, awaiting hysterectomy for dysfunctional bleeding. Cap puncture L ring finger. Hgb 9.5. Dr. Royal notified, Fe supplement ordered. _____

R. Smith, CMA

Procedure 45-8

Performing a Manual Microhematocrit Determination

Purpose: To determine the quantity of erythrocytes in a centrifuged blood specimen for diagnosis and treatment of anemia.

Equipment: Microcollection tubes, sealing clay, microhematocrit centrifuge, microhematocrit reading device

Standard:

Steps	Reason
1. Wash your hands.	
2. Assemble the equipment.	
3. Put on gloves, gown, and face shield.	
4. Draw blood into the capillary tube by one of two methods:	
A. Directly from a capillary puncture in which the tip of the capillary tube is touched to the blood at the wound and allowed to fill to three-quarters or the indicated mark (see Chapter 44).	Whole blood from a capillary puncture has not clotted and is acceptable.

Step 6. Results from the centrifuge reading device.

B. From a well-mixed EDTA tube of whole blood; again, the tip is touched to the blood and allowed to fill three-quarters of the tube. Place the forefinger over the top of the tube, wipe excess blood off the sides, and push the bottom into the sealing clay. Draw a second specimen in the same manner.	If blood from a tube is not well mixed, the reading is likely to be inaccurate. Holding the finger over the tip stops blood from dripping out the bottom. The clay seals one end of the tube to contain it during centrifugation. A second tube is necessary for duplicate testing as a quality control measure.

(continues)

Procedure 45-8   *(continued)*

Performing a Manual Microhematocrit Determination

Steps	**Reason**

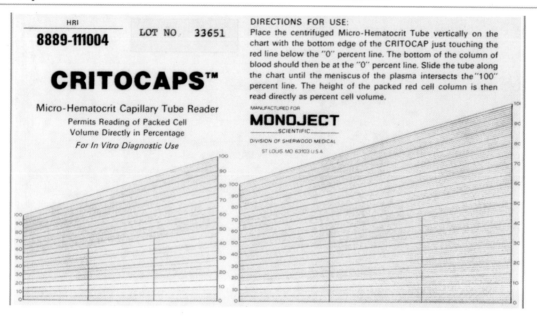

Step 6. Centrifuged tube reader.

5. Place the tubes, clay-sealed end out, in the radial grooves of the microhematocrit centrifuge opposite each other. Put the lid on the grooved area and tighten by turning the knob clockwise. Close the lid. Spin for 5 minutes or as directed by the manufacturer.	Specimens should always be placed opposite each other to balance the centrifuge. Read the manufacturer's directions for the specific centrifuge used in your facility; 5 minutes is normal.
6. Remove the tubes from the centrifuge and read the results; instructions are printed on the device. The above figure shows two methods of determining microhematocrit values. Results should be within 5% of each other. Take the average and report as a percentage.	Results greater than 5% variation have been found to offer unreliable results.
7. Dispose of the microhematocrit tubes in a biohazard container. Properly care for or dispose of other equipment and supplies. Clean the work area. Remove gloves, gown, and face shield, and wash your hands.	

Note: Some microhematocrit centrifuges have the scale printed in the machine at the radial grooves.

Charting Example

03/28/2005 4:20 P.M. Capillary tube filled from skin puncture, left ring finger. Hct: 42%. Dr. Erikson notified.
_____ M. Mays, CMA

Procedure 45-9

Wintrobe Erythrocyte Sedimentation Rate

Purpose: To determine the rate at which erythrocytes separate from plasma and settle in a tube for diagnosis of nonspecific inflammatory processes

Equipment: Anticoagulation tube, Wintrobe tube, transfer pipette, timer

Standard:

Steps	Reason
1. Wash your hands.	
2. Assemble the necessary equipment.	
3. Put on gloves, impervious gown, and face shield.	
4. Draw blood (see Chapter 44) into an EDTA lavender-stoppered anticoagulation tube.	The blood must not be allowed to clot; it must be drawn into an anticoagulation tube.
5. Fill a graduated Wintrobe tube to the 0 mark with the well-mixed EDTA whole blood using the provided transfer pipette. Be sure to eliminate any trapped bubbles and fill exactly to the 0 line.	Bubbles and incorrect filling will alter the test results.
6. Place the tube in a holder that will keep the tube vertical.	
7. Wait exactly 1 hour; use a timer for accuracy. Keep the tube straight upright and undisturbed during the hour.	Never use a shorter time and multiply the reading; less time will give inaccurate results. Tilting or disturbing the tube also will alter the results.
8. Record the level of the top of the RBCs after 1 hour. Normal results for men are 0–10 mL/hour; for women, 0–15 mL/hour.	
9. Properly care for or dispose of equipment and supplies. Clean the work area. Remove gloves, gown, and face shield. Wash your hands.	

Charting Example

02/21/2005 12:30 P.M. Pt. presented with vague aches. Specimen drawn L antecubital vein in lavender-top tube per Dr. North's order. Wintrobe ESR test results 12 mL/hour. Dr. North notified. _____ B. White, CMA

Procedure 45-10

Determining Bleeding Time

Purpose: To determine the time required for clot formation for diagnosis and treatment of clotting disorders

Equipment: Blood pressure cuff, filter paper, Simplate device, butterfly bandage, alcohol or antiseptic wipe, stop watch

Standard:

Steps	Reason
1. Wash your hands.	
2. Assemble the equipment.	
3. Greet and identify the patient. Explain the procedure. Ask for and answer any questions.	Some patients are nervous before the incision is made; reassure them that the cut is very small and will barely be felt.
4. Put on gloves, impervious gown, and face shield.	
5. Position the patient so that the arm is extended in a manner that is both comfortable and stable.	The test requires a moderate length of time and requires that the patient remain still.
6. Have the patient turn the palm upward so that the inner aspect of the arm is exposed. Select a site several inches below the antecubital area. The area should be free of lesions and with no visible veins. Clean the site with alcohol or antiseptic wipe.	The inner aspect provides a surface relatively free of hair. (Rarely, the patient's arm may have to be shaved at the site.) There are no large surface vessels at this site.
7. Apply the pressure cuff and set it at 40 mm Hg for the length of the test. Adjust it as needed throughout the test to maintain the pressure.	Placing the pressure cuff on the arm stabilizes the pressure to the arm.
8. Twist the tearaway tab on the Simplate. Make an incision 1 mm deep on the cleaned skin by placing the Simplate bleeding time device on the site and pressing the trigger button on the side. This will spring the blade to make the incision. At the same time, start the stopwatch.	A 1-mm incision is deep enough to disrupt the surface capillaries but not the underlying veins.
9. At 30-second intervals, bring the filter paper near the edge of the wound to draw off some of the accumulating blood. Avoid touching the wound with the filter paper.	Removing the blood from the wound site is essential to observe slowing of the blood flow. The filter paper should not touch the wound, because it might disrupt the platelet plug, resulting in an inaccurate measurement of bleeding time.
10. The test is complete when the blood flow stops completely. Stop the watch when the blood no longer stains the filter paper; note the time to the nearest 30 seconds.	When the blood flow stops, the platelet plug has formed.

(continues)

Procedure 45-10 *(continued)*

Determining Bleeding Time

Steps	Reason
11. Apply a butterfly bandage across the wound to keep it sealed and cover the site with a waterproof bandage. Instruct the patient to keep the site dry and not to remove the bandage for at least 24 hours.	Butterfly bandages work best to reduce scarring.
12. Properly care for or dispose of all equipment and supplies. Clean the work area. Remove gloves, gown, and face shield, and wash your hands.	

Warning! Be sure you are away from superficial veins. Puncturing superficial veins will cause a prolonged bleeding time. If the patient is having clotting problems, excessive bleeding could occur.

Note: Low platelet counts and aspirin ingestion will prolong the bleeding time. Each laboratory has a set policy for stopping the test if the flow continues for too long. Most laboratories stop the bleeding test at 15 to 30 minutes. Any testing beyond this point is not needed because it is established that the bleeding time is not normal.

Charting Example
04/23/2005 2:30 P.M. Skin puncture of L inner forearm, bleeding time test done, results 14 min. Dr. Lancaster notified. _____ S. Smith, CMA

CHAPTER SUMMARY

The medical assistant plays an important role in the hematological evaluation of the patient. Several hematology screening tests are CLIA waived and can be performed by the medical assistant in a typical physician office setting. More complex testing is performed by the hematology laboratory. The complete blood count and differential are the main procedures performed in the hematology laboratory. Anemias and infections are two conditions that can be diagnosed using this information. Other tests, such as coagulation, aid in determining the ability of a patient to maintain hemostasis.

Critical Thinking Challenges

1. A patient was taking a medication that caused him to become neutropenic. To what might he be susceptible?
2. A patient lives at a very high elevation, where there is less oxygen than at sea level. Would you expect her hemoglobin to be greater than, less than, or the same as if she lived at sea level?
3. A patient with rheumatoid arthritis has an ESR of 77 mm/hour when she has her blood tested at the doctor's office; 2 weeks later she returns, and now the rate is 31 mm/hour. With her condition in mind, would you expect that she is improving or not?

Answers to Checkpoint Questions

1. Hematopoiesis is the medical term for blood cell production. It is influenced by hormones and depends on adequate nutrients such as iron.
2. Leukopenia is a diminished number of leukocytes. It can be caused by chemical toxicity, nutritional deficiency, overwhelming or chronic infection, or certain malignancies.
3. Neutrophils defend against foreign invaders by phagocytosis.
4. Elevated eosinophils and basophils are both seen with allergic reactions.
5. A hematocrit of 20% indicates that 20% of the total blood volume consists of RBCs.
6. The two most common tests for determining how well a fibrin clot can form are prothrombin time and partial thromboplastin time.

 Websites

Beckman Coulter laboratory accreditation tools
    www.beckman.com/lars/personnel/webinars.asp
University of Minnesota Hematography
    www1.umn.edu/hema/
www.cms.hhs/clia/

46

Serology and Immunohematology

CHAPTER OUTLINE

ROLE DELINEATION

CLINICAL: FUNDAMENTAL PRINCIPLES
   • Apply principles of aseptic technique and infection
     control
   • Comply with quality assurance practices

CLINICAL: DIAGNOSTIC ORDERS
   • Collect and process specimens
   • Perform diagnostic tests

GENERAL: LEGAL CONCEPTS
   • Perform within legal and ethical boundaries
   • Document accurately
   • Comply with established risk management and safety
     procedures

GENERAL: INSTRUCTION
   • Instruct individuals according to their needs

CHAPTER COMPETENCIES

LEARNING OBJECTIVES

Upon successfully completing this chapter, you will be able to:

1. Spell and define the key terms.
2. List the indications for serological testing.
3. Describe the antigen-antibody reaction.
4. Name and describe the two most common methods of enhancing the antigen-antibody reaction for testing purposes.
5. List areas to address to ensure quality assurance and quality control in serological testing.
6. Explain the storage and handling of serological test kits.

7. List and describe serological tests most commonly encountered through the medical office.

PERFORMANCE OBJECTIVES

Upon successfully completing this chapter, you will be able to:

1. Perform an agglutination test.
2. Perform an enzyme immunoassay test.
3. Perform a mononucleosis test (Procedure 46-1).
4. Perform an HCG pregnancy test (Procedure 46-2).
5. Perform a group A rapid strep test (Procedure 46-3).

KEY TERMS

agglutination	sensitivity	false positive	external control
donor	serology	false negative	internal control
immunohematology	specificity		

SEROLOGY IS THE STUDY OF antigens and antibodies. The term *serology* refers to the source of most of the samples: the liquid part of blood, called serum, produced when whole blood is allowed to clot. Serology is used for the following:

- To identify bacterial and viral infections (e.g., streptococcus, hepatitis A, hepatitis B, human immunodeficiency virus, rubella, and Epstein-Barr virus)
- To diagnose chlamydial infections, syphilis, and Rocky Mountain spotted fever
- To detect substances such as human chorionic gonadotropin (HCG) in pregnant women, drugs in the urine, and hormones in serum

Immunohematology is the testing done in the blood bank on red blood cells (RBCs, erythrocytes) and serum to ensure that blood from a **donor** (one who contributes blood) is compatible with a recipient's blood. It includes testing for antigens on the surface of RBCs with reagents containing antibodies called antisera and for antibodies in the patient's serum with reagent RBCs. These tests are based on the attraction between antigens and antibodies.

All testing described in this chapter requires the use of standard precautions.

ANTIGENS AND ANTIBODIES

As noted in Chapter 36, antigens are substances recognized as foreign to the body that cause the body to initiate a defense response, including the production of antibodies. Antibodies are proteins produced by the body in response to a specific antigen that bind to that specific antigen to destroy it. Antibodies float freely in the bloodstream and are found in serum.

Each antibody combines with and destroys (in most instances) only one antigen; this is called specificity. It allows laboratory personnel to test the exact substance desired without interference from any other substance in serum.

Because an antibody has a particularly strong attraction for its antigen, little antigen need be present in a sample for the antibody to find it; this is referred to as sensitivity. A test is very sensitive if it can determine the presence of a substance even if only a small amount is present. Tests using antigen-antibody reactions are very specific and very sensitive. These tests can detect small amounts of a substance and pick it out of a solution, such as serum, that contains millions of other substances.

The immune system can recognize many areas or sites on a single antigen and produce several protein substances called antibodies that can combine with that one antigen. Each antibody will combine only with the specific antigen that stimulated its response in the immune system.

An antibody is named by using its specific antigen's name and adding the prefix anti-. In the blood for instance, if the antigen on the RBC's name is A, the antibody's name is anti-A. If the antigen is B, the antibody is anti-B.

Checkpoint Question

1. How would you describe a test that is both specific and sensitive?

SEROLOGY TEST METHODS AND PRINCIPLES

In serology, the substance to be tested is identified or the amount present (quantity) is measured using the binding of a specific antibody to its specific antigen. Either the antigen is detected by use of a solution containing the antibody (antisera) or the antibody is detected by using a solution containing the antigen. Usually the binding of an antigen and antibody is not visible to the naked eye. The reaction has to be enhanced or enlarged. Methods commonly used to do this:

- Agglutination (clumping) of visible particles, such as RBCs or latex particles
- Enzyme-linked immunosorbent assay (ELISA) that produces a color change from colorless to a specific color, such as blue or red

Other methods include agglutination inhibition and competitive binding assays.

Agglutination Test

Agglutination describes clumping of particles caused by binding of antibodies and antigens. For agglutination testing, only two things are necessary:

1. A reagent containing the antibody
2. The patient's sample

To perform an agglutination test, follow these steps:

1. Mix together the reagent and the patient's sample on a paper card or glass plate.
2. Gently rock the reagent and sample back and forth for a few seconds or a few minutes.
3. Observe for agglutination, or clumping of particles. If agglutination does not occur, the test solution appears smooth and milky. In most cases this is a negative finding: the sample does not contain the antibody. If agglutination does occur, the test solution appears rough and granular, with areas of clumped particles in a clear background. This is a positive finding: the sample does contain the antibody.

Some tests are designed so that agglutination must appear within a specified time to indicate a positive reaction. Agglutination tests can be used in two ways:

1. If the specific antigen is in the reagent, the patient's serum can be tested for the specific antibody. This method is used to test for infectious mononucleosis, rheumatoid arthritis, syphilis, and rubella.
2. If the manufacturer produces a reagent with the antibody attached, the patient's serum or other specimen can be tested for a specific antigen. This method is used in some tests for streptococci.

Agglutination tests are quick and easy to perform. They are also inexpensive and have a wide range of uses. Most are very sensitive and specific, reducing the incidence of **false-positive** (a positive result due to an interfering substance) or **false-negative** (failure to detect the substance in the specimen) result. The procedure for a test must be followed exactly for the result to be accurate (Box 46-1).

Enzyme-Linked Immunosorbent Assays

ELISA has more steps and more reagents than agglutination tests, but the end point is an easy-to-read color change. Agglutination, particularly if the clumps are small, can be difficult to read. Most ELISA tests come with all necessary reagents in a kit that also contains any additional necessary components for the test. Some of the newer ELISA tests require only adding the patient's sample to a cartridge containing a small filter. This filter contains all of the reagents, and as the sample migrates through the filter, the color changes if the specimen contains the specific substance in question. Be sure to follow the specific manufacturer's instructions (Box 46-2).

Box 46-1

TIPS FOR PERFORMING AGGLUTINATION TESTING

1. Start with a clean test slide that is free of fingerprints and dust.
2. Follow the times exactly.
3. View the test mixture under a direct light source.
4. Mix reagents before using.
5. Mix samples before using.
6. Do not touch reagent droppers to test area.
7. Do not smear one test mixture into another test area.

Box 46-2

TIPS FOR PERFORMING ENZYME IMMUNOASSAYS

1. Follow the times exactly.
2. Add reagents in correct order.
3. Use reagents only with other reagents from the same kit.
4. Use exact amount of reagents stated in directions.
5. Ensure that reagents and samples are at room temperature.
6. Ensure that reagents have not expired.

Checkpoint Question

2. What are two serology test methods, and how do they indicate the presence of the test substance?

REAGENT AND KIT STORAGE AND HANDLING

Most serology test reagents are manufactured as kits. These kits contain all of the reagents and often supplies, such as pipettes, tubes, and cups, needed to perform tests on a certain number of samples. **The kits must be stored at the temperature recommended on the kit box or package insert.** Some kits are stored at room temperature and some in the refrigerator; other kits have to be divided, with some reagents stored at room temperature and others in the refrigerator. Still others are stored in the refrigerator until opened and then stored at room temperature. It is important to follow the manufacturer's directions. If the kits are stored improperly, the reagents may deteriorate, and false results may be obtained.

Each kit package is marked with a lot number and expiration date. All reagents with the same lot number were made at the same time in the same manufacturing facility. **The expiration date is the day past which the reagents are no longer guaranteed to perform correctly.** Reagents from kits with different lot numbers should not be used together. The manufacturer will not guarantee that they will work correctly when components from different lots are mixed.

Reagents should never be used past their expiration date. The date of manufacture should be printed on the kit box. The date of opening and the initials of the worker who opened it should also be written on the box when the kit is opened and used for the first time. Some kits have a new expiration date starting from the day the kit is opened. Always read the package insert for details about storing and handling the reagents and supplies.

There may be specific specimen collection guidelines indicated on each kit. Be sure to read and follow the manufacturer's instructions.

Checkpoint Question

3. Why is it important to store reagent kits at specified temperatures?

FOLLOWING TEST PROCEDURES

All tests performed in serology should have written procedures. Follow these procedures each time you test a sample to ensure correct results. Test procedures typically cover these points:

- Test principle and clinical use of the test
- Reagents and materials needed to do the test
- Precautions
- Specimen collection and handling
- Controls to be run and how often
- Step-by-step procedure
- Interpretation and reporting of results
- Normal or expected values
- Test limitations

QUALITY ASSURANCE AND QUALITY CONTROL

Reagents do not always function properly even before the expiration date. Sometimes a reagent is left at room temperature when it should be refrigerated. Sometimes serum or another solution is accidentally added to a reagent, causing it to test or register incorrectly. **Kits should be tested periodically for continued stability of all reagents.** A quality control (QC) test should be performed each time the reagents are used. Other forms of QC may be performed once a day or only when a new kit is opened. Solutions used to perform some of these QC tests are called controls. Be sure to follow the facility's policies and procedures for QC when working in the laboratory.

External Controls

An external control is tested in the same manner as a patient's sample; however, its value or expected result is already known. These controls are often part of the serology kit. In some instances, separate controls can be purchased from the manufacturer.

Most serology tests necessitate use of both positive and negative controls. The positive control should give a positive reaction (agglutination, color). The negative control should give a negative reaction (no agglutination, no color). **If the controls do not give the expected result, the patient's sample findings should not be reported and the test should be repeated.** If the problem persists, it should be further investigated (Box 46-3).

Box 46-3

TEST TROUBLESHOOTING TIPS

If a serology test using a control is not producing expected results, try the following:
1. Reread the procedure to be sure a step was not omitted.
2. Check labels of reagents to be sure the correct reagents were added in the correct order.
3. Visually check reagents for signs of contamination, such as cloudiness or color change.
4. Repeat the test with new bottle of control.
5. Repeat the test with a new kit or reagent.
6. Call the manufacturer for assistance.

Internal Controls

Besides external control solutions, some serology tests have internal controls (sometimes called technique controls) built into the test packs themselves; such controls ensure that the procedure is followed correctly and that the reagents are working properly. Sometimes each test pack has positive and negative test zones. Sometimes there is only a positive test zone or a test completed zone. These zones are separate from the specimen test zone or area. The positive control zone must give a positive color reaction, and the negative control zone must give a negative (usually no color) reaction for the test to be valid and findings reported. Do not report findings if controls do not give proper reactions. Repeat the QC test for technician error. Check for outdated reagents, contaminated reagents, and compromise of the test kit (e.g., left at room temperature when it should have been refrigerated).

The positive control zone ensures that the correct reagents have been added in the proper order. The negative control zone ensures there is no nonspecific reaction of specimen and test reagents. Problems with internal controls can be investigated in the same manner as for external controls (Box 46-3). Positive and negative internal controls do not completely take the place of external control tests, which should be run daily.

SEROLOGY TESTS

There are many serological tests. Some of the more common tests performed in the physician office laboratory are discussed in the following sections.

Rheumatoid Factor and Rheumatoid Arthritis

Rheumatoid arthritis is an autoimmune progressive inflammatory disease of the joints causing pain on motion, swelling, stiffness, and subcutaneous nodules near the affected joints.

Testing

The most common tests for rheumatoid factor are based on agglutination of particles. The external controls must give appropriate reactions for the test to be valid and results to be reported. That is, the positive control must agglutinate and the negative control must not agglutinate for testing to be valid.

False-Negative and False-Positive Results

Even when the controls react appropriately, laboratory tests are not a perfect indicator of disease. Physicians use test results along with physical examination and the patient's history to make clinical decisions about disease. Sometimes findings are negative when a patient has a disease. This

is called a false-negative result. Because only 70% of patients with rheumatoid arthritis are positive for rheumatoid factor, 30% of patients with rheumatoid arthritis have a false-negative result.

Sometimes findings are positive when the patient does not have the disease. These false-positive results sometimes occur in the elderly and in patients with lupus erythematosus, syphilis, or hepatitis.

False-negative and false-positive results can occur because of biological conditions of patients. They can also be due to technical difficulty with samples or with performing the test. Testing personnel cannot control the biological conditions, but they can sometimes control the technical conditions. If testing personnel wait too long to read agglutination, the finding may be false-positive. This can be avoided by following directions carefully. Hemolyzed and lipemic samples (samples with high fat levels) can give a false-positive result. These samples must be collected again to ensure accurate testing.

Checkpoint Question

4. What is the difference between a false-negative and a false-positive test result, and why do they sometimes occur?

Infectious Mononucleosis

Infectious mononucleosis is caused by Epstein-Barr virus. It is sometimes called the kissing disease.

Testing

Tests for infectious mononucleosis include agglutination of RBCs or latex particles, or ELISA (Procedure 46-1). External or internal controls must give appropriate reactions for testing to be valid and results to be reported.

False-Negative and False-Positive Results

False-negative results can occur early in the disease, before antibodies are produced. False-positive results can be obtained by waiting too long to read agglutination tests.

Rapid Plasma Reagin Test for Syphilis

Rapid plasma reagin (RPR) is a screening test for syphilis, a sexually transmitted disease caused by a spirochete, *Treponema pallidum*.

Testing

T. pallidum does not grow in culture; the best test to demonstrate the organism is darkfield microscopy. More frequently the serum is tested for antibodies and antibody-like substances called reagins. Venereal Disease Research Laboratories (VDRL) and RPR are the most common screening tests for these nonspecific reagins. The microhemagglutination assay for *T. pallidum* (MHA-TP) and fluorescent treponemal antibody absorption test (FTA-ABS) are two confirmatory tests for the organism itself.

The RPR is an agglutination test. Reactive (positive), weakly reactive, and nonreactive (negative) controls are run with each batch of specimens. They must react appropriately for the test to be valid and results to be reported. Agglutination of the antigen solution is considered reactive for the reagin (presumptive positive test for syphilis). Even a weakly reactive agglutination is considered positive or reactive. No agglutination of the antigen solution is considered nonreactive. Determination of titer is performed on any reactive serum. This entails a serial dilution of serum to 1:2, 1:4, 1:8, 1:16, and so forth. Dilution of the serum is continued until a specimen gives a nonreactive result (no agglutination). The titer reported is the last dilution showing agglutination. If the last diluted specimen showing agglutination was the 1:8 dilution, the titer is reported as 1:8. If only the undiluted specimen showed agglutination, the titer would be reported as 1:1.

The patient's physician and the health department must be notified of all reactive results for syphilis. Serum should be sent to the state laboratory or reference laboratory for confirmation of a syphilis infection using the MHA-TP or FTA-ABS tests.

False-Negative and False-Positive Results

The RPR is reactive in 80% of cases of primary syphilis, 99% of secondary, and 1% of tertiary. The MHA-TP, in contrast, is reactive in 65% of cases of primary syphilis, 100% of secondary, and 95% of tertiary. A false-negative RPR will be obtained in 20% of primary syphilis cases. A false-negative MHA-TP will be obtained in 35% of primary syphilis cases. A false-positive RPR can be seen in patients with lupus erythematosus, infectious mononucleosis, hepatitis, rheumatoid arthritis, and in pregnancy and the elderly. Improper rotation of specimen can also cause a false-negative result.

Pregnancy Test

The test for pregnancy is based on the detection of the hormone human chorionic gonadotropin (HCG). (FIG. 46-1). Today's tests can determine pregnancy before the first missed menses. A pregnancy test is frequently used to rule out pregnancy before a medical procedure that might harm the fetus (Procedure 46-2).

Testing

Tests of HCG include agglutination and ELISA. Urine or serum is added to the test pack in the test area containing antibodies to HCG. Internal positive and negative control areas must react appropriately for results to be valid.

F I G U R E 4 6 - 1 . QuickVue Pregnancy Test. (Courtesy of Quidel, San Diego, CA.)

False-Negative and False-Positive Results

A urine specimen that is too dilute can give a false-negative reaction. The first morning urine specimen is the most likely to contain HCG if the patient is pregnant. Certain tumors (testicular and some fibroids) produce HCG and can cause a false-positive result. Therefore, don't count it strange to have an order for a pregnancy test on a male. The physician may be trying to rule out such a tumor.

Group A Streptococcus

Group A streptococcus (*Streptococcus pyogenes*) is one of the most common bacterial causes of sore throat and upper respiratory tract infections.

Testing

Group A strep infection can be diagnosed by bacterial culture or serological tests for the antigenic presence of the bacteria (FIG. 46-2). Serological tests include agglutination and ELISA (Procedure 46-3). The bacteria do not have to be alive for serology tests, as they do for culture. Serological tests are easier and more rapid (5–15 minutes) than culture, which takes 18 to 24 hours; however, culture is considered more sensitive.

False-Negative and False-Positive Results

If improper technique is used in collecting the throat swab or an inadequate specimen is obtained, a false-negative result can occur. If the test is allowed to stand too long before results are read, a false-positive result can occur. High levels of *Staphylococcus aureus* in the specimen can interfere with the interpretation of results.

F I G U R E   4 6 - 2 .   Cards QS Strep A test kit. (Courtesy of Quidel, San Diego, CA.)

 Checkpoint Question

5. What are the benefits and drawbacks of using serology tests versus cultures for group A streptococcus?

IMMUNOHEMATOLOGY

Testing in the blood bank determines whether a donor's blood is compatible with that of the recipient. If the donor's blood is compatible, the recipient's immunosurveillance will not immediately recognize it as foreign, and the RBCs may circulate in the patient's body longer after they are transfused. If the donor's blood is incompatible, the patient's body will immediately recognize the blood as foreign and begin destroying it as soon as it is transfused. This can rapidly lead to death.

Blood Group Antigens

ABO Group

Transfusion compatibility is determined by testing the antigens on RBCs (patient's and donor's) and the antibodies in the patient's serum. The main RBC antigens belong to the ABO system. Each person belongs to one of four blood groups: A, B, O, or AB. Approximately 45% are O, 40% are A, 11% are B, and 4% are AB. Consequently, some blood groups are easier to obtain, and some are more in demand than others. The ABO group of each donor and each patient who will need a transfusion is determined as described later in the chapter.

Almost every person's serum contains antibodies to the ABO antigens that he or she lacks. These antibodies occur naturally. Shortly after birth these antibodies are found in serum, even though the person has never received blood. A person in the A group has the A antigen. A person in the B group has the B antigen. A person in the O group lacks both antigens. A person in the AB group has both the A and B antigen. A person in the A group lacks the B antigen and has an antibody to B (anti-B) in serum. Someone who is B lacks the A antigen and has anti-A in serum. One who is O has both anti-A and anti-B in serum. A person who belongs to the AB group has neither antibody in serum.

These antibodies are crucial to safe transfusion of blood to a patient. They are the reason it is unsafe to give B blood to an A patient. An A patient has anti-B in the serum that would bind and destroy the B cells, causing breakdown products that are toxic and sometimes fatal. The lack of either A or B antigens on O cells makes this group the universal donor. This means type O blood may be given to patients no matter what their ABO group. If B blood is unavailable for a patient, O blood can be given safely.

Rh Type

Another group of antigens important to the blood bank is the Rh group. This includes the antigens D, E, C, e, and c. However, D is the most important. The presence of the D antigen is termed Rh positive. The absence of the D antigen is termed Rh negative. Antibodies to D do not occur naturally. A person lacking the D antigen must be exposed to the D antigen of foreign RBCs to produce antibodies. This can happen if an Rh-negative (D-negative) patient is transfused with Rh-positive (D-positive) blood. This can also happen if an Rh-negative mother is exposed to the Rh-positive cells of her baby before or during childbirth. Rh negative mothers can be prevented from producing antibodies to the Rh (D) antigen by injection of immune-D serum, or RhoGAM. This injection prevents the production of antibodies that might cause hemolytic disease of the next baby (erythroblastosis fetalis) by destroying its RBCs.

Other Blood Groups

Although the ABO blood groups and Rh types are most important to immunohematology, there are many more significant antigens and antibodies. Some other groups include Duffy, Lewis, MNS, Kidd, and Kell. These are all RBC antigens. White blood cells and platelets also have antigens. Most of these antigens belong to a system called human leukocyte antigens. Antibodies to these antigens can cause fever during transfusion of RBCs because of the presence of white blood cells (leukocytes). Antibodies to these antigens are also responsible for rejection of a transplanted organ, such as kidney, heart, or liver. Most of these antibodies do not occur naturally. A person must be exposed to foreign blood or tissue before producing antibodies.

Blood Group Testing

ABO Testing

Two reagent antisera, anti-A and anti-B, are used to test for the ABO group of a patient or blood donor. The RBCs to be tested are diluted with saline to approximately a 3% solution (3 drops of cells and about 100 drops of saline). One drop of 3% RBCs is mixed with one drop of anti-A in a glass tube labeled A. One drop of 3% RBCs is mixed with one drop anti-B in another tube labeled B. The tubes are centrifuged for 15 seconds at low speed. The RBC sediment on the bottom of the tube is gently suspended again and the solution is examined for agglutination.

The antisera will agglutinate the RBCs if the antigen is present. No agglutination will be observed if the antigen is not present. If a patient's RBCs agglutinate with anti-A but not anti-B, the patient belongs to the A group. If the RBCs agglutinate with anti-B and not with anti-A, the cells belong to the B group (FIG. 46-3). This procedure is called direct or forward typing (TABLE 46-1).

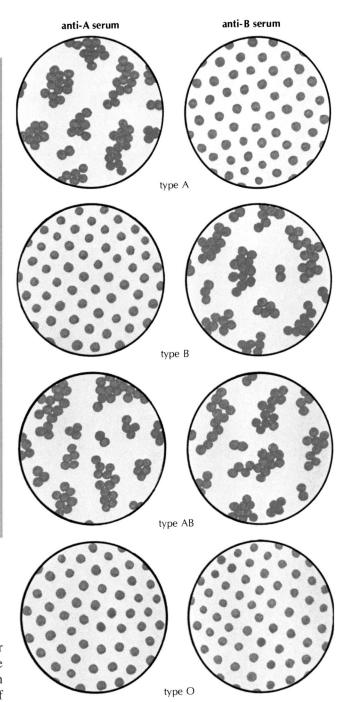

FIGURE 46-3. Blood typing. Red cells in type A blood are agglutinated (clumped) by anti-A serum; those in type B blood are agglutinated by anti-B serum. Type AB blood cells are agglutinated by both sera, and type O blood is not agglutinated by either serum.

The serum can be used to verify the ABO group of a patient or blood donor. Reagent a and b group cells are mixed with serum, centrifuged, and examined for agglutination. If a patient is A, serum will contain anti-B only. Agglutination will be observed with the b cells. This procedure using serum is called indirect or reverse typing (Table 46-1).

Table 46-1	ABO Group Testing Results			
	Reagents			**Group**
	anti-A	anti-B	a Cells	b Cells
R	1	2	2	1	**A**
E					
S	2	1	1	2	**B**
U	2	2	1	1	**O**
L					
T	1	1	2	2	**AB**

Rh Testing

Anti-D reagent is used to determine the Rh of RBCs. Add one drop of 3% cell suspension and one drop anti-D reagent in a test tube labeled D. Centrifuge for 15 seconds. Suspend the RBC button again and observe for agglutination. If agglutination is present, RBCs are Rh positive. If no agglutination is present, RBCs are Rh negative.

Many anti-D reagents require a control. One drop of 3% cell suspension and one drop of control reagent are added to a test tube labeled DC (D control). It is then centrifuged for 15 seconds, suspended again, and RBCs examined for agglutination. The control should always be negative for the test to be valid.

Checkpoint Question

6. Which ABO blood group is the universal donor? What does this mean?

BLOOD SUPPLY

Today one of the major problems facing the blood banks is obtaining sufficient supplies of safe blood and blood products to meet demand. There is a shortage of volunteer donors. The American Red Cross and other agencies collect blood from donors at bloodmobiles or sometimes at fixed sites. One donor blood unit containing about 450 mL whole blood can be divided into three products:

1. Packed RBCs, which can be stored at 2° to 8°C for 42 days and used to treat anemia

2. Plasma, which can be frozen for 1 year and used to treat bleeding caused by a lack of coagulation factors, such as fibrinogen

3. Platelet concentrates, which can be stored at room temperature for 5 days and used to treat bleeding due to low platelet count or dysfunctional platelets

Checkpoint Question

7. What three products can be obtained from 1 U whole blood, and how are they used?

WHAT IF

A patient asks you about the criteria for donating blood?

The American Red Cross bases criteria for donating blood on recommendations from government agencies and the Centers for Disease Control and Prevention and findings of research projects. In addition, each state has its own laws regulating blood donors. Generally, blood donors must meet the following criteria:

- Age 18 years or older (donors 17 years of age require a parent's permission; donors 65 years of age or older require a physician's consent)
- Weight 110 lb or more
- Hemoglobin at least 12.5 g/dL (women) or 13.5 g/dL (men)
- Pulse 50 to 110 beats per minute
- Blood pressure lower than 180/100

The donor also must provide a brief history. The entire procedure lasts approximately an hour; the actual blood donation time is about 10 minutes. Blood can be donated every 56 days. Only 1 U (pint) will be taken at a time. All blood will be tested by the American Red Cross for HIV, hepatitis, and syphilis.

Procedure 46-1

Performing a Mononucleosis Test

Purpose: To determine the presence or absence of the Epstein-Barr virus

Equipment: Patient's labeled specimen (whole blood, plasma, or serum, depending on the kit), mononucleosis kit (slide or card, controls, reagents, capillary tubes, bulb and stirrers), stopwatch or timer, saline, test tubes, pipettes (if titration is required)

Steps	Reason
1. Wash your hands.	Handwashing aids infection control.
2. Verify that the names on the specimen container and the laboratory form are the same.	
3. Assemble the equipment and ensure that the materials in the kit are at room temperature.	
4. Label the slide or card with the patient's name, positive control, and negative control. One circle or space is provided per patient and control.	This ensures accurate documentation.
5. Place the rubber bulb on the capillary tube and aspirate the patient's specimen to the marked line. Dispense the sample in the middle of the circle labeled with the patient's name. Avoid air bubbles to ensure accurate results.	
6. Gently mix the positive control. Using the capillary tube, aspirate the positive control to the marked line. Dispense the control in the middle of the circle labeled negative control. Avoid air bubbles.	These steps satisfy quality assurance and QC requirements.
7. Mix the latex reagent and add 1 drop to each circle or space (specimen, positive control, negative control). Avoid splashing the reagents, which can result in cross-contamination and incorrect results.	
8. Using a clean stirrer for each test, mix the reagent with the specimen and controls. Mix only one circle at a time, keeping within each circle. Going outside of the circle may lead to cross-contamination and incorrect results.	
9. Gently rock the slide for 2 minutes and observe for agglutination (clumping). Test time may vary if card is disposable.	
10. Verify the results of the controls before documenting the patient's results. Log controls and patient information on the worksheet.	

(continued)

Procedure 46-1   *(continued)*

Performing a Mononucleosis Test

Steps	Reason
11. Read the kit's instructions if titration is required.	
12. Clean the work area and dispose of waste properly. Wash the slide thoroughly with bleach and rinse with water before using again. Remove gown, gloves and shield. Wash your hands.	

Note: Kits vary with the manufacturer; read instructions carefully before beginning the procedure. Controls for test kits are usually done once per day or kit. Follow office policies and procedures for ensuring accuracy and QC. Controls are necessary for titration.

Charting Example

04/23/2005 10:00 A.M. Mono spot = neg on serum. _____ S. Miller, CMA

Procedure 46-2

Performing an HCG Pregnancy test

Purpose:	To detect the production of HCG to determine pregnancy
Equipment:	Patient's labeled specimen (plasma, serum, or urine depending on the kit), HCG pregnancy kit (test pack and transfer pipettes; kit contents will vary by manufacturer), HCG positive and negative control (different controls may be needed when testing urine), timer

Steps	Reason
1. Wash your hands.	Handwashing aids infection control.
2. Assemble the equipment.	
3. Verify that the names on the specimen container and the laboratory form are the same.	
4. Label the test pack (depending on type of kit) with the patient's name, positive control, and negative control. Use one test pack per patient and control.	
5. Note in the patient's information and in the control log whether you are using urine, plasma, or serum. Be sure that the kit and controls are at room temperature.	

(continued)

Procedure 46-2 *(continued)*

Performing an HCG Pregnancy test

Steps	Reason
6. Aspirate the patient's specimen using the transfer pipette and place three drops (180 mL) on the sample well of the test pack labeled with the patient's name.	
7. Aspirate the positive control using the transfer pipette and place three drops (180 mL) on the sample well of the test pack labeled positive control. Avoid splashing to eliminate cross-contamination.	This satisfies quality assurance and QC standards.
8. Aspirate the negative control using the transfer pipette, and place three drops (180 mL) on the sample well of the test pack labeled negative control. Avoid splashing to eliminate cross-contamination.	This satisfies quality assurance and QC standards.
9. Report the results when the end-of-assay window is red, after approximately 7 minutes for serum samples and 4 minutes for urine samples. Check to verify controls before reporting the results. Repeat the test if the end-of-assay window does not appear and if the controls do not work.	Waiting the appropriate amount of time ensures that testing is complete.
10. Record controls and patient's information on the worksheet and log form.	
11. Clean the work area and dispose of waste properly. Remove gown, gloves, and shield. Wash your hands.	

Note: Kits vary with the manufacturer; read instructions carefully before beginning. Controls for test kits are usually done once per day or kit. Follow office policies and procedures for ensuring accuracy and QC.

Charting Example

12/14/2005 9:30 A.M. Pt. c/o late period—LMP 11/22/05. C/o nausea in the A.M., breast tenderness. Urine sample positive for pregnancy. Dr. Wong in to examine pt. Pregnancy brochures explained to pt. RTC. _____
J. Simpson, CMA

Procedure 46-3

Performing a Group A Rapid Strep Test

Purpose: To determine the presence of Streptococcus pyogenes in the specimen

Equipment: Patient's labeled throat specimen, beta-strep agar culture (use a Culturette with two swabs provided), bacitracin disks, group A strep kit (controls may be included, depending on the kit), timer.

Steps	Reason
1. Wash your hands.	
2. Verify that the names on the specimen container and the laboratory form are the same.	
3. Label one extraction tube with the patient's name, one with the positive control, and one with the negative control.	
4. Follow the directions for the kit. Add the appropriate reagents and drops to each of the extraction tubes. Avoid splashing, and use the correct number of drops.	Following the manufacturer's instructions exactly will ensure that you adhere to the appropriate testing guidelines.
5. Insert the patient's swab (one of the two swabs) into the labeled extraction tube. If only one culture swab was submitted, first swab a beta strep agar plate, then use the swab for the rapid strep test.	This begins the test without contaminating the culture specimen.
6. Add the appropriate controls to each of the labeled extraction tubes.	This begins the chemical reaction for proper control results.
7. Set the timer for the appropriate time to ensure accuracy.	
8. Add the appropriate reagent and drops to each of the extraction tubes.	
9. Use the swab to mix the reagents. Then press out any excess fluid on the swab against the inside of the tube.	This helps deposit the maximum amount of substance to be tested.
10. Add three drops from the well-mixed extraction tube to the sample window of the strep A test unit labeled with the patient's name. Do the same for each control.	
11. Set the timer for the appropriate time.	
12. A positive result appears as a line in the result window within 5 minutes. The strep A test unit has an internal control; if a line appears in the control window, the test is valid.	
13. Read a negative result at exactly 5 minutes to avoid a false negative.	

(continued)

Procedure 46-3   *(continued)*

Performing a Group A Rapid Strep Test

Steps	Reason
14. Verify results of the controls before recording test results. Log the controls and the patient's information on the worksheet.	
15. Depending on laboratory protocol, you may have to culture all negative rapid strep screens on beta-strep agar. A bacitracin disk may be added to the first quadrant when you set up or after 24 hours if a beta-hemolytic colony appears. A culture is more sensitive than a rapid immunoassay test.	
16. Clean the work area and dispose of waste properly. Remove gown, gloves, and shield. Wash your hands.	

Note: Beta strep agar and bacitracin must come to room temperature before being used.

Kits vary with the manufacturer; read instructions carefully before beginning. Controls for test kits are usually done once per day or kit. Follow office policies and procedures for ensuring accuracy and QC.

Charting Example

05/22/2005 11:15 A.M. Pt c/o sore throat ×2 days. Group A rapid strep test positive. Dr. Harrison notified.
_____ B. White, RMA

CHAPTER SUMMARY

Serological testing addresses the reaction of antigen and antibody substances. Specimens may be serum, urine, or spinal fluid. The most common types of test are the agglutination and ELISA. QC procedures are to be adhered to each day of testing specimens. There are many types of test kits, and it is important to become familiar with the steps required for each type of testing. Because many of your physician's patients may have to undergo transfusions for various surgeries, it is imperative that you have a good understanding of the ABO blood groups and the RH types so you can answer questions and provide adequate patient education.

Critical Thinking Challenges

1. You are working for Dr. Mathers, a cardiothoracic surgeon. Dr. Mathers performs many surgeries during which patients have substantial blood loss requiring transfusions. Identify the available options for blood transfusions. How do you explain these to a patient facing elective surgery?

2. Your chapter of the American Red Cross is in great need of volunteer donors. Formulate a plan for encouraging more community members to donate blood. How can you put your plan into action?

Answers to Checkpoint Questions

1. A test that is specific and sensitive can measure a substance even if only a tiny amount is present (specificity), and it can pick that substance out of a solution containing millions of other related substances (sensitivity).

2. Two serology test methods are agglutination and ELISA. ELISA produces a color change. With agglutination tests, particles clump if the test substance is present.

3. Improper storage of the kit may result in deterioration of the reagents, hence false test results.

4. A false-negative result occurs when a patient who has a disease tests negative for it. A false-positive result occurs when a test indicates that a patient has a particular disease although he or she does not. These results can be caused by technical problems in performing the test or by the patient's biological condition.

5. Serology tests are easier to perform and provide results more quickly, but cultures are considered to be more sensitive.

6. Type O is the universal donor because it lacks A or B antigens, making it safe to give patients no matter what their ABO group.

7. A single unit of whole blood can be divided into packed RBCs (used to treat anemia), plasma (used to treat bleeding from a lack of coagulation factors), and platelet concentrates (used to treat bleeding caused by low platelet count or dysfunctional platelets).

47

Clinical Chemistry

CHAPTER OUTLINE

INSTRUMENTS AND METHODOLOGY

RENAL FUNCTION
Electrolytes
Nonprotein Nitrogenous
  Compounds

LIVER FUNCTION
Bilirubin
Enzymes

THYROID FUNCTION
Thyroid-Stimulating Hormone

CARDIAC FUNCTION
Creatine Kinase-MB
Troponin

PANCREATIC FUNCTION
Pancreatic Enzymes
Pancreatic Hormones and
  Carbohydrate Metabolism

LIPIDS AND LIPOPROTEINS
Cholesterol
Low-Density Lipoprotein
High-Density Lipoprotein
Triglycerides

ROLE DELINEATION

CLINICAL: Fundamental Principles
  • Apply principles of aseptic technique and infection
    control

CLINICAL: Diagnostic Orders
  • Collect and process specimens
  • Perform diagnostic tests

CLINICAL: Patient Care
  • Prepare patient for examinations, procedures, and
    treatments

GENERAL: Legal Concepts
  • Perform within legal and ethical boundaries
  • Document accurately

GENERAL: Instruction
  • Instruct individuals according to their needs

CHAPTER COMPETENCIES

LEARNING OBJECTIVES
Upon successfully completing this chapter, you will be able to:

1. Spell and define the key terms.
2. List the common electrolytes and explain the relationship of electrolytes to acid-base balance.
3. Describe the nonprotein nitrogenous compounds and name conditions with abnormal values.
4. List and describe the substances commonly tested in liver function assessment.
5. Explain thyroid function and the hormone that regulates the thyroid gland.
6. Describe how an assessment for a myocardial infarction is made with laboratory tests.
7. Describe how pancreatitis is diagnosed with laboratory tests.
8. Describe glucose use and regulation and the purpose of the various glucose tests.
9. Describe the function of cholesterol and other lipids and their correlation to heart disease.

PERFORMANCE OBJECTIVES
Upon successfully completing this chapter, you will be able to:

1. Determine blood glucose (Procedure 47-1).
2. Perform a glucose tolerance test (Procedure 47-2).

KEY TERMS

amylase	creatine	intracellular	lipids
bicarbonate	extracellular	ions	lipoproteins
bile	gestational diabetes	lipase	nitrogenous
body fluids			

CLINICAL CHEMISTRY entails testing for many of the chemical components found in serum, plasma, whole blood, and other **body fluids** (fluids that accumulate in the body's compartments). The chemical components can be electrically charged atoms called **ions** (K^+, Na^+, Cl^-), metabolic byproducts (urea, creatinine), proteins (albumin, globulin), or hormones (e.g., testosterone and thyroid-stimulating hormone [TSH]). Quantifying the amount of these chemicals can help the physician:

- Assess organ function (e.g., bilirubin level is an indicator of liver function)
- Gain a better understanding of the patient's overall health status (e.g., glucose and cholesterol levels can aid in assessing a patient's health)

Only a few specific chemistry tests may be performed in the physician office laboratory, but it is important for you to understand the purpose of these tests. Specimen collection, reporting, and follow-up of patient care may be your responsibility. This information is often vitally important to the treatment and recovery of the patient.

INSTRUMENTS AND METHODOLOGY

The spectrophotometer is still widely used for quantifying various substances in a patient's blood. Certain chemical substances in reaction with other chemicals will cause color formation or a color change. The concentration of the substance is determined by measuring the change in the intensity of the color.

Much chemical analysis is performed in reference laboratories on automated systems that mechanically sample, dilute, or add reagents (chemicals) to the patient's blood for quantifying components. Automation has allowed more rapid analyses, reduced operator error, and helped control the cost of testing by reducing human intervention. Small office analyzers (also called bench-top analyzers) use the color change principle to determine levels of chemicals. The normal ranges included in this text may vary among laboratories because of the use of different substrates, temperatures, and instruments.

Many chemistry tests are grouped according to body system. These are called panels or profiles. Since most of these are not performed in the physician office, this chapter does not describe them in detail. However, a basic understanding of these is necessary when taking laboratory reports by phone.

 Checkpoint Question

1. How does the physician use chemistry test results?

RENAL FUNCTION

The kidneys rid the body of waste products and help maintain fluid balance and acid-base balance. When the kidneys begin to fail, waste products, such as urea, ammonia, and creatinine, build up in the blood. The patient becomes edematous, and the delicate acid-base balance is upset. Abnormal increases or decreases in the substances that affect acid-base balance compromise health and may cause death. To assess renal function, the physician may order tests for serum measurements of electrolytes, blood urea nitrogen (BUN), creatinine, and other components. These tests, combined with information from urinalysis, can significantly aid in renal assessment.

Electrolytes

Electrolytes are **ions** (chemicals that carry an electrical charge) in blood and body fluids. They may be positively charged (cations) or negatively charged (anions). Electrolytes conduct electrical impulses across cell membranes to maintain fluid and acid-base balance and aid in the functioning of nerve cells and muscle tissue.

Electrolytes include sodium, potassium, chloride, calcium, magnesium, phosphorus, and **bicarbonate** (dissolved carbon dioxide). The renal system helps regulate electrolytes and fluid and acid-base balance. In the presence of an electrolyte imbalance, electric impulses are not transmitted properly, resulting in fluid and acid-base imbalances and impaired functioning of nervous and muscle tissue. TABLE 47-1 summarizes common electrolyte imbalances.

Sodium

Sodium (chemical symbol Na) is the major cation of the **extracellular** fluid (the fluid outside the cell). Normal serum levels range from 135 to 145 mEq/L. Hyponatremia (sodium level below 135 mEq/L), one of the most common electrolyte imbalances, can result from many factors, including gastrointestinal losses (vomiting, diarrhea), burn, cardiac or renal failure, and hypothyroidism. Symptoms of hyponatremia range in severity with the value. These may manifest as changes in energy levels and as neurological malfunctions, including seizures.

Hypernatremia (sodium level above 145 mEq/L) can be caused by drug therapy, Cushing syndrome, diabetes insipidus, and other pathologies. Typically, the kidneys help the body adjust to this more saline (salty) environment by not excreting as much water. In this way, sodium is diluted to an acceptable level. Because water is retained in hypernatremia, the patient may show signs of edema.

Potassium

Potassium (chemical symbol K) is the major cation of the intracellular fluid (fluid within the cell). Only 2% of potassium is extracellular; therefore, serum levels are much lower than those of sodium: 3.5 to 5.0 mEq/L. Hypokalemia (potassium level below 3.5 mEq/L) may occur with insulin therapy, gastrointestinal losses, and renal disease. Hyperkalemia (potassium level above 5.0 mEq/L) can occur with cell injuries and renal failure. Artifactual (caused by outside interference) hyperkalemia can result from red blood cell lysis, as with a traumatic venipuncture or the tourniquet left on the arm too long or applied too tightly. Abnormal blood levels of potassium can result in muscle weakness, paralysis, and cardiac arrhythmias.

Chloride

Chloride (chemical symbol Cl) is the major anion of the extracellular fluid. The normal range for chloride is 96 to 110 mEq/L. Hypochloremia is a condition in which the serum chloride level is below 96 mEq/L. In hyperchloremia, the serum chloride level is above 110 mEq/L. Chloride is closely associated with acid-base balance and is adversely affected in such conditions as diabetic ketoacidosis and **metabolic acidosis** (a condition of increased metabolic acids).

Calcium

Calcium (chemical symbol Ca) is a cation, with normal serum levels ranging from 8.5 to 10.5 mg/dL. Hypocalcemia (calcium level significantly below 8.5 mg/dL) may occur with acute or chronic renal failure or electrolyte imbalance due to hypoparathyroidism. Hypercalcemia (calcium level above 10.5 mg/dL) may occur in a condition such as hyperparathyroidism or excessive calcium absorption due to medication or alteration in gastrointestinal metabolism.

Magnesium

Magnesium (chemical symbol Mg) is a cation found in intracellular fluid. Normal magnesium levels range from 1.3 to 2.1 mEq/L. Hypomagnesemia (magnesium level below 1.3 mEq/L) may result from shifts in body fluids and other electrolytes. Hypermagnesemia (magnesium level above

Table 47-1	TERMS DESCRIBING ELECTROLYTE IMBALANCES
Imbalance	**Definition**
Hypernatremia	Excessive sodium in blood
Hyponatremia	Deficit of sodium in blood
Hyperkalemia	Excessive potassium in blood
Hypokalemia	Deficit of potassium in blood
Hyperchloremia	Excessive chloride in blood
Hypochloremia	Deficit of chloride in blood
Hyperphosphatemia	Excessive phosphate in blood
Hypophosphatemia	Deficit of phosphate in blood
Hypercalcemia	Excessive calcium in blood
Hypocalcemia	Deficit of calcium in blood
Hypermagnesemia	Excessive magnesium in blood
Hypomagnesemia	Deficit of magnesium in blood

2.1 mEq/L) may also result from fluid and electrolyte shifts and from impaired excretion caused by kidney failure. Symptoms of hypermagnesemia are similar to those of hyperkalemia.

Phosphorus

Phosphorus (chemical symbol P) is the major anion in the intracellular fluid. Normal phosphorus levels range from 2.5 to 4.5 mg/dL. Hypophosphatemia (phosphorus level below 2.5 mg/dL) can result from a number of factors, including inadequate absorption, gastrointestinal losses, electrolyte shifts, and endocrine disorders. Hyperphosphatemia (phosphorus level above 4.5 mg/dL) may occur with hypocalcemia, hypoparathyroidism, and renal impairment or failure. In patients with renal failure, soft tissue calcification is a long-term effect of hyperphosphatemia.

Bicarbonate

Bicarbonate (chemical symbol HCO_3) is formed when carbon dioxide dissolves in the bloodstream, forming another negatively charged ion in the extracellular fluid. Bicarbonate is the major factor in acid-base balance; increased levels result in alkalosis (the body pH is too basic), and decreased levels may result in acidosis (the body pH is too acidic).

The acid-base system is extremely sensitive and cannot tolerate large pH fluctuations. The body's normal pH range is 7.35 to 7.45, very slightly basic (neutral 7.0). The renal and respiratory systems work to regulate acid-base balance. Bicarbonate is breathed out in the form of carbon dioxide and is also excreted through the kidneys. Measurement of carbon dioxide is considered more useful for pH balance assessment than for measuring renal function, but it also aids in the overall assessment of renal function.

Checkpoint Question

2. What is hyperkalemia? Name three possible causes.

Nonprotein Nitrogenous Compounds

Three nonprotein **nitrogenous** compounds that can be increased as a consequence of impaired renal function are urea, creatinine, and uric acid. However, other diseases can also affect the concentrations of these substances, making this a relatively nonspecific indicator.

Urea

Urea is the major end product of protein and amino acid metabolism. Because urea is formed in the liver and excreted mainly by the kidneys, it can be an indicator for both liver and renal function. Typically urea, measured as BUN, ranges from 10 to 20 mg/dL. Various factors besides renal and liver function, such as dietary intake of protein and state of hydration, affect BUN levels.

Creatinine

Creatinine is a breakdown product of **creatine**, which aids in delivering energy to cells. Normal range for creatinine is 0.8 to 1.4 mg/dL, with normal ranges varying slightly among laboratories. Creatinine is more specific than BUN for assessing renal function. This is because only trace amounts of creatinine are reabsorbed in the renal tubules. Urinary excretion of this compound equals the amount produced in the body, whereas urea is reabsorbed to a certain extent. This is useful in determining the filtering ability of the kidneys.

A test called creatinine clearance is used for this purpose. A 24-hour urine sample is collected for a creatinine clearance, because excretion of creatinine varies throughout the day. (See Chapter 43.)

Uric Acid

Uric acid is a metabolic end product of proteins containing purine. For men, the normal range is 4.0 to 8.5 mg/dL, and for women, 2.7 to 7.3 mg/dL. Increased amounts of uric acid are more significant than decreased amounts. Hyperuricemia may occur with renal failure, use of diuretics (substances that promote urine formation and excretion), obesity, and atherosclerosis. Diets high in proteins (meat, legumes, and yeast) can cause mild hyperuricemia. The disease gout is characterized by high uric acid accumulation in the joints; the joints become inflamed and painful.

LIVER FUNCTION

The liver is the largest gland of the body and one of the most complex. Among its major functions are the production of **bile** (bitter yellow-green secretion), metabolism of many compounds used by the body (glucose, fats, proteins, and vitamins), processing of bilirubin, and detoxifying substances in the blood.

Bilirubin, alkaline phosphatase (ALP), alanine aminotransferase (ALT), and aspartate aminotransferase (AST) are some of the commonly tested enzymes that help determine liver function.

Bilirubin

Red blood cells live approximately 120 days; the liver and spleen remove worn-out cells from the circulation. The worn-out cells break down, and hemoglobin is released and converted to bilirubin. It travels through the bloodstream until it enters the liver and is excreted into the bile. Bilirubin is yellow-orange; if excess amounts settle into the skin and sclera, it makes the patient appear yellow (jaundiced).

WHAT IF

A patient is diagnosed with gout and asks you about dietary restrictions?

First and foremost, speak to the physician to determine whether the patient has any other medical conditions that warrant a special diet. Most patients with gout are prescribed a low-purine diet initially. Foods that are high in purine are liver, kidneys, sweetbreads, sardines, anchovies, and meat extracts. Diet and medications can often keep gout under control. Dietary retraining is usually done by the physician or a registered dietitian.

Checkpoint Question

3. Name the nonprotein nitrogenous compounds important for assessing renal function.

Enzymes

An enzyme is a protein produced by living cells that speeds up chemical reactions. The liver has many enzymes.

Alkaline Phosphatase

ALP is present in the bones, liver, intestines, kidneys, and placenta. Circulating ALP is primarily from the liver and bone. Levels of ALP rise in bone and liver disorders.

Normal values vary with age. High levels of ALP are considered normal during periods of bone growth, such as childhood growth spurts and third-trimester pregnancy.

Alanine Aminotransferase and Aspartate Aminotransferase

ALT and AST are enzymes in the liver. AST is present in many other organs as well. Increased levels of ALT and AST occur with liver damage.

Checkpoint Question

4. Name four common tests that evaluate liver function.

THYROID FUNCTION

The thyroid gland regulates metabolism by secreting the hormones triiodothyronine and thyroxine. The thyroid gland is controlled by another hormone, TSH, which is produced in the anterior pituitary gland.

Thyroid-Stimulating Hormone

In the absence of disease, when additional thyroid hormones are needed, more TSH is secreted to stimulate the thyroid gland. In the same manner, when lesser amounts of the hormones are required, less TSH is secreted and the thyroid gland reduces its production. However, many situations can cause an imbalance in this delicate endocrine system. Malfunction of the anterior pituitary gland results in oversecretion or undersecretion of TSH. If the thyroid gland is malfunctioning, it cannot be stimulated regardless of the amount of TSH secreted. TSH levels may be quite high in cases such as this.

CARDIAC FUNCTION

When a myocardial infarction occurs, the damaged heart muscle releases into the bloodstream large quantities of specific enzymes.

Creatine Kinase-MB

Creatine kinase (CK) is found almost exclusively in skeletal muscle and myocardium. CK has three isoenzymes, designated MM (muscle), MB (heart), and BB (brain). CKMB levels, along with total CK, are tested in persons who have chest pain to determine whether they have had a heart attack. Within 2 to 8 hours of a myocardial infarction, CK levels will increase. CK also increases in crushing injuries to muscles, such as those sustained in car accidents. Most of the normal levels of CK consist of the MM fraction. The MB fraction rises with myocardial infarction. A high total CK may indicate damage to either the heart or other muscles, but a high CKMB suggests that the damage was to heart muscle.

Troponin

Troponin is a protein specific to heart muscle, making it a valuable tool in the diagnosis of acute myocardial infarction. Troponin blood levels begin to rise within 4 hours of the onset of myocardial damage and stay elevated for up to 14 days, which means levels can be measured to monitor the effectiveness of thrombolytic therapy in heart attack patients.

PANCREATIC FUNCTION

The pancreas functions in both the endocrine and exocrine systems and produces many secretions. **Amylase** and **lipase**, two of its exocrine system products, are released as excretory enzymes into the intestines to aid in digestion. Insulin and glucagon, hormonal products of its endocrine function, are released into the bloodstream to regulate carbohydrate metabolism.

Pancreatic Enzymes

Amylase and Lipase

Amylase is markedly increased with pancreatitis (inflammation of the pancreas). The salivary glands also produce amylase, which accounts for the elevated levels occurring with inflammatory diseases of the salivary glands, such as mumps. **Lipase levels also rise with pancreatitis.** For a differential diagnosis of pancreatitis, it is recommended that both enzymes be measured.

Pancreatic Hormones and Carbohydrate Metabolism

Glucose is a primary energy source for the body. When foods are metabolized, nutrients including glucose are released. For glucose to be used for stored energy in the form of glycogen, it must be brought into the cells. Two hormones, insulin and glucagon, regulate this process. Blood glucose levels must be maintained within narrow limits or adverse physical effects may occur. By their actions, insulin and glucagon keep these levels within the approximate range.

Glucose-Regulating Hormones

Insulin brings the glucose used for energy into cells for immediate use or for storage. If sufficient energy is available for cell use, the glucose is stored as either glycogen (long chains of glucose) in the liver and muscles or as fat. Insulin is an important hormone; cells starve if insulin is not available or if the cells cannot bring glucose in for energy. **By facilitating glucose storage, insulin keeps glucose levels down, thereby maintaining a stable normal range.**

The hormone glucagon releases into the bloodstream glucose stored as glycogen, thereby raising glucose levels. Whenever blood glucose levels drop, glucagon acts on glycogen to break it apart so that molecules of glucose are available for cellular use.

Checkpoint Question

5. Which enzyme can assist the physician to diagnose a myocardial infarction within 3 hours of onset? Why?

Common Glucose Tests

For diagnostic usefulness, the time a blood sample is taken for glucose testing must be related to fasting or to the time of the previous meal.

The glucose reflectance photometer (glucose meter) is a quick, accurate, easy in-office procedure to measure a patient's blood glucose level. Glucose meters are sold under several names, including the Glucometer, the Accu-Chek, and the Glucosan, among others (FIG. 47-1). The testing

FIGURE 47–1. Glucose 201 hand-held glucose monitor. (Courtesy of HemoCue, Mission Viejo, CA.)

principle is application of whole blood to a reagent strip, which is read optically by the instrument after a designated time (Procedure 47-1). The amount of color change (to blue) correlates with glucose concentration and a value is reported.

Fasting Blood Glucose, or Sugar A fasting blood sugar (FBS) level can be obtained from the patient after an 8- to 12-hour fast (nothing but water is ingested during the fast). Procedure 47-1 describes obtaining an FBS level using a glucose meter. The main purpose of an FBS is to detect either diabetes mellitus or hypoglycemia. The American Diabetes Association's cutoff point for normal fasting blood glucose levels was dropped from 110 mg/dL to 100 mg/dL. A value of 100 mg/dL or above leads to a diagnosis of impaired fasting glucose, included in the term prediabetes. Prediabetes occurs when a person's glucose levels are higher than normal but not yet high enough for a diagnosis of diabetes. Studies indicate that many people in the prediabetic range go on to develop diabetes within 10 years.

Further testing by either a 2-hour postprandial glucose test or a glucose tolerance test (GTT) is used to corroborate the initial high result. Hypoglycemia is a syndrome characterized by FBS levels below 45 mg/dL and a variety of symptoms: sweating, weakness, dizziness, headache, trembling, lethargy, and other nervous manifestations.

Random Blood Glucose Although a random glucose test is not as diagnostically useful as a fasting test, it is a good screening tool. A random glucose specimen can be drawn anytime during the day; the normal range is less than 126 mg/dL.

Two-Hour Postprandial Glucose A 2-hour postprandial glucose (PP) test is used to screen for diabetes and to monitor insulin therapy of diabetic patients. The patient must eat a high-carbohydrate meal after a 12-hour fast. Patients who may not be compliant are given a glucose solution to drink as a substitute for the meal. Then, 2 hours after the meal, a blood sample is drawn and glucose is measured. Timing of the specimen collection is extremely important for this test result. "Good control" of diabetes has been defined as a 2-hour PP value of less than 140 mg/dL.

Glucose Tolerance Test   The GTT is used to diagnose diabetes and hypoglycemia. The patient is tested with a large dose of glucose; then blood glucose levels are checked at intervals to see how the body metabolizes the glucose (FIG. 47-2. A low-carbohydrate diet (less than 150 g of carbohydrate per day) prior to testing will result in an abnormal glucose tolerance study.

The GTT follows a check of the fasting glucose (Procedure 47-2). Blood is obtained 30 minutes and 1, 2, and 3 hours after the glucose has been administered. Blood sampling must occur at the precise times indicated for valid diagnosis. Urine specimens may also be collected during the timed intervals.

A serum or plasma specimen can be collected, depending on laboratory protocol. The specimen should be centrifuged and separated as soon as possible to prevent metabolism of glucose by red blood cells. Specimens collected in gray stopper tubes containing sodium fluoride are stable for up to 3 days even without centrifugation.

Interpretation of GTT Results   Medical assistants do not interpret the results of the GTT. Numerous methods are used to interpret the values obtained from a GTT. The criteria proposed by the National Diabetes Data Group and the World Health Organization and endorsed by the American Diabetes Association recommend a diagnosis of diabetes if the fasting glucose level is greater than 110 mg/dL and the 2-hour measurement is equal to or above 155 mg/dL.

Hypoglycemia can also be diagnosed by the GTT. Symptoms of hypoglycemia include headaches, weakness, shakiness, fatigue, sweating, and light-headedness. Whenever any of these occurs during a GTT, it is important to obtain a blood specimen from the patient even if it is not at an appointed time. Unfortunately, a glucose level that is lower than the normal range often does not correspond to the patient's symptoms. It is thought that emotional states and anxieties, not low glucose levels, may cause the symptoms. Frequently these same patients improve when their food intake is divided so that they eat many small meals (introducing smaller glucose loads) rather than several large ones.

  Checkpoint Question

6. What is hypoglycemia? List its signs and symptoms.

Diabetic Glucose Testing   **Although blood glucose levels are used to detect and monitor diabetic patients, the test of choice is hemoglobin A$_1$C.** This allows the physician to form an accurate picture of a diabetic's physiological condition over weeks.

Obstetric Glucose Testing   An increase of glucose intolerance has been frequently noted among pregnant patients in the second and third trimesters. Because **gestational diabetes** can endanger the fetus, the pregnant patient's glucose level must be monitored. The widely accepted screening method used for this purpose is to administer a 50-g glucose load in drink form and draw blood 1 hour later. If the value exceeds 155 mg/dL, a GTT is indicated for a diagnosis of gestational diabetes. This screen is usually done during the second trimester.

LIPIDS AND LIPOPROTEINS

Cholesterol and associated **lipids** (free fatty acids) and **lipoproteins** (substances composed of lipids and proteins) have long been implicated in heart disease. However, these compounds are important building blocks of our bodies and in proper quantities are vital to health maintenance. They are a component of every cell membrane and of the myelin sheath around the nerves. They also cushion and support organs. Testing for these quantities aids the physician in assessing the risk of heart disease (FIG. 47-3).

Cholesterol

Bile acids, partly formed by cholesterol, are produced in the liver, stored in the gallbladder and released into the intestine as needed for the digestion of fats. Vitamin D is formed from

FIGURE 47–2.   Commercial glucose tolerance test beverage, 50 g and 100 g. (Reprinted with permission from McCall R. *Phlebotomy Essentials.* Baltimore: Lippincott Williams & Wilkins, 2003.)

PATIENT EDUCATION

Using a Glucose Meter

Many diabetic patients routinely monitor glucose levels at home. As a medical assistant, you can help reinforce use of this procedure. Help the patient get familiar with the analyzer. Instruct the patient to adhere to the manufacturer's instructions. Here are points to stress:

- Teach patients about the need to test and document glucose levels regularly.
- Instruct the patient in maintaining a quality control record for the instrument using control materials within the expiration date and as directed by the manufacturer.
- Offer instructions in the proper technique for obtaining a blood sample (e.g., cleanse the area well before beginning and do not milk the finger).
- Caution patients against self-regulating with insulin. Have patients call the physician if glucose levels are abnormal.
- Alert patients to the signs and symptoms of high and low glucose levels and the treatments for each.

Most pharmacies and surgical supply stores that sell glucose meters will teach patients to use them. The strips for glucose meters are expensive and may be covered by certain insurance companies if the physician clearly documents the need.

rigid. Circulation to the organs and other areas normally supplied by these arteries is reduced. Atherosclerosis is the major cause of coronary heart disease, angina pectoris, myocardial infarction, and other cardiac disorders. As LDL values rise above the normal range, the risk of heart disease increases.

High-Density Lipoprotein

High-density lipoprotein (HDL) is the protein molecule that carries cholesterol from arterial walls back to the liver. Quantities of HDL typically are less than those of LDL. Much research has been directed along the lines of increasing HDL, because high levels of it correlate with reduction in the risk of heart disease. In contrast, decreased HDL levels correlate with increased risk of heart disease.

Triglycerides

Triglycerides store energy. They are stored in adipose tissue and muscle and released and metabolized between meals according to the body's energy demands. Adipose (fatty) tissue is composed almost entirely of triglycerides. The normal range is less than 150 mg/dL. Research identifies triglycerides as a risk factor in heart disease.

A summary of the common chemistry tests is presented in TABLE 47-2.

 Checkpoint Question

7. Which lipoprotein is beneficial? Why?

cholesterol at the skin's surface during exposure to sunlight. Various hormones, such as cortisol, testosterone, and estrogen, are also synthesized from cholesterol. Only in proportions not necessary for cell maintenance and other body functions should cholesterol be considered a health hazard.

Measurement of cholesterol is done on a 12- to 14-hour fasting blood specimen. The ideal range for cholesterol is less than 200 mg/dL (as recommended by the American Heart Association). Anyone with a cholesterol level above 200 mg/dL is considered to be at risk for developing atherosclerosis.

Low-Density Lipoprotein

Low-density lipoprotein (LDL) is a plasma protein that transports cholesterol from the liver to the walls of large and medium-sized arteries. Atherosclerotic plaques form, causing the affected vessel to thicken and become more

FIGURE 47–3. The Cholestech analyzer can perform tests for cholesterol, triglyceride, low-density lipoprotein, and high-density lipoprotein. (Cholestech, Heywood, CA.)

Table 47–2   COMMON CHEMISTRY PANEL TESTS

Test	Body Function	Normal Value	Causes of Increase	Causes of Decrease
BUN	Metabolic byproduct	7–18 mg/dL	Kidney disease, kidney obstruction, dehydration	Liver failure, malnutrition
Calcium	Structural element for bones, teeth, muscles	8.5–10.5 mg/dL	Hyperparathyroidism, hyperthyroidism, Addison disease, bone cancer, multiple myeloma, other malignancies	Hypoparathyroidism, renal failure
Chloride	Acid-base balance, component of stomach acid	98–106 mEq/L	Dehydration, Cushing syndrome, hyperven-tilation	Severe vomiting, severe diarrhea, severe burn, pyloric obstruction, heat exhaustion
Cholesterol	Building block for cell membranes, steroid hormones, bile acids	120–200 mg/dL	Atherosclerosis, heart disease, certain liver diseases with obstruction, hypothyroidism	Liver disease, hyperthy-roidism, malabsorption syndrome
Creatinine	Metabolic byproduct	0.6–1.2 mg/dL	Kidney disease, muscle disease	Muscular dystrophy
Glucose	Energy source	70–110 mg/dL	Diabetes mellitus, Cushing syndrome, liver disease	Excessive insulin, Addison disease, bacterial sepsis, hypothyroidism
Phosphorus	Used in bone, endocrine processes	2.7–4.5 mg/dL	Renal disease, hypoparathyroidism, hypocalcemia, Addison disease	Hyperparathyroidism, bone disease
Potassium	Acid-base balance	3.5–5.0 mEq/L	Kidney disease, cell damage, Addison disease	Diarrhea, starvation, severe vomiting, severe burn, some liver diseases
Sodium	Fluid balance	135–148 mEq/L	Dehydration, Cushing syndrome, diabetes insipidus	Severe burns, diarrhea, vomiting, Addison disease
Triglycerides	Energy source; lipid deposits for stored energy, organ support	Men: 40–160 mg/dL Women: 35–135 mg/dL	Atherosclerosis, liver disease, poorly controlled diabetes, pancreatitis	Malnutrition
Uric acid	Metabolic byproduct	Men: 3.5–7.2 mg/dL Women: 2.6–6.0 mg/dL	Renal failure, gout, leukemia, eclampsia	Drug therapy to lower uric acid levels

Procedure 47-1

Determining Blood Glucose

Purpose: To determine the level of glucose in the blood for diagnosis and treatment of hypoglycemia and hyperglycemia.

Equipment: Glucose meter of the physician's choice, glucose reagent strips, lancet, alcohol pad, sterile gauze, paper towel, adhesive bandage, gloves.

Steps	Reason
1. Wash your hands.	Handwashing aids infection control.
2. Assemble the equipment and supplies.	
3. Put on gloves before removing reagent strip.	Sugar residues on hands can falsely elevate glucose results if the strip is touched.
4. Turn on the instrument and ensure that it is calibrated.	Calibration of the glucose meter is essential for accurate test results.
5. Remove one reagent strip, lay it on the paper towel, and recap the container.	The strip is ready for testing. The paper towel will serve as a disposable work surface and will absorb excess blood added to the strip. The strips are sensitive to humidity and will deteriorate if allowed to absorb moisture.
6. Greet and identify the patient. Explain the procedure. Ask for and answer any questions.	
7. Have the patient wash hands in warm water.	Washing removes sugar residues from the skin, and the warm water stimulates blood flow.
8. Cleanse the selected puncture site (finger) with alcohol.	Alcohol removes bacteria from the site.

Step 8. Cleanse the site. (Reprinted with permission from McCall R: Phlebotomy Essentials. Baltimore: Lippincott Williams & Wilkins, 2003.)

(continued)

Procedure 47-1 *(continued)*

Determining Blood Glucose

Steps	Reason
9. Perform a capillary puncture, following the steps described in Chapter 44. Wipe away the first drop of blood.	

Step 9. Puncture the site with an automatic safety lancet. (Reprinted with permission from McCall R: Phlebotomy Essentials. Baltimore: Lippincott Williams & Wilkins, 2003.)

10. Turn the patient's hand palm down and gently squeeze the finger to form a large drop of blood.	Gentle squeezing obtains a blood specimen without diluting the sample with tissue fluid.

Step 10. Round blood drop forming at the puncture site. (Reprinted with permission from McCall R: Phlebotomy Essentials. Baltimore: Lippincott Williams & Wilkins, 2003.)

(continued)

Procedure 47-1 (continued)

Determining Blood Glucose

Steps	Reason
11. Bring the reagent strip up to the finger and touch the pad to the blood. Do not touch the finger. Completely cover the pad with blood.	The entire pad must be covered for accurate reading. There is no chance of contamination by oils or other residue remaining on the finger if this surface is not touched.
12. Insert reagent strip into analyzer, meanwhile applying pressure to the puncture wound with gauze. The meter will continue to incubate the strip and measure the reaction.	This allows time for the reaction.
13. The instrument reads the reaction strip and displays the result on the screen in milligrams per deciliter. If the glucose level is higher or lower than expected, refer to the troubleshooting guide provided by the manufacturer.	The reaction is now complete. The color change is photo-optically measured and reported in milligrams per deciliter.
14. Apply a small adhesive bandage to the patient's fingertip.	
15. Properly care for or dispose of equipment and supplies. Clean the work area. Remove gloves, and wash your hands.	

Note: These are generic instructions for using a glucose meter. Refer to the package insert for instructions specific to the particular instrument.

Quality assurance measure: Controls are available in the low, normal, and high range to ensure that the glucose meter is functioning properly. These controls should be run daily in accordance with the manufacturer's instructions.

Charting Example

02/12/2005 10:00 A.M. Capillary puncture right middle finger. Glucose tested with Glucometer. Results: 60 mg/dL. Dr. Peters notified. _____ M. Miller, CMA

Procedure 47-2

Glucose Tolerance Testing

Equipment/Supplies

Purpose: To determine the body's ability to metabolize a premeasured quantity of glucose over a specified time.

Equipment: Calibrated amount of glucose solution per physician's order, glucose meter equipment, phlebotomy
               equipment, glucose test strips, alcohol wipes, stopwatch, gloves

Steps	Reason
1. Wash your hands.	Handwashing aids infection control.
2. Assemble the equipment and supplies.	A stopwatch is necessary because the timing of the collections is important to the test results.
3. Greet and identify the patient. Explain the procedure. Ask for and answer any questions.	
4. Put on gloves. Obtain a fasting glucose (FBS) specimen from the patient by venipuncture or capillary puncture (see Chapter 44). It is recommended that laboratories test the blood sample before the glucose drink is administered; if the FBS exceeds 140 mg/dL, do not perform the test. Notify the physician.	Fasting glucose gives a baseline for further interpretation. Giving more glucose to a patient whose blood glucose level is already too high could cause serious harm.
5. Give the glucose drink to the patient to be taken within 5 minutes. Note the time the patient finishes the drink; this is the start of the test. Ensure that the patient remains fairly sedentary throughout this procedure; exercising will alter the glucose levels by increasing the body's demand for energy. The patient also should avoid smoking, because it may artificially increase the glucose level. Only water should be ingested. Encourage the patient to drink water to increase the blood volume and make it easier to draw blood. If the patient has any severe symptoms (e.g., headache, dizziness, vomiting), obtain a blood specimen at this time, end the test, and notify the physician. These symptoms could be the result of intolerably high or low glucose levels.	The body begins to metabolize the glucose immediately, so rapid ingestion of the drink is necessary.
6. Exactly 30 minutes after the patient finishes the glucose drink, obtain another blood specimen. Label the specimen with the patient's name and time of collection. Follow the precautions described in step 5 throughout the remainder of the test.	Precise timing of specimen collection is vital for accurate interpretation of results. Many specimens will be received from this patient, making proper notation of the sequence extremely important.
7. Exactly 1 hour after the glucose drink, repeat step 6.	
8. Exactly 2 hours after the glucose drink, repeat step 6.	

(continued)

Procedure 47-2 (continued)

Glucose Tolerance Testing

Steps	Reason
9. Exactly 3 hours after the glucose drink, repeat step 6. Unless a test longer than 3 hours has been requested, the test is complete. Otherwise continue for the specified time.	
10. If the specimens are to be tested by an outside laboratory, package as required and arrange for transportation.	Careful handling and transport help ensure accurate testing.
11. Properly care for or dispose of equipment and supplies. Clean the work area. Remove gloves and gown, and wash your hands.	

Charting Example
12/08/2005 10:30 A.M. 08:00 GTT test
08:00 FBS: 100 mg/dL glucose
08:10 Glucose drink to pt.
08:15 Glucose drink finished
08:45 Glucose 125 mg/dL
09:15 Glucose 132 mg/dL
10:15 Glucose 120 mg/dL
11:15 Glucose 110 mg/dL
Pt. tolerated procedure well, discharged by Dr. Lynch. _____ B. Smith, RMA

CHAPTER SUMMARY

Blood chemistry tests measure important substances in the blood. They can help show how well organs like the liver and kidneys are working, and can provide useful information about drug side effects. The trend continues to refer chemistry testing to regional and reference laboratories that house large automated analyzers that produce these test results at a lower cost than can be achieved in smaller laboratories. The key focus for the medical assistant is that no matter where the tests are performed, the results are only as good as the specimen submitted for testing. It is important for the medical assistant to have a basic understanding of the principles involved, proper sampling procedures required and specific handling requirements necessary for the specimen to arrive at the testing facility with the analyte to be tested intact for measurement.

Critical Thinking Challenges

1. A patient with edema is told by her physician to restrict her salt intake. Why may this help improve her condition?
2. A diabetic patient gave herself too much insulin by mistake. Would you expect her glucose to be very high or very low? Why?
3. A patient's glucose level is repeatedly normal at routine office visits, but she continues to have worsening side effects of hyperglycemia. What test might the physician request that would reflect her glucose levels over a period of weeks?
4. A medical assistant draws a red-top tube for a number of chemistry tests. Unfortunately, the tube is left on the counter for several hours before being centrifuged and refrigerated. Which chemistries may be affected by this? Why?

Answers to Checkpoint Questions

1. Physicians use chemistry test results to assess organ function and to gain a better understanding of the patient's overall health status.
2. Hyperkalemia, or elevated potassium, can occur with cell injuries, renal failure, and artifactual causes.
3. Urea, creatinine, and uric acid are important for assessing renal function.
4. Results of bilirubin, ALP, AST and ALT levels aid in the evaluation of liver function.
5. CKMB can help diagnose myocardial infarction within 3 hours of onset because CK levels increase within 2 to 8 hours of an infarction.

6. Hypoglycemia is a syndrome characterized by fasting blood sugar levels below 45 mg/dL. Symptoms include sweating, weakness, dizziness, headache, trembling, lethargy, and other nervous manifestations.
7. High-density lipoprotein is beneficial because it works to eliminate lipids via bile.

 Websites

American Diabetes Association www.diabetes.org
American Heart Association www.americanheart.org
World Health Organization www.who.int/en/

Section V

Career Strategies

Competing in the Job Market

Congratulations! You have reached a pivotal point in your medical assisting career. This unit prepares you to make the transition from student to employee. Your transition begins with an exciting externship program. Your externship is the springboard to starting your career. The remainder of Chapter 19 focuses on how to acquire the job that you have worked so hard for. You will be prepared to enter this fascinating and exciting career with confidence and professionalism and enjoy the rewards and accept the challenges that face you. Good luck on your new adventure!

48

Making the Transition: Student to Employee

ROLE DELINEATION COMPONENTS

GENERAL: Professionalism
- Display a professional manner and image
- Demonstrate initiative and responsibility
- Work as a member of the health care team
- Prioritize and perform multiple tasks
- Adapt to change
- Promote the CMA credential
- Enhance skills through continuing education
- Treat all patients with compassion and empathy
- Promote the practice through positive public relations

GENERAL: Legal Concepts
- Perform within legal and ethical boundaries
- Follow employer's established policies dealing with the health care contract

GENERAL: Communication Skills
- Recognize and respect cultural diversity
- Recognize and respond effectively to verbal, nonverbal, and written communications
- Use medical terminology appropriately
- Serve as a liaison

ADMINISTRATIVE: Administrative Procedures
- Perform basic administrative medical assisting functions

CHAPTER COMPETENCIES

LEARNING OBJECTIVES
Upon successfully completing this chapter, you will be able to:
1. Spell and define the key terms
2. Explain the purpose of the externship experience
3. List your professional responsibilities during externship
4. Understand the evaluation process for the extern student
5. List personal and professional attributes necessary to ensure a successful externship
6. Determine your best career direction based on your skills and strengths
7. Identify the steps necessary to apply for the right position and be able to accomplish those steps
8. Draft an appropriate cover letter
9. List guidelines for an effective interview that will lead to employment
10. Identify the steps that you need to take to ensure proper career advancement

PERFORMANCE OBJECTIVES
Upon successfully completing this chapter, you will be able to:
1. Write a résumé to properly communicate skills and strengths
2. Complete an employment application

KEY TERMS

externship	networking	portfolio	preceptor	résumé

Graduation from a medical assisting program is an important milestone in your life. It is normal to have conflicting emotions ranging from excitement to anxiety. The purpose of this chapter is to help you make this transition from student to employee. The first part of the chapter discusses externships. An externship is your first opportunity to use your knowledge in a clinical setting. The chapter also discusses the benefits of externship programs, how to get the most out of your externship, and the documentation that accompanies an externship. The later part of the chapter prepares you to begin searching for employment. Résumé preparation is discussed along with successful interviewing techniques. An introduction to key employment laws is also discussed.

EXTERNSHIPS

Most medical assistant programs provide an **externship** as part of the course requirement. An externship is a training program that gives you the experience of working in a professional medical office under the supervision of a preceptor or supervisor who will help you to apply the theories and procedures you learned during classroom training. This is the opportunity for you to perform and perfect the skills that you have learned during the academic portion of your program.

In an externship you will discover areas of interest in certain types of practices or health care specialties. Rotating through clinical sites will expose you to different offices you may pursue as possible opportunities for future employment. The length and schedule of your externship will depend on your school's curriculum and the medical site where you will be working.

Types of Facilities

The health care industry is diversified, with a wide variety of specialty offices and clinics. As a medical assisting student, you will experience an extensive scope of procedures during an externship in a general or family practice clinic or office. Family practices are generally referred to as primary care providers. Patients range in age from newborns to the elderly and typically have a broad range of complaints and illnesses. General practice facilities provide the best exposure to all types of procedures performed by medical assistants.

Your externship may be more limited in specialty practices. For example, staff members in obstetric offices usually do not perform electrocardiograms, nor do staff members in orthopedic offices perform gynecological examinations. Working in these types of practices, however, will give you experience in special examinations and procedures in areas that you might not observe in a general practice setting. Each specialty has advantages and disadvantages as a site, but all offer invaluable experience that cannot be adequately simulated in the classroom.

Extern Sites

Most schools have extern sites they have used for years. Based on the experience of former students, personnel in these sites know what the student must do to complete the clinical experience. An ideal site should provide a variety of experiences, both in administrative (front office) and clinical (back office) procedures.

A **preceptor** works with externship students the same as the instructor in the classroom. Preceptors typically are graduate medical assistants who have been through a similar externship program.

The school is careful to choose externship sites with preceptors who are willing to work with you and help you feel comfortable in the medical setting. They understand that all of your experience up to this point has been with fellow students in a protected classroom. They understand how nervous you are and will help you to ease the transition from classroom to the medical office. Your clinical sites are usually chosen within easy travel distance.

 Checkpoint Question

1. What is the role of the preceptor?

Benefits of Externship

Benefits to the Student

Externship is a vital part of medical assisting training. You will develop self-confidence and professionalism during the externship portion of your training. No amount of classroom training can compare with the experience of applying skills and knowledge in a medical facility. An externship also allows you to broaden your knowledge base by learning new and different techniques.

Benefits to the Medical Assisting Program

As you gain experience from the externship, the school also benefits from the affiliation, or connection, with the medical community. Many sites have a long history of training students. Schools rely on good training sites to enhance the medical assisting curriculum. Medical assisting programs also rely on the medical profession to aid in updating and revising the curriculum and course content to ensure that the methods and procedures presented to the students from year to year are current.

The school, the program director, and externship preceptors review students' extern experiences to change the program to reflect the needs of the community and the profession as health care constantly changes, such as with new technology. If students are routinely required to perform a procedure or examination that is not a part of the curriculum, for example, this will usually be considered for an addition to future lectures and laboratory sessions. If the accepted practice of a procedure has changed, changes will be made in the way it is taught to ensure that students are kept abreast of health care advances.

Benefits to the Externship Site

The student and the school are not the only ones to benefit from the externship period. The site also gains information about how well different areas of the facility are functioning. Site personnel may discover through the presence and questions of students that they should review certain policies or add others to help the office run more smoothly. Medical facilities must be updated on a continuing basis. Items may be deleted or added to policy, and procedure manuals or parts may have to be revised to provide clearer instructions.

As a student, you will be looking at the office as a newcomer, with a fresh perspective, and you may have many questions for the staff. As you become more familiar with the office routine, you will be more comfortable asking questions without the fear of appearing inexperienced. These questions may help point out to the office personnel things that should be changed or clarified.

Responsibilities of Externship

Responsibilities of the Student

You will develop many attributes, or characteristics, of a professional health care worker during the externship program. You should foster characteristics during this time to ensure that you continue to grow professionally and are an asset to the profession.

You must be dependable. Dependability is a good sign of maturity. Students who are not at the site on time, who take excessive numbers of breaks, or who do not follow through on assignments cannot properly provide for the needs of the patients who rely on the medical staff of the facility.

You must act in a professional manner. All concepts of professionalism include a positive, pleasant, confident attitude with a sincere desire to help the physician, the patient, and the staff.

You must be well groomed and meet the program's dress code. If the medical facility requires clothing that differs from your school's requirements, you are usually asked to comply with the site's requirements.

Checkpoint Question

2. List three responsibilities that you have during your externship.

Responsibilities of the Medical Assisting Program

The primary responsibility of the program is to arrange for the best possible clinical experience for students. The pro-

gram usually has a coordinator who matches students to appropriate sites. Once a site has been chosen, you will meet with the clinical coordinator to discuss the particulars of the medical facility. An interview is sometimes held to acquaint you with your preceptor before the externship begins.

After your site rotation has begun, the program's clinical coordinator will visit or call frequently to follow your progress. If either you or the site has concerns, the coordinator will mediate to eliminate problems or concerns as they arise.

The clinical coordinator will make an evaluation, or appraisal, of your progress at the site. Sites evaluations are usually completed on a form that contains detailed areas to be graded; these are equivalent to grades on a test or examination. These evaluations will be used to determine whether you are prepared for the profession or your skills are deficient and need more reinforcement. The clinical coordinator is responsible for compiling evaluations and keeping you abreast of your progress. Frequent conferences with your coordinator usually help accomplish this.

The school is also responsible for maintaining liability insurance for students during clinical hours. Students are required in most instances to provide proof of general immunizations and vaccination for hepatitis B. Some schools may provide the vaccine for students. Most programs require a current physical examination, a serology profile, and a tuberculin skin test before students are admitted to the program or before they make contact with patients.

Responsibilities of the Externship Site

The medical facility is, of course, responsible for providing opportunities for training. The staff will help orient you to the office and its policies. In some sites, students are allowed only to observe certain procedures but are given permission to perform some basic or routine procedures. Even if you are not allowed to perform specific procedures, the opportunity to observe and ask questions will be useful. In this way, you will become as familiar as possible with all clinical areas and functions.

Guidelines for a Successful Externship

Success in your externship is important for you to obtain employment. Your success in your externship is evaluated according to certain standards, or criteria. The person or persons evaluating you during your externship are professional medical personnel who know the standards for the health care field as they relate to medical assisting. These areas include the following:

- Procedural performance
- Preparedness
- Attendance
- Appearance
- Attitude

Procedural Performance

You will be judged on your ability to measure up to the standard of care for an entry-level medical assistant. This means you are expected to perform at the level of a new employee in the field. Your preceptor is there to assist you, not to teach you the basics that you should have learned in the classroom. Come to your externship prepared. Ask questions, when in doubt, before starting any procedure. Ask questions outside the patient's room. Never perform a procedure alone, unless otherwise directed by your instructor.

Preparedness

Preparation is the best insurance for success, regardless of the goal. Personal preparation for the externship helps prevent losing time because of other extracurricular obligations. Make sure in advance that you have prepared:

- Reliable transportation
- Reliable day care services
- Backup systems for a sick child, snow cancellations of school, or early dismissals from school
- Financial coverage and support for any hours that you are unable to work at your usual job because of your extern site hours.

Attendance

If you have planned well for transportation, family considerations, and finances, you are more likely to attend all sessions at the clinical sites. You must also be healthy. A good diet, regular exercise, and proper rest help you maintain good health. Careful attention to hygiene and medical asepsis help ensure that you do not bring illnesses home from the clinical sites.

If at any time you will be late or will not be able to attend the site for any reason, you must notify both the clinical coordinator and the site preceptor. Never be a no-call or no-show. Almost all sites have an answering service for leaving messages, as do most schools. There is no excuse for not notifying all parties involved if you will be unavoidably late or will not be able to attend the scheduled session.

Office hours vary from site to site; it is always a good practice, however, to arrive a few minutes before the scheduled opening. This allows time to check for telephone messages, arrange the day's appointments, turn on office equipment, and generally get into the routine of the office. Plan your transportation, leaving plenty of time for any problems that may occur. Arriving in a flurry, frustrated by traffic or home problems, with no time to ease into your day causes a high level of tension and anxiety. It is more difficult to have the caring and compassionate attitude necessary to deal with the complex problems in the medical office.

Appearance

You have only one opportunity to make a first impression, which is usually based on appearance. Appearance is much more than looks. A beautiful face on a poorly groomed person is not seen as professional and does not inspire trust and confidence in patients or coworkers. The key to a professional appearance is careful preparation and planning.

If you wear a uniform for your externship, it must be freshly laundered and pressed; clean but wrinkled is not acceptable. Plan your wardrobe for ease of care and a professional appearance. Fad or trendy clothing, suggestive clothing, and flashy clothing are not appropriate for clinical sites. All clothing should be in good repair, with no missing buttons, hanging hems, tears, rips, or stains. Duty shoes should be clean, polished frequently, and kept in good condition. Laced shoes look better with fresh, clean shoelaces. Check nylon hosiery for runs and snags and replace them as needed. You may wear laboratory coats in some programs; uniforms may be worn in others. The clinical preceptor or the clinical coordinator will inform you of the dress code in advance.

Professional appearance includes hair and makeup. Your hair should be conservatively styled, and long hair must be kept away from the face. Wash it frequently so that it is fresh and clean. Makeup should be minimal and tastefully applied. Never use perfume or cologne, which may be irritating to coworkers and patients. Keep fingernails short to avoid transferring pathogens or ripping gloves when you perform procedures.

Wear only minimal, tasteful jewelry. Rings can puncture gloves, possibly causing exposure to a pathogen. Therefore, it is a good idea to avoid wearing them in the clinical site.

Checkpoint Question

3. Describe the proper attire for your externship.

Attitude

Attitude is also part of appearance. Most patients and coworkers will easily see your emotions revealed by facial expressions and body language. A person who looks eager is usually perceived as a good, diligent worker.

Much attitude is determined by how well you handle change and direction and how adaptable and flexible you are during difficult assignments.

The medical profession is constantly changing, making it imperative for all professionals to stay flexible. In the classroom, you learn generic methods for treatments and procedures. Because of the constantly changing technology, you may have to adjust to other methods in the field. If you learned a procedure one way in the classroom training but find that it is performed differently in the clinical site, the new method must be accepted and performed as well as possible. Frequently, there is more than one right way to do a procedure, and the classroom method you learned may be just one of the accepted methods. The next physician or clinical site may use yet another equally correct procedural method.

Your attitude determines your altitude. Students who work with a positive attitude during their externship are likely to reach higher levels of the profession than those who see the externship as an imposition or a burden. Box 48-1 offers some additional suggestions.

Externship Documentation

Time Records

Most programs use a time sheet or record of some sort to document your hours in the externship (Fig. 48-1). The beginning and ending hours of each day are recorded. How breaks are handled depends on the clinical coordinator, program requirements, and specific site. Some sites allow half an hour for lunch, and others allow an hour; some close for an hour or more midday, while others are open and staffed from morning until evening. Some programs make students responsible for time sheet signatures; others delegate the responsibility to the site preceptor. However the form is handled, it is used to validate your time in the externship and is a requirement for completion of most programs.

Site Evaluation

Most schools use a site evaluation form to gather impressions of the site and externship experience (Fig. 48-2). This form helps determine the effectiveness of the site for training and whether any issues should be addressed before assigning other students. Be objective and honest in your evaluation of the site. When completing a site evaluation, consider these questions:

- Was the overall experience positive or negative?
- Were opportunities for learning abundant and freely offered or hard to obtain?
- Were staff personnel open and caring or unwelcoming?
- Was the preceptor available and easily approachable or preoccupied and distant?

If the site is not providing a positive learning experience, the program should discontinue using it.

Self-Evaluation

The self-evaluation form helps you determine what personal and professional skills you still need to develop or enhance. These forms encourage introspection and personal honesty as you begin a lifelong program of self-improvement. They usually include components that encourage you to outline the things you performed well and are proud of and areas that can use some improvement.

Checkpoint Question

4. What three types of documentation are often required in extern programs?

ESTABLISH THE JOB FOR YOU

Setting Employment Goals

Once your externship is complete, you are one step closer to getting the job that you desire. Before beginning to search for a job, decide what you want and need from a job and make that your goal. People who do not set employment goals too often accept only what is presented to them. They often end up unhappy in their work because they did not choose their job in the first place. The average person approaches the job search with the attitude, "I wonder what is available," rather than, "Here is what I would like to do, and here is the facility where I would like to work." *That* is setting a goal. It is also a positive, proactive approach to the job market rather than a reactive position to what is available. In general, the medical field is looking for proactive people. You will work harder and more enthusiastically if you choose your workplace.

The best way to set a goal and eventually get what you want is to study your strengths and weaknesses and from that self-knowledge design the best job for you. Goal setting means describing the ideal job for you and deciding that this is the job that you will someday have.

On a sheet of paper, describe the best job for you if you had your choice. For example, you might describe these elements:

CLINICAL EXPERIENCE
STUDENT'S TIME REPORT

To obtain proper credit, an account of time and days in attendance must be recorded by each intern student. This report must be verified by the job supervisor and attached to the final 55-day roster. This information is kept strictly confidential.

Student's Name: _____   Course No.: _____

Program: _____   Course Title: _____

Minimum Contact Hrs. Required: _____   Quarter/Year: _____

WEEK OF (DATES)	M	T	W	TH	F	S	TOTAL HOURS	SITE SUPERVISOR

TOTAL HOURS FOR QUARTER: _____

I certify that the above time report is a true statement of the hours worked.

I approve this statement of hours in attendance for the quarter covered.

_____   _____
Student's Signature   Date

_____   _____
Curriculum Coordinator's Signature   Date

FIGURE 48–1.   Sample student time report.

- Specialty area (e.g., obstetrics, pediatrics, surgery)
- Duties (clinical or administrative)
- Type of employer and supervisor
- Other employees and coworkers
- Type of facility
- Desired atmosphere (casual or formal)
- Ideal hours
- Availability of flextime (a system of scheduling that allows for a personal choice in hours or days worked)

Next, write down where you expect to be in 2 years and in 5 years, in terms of both position and income. Now you are more focused on where you want to work, what you want to do, and the direction you want to be going. The next question is how to get there.

To win the position you want, you have to learn to sell yourself. Generally, employers will not come looking for you; you will have to go to them. They will compare you with all of the other equally well qualified candidates who are interested in the same position. If 25 people interview for a job, even if you are second best, you still lose. The one who is chosen is the one who interviews best. The one who is best suited for a job does not necessarily get it; instead, frequently the one who performs best in the interview does. To market yourself takes real effort.

Self-Analysis

A good presentation of your qualifications begins with self-analysis. You must know what strengths you have to offer a potential employer as well as your weaknesses. Make an honest list of your strengths and weaknesses. (If you skipped this exercise, one of your weaknesses is likely a failure to follow through, taking short cuts, and perhaps procrastination.)

Each of your strengths presents an opportunity to sell yourself and your value as an employee. When you are interviewing for a position, concentrate on projecting your strengths to the interviewer.

Just as your strengths give you a special advantage, each weakness is a reason someone may not want to offer you the position. Recognize and work to resolve your weaknesses. Recognizing your weaknesses as a threat to securing the position you want will help you develop strategies to eliminate these problems or turn them into strengths. As long as you are aware of your weaknesses, you are better prepared to handle them.

Once you know the type of job you want and have identified your positive and negative qualities, it is time to begin to look for the right job.

 Checkpoint Question

5. What is the purpose of self-analysis?

FINDING THE RIGHT JOB

Everybody begins with the newspaper, and you should too. But other opportunities too might work for you. Keep in

---

CLINICAL SITE EVALUATION
STUDENT QUESTIONNAIRE

Name of Clinical Site: _____

Department/Unit Worked: _____

Dates Worked: From _____   To _____

Name of Preceptor _____

SCALE CODES: 1 = Disagree; 2 = Agree; 3 = No opinion

1. The clinical experience was worthwhile.

    1   2   3

    Comments: _____

2. The objectives of the clinical experience seemed adequately understood and followed by the clinical site.

    1   2   3

    Comments: _____

3. Would you recommend this clinical site for future externs?

    1   2   3

    Comments: _____

4. Was the preceptor helpful?

    1   2   3

    Comments: _____

5. The routines of the department/unit were clearly explained throughout the clinical experience.

    1   2   3

    Comments: _____

6. The clinical site provided sufficient educational experiences.

    1   2   3

    Comments: _____

7. Did you receive constructive feedback, both verbal and written, on your clinical performance?

    1   2   3

    Comments: _____

8. What part of the clinical experience did you like the best?

    Comments: _____

9. What part of the clinical experience did you like the least?

    Comments: _____

10. What changes would you recommend for future clinical experiences at this clinical site?

    Comments: _____

11. Upon completion of your clinical experience, did you feel like a part of the team?

    Comments: _____

12. Were you offered a position at this site?

    Yes _____   No _____

    If yes, fill in the blank spaces.

    FT_____   PT_____   Starting salary _____

Date Completed: _____   Signature: _____

FIGURE 48–2. Sample site evaluation form.

mind that many of the most desirable job openings are never advertised; they are posted internally and filled from within.

Many studies show that most positions are never advertised in the media. Open positions that are posted internally are often filled with current employees or by referrals from current employees. Any organization that looks within and obtains a recommendation from a current employee to fill an available position accomplishes two things: (1) it saves the cost of advertising, and (2) the recommendation itself is usually a good one because it comes from someone who presumably knows the demands and special needs of that particular organization.

It is important for someone seeking employment in the medical field to build as many contacts within the field as possible. These contacts help you with **networking**. Networking is using friends, family members, and professional colleagues to advance or obtain information in the workplace. It is impossible to have too many contacts. Everyone with whom you associate should know that you are looking for employment. Friends and acquaintances cannot tell you about a job or recommend you for a job if they do not know that you are searching.

Traditional sources of information for job openings:

- *Local, state, or federal government employment offices.* These agencies are designed to find work for the unemployed. They frequently have listings of positions that are not found anywhere else. Rather than calling the office with inquiries, make an appointment to visit. Register with the service. Get to know the contact person with whom you will be contacting frequently.
- *School placement office.* If your school has a placement office, contact the coordinator or personnel officer and outline what you are looking for and where you want to work. Their job is to assist you in securing the position you want. If you establish a working relationship with a contact person, you will probably have better results.
- *Medical facilities.* Do not wait for an advertisement. Go to the office or facility where you would like to work and leave a résumé—a document summarizing your professional qualifications—and a cover letter explaining how much you want to work there. Find out the name of the office manager or personnel officer and call first for an appointment. This shows better planning and foresight and is more professional than dropping by unannounced.
- *Private agencies.* Many medical facilities solicit privately to avoid being swamped by applications from unqualified applicants. A fee is charged for the service but is usually paid by the employer. Call the agency to make an appointment with a representative who will interview you and tell you what steps to follow.
- *Temporary services.* These agencies fill short-term vacancies for medical offices. If you are new in an area, this is a good way to learn which facilities would be good choices for you. You may be assigned for several

days or several weeks. If you work well as a temporary replacement and like the site, leave your résumé and let the appropriate individuals know that you would like to work in this place if an opening occurs. Check with the temporary agency regarding any fees that you may be charged or that the medical office may have to pay if it hires you, often called a finder's fee.

Checkpoint Question

6. List four resources that you may use to identify potential job opportunities.

APPLYING FOR THE JOB

Answering Newspaper Advertisements

When responding to a newspaper advertisement, be sure to do exactly what the advertisement asks you to do; one of the qualities that many interviewers look for is the ability to follow directions. At the same time, try to make your response more distinctive (yet still professional) than others they may receive. The medical profession rarely responds well to those who do not fit its image and almost never accepts someone who does not conform at the entry level. Most employers will require you to submit a résumé. A well-prepared résumé and cover letter are essential to job hunting.

Preparing Your Résumé

Many resources can help you write your **résumé**. Start with your school library. Most schools have books on how to create résumés. Numerous websites also offer this information. Caution: many websites have free information, but some charge fees. Focus on free resources before paying for these services. Many word processing programs have templates for résumés. Put your résumé on a computer disk and be sure to personalize it for the position you are seeking. For example, if you give a career objective, try putting in the title a description of the particular job you are seeking. Keep changing this for every different position so that your résumé is personalized for each interview.

The résumé is a flash picture of yourself; if it is neat and professional, the reviewer will presume that it is a reflection of you. Remember these guidelines as you prepare to capture the reviewer's interest:

1. Evaluate your skills, goals, and what you have to offer. With this list in hand, you can better concentrate on highlighting your strengths.
2. Confine your résumé to one page, selecting carefully what you want to include. The résumé must state just what the reviewer needs to know and no more.
3. Include the following key information:
   - Name, address, and telephone number: Include these at the top of your résumé (usually centered).

(Because you are including your telephone number, you should expect calls from prospective employers. Box 48-2 offers some tips for handling such calls.)

Box 48-2

HANDLING CALLS FROM PROSPECTIVE EMPLOYERS

Here are some tips for handling calls from prospective employers:

- Tell family members or other household members that you are expecting important telephone calls.
- Keep a pen and paper with telephone.
- Instruct people to take a complete message. Ask them to write down the person's name, phone number, message, and what time the call was received.
- Leave a professional message on your answering machine. Avoid leaving cute or silly messages.

- Education: Start with the most recent and work backward.
- Affiliations or volunteer work (if appropriate): If this information shows that you have good organizational skills or have held an office for the group, you should include it.
- Experience: This may be listed in either of two standard forms: functional or chronological. A functional résumé focuses on skills and qualifications rather than employment and works well for those who recently graduated or who are reentering the job market after a period of years (Fig. 48-3). A chronological résumé is useful for those who have an employment history, particularly if the history is relevant to the position be-

FIGURE 48–3. Sample functional résumé.

Tina Elmwood C.M.A.
22 Brandy Drive
Dayton, Ohio 00000
444-777-6666

Employment Objective: To use my medical assisting skills in a challenging position. My goal is to work with children. (*Change this sentence to reflect the type of office that you are applying to.*)

Experience:

Externship (160 hours) at Family Practice Associates, Bayview Drive, Dayton, Ohio (*If you have a positive evaluation from your preceptor, bring it with you to the interview. Do not attach it to the resume.*)

Education:

Medical Assisting Program, Diploma. Graduated June 2003. West County Community College, Dayton Ohio (*Bring a copy of your diploma and transcripts to the interview. Do not attach them unless employer has specifically requested them.*)
Dayton High School, Diploma. Graduated June 2001. Dayton, Ohio

Skills:

Clinical and Laboratory skills listed on Role Delineation for Medical Assisting

Administrative skills listed on Role Delineation for Medical Assisting

Comfortable using all types of standard office equipment

Familiar with XYZ software programs (*List software programs that you are comfortable with. If you know what type of software the office uses, list that as well.*)

Certifications:

Certified Medical Assistant, American Association of Medical Assistants (*Bring copy to interview or attach to résumé.*)
Cardiopulmonary Resuscitation, American Heart Association (*Bring copy to interview or attach to résumé.*)

FIGURE 48–4. Sample chronological résumé.

Beatrice Meza C.M.A.
123 Main Street
West Harford, CT 00000
888-999-6666

Employment Objective: To use my medical assisting skills in a challenging position. My goal is to work in an obstetrical office. (*Change this sentence to reflect the type of office that you are applying to.*)

Education:

2002–2003 Medical Assisting Program; Mountain Laurel Community College, West Hartford, Connecticut (*Bring a copy of your diploma and transcripts to the interview. Do not attach them unless employer has specifically requested them.*)

Externship:

July 2003–(160 hours) Women's Health Care Center, Hartford, Connecticut (*If you have a positive evaluation from your preceptor, bring it with you to the interview. Do not attach it to the résumé.*)

Work Experience:

July 2002–present Receptionist, Dermatology Consultants, West Hartford, Connecticut. Worked part time while I was in school. Answered and triaged telephone calls. Assisted with various other medical administrative responsibilities. (*If you have a reference letter from this employer, bring it with you to the interview. Be prepared to answer questions about why you are leaving this position.*)
May 1999–July 2002 Cashier/Clerk for SuperMarket Grocers, West Hartford, Connecticut. Worked part time. Responsible for training new employees. Promoted to senior cashier.

Skills:

Clinical and Laboratory skills listed on the Role Delineation for Medical Assisting

Administrative skills listed on the Role Delineation for Medical Assisting

Comfortable using all types of standard office equipment

Familiar with XYZ software programs (*List software programs that you are comfortable with. If you know what type of software the office uses, list that as well.*)

Activities/Honors

Student Government representative

Most Improved Medical Assisting Student in 2002

ing sought. Start with the most recent employment and work backward. Include your title, position, and a few of your key responsibilities (Fig. 48-4). Explain any gaps such as pregnancy, schooling, relocations, and so on.

- References: You may or may not include your references on a separate sheet. When you have chosen the people you want to use as references, be sure to ask their permission. Start by asking your instructors if you can use them as references. Other medical professionals (physicians or nurses) will also make strong references. Previous employers also make very good references. You should have a minimum of three references. Do not bring a list of more than five people. Prospective employers are not interested in your neighbors or pastor and are certainly not interested in your relatives as references.

4. Do not include hobbies and personal interests unrelated to work. It is not relevant that you play the guitar, but it would be impressive to know that you volunteer at a free clinic.

5. Use action words (Box 48-3).

6. Center the résumé on white or off-white heavy bond or high rag content paper, 8.5 by 11 inches. (Colors are not acceptable, and cheap paper will not convey the professional impression you hope to make.) Keep a 1-inch margin around the text. Single-space within the sections of information but leave a blank line between the sections.

7. Use regular type. Avoid fonts that are cute or fancy. Use black ink. Do not print your résumé in color.

Box 48-3

ACTION WORDS

Achieved	Established	Planned
Attained	Filed	Prepared
Assisted	Handled	Processed
Conducted	Generated	Scheduled
Completed	Implemented	Selected
Composed	Maintained	Systemized
Created	Organized	Screened
Developed	Operated	Solved
Directed	Participated	Wrote
Ensured	Performed	

8. Have someone proofread your work. It is difficult to find your own errors or see areas that are not clearly worded.
9. Print your résumé on a letter-quality printer. A dot matrix printer is not acceptable.
10. Mail the résumé in an 8.5 by 11 inch manila envelope. This will present the interviewer with a résumé and cover letter that are smooth, with no fold lines. Many prefer to work with résumés that have not been folded for an envelope.
11. **Be honest.** Do not embellish your résumé or add fictional information. This could get you fired.

Checkpoint Question

7. What is the difference between a functional and a chronological résumé?

Preparing Your Cover Letter

When contacting a prospective employer about a job, you need to send a résumé along with a cover letter. Keep your cover letter brief and meaningful. You want it to be read, and you want the reader to be impressed by what it says. Be sure that you mention the job itself in your letter. You may even consider a statement such as, "This is the type of position I would prefer." If you are applying to a pediatrician's office, you may write, "My goal is work with children." If you know something favorable about the facility, include that in your letter. If you know anyone who works for the company, mention it. *Do not* mention the person by name unless you have secured his or her permission.

Make sure you address your letter to the right person. Call the personnel department or office manager and ask the name of the person handling the applications. Determine the correct spelling of the name and the preferred honorific, such as Mr., Ms., or Mrs.

The standard form for a cover letter has three brief paragraphs:

- First paragraph: State the position for which you are applying.
- Second paragraph: Stress your skills. Do not be redundant, since you will also send a résumé, but mention or highlight specifically the skills needed for this job.
- Third paragraph: Request an interview. Offer to call in a week to set up an interview (then do so). Keep a copy of your letter to refer to when calling.

Use the same good quality paper for the cover letter that you use for your résumé. Include your name, address, and telephone number at the top of the page, centered or in block form. Single-space the letter and double-space between paragraphs. Either block or modified block form is acceptable.

Completing an Employment Application

Some sites will have you fill out an employment application while you wait for your interview; others may mail one to you to be filled out and taken to the interview. Although résumés have their place and are indispensable, many facilities rely more on an application form.

Follow these guidelines when completing an application:

1. Read through completely before beginning.
2. Follow the instructions exactly. Prospective employers notice neatness, erasures, evasions, and indecision.
3. Answer every question. If the question does not apply to you, draw a line or write N/A so that the interviewer will know that you did not overlook the question.
4. In the line for wage or salary desired, write "negotiable" or find out before the interview what is usual for the area for this type of position.
5. In spaces requesting your reason for leaving a previous position, try to sound positive. Answers such as "to explore a new career direction" are general enough to fill many needs. If the reason for leaving was relocation, schooling, or pregnancy, say so.
6. Write your very best, being as neat as possible.
7. Use a black or blue pen. Never use a pencil or colored pen (red, green, purple) to complete the application. It does not portray a professional image.

You may attach your résumé to the application if you did not mail one already.

INTERVIEWING

Interviewing well is a skill that takes effort to develop. As with any skill, if you want to stay proficient and keep your skills in good working order, you have to practice. Ask friends or family members to work with you to develop a relaxed approach to answering the questions most often asked during an interview. Have them try to trip you up or confuse you by throwing in tricky questions. Although the effect will not be the same with a friend or family member as with an interviewer, this practice can make a difference between getting the job and losing the chance. You can also rehearse in front of a mirror.

Usually, the person who interviews best is hired for the position. An excellent interview is absolutely crucial for obtaining any job. It is highly unlikely that you will get the job you want without doing well in the interview.

Preparing for the Interview

Before the day of the interview, find out all you can about the facility. What is its reputation? Does it have a big turnover of employees? Review your textbooks that cover the specialty so that you can ask informed questions about procedures performed at the site. Think of questions to ask and write them down. Anticipate questions that might be asked of you. Find out the name of the interviewer; if it is a difficult name, practice saying it. Go to the site ahead of time to be sure of its location and time the trip so that you will not be late for your appointment. Do this ideally at the same time of day as your appointment to judge traffic delays, parking problems, and so on.

Dress appropriately for the interview. The general rule is to dress one step above what is required for the job. Do not overdress, as if for a party; make sure your outfit is professional. Your personal hygiene must be above reproach. If you normally smoke, avoid smoking before the interview. Those who do not smoke are acutely aware of the odor of smoke on one's clothes and breath. Avoid large jewelry and apply makeup carefully. Avoid perfumes; some people are very sensitive to scents.

Arrive on time or a few minutes early. Go alone; do not take a friend or family member for moral support. When you are introduced to the interviewer, offer your hand for a handshake and sit only when and where you are directed. Do not fidget, swing your foot, play with your hair, or tap your fingers on the chair arm. Make eye contact when the interviewer speaks with you and when you respond to the questions (Fig. 48-5). Sit up straight but relaxed, with your portfolio on your lap. A **portfolio** is a folder containing all of the information you will need to impress the interviewer. If you do not have a special folder or briefcase, a neat, new manila folder will be adequate. This folder or portfolio will contain items crucial to your interview (Box 48-4.)

Crucial Interview Questions

Every interviewer must have the answers to three basic questions. When you respond to the interviewer's questions, keep these in mind:

1. Do you have the necessary skills to do the job? (Don't forget to include any foreign language skills (Box 48-5)).

FIGURE 48–5. During an interview, be sure to use correct posture and to make eye contact with the interviewer.

Box 48-4

PORTFOLIO BOX

Take these items with you to the interview:
- Two pens
- A notepad
- Your Social Security card
- Verification or at least the dates of immunizations (hepatitis B, TB test)
- Two copies of your résumé
- Two letters of reference
- Copies of awards received
- Typed list of three references including names, phone numbers, and addresses
- Documentation of any special projects

Box 48-5

KNOWLEDGE OF A FOREIGN LANGUAGE

If you are applying for a position that encourages bilingual applicants, be prepared for questions during the interview regarding your ability to speak another language. Know what languages are commonly spoken in your community. Whether it is Spanish, Polish, Italian, or any other language, take the time to become familiar with simple greetings: "Hello." "What is your name?" "Can I help you?" Tell the interviewer that you know a few words but are not fluent. It is not fair to the employer or to the patients to pretend otherwise if you are unable to communicate effectively. Most community colleges offer language courses. A local hospital may offer these courses with a focus on medical terms. Finally, the best way to learn a new language is to use it. If your classmates speak another language, ask them to tutor you. Being bilingual in the medical profession is always an asset.

2. Do you have the necessary drive, energy, and commitment to get the job done?
3. Will you work well with the rest of the team?

A positive answer to all of these questions is not a guarantee that you will be offered the job, but a negative answer to any one of these will most assuredly mean that you will *not* get the job. Make sure that your comments make a positive impression regarding these three questions. In the medical field, the interviewer will need to establish your professionalism and ability to keep confidentiality. The interviewer will also want to know how interested you are in increasing and continuing your education and skills. Be sure that your answers will satisfy the interviewer.

Many interviewers use a prepared list of questions to direct the flow of the interview. Table 48-1 contains some commonly asked interview questions and guidance for responses. Be prepared with answers that will reflect well on your professionalism and qualifications.

When the interviewer finishes asking questions, he or she will usually ask if you have any questions. Refer to your notepad, on which you have listed questions such as these:

- What are the responsibilities of the position offered?
- If it is not personal, why is the current employee leaving?
- What are the opportunities for future advancement?
- How long is the training or probation period?

Table 48-1 INTERVIEW QUESTIONS AND RESPONSES

Common Interview Questions	Possible Responses and Points to Mention
1. Tell me about yourself.	"I enjoy working with other people." Stress the good points you wrote on your self-analysis. Keep the comments professional. Do not give long explanations about personal topics. ("I have three brothers." "I like basketball.")
2. What are your strengths?	"My strengths are honesty and dependability." List any clinical or administrative skills that you excel at.
3. What are your weaknesses?	Be honest; everyone has a weakness. "My weakness is phlebotomy skills," and add, "but I have improved my skills by reading magazine articles about blood drawing and by practicing in the school laboratory." Do not say, "I am perfect" or "I have no weaknesses." State one weakness and explain how you are trying to improve it.
4. Why do you want this position?	"I like this office setting." "I always wanted to work for [as an example] a cardiologist." Mention that you are aware of the office's good reputation in the community, and if the location of the office is convenient, say so.
5. What are your goals?	List two or three immediate goals: "My priority is to acquire a medical assisting position that will be challenging and rewarding." Have at least two goals in your mind for where you want to be in 5 years.
6. Why did you leave your last position?	Always place a positive spin on why you left: "Looking for new challenge." Never criticize past employers, their offices, or your coworkers.
7. What salary rate are you looking for?	Know the average pay in your area. Check with your placement office if you are unsure of the typical salaries. Never demand a certain pay rate.
8. How do you handle pressure?	Possible explanations can include, "I set priorities" and "I remain calm and well organized." Avoid comments such as "I hate stress" or "I panic when I feel pressured."
9. Do you work better alone or as a team?	Stress that you can work as a team member but that you can also function independently.
10. Who was your best supervisor and why?	Possible remarks may include phrases such as "always fair," "supportive," and "encouraging." Avoid comments such as "She gave us long lunch breaks" or "She didn't make us work hard."
11. How do you handle conflict?	Indicate that you begin trying to resolve any problems in a professional manner. Indicate that you are always open to constructive criticism.
12. How would your classmates describe you?	Include remarks such as "good student," "team worker," and "helpful."
13. I noticed your grades in computer class were poor. Why?	Be honest: " It was a tough course" or "Although my grade was poor, I have restudied the course material, and my computer skills have improved." If you have taken any additional studies or tutoring to help in this subject area, mention that. Never say the teacher was unfair, the class was boring, or you didn't care about the class.
14. Describe the term *confidentiality* and how you would use it in our office.	Review the term. Stress to the interviewer that you know how important patient confidentiality is from a legal and ethical viewpoint.

- How does the facility feel about continuing education? Is time off offered to employees to upgrade their skills? Does the facility subsidize the expense?
- Is there a job performance or evaluation process?
- What is the benefit package? Is there access to a 401(k) plan or other retirement plan? Health insurance? Life insurance?

Make notes of the answers for future reference. Avoid asking about time off or vacations during the interview. These questions imply that you are more interested in being paid to avoid work than you are in contributing to the work at hand.

Make sure the interviewer knows how important continuing education is to you. Talk about the types of continuing education courses you would like to attend and the subjects you would like to study. Show that you realize that the only constant in medicine is change and that you expect to keep abreast of the information in your area. Thank the interviewer for the opportunity to apply for the position and ask the time frame for a decision. As you leave, offer your hand for a handshake and ask if you may call again before the decision date to clear up any questions that the interviewer may have during the decision-making process.

FOLLOW-UP

The day of the interview or no later than the day after, write a short thank-you note for the opportunity to be interviewed and restate how interested you are in the job (Fig. 48-6). Remind the interviewer that you are available for additional questions.

Call several days after the interview. Reintroduce yourself politely and add any new information or ask any questions

Maria Sefferin C.M.A.
11 Jersey Road
Fredericksburg, VA 00000
888-555-4444

Ms. Joan Brown
Office Manager
Middletown Cardiology Consultants
24 Main Street
Williamsburg, VA 00000

October 22, 2003

Dear Ms. Brown:

Thank you for giving me the opportunity to interview for the position of Medical Assistant in your office. I enjoyed meeting you and touring your facility.

I feel I would be an asset to your office for many reasons. I have a strong knowledge of medical terminology, anatomy and physiology, and cardiac diseases. I have solid clinical and administrative skills. I believe that this position will offer me an opportunity to use the education and training that I have received in my medical assisting courses.

I am very interested in this position. This is the type of career opportunity that I had hoped to find. If you have any questions, please feel free to call me at 888-555-4444.

Sincerely,

Maria Sefferin, C.M.A.

FIGURE 48-6. Sample follow-up letter.

WHAT IF

You become tongue-tied during an interview. What should you do?

It's not unusual to feel nervous during the interview. To stay calm, take a deep breath and count to three before answering a question. Doing this also gives you time to think before you speak. Remember: Believe in yourself and your skills. Say to yourself, "I am going to get this job." Rehearse your answers to the common interview questions. Doing this exercise in front of a mirror is beneficial. Visit the websites listed in this chapter. Some of these sites offer virtual interviewing skills and have excellent tips for interviewing. Finally, arrive prepared and relaxed. Avoid excessive caffeine ingestion before the interview. Caffeine will increase your anxiety level.

that might have occurred to you after the interview. Thank the interviewer again for this opportunity.

Why Some Applicants Fail to Get the Job

The first reason not to be hired is simple: lack of the necessary abilities (Box 48-6). Every employer is looking for something special from each employee. Medicine has special needs. The employer must believe that you possess a number of skills necessary to do the job:

- *Technical skills.* You must have the necessary proficiency to get the job done.
- *Confidentiality.* In medicine you are exposed to sensitive information about patients. Is the interviewer convinced that you can be relied on to keep those confidences?
- *Human relations skills.* Will you get along with the others in the workplace?
- *Communication skills.* Do you have the verbal and writing skills that the job demands? Remember the importance of correct English. You will not be hired if your English and grammar are not exemplary.

If you fail to impress the interviewer with your grasp of these skills, you will never be considered for the position.

Another major reason an applicant is not hired is lack of professionalism. Watch the way you dress and speak. The interviewer knows that whatever you display in the interview will also be displayed to the patients.

KEEP THE JOB OR MOVE ON?

Almost everyone comes to this question at some point in his or her career. Should I look for a new place to work and leave this place where I am safe and comfortable? Would another job be better or more satisfying? Would benefits be better?

An important factor in many relocations is salary. In addition to the financial aspects, however, employees today are looking for other elements that contribute to job satisfaction:

- A sense of achievement
- Recognition
- Opportunity for growth and advancement
- Harmonious peer group relationships
- A good working relationship with supervisors
- Status
- Job security
- Comfortable working conditions
- Fair company policies

If you are no longer happy in your job, the reason probably lies in one or more of these elements. Before you make the decision to change jobs, do some internal soul searching to determine exactly what type of position would make you happy. If you decide to leave, you must leave with positive feelings all around. Box 48-7 offers some guidelines for leaving your job.

EMPLOYMENT LAWS

Many state and federal laws regulate employers. The U. S. Equal Employment Opportunity Commission (EEOC) enforces many of these laws. Under Title VII, Americans with Disabilities Act (ADA), and the Age Discrimination in Employment Act (ADEA), it is illegal to discriminate in any as-

---

Box 48-6

NO HIRE

Here are several reasons a person may not be hired:
- Poor personal appearance
- Inappropriate demeanor, such as unenthusiastic, overly aggressive
- Displayed lack of purpose or direction
- Lack of tact and diplomacy
- Inappropriate humor
- Failure to research the type of office setting or practice
- Failure to make eye contact
- Poorly completed application, messy application, spelling errors on application
- Overemphasis on need for time off or higher wages

pect of employment. For example, it is illegal to discriminate in areas such as hiring, firing, transfers, promotion, recruitment, training, benefits, pay, retirement plans, and disability leave of employees. All employees must be treated fairly in all areas.

It is illegal to discriminate against an employee for any of these reasons:

- Race
- Color
- National origin
- Religion or religious beliefs
- Sex
- Age (age limits can be specified only when there is a bona fide occupational qualification)
- Disability
- Martial status
- Political affiliation
- Sexual orientation
- Pregnancy

The Equal Pay Act prohibits pay discrepancies on the basis of sex. In other words, a man and a woman who perform the same job with the same experience level must be paid the same and have the same benefits. The law also protects you against sexual harassment in the workplace. If you feel that you are being discriminated against in the workplace, you should contact your local EEOC district office.

Box 48-7

LEAVING A JOB

Always follow these steps when you decide to leave your position:

- Always give adequate notice (minimum 2 weeks, optimal a month).
- Write a resignation letter. Keep the letter positive: "I am leaving this position to explore new opportunities." This is often the last item in your personnel file.
- Be positive during your exit interview. Do not criticize employees or the position.
- Clean and empty your locker, desk, and any other assigned space.
- Return your pager and any other equipment that has been assigned to you.
- Finish all duties and tie up any loose ends.
- Alert your supervisor to any unfinished business.
- Ask for a letter of reference.

CHAPTER SUMMARY

Your externship is the transition from classroom to employment. A successful externship helps lead to your ultimate goal—employment. During your externship you will work with a preceptor who will help you perform your skills in the workplace. After your externship is complete, do a self-analysis and write your résumé. Many resources can help you locate job openings. A job should be fulfilling and rewarding in ways beyond just the income. Learn how to promote yourself and earn the position you want. Know the laws that protect your rights as an employee. You will work hard, but there are many rewards. Welcome to the world of medical assisting!

Critical Thinking Challenges

1. You notice that your preceptor does not follow standard precautions on several occasions. Why is this dangerous? Whom should you tell? Would you tell your instructor at school? Why or why not? How would you discuss this with your preceptor?

2. Read the classified section of the Sunday newspaper and select a job advertisement that interests you. Write a cover letter and résumé tailored to this position. Assume you have been called for an interview. What questions do you ask the prospective employer? What questions do you expect to be asked? Explain your responses.

3. Obtain two employee application forms from the human resources department of your local hospital. Complete one application form yourself and invite a fellow student to complete the other. Swap applications and evaluate each other's work. Determine which areas are appropriately addressed and which need further attention.

4. Visit the EEOC website. What is the purpose of the EEOC? Where is your nearest EEOC district office? Would you talk to your supervisor if you felt that you were discriminated against? Why or why not?

5. Suppose you were just hired into your dream position. On day 2, you overhear your supervisor telling another employee, "Don't report that billing error to Medicare. They won't catch us." What would you do? Whom would you tell, or would you pretend you didn't hear it? Would you report to Medicare? Why or why not?

Answers to Checkpoint Questions

1. The preceptor acts as the instructor in the clinical site, providing supervision and technical direction to medical assisting students.
2. You must be dependable, professional, and well groomed.
3. The proper attire includes a freshly laundered uniform, clean shoes, neatly groomed hair, limited makeup, and jewelry kept to a minimum.
4. Documentation includes times sheets, a site evaluation, and a self-evaluation.
5. A self-analysis helps you identify your strengths and weaknesses.
6. Sources of job information include government employment offices, your school placement office, medical facilities, private agencies, and temporary services.

7. A functional résumé stresses skills and qualifications rather than employment history. A chronological résumé lists positions held, starting with the most recent and working backward.

 Websites

Careerspan.com
Resume.com
Resumewriters.com
Seekingsuccess.com
10minuteresume.com
U. S. Equal Employment Opportunity Commission
   www.eeoc.gov

Appendices

APPENDIX A

MEDICAL ASSISTING ROLE DELINEATION CHART

Administrative

Administrative Procedures

- Perform basic administrative medical assisting functions
- Schedule, coordinate, and monitor appointments
- Schedule inpatient/outpatient admissions and procedures
- Understand and apply third-party guidance
- Obtain reimbursement through accurate claims submission
- Monitor third-party reimbursement
- Understand and adhere to managed care policies and procedures
  —*Negotiate managed care contracts*

Practice Finances

- Perform procedural and diagnostic coding
- Apply bookkeeping principles
- Manage accounts receivable
  —*Manage accounts payable*
  —*Process payroll*
  —*Document and maintain accounting and banking records*
  —*Develop and maintain fee schedules*
  —*Manage renewals of business and professional insurance policies*
  —*Manage personnel benefits and maintain records*
  —*Perform marketing, financial, and strategic planning*

Clinical

Fundamental Principles

- Apply principles of aseptic technique and infection control
- Comply with quality assurance practices
- Screen and follow up patient test results

Diagnostic Orders

- Collect and process specimens
- Perform diagnostic tests

Patient Care

- Adhere to established patient screening procedures
- Obtain patient history and vital signs
- Prepare and maintain examination and treatment areas
- Prepare patient for examinations, procedures, and treatments
- Assist with examinations, procedures, and treatments
- Prepare and administer medications and immunizations
- Maintain medication and immunization records
- Recognize and respond to emergencies
- Coordinate patient care information with other health care providers
- Initiate IVs and administer IV medications with appropriate training and as permitted by state law

General

Professionalism

- Display a professional manner and image
- Demonstrate initiative and responsibility
- Work as a member of the health care team
- Prioritize and perform multiple tasks
- Adapt to change
- Promote the CMA credential
- Enhance skills through continuing education
- Treat all patients with compassion and empathy
- Promote the practice through positive public relations

Communication Skills

- Recognize and respect cultural diversity
- Adapt communications to individual's ability to understand
- Use professional telephone technique
- Recognize and respond effectively to verbal, nonverbal, and written communications
- Use medical terminology appropriately
- Utilize electronic technology to receive, organize, prioritize and transmit information
- Serve as a liaison

Legal Concepts

- Perform within legal and ethical boundaries
- Prepare and maintain medical records
- Document accurately
- Follow employer's established policies dealing with the health care contract
- Implement and maintain federal and state health care legislation and regulations
- Comply with established risk management and safety procedures
- Recognize professional credentialing criteria
  —*Develop and maintain personnel, policy, and procedures manuals*

Instruction

- Instruct individuals according to their needs
- Explain office policies and procedures
- Teach methods of health promotion and disease prevention
- Locate community resources and disseminate information
  —*Develop educational materials*
  —*Conduct continuing education activities*

Operational Functions

- Perform inventory of supplies and equipment
- Perform routine maintenance of administrative and clinical equipment
- Apply computer techniques to support office operations
  —*Perform personnel management functions*
  —*Negotiate leases and prices for equipment and supply contracts*

APPENDIX B

KEY ENGLISH-TO-SPANISH HEALTH CARE PHRASES

Although English is the major language spoken in North America, a variety of languages are used in certain areas. Prominent among them is Spanish, representing Spain, the Caribbean Islands, Central and South America, and the Philippines. Rapport can be more easily established, and the patient and family will be at ease and feel more relaxed, if someone on the staff speaks their language. Some health care facilities, especially in areas with a large population of Spanish-speaking people, provide interpreters. In smaller hospitals or smaller communities this may not be possible.

It is to your advantage to learn the second most prominent language in your community. For this reason, the following table of English-to-Spanish phrases has been prepared. Instructions for using it are simple. Look for the phrase in English in the first column of the table. The second colulmn gives the phrase in Spanish. You can write this or point to it. The third column gives a phonetic pronunciation. The syllable in each word to be accented is printed in italic type. Even if you are not proficient in English-to-Spanish, your Spanish-speaking patients will appreciate your trying to converse in their language. Begin with "Buenos días. ¿Cómo se siente?" And remember "por favor."[a]

Introductory Phrases

please[a]	por favor	por fah-*vor*
thank you	gracias	*grah*-see-ahs
good morning	buenos días	*bway*-nos *dee*-ahs
good afternoon	buenas tárdes	*bway*-nas *tar*-days
good evening	buenas noches	*bway*-nas *noh*-chays
my name is	mi nombre es	me *nohm*-bray ays
yes/no	si/no	see/no
What is your name?	¿Cómo se llama?	¿Koh-moh say *jah*-mah?
How old are you?	¿Cuántos años tienes?	¿*Kwan*-tohs ahn-yos tee-*ayn*jays?
Do you understand me?	¿Me entiende?	¿Me ayn-tee-*ayn*-day?
Speak slower.	Habla más despacio.	*Ah*-blah mahs days-*pah*-see-oh
Say it once again.	Repítalo, por favor.	Ray-*pee*-tah-loh, por fah-*vor*
How do you feel?	¿Cómo se siente?	¿*Kob*-moh say see-*ayn*-tay?
good	bien	bee-ayn
bad	mal	*mah*l
physician	médico	*may*-dee-koh
hospital	hospital	*ooh*-spee-tall
midwife	comadre	koh-*mah*-dray
native healer	curandero	ku-ren-*day*-roh

General

zero	cero	*se*-roh
one	uno	*oo*-noh
two	dos	dohs
three	tres	trays
four	cuatro	*kwah*-troh
five	cinco	*sin*-koh
six	seis	says
seven	siete	see-*ay*-tay
eight	ocho	oh-choh

From Rosdahl, C.B. [1995]. Textbook of Basic Nursing, 6th ed. Philadelphia: J.B. Lippincott.
[a] You should begin or end any request with the word PLEASE (POR FAVOR).

nine	nueve	new-*ay*-vay
ten	diez	*dee*-ays
hundred	ciento, cien	see-*en*-toh, see-*en*
hundred and one	ciento uno	see-*en*-toh *oo*-noh
Sunday	domingo	doh-*ming*-goh
Monday	lunes	*loo*-nays
Tuesday	martes	*mar*-tays
Wednesday	miércoles	mee-*er*-cohl-ays
Thursday	jueves	*hway*-vays
Friday	viernes	vee-*ayr*-nays
Saturday	sábado	*sah*-bah-doh
right	derecho	day-*ray*-choh
left	izqierdo	ees-kee-*ayr*-doh
early in the morning	temprano por la mañana	tehm-*prah*-noh por lah mah-*nyah*-na
in the daytime	en el dìa	ayn el *dee*-ah
at noon	a mediodía	ah meh-dee-oh-*dee*-ah
at bedtime	al acostarse	al ah-kos-*tar*-say
at night	por la noche	por la *noh*-chay
today	ñoy	oy
tomorrow	mañana	mah-*nyah*-nah
yesterday	ayer	ai-*yer*
week	semana	say-*may*-nah
month	mes	mace

Parts of the Body

the head	la cabeza	la kah-*bay*-sah
the eye	el ojo	el *o*-hoh
the ears	los oídos	lohs o-*ee*-dohs
the nose	la nariz	la nah-*reez*
the mouth	la boca	lah *boh*-kah
the tongue	la lengua	la *len*-gwah
the neck	el cuello	el koo-*eh*-joh
the throat	la garganta	lah gar-*gan*-tah
the skin	la piel	la pee-el
the bones	los huesos	lohs hoo-*ay*-sos
the muscles	los músculos	lohs *moos*-koo-lohs
the nerves	los nervios	lohs *nayhr*-vee-ohs
the shoulder blades	las paletillas	lahs pah-lay-*tee*-jahs
the arm	el brazo	el *brah*-soh
the elbow	el codo	el *koh*-doh
the wrist	la muñeca	lah moon-*yeh*-kah
the hand	la mano	lah *mah*-noh
the chest	el pecho	el *pay*-choh
the lungs	los pulmones	lohs puhl-*moh*-nays
the heart	el corazón	el koh-rah-*son*
the ribs	las costillas	lahs kohs-*tee*-jahs
the side	el flanco	el *flahn*-koh
the back	la espalda	lay ays-*pahl*-dah
the abdomen	el abdomen	el ahb-*doh*-men
the stomach	el estómago	el ays-*toh*-mah-goh
the leg	la pierna	lah pee-ehr-nah
the thigh	el muslo	el *moos*-loh
the ankle	el tobillo	el toh-*bee*-joh
the foot	el pie	el *pee*-ay
urine	urino	u-*re*-noh

Diseases

allergy	alergia	ah-*layr*-hee-ah
anemia	anemia	ah-*nay*-mee-ah
cancer	cancer	kahn-sayr
chickenpox	varicela	vah-ree-*say*-lah
diabetes	diabetes	dee-ah-bay-tees
diphtheria	difteria	deef-*tay*-ree-ah
German measles	rubéola	roo-*bay*-oh-lah
gonorrhea	gonorrea	gun-noh-*ree*-ah
heart disease	enfermedad del corazón	ayn-*fayr*-may-*dahd* dayl koh-rah-*sohn*
high blood pressure	presión alta	pray-see-*ohn al*-ta
influenza	gripe	*gree*-pay
lead poisoning	envenenamiento con plomo	ayn-vay-nay-nah-mee-*ayn*-toh kohn *ploh*-moh
liver disease	enfermedad del hígado	ayn-*fayr*-may-dahd del *ee*-gah-doh
measles	sarampión	sah-rahm-pee-*ohn*
mumps	paperas	pah-*pay*-rahs
nervous disease	enfermedades nerviosa	ayn-fayr-may-*dahd*-days nayr-vee-oh-sah
pleurisy	pleuresía	play-oo-ray-*see*-ah
pneumonia	pulmonía	pool-moh-*nee*-ah
rheumatic fever	reumatismo (fiebre reumatica)	ray-oo-mah-*tees*-moh (fee-*ay*-bray ray-oo-*mah*-tee-kah)
scarlet fever	escarlatina	ays-kahr-lah-*tee*-nah
syphilis	sífilis	*see*-fee-lees
tuberculosis	tuberculosis	too-*bayr*-koo-lohs-sees

Signs and Symptoms

Do you have stomach cramps?	¿Tiene calambres en el estómago?	¿Tee-*ay*-nay kah-*lahm*-brays ayn el ays-*toh*-mah-goh?
chills?	escalofrios?	ays-kah-loh-*free*-ohs?
an attack of fever	un ataque de fiebre?	oon ah-*tah*-kay day fee-*ay*-bray?
hemorrhage?	hemoragia?	ay-moh-*rah*-hee-ah?
nosebleeds?	hemoragia por la nariz?	ay-moh-*rah*-hee-ah por-lah nah-*rees*?
unusual vaginal bleeding?	hemoragia vaginal fuera de los periodos?	ay-moh-*rah*-hee-ah *vah*-hee-nahl foo-*ay*-rah day lohs pay-ree-*oh*-dohs?
hoarseness?	ronquera?	rohn-*kay*-rah?
a sore throat?	le duele la garganta?	lay doo-*ay*-lay lah gahr-*gahn*-tah?
Does it hurt to swallow?	¿Le duele al tragar?	¿Lay doo-ay-lay ahl trah-gar?
Have you any difficulty in breathing?	¿Tiene difficultad al respirar?	¿Tee-*ay*-nay dee-fee-kool-*tahd* ahl rays-*pee*-rahr?
Does it pain you to breathe?	¿Le duele al respirar?	¿Lay doo-*ay*-lay ahl rays-*pee*-rahr?
How does your head feel?	¿Cómo siente la cabeza?	¿*Koh*-moh see-*ayn*-tay lah kah-*bay*-sah?
Is your memory good?	¿Es buena su memoria?	¿Ays *bway*-nah soo may-*moh*-ree-ah?
Have you any pain the head?	¿Le duele la cabeza?	¿Lay doo-*ay*-lay lah Kah-*bay*-sah?
Do you feel dizzy?	¿Tiene usted vértigo?	¿Tee-ay-nay ood-*stayd vehr*-tee-goh?
Are you tired?	¿Está usted cansado?	¿Ay-*stah* ood-*stayd* kahn-sah-doh?
Can you eat?	¿Puede comer?	¿*Pway*-day koh-*mer*?
Have you a good appetite?	¿Tiene usted buen apetito?	¿Tee-*ay*-nay ood-*stayd* bwayn ah-pay-*tee*-toh?

How are your stools?	¿Cómo son sus heces fecales?	¿*Kog*-moh sohn soos *bay*-says fay-*kal*-ays?
Are they regular?	¿Son regulares?	¿Sohn ray-goo-*lah*-rays?
Are you constipated?	¿Está estreñido?	¿Ay-*stah* ays-trayn-*yee*-do?
Do you have diarrhea?	¿Tiene diarrea?	¿Tee-*ay*-nay dee-ah-*ray*-ah?
Have you any difficulty passing water?	¿Tiene dificultad en orinar?	¿Tee-*ay*-nay dee-fee-kool-*tahd* ayn oh-ree-*nahr*?
Do you pass water involuntarily?	¿Orina sin querer?	¿Oh-*ree*-nah seen kay-rayr?
How long have you felt this way?	¿Desde cuándo se siente asi?	¿*Days*-day *Kwan*-doh say see-*ayn*-tay ah-see?
What diseases have you had?	¿Qué enfermedades ha tenido?	¿Kay ayn-fer-may-*dah*-days hah tay-*nee*-doh?
Do you hear voices?	¿Tiene los voces?	¿Tee-*ay*-nay los *vo*-ses?

Examination

Remove your clothing.	Quítese su ropa.	*Key*-tay-say soo *roh*-pah.
Put on this gown.	Pongáse la bata.	Phon-*gah*-say lah *bah*-tah.
We need a urine specimen.	Es necesário una muestra de su orina.	Ays nay-*say*-sar-ee-oh oo-nah moo-*ay*-strah day oh-*ree*-nah.
Be seated.	Siéntese.	See-*ayn*-tay-say.
Recline.	Acuestése.	Ah-*cways*-tay-say.
Sit up.	Siéntese.	See-*ayn*-tay-say.
Stand.	Parése.	*Pah*-ray-say.
Bend your knees.	Doble las rodíllas.	*Doh*-blay lahs roh-*dee*-yahs.
Relax your muscles.	Reláje los músculos.	Ray-*lah*-hay lohs *moos*-koo-lohs.
Try to . . .	Atente . . .	Ah-*tayn*-tay . . .
Try again.	Atente ótra vez.	Ah-*tayn*-tay *oh*-tra vays.
Do not move.	No se muéva.	Noh say moo-*ay*-vah.
Turn on (or to) your left side.	Voltese a su lado izquierdo.	Vohl-*tay*-say ah soo *lah*-doh is-key-*ayr*-doh.
Turn on (or to) your right side.	Voltése a suládo derécho.	Vohl-*tay*-say ah soo *lah*-doh day-*ray*-choh.
Take a deep breath.	Respíra profúndo.	Ray-*speer*-rah pro-*foon*-doh.
Hold your breath.	Deténga su respiración.	Day-*tayn*-gah soo ray-speer-ah-see-*ohn*.
Don't hold your breath.	No deténga su respiración.	Noh day-tayn-gah soo ray-speer-ah-see-*ohn*.
Cough.	Tosa.	*Toh*-sah.
Open your mouth.	Abra la boca.	*Ah*-brah lah *boh*-kah.
Show me . . .	Enséñeme . . .	Ayn-*sayn*-yay-may . . .
Here?	¿Aqui?	¿Ah-*kee*?
There?	¿Allí?	¿Ah-*jee*?
Which side?	¿En qué lado?	¿Ayn kay *lah*-doh?
Let me see your hand.	Enséñeme la mano.	Ayn-*sehn*-yay-may lah *mah*-noh.
Grasp my hand.	Apriete mi mano.	Ah-*pree*-it-tay mee *mah*-noh.
Raise your arm.	Levante el brazo.	Lay-*vahn*-tay el *brah*-soh.
Raise it more.	Más alto.	Mahs *ahl*-toh.
Now the other.	Ahora el otro.	Ah-*oh*-rah el *oh*-troh.

Treatment

It is necessary.	Es necesario.	Ays neh-say-*sah*-ree-oh.
An operation is necessary.	Una operación es necesaria.	Oo-nah oh-peh-rah-see-*ohn* ays neh-say-*sah*-ree-ah.
a prescription	una receta	*oo*-na ray-say-tah
Use it regularly.	Tómelo con regularidad.	*Toh*-may-loh kohn ray-goo-*lah*-ree-dad.
Take one teaspoonful three times daily (in water).	Toma una cucharadita tres veces al dia, con agua.	*Toh*-may oo-na koo-chah-rah-*dee*-tah trays *vay*-says ahl *dee*-ah, kohn ah-gwah.
Gargle.	Haga gargaras.	*Ah*-gah gar-*gah*-rahs.
Use injection.	Use una inyección.	*Oo*-say *oo*-nah in-*yek*-see-ohn.
oral contraceptives	una pildora	*oo*-nah peel-*doh*-rah
a pill	una pastilla	*oo*-nah pahs-*tee*-yah
a powder	un polvo	oon *pohl*-voh
before meals	antes de las comidas	*ahn*-tays day lahs koh-*mee*-dahs
after meals	despues de las comidas	*days*-poo-ehs day lahs koh-mee-dahs
every day	todos los día	*toh*-dohs lohs *dee*-ah
every hour	cada hora	*kah*-dah *oh*-rah
Breathe slowly—like this (in this manner).	Respire despacio—asi.	Rays-*pee*-ray days-*pah*-see-oh—ah-*see*.
Remain on a diet.	Estar a dieta.	Ays-*tar* a dee-*ay*-tah.

General

How do you feel?	¿Cómo se siénte?	¿*Koh*-moh say see-*ayn*-tay?
Do you have pain?	¿Tiéne dolor?	¿Tee-*ay*-nay doh-*lorh*?
Where is the pain?	¿Adónde es el dolor?	¿Ah-*dohn*-day ays ayl doh-*lorh*?
Do you want medication for your pain?	¿Quiére medicación para su dolor?	¿Kay-*ay*-ray may-dee-kah see-*ohn* pak-rah soo doh-*lorh*?
Are you comfortable?	¿Está confortáble?	¿Ay-*stah* kohn-for-*tah*-blay?
Are you thirsty?	¿Tiéne sed?	¿Tee-*ay*-nay sayd?
You may not eat/drink.	No cóma/béba.	Noh *koh*-mah/bay-*bah*.
You can only drink water.	Solo puede tomar agua.	Soh-loh *pway*-day toh-mar *ah*-gwah.
Apply bandage to . . .	Ponga una vendaje a . . .	*Pohn*-gah *oo*-nah vehn-*dah*-hay ah . . .
Apply ointment.	Aplíquese unguento.	Ah-*plee*-kay-say oon-goo-*ayn*-toh.
Keep very quiet.	Estese muy quieto.	Ays-*tay*-say moo-ay key-*ay*-toh.
You must not speak.	No debe hablar.	Noh *day*-bay ha-*blahr*
It will be uncomfortable.	Séra incomódo.	*Say*-rah een-koh-*moh*-doh.
It will sting.	Va ardér.	Vah ahr-*dayr*.
You will feel pressure.	Vá a sentír presión.	Vah ah sayn-*teer* pray-see-*ohn*.
I am going to . . .	Voy a . . .	Voy ah . . .
Count (take) your pulse.	Tomár su púlso.	Toh-*marh* soo *pool*-soh.
Take your temperature.	Tomár su temperatúra.	Toh-*marh* soo taym-pay-rah-*too*-rah.
Take your blood pressure.	Tomar su presión.	Toh-*mahr* soo pray-see-*ohn*.
Give you pain medicine.	Dárle medicación para dolór.	*Dahr*-lay may dee-kah-see-*ohn* pah-rah doh-*lohr*.
You should (try to) . . .	Trate de . . .	*Tray*-tay day . . .
Call for help/assistance.	Llamar para asisténcia.	Yah-*marh* pah-rah ah-sees-*tayn*-see-ah.
Empty your bladder.	Orinar.	Oh-ree-*narh*.
Do you still feel very weak?	¿Se siente muy débil todavía?	¿Say see-*ayn*-tay moo-ee *day*-beel toh-dah-*vee*-ah?
It is important to . . .	Es importánte que . . .	Ays eem-por-*tahn*-tay Kay . . .
Walk (ambulate).	Caminar.	Kah-mee-*narh*.
Drink fluids.	Beber líquidos.	Bay-*bayr* lee-kay-dohs.

APPENDIX C

TWO-LETTER POSTAL ZIP CODE ABBREVIATIONS

Alabama	AL	Nebraska	NE
Alaska	AK	Nevada	NV
Arizona	AZ	New Hampshire	NH
Arkansas	AR	New Jersey	NJ
American Samoa	AS	New Mexico	NM
California	CA	New York	NY
Colorado	CO	North Carolina	NC
Connecticut	CT	North Dakota	ND
Delaware	DE	Northern Mariana Islands	MP
District of Columbia	DC	Ohio	OH
Federated States of Micronesia	FM	Oklahoma	OK
Florida	FL	Oregon	OR
Georgia	GA	Palau	PW
Guam	GU	Pennsylvania	PA
Hawaii	HI	Puerto Rico	PR
Idaho	ID	Rhode Island	RI
Illinois	IL	South Carolina	SC
Indiana	IN	South Dakota	SD
Iowa	IA	Tennessee	TN
Kansas	KS	Texas	TX
Kentucky	KY	Utah	UT
Louisiana	LA	Vermont	VT
Maine	ME	Virginia	VA
Marshall Islands	MH	Virgin Islands	VI
Maryland	MD	Washington	WA
Massachusetts	MA	West Virginia	WV
Michigan	MI	Wisconsin	WI
Minnesota	MN	Wyoming	WY
Mississippi	MS	Armed Forces of the Americas	AA
Missouri	MO	Armed Forces Europe	AE
Montana	MT	Armed Forces Pacific	AP

APPENDIX D

ABBREVIATIONS COMMONLY USED IN DOCUMENTATION

Abbreviation	Meaning	Abbreviation	Meaning
ā	before	NKDA	no known drug allergies
abd	abdomen	noct.	nocturnal
ac	before meals	NPO	nothing by mouth
ADL	activities of daily living	os	mouth
ad lib	as needed	OOB	out of bed
adm	admitted, admission	oz	ounce
amp	ampule	p̄	after
ant.	anterior	p.c.	after meals
AP	anterior-posterior	post	posterior
ax.	axillary	prep	preparation
b.i.d.	twice a day	pm	when necessary
BP	blood pressure	p.r.n.	as needed
BR	bed rest	pt.	patient
BRP	bathroom privileges	q̄, q	every
C	Celsius	q̄ 2 (3, 4, etc.) hours	every 2 (3, 4, etc.) hours
c̄	with	qd	every day
caps	capsule	qh	every hour
CC	chief complaint	q.i.d.	four times a day
cc	cubic centimeter (1 cc = 1 mL)	q.o.d.	every other day
c/o	complains of	q.s.	quantity sufficient
CVP	central venous pressure	R	right
CPX	complete physical examination	R/O	rule out
Cx	canceled	ROM	range of motion
D/C	discontinue	r/s	rescheduled
disch; DC	discharge	s̄	without
drsg	dressing	SBA	stand by assistance
dr	dram	SC	subcutaneous
elix	elixir	SL	sublingual
ext	extract or external	SOB	shortness of breath
F	Fahrenheit	sol, soln	solution
Fx	fracture, fractional	spec	specimen
gm	gram	s/p	status post
gr	grain	sp. gr.	specific gravity
gt/gtt	drop/drops	S.S.E.	soapsuds enema
"H," SC, or sub q	hypodermic or subcutaneous	ss	one-half
h	hour	STAT	immediately
HOB	head of bed	tab	tablet
h.s.	bedtime (hour of sleep)	t.i.d.	three times a day
Hx	history	tinct or tr.	tincture
I & O	intake & output	TKO	to keep open
IM	intramuscular	TPN	total parenteral nutrition hyperalimentation
IV	intravenous		
kg	kilogram	TPR	temperature, pulse, respiration
KVO	keep vein open	tsp	teaspoon
L	left, liter	TO	telephone order
lat	lateral	TWE	tap water enema
MAE	moves all extremities	VO	verbal order
mg	milligram	VS	vital signs
ml, mL	milliliter (1 mL = 1 cc)	VSS	vital signs stable
NAD	no apparent distress	W/C	wheelchair
NG	nasogastric	WNL	within normal limits

Abbreviation	Meaning

Selected Abbreviations Used for Specific Descriptions

AKA	above-knee amputation
ASCVD	arteriosclerotic cardiovascular disease
ASHD	areteriosclerotic heart disease
BKA	below-knee amputation
ca	cancer
chest clear to A & P	chest cleart to auscultation & percussion
CMS	cirulation movement sensation
CNS	central nervous system
DJD	degenerative joint disease
DOE	dyspnea on exertion
DTs	delirium tremens
D_5W	5% dextrose in water
FUO	fever of unknown origin
GB	gallbladder
GI	gastrointestinal
GYN	gynecology
H_2O_2	hydrogen peroxide
HA	hyperalimentation headache
HCVD	hypertensive cardiovascular disease
HEENT	head, ear, eye, nose, throat
HVD	hypertensive vascular disease
ICU	intensive care unit
I & D	incision and drainage
LLE	left lower extremity
LLQ	left lower quadrant
LOC	level of consciousnesss; laxatives of choice
LMP	last menstrual period
LUE	left upper extremity
LUQ	left upper quadrant
MI	myocardial infarction
Neuro	neurology; neurosurgery
NS	normal saline
Nys.	nursery
NWB	non–weight-bearing
O.D.	right eye
O.S.	left eye
O.U.	each eye
OPD	outpatient department
ORIF	open reduction internal fixation
Ortho	orthopedics
OT	occupational therapy
PE	physical examination
PERRLA	pupils equal, round, & react to light and accomodation
PID	pelvic inflammatory disease
PI	present illness
PM & R	physical medicine & rehabilitation
Psych	psychology; psychiatric

Abbreviation	Meaning
PT	physical therapy
RL (or LR)	Ringer's lactate; lactated Ringer's
RLE	right lower extremity
RLQ	right lower quadrant
RR, PAR, PACU	recovery room, post-anesthesia room, post-anesthesia care unit
RUE	right upper extremity
RUQ	right upper quadrant
Rx	prescription
SOB	short of breath
STD	sexually transmitted disease
STSG	split-thickness skin graft
Surg	surgery, surgical
T & A	tonsillectomy & adenoidectomy
THR, TJR	total hip replacement; total joint replacement
URI	upper respiratory infection
UTI	urinary tract infection
vag	vaginal
WNWD	well-nourished, well-developed

Selected Abbreviations Related to Common Diagnostic Tests

BE	barium enema
B.M.R	basal metabolism rate
Ca^{++}	calcium
CAT	computed axial tomography
CBC	complete blood count
Cl^-	chloride
C & S	culture & sensitivity
Dx	diagnosis
ECG, EKG	electrocardiogram
EEG	eletroencephalogram
FBS	fasting blood sugar
hct	hematocrit
Hgb	hemoglobin
IVP	intravenous pyelogram
K^+	potassium
LP	lumbar puncture
MRI	magnetic resonance imaging
Na^+	sodium
RBC	red blood cell
UGI	upper gastrointestinal x-ray
UA	urinalysis
WBC	white blood cell

Commonly Used Symbols

$>$	greater than
$<$	less than
$=$	equal to
$\approx$	approximately equal to
$\leq$	equal to or less than
$\geq$	equal to or greater than

Abbreviation	Meaning	Abbreviation	Meaning
↑	increased	±	positive or negative
↓	decreased	F_1	first filial generation
♀	female	F_2	second filal generation
♂	male	PO_2	partial pressure of oxygen
°	degree	PCO_2	partial pressure of carbon dioxide
#	number or pound	:	ratio
×	times	∴	therefore
@	at	%	percent
+	positive	$2°$	secondary to
−	negative	△	change

From Craven, R.F., and Hirnle, C.J. (1996). Human Health and Function, 2nd ed. Philadelphia: Lippincott-Raven.

APPENDIX E

COMMONLY MISUSED WORDS

Because these words have similar spellings and pronunciation, they can easily be confused or misused. Watch your spelling carefully! Always proofread all business letters for accuracy and grammar.

Word	Example of Correct Use
adverse (harmful) averse (opposed to)	Some adverse reactions can be life threatening. I am not averse to working on Mondays.
affect (verb, to influence, change) effect (noun, result)	The protesters will not affect the outcome. The effect of the antibiotics has been beneficial.
already (previously) all ready (prepared, all set)	We already tried that approach. Are we all ready to go?
anoxia (without oxygen) anorexia (without appetite)	Anoxia will cause the brain cells to die quickly. Anorexia is a serious illness that faces teenagers.
aphagia (without swallowing) aphasia (without speech)	A feeding tube is needed because of her aphagia. Her stroke caused aphasia.
appendices (end of book) appendicitis (inflammation of appendix)	There are five appendices at the end of book. The patient was treated for appendicitis.
biannual (twice a year) biennial (occurring every 2 years)	Productivity reports are printed on a biannual basis. Staff contracts are renewed on a biennial basis.
bite (grip with teeth) byte (character)	The patient's bite is poorly aligned. Buy a computer with enough bytes for future growth.
bowl (container) bowel (intestines, colon)	The jelly beans are in the bowl. Instruct the patient to complete the bowel preparation.
emphysema (chronic lung disease) empyema (accumulation of pus)	Smoking causes emphysema. Empyema most commonly occurs in the pleural cavity.
ensure (be certain) insure (protect against risk) assure (provide confidence)	Call this patient to ensure that he comprehends the instructions. Please insure this package for $200. I assure you that he is getting the correct treatment.
everyday (adjective, routine, ordinary) every day (adverbial phrase, each day)	Quality checks are an everyday procedure. There can be legal ramifications if this is not done every day.
except (exclude) expect (anticipate) accept (agree)	All antibiotics except penicillin will work. I expect this work to be completed by noon. I accept this challenge.
farther (greater distance) further (greater degree)	It is 1 mile farther down the road. The process needs further refinement.

Word	Example of Correct Use
fundus (pertains to hollow organ)	The fundus was firm after the baby's delivery.
fungus (organism that can lead to infection)	A fungus was growing under her nails.
its (possessive pronoun)	The pharmacy must protect its supply of opioids.
it's (contraction of it and is)	It's time to take a break.
lactose (type of sugar in milk)	I have a lactose allergy.
lactase (enzyme)	Lactase is responsible for dissolving lactose.
libel (written defamatory statement)	The statements about John Roberts were libel.
liable (legally responsible)	You are liable for your actions.
may be (compound verb)	Dr. Rogers may be in surgery this afternoon.
maybe (adverb, perhaps)	Maybe it will snow tomorrow.
metatarsals (bones in foot)	Crutches are often needed when the metatarsals are fractured.
metacarpals (bones in palm)	Typing is difficult for patients with a metacarpal fracture.
mucus (substance that is secreted)	The patient had a mucus plug.
mucous (membrane that secretes)	The mucous membrane secretes the mucus.
parental (pertaining to parent)	Follow parental guidelines for TV use.
parenteral (not by mouth)	Parenteral feedings will start on Monday.
postnatal (after birth)	Complications can occur in the postnatal period.
postnasal (behind nose)	Postnasal drainage can be uncomfortable.
principle (noun, law)	A key principle of economics is understanding cash flow.
principal (noun, leader; adjective, most important)	The principal's name is Tina Sefferin; her experience is the principal reason she was hired.
rubella (German measles)	You need a rubella vaccination.
rubeola (14-day measles)	There is a outbreak of rubeola at the middle school.
serum (watery component of blood)	The patient's serum is used for various tests.
sebum (oily substance secreted by the sebaceous glands)	Sebum helps to lubricate the skin surface.
tact (behavior)	He handled his child with great tact.
tack (different direction)	A new tack may be needed for us to win that bid.
than (to show comparison)	Salaries are higher now than they were a year ago.
then (next)	Clean room 2; then go to lunch.
there (place, point)	You need to be there at 2 PM.
their (possessive pronoun)	Leaving their bikes on the road caused the accident.
they're (pronoun plus verb)	They're going to be late.
uvula (soft tissue at back of palate)	The patient's uvula was swollen.
vulva (external female organ)	A laceration of the vulva was noted during the gynecological examination.
weather (climate)	The weather is unpredictable.
whether (indicating a possibility)	I wonder whether it will rain or snow.

APPENDIX F

METRIC MEASUREMENTS

Unit	Abbreviation	Metric Equivalent	U.S. Equivalent
Units of weight			
Kilogram	kg	1000 g	2.2 lb
Gram*	g	1000 mg	0.35 oz.; 28.5 g/oz
Milligram	mg	1/1000 g; 0.001 g	
Microgram	μg	1.1000 mg; 0.001 mg	
Units of length			
Kilometer	km	1000 meters	0.62 miles; 1.6 km/mile
Meter*	m	100 cm; 1000 mm	39.4 inches; 1.1 yards
Centimeter	cm	1/100 m; 0.01 m	0.39 inches; 2.5 cm/inch
Millimeter	mm	1/1000 m; 0.001 m	0.039 inches; 25 mm/inch
Micrometer	μm	1/1000 mm; 0.001 mm	
Units of volume			
Liter*	L	1000 mL	1.06 qt
Deciliter	dL	1/10 L; 0.1 L	
Milliliter	mL	1/1000 L; 0.1 L	0.034 oz., 29.4 mL/oz
Microliter	μL	1/1000 mm; 0.001 mL	

*Basic unit

(From Memmler, R.L., Cohen, B.J., and Wood, D.L. [1996], The Human Body in Health and Disease, 8th ed. Philadelphia: Lippincott-Raven.)

APPENDIX G

CELSIUS–FAHRENHEIT TEMPERATURE CONVERSION SCALE

Celsius to Fahrenheit

Use the following formula to convert Celsius readings to Farenheit readings:

$$°F = 9/5 \ °C + 32$$

For example, if the Celsius reading is 37°:

$$°F = (9/5 \times 37) + 32$$
$$= 66.6 + 32$$
$$= 98.6°F \text{ (normal body temperature)}$$

Fahrenheit to Celsius

Use the following formula to convert Fahrenheit readings to Celsius readings:

$$°C = 5/9 \ (°F - 32)$$

For example, if the Fahrenheit reading is 68°:

$$°C = 5/9(68 - 32)$$
$$= 5/9 \times 36$$
$$= 20°C \text{ (a nice spring day)}$$

temperature
conversion
scale

(From Memmler, R.L., Cohen, B.J., and Wood, D.L. [1996], The Human Body in Health and Disease, 8th ed. Philadelphia: Lippincott-Raven.)

APPENDIX H

LABORATORY TESTS

■ TABLE I ROUTINE URINALYSIS

Test	Normal Value	Clinical Significance
General characteristics and measurements		
Color	Pale yellow to amber	Color change can be due to concentration or dilution, drugs, metabolic or inflammatory disorders
Odor	Slightly aromatic	Foul odor typical of urinary tract infection, fruity odor in uncontrolled diabetes mellitus
Appearance (clarity)	Clear to slightly hazy	Cloudy urine occurs with infection or after refrigeration; may indicate presence of bacteria, cells, mucus, or crystals
Specific gravity	1.003–1.030 (first morning; routine is random)	Decreased in diabetes insipidus, acute renal failure, water intoxication; increased in liver disorders, heart failure, dehydration
pH	4.5–8.0	Acid urine accompanies acidosis, fever, high protein diet; alkaline urine in urinary tract infection, metabolic alkalosis, vegetarian diet
Chemical determinations		
Glucose	Negative	Glucose present in uncontrolled diabetes mellitus, steroid excess
Ketones	Negative	Present in diabetes mellitus and in starvation
Protein	Negative	Present in kidney disorders, such as glomerulonephritis, acute kidney failure
Bilirubin	Negative	Breakdown product of hemoglobin; present in liver disease or in bile blockage
Urobilinogen	0.2–1.0 Ehrlich units/dL	Breakdown product of bilirubin; increased in hemolytic anemias and in liver disease; remains negative in bile obstruction
Blood (occult)	Negative	Detects small amounts of blood cells, hemoglobin, or myoglobin; present in severe trauma, metabolic disorders, bladder infections
Nitrite	Negative	Product of bacteria breakdown of urine; positive result suggests urinary tract infection and need to be followed up with a culture of the urine.
Microscopic		
Red blood cells	0–3 per high-power field	Increased due to bleeding within the urinary tract from trauma, tumors, inflammation, or damage within the kidney
White blood cells	0–4 per high-power field	Increased in infection of the kidney or bladder
Renal epithelial cells	Occasional	Increased number indicates damage to kidney tubules
Casts	None	Hyaline casts normal; large number of abnormal casts indicates inflammation or a systemic disorder
Crystals	Present	Most are normal; may be acid or alkaline
Bacteria	Few	Increased in infection of urinary tract or contamination from infected genitalia
Others		Any yeasts, parasites, mucus, spermatozoa, or other microscopic findings would be reported here

■ TABLE 2 COMPLETE BLOOD COUNT (CBC)

Test	Normal Value*	Clinical Significance
Red blood cell count (RBC)	Men: 4.2–5.4 million/μL Women: 3.6–5.0 million/μL	Decreased in anemia; increased in dehydration, polycythemia
Hemoglobin (HGB)	Men: 13.5–17.5 g/dL Women: 12–16 g/dL	Decreased in anemia, hemorrhage and hemolytic reactions; increased in dehydration, heart and lung disease
Hematocrit (HCT) or packed cell volume (PCV)	Men: 40%–50% Women: 37%–47%	Decreased in anemia; increased in polycythemia, dehydration
Red blood cell indices (examples)		These values, calculated from the RBC, HGB, and HCT, give information valuable in the diagnosis and classification of anemia
Mean corpuscular volume (MVC)	87–103 μl/red cell	Measures the average size or volume of each red blood cell: Small size (microcytic) in iron-deficiency anemia; large size (macrocytic) typical of pernicious anemia
Mean corpuscular hemoglobin (MCH)	26–34 pg/red cell	Measures the weight of hemoglobin per red blood cell; useful in differentiating types of anemia in a severely anemic patient
Mean corpuscular hemoglobin concentration (MCHC)	31–37 g/dL	Defines the volume of hemoglobin per red blood cell; used to determine the color or concentration of hemoglobin per red cell
White blood count (WBC)	5,000–10,000/μL	Increased in leukemia and in response to infection, inflammation, and dehydration; decreased in bone marrow suppression
Platelets	150,000–350,000/μL	Increased in many malignant disorders; decreased in disseminated intravascular coagulation (DIC) or toxic drug effects; spontaneous bleeding may occur at platelet counts below 20,000
Differential (Peripheral blood smear)		A stained slide of the blood is needed to perform the differential. The percentages of the different white cells are estimated, and the slide is microscopically checked for abnormal characteristics in WBCs, RBCs, and platelets.
White cells		
Segments neutrophils (SEGs, POLYs)	40%–74%	Increased in bacterial infections; low numbers leave person very susceptible to infection
Immature neutrophils (BANDs)	0%–3%	Increase when neutrophil count increases
Lymphocytes (LYMPHs)	20%–40%	Increased in viral infections; low numbers leave a person dangerously susceptible to infection
Monocytes (MONOs)	2%–6%	Increased in specific infections
Eosinophils (EOs)	1%–4%	Increased in allergic disorders
Basophils (BASOs)	0.5%–1%	Increased in allergic disorders

*Values vary depending on instrumentation and type of test.

■ TABLE 3   BLOOD CHEMISTRY TESTS

Test	Normal Value	Clinical Significance
Basic panel: An overview of electrolytes, waste product management, and metabolism		
Blood urea nitrogen (BUN)	7–18 mg/dL	Increased in renal disease and dehydration; decreased in liver damage and malnutrition
Carbon dioxide (CO_2) (includes bicarbonate)	23–30 mmol/L	Useful to evaluate acid-base balance by measuring total carbon dioxide in the blood: Elevated in vomiting and pulmonary disease; decreased in diabetic acidosis, acute renal failure, and hyperventilation
Chloride (Cl)	98–106 mEq/L	Increased in dehydration, hyperventilation, and congestive heart failure; decreased in vomiting, diarrhea, and fever
Creatinine	0.6–1.2 mg/dL	Produced at a constant rate and excreted by the kidney; increased in kidney disease
Glucose	Fasting: 70–110 mg/dlL Random: 85–125 mg/dL	Increased in diabetes and severe illness; decreased in insulin overdose or hypoglycemia
Potassium (K)	3.5–5.0 mEq/L	Increased in renal failure, extensive cell damage and acidosis; decreased in vomiting, diarrhea, and excess administration of diuretics or IV fluids
Sodium (Na)	135–148 mEq/L	Increased in dehydration and diabetes insipidus; decreased in overload of IV fluids, burns, diarrhea, or vomiting
Additional blood chemistry tests		
Alanine aminotransferase (ALT)	Men: 7–24 U/L Women: 7–17 U/L	Used to diagnose and monitor treatment of liver disease and to monitor the effects of drugs on the liver, increased in myocardial infarction
Albumin	3.8–5.0 g/dL	Albumin holds water in blood; decreased in liver disease and kidney disease
Albumin-globulin ratio (A/G ratio)	Greater than 1	Low A/G ratio signifies a tendency for edema because globulin is less effective than albumin at holding water in the blood.
Alkaline phosphatase (ALP)	20–70 U/L (varies by method)	Enzyme of bone metabolism; increased in liver disease and metastatic bone disease
Amylase	21–160 U/L	Used to diagnose and monitor treatment of acute pancreatitis and to detect inflammation of the salivary glands
Aspartate aminotransferase (AST)	0–41 U/L (varies)	Enzyme present in tissues with high metabolic activity; increased in myocardial infarction and liver disease
Bilirubin, total	0.2–1.0 mg/dL	Breakdown product of hemoglobin from red blood cells; increased when excessive RBCs are being destroyed or in liver disease
Calcium (Ca)	8.8–10.0 mg/dL	Increased in excess parathyroid hormone production and in cancer; decreased in alkalosis, elevated phosphate in renal failure, and excess IV fluids
Cholesterol	120–200 mg/dL desirable range	Screening test used to evaluate risk of heart disease; levels of 200 or above indicate increased risk of heart disease and warrant further investigation
Creatinine phosphokinase (CPK or CK)	Men: 38–174 U/L Women: 96–140 U/L	Elevated enzyme level indicates myocardial infarction or damage to skeletal muscle. When elevated, specific fractions (isoenzymes) should be tested

continued

■ TABLE 3 BLOOD CHEMISTRY TESTS *(Continued)*

Test	Normal Value	Clinical Significance
Gamma glutamyl transferase (GGT)	Men: 6–26 U/L Women: 4–18 U/L	Used to diagnose liver disease and test for chronic alcoholism
Globulins	2.3–3.5 g/dL	Proteins active in immunity; help albumin keep water in blood
Iron, serum (Fe)	Men: 75–175 μg/dL Women: 65–165 μg/dL	Decreased in iron deficiency and anemia; increased in hemolytic conditions
High-density lipoproteins (HDLs)	Men: 30–70 mg/dL Women: 30–85 mg/dL	Used to evaluate the risk of heart disease
Lactic dehydrogenase (LDH or LD)	95–200 U/L (normal ranges vary greatly)	Enzyme released in many kinds of tissue damage; including myocardial infarction, pulmonary infarction, and liver disease
Lipase	4–24 U/L (varies with test)	Enzyme used to diagnose pancreatitis
Low-density lipoproteins (LDLs)	80–140 mg/dL	Used to evaluate the risk of heart disease
Magnesium (Mg)	1.3–2.1 mEq/L	Vital in neuromuscular function; decreased levels may occur in malnutrition, alcoholism, pancreatitis, diarrhea
Phosphorus (P) (inorganic)	2.7–4.5 mg/dL	Evaluated in response to calcium; main store is in bone: elevated in kidney disease; decreased in excess parathyroid hormone
Protein, total	6–8 g/dL	Increased in dehydration, multiple myeloma; decreased in kidney disease, liver disease, poor nutrition, severe burns, excessive bleeding
Serum glutamic oxalacetic transaminase (SGOT)		See aspartate aminotransferase (AST)
Serum glutamic pyruvic transaminase (SGPT)		See alanine aminotransferase (ALT)
Thyroxin (T_4)	5–12.5 μg/dL (varies)	Screening test of thyroid function; increased in hyperthyroidism; decreased in myxedema and hypothyroidism
Thyroid stimulating hormone (TSH)	0.5–6 mIU/L	Produced by pituitary to cause thyroid gland to function; elevated when thyroid gland is not functioning
Triiodothyronine (T_3)	120–195 mg/dL	Elevated in specific types of hyperthyroidism
Triglycerides	Men: 40–160 mg/dL Women: 35–135 mg/dL	An indication of ability to metabolize fats; increased triglycerides and cholesterol indicate high risk of atherosclerosis
Uric acid	Men: 3.5–7.2 mg/dL Women: 2.6–6.0 mg/dL	Produced by breakdown of ingested purines in food and nucleic acids; elevated in kidney disease, gout, and leukemia

From Memmler, R.L., Cohen, B. J., and Wood, D.L. [1996]. The Human Body in Health and Disease, 8th ed. Philadelphia: Lippincott-Raven.)

APPENDIX I

Performing Cardiopulmonary Resuscitation (CPR)

Purpose:	Perform chest compressions and rescue breathing to maintain or restore cardiopulmonary function until advanced emergency medical services are available.
Equipment:	Mouth-to-mouth barrier device, clean examination gloves
Standard:	Demonstration of competency depends upon the individual student and the structured educational protocol.

Steps	Reason
1. Determine patient's level of unresponsiveness by shaking the patient and shouting, "Are you okay?"	Establishing unresponsiveness prevents rescue measures for a patient who does not need them.
2. If the patient does not respond and no neck injury is suspected, assess for airway patency and respirations using the head tilt–chin lift maneuver. Instruct another staff member to obtain the physician and the emergency medical cart. If gloves are easily accessible, put clean gloves on both hands.	The patient must be supine before the airway can be assessed. If a neck injury is suspected, roll the patient carefully to the back without twisting or moving the neck and use the jaw thrust method to open the airway.
3. After opening the airway, assess for breathing by placing the side of your face 2 to 3 inches in front of the patient's mouth to feel for air movement while watching the chest for rise and fall.	Determining breathlessness avoids giving respirations to a patient who is breathing.
4. If the patient is breathing adequately, place the patient in the recovery position until consciousness returns or EMS arrives.	The recovery position (side-lying) facilitates respirations and prevents aspiration of emesis in the event that the patient vomits.
5. If the patient is not breathing adequately, instruct a staff member to notify EMS and begin rescue breathing by placing a barrier device over the patient's mouth and nose and giving 2 slow breaths, causing the chest to rise without overfilling the lungs.	Quick access to EMS increases the patient's chance for survival. Slow breaths provide oxygen without overfilling the lungs causing gastric distention and vomiting.
6. Check for cardiac function by palpating the carotid pulse on the side of the neck.	
7. If a pulse is present, continue rescue breathing as needed.	During rescue breathing, periodically check for a pulse and be prepared to begin chest compressions if needed. If the patient resumes adequate respirations, put the patient in the recovery position until EMS arrives.
8. If no pulse is present, follow these steps to perform chest compressions:	
A. Place the palm of one hand on the sternum, 2 fingers above the xiphoid process at the lowest end of the sternum.	Avoid pressing directly on the xiphoid process to prevent injury to internal structures if this structure breaks off.
B. Place the palm of the other hand on top of the correctly placed hand, lacing the fingers.	

(continued)

Appendix I *(continued)*

Performing Cardiopulmonary Resuscitation (CPR)

Steps	Reason
C. With your upper body perpendicular to the patient's chest, lock the elbows and press straight down, compressing the sternum 1.5 to 2 inches.	
D. Keep your hands in position during the upstroke, but allow the patient's chest to expand completely before the next compression. Give cycles of 15 chest compressions and 2 breaths.	
9. After about 1 minute, check the carotid pulse. If no pulse is present, continue the cycle, beginning with chest compressions. Continue until help arrives or until a pulse is palpated during the periodic pulse check. If the pulse returns but respirations do not, continue giving breaths at 14 to 16 per minute until EMS arrives.	

EMS, emergency medical service.

Note: In the clinical situation, respiratory barrier devices and gloves will be available to protect you from the patient's oral secretions and should be used appropriately. In the out-of-office situation, these devices may not be at hand.

All health care professionals should receive training for proficiency in CPR in an approved program. The procedure described here is not intended to substitute for proficiency training with a mannequin and a structured protocol.

Charting Example

10/14/2005 10:30 A.M. Pt. arrived c/o chest pain. Skin diaphoretic, color pale. Pulse 125 and regular, BP 88/54 (L). Collapsed in exam room, Dr. Barton notified. Pulse and respirations absent, CPR started. EMS notified. _____ S. Pencil, CMA

10/14/2005 10:40 A.M. CPR continued per EMS. Pt. transported to General Hospital. _____ S. Pencil, CMA

Using an Automatic External Defibrillator (AED)

Purpose:	Use an automatic external defibrillator to restore normal cardiac function after cardiac arrest.
Equipment:	An automatic external defibrillator (AED), chest electrodes with connection wire for use with the AED, mouth-to-mouth barrier device
Standard:	Demonstration of competency depends on the student and the structured educational protocol.

Steps	Reason
1. Determine patient level of unresponsiveness by shaking the patient and shouting, "Are you okay?"	Establishing unresponsiveness prevents rescue measures for a patient who does not need them.
2. Follow the procedure for assessing airway patency and respirations, giving 2 rescue breaths, and checking for a carotid pulse (Appendix G). Instruct another staff member to notify the physician, obtain the emergency cart and AED, and phone EMS.	Quick access to an AED and EMS increases the patient's chances for survival.
3. Begin CPR in absence of adequate respirations or a carotid pulse.	
4. When the AED is available, the second rescuer removes the patient's shirt and prepares the chest for the electrodes while the first rescuer continues CPR.	The skin on the chest must be dry to allow for adequate contact of the electrodes. Any excess hair must be shaved before the electrodes are placed. Medication patches that interfere with placement of the electrodes must be removed and the medication wiped away.
5. After removal of the sticky paper backing, apply the chest electrodes, one on the upper right chest and the other on the lower left chest.	The front of the electrodes depicts placement as a reminder. Chest compressions are not possible during application of the electrodes.
6. Once the electrodes are in place, connect the wire from the electrodes to the AED and the AED turned on.	
7. Follow the instructions given by the AED as the heart rhythm is analyzed. Do not touch the patient during the analysis, including performing CPR. If no shock is indicated, the AED will indicate this and instruct you to resume CPR. Begin by checking the patient for respirations and a carotid pulse. If not present, resume CPR.	
8. If the AED indicates that an electrical shock is necessary, the second rescuer makes sure that no person is touching the patient or the examination table before delivering the electrical shock by pressing the appropriate button on the AED.	If another person is touching the patient or the examination table when an electrical shock is delivered, the shock will be transferred to that person as well as the patient.

(continued)

Appendix J *(continued)*

Using an Automatic External Defibrillator (AED)

Steps	Reason
9. After delivering the shock, the AED will again analyze the patient's heart rhythm. The patient must not be touched during this process.	
10. After the second analysis of the heart rhythm, the AED will instruct you to resume CPR or deliver another electrical shock. Continue to follow the instructions given by the AED, being prepared to perform CPR if needed, until the EMS arrives.	

Note: All health care professionals should take an approved training course in CPR and use of an AED. This procedure is not intended to substitute for proficiency training with a mannequin in a structured educational protocol.

Charting Example

11/15/2005 3:15 P.M. Pt. became unresponsive while waiting in reception area; no pulse or respiratory effort. Dr. Barton and EMS notified. CPR started. _____ J. Crete, CMA

11/15/2005 3:20 P.M. AED applied, 2 electrical shocks delivered, pulse returned, no respiratory effort. Rescue breathing resumed. _____ J. Crete, CMA

11/15/2005 3:25 P.M. EMS here. Pt. transported to General Hospital. _____ J. Crete, CMA

Managing a Foreign Body Airway Obstruction

Purpose:	To restore airway patency by removing a foreign body obstruction.
Equipment:	Mouth-to-mouth barrier device, clean examination gloves.
Standard:	Demonstration of competency depends on the student and the structured educational protocol.

Steps	Reason
1. Ask the patient, "Are you choking?" If the patient can speak or cough, the obstruction is not complete. Observe the patient for increased distress and assist as needed, but do not perform thrusts.	The patient who is coughing or speaking can breathe and may be able to remove the obstruction without assistance. Performing abdominal thrusts on a patient who is not in need of assistance may cause injury.
2. If the patient cannot speak or cough and is displaying the universal sign of distress (grasping the throat with both hands), follow these steps to perform abdominal thrusts and have a coworker notify the physician and EMS according to office policy:	
A. Stand behind the patient and wrap your arms around his or her waist.	
B. Make a fist with your nondominant hand, thumb side against the patient's abdomen between the navel and the xiphoid process.	
C. Grasp your fist with your dominant hand and give quick upward thrusts. Completely relax your arms between each thrust and make each thrust forceful enough to dislodge the obstruction.	
3. Repeat the thrusts until the object is expelled and the patient can breathe or the patient becomes unconscious.	Several thrusts may be necessary to expel the object.
4. If the patient is unconscious or becomes unconscious, perform a tongue–jaw lift followed by a finger sweep to remove the object.	Before performing the tongue–jaw lift and finger sweep, apply clean examination gloves if available to avoid contact with the patient's oral secretions.
5. Open the airway and try to ventilate. If the airway is still obstructed, reposition the patient's head and try to give rescue breaths again. Use a barrier device if available.	Repositioning the patient's head ensures that the airway obstruction is not caused by improper head position.
6. If rescue breaths continue to be obstructed, begin abdominal thrusts:	
A. Straddle the patient's hips.	
B. Place the palm of one hand between the patient's navel and the xiphoid process.	
C. Lace your fingers with the other hand against the back of the properly positioned hand.	

(continued)

Appendix K *(continued)*

Managing a Foreign Body Airway Obstruction

Steps	Reason
7. Give 5 abdominal thrusts, perform the tongue–jaw lift and finger sweep, and attempt rescue breaths. If rescue breaths ventilate the lungs, continue rescue breaths until the patient resumes breathing or EMS arrives. Periodically check for a carotid pulse and be prepared to start CPR if necessary.	
8. If no object is removed after the finger sweep or the lungs cannot be inflated during rescue breaths, continue the cycle of abdominal thrusts, tongue–jaw lift and finger sweep, and rescue breaths until EMS arrives.	

Notes: Obese or pregnant patients require chest thrusts rather than abdominal thrusts.

Children over age 8 years are considered to be adults for the purpose of foreign body airway obstruction.

All health care professionals should be trained for proficiency in CPR and managing foreign body airway obstructions in an approved program. This procedure is not intended to substitute for proficiency training with a mannequin and a structured protocol.

Charting Example
07/09/2005 2:15 P.M. Pt. choked on a throat lozenge in exam room. Abdominal thrusts x6 administered; lozenge removed. Dr. Kramer notified. Pulse 104, Respirations 26, BP 160/98 (R). _____ R. Lent, CMA

GLOSSARY OF KEY TERMS

A

abandonment withdrawal by a physician from a contractual relationship with a patient without proper notification while the patient still needs treatment.

abdominal regions divisions of the abdomen into nine regions by two horizontal and two vertical lines; used to identify specific locations.

ablation removal or excision of a part; laser ablation is destruction/removal of tissue by use of laser.

abortion termination of pregnancy or products of conception prior to fetal viability and/or 20 weeks gestation.

abscess inflamed cavity filled with pus as a result of infection.

accounting cycle a consecutive 12-month period for financial record keeping following either a fiscal year (starting on a specified date) or the calendar year (January to December).

accounts payable a record of all monies owed.

accounts receivable a record of all monies due.

accreditation a nongovernmental professional peer review process that provides technical assistance and evaluates educational programs for quality based on preestablished academic and administrative standards.

acquired immunodeficiency syndrome (AIDS) acquired immunodeficiency syndrome: cluster of disorders caused by HIV that specifically destroys cell-mediated immunity.

acrosome the superior surface of the head of the spermatozoon.

activities of daily living (ADL) activities usually performed in the course of the day, i.e., bathing, dressing, feeding oneself.

acute abrupt in onset

Addison's Disease partial or complete failure of the adrenal cortex functions, causing general physical deterioration.

adenosine triphosphate (ATP) the energy currency used by the body; breaking down the phosphate bond of the compound releases high energy potential.

adipose of or pertaining to fat.

adjustments changes in a posted account.

administrative pertaining to administration (e.g., office procedures and nonclinical tasks that a medical assistant will perform).

adnexa any part added to a main structure; an accessory part.

advance beneficiary notice document that informs covered patients that Medicare may not cover a certain service and the patient will be responsible for the bill.

advance directive a statement of a patient's wishes regarding health care prior to a critical medical event.

aerobe microorganism that requires oxygen to live and reproduce.

aerosol suspended particles in gas or air.

afebrile body temperature not elevated above normal.

afferent carrying impulses towards the center.

affiliation to connect or associate with, as a medical site would associate with a school to assist in completion of student training.

agar a type of seaweed or algae that helps solidify culture media; the media may be referred to as agar.

age of majority age at which an individual is considered to be an adult (usually 18–21 years of age).

agenda a brief outline of the topics to be discussed at a meeting.

agglutination clumping of cells due to the presence of antibodies called agglutinins.

aging schedule a form used to track outstanding balances.

agranulocytes white blood cells that do not contain visible granules when stained.

allergen any substance that causes manifestations of an allergy, usually a protein to which the body has built antibodies.

allergy acquired abnormal response to a substance (allergen) that does not ordinarily cause a reaction.

alopecia baldness.

alphabetic filing arranging of names or titles according to the sequence of letters in the alphabet.

alphafetoprotein substance produced by the embryonic yolk sac.

alternative an option or substitute to the standard medical treatment plan, e.g. herbal therapies, acupuncture, hypnosis.

alveolar-capillary membrane the structure in the lung fields through which oxygen and carbon dioxide diffuse during the respiratory process.

amenorrhea condition of not menstruating, without menses.

American Association of Medical Assistants (AAMA) professional organization for medical assistants.

American Medical Technologist Institute for Education (AMTIE) professional organization for medical assistants, medical laboratory technicians, and dental technicians.

Americans With Disabilities Act (ADA) a law designed to meet the needs of people with physical and mental challenges.

ammonia a substance produced by decomposition of organic matter containing nitrogen.

amniocentesis puncture of the amniotic sac in order to remove fluid for testing.

amphiarthroses slightly movable joints.

ampule   small glass container that must be broken at the neck to aspirate the solution into the syringe.

anacusis   complete hearing loss.

anaerobe   bacterium that does not require oxygen for growth and reproduction.

analogue   pertains to use of dictation machine with a hand-held microphone to tape a report of a patient encounter or other correspondence.

anaphylactic shock   severe allergic reaction within minutes to hours after exposure to a foreign substance.

anaphylaxis   severe allergic reaction that may result in death.

anatomical position   a position used for reference in which the subject is standing erect, facing forward, feet are slightly apart and pointing forward, the hands are down at the sides with palms forward and thumbs outward.

anatomy   the study of the structure of the body.

aneroid   sphygmomanometer that measures blood pressure without using mercury.

aneurysm   local dilation in a blood vessel wall.

angina pectoris   paroxysmal chest pain usually caused by a decrease in blood flow to the heart muscle due to coronary artery occlusion.

angiotensin   a substance occurring in the blood that works with renin to affect the blood pressure, usually increasing the pressure by vasoconstriction.

anisocytosis   blood abnormality in which red blood cells are not equal in size (aniso = unequal).

ankylosing spondylitis   stiffening of the spine with inflammation.

annotation   the process of reading, highlighting and summarizing a document for another person.

anorexia   loss of appetite.

anovulation   condition of not ovulating.

antagonism   mutual opposition or contrary action with something else; opposite of synergism.

antagonist   any muscle that opposes the action of the prime mover to balance movement. (Example: When the biceps contract and pull the forearm upward, the triceps oppose the motion and relax.)

antecubital space   inner surface of the bend of the elbow where the major veins for venipuncture are located.

antepartum   period of time prior to labor.

anthropometric   pertaining to measurements of the human body.

antibiotic   a drug that inhibits or destroys pathogenic microorganisms.

antibodies   complex glycoproteins produced by B lymphocytes in response to an antigen.

anticoagulant   anything that prevents or delays the clotting of blood.

antigen   protein markers on cells that cause formation of antibodies and react specifically with those antibodies.

antihistamine   medication that opposes the action of a histamine.

antiseptic   any substance that inhibits the growth of bacteria; used on skin before any procedure that breaks the integumentary barrier.

anuria   failure of the kidneys to produce urine.

apothecary system of measurement   old system that uses grains, minims, and drams.

appeal   process by which a higher court reviews the decision of a lower court.

appendicular skeleton   the parts of the skeleton added to the axial skeleton, including the shoulder and pelvic girdles and all of the bones of the upper and lower extremities.

applicator   device for putting applying local treatments and tests.

approximate   bring tissue surfaces as close as possible to their original positions.

arachnoid   web-like membrane covering the brain and spinal cord.

arrector pili   involuntary muscle attached to the hair follicle that when contracted causes "goose bumps."

arteriole   a small arterial branch that joins a capillary to an artery.

arthrogram   x-ray of a joint.

arthroplasty   surgical repair of a joint.

arthroscopy   examination of the inside of a joint through an arthroscope.

artifact   activity recorded in an electrocardiogram caused by extraneous activity such as patient movement, loose lead, or electrical interference.

artifactual   something added to a substance or structure, not belonging to it; in medicine, generally implies a negative connotation.

artificial insemination   the insertion of sperm into a woman's vagina by artificial means.

ascites   accumulation of serous fluid in the peritoneal cavity.

asepsis   a state of being sterile; a condition free from germs, infection, and any form of life, including spore forms.

aspiration   drawing in or out by suction; as in breathing objects into the respiratory tract or suctioning substances from a site.

assault   an attempt or threat to touch another person without his or her consent.

assessment   process of gathering information about the patient and the presenting condition.

assignment of benefits   transfer of the patient's legal right to collect third-party benefits for medical expenses to the provider of the services.

astigmatism   unfocused refraction of light rays on the retina.

asymmetry   lack or absence of symmetry; inequality of size or shape on opposite sides of the body.

asymptomatic   without any symptoms.

atelectasis collapsed lung fields; incomplete expansion of the lungs, either partial or complete.

atherosclerosis buildup of fatty plaque on the interior lining of arteries.

atraumatic without injury; may pertain to treatments or instruments that are not likely to cause further damage.

atria (plural) the upper chamber of each half of the heart; the atria receive blood from the great vessels (singular; atrium).

atrioventricular (AV) node located on the floor of the right atrium on or close to the septum; receives the electrical impulse from the SA node after it is transmitted through the upper half of the heart; transmits the impulse to the bundle of His.

attenuated diluted or weakened; pertaining to reduced virulence of a pathogenic microorganism.

attitude a state of mind; how a person feels about a given subject or at a given time.

attribute a characteristic or quality of a person; usually considered a positive feature.

audit a review of an account.

audits inspection of records to determine compliance and to detect fraud.

auscultation act of listening for sounds within the body, usually with a stethoscope, such as to evaluate the heart, lungs, intestines, or fetal heart tones.

autoclave appliance used to sterilize medical instruments with steam under pressure.

autolet small, sharp, spring-loaded instrument for quick capillary puncture.

autonomic self controlling, spontaneous.

autonomous existing or functioning independently.

axial skeleton the bones forming the main skeleton around which the appendicular skeleton moves, including bones of the head, thorax, and trunk.

axon part of the neuron that transmits impulses away from the cell body.

Azidothymidine (AZT) a drug used to treat AIDS by blocking the growth of the virus after it enters the T-cell lymphocyte.

azotemia from the Latin azote meaning nitrogen plusemia, meaning blood; the condition of having excessive amounts of nitrogen in the blood.

B

Babinski reflex reflex (dorsiflexion of the great toe and extension and fanning of the other toes upon stroking the sole of the foot) exhibited normally by infants. This reflex is abnormal in children and adults.

bacilli rod-shaped or cylindrical organisms.

back-up (noun) a duplicate file made to a separate disk to protect information; (verb) to make a duplicate file.

bactericidal substance that kills or destroys bacteria.

bacteriology the science and study of bacteria.

balance equality between the debit and credit sides of an accounting equation; that which is left over after additions and subtractions have been made to an account; remainder; amount due.

balance billing billing the patient for the balance or difference between the physician's charges and the Medicare-approved charges; prohibited by most managed care contracts.

bandage *noun*, soft material applied to a body part for hold a dressing in place, immobilize a body part, or aid in controlling bleeding; *verb*, to apply a wrapping material for treatment.

Bartholin's glands small mucous glands bilaterally in the vaginal vestibule.

basal ganglia pertaining to the gray matter in the cerebral hemispheres.

basal metabolic rate the amount of energy used in a unit of time to maintain vital functions by a fasting, resting subject.

baseline original or initial measure with which other measurements will be compared.

battery actual touching of a person without his or her consent.

B-cells lymphoid stem cells from the bone marrow that migrate to and become mature antigen-specific cells in the spleen and lymph nodes.

beliefs ideas that are held to be true.

bench trial trial in which the judge hears the case and renders a verdict; no jury is present.

benign tumor tumor that is not malignant.

benign not cancerous or malignant.

bias formation of an opinion without foundation or reason; prejudice.

bibulous very absorbent.

BiCaps words or phrases with unusual capitalization.

bicarbonate the dissolved form of carbon dioxide; it combines with water to make carbonic acid, H_2CO_3. Carbonic acid loses one of its hydrogen (H) ions to then form bicarbonate, HCO_3-.

bile a bitter, yellow-green secretion of the liver stored by the gallbladder; derived from bilirubin, cholesterol, and other substances. Emulsifies fats in the small intestine so they can be further digested and absorbed.

biliary obstruction blockage of one of the bile ducts (the tubes leading from liver and gallbladder into duodenum); common causes include cysts, tumors, and stones.

bilirubinuria bilirubin in the urine.

bimanual pertaining to the use of both hands; an examination performed with both hands.

bioethics moral issues and concerns that affect a person's life.

biohazard substance that is a risk to the health of living organisms.

biotransform convert the molecules of a substance from one form to another, as in medications within the body.

biotransforming   conversion of the molecules of a substance from one form to another, as in medications within the body.

birthday rule   determination of which policyholder's insurance is the first to pay when a patient is covered by two policies. The policyholder whose birth month and day comes first in the calendar is primary.

blister   a collection of fluid in or beneath the epidermis; a vesicle.

block   a type of letter format in which the date, subject line, closing and signatures are to the right margin; all other lines are justified left.

blood-borne pathogens   viruses that can be spread through direct contact with blood or body fluids from an infected person.

blood urea nitrogen   blood test to determine amount of nitrogen in blood in form of urea, a waste product normally excreted in urine.

body fluids   any of the fluids that accumulate in the compartments of the body, such as the blood plasma, and the intracellular and extracellular spaces.

boil   an abscess of the subcutaneous tissues of the skin; a furuncle.

bolus   a mobile mass, for instance, a mass of food that passes into the upper gastrointestinal tract in one swallow, or a dose of medication injected intravenously.

bookkeeping   organized and accurate record keeping for financial transactions.

boot   to start up the computer.

bradycardia   heart rate of less than 60 beats per minute.

bradykinesia   abnormally slow voluntary movements.

Braxton-Hicks contractions   uterine contractions during pregnancy.

breach   an infraction, such as breach of contract, in which the agreed-on terms are violated.

bruit   abnormal sound or murmur in the blood vessels during auscultation.

buccal medication   medication administered between the cheek and gum of the mouth.

budget   financial planning tool that helps an organization estimate its anticipated expenditures and revenues.

buffer   extra time to accommodate emergencies, walk-ins, and other demands on the provider's daily time schedule that are not considered direct patient care

bulla   large blister or vesicle.

BUN   abbreviation for blood urea nitrogen.

bundle of His   a band of specialized cardiac muscle fibers that receive the electrical impulse from the AV node and transmit it through right and left branches to the Purkinje fibers.

bursae   small sacs filled with clear synovial fluid that surround some joints.

byte   a unit of symbolic transfer; each character equals one byte.

C

caduceus   a symbol using a wand or staff with two serpents coiled around it; sometimes used as the sign of the medical profession (the more appropriate symbol has only one snake).

calibrated   marked in units of measurement, as a thermometer calibrated in Celsius.

calibrations   measurements for size or volume, as in calibrations on a syringe or pipette.

callus   in the musculoskeletal system, a deposit of new bone tissue that forms between the healing ends of broken bones; in the integumentary system, a thickened area of the epidermis caused by pressure or friction.

calyx (pl. calyces)   a cup-like collecting structure of the kidney.

cancellous   porous, spongy bone inside the medulla of the bone, usually filled with marrow.

capillary action   the raising or lowering of a liquid at the point of contact with a solid; used to pull blood into a capillary tube or small pipette.

capitation   managed care plan that pays a certain amount to a provider over a specific time for caring for the patients in the plan regardless of what or how many services are performed.

carbohydrates   chemical elements in food that convert to sugar, providing energy.

carbuncle   infection of interconnected group of hair follicles or several furuncles forming a mass.

cardiac cycle   period from the beginning of one heartbeat to the beginning of the next; includes systole and diastole.

cardiac output   the amount of blood ejected from either ventricle per minute, either to the pulmonary or to the systemic circulation.

cardinal signs   usually, vital signs; signifies their importance in assessment.

cardiogenic shock   type of shock in which the left ventricle fails to pump enough blood for the body to function.

cardiomegaly   enlarged heart muscle.

cardiomyopathy   any disease affecting the myocardium.

carina   a ridge-like structure; that part of the trachea that projects from the lower end of the trachea.

carrier   person infected with a microorganism but without signs of disease; a company that assumes the risk of an insurance company.

cassette   light-proof holder in which x-ray film is exposed.

catalyzes   increases the rate at which a chemical reaction takes place. Example: Amylase found in saliva catalyzes (speeds up) the rate at which starches are broken down.

cataracts   progressive loss of transparency of the lens of the eye, resulting in opacity and loss of sight.

catheterization   procedure for introducing a flexible tube into the body; urinary catheterization is for removal of urine from the bladder.

cautery   means, device, or agent that destroys or coagulates tissue; may be electrical current, freezing or burning agent, or chemical solution (caustic).

cell   the most basic unit of all living organisms.

cellular telephone   a telephone that works by electronic signals and does not require attachment to a telephone plug.

cellulitis   inflammation or infection of the skin and deeper tissues that may result in tissue destruction if not treated properly.

Celsius, centrigrade (C)   a temperature scale on which 0 degrees is the freezing point of water and 100 degrees is the boiling point of water at sea level.

censure   a verbal or written reprimand from a professional organization regarding a specific incident.

Centers for Medicare & Medicaid   federal agency that regulates Medicare and Medicaid along with the Clinical Laboratory Improvement Amendments Act and Health Insurance Portability and Accountability Act.

centesis   surgical puncture made into a cavity.

central processing unit (CPU)   circuitry imprinted on a silicon chip that processes information; the "brain" of the computer.

centrifugal force   a spinning motion to exert force outward, heavier components of a solution are spun downward.

cephalagia   headache.

cerebellum   located in the posterior part of the brain, responsible for balance and muscle coordination.

cerebrovascular accident (CVA)   ischemia of the brain due to an occlusion of the blood vessels supplying the brain, resulting in varying degrees of debilitation.

cerebrum   largest part of the brain, divided into two hemispheres, responsible for thought processes, sensory and motor functions, speech, writing, memory, and emotions.

certification   voluntary process that involves a testing procedure to prove an individual's baseline competency in a particular area.

cerumen   yellowish or brownish waxlike secretion in the external ear canal; earwax.

Chadwick's sign   sign of early pregnancy in which the vaginal, cervical, and vulvar tissues develop a bluish-violet color.

challenge   a method of testing a patient's sensitivity or response to a substance by introducing it into the body and watching its effects.

chancre   a hard ulcer that appears two to three weeks after exposure to syphilis, near the site of infection.

charge slip   a preprinted three-part form that can be placed on a day sheet to record the patient's charges and payments along with other information in an encounter form.

check register   place to record checks that have been written.

check stub   indicates to whom a check was issued, in what amount, and on what date.

chemical name   exact chemical descriptor of a drug.

chief complaint   main reason for the visit to the medical office.

chlamydia   a parasitic microorganism with properties common to bacteria but unable to sustain life without a host, in the manner of a virus.

chronic   long-standing.

chronic obstructive pulmonary disease (COPD)   progressive, irreversible condition with diminished respiratory capacity.

chronological order   placing in the order of time; usually the most recent is placed foremost.

chyle   milky, fatty product of digestion absorbed through the small intestines and returned to circulation by the lymphatics.

chyme   the thick, semi-liquid mass of ingested food mixed with gastric juices as it passes from the stomach.

cilia   hair-like projections on cells that either propel the cell or objects that come in contact with the cell.

circumcision   surgical removal of the prepuce.

civil law   a branch of law that focuses on issues between private citizens.

claims   requests to an insurance company for reimbursement of costs.

claims administrator   an individual who manages the third-party reimbursement policies for a medical practice.

clarification   explanation; removal of confusion or uncertainty.

climacteric period   menopause; developmental phase in which a woman's reproductive ability ceases.

Clinical Laboratory Improvement Amendments (CLIA)   guidelines established by Congress in 1988 to standardize and improve laboratory testing.

clinical   pertaining to direct patient care (e.g., nonadministrative tasks that a medical assistant will perform).

cloning   genetically identical replication of cells, an organ, or an organism in the laboratory.

closing   a one to two word phrase that precedes the sender's signature and indicates the end of the letter.

closed captioning   printed words displayed on a television screen to help people with hearing disabilities or impairments.

clustering   grouping patients with similar problems or needs.

coagulate   change from a liquid to a solid or semi-solid mass.

coerce   to force or compel a person to do something against his or her wishes.

coinsurance   the agreed-upon amount paid to the provider by a policyholder. Also called co-payment.

collagen   protein substance that gives structure to the connective tissue.

collection   a process of acquiring funds that are due.

colpocleisis   surgery to occlude the vagina.

colporrhaphy suturing of the vagina.

colposcopy visual examination of the vagina and cervix under magnification.

comedo blackhead.

common law traditional laws that were established by the English legal system.

comparative negligence a percentage of damage awards based on the contribution of negligence between two parties.

complement group of proteins in blood that influence the inflammatory process; primary mediator in the antigen–antibody reactions of the B cell–mediated response.

compliance willingness of a patient to follow a prescribed course of treatment.

compliance officer person charged with ensuring that a facility follows laws, policies, and protocols.

concussion injury to the brain due to trauma.

conference call a telephone call between two or more people that occurs at a designated time and is used for discussing a topic of mutual concern.

confidentiality protection of patient data from unauthorized personnel.

congenital anomaly abnormality, either structural or functional, present at birth.

congestive heart failure condition in which the heart cannot pump effectively.

conjugate joined or paired.

consent an agreement between a patient and physician to do a given medical procedure.

consideration the exchange of fees for a service.

constellation of symptoms a group of clinical signs indicating a particular disease process.

continuing education units credits awarded for attendance at approved local and state AAMA meetings and seminars, completion of guided study courses, and journal articles designed to submit a posttest for CEU credit.

consultation request for assistance from one physician to another.

contract an agreement between two or more parties for a given act.

contracture abnormal shortening of muscles around a joint caused by atrophy of the muscles and resulting in flexion and fixation.

contraindication situation or condition that prohibits the prescribing or administering of a drug or medication.

contrast medium substance ingested or injected into the body to facilitate imaging of internal structures.

contributory negligence a defense strategy in which the defendant admits to negligence but claims that the plaintiff assisted in promoting the damages.

contusion collection of blood in tissues after an injury; a bruise

conventions general notes, symbols, typeface, format, and punctuation that direct and guide the coder to the most complete and accurate ICD-9 code.

convoluted tubules the twisted portion of the nephron that connects the glomerulus to the collecting tubules; consists of a proximal and a distal portion connected by the Loop of Henle.

convulsion sudden, involuntary muscle contraction of voluntary muscle group.

cookies tiny files that are left on your computer's hard drive by a website without your permission.

coordination of benefits the method of designating the order in which multiple carriers pay benefits to avoid duplication of payment.

co-payments that part of an insured service the patient must pay.

coping mechanisms unconscious methods of alleviating intense stressors.

coronary artery bypass graft surgical procedure that increases the blood flow to the heart by bypassing the occluded or blocked vessel with a graft.

corpora cavernosa the erectile bodies of the penis or clitoris.

corpus spongiosum erectile tissue around the male uretrha.

corticoid any of the hormonal steroid substances obtained from the adrenal cortex.

cortisol a naturally occurring steroidal hormone that regulates metabolism and acts as an anti-inflammatory agent.

coumarin an anticoagulant prescribed for persons likely to form blood clots, such as valve replacement recipients; also called Coumadin (trade name) or warfarin.

cranium the portion of the skull that encloses the brain.

crash "lock up" of the computer central processing unit as a result of a system breakdown.

creatine a chemical compound in the body that adds phosphorus to ADP (adenosine diphosphate) to make ATP (adenosine triphosphate) that is the energy currency of the body.

creatinine the substance formed when creatine (an important compound in metabolic processes) is used.

credit balance in one's favor on an account; promise to pay a bill at a later date; record of a payment received.

cretinism severe congenital hypothyroidism; signs include dwarfism, low intelligence, puffy features, dry skin, macroglossia, and poor muscle tone.

criteria the standard, rule, or test by which something or someone can be judged.

cross examination questioning of a witness by the opposing attorney.

cross-reference notation in a file telling that a record is stored elsewhere and giving the reference; verification to another source; checking the tabular list against the alphabetic list in ICD-9 coding.

crossover claim a claim that crosses over automatically from one coverage to another for payment.

cul-de-sac blind pouch or cavity, as in the cul-de-sac that lies between the rectum and the posterior uterus.

culdocentesis   surgical puncture of and aspiration of fluid from the vaginal cul-de-sac for diagnosis or therapy.

culture   a laboratory process whereby microorganisms are grown in a special medium often for the purpose of identifying a causative agent in an infectious disease; also means the way of life, including commonly held beliefs, of a group of people.

curettage   scraping of a body cavity, such as the uterus.

Current Procedural Terminology (CPT)   a comprehensive list of codes used by physicians to bill for procedures and services

cursor   flashing line on the monitor indicating where data input will occur.

cyanotic   a bluish discoloration of the skin due to the lack of oxygen.

cyst   sac of fluid or semisolid material under the skin.

cystocele   herniation of the urinary bladder into the vagina.

cystoscopy   direct visualization of the urinary bladder through a cystoscope inserted through the urethra.

cytology   study of cells.

D

DACUM   a code of educational standards for medical assisting students developed by the American Association of Medical Assistants.

damages   the resulting injury or suffering that resulted from negligence.

data   information that is stored and processed by the computer.

database   accumulation of files on the computer

day sheet/daily journal   a daily business record of charges and payments.

debit   a charge or money owed on an account.

decibel (db)   unit of intensity of sound.

deciduous   to fall or shed; deciduous teeth: the set of 20 teeth appearing during infancy and shedding during childhood.

decongestant   substance that reduces congestion or swelling.

deductible   a specified amount paid by the policyholder before the carrier begins paying.

defamation of character   making false or malicious statements about a person's character or reputation.

defendant   the party that is accused.

degenerative joint disease (DJD)   also known as osteoarthritis; arthritis characterized by degeneration of the bony structure of the joints, usually noninflammatory.

deglutition   the act of swallowing.

dehiscence   separation or opening of the edges of a wound.

demeanor   the way a person looks, behaves, and conducts himself or herself.

dementia   progressive organic mental deterioration with loss of intellectual function.

demographic   relating to the statistical characteristics of populations.

dendrite   part of the neuron that transmits impulses toward the cell body.

denial   saying that something is not true; refusing to acknowledge.

dentin   the main component of the tooth structure, surrounds the inner pulp and lies just below the enamel.

dependent   spouse, children, and sometimes other individuals designated by the insured who are covered under a health care plan.

depolarization   progressive wave of stimulation causing contraction of the myocardium.

deposition   a process in which one party questions another party under oath.

dermatitis   inflammation of the skin.

dermatophytosis   fungal infection of the skin.

dermis   layer of skin under the epidermis.

descriptor   description of a service listed with its code number.

detoxification   clearing of drugs from the body and treating the withdrawal symptoms.

dextrocardia   the condition of having the heart in the right side of the thoracic cavity.

diabetes insipidus   a disorder of metabolism characterized by polyuria and polydipsia; caused by a deficiency in ADH or an inability of the kidneys to respond to ADH.

diagnosis   identification of a disease or condition by evaluating physical signs and symptoms, health history, and laboratory tests; a disease or condition identified in a person.

Diagnostic Related Group (DRG)   categories used to determine hospital and physician reimbursement for Medicare patients' inpatient services.

dialysis   removal of waste in blood not filtered by kidneys by passing fluid through a semipermeable barrier that allows normal electrolytes to remain, either with a machine with circulatory access or by passing a balanced fluid through the peritoneal cavity.

diaphoresis   profuse sweating.

diaphragmatic excursion   the movement of the diaphragm during respiration.

diarthroses   freely-movable joints; also called synovial joints.

diastole   relaxation phase of the cardiac cycle.

diazo   a double nitrogen compound that reacts with bilirubin.

diction   the style of speaking and enunciating words.

dideoxycytidine (ddC)   a drug used to treat AIDS by blocking the growth of the virus after it enters the T-cell lymphocytes.

dideoxyinosine (ddI)   a drug used to treat AIDS by blocking the growth of the virus after it enters the T-cell lymphocytes.

diencephalon   part of the brain lying beneath the hemispheres, containing the thalamus and hypothalamus.

digital   pertaining to, resembling, or performed with a finger; expressed in digits (0–9).

diluent specified liquid used to reconstitute powder medications for injection

diplococci spherical microorganisms in pairs.

diplomacy the art of handling people with tact and genuine concern.

direct examination questioning of a witness by the attorney for the individual the witness is representing.

directory a "table of contents" of a file system.

discrimination making a difference in favor of or against someone.

disease definite pathological process having a distinctive set of symptoms and course of progression.

disinfectant a chemical that can be applied to objects to destroy microorganisms; will not destroy bacterial spores.

disinfection killing or rendering inert most but not all pathogenic microorganisms.

disk drive a device that gets information on and off a floppy disk.

diuretics substances that promote the formation and excretion of urine.

documentation the process of recording patient information.

donor one who contributes something to another.

double booking the practice of booking two patients for the same period with the same physician

dowager's hump exaggerated cervical curve with prominence of the top thoracic vertebrae found in some osteoporotic elderly women; a type of kyphosis.

downloading transferring information from an outside location to your computer.

downtime computer malfunction or any time when the machine is not operational.

dress to apply a covering to a wound.

dressing covering applied directly to a wound to apply pressure, support, absorb secretions, protect from trauma or microorganisms, stop or slow bleeding, or hide disfigurement.

drug any substance that may modify one or more of the functions of an organism.

due process a formal proceeding in which the accused is considered not guilty until a verdict is reached.

dura mater the outer covering of the brain.

durable power of attorney a legal document giving another person the authority to act in one's behalf.

duress the act of compelling or forcing someone to do something that they do not want to do.

dwarfism (endocrine or pituitary) abnormal underdevelopment of the body with extreme shortness but normal proportions; achondroplastic dwarfism is an inherited growth disorder characterized by shortened limbs and a large head but almost normal trunk proportions.

dysmenorrhea painful menstruation.

dyspareunia painful coitus or sexual intercourse.

dysphagia inability to swallow or difficulty in swallowing.

dysphasia difficulty speaking.

dysphonia impairment of voice; hoarseness.

dyspnea difficulty breathing.

dysuria painful or difficult urination.

E

E-codes codes indicating the external cause or reason for an injury or illness.

ecchymosis characteristic black and blue mark that results from blood as it accumulates under the skin.

eczema superficial dermatitis.

edema an accumulation of fluid within the tissues.

efferent carrying impulses away from the center.

elastin protein substance that gives elasticity and flexibility to the connective issues.

electrocardiography procedure that produces a record of the electrical activity of the heart.

electrode medium for conducting or detecting electrical current.

electroencephalogram (EEG) tracing of the electrical activity of the brain.

electrolytes certain chemical substances dissolved in the blood and having numerous basic functions such as conducting electrical currents; the principal electrolytes are sodium, potassium, chloride, and bicarbonate.

electromyography recording of electrical nerve transmission in skeletal muscles.

electronic medical records (EMR) information about patients that is recorded and stored on computer

element a substance that cannot be separated or broken down into substances with properties other than its own; a primary substance.

ELISA enzyme-linked immunosorbent assay: test to screen blood for antibody to the AIDS virus.

eligibility the determination of an insured's right to receive benefits from a third-party payer based on such criteria as payment of premiums and date of start of coverage.

elliptocytosis a condition in which all or almost all of the red blood cells are elliptical or oval in shape; typically asymptomatic.

emancipated minor a patient under the age of majority but who is legally considered to be an adult.

embolus mass of matter (thrombus, air, fat globule) freely floating in the circulatory system.

emergency medical service (EMS) a group of health care providers working as a team to care for sick or injured patients before they arrive at the hospital.

empathy the ability to understand or to some extent share what someone else is feeling.

employee a person hired to perform given duties in return for financial compensation.

emulsify to disperse a liquid into another, usually incompatible, liquid.

enclosure indication for the reader that an item is accompanying the letter.

encounter form   a preprinted statement that lists codes for basic office charges and has sections to record charges incurred in an office visit, the patient's current balance, and next appointment.

encryption   scrambling E-mail messages as they leave one site and unscrambling them when they arrive at the designated address.

endemic   a disease that occurs continuously in a particular population but has a low mortality; used in contrast to epidemic.

endocarditis   inflammation of the inner lining of the heart.

endocardium   the innermost part of the heart wall; it lines the heart chamber and covers the connective tissue skeleton of the heart valves.

endogenous   having its origin within an organism.

endotracheal tube   a large instrument usually inserted through the mouth (may use the nose) and into the trachea to the point of the tracheal division to deliver oxygen under pressure.

enumerated   counted.

enuresis   bed wetting.

enzyme   a protein that begins (catalyzes) a chemical reaction.

epicardium   the inner or visceral layer of the pericardium that forms the outermost layer of the heart wall.

epidermis   outer layer of the skin.

epiglottis   the leaf-like flap that closes down over the glottis during swallowing.

epiphyseal end plate   a thin layer of cartilage at the end of long bones where new growth takes place.

episiotomy   incision of the perineum to accommodate vaginal delivery of fetus.

eponym   word derived from a personal name, e.g., *Alzheimer* disease.

ergonomic   describes a workstation designed to prevent work-related injuries and to promote work efficiency.

Erlich units   a unit of measurement for urobilinogen.

erythema   redness of the skin.

erythematous   characterized by redness (erythema).

erythropoietin   a hormone produced mainly by the kidney in response to lowered oxygen levels; stimulates the production of red blood cells to increase blood oxygen levels.

ester   compound formed by combining alcohol and acid; fats are esters.

esterase   an enzyme that splits esters.

Ethernet   system that allows the computer to be connected to a cable or DSL system.

ethics   guidelines for moral behavior that are enforced by peer groups.

ethylene oxide   gas used to sterilize surgical instruments and other supplies.

etiology   cause of disease.

eunuchoidism   deficient production of male hormone by the testes, resulting in loss of the secondary male characteristics.

eustachian tubes   a mucous membrane-lined tube between the nasopharynx and the middle ear bilaterally that equalizes the internal and external otic air pressure.

euthanasia   allowing a patient to die with minimal medical interventions.

evaluation   the process of indicating how well the patient or person is progressing toward a particular goal; to appraise; to determine the worth or quality of something or someone.

exercise   performed activity of the muscles, voluntary or otherwise, to maintain fitness.

exogenous   having its origin outside of the organism; its opposite is endogenous.

exophthalmic goiter   abnormal protrusion of the eyeballs accompanied by goiter.

expected threshold   a numerical goal.

expert witness   a professional who testifies on the standard of care in a trial.

explanation of benefits (EOB)   a statement that accompanies a payment from an insurance carrier and outlines which dates and services are being paid.

exposure control plan   written plan required by the Occupational Safety and Health Administration that outlines an employer's system for preventing infection.

exposure risk factors   conditions that tend to put employees at risk for contact with biohazardous agents such as blood-borne pathogens.

expressed consent   a statement of approval from the patient for the physician to perform a given procedure after the patient has been educated about the risks and benefits of the particular procedure; also referred to as informed consent.

expressed contracts   formal agreements between two or more people.

expulsion   formal discharge from a professional organization.

externship   an educational course that allows the student to obtain hands-on experience.

extracellular   outside of the cell.

extraocular   outside the eye, as in extraocular eye movement.

exudate   drainage.

F

familial disorder   disorder that tends to occur more often in a family than would be anticipated solely by chance.

Family and Medical Leave Act   a law designed to allow an employee up to 12 weeks of unpaid leave from his or her job to meet family needs.

fascia   fibrous membrane tissue that covers and supports the muscles and joins the skin with underlying tissue.

febrile   having above-normal body temperature.

federal unemployment tax   tax is used to finance all administrative expenses of the federal/state unemployment insurance system and the federal costs involved in extended benefits.

fee-for-service   an established set of fees charged for specific services and paid by the patient or insurance carrier.

fee-splitting   sharing of fees between physicians for patient referrals.

fee schedule   a list of preestablished fee allowances set for specific services and procedures performed by a provider.

feedback   in communication, the response to input from another.

femtoliter   one quadrillionth of a liter.

FICA   Federal Insurance Contributions Act; the law that established Social Security and that mandates Social Security tax payments and benefits.

file   grouping of data that is given a name for easy access.

filing system   a method for organizing records so that they can be found when needed.

film   raw material on which x-rays are projected through the body; prior to processing does not contain a visible image (similar to photographic film).

filtration   removal of particles from a solution by passing the solution through a membrane.

fissure   crack in skin or mucous membrane.

fixative   a chemical substance used to bind, fix or stabilize specimens of tissue to slides for later examination.

flagella   hair-like extremity of a bacterium or protozoan; used to facilitate movement.

flextime   a system of scheduling that allows for a personal choice in hours or days worked.

flocculation   condition of having a consistency of loose woolly masses.

floppy disk   thin magnetic film on which to store data.

flow sheet   color-coded sheets that allow information to be recorded in graphic or tabular form for easy retrieval.

fluorescein angiography   intravenous injection of fluorescent dye; photographing blood vessels of the eye as dye moves through them.

fluoroscopy   special x-ray technique for examining a body part by immediate projection onto a fluorescent screen.

folate   a salt of folic acid; it acts to help enzymes that build structures such as blood cells.

folliculitis   inflammation of hair follicles.

font   a typeface; affects the way written messages look.

forced expiratory volume (FEV)   volume of air forced out of the lungs.

forceps   surgical instrument used to grasp, handle, compress, pull, or join tissues, equipment, or supplies.

fraud   a deceitful act with the intention to conceal the truth.

fructose   a simple sugar; a monosaccharide.

fulgurate   destroy tissue by electrodessication.

full block   a type of letter format in which all letter components are justified left.

full-thickness burn   burn that has destroyed all skin layers.

furuncle   infection in a hair follicle or gland; characterized by pain, redness, and swelling with necrosis of tissue in the center.

G

gait   manner or style of walking.

galactosuria   condition in newborns lacking an enzyme that metabolizes galactose; increased levels of galactose appear in the blood and urine (if proper therapy is not initiated, mental retardation and other difficulties will occur).

gastroenteritis   inflammation of the gastrointestinal tract caused by bacteria or viruses.

gauge   diameter of a needle lumen

gel separator   a nonreacting substance located in an evacuated tube that forms a physical barrier between the cells and serum or plasma after the specimen has been centrifuged.

generic name   official name given to a drug whose patent has expired.

generic   the official name given to a drug that is no longer owned by the company that developed it.

germicide   chemical that kills most pathogenic microorganisms; disinfectant.

gerontologist   specialist who studies aging.

gestation   period of time from conception to birth; usually 37–41 weeks.

gestational diabetes   a disorder characterized by an impaired ability to metabolize carbohydrates, usually due to insulin deficiency occurring in pregnancy and usually disappearing after delivery.

gigantism   excessive size and stature caused most frequently by hypersecretion of the Human Growth Hormone (HGH).

gingiva   the gums; the mucous membrane covered tissues that support the teeth.

glaucoma   abnormal increase in the fluid in the eye, usually as a result of obstructed outflow, resulting in degeneration of the intraocular components and blindness.

glomerulus   a small cluster of blood vessels within the Bowman's Capsule.

glucocorticoid   an adrenal cortex hormone that increases the conversion of fatty acids and proteins to glucose for energy.

glycosuria   the presence of glucose in the urine.

goiter   an enlargement of the thyroid gland.

gonads   a generic term referring to the sex glands of both sexes, either ovaries or testes.

goniometer   instrument used to measure the angle of joints for range of motion.

Goodell's sign   softening of the cervix early in pregnancy.

granulocytes   white blood cells that have visible granules when stained.

Grave's disease   pronounced hyperthyroidism with signs of enlarged thyroid and exophthalmos.

gravid   pregnant.

gravida   pregnant woman.

gravidity   pregnancy

grief   great sadness caused by loss.

gross income   the amount of money earned by an employee before taxes are withheld.

group member   a policyholder who is a member of a group and covered by the group's insurance carrier.

guaiac   substance used in laboratory tests for occult blood in the stool.

gyri   the convolutions of the brain tissue.

H

hard copy   printed copy on paper.

hard drive   a place where the computer stores programs and data files.

hardware   equipment on the computer system, e.g., keyboard, disk drive, monitor, printer.

HCFA   see Health Care Financing Administration

HCPCS   see Health Care Financing Administration Common Procedures Coding System.

Health Care Financing Administration (HCFA)   a federal agency that regulates health care financing and the procedural classification (Volume 3 of the ICD-9-CM coding book).

Health Care Financing Administration Common Procedures Coding System (HCPCS)   a numerical system used by HCFA for services not covered by the CPT coding system.

Health Insurance Portability and Accountability Act   federal law that requires all health care settings to ensure privacy and security of patient information. Also requires health insurance to be accessible for working Americans and available when changing employment.

health maintenance organization (HMO)   an organization that provides a wide range of services through a contract with a specified group at a predetermined payment.

Healthcare Common Procedure Coding System   AMA's coding system based on CPT-4; assigns alphabetic and numeric codes to items such as ambulance service, wheelchairs, and injections.

healthcare surrogate   a patient's representative who makes health care decisions for the patient.

heat exhaustion   a type of hyperthermia that causes an altered mental status due to inadequate fluid replacement.

heat cramps   type of hyperthermia that causes muscle cramping resulting from high-sodium heat exhaustion; hyperthermia resulting from physical exertion in heat without adequate fluid replacement.

heat stroke   most serious type of hyperthermia; body is no longer able to compensate for elevated temperature.

hematemesis   vomiting blood or bloody vomitus.

hematocytometer (hemocytometer)   device for counting blood cells.

hematemesis   vomiting blood or bloody vomitus.

hematoma   blood clot that forms at an injury site.

hematuria   blood in the urine.

hemoglobin C disease   a genetic blood disorder in which the red blood cells contain an abnormal hemoglobin C, which reduces the elasticity of the red cells causing them to hemolyze easily.

hemoglobinuria   presence of free hemoglobin in urine.

hemolysis   rupture of erythrocytes with the release of hemoglobin into the plasma or serum causing the specimen to appear pink or red in color.

hemolytic anemia   a disorder characterized by premature destruction of the red cells; this may be brought on by an infectious process, inherited red cell disorders, or as a response to certain drugs or toxins.

hemoptysis   coughing up blood from the respiratory tract.

hemostat   surgical instrument with slender jaws used for grasping blood vessels.

hemostasis   process that results in control of bleeding after an injury.

heparin   a naturally occurring anticoagulant given to prevent clot formation.

hepatomegaly   enlarged liver.

hepatotoxin   substance that can damage the liver.

hereditary traits   traits or disorders that are transmitted from parent to offspring.

hernia   protrusion of an organ through the muscle wall of the cavity that normally surrounds it.

herpes simplex   infection caused by the herpes simplex virus.

herpes zoster   infection caused by reactivation of varicella zoster virus, which causes chickenpox.

hiatus   an opening or gap; hiatal hernia: a protrusion of part of the stomach upward through the diaphram.

HIPAA   federal law, originally passed as the Kassebaum-Kennedy Act, whose several components include protecting private health information.

Hippocratic Oath   a code of ethics written by Hippocrates.

hirsutism   abnormal or excessive growth of hair in women.

histamine   substance found normally in the body in response to injured cells, producing the inflammatory process: dilation of capillaries, increased gastric secretions, contraction of smooth muscles.

homeopathic medicine   alternative type of medicine in which patients are treated with small doses of substances that produce similar symptoms and use the body's own healing abilities.

homeostasis   maintaining a constant internal environment by balancing positive and negative feedback.

hormone   a substance that is produced by an endocrine gland and travels through the blood to a distant organ or gland where it acts to modify the structure or function of that gland or organ.

human chorionic gonadotropin (HCG)   hormone secreted by the placenta and found in the urine and blood of a pregnant female.

humidifier   appliance that increases the moisture content in the air.

hydrogen ion   hydrogen that is missing an electron and therefore readily binds with substances having extra electrons; it is an important constituent of acids.

hypercalcemia   an excessive amount of calcium in the blood.

hyperglycemia   an increase in blood sugar, as in diabetes mellitus.

hyperopia   farsightedness.

hyperosmolarity   a condition of having increased numbers of dissolved substances in the plasma.

hyperplasia   excessive proliferation of normal cells in the normal tissue arrangement of an organism.

hyperpyrexia   dangerously high temperature, 105° to 106°F

hypertension   morbidly high blood pressure.

hyperthermia   general condition of excessive body heat.

hypoglycemia   deficiency of sugar in the blood.

hypothalamus   part of the diencephalon; activates and controls the peripheral nervous system, endocrine system, and certain involuntary functions.

hypothermia   below-normal body temperature.

hypovolemic shock   shock caused by loss of blood or other body fluids.

hysterosalpingogram   radiograph of the uterus and fallopian tubes after injection with a contrast medium.

hysteroscopy   visual examination with magnification of the uterus.

I

iatrogenic   a condition caused by treatment or medical procedures.

identification line   a series of initials indicating who dictated the letter and who composed it.

idiopathic   unknown etiology.

immune globulins   proteins produced by plasma cells in response to foreign antigens; provide immediate antibody protection for a few weeks to a few months.

immunity   lack of susceptibility to a disease.

immunization   act or process of rendering an individual immune to specific disease.

immunohematology   the study of the antigen-antibody reaction including the study of autoimmunity.

impetigo   highly infectious skin infection causing erythema and progressing to honey-colored crusts.

implementation   the process of initiating and carrying out an action such as a teaching plan or patient treatment

implied consent   an informal agreement of approval from the patient to perform a given task.

implied contracts   contracts between physician and patient not written but assumed by the actions of the parties.

impotence   inability to achieve or maintain an erection.

incident report   a form used by an organization to document an unusual occurrence to a patient, visitor or employee.

incontinence   inability to control elimination, either urine or feces or both.

independent practice association (IPA)   several independently practicing physicians contracted with a health maintenance organization to provide services to HMO members.

indices (sing. index)   numbers expressing a property or ratio

induration   hardened area at the injection site after an intradermal screening test for tuberculosis

infarction   death of tissues due to lack of oxygen.

infection   invasion by disease-producing microorganisms.

infiltration   leakage of intravenous fluids into surrounding tissues.

informed consent   a statement of approval from the patient for the physician to perform a given procedure after the patient has been educated about the risks and benefits of the procedure; also referred to as expressed consent.

inguinal   pertaining to the regions of the groin.

inpatient   a medical setting in which patients are admitted for diagnostic, radiographic, or treatment purposes.

insertion   a place of attachment, usually the freely movable portion of a muscle.

inspection   visual examination.

installment   partial payment of a bill.

institutional review board   internal committee that reviews ethical issues.

instrument   a surgical tool or device designed to perform a specific function, such as cutting, dissecting, grasping, holding, retracting, or suturing.

insufflator   device for blowing air, gas, or powder into a body cavity.

insula   fifth lobe of the cerebrum.

insulin dependent diabetes mellitus (IDDM)   a deficiency in insulin production that leads to an inability to metabolize carbohydrates.

insurance   a policy that promises to pay some or all of a customer's medical bills.

insured   an individual who owns a policy that promises to pay some or all of his or her medical bills.

intentional tort   an act that takes place with malice and with the intent of causing harm; a deliberate violation of another person's legal rights.

interaction   effects, positive or negative, of two or more drugs taken by a patient.

intercaps   words or phrases with unusual capitalization.

interferon   group of proteins released by white blood cells and fibroblasts when the invading microorganism is a virus.

intermittent   occurring at intervals.

Internal Revenue Service (IRS)   a federal agency that regulates and enforces various taxes.

International Classification of Diseases (ICD)   a classification system used to assign a numerical code to a disease.

International Classification of Diseases, Ninth Revision, Clinical Modification   a system for transforming verbal descriptions of disease, injuries, conditions, and procedures to numeric codes.

Internet   global system used to connect one computer to another.

interosseous   between bones.

interstitial   the spaces between the cells.

intracellular   inside of the cell.

intranet   a private network system of computers.

intraocular pressure   pressure within the eyeball.

intrauterine pregnancy (IUP)   pregnancy located in the uterus.

intravascular coagulation   clot formation within the vessels; strands of fibrin may form from one wall of the vessel to the other and shear red cells as they pass by.

intravenous pyelogram (IVP)   radiography using contrast medium to evaluate kidney function.

intrinsic   found within a structure.

introitus   vaginal orifice.

invoice   a statement of debt owed; a bill.

iodine   an element that is an essential micronutrient used in the thyroid gland to manufacture its hormones; present in seafood, foods grown in iodized soil, iodized salt and some dairy products.

ion   an atom or group of atoms that has become electrically charged by the loss or gain of one or more electrons

iontophoresis   introduction of various chemical ions into the skin by means of electrical current.

ischemia   decrease in oxygen to tissues.

J

job description   a statement that informs an employee about the duties and expectations for a given job.

Joint Commission on Accreditation of Health Care Organizations (JCAHO)   a voluntary organization that sets and evaluates the standards of care for health care institutions; based on the JCAHO evaluation, an accreditation title will be given to the organization.

K

Kaposi sarcoma   cancer of the skin that is extremely rare except in AIDS patients

Kegel exercises   isometric exercises in which the muscles of the pelvic floor are voluntarily contracted and relaxed while urinating.

keratin   a tough, insoluble protein substance of the stratum corneum, hair and nails.

keratoses (senile)   premalignant overgrowth or thickening of the upper layer of epithelium or horny layer of the skin.

keratosis   skin condition characterized by overgrowth and thickening.

ketoacidosis   acidosis accompanied by an accumulation of ketones in the body.

ketones   the end products of fat metabolism.

key component   the criteria or factors on which the selection of a CPT-4 evaluation and management is based.

kinesics   a form of non-verbal communication including gestures, body movements, facial expressions.

Krebs cycle   a sequence of reactions within cells that metabolizes sugars and other energy sources, such as carbo-hydrates, proteins and fats, into carbon dioxide, water and ATP.

kyphosis (dowager's hump)   abnormally deep dorsal curvature of the thoracic spine; also known as humpback or hunchback.

L

labor   involuntary contractions of the uterine muscle resulting in cervical dilation and effacement (thinning) of the cervix; prelude to childbirth.

laboratory   a place where research, investigation, or scientific testing takes place.

laparoscopy   process of viewing the internal abdominal cavity and its contents through a specialized endoscope.

laparotomy   incision of the abdominal cavity.

laryngectomy   surgical removal of the larynx.

laser ablation   destruction or removal of tissue by use of laser.

late effects   conditions that result from another condition. For example, left-sided paralysis may be a *late effect* of a stroke.

lead   electrode or electrical connection attached to the body to record electrical impulses in the body, especially the heart or brain.

learning objectives   steps that needed to be achieved to accomplish the learning goal.

learning goal   an agreed upon outcome of the teaching process.

ledger card   a record of the patient's financial activities.

ledger   a continuous record of business transactions with debits and credits.

legally required disclosure   reporting of certain events to governmental agencies without the patient's consent.

lentigines   brown skin macules occurring after exposure to the sun; freckle.

lentigines   tan or brown macules found on elderly skin after prolonged sun exposure; also known as liver spots.

leukocytosis   abnormal increase of leukocytes (white blood cells).

leukoplakia   white, thickened patches on the oral mucosa or tongue that are often precancerous.

liabilities   amounts the practice owes.

libel   written statements that defame a person's reputation or character.

licensure   the strictest form of professional accreditation.

ligament   a flexible band of tissue that holds joints together.

lightening   the descent of the fetus in the pelvis.

lipase   any of several enzymes that begin the breakdown of fats in the digestive tract.

lipids   any of the free fatty acids (fats) in the body.

lipoproteins   a substance made up of a lipid and a protein.

literary search   finding professional journal articles on a given subject.

lithotripsy   crushing of a stone with sound waves.

litigation   process of filing or contesting a lawsuit.

lochia   uterine discharge following childbirth, composed of some blood, mucus and tissue.

locum tenens   a substitute physician.

login   use of a password to gain access to the computer.

loop of henle   a portion of the renal tubule, shaped like a U and consisting of a thick ascending and thin descending vessels.

lordosis   abnormally deep ventral curve at the lumbar flexure of the spine; also known as swayback.

lubricant   agent that reduces friction.

Luer adapter   a device for connecting a syringe or evacuated holder to the needle to promote a secure fit.

lyse   to cause disintegration; i.e., destruction of adhesions, or the breakdown of red blood cells.

M

macrophage   a monocyte that has left the circulation and settled and matured in tissue; macrophages process antigens and present them to T-cells, activating the immune specific response.

macule   small, flat discoloration of the skin.

magnetic resonance imaging   imaging technique that uses a strong magnetic field.

main terms   words in a multiple-word diagnosis that a coder should locate in the alphabetic listing. They represent the condition (not the location) to be coded.

mainframe   central computer to which individual computers are connected; used in large institutions.

malaise   general feeling of illness without specific signs or symptoms.

malignant   cancerous.

malignant tumor   tumor or growth that is cancerous and may spread to other tissues.

malocclusion   abnormal contact between the teeth in the upper and lower jaw.

malpractice   a tort in which the patient is harmed by the actions of a health care worker.

managed care   the practice of third-party payers to control costs by requiring physicians to adhere to specific rules as a condition of payment.

manipulation   skillful use of the hands in diagnostic procedures.

Mantoux   intradermal injection screening test for tuberculosis.

margin   the blank space around the edges of a piece of paper, such as a letter or page of a book.

masticate   the act of chewing or grinding, as in chewing food.

Material Safety Data Sheet (MSDS)   a detailed record of all hazardous substances kept within a site.

matrix   a system for blocking off unavailable patient appointment times.

mediastinum   the mid-portion of the thoracic cavity containing the heart, the great vessels, the upper esophagus and the trachea.

medical asepsis   removal or destruction of microorganisms.

medical assistant   a multiskilled health professional who performs a variety of clinical and administrative tasks in a medical setting.

medical history   record containing information about a patient's past and present health status.

medical necessity   a determination made by a third party that a certain service or procedure was necessary based on sound medical practice.

medical setting   a place that is designed to meet the health care needs of patients; may be inpatient or outpatient.

Medicare   Social Security–established health insurance for the elderly.

medulla oblongata   part of the brain that controls breathing, heart rate, and blood pressure.

megabyte   one million bytes; a way to measure the quantity of computer information that a particular device can hold.

megaloblastic anemia   a disorder characterized by production of large, dysfunctional erythrocytes; folate deficiency is considered a cause.

meiosis   the cell division specific to sperm and ova that results in 23 chromosomes rather than 46 (23 pairs).

melanin   dark pigment that gives color to the skin, hair and eyes.

melanocyte   cell that produces melanin.

melena   black, tarry stools caused by digested blood from the gastrointestinal tract.

memorandum   a type of written documentation used for interoffice communication.

menarche   onset of first menstruation.

meninges   membranes of the spinal cord and brain.

meningocele   meninges protruding though the spinal column.

meniscus   the curved upper surface of a liquid in a container.

menorrhagia   excessive bleeding during menstruation.

menses   menstruation; bloody discharge monthly or cyclically in the female when fertilization has not occurred.

mensuration   the act or process of measuring.

message   words sent from one person to another; information sent through spoken, written, or body language.

metabolic acidosis   an acidic condition of the body caused when excess acids are produced in the body's fluids (as in the metabolism of fats instead of glucose) or when the body's natural bicabonates are lost or diminished.

metabolism   sum of chemical processes that result in growth, energy production, elimination of waste, and body functions performed as digested nutrients are distributed.

metric system   system of measurement that uses grams, liters, and meters.

metrorrhagia   irregular uterine bleeding.

microbiology   the study of microscopic organisms.

microfiche   sheets of microfilm.

microfilm   photographs of records in a reduced size.

microorganisms   microscopic living organisms.

microprocessor   a chip that allows the computer to function.

micturition   also known as voiding or urination.

midbrain   part of the brain stem, responsible for relaying messages.

migraine   type of severe headache, usually unilateral; may appear in cluster.

mission statement   a statement describing the goals of the medical office and those it serves.

modem (modulator/demodulator)   a communication device that connects a computer to the standard telephone system, allowing information exchange with other computers off site.

modifiers   letters or numbers added to a code to clarify the service or procedure.

monitor   visual display terminal (VDT) that shows information being input via the keyboard.

monosaccharide   a simple sugar that cannot be broken down further.

mordant   a substance used to fix, or bind, dyes or stains.

morphology   description of the physical characteristics of blood cells.

motherboard   fiberglass board that contains the central processing unit (CPU), memory, and other pieces of circuitry.

mourning   to demonstrate signs of grief; grieving.

mouse   a device that allows the user to control cursor movement on the monitor.

multidisciplinary   involving many disciplines; a group of healthcare professionals from various specialties brought together to meet the patient's needs.

multimedia   various forms of communication available on the computer, e.g., stereophonic sound, animation, full-motion video, photographs.

multipara   woman who has given birth to more than one viable fetus.

multiskilled health professional   an individual with versatile training in the healthcare field.

muscular dystrophies   a group of genetically transmitted diseases characterized by progressive atrophy of skeletal muscles.

mycology   the science and study of fungi.

myelofibrosis   a disorder in which bone marrow tissue develops in abnormal sites such as the liver and spleen; signs include immature cells in the circulation, anemia, and splenomegaly.

myelogram   invasive radiological test in which dye is injected into the spinal fluid.

myelomeningocele   protrusion of the spinal cord through the spinal defect; spina bifida.

myocardial infarction (MI)   death of cardiac muscle due to lack of blood flow to the muscle; also known as heart attack.

myocarditis   inflammation of the myocardial layer of the heart.

myocardium   the middle layer of the walls of the heart, composed of cardiac muscle.

myofibrils   a slender light/dark strand of muscle tissue in striated muscle.

myopia   nearsightedness.

myringotomy   incision into the tympanic membrane to relieve pressure.

myxedema   the most severe form of hypothyroidism; signs include edema of the extremities and the face.

N

narrative   a paragraph indicating the contact with the patient, what was done for the patient, and the outcome of any action.

nasal septum   wall or partition dividing the nostrils.

National Committee for Clinical Laboratory Standards (NCCLS)   a committee appointed to establish rules to ensure the safety, standards and integrity of all testing performed on human specimens.

nebulizer   device for administering respiratory medications as a fine inhaled spray

needle holder   type of surgical forceps used to hold and pass suture through tissue.

negative feedback   a decrease in function in response to a stimulus.

negative stress   stress that does not allow for relaxation periods.

negligence   performance of an act that a reasonable health care worker would not have done or the omission of an act that a reasonable person would have done.

neonatologist   physician who specializes in the care and treatment of newborns.

neoplasm   abnormal growth of new tissue; tumor.

nephron   the portion of the kidney responsible for the production of urine.

nephrostomy   placement of a catheter in the kidney pelvis to drain urine from an obstructed kidney.

net pay   the amount of money an employee is paid after all taxes are withheld.

networking   a system of personal and professional relationships through which to share information.

neurogenic shock   shock that results from dysfunction of nervous system following spinal cord injury.

neuron   a nerve cell.

neurotransmitter   chemical needed to transmit a message between synapses.

nitrogenous   pertaining to or containing nitrogen, usually the end-product of protein metabolism.

nitroprusside   a nitrogen cyanic compound that reacts with ketones.

nocturia   excessive urination at night.

nodule   small node, mass, or swelling.

non compos mentis   mental incompetence.

non-insulin dependent diabetes mellitus (NIDDM)   a type of diabetes in which patients do not require insulin to control the blood sugar.

noncompliance   the patient's inability or refusal to follow prescribed orders.

noncompliant   describes a patient who refuses or is unable to follow prescribed orders.

nonlanguage   not expressed in spoken language, e.g., laughing, sobbing, grunting, sighing.

normal value   acceptable range as established for an age, a population, or a sex; variations usually indicate a disorder.

normal flora   microorganisms normally found in the body; also known as resident flora.

nosocomial infection   infection acquired in a medical setting, generally presumed to be in a hospital setting but may also refer to the medical office.

nuclear medicine   branch of medicine that uses radioactive isotopes to diagnose and treat disease.

nulligravida   woman who has never been pregnant.

nullipara   woman who has never given birth to a viable fetus.

numeric filing   arranging files by a numbered order.

nutrition   the study of food and how it is used for growth, nourishment, and repair.

O

obligate   to require; a parasite that has no choice but to attach to a living organism.

obstipation   extreme constipation.

obturator   smooth, rounded, removable inner portion of a hollow tube, such as an anoscope, that allows for easier insertion.

occult   hidden or concealed from observation.

Occupational Safety and Health Administration   a federal agency with a mission to protect employees from work related hazards.

olecranon fossa   the depression in the posterior surface of the humerus that allows the arm to extend by receiving the olecranon process.

olecranon process   the proximal end of the ulna that becomes the point of the elbow that fits into the olecranon fossa.

oliguria   scanty urine production.

on-line   direct link to off-site computers.

oophorectomy   excision of an ovary.

operating system   the program that tells the computer how to interface with hardware and software.

ophthalmic medication   medication instilled into the eye

ophthalmologist   physician who specializes in treatment of disorders of the eyes.

ophthalmoscope   lighted instrument used to examine the inner surfaces of the eye.

opportunistic infection   infection resulting from a defective immune system that cannot defend against pathogens normally found in the environment.

optician   specialist who grinds lenses to correct errors of refraction according to prescriptions written by optometrists or ophthalmologists.

optometrist   specialist who can measure for errors of refraction and prescribe lenses but who cannot treat diseases of the eye or perform surgery.

organ   the source or starting point; (muscle) any part that is made up of cells and tissues that cause it to perform its specified function in conjunction with a body system.

organizational chart   a flow sheet depicting the members of a team in a structured or hierarchical manner.

origin   the source or starting point; (muscle) the more fixed end of a muscle, usually the proximal end.

OSHA   Occupational Safety and Health Administration. The federal agency that oversees working conditions.

osteoporosis   abnormal porosity of the bone, most often found in the elderly, predisposing the affected bony tissue to fracture

otic medication   medication instilled into the ear

otolaryngologist   physician who specializes in treatment of diseases and disorders of the ears, nose, and throat.

otoscope   instrument used for visual examination of the ear canal and tympanic membrane.

outcomes   final results of patient care.

outlier   a patient whose hospital stay is longer than allowed by the DRG.

outpatient   a medical setting in which patients receive care but are not admitted.

over-the-counter   available without a prescription; includes herbal and vitamin supplements.

overdraft protection   protection against having insufficient funds to cover checks.

ovulation   the periodic rupture of the mature ovum from the ovary.

ovum (pl. ova)   the female reproductive cell; sex cell or egg.

P

packing slip   a document that accompanies a supply order and lists the enclosed items.

Paget's disease   degenerative bone disease usually in older persons with bone destruction and poor repair

palliative   easing symptoms without curing.

palmar   the palm surface of the hand.

palpation   technique in which the examiner feels the texture, size, consistency, and location of parts of the body with the hands.

palpitations   feeling of an increased heart rate or pounding heart that may be felt during an emotional response or a cardiac disorder.

pancreatitis   an inflammation of the pancreas that may be brought on by alcohol, trauma, infection, or certain drugs.

Papanicolaou (Pap) test or smear   smear of tissue cells examined for abnormalities including cancer, especially of the cervix; named for George N. Papanicolaou, a physician, anatomist, and cytologist.

papilla (pl. papillae)   a small nipple shaped projection.

papillae lingua   the taste buds.

papilloma   benign skin tumor.

papilloma virus   benign skin tumor caused by a virus.

papule   small, red elevation of the skin.

paralanguage   factors connected with, but not essentially part of language, e.g., tone of voice, volume, pitch.

parameters   values used to describe or measure a set of data representing a physiologic function or system.

paraphrasing   restating what you heard using your own words.

parasitology   the science and study of parasites.

parasympathetic   the part of the autonomic nervous system involved in periods free from stress.

parenteral medication   medication administered by any method other than orally

parity   pregnancy that resulted in a viable birth.

partial-thickness burn   burn that involves epidermis and varying levels of the dermis.

participating providers   those who agree to participate with managed care contracts and other third-party payers in exchange for building a solid patient base.

particulate matter   a material composed of particles.

passive range of motion   assisted range-of-motion movements.

pathogens   disease-causing microorganisms.

patient co-payment   the part of an insured service that the patient must pay.

patient education   active participation of the patient in a process that will yield a change in behavior.

payroll   the process of calculating employee salary.

payroll journal   a method for keeping track of payroll data using the pegboard system.

payroll   the process of calculating employee salary.

peer review organization   a group of physicians and specialists that conducts a review of a disputed case and makes a final recommendation.

pediatrician   physician who specializes in the care of infants, children, and adolescents.

pediatrics   specialty of medicine that deals with the care of infants, children and adolescents.

pediculosis   infestation with parasitic lice.

percussion   striking with the hands to evaluate the size, borders, consistency, and presence of fluid or air.

percutaneous transluminal coronary angioplasty (PTCA)   procedure that improves blood flow through a coronary artery by pressing the plaque against the wall of the artery with a balloon on a catheter, allowing for more blood flow.

pericarditis   inflammation of the sac that covers the heart.

pericardium   the double-layered serous, membranous sac that encloses the heart and the origins of the great vessels.

peripheral   pertaining to or situated away from the center.

peristalsis   contraction and relaxation of involuntary muscles of the alimentary canal producing wavelike movement of products through the digestive system.

PERRLA   abbreviation used in documentation to denote *p*upils *e*qual, *r*ound, *r*eactive to *l*ight and *a*ccommodation if all findings are normal; refers to the size and shape of the pupils, their reaction to light, and their ability to adjust to distance.

personal protective equipment   equipment used to protect a person from exposure to blood or other body fluids.

pessary   device that supports the uterus when inserted into the vagina.

petri plate   a shallow glass or plastic dish with a lid to hold solid media for cultures.

pH   abbreviation for potential hydrogen, pH is a scale representing the relative acidity or alkalinity of a substance in which 7.0 is neutral; numbers lower than 7.0 are acid and numbers above 7.0 are basic.

phagocyte   a cell that has the ability to ingest and destroy particular substances such as bacteria, protozoa, cells and cell debris by ingesting them.

phagocytosis   the process by which certain cells engulf and dispose of microorganisms; to eat or ingest.

pharmacodynamics   study of how drugs act within the body.

pharmacokinetics   study of the action of drugs within the body from administration to excretion.

pharmacology   study of drugs and their origin, nature, properties, and effects upon living organisms.

phimosis   narrowing or tightening of the prepuce that prevents retraction over the glans penis.

phonophoresis   ultrasound treatment used to force medications into tissues.

phosphates   a compound containing phosphorus and oxygen; they are very important in living organisms, especially for the transfer of genetic information.

physician hospital organization   a coalition of physicians and a hospital contracting with large employers, insurance carriers, and other benefits groups to provide discounted health services.

physiology   the study of the function of the body.

pia mater   thin vascular covering that adheres to the surface of the brain.

placebo   the power of believing that something will make you better without any chemical reaction that warrants improvement, e.g., sugar pills.

plaintiff   the party who initiates a lawsuit.

plan maximum   the highest amount paid by a third-party payer for any given service.

planes   a point of reference made by a straight cut through the body at any given angle.

planning   the process of using information gathered during the assessment phase to organize learning or patient care objectives in order to accomplish the specific learning or treatment goal.

pleura   the serous membrane enclosing the lungs; (visceral pleura: the layer that covers the lungs most closely; parietal pleura: the layer that follows the contours and lines the chest wall, the diaphragm, and the mediastinum).

poikilocytosis   abnormal variations in the shapes of red blood cells (poikilo = variation).

policy a statement that reflects the organization's rules on a given topic.

polydipsia excessive thirst.

polymenorrhea abnormally frequent menstrual periods.

polyphagia abnormal hunger.

polyuria excessive excretion and elimination of urine.

pons part of the brain stem, responsible for communication withn the central nervous system.

portfolio a portable case containing documents.

positive stress stress that allows a person to perform at peak levels and then relax afterward.

positive feedback an increase in function in response to a stimulus.

positron emission tomography (PET) computerized radiography using radioactive substances to assess metabolic or physiological functions within the body rather than anatomical structures.

postexposure testing laboratory tests that may be performed after a person comes into contact with a biohazard.

posting listing financial transactions in a ledger.

postural hypotension sudden drop in blood pressure upon standing.

potentiation describes the action of two drugs taken together in which the combined effects are greater than the sum of the independent effects.

precedent the use of previous court decisions as a legal foundation.

preceptor a teacher; one who gives direction, as in a technical matter.

precertification approved documentation prior to referrals to specialists and other facilities

precipitation the settling out of a substance in a solution.

preexisting condition medical problem treated by a physician before an insurance plan's effective date. A third-party payer may exclude coverage for preexisting conditions.

preferred provider organization (PPO) an organization whose purpose is to contract with providers, then lease this network of contracted providers to health care plans.

prepuce a fold of skin that forms a cover.

presbyacusis loss of hearing associated with aging.

presbycusis loss of hearing associated with aging.

presbyopia vision change (farsightedness) associated with aging.

present illness a specific account of the chief complaint, including time frames and characteristics.

preservative substance that delays decomposition.

primary diagnosis the condition or chief complaint that brings a person to a medical facility for treatment.

primary survey an initial assessment of an emergency patient for life-threatening problems.

prime mover the muscle most responsible for the desired muscle action or movement.

primigravida woman who is pregnant for the first time.

primipara woman who has given birth to one viable infant.

printer a device that transfers information on the computer into hard copy.

problem-oriented medical record (POMR) a common method of compiling information that lists each problem of the patient, usually at the beginning of the folder, and references each problem with a number throughout the folder.

procedure a series of steps required to perform a given task; a medical service or test that is coded for reimbursement.

professional courtesy a discount fee given to healthcare professionals.

profit-and-loss statement statement of income and expenditures; shows whether in a given period a business made or lost money and how much.

proofreading a part of editing a document in which the writer reads the draft for accuracy and clarity and corrects errors.

proprietary private school with preset curricula.

prostate-specific antigen normal protein produced by the prostate that usually elevates in the presence of prostate cancer.

prosthesis any artificial replacement for a missing body part, such as false teeth or an artificial limb.

protinuria the presence of large quantities of protein in the urine; usually a sign of renal dysfunction.

protocol a code of proper conduct; a treatment plan.

providers a health care worker who delivers medical care.

proxemic having to do with the degree of physical closeness tolerated by humans.

pruritus itching.

psoriasis chronic skin disorder that appears as red patches covered by thick, dry, silvery scales.

psychogenic of psychological origin.

psychomotor describes a physical task.

psychosocial relating to mental and emotional aspects of social encounters.

puerperium period of time (about 6 weeks) from childbirth until reproductive structures return to normal.

purchase order a document that lists the required items to be purchased.

Purkinje fibers extensions of the Bundle of His that branch through the myocardium to end the transmission of the electrical impulse and cause the ventricles to contract.

purulent describes drainage that is white, green, or yellow; characteristic of an infection.

pustule vesicle filled with pus.

pyosalpinx pus in the fallopian tube(s).

pyrexia body temperature of 102°F or higher rectally or 101°F or higher orally.

pyuria pus in the urine.

Q

quadrants a division of the abdomen into four equal parts by one horizontal and one vertical line dissecting at the umbilicus.

quality assurance (QA) an evaluation of health care services as compared to accepted standards.

quality control (QC) method to evaluate the proper performance of testing procedures, supplies or equipment in a laboratory.

quality improvement a plan that allows an organization to scientifically measure the quality of its product and service.

quantification the process of ascertaining the amount of something.

quantitative the measuring of an amount.

Queckenstedt test test to determine presence of obstruction in the CSF flow performed during a lumbar puncture.

R

radiograph processed film that contains a visible image.

radiographer technical specialist who works to assist the radiologist in the performance of procedures and who is responsible for producing routine examination images for the radiologist to interpret.

radiography art and science of producing diagnostic images with x-rays.

radioimmunoassay (RIA) the introduction of radioactive substances into the body to determine the concentration of a substance in the serum, usually the concentration of antigens, antibodies, or proteins.

radiologist physician who specializes in radiology; performs some procedures and interprets images to provide diagnostic information.

radiology branch of medicine including diagnostic and therapeutic applications of x-rays.

radiolucent permitting the passage of x-rays.

radionuclide radioactive material with a short life that is used in small amounts in nuclear medicine studies.

radiopaque not permeable to passage of x-rays.

random access memory (RAM) temporary memory; data is lost when the computer is turned off if it is not backed up on disk.

range of motion (ROM) range in degrees of angle through which a joint can be extended and flexed.

ratchet notched mechanism, usually at the handle end of an instrument, that clicks into position to maintain tension on the opposing blades or tips of the instrument.

read only memory (ROM) permanent memory inside the computer.

reagent a substance used to react in a certain manner in the presence of specific chemicals to obtain a diagnosis.

receptionist a person who greets patients as they arrive at a medical office and performs various administrative tasks.

recertification certification renewed either by taking the examination again or by completing a specified number of continuing education units in a 5-year period.

rectocele herniation of the rectum into the vaginal area.

rectovaginal pertaining to the rectum and vagina.

reduction correcting a fracture by realigning the bones; may be closed (corrected by manipulation) or open (requires surgery).

reference value a range established for test results assumed to be typical for a population asymptomatic for disease processes.

referral instruction to transfer a patient's care to a specialist

reflecting repeat what one heard using open-ended questions.

reflux a return or backward flow of fluid.

refraction bending of light rays that enter the pupil to reflect exactly on the fovea centralis, the area of greatest visual acuity.

registered indicates that a professional has met basic requirements, usually for education; has passed standard testing; and has been approved by a governing body to perform given tasks within a state.

relapsing fever fever that returns after extended periods of being within normal limits.

remittent fluctuating.

remittent fever fever that is fluctuating.

renal pelvis the funnel-shaped upper portion of the ureters that collects urine from the kidneys.

renal cortex the portion of the kidney that contains the structures that form urine.

renal medulla the inner portion of the kidney that contains the collecting structures.

renal pyramids situated in the renal medulla, part of the collecting structures.

renin enzyme formed in the kidney that works with angiotensin to affect the blood pressure.

repolarization the active process of restoring the cardiac fibers to the resting (polarized) state. Re-establishment of the electrical polarized state in a muscle or nerve fiber following contraction or conduction of a nerve impulse.

res ipsa loquitur "the thing speaks for itself".

res judicata "the thing has been decided".

resident flora microorganisms normally found in the body; also known as normal flora.

resistance body's immune response to prevent infections by invading pathogenic microorganisms.

Resource-Based Relative Value Scale (RBRVS) a value scale designed to decrease Medicare Part B costs and establish national standards for coding and payment.

respiration the exchange of oxygen and carbon dioxide (external respiration: the exchange between the alveoli and the bloodstream; internal respiration: the exchange between the cells and the bloodstream).

respondent superior "let the master answer".

restrain control or confine movement.

résumé document summarizing individual's work experience or professional qualifications.

retinal degeneration pathological changes in the cell structure of the retina that impair or destroy its function, resulting in blindness.

retrograde pyelogram an x-ray of the urinary tract using contrast medium injected through the bladder and ureters; useful in diagnosing obstructions.

retroperitoneal   the space behind the peritoneal cavity that contains the kidneys.

retrovirus   virus containing reverse transcriptase, which allows the viral cell to replicate its DNA in the DNA of the host cell, thereby taking over the substance of the cell.

returned check fee   amount of money a bank or business charges for a check written with insufficient funds.

reverse chronological order   items placed with oldest first.

rickettsia   organism that is smaller than bacteria, larger than viruses.

ringworm   lay term for tinea, a group of fungal diseases.

risk factors   any issue that possesses a safety or liability concern for an organization.

role delineation chart   a list of the areas of competence expected of the graduate

Romberg test   test for inability to maintain body balance when eyes are closed and feet are together, indication of spinal cord disease.

rugae   ridges or folds in the skin or mucous membranes that allow for expansion of a part.

rule of nines   the most common method of determining the extent of burn injury; the body surface is divided into sections of 9% or multiples of 9%.

S

salpingectomy   excision of the fallopian tube.

salpingo-oophorectomy   surgical excision of both the fallopian tube and the ovary.

salutation   an introductory phrase that greets the reader of a letter.

sanitation   maintenance of a healthful, disease-free environment.

sanitization   processes used to lower the number of microorganisms on a surface by cleansing with soap or detergent, water, and manual friction.

sanitize   reduce the number of microorganisms on a surface by use of low-level disinfectant practices.

sanitizing   the practice of lowering the number of microorganisms on a surface by use of low-level disinfectant practices.

scale   a thin, dried flake of skin.

scalpel   small, pointed knife with a convex edge for surgical procedures.

scanner   a piece of office equipment that transfers a written document into a computer.

scissors   sharp instrument composed of two opposing cutting blades, held together by a central pin on which the blades pivot.

sclera   white fibrous tissue that covers the eye.

sclerotherapy   use of chemical agents to treat esophageal varices to produce fibrosis and hardening of the tissue.

scoliosis   lateral curve of the spine, usually in the thoracic area, with a corresponding curve in the lumbar region, causing uneven shoulders and hips.

screening   a preliminary procedure, such as a test or exam, to detect the more characteristic signs of a disorder.

search engine   program that allows you to find information on the Internet rapidly and effectively.

sebaceous gland   oil gland.

seborrhea   overproduction of sebum by the sebaceous glands.

sebum   fatty secretion of the sebaceous gland.

secondary survey   an assessment of an emergency victim for head to toe injuries.

seizure   abnormal discharge of electrical activity in the brain, resulting in involuntary contractions of voluntary muscles.

semi-block   a type of letter format that is styled the same as block, except the first sentence of each paragraph is indented five spaces.

senility   general mental deterioration associated with aging.

sensitivity   susceptibility to a certain substance.

sentinel event   an unexpected occurrence or event that results in death or serious physical or psychological injury.

septic shock   shock that results from general infection in the bloodstream.

septicemia   presence of pathogenic bacteria in the blood.

serology   the study of the nature and properties of serum.

serration   groove, either straight or criss-cross, etched or cut into the blade or tip of an instrument to improve its bite or grasp.

service   medical interventions completed by a provider.

service charge   a charge by a bank for various services.

sesamoid   resembling the shape of a sesame seed.

shock   lack of oxygen to individual cells of the body.

sick child visit   a pediatric visit for the treatment of illness or injury.

sickle cell anemia   a condition in which the patient has both copies of the gene for hemoglobin S; the red cells become sickle shaped and non-flexible causing obstruction of small vessels and capillaries. Necrosis due to tissue hypoxia occurs beyond the obstruction. Most commonly seen in African-Americans.

signs   objective indications of disease or bodily dysfunction as observed or measured by the health care professional.

sinoatrial (SA) node   considered the pacemaker of the heart, located in the upper portion of the right atrium; a specialized group of cells that initiate the electrical impulse of the heart.

slander   oral statements that defame a person's reputation or character.

smegma   a cheesy secretion of the sebaceous glands either in the labia or prepuce.

SOAP   a style of chanting that includes subjective, objective, assessment, and planning notes.

software   application programs that direct the hardware to perform given tasks.

sound   long instrument for exploring or dilating body cavities or searching cavities for foreign bodies.

specialty   a subcategory of medicine, such as pediatrics, studied after completion of medical school.

specific gravity   density of a liquid, such as urine, compared with water.

specificity   relating to a definite result.

specimen   a small portion of anything used to evaluate the nature of the whole.

speculum   instrument that enlarges and separates the opening of a cavity to expose its interior for examination.

spherocytosis   a condition where all or almost all of the red cells are spherocytes; typically asymptomatic.

sphygmomanometer   device used to measure blood pressure

spicules   sharp points.

spina bifida occulta   congenital defect in the spinal column caused by lack of union of the vertebrae.

spinal   pertaining to the spine.

spirochete   long, flexible, motile microorganisms.

splint   device used to immobilize a sprain, strain, fracture, or dislocated limb.

spore   bacterial life form that resists destruction by heat, drying, or chemicals. Spore-producing bacteria include botulism and tetanus.

staff privileges   hospital approval for a physician to admit patients for treatment.

stagborn   stone formation in the renal pelvis that fills the chamber and assumes the shape of the calyces.

standard precautions   usual steps to prevent injury or disease.

staphylococci   spherical microorganism found in grapelike clusters.

Staphylococcus   genus of bacteria, some of which can cause skin infections.

stare decisis   "the previous decision stands".

STAT   immediately.

status asthmaticus   asthma attack that is not responsive to treatment.

statute of limitations   a legal time limit; e.g., the length of time in which a patient may file a lawsuit.

statutes   laws that are written by federal, state or local legislators.

stereotyping   to place in a fixed mold, without consideration of differences.

sterile field   a specific area, such as within a tray or on a sterile towel, that is considered free of microorganisms.

sterilization   process, act, or technique for destroying microorganisms using heat, water, chemicals, or gases.

stoma   an opening to the surface; suggests that it is surgically created.

stomatitis   inflammation of the mucous membranes of the mouth.

stratum corneum   outer layer of the epidermis.

stratum germinativum   innermost layer of the epidermis.

streaming   a method of allotting time for appointments based on the needs of the individual patient to minimize gaps in time and backups

Streptococcus   genus of bacteria commonly implicated in infections of the skin.

stress   a factor that induces body tension; can be positive or negative.

striated   having a striped appearance with alternating light and dark bands.

subcutaneous   beneath the skin.

subject filing   arranging files according to their title, grouping similar subjects together.

sublingual medication   medication administered under the tongue

subpoena duces tecum   a court order requiring medical records to be submitted to the court at a given date and time.

subpoena   a court order requiring an individual to appear at court at a given date and time.

substrate   an underlying layer; a substance acted upon, as by an enzyme or reagent.

sudoriferous gland   sweat gland.

sulci   a groove in the brain tissue.

sulfosalicylic acid   an acid used to test for protein.

summarizing   briefly review the information discussed to determine the patient's comprehension.

summation report   any report that provides a summary of activities, such as a payroll report or a profit-and-loss statement.

superbill   preprinted patient bill that lists a variety of procedures.

superficial burn   burn limited to the epidermis.

surfing   navigating the Internet.

surgical asepsis   destruction of organisms before they enter the body.

surrogate mother   a woman who carries a baby to term for another female who is unable to carry a pregnancy to term.

suspension   temporary removal of privileges.

sustained fever   fever that is constant or not fluctuating

swab (noun)   stick topped with cotton or other absorbent man-made fiber for cleaning areas, applying treatments or for obtaining specimens.

swab (verb)   to wipe with a swab.

swaged needle   metal needle fused to suture material.

symmetry   equality in size or shape or position of parts on opposite sides of the body.

sympathetic   the part of the autonomic nervous system involved in stress reaction.

sympathy   feeling sorry for or pitying someone.

symptoms   subjective indications of disease or bodily dysfunction as sensed by the patient.

synapse   the junction of two neurons.

synarthroses   immovable joints.

syncope   sudden fall in blood pressure or cerebral hypoxia resulting in loss of consciousness.

synergism   harmonious action of two agents, such as drugs or organs, producing an effect that neither could produce alone or that is greater than the total effects of each agent operating by itself.

synergist   muscles that work together for more efficient movement.

system   a collection of organs that perform a certain function.

systole   contraction phase of the cardiac cycle.

T

T cells   lymphoid cells from bone marrow that migrate to the thymus gland where they mature into differentiated lymphocytes that circulate between blood and lymph.

tab   the projection on a file folder on which the patient name or title is written.

tachycardia   heart rate of more than 100 beats per minute.

tactile   pertaining to the sense of touch.

task force   a group of employees that works together to solve a given problem.

tax withholding   the amount of tax that is withheld from a paycheck

teleradiology   use of computed imaging and information systems to transmit diagnostic images to distant locations.

teletypewriter (TTY)   a special machine that allows communication on a telephone with a hearing-impaired person.

template   a skeleton of a letter or document with preset and prespaced elements.

tendons   tough, flexible fibers that bind muscle to bone.

tetany   severe cramping, convulsions or muscle spasms due to an abnormality of calcium metabolism.

thalamus   part of the diencephalon, responsible for sorting messages.

thalassemia   a hemolytic anemia caused by deficient hemoglobin synthesis; more commonly found in those of Mediterranean heritage.

therapeutic   having to do with treating or curing disease; curative.

third-party administrator   administrator who processes claims for the sponsor of self-funded benefit planning.

thoracentesis   surgical puncture into the pleural cavity for aspiration of serous fluid or for injection of medication.

thromboplastin   a complex substance found in blood and tissues that aids the clotting process.

thyrotoxicosis   excess quantities of thyroid hormone in the tissues.

tickler file   a file that provides a reminder to do a given task at a particular date and time.

tidal volume   amount of air inhaled and exhaled during a normal respiration.

tine test   skin test for exposure to tuberculosis, involves pricking the skin with sharp tines coated with the tuberculin bacillus.

tinnitus   an extraneous noise heard in one or both ears, described as whirring, ringing, whistling, roaring, etc.; may be continuous or intermittent.

tissues   a group of cells that function together for a specific purpose.

titer   measure of the amount of an antibody in serum.

tomography   procedure in which the x-ray tube and film move in relation to each other during exposure, blurring out all structures except those in the focal plane.

tonometry   measurement of intraocular pressure using a tonometer.

tonsils   a small mass of lymphoid tissue; includes the palatine, nasopharyngeal and lingual tonsils.

tonus   the steady, partial contraction of skeletal muscles that allows the body to remain upright.

topical medication   medication applied directly to the skin or mucous membranes

tort   the righting of wrongs or injuries suffered by someone because of another person's wrongdoing.

toxoid   toxin treated to destroy its toxicity but still capable of inducing formation of antibodies.

tracheostomy   permanent surgical stoma in the neck with an indwelling tube.

tracheotomy   incision into the trachea below the larynx to circumvent a blockage superior to this point; suggests an emergency situation and a reversible procedure.

trade name   name given to a medication by the company that owns the patent.

transcription   the process of typing a dictated message.

transient flora   microorganisms that do not normally reside in a given area; transient flora may or may not produce disease.

transient ischemic attack (TIA)   acute episode of cerebrovascular insufficiency, usually a result of narrowing of an artery by atherosclerotic plaques, emboli, or vasospasm; usually passes quickly but should be considered a warning for predisposition to cerebrovascular accidents.

transillumination   passage of light through body tissues for the purpose of examination.

transition   passing from one place or activity to another.

traumatic   causing or relating to tissue damage.

triage   sorting of patients into categories based on their level of sickness or injury; to ensure that life-threatening medical conditions are treated immediately.

trigone   the triangle formed in the base of the bladder by the entrance of the two ureters and the exit of the urethra.

truss   a device of pressing against a hernia to keep it in place.

turbid   cloudy.

turbinates   mucous membrane-covered conchae, the three scroll-shaped bones that project into the nasal cavity bilaterally from the lateral walls, each covers a sinus meatus.

turgor   normal tension in a cell or the skin; normal skin turgor resists deformation and will resume its former position after being grasped or pulled.

tympanic membrane thin, semitransparent membrane in the middle ear that transmits sound vibrations; the eardrum.

tympanic thermometer device for measuring the temperature using the blood flow through the tympanic membrane, or eardrum.

U

ultrasound imaging technique that uses sound waves to diagnose or monitor various body structures.

unbundling the practice of submitting a claim with several separate procedure codes rather than a single code that represents the services performed.

unemployment tax federal tax paid by the employer based on each employee's gross income.

unintentional tort describes an honest mistake by a person operating in good faith.

unit each part of a name or title that is used in indexing; a quantity of a standard measurement.

upcoding billing more for a patient care service than it is worth by selecting a code that is higher on the coding scale; this is an illegal practice.

upper respiratory infection (URI) infection of the nasopharynx, throat, and bronchi.

urates a nitrogenous compound derived from protein use and is excreted in the urine.

urea the final product of protein metabolism in the body and the main nitrogenous component in the urine.

uremic frost a frost-like deposit of uremic compounds on the skin of patients whose kidneys are no longer functional.

ureterostomy surgical opening to the outside of the body from the ureter to facilitate drainage of urine from an obstructed kidney.

ureters the pair of tubes designed to carry urine from the kidneys to the bladder.

urethra the short tube that carries urine from the bladder to the outside of the body.

URI upper respiratory infection.

uric acid a by-product of protein metabolism present in the blood and excreted by the kidneys.

urinalysis examination of the physical, chemical, and microscopic properties of urine.

urinary frequency the urge to urinate occurring more often than is required for normal bladder elimination.

urticaria hives.

usual, customary, and reasonable (UCR) the basis of a physician's fee schedule, the usual and customary cost of the same service or procedure in a similar geographic area and under the same or similar circumstances.

utilization review an analysis of individual cases by a committee to make sure services and procedures being billed to a third-party payer are medically necessary and to ensure compliance with its rules and regulations regarding reimbursement.

V

V-codes codes assigned to patients who receive service but have no illness, injury, or disorder, e.g., a vaccination or a screening mammogram.

vaccine suspension of infectious agents or some part of them, given to establish resistance to an infectious disease.

values establishd ideals of life, conduct, customs, etc., of an individual person or members of a society.

varicella zoster viral infection manifested by characteristic rash of successive crops of vesicles that scab before resolution; also called chicken pox.

vasopressin a hormone formed in the hypothalamus and transported to the posterior lobe of the pituitary through the hypothalamo-hypophyseal tract. It has an antidiuretic and a pressor effect that elevates the blood pressure.

vector (biological) a living, nonhuman carrier of disease, usually an arthropod; (mechanical) a carrier of disease that does not support growth; examples include contaminated inanimate objects.

ventricle either of the two lower chambers of the heart that when filled with blood contract to propel it into the arteries.

venule the small vessel that joins a capillary to a vein.

verdict a decision of guilty or not guilty based on evidence presented in a trial.

verruca wart.

vertigo sensation of whirling of oneself or the environment; dizziness.

vesicle skin lesion that appears as a small sac containing fluid; a blister.

viable capable of growing and living.

vial glass or plastic container sealed at the top by a rubber stopper

villus (pl. villi) tiny, almost microscopic projections in the mucous membrane of the small intestines.

virology the science and study of viruses.

virtual a paperless system or chart on your computer.

virulent highly pathogenic and disease producing; describes a microorganism.

virus a harmful invader that can damage your computer.

visualization a relaxation technique that allows the mind to wander and the imagination to run free and focus on positive and relaxing situations.

W

wave scheduling a flexible scheduling method that allows time for procedures of varying lengths and the addition of unscheduled patients, as needed.

well-child visit visit to the medical office for administration of immunizations and evaluation of growth and development.

Western blot specific confirmatory antibody test for presence of HIV in blood.

wheal small, round itchy elevation of the skin with a white center and a red border; a hive.

whorls   a spiral arrangement, as in the ridges on the finger that make up a fingerpoint.

withdrawing   the act of terminating a medical treatment that has already been initiated.

withholding   not initiating certain medical treatments.

Wood's light   ultraviolet light used to detect fungal diseases.

workers' compensation   employer insurance for treatment of an employee's injury or illness related to the job.

write off   cancellation of an unpaid debt.

x-rays   invisible electromagnetic radiation waves used in diagnosis and treatment of various disorders.

yolk sac   a structure that develops in the inner zygotic cell mass and supplies nourishment for the embryo until the seventh week when the placenta takes over the function.

ESL GLOSSARY

KAREN A. SANTIAGO
Director of English as a Second Language
Nueva Esperanza, Inc.
Philadelphia, PA

This glossary has been provided to help students whose first language is not English. It does not contain technical words. It has other verbs, adverbs, nouns, and adjectives that you may not know but that are used in this text. Definitions provided relate to use of the word in the text. There may be other definitions of the same word when used in a different context and the same words may be used as different parts of speech. For other definitions of the same word, please consult a dictionary.

Term	Part of Speech	Meaning
Abraded	Adjective	Hurt
Abrupt	Adjective	Quick
Accurate	Adjective	Exact, all information is correct
Acutely	adverb	sharply, severely
Adhere	verb	stick to, follow completely
Adhere	verb	stay with, stick
Adhere to	Verb	Always follow
Adjunct	Noun	Help
Advent	noun	coming, arrival
Adverse	adjective	negative, bad, undesirable
Adversely	Adverb	Negatively, badly
Allay	Verb	Relieve, reduce, do away with (fears), calm
Alleged	adjective	said to have happened but not proved
Allied	adjective	joined, united
Alleviate	Verb	Relieve, make less
Alter	verb	change
Altered	Adjective	Changed
Angled (at an angle)	adjective	not directly facing
Anticipate	Verb	Being ready by thinking ahead to the next action
Appropriate	adjective	right, correct
Arise	verb	come up

Term	Part of Speech	Meaning
Arrears	noun	overdue payment or debt not settled
Aspirated	Verb	Pulled, sucked
Assault	noun, verb	attack
Asset	noun	advantage, highly valued person
Attained	Verb	Gotten, reached
Attempt	Verb	Try
Attuned	adjective	sensitive to or aware of
Barrier (defenses)	Adjective	Blocking
Batch	noun	group
Belittle	verb	disparage; make a person feel unimportant
Bends	Noun	Places that are not straight
Bias	noun	prejudice, personal opinion
Blatant	adjective	obvious
Blows	Noun	Hits
Blurred	adjective	not clear
Breach	noun	break, split
Breached	Verb	Broken
Bruise	noun	contusion; dark mark on the skin from an injury
Bubbles	Noun	Small amounts of air trapped in the medication
Bulk	Adjective	Having many in one place
Bunching	Verb	Pushing together
Burden	noun	trouble, problem
Buzz	noun	sound of zzzzzz, as a bee makes
Carcinogen	noun	substance that causes cancer
Cast	verb	throw, as cast a glance at
Cessation	Noun	The stopping of an action
Chain of events	Noun phrase	What happened that caused the patient to make the appointment
Charge	noun	accusation
Chief	Adjective	Main, most important
Cliché	noun	a saying that is so generally understood to be true that it is unnecessary to repeat it
Clues	Noun	Signs

Term	Part of Speech	Meaning
Compassion	Noun	Feelings
Complexity	noun	amount of complication
Compliance	noun	the act of following the rules
Comply	Verb	Follow
Compressed	Adjective	Squeezed, pressed together
Compromise	verb	find middle ground in a dispute or conflict
Conglomerate	noun	very large company with many products, services, and locations
Consensus	noun	general agreement
Contamination	noun	presence of unclean substances
Convey	verb	literally transport; explain, make clear
Core	adjective	basic, most important
Cornerstone	Noun	Foundation, basis
Countersue	verb	respond to a lawsuit with lawsuit
Creed	noun	a statement of beliefs
Crucial	Adjective	Extremely important
Crutches	noun	supports used by people with leg or foot injuries to help them walk
Cues	Noun	Signs, signals, (physical) movement
Damp	Adjective	Not dry
Daunting	adjective	frightening
Debilitated	Adjective	Weak, not strong
Deem	verb	decide, conclude
Deformity	Noun	Something not made correctly or that doesn't look right
Demeanor	noun	behavior
Denigrate	verb	make someone feel unimportant, lower
Depressed	Adjective	Pushed in, lower in the middle than the edges
Deprived	Verb	Not given
Dereliction	noun	failure to carry out a duty or responsibility
Deterrent	noun	action or object that stops a person from doing something
Diluted	Verb	To dilute is to make weaker by adding a liquid
Discard	Verb	Throw away
Discernible	Adjective	Able to be noticed or seen
Discomfort	Noun	Not feeling good or comfortable

Term	Part of Speech	Meaning
Dislodged	Verb	Moved from its original place
Disposable	Adjective	Can be thrown away after being used
Disrobing	Noun	Action of taking off clothes
Disrupt	Verb	Block, interrupt, change
Distended	Adjective	Sticks out too far
Distort	verb	make appear different from reality, change
Distract	Verb	Change a person's attention
Distractions	Noun	Things that the patient would want to look at
Distressed	adjective	upset, not calm
Diversity	Noun	Many different races, colors and religions of patients
Dormant	Adjective	Not active, like sleeping
Doubt	noun	uncertainty; lack of belief
Drainage	Noun	Liquid that comes out of wound
Dressing	noun	bandage, protective cover on wound
Drive	verb	power, transport by car or bus
Droops	Verb	Hangs, does not stay upright or erect
Drowsiness	Noun	When a person feels sleepy
Dust mite	Noun	Microscopic spider-like insect that lives in household items
Ease	Noun	Relaxed, not nervous
Efficacy	noun	level of efficiency or usefulness
Elderly	adjective	old
Elective	noun	a choice, the thing chosen
Elicit	verb	bring out, encourage
Eliminate	Verb	Remove, destroy
Empathy	Noun	Understanding the feelings of the patient
Enhance	Verb	Make better
Enlightenment	noun	the awakening of new ideas
Entitled	adjective	allowed, authorized
Ethical	Adjective	Moral
Enunciate (well)	verb	say words very clearly
Escalate	verb	to become greater
Euphoria	noun	a feeling that everything is great

Term	Part of Speech	Meaning
Evolve	verb	develop
Exacerbation	noun	thing that makes something worse
Extraneous	adjective	extra, unnecessary
Face	Verb	Stand so you can see it
Fasting	Verb	To fast: to not eat or drink
Felon	noun	person guilty of one or more major crimes
Fidget	verb	move parts of the body, such as hands, feet, indicating nervousness
Field of vision	Noun phrase	Area that you can see
Fines	Noun	Money paid for something done incorrectly or illegally
Fiscal	adjective	related to money management, especially governmental spending
Flatware	Noun	Utensils used in the home for eating: knives, forks, spoons
Flight of ideas	phrase	many ideas spoken quickly
Flipped	Verb	To flip: to use a quick movement of the hand causing an item to move from one place to another
Flow (of traffic)	noun	the pattern people walk through an office area
Follow-up	Adjective	Actions taken to check something you have done or that has happened
Foster	verb	support or encourage
Foul	Adjective	Very bad
Fraudulent	adjective	deceptive and illegal
Freestanding	adjective	not connected to a larger institution
Gait	Noun	The way a person walks
Gatekeeper	noun	a controller
Gather	verb	to collect into one place
Gear (up)	verb	equip, prepare
Germicide	noun	something that kills germs
Given (a given)	noun	something definite and expected, taken for granted
Good Samaritan	noun	someone who takes care of people in need
Gowning	Noun	Putting on the covering (gown) for an examination or operation
Gradual	Adjective	Slow
Grafting	Adjective	Taking skin or tissue from one place on the body and putting it on another one to fix a problem
Grimace	noun	movement of the face that indicates dislike or pain
Grossly	adverb	greatly

Term	Part of Speech	Meaning
Ground	Verb	To make it so that the patient doesn't get burned by the electricity
Gross breach	noun	very serious illegal act
Grunt	verb	make a sound deep in the throat that can show hard work, disgust, or boredom
Guidelines	Noun	Rules, restrictions
Hacker	noun	person who finds a way into a private computer system to take information or cause damage
Hailed	adjective	praised as something good
Halt	verb	stop
Handle	verb	take care of
Harsh	adjective	irritating, as *bright, harsh light*
Hazards	Noun	Dangers
Higher	adjective	more powerful
Hinder	verb	to slow or stop an action or idea
Hoarseness	Noun	The voice is not clear
Hose	noun	stockings, pantyhose
Hospice	noun	a center or program to care for people who are dying
Horny	Adjective	Not smooth
Humming	Adjective	A low, steady continuous sound
Image	Noun	The way you look
Imbedded	Adjective	Dirt and other items that are stuck inside the wound
Immersion	Noun	Being completely covered
Immunity	noun	protection from punishment
Impacted	Adjective	Stuck, cannot move
Impair	Verb	Bother, block, make less
Impairment	noun	malfunction, handicap, diminished ability as a result of an injury
Impartial	adjective	having no opinion or preference before the action
Impeccably	Adjective	Perfectly
Impassive	adjective	not showing emotion
Impede	Verb	Block, get in the way
Impending doom	Noun phrase	The feeling that something bad is going to happen
Imperative	Adjective	A command, something you must do
Inappropriate	adjective	not right or correct for the situation

Term	Part of Speech	Meaning
Incur	verb	cause, bring on oneself
Index cards	Noun phrase	Small card that usually measures 3 inches by 5 inches
Indigent	noun	poor, in poverty
Infinite	Adjective	Too many to count
Infraction	noun	breach of a rule or law
Ingested	Verb	Taken in by the mouth
Initial	Adjective	First
Innermost	Adjective	Inside
Insanity	noun	mental illness
Integrity	noun	honesty, steadfast morality, trustworthiness
Intermediary	noun	person or organization that communicates between two groups
Intermingled	adjective	mixed
Intervals	Noun	Regular periods of time
Intimidating	adjective	causing fear
Introspection	noun	thoughts about oneself
Invasive	adjective	entering or cutting into the body
Irate	verb	angry
Jargon	noun	slang; special words understood by specific group of people, as *medical jargon*
Jeopardize	noun	put in danger
Jeopardize	Verb	To put in danger, to make it fail
Jump start	noun	a quick beginning
Kin	noun	family, relatives
Laundering	Noun	The cleaning/washing of the linens
Lethal	adjective	deadly, causing death
Lethargy	Noun	Not very active, slow and tired
Levy	verb	ask for, require
Liable	noun	responsible
Liaison	Noun	A helper or person who helps
Likelihood	noun	probability
Loads	Noun	The articles you are sterilizing
Lodged	Adjective	Stuck. Won't come out easily
Lot	noun	group; large amount

Term	Part of Speech	Meaning
Lower	adjective	less powerful
Low-key	adjective	not exciting or loud
Malicious	adjective	causing pain, injury, or distress
Malpractice suit	noun, verb	a legal action saying a doctor or medical facility did something wrong
Mandate	verb	command, as in a law
Manslaughter	noun	killing someone by accident
Meticulous	adjective	careful
Mode	Noun	Way or method
Moisture	Noun	Water or liquid
Mound	noun	a large quantity; literally a heap
Mounted	Verb	To mount: to put or secure permanently
Mute	adjective	not able to talk
Nicks	Noun	Having little pieces missing
Nourish	Verb	Feed
Obese	Adjective	Fat, weigh too much
Obstructed	Adjective	Blocked, cannot go through
Omit	verb	leave out, not do
Onset	Noun	Beginning of the problem or condition
Open-ended	adjective	with no definite answer or choice of answers
Opt	verb	choose
Optimal	noun	the best, most nearly perfect
Optimum	Adjective	The best possible
Options	noun	possibilities
Outburst	noun	a sudden loud expression or action
Outlay	noun	money spent
Outline	verb	describe, especially in a list
Overlooked	Verb	Not done or seen
Overpowered	Verb	More than can be defended
Overwhelm	Verb	To have too much of something
Peeling	Noun	Removing the surface
Penetrate	Verb	To go into
Perceive	verb	see, understand

Term	Part of Speech	Meaning
Perceived	adjective	understood
Permeability	Noun	Ability to pass through
Persistent	Adjective	Doesn't go away easily, not easy to cure
Pertinent	adjective	related to, relevant
Pet dander	Noun	The substance produced on the skin of an animal that some people are allergic to
Phone tag	noun	sequence of unanswered phone calls between two people who keep leaving messages
Physically challenged	adjective	having physical problems making it hard to walk or perform other activities of daily living
Piece	noun	part, fragment of a whole
Pitch	noun	the way the voice goes up and down
Pitted	Adjective	Not smooth, having little holes in the surface
Pleasant	adjective	nice
Polarized	adjective	opposite; having opposite opinions or ideas
Pools	Verb	To collect or go to one place
Pose (a question)	verb	ask, raise
Posted	Verb	To post: to display, to put
Potential	noun	the possibility of an act or event
Pouches	Noun	Like pockets or little bags
Predisposed	Adjective	Not having defenses against other diseases
Prelude	noun	something that comes before the main event
Prerequisite	noun	requirement before doing something
Prescription	noun	a paper from a doctor that you take to the pharmacy to get medicine; an order for treatment
Prevent	Verb	To make it impossible to happen or occur
Prior	Adjective	Before
Prioritize	Verb	Put actions or items in the order of importance
Probe	Verb	Look, search
Procrastination	noun	waiting to do something instead of doing it immediately
Proficient	Adjective	Very good, exact
Prone	Adjective	Get this condition easily
Protocol	noun	the right way to do something
Protrudes	Verb	Sticks out

Term	Part of Speech	Meaning
Raising the voice	Noun phrase	To speak louder
Range	noun	how high or how low a voice goes
Rape	verb	to force someone to have sex
Rapport	Noun	Pleasant, agreeable relationship
Recurrence	Noun	Happen again
Red flag	noun	sign that something is wrong, not good
Reimburse	verb	pay money owed
Relay	verb	tell, pass on to another person
Render	verb	provide
Repel	verb	force away
Residency	adjective	the final hospital training for a doctor
Restitution	noun	payment to someone for harm or damage
Restore	Verb	Make good again
Retain	verb	keep
Retained	Verb	To retain: to keep
Retrievable	adjective	able to get or obtain again
Retroactive	adjective	going back in time
Reveal	Verb	To show
Review	noun	the process of checking something
Rhythmic	Adjective	Regular
Risk	noun	danger
Risks	Noun	Dangers
Rolled	Adjective	Turned over on itself
Rough handling	Noun phrase	Not being gentle and careful
Run the spectrum	phrase	go from one extreme to the other
Safeguard	Verb	Protect
Sanction	noun	a law that punishes for not following the rules
Scan	Verb	To look very quickly
Scope	noun	range; set of limitations
Scribble over	verb	make marks on paper, not words, to cover incorrect information; cross out heavily
Scrupulously	adverb	very carefully

Term	Part of Speech	Meaning
Scrutinize	verb	look very carefully
Sedentary	Adjective	Not active
Sequential	adjective	in order
Setback	noun	thing or action that stops progress
Shelf life	Noun phrase	How long an item is still good
Shift	verb	change
Shift	noun	time of day when a person works, such as day shift
Shuffling (papers)	Verb	To move papers around
Sibling	noun	brother or sister
Side effects	Noun	Conditions that the medicine may cause
Sigh	verb	let air out of the mouth, meaning the person is tired or feeling a strong emotion
Simulate	verb	imitate, fake
Skyrocket	verb	go up quickly
Sluggish	adjective	slow moving, not alert
Slurred	Adjective	Not speaking words clearly
Snags	Noun	When closing the scissors it sticks and doesn't close easily and doesn't cut correctly
Snap	noun	a quick, strong reaction, usually negative
Snapshot	noun	a quick look or understanding, like a photograph taken casually
Snoring	Adjective	A noisy breathing sound some people make when sleeping
Snugly	Adverb	Tightly, not loose
Soar	verb	go up quickly
Sob	verb	cry, weep
Soiled	Adjective	Not clean
Sole	adjective	only
Solid	adjective	firm, hard
Sophisticated	adjective	very complex or complicated
Spatial	adjective	related to space, room, area
Spread	Verb	To become widely known or suffered
Stake	noun	interest
Stalled	adjective	stopped by something
Stark	adjective	bare, blunt, extreme

Term	Part of Speech	Meaning
Stat.	adverb, abbreviation	immediately; from Latin *statim*
Statute	noun	law
Stipulate	verb	say what is required
Stirrups	noun	set of foot rests used to keep legs up and apart for female internal examination
Stoic	adjective	not showing emotion or reaction
Store	Verb	Keep
Streamline	verb	to make efficient
Strict adherence	Noun phrase	Complete following
Strive	verb	try, attempt, work hard
Stuff	verb	put papers in envelopes
Stumble	verb	walk unsteadily, without balance; trip over something
Stuttering	noun	speech that is greatly slowed by elongation or repetition of sounds
Subpoena	noun	an order to speak or be present in a court
Substantial	adjective	large
Suction	Adjective	Using air pressure to remove liquid/tissue with a pulling action
Summon	Verb	Call for
Surrogate	noun	replacement for a person or thing
Surveillance	noun	continuous watch on something or someone
Survey	Verb	Look at carefully
Suspicions	Noun	Thoughts, guesses
Suture	noun	stitch
Suture	adjective	used in sewing
Suture	verb	close a wound by sewing
Swallowed	Verb	Taken in by the mouth
Swelling	Noun	Accumulation of fluid under the skin
Tact	noun	politeness, consideration of others' feelings
Tailored	adjective	made to fit something or someone specific
Tally	noun	a record, a summary, a total
Tally	verb	to add up, to figure, to total
Tamper	verb	to interfere harmfully
Tangled	Verb	Mixed up together

Term	Part of Speech	Meaning
Target	verb	focus on, aim at
Taut	Adverb	Tight
Terminate (employment)	verb	fire, tell a person he or she can no longer work for you
Thorough	Adjective	Careful
Threat	noun	danger or warning of danger
Threshold	noun	starting place
Tickler	noun	reminder
Tickler file	Noun phrase	A file which reminds the staff to do certain things at certain times or on certain dates
Time consuming	phrase	taking a lot of time
Time frame	noun	the time for doing something
Tone (of voice)	noun	feeling, mood, loudness, or nature of the voice
Tossed	Verb	To toss: to throw
Track	verb	check progress, record changes
Tracking form	Noun phrase	A paper that shows all actions
Transmitted	Verb	To go from one person to another
Trend	noun	pattern
Trend	verb	make a pattern
Trigger	noun	something that causes something else to happen
Twitching	Noun	Quick movements or contractions
Underlying	Adjective	The condition causing the condition
Undetected	Adjective	Not noticed, not seen or observed
Utmost	adjective	the greatest
Vague	adjective	not clear, not specific
Vehicle	noun	method, carrier
Verifying	Verb	To verify: to make sure the information is correct
Veteran	adjective	having much experience
Vigilant	Adjective	Watching carefully
Viselike	Adjective	Extreme squeezing or pressure
Wail	verb	cry loudly
Wand	noun	hand-held electronic scanner; reads information such as bar codes
Welfare	noun	condition

Term	Part of Speech	Meaning
Whirr	noun	sound of something spinning quickly
Wicking	Adjective	Drawing of liquid from one object to another
Willfully	adverb	deliberately, on purpose
Wincing	Verb	To wince: movement of the face made when a person has a pain
Woe	noun	problem, trouble
Wringing hands	phrase	moving hands as if washing them; sign of worry or tension
Wrung	Verb	To wring: to remove liquid by twisting the material

INDEX

Page numbers in *italics* denote figures, those followed by a "t" indicate tables, those followed by a "b" indicate boxes, those followed by a "p" indicate procedures.